Paediatric Cardiology

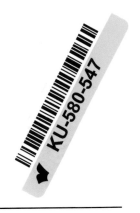

EDITED BY

Robert H. Anderson

BSc MD FRCPath

Joseph Levy Professor of Paediatric Cardiac Morphology, Cardiothoracic Institute, London; Honorary Consultant, Brompton Hospital, London, UK

Fergus J. Macartney

MA FRCP FACC

Vandervell Professor of Paediatric Cardiology and Honorary Consultant Paediatric Cardiologist, Hospital for Sick Children, Great Ormond Street, London, UK

Elliot A. Shinebourne

MD FRCP

Consultant Paediatric Cardiologist, Brompton Hospital, National Heart and Chest Hospitals, London, UK

Michael Tynan

MD FRCP

Joseph Levy Professor of Paediatric Cardiology, United Medical and Dental Schools of Guy's and St Thomas's Hospitals, London, UK

VOLUME ONE

CHURCHILL LIVINGSTONE
EDINBURGH LONDON MELBOURNE AND NEW YORK 1987

CHURCHILL LIVINGSTONE
Medical Division of Longman Group UK Limited

Distributed in the United States of America by Churchill
Livingstone Inc., 1560 Broadway, New York, N.Y. 10036, and
by associated companies, branches and representatives
throughout the world.

First published 1987

ISBN 0 443 02105 8 (2 vols)

British Library Cataloguing in Publication Data
Paediatric cardiology.
   1. Pediatric cardiology
   I. Anderson, Robert H. (Robert Henry), *1942–*
618.92′19   RJ421

Library of Congress Cataloging in Publication Data
Paediatric cardiology.
   Includes bibliographies and index.
   1. Pediatric cardiology.   I. Anderson, Robert Henry.
[DNLM: 1. Heart Defects, Congenital.   2. Heart Diseases –
in infancy & childhood. WS 290 P126]
RJ421.P333   1987   618.92′12   86-24505

Printed and bound in Great Britain by
Butler & Tanner Ltd, Frome and London

Preface

Ten years ago, when we started our collaboration concerning the naming of congenitally malformed hearts, a book such as this was in our minds. Initially it was conceived as a compilation of the work from several centres concerned with the diagnosis and treatment of childhood heart disease in the UK. When a publisher was found, it was decided that a comprehensive account would require a worldwide authorship. We have been most fortunate in obtaining the collaboration of many friends who are also leading authorities in their fields. All those invited accepted. We thank them for their efforts on our behalf.

A review of the table of contents will show that we have attempted to make the book comprehensive and applicable throughout the world. For example, we are happy to include a chapter on tropical heart disease, while our pleasure in incorporating an extensive chapter on rheumatic heart disease is clouded by the untimely death of its author, Professor I. P. Sukumar. Apart from innovations such as the chapter on ethical considerations, the general sections of the book follow the familiar pattern. Our major departure is in the organisation of the section dealing with congenital malformations. In this we have arranged the chapters in accord with our approach to nomenclature. We have felt this necessary since the study of congenital heart disease has moved on from 'syndromal' accounts to a more detailed and yet generalised understanding of the underlying anatomy and physiology. Although we have not yet achieved the ideal proposed by Moran Campbell (1977) of being able to ascribe causes to most of the individual malformations, our knowledge even in this respect has deepened in the past decade. Our attempt to integrate the individual congenital anomalies in a sequential segmental fashion will, we hope, remove much of the confusion inherent in describing them as isolated syndromes.

The basis of our approach to diagnosis, description and treatment has been an understanding of the anatomy as it is observed. Here a major advance in the past decade has been the ability to study this three-dimensional anatomy in exquisite detail using cross-sectional echocardiography. We were fortunate that the technique arrived just before we began thinking about the book and has matured during its gestation. Today, this technique is the cornerstone of diagnosis. This is the first major textbook which has been able to accord it its rightful place.

The nomenclature found throughout the book reflects the renaissance of Old World thinking of which we have been major protagonists. We make no apologies for proposing these changes, radical though they may appear to those who were nurtured on more traditional works. The confusion which arises when scientific advances are not matched by complementary changes in nomenclature has been highlighted by Scadding (1967). That such confusion exists in the study of congenital heart diseases is undoubted. It is our hope that taking the naming of congenital lesions of the heart out of the arena of embryological and morphogenetic speculation will result in easier understanding for the clinician and will liberate embryologists and morphologists.

So much for the philosophy. Writing and editing a multiauthor textbook turned out to be a far more difficult task than any of us imagined, even in our worst nightmares. We cannot conclude this brief preface without a catalogue of thanks. First we thank all of our contributors. We edited their texts extensively but with their agreement. We give them credit for the strengths of the book, and take responsibility for any shortcomings. We thank our wives and families for their forebearance. Most of the chapters and references were compiled by Christine Anderson, Anne Kruger, Dorothy Lewis and Rachel Green. The considerable task of providing uniform illustrations was willingly undertaken by Siew Yen Ho and Anita Hegerty. Throughout the preparation of our own chapters we drew heavily on ideas and contributions from our colleagues. In many cases these colleagues appear as co-authors. We sincerely thank all those who do not.

London, 1986

R. H. A.   F. J. M.
E. A. S.   M. T.

Campbell E J M 1977 The science of diagnosis. In: Phillips C I, Wolfe J N (eds) Clinical practice and economics. Pitman, London, pp 101–112

Scadding J G 1967 Diagnosis: the clinician and the computer. Lancet 2: 877–882

Contributors

Lindsey D. Allan MD MRCP
Senior Lecturer in Paediatric Cardiology, Guy's Hospital, London, UK

Robert H. Anderson BSc MD FRCPath
Joseph Levy Professor of Paediatric Cardiac Morphology, Cardiothoracic Institute, London; Honorary Consultant, Brompton Hospital, London, UK

Edward J. Baker MA MRCP
Senior Lecturer in Paediatric Cardiology, Guy's Hospital, London, UK

Anton E. Becker MD FACC FCCC
Professor of Pathology, University of Amsterdam, Academic Medical Centre, Netherlands

Lee B. Beerman MD
Associate Professor of Pediatrics, University of Pittsburgh School of Medicine, Pennsylvania, USA

Arnon Bentovim FRCPsych DPM
Consultant Psychiatrist, Hospital for Sick Children, Great Ormond Street, and the Tavistock Clinic, London, UK

Edmond Bertrand MD
Professor, Faculty of Medicine, University of Abidjan; Director, Abidjan Institute of Cardiology, Ivory Coast

John Burn BMedSci MRCP
Consultant Clinical Geneticist, Royal Victoria Infirmary, Newcastle, UK

Andrew Bush MA MRCP
British Heart Foundation Research Fellow, Departments of Paediatric Cardiology and Clinical Pharmacology, Brompton Hospital, London, UK

Cyril Chantler MA MD FRCP
Professor of Paediatric Nephrology, Evelina Children's Hospital, United Medical and Dental Schools of Guy's and St Thomas's Hospitals, London, UK

A. Chrispin FRCP DMRD
Consultant Radiologist, City Hospital and University Hospital, Nottingham; Clinical Teacher, University of Nottingham, UK

Gordon K. Danielson MD
Professor of Surgery, Mayo Medical School, Rochester, Minnesota; Consultant in Thoracic and Cardiovascular Surgery, Mayo Clinic/Foundation, Rochester, Minnesota, USA

J. E. Deanfield MRCP
Consultant Cardiologist, Hospital for Sick Children, Great Ormond Street, London; Senior Lecturer, Institute of Child Health, London, UK

William D. Edwards MD
Consultant, Department of Pathology, Mayo Clinic, Rochester, Minnesota; Associate Professor of Pathology, Mayo Medical School and Mayo Graduate School of Medicine, Rochester, Minnesota, USA

José A. Ettedgui Médico Cirujano (Venezuela)
Fellow in Paediatric Cardiology, Guy's Hospital, London, UK

Donald R. Fischer MD
Assistant Professor of Pediatrics, Division of Pediatric Cardiology, University of Pittsburgh, Pennsylvania, USA

Robert M. Freedom MD FRCP(C) FACC
Professor of Paediatrics and Pathology, University of Toronto Faculty of Medicine, Ontario; Senior Staff Cardiologist, The Hospital for Sick Children, Toronto, Ontario, Canada

F. Jay Fricker MD
Associate Professor of Pediatrics, University of Pittsburgh, Children's Hospital of Pittsburgh, Pennsylvania, USA

Valentin Fuster MD
Arthur M. & Hilda A. Master Professor of Medicine, and Chief, Division of Cardiology, Mount Sinai Medical Center, New York, USA

Arthur Garson Jr MD
Professor of Pediatrics and Medicine, Baylor College of
Medicine, Houston, Texas, USA

D. G. Gibson FRCP
Consultant Cardiologist, Brompton Hospital, London,
UK

Paul C. Gillette MD
Director, Pediatric Cardiology, South Carolina Children's
Heart Center, Medical University of South Carolina,
Charleston, South Carolina, USA

Danya Glaser DCH MRCPsych
Consultant Child Psychiatrist, Guy's Hospital and Forest
Hill Child Guidance Unit, London, UK

S. Godfrey MD PhD FRCP
Chairman, Department of Paediatrics, Hadassah
University Hospital, Jerusalem, Israel

Sheila G. Haworth MD MRCPath FRCP FACC
Reader in Paediatric Cardiology, Institute of Child
Health, London; Honorary Consultant Cardiologist,
Hospital for Sick Children, Great Ormond Street,
London, UK

Julian I. E. Hoffman BSc MD FRCP
Professor of Pediatrics and Psychology and Senior
Member of Cardiovascular Research Institute, University
of California, San Francisco, California, USA

Albert R. Jonsen PhD
Professor of Ethics in Medicine, and Chief, Division of
Medical Ethics, School of Medicine, University of
California, San Francisco, California, USA

Marc de Leval MD
Consultant Cardiothoracic Surgeon, Hospital for Sick
Children, Great Ormond Street, London, UK

Tom G. Losekoot MD PhD
Professor of Paediatrics, University of Amsterdam,
Academic Medical Centre, Netherlands

Paul R. Lurie AB MD
Professor of Pediatrics, Albany Medical College of Union
University, Albany, New York; Emeritus Professor of
Pediatrics, University of Southern California, USA

Fergus J. Macartney MA FRCP FACC
Vandervell Professor of Paediatric Cardiology and
Honorary Consultant Paediatric Cardiologist, Hospital for
Sick Children, Great Ormond Street, London, UK

Dan G. McNamara MD
Chief, Pediatric Cardiology, and Professor of Pediatrics,
Baylor College of Medicine, Houston, Texas, USA

Douglas D. Mair MD
Professor of Pediatrics, Mayo Foundation and Mayo
Medical School, Rochester, Minnesota, USA

Dominique Metras MD
Professor of Thoracic and Cardiovascular Surgery and
Chief of Unit of Cardiac Surgery, Children's Hospital,
Marseille, France

Peter M. Olley FRCP(C) FRCP
Professor and Chairman, Department of Paediatrics,
Walter Mackenzie Health Sciences Centre, University of
Alberta, Edmonton, Canada

Sang C. Park MD
Professor of Pediatrics, University of Pittsburgh School
of Medicine, Pennsylvania, USA

Co-burn J. Porter MD
Senior Associate Consultant, Mayo Clinic, Rochester,
Minnesota; Assistant Professor of Pediatrics, Mayo
Medical School, Rochester, Minnesota, USA

Michael L. Rigby MD MRCP
Consultant Paediatrician and Cardiologist, and Honorary
Senior Lecturer, Brompton Hospital and Cardiothoracic
Institute, London, UK

David W. Sapire Dip Paed FCP(SA)Paed
Professor of Pediatrics, and Chief, Division of Pediatric
Cardiology, University of Texas Medical Branch,
Galveston, Texas, USA

James B. Seward MD FACC
Associate Professor of Internal Medicine and Pediatrics,
Mayo Medical School, Rochester, Minnesota; Consultant,
Department of Internal Medicine and Pediatric
Cardiology, Mayo Clinic, Rochester, Minnesota, USA

Elliot A. Shinebourne MD FRCP
Consultant Paediatric Cardiologist, Brompton Hospital,
National Heart and Chest Hospitals, London, UK

David Silverman BSc MA PhD
Reader in Sociology, Goldsmiths' College, University of
London, UK

Jeffrey F. Smallhorn FRACP FRCP(C)
Associate Professor of Paediatrics, University of Toronto,
Ontario; Director of Cardiac Ultrasound, The Hospital
for Sick Children, Toronto, Ontario, Canada

Jane Somerville MD FRCP
Consultant Physician in Charge, Paediatric and
Adolescent Unit, National Heart Hospital, London;
Honorary Consultant Physician, Thoracic Unit, Hospital
for Sick Children, Great Ormond Street, London, UK

David John Spiegelhalter PhD
Biostatistician, Biostatistics Unit, Medical Research
Council, Shaftesbury Road, Cambridge, UK

The late I. P. Sukumar DM FRCP FACC FAMS FIMSA
Professor and Head, Cardiology Department, Christian Medical College and Hospital, Vellore; Paediatric Cardiologist, Christian Medical College and Hospital, Vellore, India

Michael de Swiet MD FRCP
Consultant Physician, Queen Charlotte's Hospital, London; Senior Lecturer, Cardiothoracic Institute, London, UK

Michael Tynan MD FRCP
Joseph Levy Professor of Paediatric Cardiology, United Medical and Dental Schools of Guy's and St Thomas's Hospitals, London, UK

Arnold C. G. Wenink MD PhD
Senior Lecturer in Anatomy, State University, Leiden, Netherlands

James L. Wilkinson FRCP
Consultant Paediatric Cardiologist, Royal Liverpool Children's Hospital; Honorary Research Fellow, University of Liverpool, UK

J. R. Zuberbuhler MD
Professor of Pediatrics, University of Pittsburgh, Pennsylvania; Director of Pediatric Cardiology, Children's Hospital of Pittsburgh, Pennsylvania, USA

Contents

VOLUME ONE

SECTION ONE General Considerations

1 Incidence, mortality and natural history 3
J. I. E. Hoffman

2 The aetiology of congenital heart disease 15
J. Burn

3 Terminology 65

4 Embryology of the heart 83
A. C. G. Wenink

5 Fetal circulation and circulatory changes at birth 109

6 Pulmonary vasculature 123
S. G. Haworth

7 Ventricular function 159
D. Gibson

SECTION TWO General Clinical Topics

8 History and physical examination 183

9 Clinical presentation of heart disease in infants and children 191

10 Imaging the heart and chest 201
A. Chrispin E. J. Baker

11 Electrocardiography 235
A. Garson

12 Echocardiography 319
Written in collaboration with J. Smallhorn M. L. Rigby J. E. Deanfield

13 Prenatal detection of congenital heart disease 351
L. D. Allan

14 Cardiac catheterisation and angiocardiography 363

15 Exercise and pulmonary function 395
S. Godfrey

SECTION THREE Management

16 Medical management 421
Written in collaboration with D. J. Spiegelhalter M. L. Rigby

17 Principles of surgical treatment 443
M. de Leval

18 The asymptomatic child with a murmur 465

SECTION FOUR Specific Conditions

19 Atrial isomerism 473
Written in collaboration with D. W. Sapire

20 Anomalous systemic venous return 497
D. R. Fischer J. R. Zuberbuhler

21 Pulmonary venous abnormalities 509

22 Atrial septal defect 541
L. B. Beerman J. R. Zuberbuhler

23 Partitioning of atrial chamber ('cor triatriatum') 563

24 Atrioventricular septal defects 571

25 Ventricular septal defect 615

Index I1

VOLUME TWO

26 Double inlet ventricle 643

27 Tricuspid atresia 675

28 Straddling atrioventricular valves 697

29 Pulmonary atresia with intact ventricular septum 711
F. J. Fricker J. R. Zuberbuhler

30 Ebstein's malformation and related lesions of the tricuspid valve   721

31 Atresia or hypoplasia of the left atrioventricular and/or ventriculo-arterial junction   737
R. M. Freedom

32 Fallot's tetralogy   765

33 Pulmonary atresia with ventricular septal defect   799

34 Complete transposition   829

35 Discordant atrioventricular connexion and congenitally corrected transposition   867
T. G. Losekoot   A. E. Becker

36 Double outlet ventricle   889
J. L. Wilkinson

37 Truncus arteriosus and aortopulmonary window   913
D. D. Mair   W. D. Edwards   V. Fuster
J. B. Seward   G. K. Danielson

38 The ductus arteriosus, its persistence and its patency   931
P. M. Olley

39 Pulmonary stenosis   959

40 Aortic stenosis and incompetence   977
J. Somerville

41 The child with a continuous murmur   1001
Written in collaboration with A. Bush

42 Mitral valve anomalies and supravalvar mitral ring   1023

43 Abnormal positions and relationships of the heart   1057

44 Anomalies of the coronary arteries   1073
P. R. Lurie

45 Coarctation and interrupted aortic arch   1087

46 Vascular ring and pulmonary sling   1123
S. C. Park   J. R. Zuberbuhler

47 Hypertrophic cardiomyopathy   1137
T. G. Losekoot   A. E. Becker

48 Cardiac tumours   1153
A. E. Becker   T. G. Losekoot

SECTION FIVE General Paediatric Cardiological Disease

49 Non-rheumatic inflammatory heart disease   1165
T. G. Losekoot   A. E. Becker

50 Acute and chronic rheumatic heart disease   1179
I. P. Sukumar

51 Primary endocardial fibroelastosis   1223
T. G. Losekoot   A. E. Becker

52 Infective endocarditis   1229

53 Cardiological aspects of systemic disease   1245
Written in collaboration with J. A. Ettedgui

54 Arrhythmias   1273
P. C. Gillette   A. Garson   C. J. Porter
D. G. McNamara

55 Systemic hypertension   1293
C. Chantler

56 Paediatric cardiology in the tropics   1321
Ed. Bertrand   D. Metras

SECTION SIX Risk Factors and Follow-up

57 Cardiovascular risk factors in infancy and childhood   1345
M. de Swiet

58 Management of congenital heart disease in pregnancy   1355
M. de Swiet

59 The fate of survivors of surgery for congenital heart disease   1363

SECTION SEVEN Psychosociological Problems

60 Psychological aspects of congenital heart disease   1373
D. Glaser   A. Bentovim

61 Social aspects of congenital heart disease   1385
D. Silverman

62 Ethical issues in paediatric cardiology   1399
A. R. Jonsen

Index   I1

General Considerations

Incidence, mortality and natural history

INCIDENCE

Knowledge of the incidence of congenital heart disease is useful for two main purposes. The frequency of occurrence of various congenital heart lesions, no matter how mild, may ultimately yield insight into their causes, especially if clusters of specific lesions are observed in certain places, at certain times or associated with certain external agents. On the other hand, information about the frequency of occurrence of clinically significant congenital heart lesions is a factor in assessing their economic impact and planning medical services.

Definitions

The *incidence* of a disease is a rate that specifies the number of new occurrences of the disease in a given population in a given time period. It must be distinguished from the *prevalence* of the disease which is a rate that specifies the number of people with that disease at any one time in a given population; this rate includes all survivors of that disease, no matter how long they have had it. A *cohort* is a group with a common characteristic (for example, being born in the same year) that is followed longitudinally to determine the outcome. By contrast, a *cross-sectional* survey that examines all patients with a certain disease at a given time will be examining the survivors of several successive yearly cohorts.

Effect of prenatal death on incidence rates

The incidence of congenital heart disease is usually given as the number of children born with congenital heart lesions in a given number of total births, for example, per 1000, 10 000 or 100 000. The number born with heart disease usually refers to those who are liveborn. This convention, however, ignores the fact that the incidence of congenital heart disease is about 10 times higher in stillborn than in liveborn infants (Richards et al, 1955; Feldt et al, 1971; Mitchell et al, 1971a; Bound & Logan, 1977;

Hoffman & Christianson, 1978). Because in stillborn infants the diagnosis of congenital heart disease depends on careful autopsy examination of an unmacerated fetus, accurate data are seldom available. The incidence of congenital heart disease may well be higher in abortuses, defined as products of conception that die or are expelled from the uterus before 20 weeks of gestation in the USA or before 28 weeks of gestation in the UK, but there are no systematic studies of congenital heart disease in abortuses.

The inclusion of intra-uterine deaths leads to a much greater figure for the incidence of congenital heart disease than is generally appreciated. For example, out of 100 000 pregnancies that last at least 4 weeks there are likely to be 21 800 spontaneous abortions, 1900 stillbirths and 76 300 live births (Bierman et al, 1965). If the incidence of congenital heart disease in each group respectively is 20% (assumed), 10% and 1% (the latter incidences from Hoffman & Christianson, 1978), then the total incidence of congenital heart disease in 100 000 pregnancies will be 4360 + 190 + 763 = 5313. This is 5 times the incidence that is based on live births alone. Since abnormalities of genetic and chromosomal origin are more common in abortuses and stillborn infants than in liveborn infants (Boue & Boue, 1968; Poland & Lowry, 1974), failure to consider prenatal deaths when studying congenital heart disease will lead to an underestimate of the importance of genetic and chromosomal factors.

Early studies of incidence rates

The completeness of ascertainment of the incidence of congenital heart disease in a population varies widely depending on the methods used to detect and diagnose these patients. By virtue of how they present, some congenital heart lesions are more likely to be detected and diagnosed than are others. For example, cyanotic heart disease is almost certain to be detected early, and with available methods is likely to be diagnosed accurately. On the other hand, small atrial and ventricular septal defects, mild pulmonary stenosis and bicuspid aortic valves cause no symptoms and are often inconspicuous. Unless they are detected during a routine examination, these patients may never be registered in any series so that the incidence of these particular lesions and of congenital heart disease as a whole will be underestimated.

Large populations can be investigated inexpensively by examining birth certificates, but this is very inaccurate, mainly because heart disease is often not manifest by the time the birth certificate is filled in. For example, in groups of children subsequently shown to have congenital heart disease, only 43.5–51% were suspected of or diagnosed as having heart disease within the first week after birth (Benson et al, 1961; Feldt et al; 1971, Hoffman & Christianson, 1978); in the large Liverpool series only 51.6% presented within one month after birth (Dickinson et al, 1981b). Furthermore, even known cardiac disease may not be recorded on birth certificates; two studies have found that only one-third or fewer of known congenital malformations were listed on the birth certificates (Lilienfeld et al, 1951; Bierman et al, 1965).

Death certificates may also be inaccurate (Feldt et al, 1971; Hook et al, 1977), particularly because the causes of deaths in newborn infants are often inaccurately diagnosed in the absence of an autopsy (Neel, 1958; Landtman, 1971). Furthermore, because most congenital heart lesions do not cause early death, retrospective detection of cohorts of children born in a given region with congenital heart disease by examining death certificates is wellnigh impossible.

Better information has come from registry studies done in a city or a region. Early studies of the incidence of congenital heart disease reported to Registries of Congenital Malformations, however, yielded falsely low incidence rates of 3.2–4.7 per 1000 live births (Hoffman, 1968). These registries were active between 1940 and 1960 when surgical treatment for most congenital heart lesions was lacking and interest in congenital heart disease was relatively low. Furthermore, paediatricians were not skilled in diagnosing these lesions, there were few paediatric cardiologists, and diagnostic techniques were not generally available for infants with heart disease.

Intensive studies of incidence

More intensive studies in which paediatric cardiologists played a large part have reported incidences of congenital heart disease per 1000 live births that vary from 5.5–8.6 (Table 1.1). The series are more notable for their similarities than their differences. The incidence rate does not appear to vary much from country to country, nor from earlier to later periods. Thus the two consecutive decades studied in Gothenburg by Carlgren (1959, 1969) are remarkably alike, and Bound & Logan (1977) noted no changes in incidence in three successive 5-year periods in Blackpool. Where there are differences, these are due usually to failure to include children with minimal congenital heart disease. For example, Carlgren (1959, 1969) observed an increase in the incidence of ventricular septal defects in the second decade of his study, and attributed this increase to failure to include in the first decade small ventricular septal defects that closed early by themselves. Laursen (1980) included ventricular septal defects only if they had at least grade 4 murmurs, thereby excluding many with small defects. These common small ventricular septal defects are also under-represented in the studies from Blackpool (Bound & Logan, 1977) and Liverpool (Dickinson et al, 1981b), as are those children with mild pulmonary stenosis, defined as having less than a 25 mmHg systolic pressure difference between the right ventricle and the pulmonary trunk. In fact, it is doubtful if any study will detect all children with small atrial or ventricular septal

Table 1.1 Incidence of congenital heart disease in liveborn infants

Years of birth	Place of study	Total live births	Congenital heart disease	Congenital heart disease/ 1000 live births
1946–1953	New York City	5 628	43	7.64
1941–1950	Gothenburg, Sweden	58 105	363	6.25
			(388)+	(6.68)+
1951–1960	Gothenburg, Sweden	58 314	450	7.72
1952–1961	Uppsala, Sweden	48 500°	291	6.0
1958	Leiden, Netherlands	1 817	15	8.25
1950–1969	Olmsted County, Minnesota	32 393	186	5.74
1959–1967	USA 12 centres	54 765	420	7.67
1957–1971	Blackpool, England	56 982	338	5.95
1959–1966	East Bay, California	19 044	163	8.56
			(199)*	(10.45)*
1960–1969	Liverpool & Bootle, England	160 480	884	5.51
1963–1973	Denmark	854 886	5 249	6.14

+ Including patients detected after the initial report; °Estimated; *Including possible heart disease as well.

References. New York City – Richards et al, 1955; Gothenburg – Carlgren, 1959 and Carlgren, 1969; Uppsala – Michaëlsson, 1965; Leiden – Kerrebijn, 1966; Minnesota – Feldt et al, 1971; USA multicentre study – Mitchell et al, 1971a; Blackpool – Bound & Logan, 1977; California – Hoffman & Christianson, 1978; Liverpool – Dickinson et al, 1981b; Denmark – Laursen, 1980.

defects, or with mild pulmonary stenosis, so that the true incidence of congenital heart disease in liveborn infants could be much higher than any incidence reported hitherto. These added patients with minor lesions are of almost no consequence in terms of clinical management, but their absence distorts epidemiological data used to make inferences about the aetiology of congenital heart disease.

Two prominent omissions deserve mention. Congenitally bicuspid aortic valves are thought to occur in at least 2% of the population (Roberts, 1970) so that this single lesion occurs more than twice as often as do all the other types of congenital heart disease put together. It is not listed in any of the series in Table 1.1. Secondly, patency of the arterial duct in premature infants is also not usually recorded in any of the reports listed in Table 1.1. With advances in treatment over the last fifteen years there has been a high survival rate of small preterm infants who often manifest a patent arterial duct. Given the average incidence of prematurity, there may be born each year as many premature infants with a patent arterial duct as there are liveborn infants with all other forms of congenital heart disease.

Incidence of specific lesions

Table 1.2 gives the available information about congenital heart lesions in stillborn infants. The most common lesions are ventricular septal defects which form the same proportion of all congenital heart lesions in both stillborn and liveborn infants. There is a lower than expected proportion of aortic and pulmonary stenosis and a higher than expected proportion of complex lesions like double inlet ventricle, hypoplastic left heart syndrome, and complete transposition. The high incidence of coarctation of the aorta is also noteworthy, but descriptions provided in the original articles are not adequate to determine the type of coarctation or its associated lesions. There is no reason to believe that any of these cardiac lesions cause intra-uterine death, and the factors responsible for their high incidence in stillborn infants are unknown.

The incidence of various congenital heart lesions in liveborn infants is given in Table 1.3. There is rough agreement among different series for the more common lesions, and the greater variability of incidence among the less frequent lesions is likely to be due to sampling variation. The slightly lower incidence of ventricular septal defects in the first series of Carlgren (1959) and the more recent series of Bound & Logan (1977) is probably due to the omission of patients with very small ventricular septal defects. A similar deficiency may explain the lower proportion of ventricular septal defects in the Danish series reported by Laursen (1980). The incidence of pulmonary stenosis varies markedly, probably because children with mild pulmonary stenosis may not be diagnosed or even referred to a cardiologist, and the same explanation may apply to the variable incidence reported for aortic stenosis.

Atrioventricular septal ('endocardial cushion') defects also show variability of incidence that may reflect differences in maternal age, since older mothers have an increased risk of having children with trisomy 21 (Hook, 1976). These children with Down's syndrome have a high incidence of congenital heart disease which has been reported to occur

Table 1.2 Distribution of congenital heart lesions among affected stillborn infants

Lesion	New York	Minnesota	London Birmingham	Hamburg	USA multicentre	Blackpool	California	Pooled percentage frequency
VSD	17	7	11	28	9	15	5	34.7
ASD	1	1	3	3	3	13	3	10.2
AVSD	0	0	7	2	5	4	0	6.8
PS	0	0	0	0	1	0	2	1.1
AS	0	0	0	0	0	0	0	0.0
Coarc	0	0	2	12*	2	6	3	9.4
TGA	2	0	4	17	0	1	0	9.1
T of F	0	1	3	1	1	3	0	3.4
CAT	0	2	4	4	2	4	0	6.0
HLH	0	0	0	2	2	2	2	3.0
HRH	0	0	0	0	2	0	1	1.1
DIV	0	1	2	8	1	5	0	6.4
SA	0	0	1	3	0	0	1	1.9
DORV	0	0	0	0	1	0	0	0.4
Misc	0	1	3	0	9	4	0	9.4
Total	*20*	*13*	*40*	*80*	*38*	*57*	*17*	

*With ventricular septal defect

Abbreviations. VSD – ventricular septal defect; ASD – atrial septal defect; AVSD – atrioventricular septal (cushion) defect; PS – pulmonary stenosis; AS – aortic stenosis; Coarc – coarctation of aorta; TGA – complete transposition of the great arteries; T of F – tetralogy of Fallot; CAT – common arterial trunk; HLH – hypoplastic left heart; HRH – hypoplastic right heart (pulmonary or tricuspid atresia, Ebstein's syndrome); DIV – double inlet ventricle; SA – single atrium; DORV – double outlet right ventricle; Misc – miscellaneous lesions.

Sources cited. New York – Wilson & Lubschez, 1942; Minnesota – Clawson, 1944; London, Birmingham – Berg et al, 1960; Hamburg – Hoffheinz et al, 1964; USA multicentre – Mitchell et al, 1971a; Blackpool – Bound & Logan, 1977; California – Hoffman & Christianson, 1978.

Table 1.3 Percentage distribution of types of congenital heart disease in liveborn infants

Lesion	Gothenburg	Toronto	Minnesota	USA multicentre	Blackpool	California	Denmark	Liverpool
VSD	27.1	31.0	34.6	32.1[1]	28.1	31.3	24.0	32.5
PAD	9.5	7.1	10.6	8.3	6.5	5.5	12.6	11.9
ASD	4.3	11.2	7.3	7.4	8.3	6.1	9.4[4]	5.9
AVSD	3.0		4.5	3.6	7.4	3.7	2.6	2.4
PS	3.8	10.8	5.0[2]	8.6	2.7	13.5	5.9	7.6
AS	5.4	8.4	6.1	3.8	4.1	3.7	4.7	5.1
Coarc	9.8	3.4	5.6	6.7[3]	5.6	5.5	7.0	6.3
TGA	6.0	2.6	7.8	2.6	5.6	3.7	4.8	5.0
T of F	4.1	8.0	5.0	3.8	8.6	3.7	5.8	5.9
CAT	1.4	0.0	0.0	1.7	1.2	2.5	1.4	1.1
HLH	0.8	0.0	4.5	3.1	3.3	0.6	3.0	2.8
HRH	2.4	1.1	3.4	2.4	1.5	0.6	1.8	2.5
DIV	0.0	0.0	0.0	0.7	1.5	0.6	1.5	1.7
DORV	0.0	0.0	0.0	1.0	0.0	0.6	0.0	0.0
TAPVC	0.8	0.0	2.8	0.0	2.1	0.6	1.4	0.8
Misc	21.7	16.4	2.8	13.8	13.6	17.8	15.7	8.0
Total	*369*	*464*	*179*	*420*	*338*	*163*	*5 249*	*884*

Abbreviations. PAD – patency of arterial duct; TAPVC – total anomalous pulmonary venous connection; other abbreviations as in Table 1.2. [1]Eleven with pulmonary stenosis; [2]includes pulmonary atresia; [3]seven with ASD or VSD; [4]includes ostium primum.
Sources cited. Gothenburg – Carlgren, 1959; Toronto – Rose et al, 1964; Minnesota – Feldt et al, 1971; USA multicentre – Mitchel et al, 1971a; Blackpool – Bound & Logan, 1977; California – Hoffman & Christianson, 1978; Denmark – Laursen, 1980; Liverpool – Dickinson et al, 1981b.

in 23–56% of them (Liu & Corlett, 1959; Berg et al, 1960; Rowe & Uchida, 1961; Mitchell et al, 1971b; Kenna et al, 1975; Hoffman & Christianson, 1978). Conversely, in a series of children born with congenital heart disease, trisomy 21 occurs in 3.2–8.7% (Carlgren, 1959, 1969; Cullum & Liebman, 1969; Feldt et al, 1971; Mitchell et al, 1971b; Greenwood et al, 1975; Kenna et al, 1975; Bound & Logan, 1977; Hoffman & Christianson, 1978). The estimate of 8.7% in the first series reported by Carlgren (1959) is falsely high, due to exclusion of many children with small ventricular septal defects from that series; when these were included in his second series (1969) the proportion of children with trisomy 21 fell to 6.0%. About 25–50% of children with trisomy 21 and congenital heart disease have atrioventricular septal defects (Berg et al, 1960; Rowe & Uchida, 1961; Cullum & Liebman, 1969; Landtman, 1971; Shaher et al, 1972; Greenwood et al, 1975; Hoffman & Christianson, 1978). Thus slight

increases in the average age of mothers of children with congenital heart disease in any series will increase the proportion of atrioventricular septal defects observed in it.

It is more difficult to account for the variations in incidence of lesions like coarctation of the aorta, complete transposition of the great arteries or tetralogy of Fallot, although because many coarctations are asymptomatic there is often delay in their detection and referral to a cardiologist. With exception of coarctation of the aorta, mild aortic stenosis and some atrial septal defects, differences of incidence in various series cannot be attributed to too short a follow-up, because most children with congenital heart lesions are detected by two years of age (Table 1.4).

Data on the relative incidence of various types of congenital heart disease in different racial groups in Asia and Africa are lacking because no intensive population studies have been done. Ascertainment is incomplete,

Table 1.4 Cumulative percentage frequency of detection of congenital heart disease by age

	Age								
		Months			Years				
	1 week	1	3	6	1	2	3	4	5
New York			83	95					
Minnesota	44	50	68		86	90		94	
Blackpool			74		82		90		
California	46	60	74		88	93	97	99	100
Denmark		36		63					
Liverpool		52		76					90

Sources cited. New York – Richards et al, 1955; Minnesota – Feldt et al, 1971; Blackpool – Bound & Logan, 1977; California – Hoffman & Christianson, 1978; Denmark – Laursen, 1980; Liverpool – Dickinson et al, 1981b.
Age listed refers to total duration after birth; thus '2 years' refers to all patients identified by their second birthday.

Table 1.5 Prevalence of congenital heart disease in Africa and Asia

	Durban	Capetown	Uganda	Nigeria	India	Ceylon	Singapore[1]	Taiwan	Minnesota[2]
VSD	18.8	21.8	36.4	38.8	29.0	17.6	27.0	33.7	33.8
PDA	25.6	16.1	27.2	20.9	11.0	14.8	11.4	12.2	7.4
ASD	6.0	17.0			12.0	31.9	11.2	3.7	13.2
AVD	2.6		4.5	9.0		rare	3.9	4.3	1.5
PS	6.8	9.2		6.0	7.0	12.6	8.0	4.3	13.2
AS		4.4	2.3	3.0	2.5		2.4		2.9[3]
Coarc	0.9	6.1			2.0	0.7	4.6	1.2	1.5
TGA		1.8	4.5	1.5	4.5	0.4	5.1	4.8	1.5
T of F	21.4	12.2	2.3	3.0	17.0	7.5	10.2	16.0	7.4
CAT	2.6	0.7				5.9	2.9	0.9	
HLH			2.3	1.5				0.9	
HRH	5.1	3.7	6.8	4.5		1.0	1.9	0.9	1.5
DIV	1.7	0.7[4]	2.3				3.9		
DORV	0.9							2.2	
TAPV		0.5		1.5				0.5	1.5
Misc	7.7	6.5	11.4	10.4	15.0		7.3	14.6	14.7
Total	117	1 439	44	67	200	55	411	588	68

[1]Autopsy series – 97% Chinese; [2]American Indians only; [3]Includes one with associated coarctation of the aorta; [4]double inlet ventricle with common arterial trunk combined form 0.7% of series.
Sources cited. Durban – van der Horst et al, 1968; Capetown – Schrire, 1963; Uganda – Caddell & Conner, 1966; Nigeria – Caddell & Morton, 1967; India – Pai & Varkey, 1974; Ceylon – Wallooppillai & Jayasinghe, 1970; Singapore – Muir, 1966; Taiwan – Shann, 1969; Minnesota – Anderson, 1977.

partly because access to medical care is limited and partly because racial customs may not bring infants to receive care or may not permit autopsies. As a result the more serious lesions that present in infancy are likely to be under-represented, and reported series thus contain excessive proportions of patients with lesions that do not cause early disability and death. Despite these difficulties, the prevalence data given in Table 1.5 show good general agreement with the more intensively studied groups listed in Table 1.3. Perhaps the most interesting features of this table are the relatively low proportions of coarctation of the aorta and aortic stenosis, a deficit commented on by Anderson (1977) who cited similar low proportions of these lesions reported from Japan, Korea, and Thailand. He regarded the low proportions of these two lesions as indicating some common genetic feature, but it is more likely that inadequate ascertainment is responsible for the apparent deficiency (van der Horst & Gotsman, 1972). Coarctation of the aorta is not rare in Japan: Sakakibara (1964) believed that the low incidence of congenital heart disease in general and coarctation of the aorta in particular in Japan was due to delayed or inadequate diagnosis, and Momma et al (1982) described 154 patients with coarctation of the aorta seen in one Japanese hospital from 1966–1980. In fact, even today in the USA the diagnosis of coarctation of the aorta was made prior to referral to a cardiologist in only 14% of the affected patients (Strafford et al, 1982).

NATURAL HISTORY

The true natural history of any disease is determined by following large numbers of people with that disease who are never treated. For congenital heart disease this determination is not possible because surgical treatment and accurate diagnostic methods developed at about the same time, so that there was never a long period during which these lesions could be diagnosed and followed but not treated. Furthermore, treatment for congestive heart failure has long been available and it presumably alters the natural course of some lesions.

Mortality in childhood

The most important complication of congenital heart disease is premature death. Because most deaths from congenital heart disease occur early, it is possible to obtain accurate mortality figures: most of those who died had autopsy confirmation of the diagnoses, and surgical treatment of these infants was not readily available when most of the studies were done, so that outcomes without treatment could be assessed.

The total death rate in children with congenital heart disease as determined by several intensive studies is given in Table 1.6. By 15 years of age, 26–48% of all these children had died, as compared with 5% for all liveborn children. In general, the lower mortality rates reflect studies in which attempts were made to include even minor congenital heart lesions; for example, including children with small ventricular defects accounts for the fall of mortality rate from 37 to 29% in the two consecutive decades studied by Carlgren in Gothenburg (1959, 1969). The high rate in Minnesota (Feldt et al, 1971), however, and the low rate in Liverpool (Dickinson et al, 1981b) cannot be so explained. The high mortality rate in Denmark (Laursen, 1980) was much lower in the second than in the first 5-year period.

Table 1.6. Percentage survival of liveborn children with congenital heart disease

			Months			Years										
	1 day	1 week	1	3	6	1	2	3	4	5	6	7	8	9	10	15
New York	88		77			67	62									
Gothenburg 1		87	79		71	68		65			64					63
Gothenburg 2																71
The Netherlands	89*	84*			74			70							67	
Minnesota	92	76	69	63	62	59				56						
USA multicentre		81			70											
California			87			77					73					
Liverpool																
Denmark			75							58						52
USA (all children)			98.4			96.1				95.7						

Sources cited. New York – Richards et al, 1955; Gothenburg 1 – Carlgren, 1959; Gothenburg 2 – Carlgren, 1969; The Netherlands – Kerrebijn, 1966; Minnesota – Feldt et al, 1971; USA multicentre – Mitchell et al, 1971a; California – Hoffman & Christianson, 1978; Liverpool – Dickinson et al, 1981b; Denmark – Laursen, 1980; USA (all children) – US Bureau of the Census, 1970.

Table 1.7 indicates the cumulative percentages of deaths by age from 1 day to 15 years for a number of prospective hospital and registry studies. It also includes three autopsy studies done in hospitals where it is likely that the population and referral patterns did not change during the period of the study, so that the results of cross-sectional studies should be similar to those of cohort studies. In general, about 50% of all deaths in children with congenital heart disease occur at or under 1 month of postnatal age, whereas for all childhood deaths (which are proportionally much fewer – see Table 1.6) the 50th percentile is reached at about 6 months of age.

It is often difficult to decide whether death was due to the congenital heart lesion or to associated defects and dis-eases. Richards et al (1955) adjudged that only 6/10 deaths in neonates were due to the congenital heart lesion whereas all 6 deaths in older children were from their heart disease. Carlgren (1959) thought that only one-third of all deaths in these children under 1 month of age could be ascribed to their congenital heart lesions. Mitchell et al (1971a) concluded from autopsy studies that death was due to the heart lesions in 36/76 (47%) of the neonates, 32/45 (71%) of the infants from 1–12 months of age and in 14/20 (70%) of the older children. Similarly, Hoffman & Christianson (1978) regarded death as being related to the heart disease in only 6/21 (29%) of the neonates but in 16/22 (73%) of the older children. Finally, Dickinson et al (1981b), in the largest reported study to date, concluded that of the 297 children

Table 1.7 Cumulative percentage mortality rate versus age for deaths in childhood from congenital heart disease

			Months			Age Years										
	1 day	1 week	1	3	6	1	2	3	4	5	6	7	8	9	10	15
Singapore		19	31		72	83										
New York	31		62			88	100									
Gothenburg 1	12	36	56		78	86		92				97				100
Gothenburg 2		30	52			83							98			100
New Zealand			45			85			94							
Netherlands		33*	50*			80		92								100
Minnesota	17	54	70	84	88	95				100						
Finland	32	53	66	78	86		92		94				97		100	
USA multicentre			53			86										
Upstate New York						75		92					96			99
California			49			82	87									100
Denmark			52						87.5							100
USA (all deaths)			36			84				93				97		100

*estimated by author.

Sources cited. Singapore – Muir, 1966; New York – Richards et al, 1955; Gothenburg 1 – Carlgren, 1959; Gothenburg 2 – Carlgren, 1969; New Zealand – McGeorge & Rodda, 1963; Netherlands – Kerrebijn, 1966; Minnesota – Feldt et al, 1971; Finland – Landtman, 1971; USA multicentre – Mitchell et al, 1971a; Upstate New York – Hook et al, 1977; California – Hoffman & Christianson, 1978; Denmark – Laursen, 1980; United States (all deaths) – US Bureau of the Census, 1970.

United States (all deaths) refers to deaths in 1967 from any cause, not only congenital heart disease.

who died, 177 (60%) died from their heart disease, 55 (19%) died from non-cardiac causes and another 65 (22%) died after cardiac surgery; distinction by age-group was not reported.

One of the principle causes for the high non-cardiac mortality rate is that in children born with congenital heart disease severe single or multiple extracardiac malformations are common; these are reported in 16–31% of live-born infants with congenital heart disease (Richards et al, 1955; Carlgren 1959; Mitchell et al, 1971a; Feldt et al, 1971; Greenwood et al, 1975; Kenna et al, 1975; Hoffman & Christianson, 1978). In part, differences in the reported frequencies of these extracardiac malformations are likely to be due to defining which malformations should be included (Hoffman & Christianson, 1978). These extracardiac lesions greatly influence mortality rates for congenital heart disease. Thus mortality rates with and without associated extracardiac malformations were respectively 67% and 40% (Carlgren, 1969), 58% and 23% (Mitchell et al, 1971a), and 57% and 39% (Greenwood et al, 1975).

The extracardiac lesions described involved all systems, but most commonly affected musculoskeletal, central nervous and renal-urinary systems; specific genetic or chromosomal syndromes were reported in about 7% of the children studied (Greenwood et al, 1975). Although extracardiac anomalies could be associated with any congenital heart lesion, they were most frequently noted with the left-to-right shunt lesions, coarctation of the aorta, tetralogy of Fallot, malpositions and with univentricular atrioventricular connexion. By contrast, extracardiac anomalies were relatively uncommonly associated with complete transposition, pulmonary stenosis or atresia, hypoplastic left heart syndrome, common arterial trunk or total anomalous pulmonary venous connexion (Greenwood et al, 1975).

Natural history of specific lesions

Mortality rates

Mortality rates of individual lesions vary widely, and again it is important to separate cardiac from non-cardiac causes of death, as well as to make some allowance for those who died after cardiac surgery or who would have died but for cardiac surgery. In Table 1.8 the available data are set out. The 1959 report by Carlgren includes 49 surgical procedures (mostly in patients with patent arterial duct, atrial septal defect and tetralogy of Fallot) with only 2 deaths. His figures for mortality rates of individual lesions resemble those reported in 1971 by Mitchell et al (1971a) in which there were only 13 deaths related to cardiac surgery. The biggest differences between mortality rates for individual lesions in these two series are found for aortic stenosis, perhaps because surgery for infants with this disease was not available in Gothenburg at that time, and in coarctation of the aorta which was divided into simple postductal and complex preductal groups only in the series of Mitchell et al (1971a). In the data from Denmark, Laursen (1980) noted that for almost all lesions the mortality rate was lower from 1969–1973 than from 1963–1968; for all lesions combined, the mortality rate decreased from 56% in the first period to 35% in the second

Table 1.8 Percentage mortality of specific congenital heart lesions in childhood

	Gothenburg	USA multicentre	Denmark	Liverpool Cardiac	Non-cardiac	Surgery	New England Medical	Surgical
VSD	22	12	20	5	8	3	7	7
PAD	3	34	31	7	7	3	5	31
ASD	33	23	30	4	12	2	9	1
AVSD	60	47	68	43	0	14	28	14
PS	22	14	7	3	0	0	1	19
AS	50	0	20	11	2	0		
Coarc	86	94(9)*	56	32	7	9	23	30
TGA	91	82	72	57	2	30	11	29
T of F	27	31	39	23	10	33	9	20
CAT	80	86	95	90	0	0	70	
HLH	100	100	100	100	0	0	78	15
P at	100	100	97	100	0	0	17	77
T at	33	80	76	73	7	13	15	26
DIV		67	83	33	13	13	47	
TAPVC	100		51	67	0	33	24	32
Misc	36	61	35	36	10	14		
Undiag			47	7	0	0		

Abbreviations. P at – pulmonary atresia with intact ventricular septum : T at – tricuspid atresia; Undiag – undiagnosed; others as in Table 1.2.
Sources cited. Gothenburg – Carlgren, 1959; USA multicentre – Mitchell et al, 1971a; Liverpool – Dickinson et al, 1981b; New England – Fyler et al, 1980; Denmark – Laursen, 1980.
In Liverpool studies, percentages are of total number of children with a given lesion; thus sum of all percentages is total childhood mortality for that lesion. The same applies to the New England studies.
*9 refers to uncomplicated coarctations; 94 refers to complicated preductal coarctations.

period. Subsequently the large and carefully studied series by Dickinson et al (1981b) was published. This series distinguishes among deaths due to the cardiac lesion, due to cardiac surgery and to non-cardiac causes. From these three studies it is clear that deaths in early childhood are infrequent in the left-to-right shunt lesions except for atrioventricular septal defects and are infrequent in the obstructive lesions except for coarctation of the aorta. By contrast, mortality rates are very high for all the cyanotic heart lesions except for tetralogy of Fallot. Finally, Table 1.8 shows for comparison data reported by the New England Regional Infant Care Program (Fyler et al, 1980). This study was designed to detect and treat all serious congenital heart disease in the New England region, so that their data do not give information about any children with mild congenital heart disease, who would be expected to do well in childhood, but give excellent information on the more severe forms of left-to-right shunts and obstructive lesions, as well as for all children with cyanotic heart disease.

Although Fyler et al did not specifically identify non-cardiac causes of death, they did make allowance for severe extracardiac malformations and very low birth weight (under 2.0 kg). Adjustment for these risk factors reduced mortality in all groups in which it was done.

Natural history of those surviving early childhood

Cyanotic heart disease

As shown in Table 1.8, untreated cyanotic heart disease is seldom compatible with survival beyond childhood, except for tetralogy of Fallot. Studies of individual lesions support this conclusion. Thus, if untreated, 90% of children with complete transposition die by 1 year of age and 95% by 5 years of age (Liebman et al, 1969; Kidd et al, 1971; Shaher, 1973). The same bleak outlook applies to most other forms of cyanotic congenital heart disease, as indicated by the very young age at death reported in the surveys by Fontana & Edwards (1962) and Campbell (1972). Even tetralogy of Fallot, which untreated has the most favourable prognosis of all cyanotic heart lesions, does not produce many who enter adult life. Their median age at death has been found to range from 2.5–7 years of age, and only about 10% of untreated patients live more than 20 years (Rowe et al, 1955; Rygg et al, 1971).

Ventricular septal defects

Unlike the cyanotic lesions, these commonest of congenital heart lesions range from the small and trivial to the large and fatal. One major determinant of outcome in this lesion is the size of the defect. As a general rule, those who are asymptomatic are likely to have small defects. Two studies have estimated that these relatively small, asymptomatic

ventricular septal defects occur in about 70% of all children born with these defects (Hoffman & Rudolph, 1965; Dickinson et al, 1981a). The other major determinant of outcome is the presence of associated severe extracardiac malformations. These occurred in 20% of the patients studied by Dickinson et al (1981a) and 33% of the patients studied by Fyler et al (1980). About 50% of the deaths in the series of Dickinson et al (1981a) were related to these malformations and not to the ventricular septal defect alone.

Spontaneous closure of the defect has been regarded as frequent. As expected, it occurs most often in those with small defects; closure has been described in 17–60% of children with ventricular septal defects (Evans et al, 1960; Hoffman & Rudolph, 1965; Campbell, 1971; Keith et al, 1971; Corone et al, 1977; Weidman et al, 1977; Dickinson et al, 1981a). Interestingly enough, closure has also been seen in patients who have large defects with significant symptoms (Hoffman & Rudolph, 1965; Fyler et al, 1980) even though the frequency of closure may be only 10–12%. However, in addition to those that close, there are probably many more that become smaller and cease to be haemo-dynamically or clinically significant (Hoffman & Rudolph, 1965; Dickinson et al, 1981a). Data about spontaneous closure of these defects in adult life are inadequate, but some studies suggest that closure may be frequent (Bloomfield, 1964; Hoffman, 1968).

If the defects do not close and the patient does not die in childhood from heart failure or a non-cardiac cause, then several outcomes can occur: development of aortic incompetence, infective endocarditis, complications of a ventricular septal aneurysm, infundibular pulmonary stenosis or pulmonary vascular disease. The first three complications can occur with defects of any size, the last two only with large defects. In the whole population of ventricular septal defects these complications are each infrequent, and most patients will lead normal lives (Bloomfield, 1964; Campbell, 1971; Corone et al, 1977; Gersony & Hayes, 1977; Weidman et al, 1977).

Patency of the arterial duct

This lesion in full-term infants has been known to close spontaneously, but not very often (Campbell, 1968a). Apart from the very large ducts that cause early death (Table 1.8) most affected people survive to adult life. Campbell (1968a) concluded that, if not treated, about 80% of these patients survive to thirty years of age but only 40% to sixty years of age.

Atrial septal defect

This lesion seldom causes difficulties in childhood and most affected people become adults. With age an increasing proportion of patients develop severe symptoms, atrial flutter or fibrillation or pulmonary vascular disease (Bedford & Sellors, 1960; Hamilton et al, 1979). Siltanen (1968) found in a large personal series that the average age at death in patients with large atrial septal defects was 40 years and that those over 50 years old were disabled. Confirmatory data can be found in the series reported by Fontana & Edwards (1962), Craig & Selzer (1968) and Campbell (1970b).

Atrioventricular septal defects

These have a much higher mortality in childhood (Table 1.8). Some 50–70% survive to adult life (Somerville, 1965; Dickinson et al, 1981b) but in general not as long as do those with atrial septal defects within the oval fossa.

Coarctation of the aorta

Information about this lesion is often confusing because some studies in infants do not distinguish between complex preductal coarctations, which have a high early death rate, and the more benign simple juxtaductal coarctations. Even these, if untreated, have an appreciable early mortality. Beyond infancy there may be an asymptomatic period, but the mean age at death was found to be 35 years by Reifenstein et al (1947), and this was confirmed by the study of Campbell (1970a) of patients surviving the first year of life. Few of these patients will live beyond 50 years of age, in contradistinction to the bulk of the population.

Aortic and pulmonary stenosis

These lesions do not commonly cause death in childhood. Because aortic stenosis tends to become more severe with age, even in childhood (Hoffman, 1969; Wagner et al, 1977) it is not surprising that Campbell (1968b) found a median age at death of under 40 years in untreated patients. Even the majority of people with bicuspid aortic valves will eventually develop stenosis or incompetence (Fenoglio et al, 1977), the latter due mainly to infective endocarditis. Pulmonary stenosis appears to have a better prognosis (Hoffman, 1969; Danilowicz et al, 1975), although there have been no good long-term studies of this disease in adults. Campbell (1969) thought that the prognosis was not as good in this lesion as in coarctation of the aorta but his outlook may be too pessimistic since he probably did not have many people with mild pulmonary stenosis in his series.

Prevalence of congenital heart disease in childhood

In any year the total number of people under 20 years of age who have congenital heart disease represents the total number born with congenital heart disease over the past 20 years less those who have died or have cured themselves spontaneously. The affected people will consist of those who need observation but no surgery, are awaiting surgery, or have had surgery; these, in turn, include some with little need for further medical care (for example, after closure of a patent arterial duct), others who need prolonged medical supervision (for example, after surgery for tetralogy of Fallot or aortic stenosis), and still others who need further surgical procedures (for example, changing a conduit or a prosthetic valve). The prevalence figures in any country are useful for planning medical services but are subject to fluctuations as the birth rate varies, the indications for surgery change, or new forms of treatment with a lower mortality rate are introduced. Thus whereas the numbers of surviving patients with complete transposition used to be low, the advent of successful surgical procedures has greatly increased their prevalence.

An attempt to assess the prevalence of major congenital heart lesions in the USA was made by Roberts & Cretin (1980). Beginning with figures for the incidence of congenital heart disease estimated for 1975, they projected the numbers of live births and congenital heart disease to 1995, and then devised rough life tables for each of the seven selected lesions. Their estimates of surgical mortality, although taken from reported data, would be regarded as too high in most major centres today. They concluded that in 1995 in the USA there will be nearly 300 000 children under 21 years old with congenital heart disease, 38% of whom would have had one or more surgical procedures. For England and Wales the total number of children with congenital heart disease might be 60 000. As surgical mortality falls, the number of surviving children will rise, thereby increasing the numbers of consumers of cardiological services. Table 1.9, adapted from their article, indicates the prevalence and surgical experience for each lesion.

ECONOMIC IMPLICATIONS

Dickinson et al (1981b) estimated that the total number of cardiac surgical procedures needed in England and Wales would be 3759 per million live births, a value similar to that suggested in the USA in 1971 by Engle et al. A larger estimate was derived in an unpublished task force study done by the National Heart, Lung and Blood Institute of the US Public Health Service but this was inflated by not allowing for deaths due to cardiac or non-cardiac causes before surgery. Dickinson et al (1981b) also attempted to estimate which children would need surgery before one year of age, and decided that about one-third, or 1383 per million live births, would need surgery as infants. This is similar to the infant surgery rate of 1409 per million live births observed in the New England Regional Infant Care Program (Macartney, 1979; Fyler et al, 1980). The cardiac catheterisation rate in infancy was 2500 per million live births in Liverpool (Dickinson et al, 1981b) and 2700 per

Table 1.9 Estimated prevalence of congenital heart disease for 1995 in the USA (after Roberts & Cretin, 1980)

	Prevalence			Percentage of survivors who have had surgery			
	Total	Under 1 year	1–20 years	Total	Under 1 year	1–5 years	5–20 years
VSD	64 173	9 623	54 550	25.3	0.9	5.8	38.3
PS	57 957	3 319	54 638	28.3	3.3	11.1	35.2
ASD	34 593	1 921	32 672	40.4	0.8	8.6	52.5
PAD	32 239	2 226	30 013	65.2	31.4	48.0	73.5
Coarc	16 450	1 064	15 386	64.6	23.0	29.0	78.8
T of F	16 312	1 084	15 228	60.0	3.5	16.7	78.7
AS	21 857	1 221	20 636	24.3	2.7	7.3	30.8
Misc	52 560	5 743	46 817	34.1	4.3	15.1	45.1
Total	296 141	26 201	269 940	37.6	5.6	15.3	48.6

Abbreviations as in Table 1.2.

million live births in New England (Macartney, 1979). The crude estimate for the USA by the Task Force for cardiac catheterisations at all ages in childhood was 5737 per million live births, which fits fairly well with the data for infants. What the actual rate of all cardiac catheterisations will be eventually is uncertain. On the one hand, many children require more than one such study, particularly when the cardiac lesion is complex. On the other hand, non-invasive methods are beginning to replace cardiac catheterisation and will probably do so to a greater extent in the future.

To these numbers must be added the cardiac catheterisations and cardiac surgery necessary to diagnose and treat aortic stenosis that is secondary to a bicuspid aortic valve but presents only in adult life. If, as some estimate, one-half of the people who have bicuspid aortic valves will eventually develop significant aortic stenosis, then each year there will be another 10 000 cardiac catheterisations and cardiac surgical procedures per million live births in these adults.

The financial cost of congenital heart disease based on these numbers is considerable. In the New England study (Fyler et al, 1980) the average figure for the cost of treatment in 1975 was $6600; this included all hospital costs, such as costs of cardiac catheterisation, surgery, intensive care and general hospitalisation. To this ought to be added another $2200 or so for professional fees to give a total of $8800. In 1984 the costs might be about two to three times this amount. To estimate total yearly costs in 1981 for managing congenital heart disease, multiply the number of cardiac catheterisations per million live births by the crudely estimated costs of about $1500 per cardiac catheterisation (total of all costs) and multiply the number of cardiac surgical procedures per million live births by $20 000 per procedure. Then, per million live births, cardiac catheterisation will have an annual cost in the USA of $24 000 000 and cardiac surgery will have an annual cost of $280 000 000. Because the birth rate is about 3.4 million per year in the USA, yearly costs will total $82 000 000 for cardiac catheterisation and $952 000 000 for cardiac surgery. These figures combine all congenital heart diseases, including adult aortic stenosis. For children alone, the totals come to $31 000 000 for cardiac catheterisation and $272 000 000 for cardiac surgery. In the UK costing is not comparable, but as the birth rate was about 640 000 in England and Wales in 1979 the equivalent costs will be (0.64/3.4) × 100 or about 20% of the costs in the USA. These figures are at best very crude estimates, and in particular will vary widely depending on the price structure in any country at any given time. They do, however, give a rough idea of how vast the cost of congenital heart disease may be.

To offset some of the gloom that the thought of such an expenditure might bring, one must consider first of all that most children with congenital heart disease can be brought by medical and surgical management to lead reasonably healthy and productive lives. Few of these children will be completely normal, and they may not all live a full life span, but most will survive to be productive in society. Secondly, in any assessment of costs of disease the loss of earnings must be considered. This can be done actuarially (Cooper & Rice, 1976), and one estimate of the loss of earnings of children with congenital heart disease based on estimated age at death in the USA came to a figure of $720 000 000 in 1975 (Task Force). Since this referred to children alone, it should be compared to the costs of congenital heart disease, which total some $300 000 000. In other words, not only does successful treatment decrease human suffering and prolong life, but it also pays society in economic terms to produce healthy wage-earners.

One final comment should be made about the medical and economic burden of congenital heart disease. Although the incidence of coronary heart disease is greater by far than the incidence of congenital heart disease, those affected by coronary disease usually become ill after the fourth decade of life, often not until the sixth or seventh decades. Their remaining life span is certainly shorter than that hoped for by the child with heart disease, so that the disproportion between the two groups of diseases in patient years of medical care is less by a factor of 3 or 4 than the disparity between their incidences suggests. Furthermore, it is likely that in the next twenty years the incidence of cardiovascular disease from coronary heart disease and hypertension will decline, whereas the incidence of congenital heart disease is likely to increase slowly as survivors produce their own families. As a result, in the foreseeable future, congenital heart disease is likely to consume increasing cardiovascular services and costs.

REFERENCES

Anderson R C 1977 Congenital heart malformations in North American Indian children. Pediatrics 59: 121–123

Bedford D E, Sellors T H 1960 Atrial septal defect. In: Jones A M (ed) Modern trends in cardiology. Butterworths, London, p 138

Benson P F, Bonham-Carter R E, Smellie J M 1961 Transient and intermittent systolic murmurs in newborn infants. Lancet 1: 627–630

Berg J M, Crome L, France N E 1960 Congenital malformations in mongolism. British Heart Journal 22: 331–346

Bierman J M, Siegel E, French F E, Simonian K 1965 Analysis of the outcome of all pregnancies in a community: Kauai pregnancy study. American Journal of Obstetrics and Gynecology 91: 37–45

Bloomfield D K 1964 Natural history of ventricular septal defect in patients surviving infancy. Circulation 29: 914–955

Boue J, Boue A 1968 Chromosome aberrations in human spontaneous abortion. Mammalian Chromosome Newsletter 9: 246–248

Bound J P, Logan W F W E 1977 Incidence of congenital heart disease in Blackpool 1947–1971. British Heart Journal 39: 445–450

Caddell J L, Conner D H 1966 Congenital heart disease in Ugandan children. British Heart Journal 28: 766–767

Caddell J L, Morton P 1967 Pattern of congenital heart disease in Yoruba children of Western Nigeria. American Heart Journal 73: 431–432

Campbell M 1968a Natural history of persistent ductus arteriosus. British Heart Journal 30: 4–13

Campbell M 1968b The natural history of congenital aortic stenosis. British Heart Journal 30: 514–526

Campbell M 1969 The natural history of congenital pulmonic stenosis. British Heart Journal 31: 394

Campbell M 1970a Natural history of coarctation of the aorta. British Heart Journal 32: 633–640

Campbell M 1970b Natural history of atrial septal defect. British Heart Journal 32: 820–826

Campbell M 1971 Natural history of ventricular septal defect. British Heart Journal 33: 246–257

Campbell M 1972 Natural history of cyanotic malformations and comparison of all common cardiac malformations. British Heart Journal 34: 3–8

Carlgren L-E 1959 The incidence of congenital heart disease in children born in Gothenburg 1941–1950. British Heart Journal 21: 40–50

Carlgren L-E 1969 The incidence of congenital heart disease in Gothenburg. Proceedings of the Association of European Paediatric Cardiologists 5: 2–8

Clawson B J 1944 Types of congenital heart disease in 15 597 autopsies. Lancet 64: 134–136

Cooper B S, Rice D P 1976 The economic cost of illness revisited. Social Security Bulletin 39: 21–36

Corone P, Doyon F, Gaudeau S, Guérin F, Vernant P, Ducam H, et al 1977 Natural history of ventricular septal defect. A study involving 790 cases. Circulation 55: 908–915

Craig R J, Selzer A 1968 Natural history and prognosis of atrial septal defect. Circulation 37: 805–815

Cullum L, Liebman J 1969 The association of congenital heart disease with Down's syndrome (mongolism). American Journal of Cardiology 24: 354–347

Danilowicz D, Hoffman J I E, Rudolph A M 1975 Serial studies of pulmonary stenosis in infancy and childhood. British Heart Journal 37: 808–818

Dickinson D F, Arnold R, Wilkinson J L 1981a Ventricular septal defect in children born in Liverpool 1960 to 1969. Evaluation of natural course and surgical implications in an unselected population. British Heart Journal 46: 47–54

Dickinson D F, Arnold R, Wilkinson J L 1981b Congenital heart disease among 160 480 liveborn children in Liverpool 1960 to 1969. Implications for surgical treatment. British Heart Journal 46: 55–62

Engle M A, Adams F H, Betson C, et al 1971 Resources for the optimal acute care of patients with congenital heart disease. Circulation 43: A123–A133

Evans J R, Rowe R D, Keith J D 1960 Spontaneous closures of ventricular septal defects. Circulation 22: 1044–1054

Feldt R H, Avasthey P, Yoshimasu F, Kurland L T, Titus J L 1971 Incidence of congenital heart disease in children born to residents of Olmsted County, Minnesota, 1950–1969. Mayo Clinic Proceedings 46: 794–799

Fenoglio J J Jr, McAllister H A Jr, De Castro C M, Davia J E, Cheitlin M D 1977 Congenital bicuspid aortic valve after age 20. American Journal of Cardiology 39: 164–169

Fontana R S, Edwards J E 1962 Congenital cardiac disease: A Review of 357 cases studied pathologically. Saunders, Philadelphia

Fyler D C, Buckley L P, Hellenbrand W E, Cohn H E 1980 Report of the New England Regional Infant Care Program. Pediatrics 65 (Suppl): 375–461

Gersony W M, Hayes C J 1977 Bacterial endocarditis in patients with pulmonary stenosis, aortic stenosis, or ventricular septal defect. Circulation 56 (Suppl I): 84–87

Greenwood R D, Rosenthal A, Parisi L, Fyler D C, Nadas A A 1975 Extracardiac anomalies in infants with congenital heart disease. Pediatrics 55: 485–492

Hamilton W T, Haffajee C I, Dalen J E, Dexter L, Nadas A S 1979 Atrial septal defect secundum: Clinical profile with physiologic correlates in children and adults. In: Roberts W C (ed) Congenital heart disease in adults. Davis, Philadelphia, p 267

Hoffheinz H J, Glaser E, Rodewald G 1964 Über die Häufigkeit angeborener Herzfehler in Hamburger Sektionsgut. Zentralblatt fur Chirurgie 89: 326–340

Hoffman J I E 1968 Natural history of congenital heart disease. Problems in its assessment with special reference to ventricular septal defects. Circulation 37: 97–125

Hoffman J I E 1969 The natural history of congenital isolated pulmonic and aortic stenosis. Annual Review of Medicine 20: 15–28

Hoffman J I E, Christianson R 1978 Congenital heart disease in a cohort of 19 502 births with long-term follow-up. American Journal of Cardiology 42: 641–647

Hoffman J I E, Rudolph A M 1965 Natural history of ventricular septal defects in infancy. American Journal of Cardiology 16: 634–653

Hook E B 1976 Estimates of maternal age-specific risks of a Down's syndrome birth in women aged 34–41. Lancet 2: 33–34

Hook E B, Farina M A, Hoff M B 1977 Death certificate reports of cardiovascular disorders in children: comparison with diagnoses in a pediatric cardiology registry. Journal of Chronic Diseases 30: 383–391

van der Horst R L, Gotsman M S 1972 Racial incidence of coarctation of the aorta. British Heart Journal 34: 289–294

van der Horst R L, Winship W S, Pittaway D, Gibb B H, Lapinsky G B 1968 Congenital heart disease in the South African Bantu: a report of 117 cases. South African Medical Journal 42: 1271–1273

Keith J D, Rose V, Collins G, Kidd B L S 1971 Ventricular septal defect. Incidence, morbidity and mortality in various age groups. British Heart Journal 33 (Suppl): 81–87

Kenna A P, Smithells R W, Fielding D W 1975 Congenital heart disease in Liverpool: 1960–69. Quarterly Journal of Medicine 173: 17–44

Kerrebijn K F 1966 Incidence in infants and mortality from congenital malformations of the circulatory system. Acta Paediatrica Scandinavica 55: 316–320

Kidd B S L, Tyrell M J, Pickering D 1971 Transposition 1969. In: Kidd B S L, Keith J D (eds) The natural history and progress in treatment of congenital heart defects. Thomas, Springfield, p 127

Landtman B 1971 Clinical and morphological studies in congenital heart disease. Acta Paediatrica Scandinavica (Suppl) 213: 1–27

Laursen H B 1980 Some epidemiological aspects of congenital heart disease in Denmark. Acta Paediatrica Scandinavica 69: 619–624

Liebman J, Cullum L, Belloc N B 1969 Natural history of transposition of the great arteries. Circulation 40: 237–262

Lilienfeld A M, Parkhurst E, Patton R, Schlesinger E R 1951 Accuracy of supplemental medical information on birth certificates. United States Public Health Reports 66: 191–198

Liu M C, Corlett K 1959 A study of congenital defects in mongolism. Archives of Disease in Childhood 34: 410–419

Macartney F 1979 A better deal for newborns with congenital heart disease. Archives of Disease in Childhood 54: 268–270

McGeorge M, Rodda R (1963) Deaths from congenital cardiac malformations in infancy and childhood. New Zealand Medical Journal 62: 261–269

Michaëlsson M 1965 Congenital heart disease – some data on the relative incidence, natural history and operability. Acta Paediatrica Scandinavica 154 (Suppl 159): 154–155

Mitchell S C, Korones S B, Berendes H W 1971a Congenital heart disease in 56 109 births. Incidence and natural history. Circulation 43: 323–332

Mitchell S C, Sellmann A H, Westphal M C, Park J 1971b Etiologic correlates in a study of congenital heart disease in 56 109 births. American Journal of Cardiology 28: 653–657

Momma K, Takao A, Ando M 1982 Angiocardiographic study of coarctation of the aorta – morphology and morphogenesis. Japanese Circulation Journal 46: 174–183

Muir C S 1966 Incidence of congenital heart disease in Singapore. British Heart Journal 22: 243–254

Neel J V 1958 A study of major congenital defects in Japanese infants. American Journal of Human Genetics 10: 398–445

Pai B V, Varkey C C (1974) Spectrum of congenital heart disease in a general hospital. Study of 200 cases. Indian Journal of Pediatrics 41: 317–321

Poland B J, Lowry R B 1974 The use of spontaneous abortions and stillbirths in genetic counseling. American Journal of Obstetrics and Gynecology 118: 322–326

Reifenstein G H, Levine S A, Gross R E 1947 Coarctation of the aorta. A review of 104 autopsied cases of the 'adult type', 2 years of age or older. American Heart Journal 33: 146–168

Richards M R, Merritt K K, Samuels M H, Langmann A G 1955 Congenital malformations of the cardiovascular system in a series of 6053 infants. Pediatrics 15: 12–29

Roberts N K, Cretin S 1980 The changing face of congenital heart disease. A method for predicting the influence of cardiac surgery upon the prevalence and spectrum of congenital heart disease. Medical Care 18: 930–939

Roberts W C 1970 The congenitally bicuspid aortic valve. A study of 85 autopsy cases. American Journal of Cardiology 26: 72–83

Rose V, Boyd A R J, Ashton T E 1964 Incidence of heart disease in the city of Toronto. Canadian Medical Association Journal 91: 95–100.

Rowe R D, Uchida I A 1961 Cardiac malformation in mongolism. American Journal of Medicine 31: 726–735

Rowe R D, Vlad P, Keith J D 1955 Experiences with 180 cases of tetralogy of Fallot in infants and children. Canadian Medical Association Journal 73: 23–30

Rygg I H, Olesen K, Boesen I 1971 The life history of tetralogy of Fallot. Danish Medical Bulletin 18 (Suppl 2): 25–30

Sakakibara S 1964 Surgical treatment of congenital cardiac lesions in infants younger than 2 years of age. Japanese Heart Journal 5: 297–300

Schrire V (1963) Experience with congenital heart disease at Groote Schuur hospital, Cape Town. South African Medical Journal 37: 1175–1180

Shaher R M 1973 Complete transposition of the great arteries. Academic Press, New York & London

Shaher R M, Farina M A, Porter I H, Bishop M 1972 Clinical aspects of congenital heart disease in mongolism. American Journal of Cardiology 29: 497–503

Shann M K M 1969 Congenital heart disease in Taiwan, Republic of China. Circulation 39: 251–258

Siltanen P 1968 Atrial septal defect of secundum type in adults. Academic dissertation, University of Helsinki, Finland

Somerville J 1965 Ostium primum defect: factors causing deterioration in the natural history. British Heart Journal 27: 413–419

Strafford M A, Griffiths S P, Gersony W M 1982 Coarctation of the aorta: a study in delayed detection. Pediatrics 69: 159–163

US Bureau of the Census 1970 Statistical abstract of the United States; 91st edn. Washington

Wagner H R, Ellison R C, Keane J F, Humphries J O, Nadas A S 1977 Clinical course in aortic stenosis. Circulation 56 (Suppl I): 47–56

Wallooppillai N J, Jayasinghe M de S 1970 Congenital heart disease in Ceylon. British Heart Journal 32: 304–306

Weidman W H, Blount S G Jr, DuShane J W, Gersony W M, Hayes C J, Nadas A S 1977 Clinical course in ventricular septal defect. Circulation 56 (Suppl I): 57–69

Wilson M G, Lubschez R 1942 Prognosis for children with congenital anomalies of the heart and central vessels. Journal of Pediatrics 21: 23–30

The aetiology of congenital heart disease

Ectopia cordis was known to the Babylonians, who regarded it as a portent of national disaster (Taussig, 1982). It is almost certain that the ancients also recognised cyanosis. Nonetheless, 'modern' studies of congenital heart defects date from the Renaissance. The earliest scientific record is credited to Leonardo da Vinci who, in 1513, described an atrial septal defect in a necropsy specimen (Rashkind, 1972). The following four centuries saw the delineation of the spectrum of congenital heart defects, but there was little progress in the understanding of their causes.

As with other congenital malformations, a variety of environmental insults were suspected. Observations of families with more than one affected member raised the possibility of hereditary factors. The recognition of rubella embryopathy gave credence to the environmental lobby, while a search for heart defects which followed Mendelian patterns of inheritance yielded examples such as Ellis van Creveld syndrome (1940) (see below). Systematic analyses of large groups of patients with heart defects (McKeown et al, 1953; Polani & Campbell, 1955), however, failed to produce evidence for either obvious environmental factors or a single gene defect in most patients. It was concluded that a complex interaction of genes and environment was responsible for most congenital heart defects. The discovery of trisomy 21 in 1959, and the subsequent rapid progress of clinical cytogenetics, permitted the definition of the important minority in which heart development is disordered by a major chromosomal defect.

It has become customary to divide reviews of the aetiology of congenital heart disease into four categories – chromosome defects, environmental causes, genetic causes, and mutifactorial causes. It is reasonable to discuss separately the chromosome disorders, since the high incidence of heart defects in such patients probably results solely from a major disruption of genetic control. The other 'categories' imply clear divisions where often none exist. Therefore, instead I review in the second part of the chapter those defects known to be produced by teratogens and malformation syndromes respectively. The principles of polygenic inheritance and the multifactorial model are reviewed in the third section. Persistent patency of the arterial duct is used to illustrate how this model fits in with single gene defects and specific teratogens. In the fourth part I review the roles of epidemiology, twin studies and family studies as applied to isolated or 'non-syndromic' heart defects so as to assess the relevance of the different hypotheses.

CHROMOSOME DEFECTS (ANEUPLOIDY)

Each body cell contains, in its nucleus, 46 chromosomes – its own copy of the body's blueprint. Of these, 44 chromosomes are common to males and females – the 22 pairs of autosomes. The remaining two are the sex chromosomes, X and Y. 'Aneuploidy' is a generic term for any disturbance of the chromosome complement other than the addition of whole extra sets, polyploidy. Translated literally, 'aneuploidy' means 'not good set', and may be defined as the loss or gain of all or part of a chromosome.

Autosomal aneuploidy

Autosomal aneuploidy, that is, any disturbances of chromosomes other than X or Y, causes major disturbances of embryonic development, with the result that most are spontaneously aborted. Among the survivors, the commonest form of aneuploidy is trisomy. This is the addition of one whole extra chromosome. Most cases are the result of non-disjunction at meiosis. When the primordial cell divides to produce an egg or sperm, the matching pairs of chromosomes separate, so that the gamete contains one of each (23 in all – a haploid set). The fusion of an egg and sperm restores the number to 46. If a chromosome pair fails to separate at meiosis, the gamete (and hence the embryo) will have either one too many or one too few. The latter group abort, as do most of the former, particularly when large chromosomes are involved. Fetuses with trisomy for the smaller chromosomes may reach term, in particular trisomy 13, 18 or 21.

Trisomy 21

One in 20 children born with a heart defect has trisomy 21 (Kenna et al, 1975). It is, therefore, the largest specific aetiological category. The term 'mongolian idiot' was first used by John Langdon Down in 1866 in his classic description of the syndrome, on the incorrect premise that these children look like members of the Mongolian race. In 1959 Lejeune et al identified the presence of an extra small chromosome designated number 21. Figure 2.1a shows the appearance using modern banding techniques. The characteristic dysmorphic features are easily recognised (Fig. 2.1b). Intelligence is rarely in the normal range, the mean quotient being about 50. Such children have an increased incidence of malformation and disease (duodenal atresia, Hirschsprung's disease and anal atresia, leukaemia and immune system defects). Those who reach

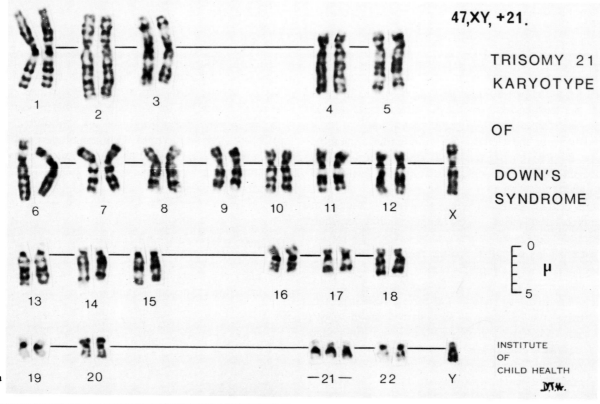

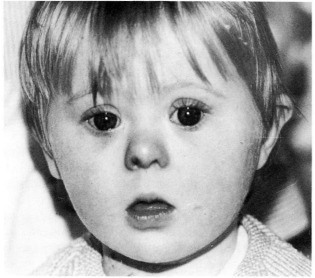

Fig. 2.1 The chromosomal and facial appearance of trisomy 21.
(a) Karyotype of trisomy 21 using modern banding techniques.
(b) Facial appearance.

Table 2.1 Down's syndrome – facts and figures.

1. Down's syndrome affects 1 in 700 children born.

2. Trisomy 21 accounts for 1 in 20 of all children with a heart defect.
   92% due to non-disjunction.
   5% due to Robertsonian translocation.
   3% due to parental mosaicism.

3. A cardiovascular malformation is present in 40% of affected infants.

4. Nature of heart defect.
   43% atrioventricular septal defect.
   32% ventricular septal defect.
   10% atrial septal defect within oval fossa.
   6% tetralogy of Fallot.
   4% isolated persistent patency of arterial duct.
   5% other.

5. In non-disjunction trisomy 21, 25% are of paternal origin.

adulthood tend to age prematurely. Of particular interest here is the frequency of heart malformation; Rowe & Uchida (1961) found 70 of a prospective series of 174 cases (40%) to have a defect of the heart and/or great vessels. Of these, 24 (36%) had an atrioventricular septal defect and 23 (33%) had a ventricular septal defect. In a review of 251 infants with trisomy 21 who had a heart defect, Park et al (1977) found 43% to have an atrioventricular septal defect (Table 2.1). 30% had multiple anomalies, with persistence of the arterial duct being the second most common lesion (affecting 16%). In a review of necropsy series, Warkany et al (1966) found 140 of 272 infants with Down's syndrome to have a heart malformation. 64% had an atrioventricular septal defect.

The strong association of atrioventricular septal defect with trisomy 21 is not seen with other chromosome anomalies. It prompts the speculation that some important function of endocardial cushion growth or adhesion is determined by genes on chromosome 21.

From a practical viewpoint the presence of left axis deviation in a neonate with the features of Down's syndrome makes an atrioventricular septal defect very likely. Conversely, the frequent association of congenital heart defects and trisomy 21 makes it important to consider Down's syndrome in any neonate presenting with a probable heart malformation. The diagnosis may be difficult in a sick, intubated infant. In this situation the flat occiput, short curved little fingers with single flexion creases and single palmar creases are helpful. It should be remembered that the latter occur as a unilateral feature in 1 in 25 children with non-syndromic heart defects, but in only 1 in 75 is it a bilateral feature. This is one of the few situations where bedside dermatoglyphic examination may be of practical use. 'Finger-print' patterns are under strong genetic control and reveal a disturbance in chromosome disorders. Figure 2.2 shows how to identify and interpret the relatively characteristic features in Down's syndrome, namely a distal axial triradius, and a high frequency of ulnar loops on the finger tips.

A further useful sign is the wide first toe cleft. Associated with this is a variant of the dermatoglyphic pattern over the first metatarsal head. 75% of children with Down's syndrome have a tibial arch. This feature is seen in only 0.3% of the normal population.

It is always important to remember that normal individuals can possess these features. So the distal axial triradius can occur in up to 10% of the normal population and ulnar loops occur on the right first finger in about 30%. Therefore, their main value is negative. If they are absent, this is against the diagnosis of Down's syndrome, but their presence cannot be regarded as an absolute confirmation. David (1981) examined the dermatoglyphics of 800 heart patients and compared them to 1000 controls. He could not confirm earlier claims that non-syndromic heart defects are associated with abnormal dermatoglyphics.

Mosaic Down's syndrome. About 3% of children with trisomy 21 have a parent who is a mosaic. This means that some of the cells of the parents have an extra chromosome 21, and this involves one or both gonads. If mosaicism is identified in the parent, the recurrence risk is greater than 10% (Harris et al, 1982). It is the existence of such families which accounts for part of the 1% recurrence risk in sibs of a child with trisomy 21. In addition, some parents seem to have an increased risk of non-disjunction, since recurrences of trisomy involving chromosomes other than 21 have been described.

Translocation Down's syndrome. Trisomy 21 in 3–6% of children with Down's syndrome is associated with a Robertsonian translocation. About one-quarter are inherited from a parent, usually the mother. The other three-quarters are new mutations. (Speed et al, 1976, Albright & Hook, 1980). A carrier of a balanced Robertsonian translocation is entirely normal but has only 45 chromosomes in each cell because one number 21 chromosome is fused to another. The other chromosome is usually a number 14 which is also acrocentric (i.e. has negligible short arms which may be lost in the fusion). At gamete formation the 14s determine migration. The other unpaired number 21 chromosome may go either way, so that up to 50% of gametes contain either two 21 chromosomes or no number 21. The latter produces an embryo which is monosomic for 21 and is not viable. The former results in trisomy 21. The other possibilities are normal or carrier, so one-third of a carrier's surviving offspring should have Down's syndrome. In practice the risk is less than 1% if father is a carrier and 10% if mother is the carrier. Presumably this is because an unbalanced translocation has a deleterious effect on the gamete or on the embryo. A karyotype should be obtained in all babies with Down's syndrome. If an unbalanced translocation is found, the parents should be checked for carrier status. If the translocation involves fusion of both 21 chromosomes in the parent, all surviving offspring will have Down's syndrome.

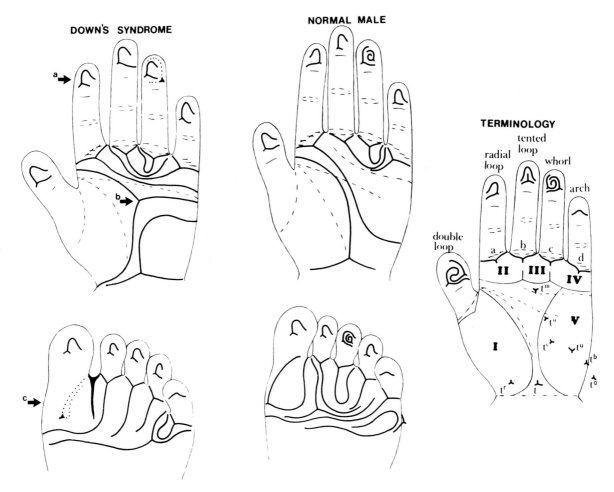

Fig. 2.2 Dermatoglyphics in Down's syndrome. The dotted lines illustrate the palmar creases. The solid lines illustrate the fine ridge patterns. Examination is possible with the naked eye, but is easier with an auroscope without earpiece or ophthalmoscope using a plus 20 lens. To support a diagnosis of trisomy 21, first check with naked eye for absence of the distal flexion crease on the fifth finger and single ('simian') palmar creases. Then, with a lens, examine the index finger of the right hand for an ulna loop (a) which occurs in over 90% of children with trisomy 21. If time permits examine the other fingers. There should be 8–10 ulnar loops whereas normally there are less than 7. Next follow the ridge pattern from the thenar eminence across the palm to identify the triradius where it meets the ridge pattern from the wrist, and that from the hypothenar eminence. The triradius should be distally placed (b). Finally, check the pattern over the head of the first metatarsal. There should be a tibial arch – the ridge pattern crosses to the medial border without forming a triradius. (Reproduced by kind permission of Pedro Saldana-Garcia.)

When patients with Down's syndrome reach puberty, parents become concerned at the possibility of them having children. Males with trisomy 21 are almost invariably sterile. Females have reduced fertility but are able to bear children. A review of 21 such cases (Masterson et al, 1970) found 33% of the children to have Down's syndrome. Table 2.2 summarises the figures needed when counselling the parents of a child with Down's syndrome.

Trisomy 18 (Edward's syndrome)

Trisomy 18 affects 1 in 3500 newborn. Early death is almost invariable due to multiple malformations. Survivors are severely retarded. Typical features are a prominent occiput, low set malformed ears and micrognathis (Fig. 2.3), though the appearance is less characteristic than that seen with trisomy 21 or 13. Two additional clinical signs of great value are the unusual clenched fists (Fig. 2.3) and rockerbottom feet. Heart defects are present in the majority, most being persistent patency of the arterial duct or ventricular septal defects. A bedside diagnosis is strengthened by examination of dermatoglyphic patterns. A distal axial triradius and simple arches on 3 or more digits are characteristic but are not unique to this abnormality.

Trisomy 13 (Patau's syndrome)

One in 7000 newborn infants have Patau's syndrome. The majority die as neonates. Survival beyond the first year is exceptional. The characteristic clinical features are polydactyly, cleft lip and palate, often bilateral and severe, and

Table 2.2 Genetic counselling for Down's syndrome.

Risk increases with

a. **Maternal age at delivery**		35	36	37	38	39	40	41	42	43
Risk of affected live birth (based on Hook & Lindsjo, 1978)	*one in*	398	305	234	179	137	105	80	61	47
Risk of positive aminocentesis (based on Ferguson-Smith & Yates, 1984)	*one in*	263	204	159	124	96	75	58	46	36

b. **Previous trisomic child** – about 10%

c. **Mosaicism in one parent** – to about 10%

d. **Robertsonian translocation** e.g. 14/21
   Parents' karyotypes normal   – 'age' risk only
   Father carrier   – 'age' risk + 1%
   Mother carrier   – 10%

e. **21/21 Translocation**
   Balanced form in either parent – all offspring affected

f. **Full trisomy 21 in mother** – risk 33%

AMNIOCENTESIS – performed at 16 weeks
                         – results in 2–4 weeks
                         – termination of affected pregnancy at about 20 weeks
Risk of procedure   – miscarriage in 1 in 200
                         – fetal and maternal morbidity negligible

hypotelorism associated with malformation of the frontal lobes of the brain (holoprosencephaly – Fig. 2.4). There is a high incidence of cardiac defects, in particular atrial and ventricular septal defects. Abnormalities of cardiac position are relatively frequent (Schinzel, 1983), perhaps indicating atrial isomerism. As with atrioventricular septal defects and trisomy 21, the high incidence of disturbed cardiac position in trisomy 13 may reflect a specific role for this part of the genome in the determination of laterality.

Other defects of the autosomes

An increasing number of syndromes have been assigned to specific autosomal anomalies since the introduction of G banding in the early 1970s permitted the recognition of individual chromosomes and parts thereof (Schinzel, 1983). There are a number of characteristic features common to most infants in this group. The most notable are low birth weight, mental retardation, short stature, microcephaly, dysmorphic features, cerebral and urogenital malformation and congenital heart defects.

Figure 2.5a shows a 2-year-old child treated surgically as a neonate for absent right atrioventricular connexion (tricuspid atresia). At 2 years, developmental delay, short stature and dysmorphic facies prompted examination of the karyotype. This revealed extra material on the long arm of chromosome 13. The karyotype of the other family

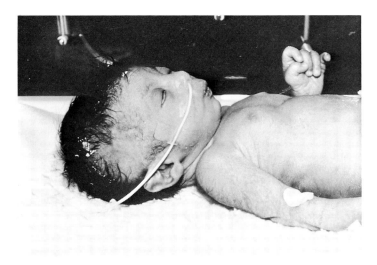

Fig. 2.3 The features of a patient with trisomy 18. Note the prominent occiput, small mandible, short sternum and unusual clenched fist with fingers 2 and 5 over 3 and 4.

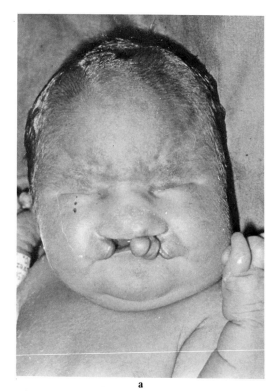

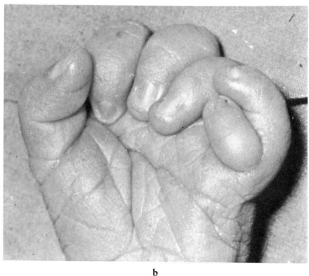

Fig. 2.4 Features of trisomy 13 – Patau's syndrome. (a) Severe facial clefting. (b) An example of typical ulnar polydactyly.

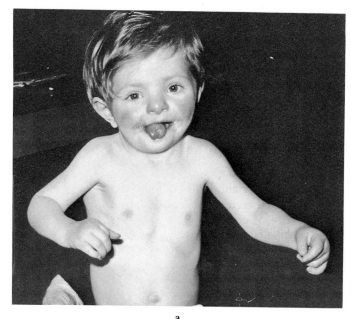

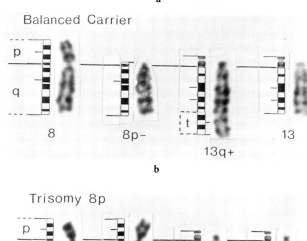

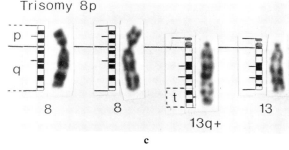

Fig. 2.5 (a) 2-year-old child with dysmorphic features, absent right atrioventricular connexion and developmental delay due to trisomy for the short arm of chromosome 8. (b) Chromosome appearance in carrier father. (c) Chromosome appearance in affected child (trisomy 8p).

members showed this to be part of the short arm of chromosome 8 (Fig. 2.5b). Father carried a balanced 8; 13 translocation; this child had resulted from the fertilisation of a normal egg containing one 8 and one 13 chromosone, with a sperm containing a normal 8 and the elongated 13. As a result, she had 3 short arms of 8, designated trisomy 8p. Her brother was a carrier like father (Burn et al, 1984).

The recurrence risk in such families, ascertained through the birth of a child with an unbalanced karyo-type, is just under 1 in 5 (Boue, 1981). Unlike carriers of Robertsonian translocations, male and female carriers of reciprocal translocations seem equally likely to transmit the unbalanced form.

In practice, chromosome analysis is not indicated when a heart defect is present in isolation, or, in the older child, when intelligence is normal. It is indicated in any neonate likely to die from a heart defect who has additional malformations, or in an older child who shows significant developmental delay. If necessary a cardiac aspiration should be performed after death. In some centres an urgent chromosome count may be carried out when indicated on bone marrow aspirate, though this method can exclude only full trisomy.

It is likely that a substantial number of cases are not recognised at present. Minor dysmorphic features are often difficult to evaluate, and it is not difficult to attribute short stature and developmental delay to the impact of physical illness. Recognition of chromosomal aneuploidy is, however, important. If a familial reciprocal translocation is recognised, recurrence of malformation may be avoided. Conversely, if normal karyotypes in the parents show the child's anomaly to have arisen 'de novo' it is possible to offer an explanation for the heart malformation, and reassure the parents that there is no increased risk to their future offspring.

Sex chromosome aneuploidy

The female has two X chromosomes in each cell. The male has one X and the small Y chromosome. The latter determines maleness. The normal development of males shows that only a single 'copy' is required for genes on the X chromosome. Females avoid having excess by inactivating one of the two X chromosomes in each cell (lyonisation), between the 16 and 1000 cell stage of embryonic life. When an excess of X chromosomes are present in each cell, all but one are switched off. An embryo can therefore tolerate chromosome complements which contain three, four or five X chromosomes with relatively little disturbance of development. Apart from the frequent occurrence of persistent patency of the arterial duct in the penta-X group, heart development is not affected. This is not the case when a single sex chromosome is present from the start, 45X.

45X Turner's syndrome

Though first described by Ullrich (1930), the resultant syndrome is associated with the name of the American physician Turner (1938). Despite being mild relative to most other forms of chromosome aneuploidy, Turner's syndrome is associated with particularly heavy prenatal loss. Based on studies of aborted fetuses, it is estimated that the 1 in 10 000 birth frequency represents only 1% of conceptions with the 45X karyotype (Polani, 1982). Figure 2.6 shows the typical features. Failure of sexual maturation, and short stature are associated often with a webbed neck (also known as 'pterygium colli'), 'shark' mouth, down-slanting palpebral fissures and low set ears. The strong association with aortic coarctation is well known. Aortic stenosis is the commonest of a wide variety of other heart defects seen rarely in patients with Turner's

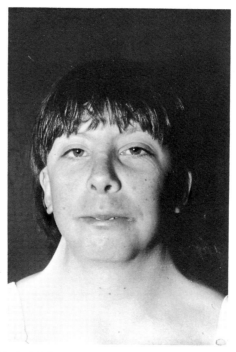

Fig. 2.6 Typical facies and webbed neck appearance of a patient with 45X Turner's syndrome.

syndrome. The prevalence of heart defects among 45X individuals cannot be established easily because of the difficulty in ascertaining an unbiased sample. Simpson (1976) reviewed reports of heart defects with 45X identified through surveys of gonadal dysgenesis, amenorrhoea or chromosome screening. Of 228 pooled cases, 22 cases of heart defects were noted, though heart defects were excluded in only 119 of these. This gives a risk of 10–16%. Miller et al (1983) identified 80 45X girls in a paediatric endocrinology clinic, 13 of whom had coarctation. In a consecutive sample of 35 not known to have a heart defect, detailed echographic examination revealed evidence of bicuspid aortic valve in 12, mitral valve prolapse in 2, and idiopathic aortic root dilation in 2. Conversely, heart defects are uncommon among 45X patients diagnosed in gynaecology clinics (Simpson, 1976). An association between cardiovascular anomalies and the more obvious Turner stigmata (such as neck webbing and lymphoedema) which prompt early referral would account for the disparity. A reasonable working figure would be that 10% of 45X children have a significant cardiovascular disorder and perhaps a further 10% have minor valve anomalies on echocardiography.

The 'buccal smear' reveals absence of Barr bodies, the condensed inactivated X chromosome lying by the nuclear membrane. This test continues to be used in some centres as a rapid confirmation of diagnosis but should not now be regarded as a substitute for detailed chromosome examination.

It might be asked why a 45X karyotype is such a disadvantage when all males have only one X chromosome. In the ovaries, both X chromosomes are active and are essential to development of the gonad. In other tissues inactivation of one X chromosome is not complete. It is now known that several genes near the end of the short arm of the X chromosome (including the Xg blood group locus) remain functional after 'lyonisation', and that the Y chromosome carries equivalent genes. The 45X individual has only a single copy of these genes. It is this deficiency which probably accounts for several stigmata of Turner's syndrome.

XXY syndrome (Klinefelter's syndrome) does not have a high incidence of heart disorder. Rosenthal (1972) found cases of XXY syndrome with tetralogy of Fallot, persistent patency of the arterial duct and septal defects, but the prevalence of heart defects differed little from the general population. More recently an excess of cases with the floppy mitral valve syndrome has been noted (Fricke et al, 1981).

SINGLE GENES, MAJOR TERATOGENS AND SYNDROMES

Nine-tenths of liveborn children with heart defects have normal karyotypes. This does not exclude a genetic basis, since individual genes are far beyond the resolution of the microscope. Each chromosome contains a single molecule of DNA, condensed by tight coiling. The smallest band on chromosome 1 contains enough DNA for 2000–3000 genes. In practice there may be only 50 or so, as the majority of chromosomal DNA is intergenic (that is, it contains no apparently useful information). If an abnormality in one gene pair results in malformation of the heart, the term 'single gene defect' is applied. These obey the basic Mendelian rules of inheritance, and may be divided into three categories: autosomal recessive, autosomal dominant and X-linked. In a proportion of families the family history and/or the presence of distinctive extracardiac features permit recognition of a 'single gene defect'. These are discussed first.

Single gene defects

A gene or allele is a piece of DNA which includes the code for a single polypeptide chain. The position of the allele on a chromosome is the 'gene locus'. As all chromosomes (except the sex chromosomes) are present in matching pairs, each locus on the autosomes has two alleles. Each allele contributes an equal amount to the gene product in the cell. If trisomy occurs, there are three alleles at each locus on the chromosome involved. This causes a 50% increase in production of polypeptide chains from these loci.

The genetic code is written using 4 bases : adenine (A), guanine (G), cytosine (C) and thymine (T). The bases are 'read' in blocks of three with a triplet representing one amino acid residue in the polypeptide chain. There are 64 possible combinations of the 4 letters, so most of the amino acids have more than one code. Other triplets act as breaks or full stops. Typically, genes (alleles) have intervening sequences. These are sequences of letters with no apparent meaning which are removed during the transcription to messenger RNA.

If the two alleles at a locus have exactly the same sequence of bases, the individual is homozygous for that allele. If there are differences, the individual is a heterozygote. While each person has only two alleles, there may be dozens, or even hundreds, of variant alleles in a population. In a few, the variation in the gene results in a defective gene product. When a single abnormal allele is present at a locus, the normal allele continues to generate 50% of the normal polypeptide. If this is sufficient for the needs of the body, heterozygotes remain healthy and are referred to as carriers. Only when two defective alleles are present at the locus does the disease occur. It is then referred to as an 'autosomal recessive' disease; that is, the 'disease' gene is recessive to the 'normal gene'. Among recessive disorders involving the heart, a good example is Pompe's disease (glycogen storage disease type IIa; Pompe, 1933; Fig. 2.7). In this case the gene product involved is the enzyme 1α-glucosidase, or acid maltase, a lysosomal enzyme providing an important secondary pathway for the breakdown of glycogen. Pompe's disease is an 'inborn error of metabolism'. It is rare, affecting about 1 in 125 000 (Loonen, 1979). From this figure, it may be deduced that, in the whole population, 1 in 350 alleles are of 'Pompe's type'. (q is the frequency of the abnormal gene in the population. q^2 is the probability of two such alleles occurring in the same person, that is, the homozygote frequency. Therefore the gene frequency is the square root of the disease incidence.) As each individual has two alleles at this locus, there are two chances of having at least one abnormal allele, so the carrier frequency is 1 in 175.

Having had one affected child, the parents may be regarded as proven heterozygotes. In subsequent pregnancies the recurrence risk is 1 in 4; there is a half chance of the sperm receiving the chromosome with the defective allele and similarly a half chance of an 'affected' ovum. If either parent has children with another consort the risk falls to 1 in 350 (1/2 × 1/175). Therefore, artificial insemination by donor may be offered as a means of prevention. Alternatively, prenatal diagnosis is effective, either looking for vacuoles in the fibroblasts on electron microscopy or identifying acid maltase deficiency in the cultured fibroblasts. Polani et al (1979) reported that, over a 10-year period, 6 amniotic fluid samples were tested for this condition at Guy's Hospital. One infant was shown to be

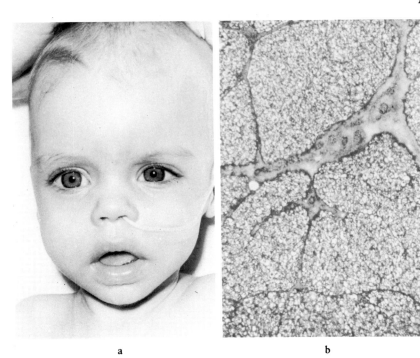

a   b

Fig. 2.7 Pompe's disease – autosomal recessive cardiomyopathy. Hypotonia, cardiomegaly and macroglossia due to the deposition of glycogen in muscle lysosomes. Echocardiography reveals marked thickening with a short PR interval of 0.05–0.09 seconds. Vacuolated lymphocytes are seen on the blood film. Death is invariable, usually occurring in the first twelve months of life. (a) A patient with typical hypotonic facies. (Reproduced by kind permission of Dr H. Bain.) (b) Glycogen deposits in skeletal muscle. (Reproduced by courtesy of Dr P. Hudgson.)

affected and pregnancy was terminated. The other 5 produced normal children.

In most autosomal recessive disorders no biochemical disorder is recognised and the inheritance pattern is recognised by the occurrence of the same pattern of malformation in several members of the same sibship with normal parents. Consanguinity (cousin marriage) in the parents is another clue. A good example of a well-recognised autosomal recessive syndrome is Ellis van Creveld syndrome (Fig. 2.8).

If some or all cells in the body need both alleles at a locus to be functioning normally, a heterozygote with one defective allele will fall below normal requirement, and disease will result. This is typically seen with structural proteins. Marfan's syndrome is the classic example in cardiology. Because the heterozygote has features of the disease (aortic and mitral valve regurgitation, aortic aneurysm, arachnodactyly, lens dislocation and joint laxity), we regard this as an autosomal dominant condition. When an individual suffering from Marfan's syndrome has childen, there is a 50% chance that the patient's egg or sperm will contain the defective allele. Since this is enough to cause disease, the recurrence risk in offspring is 50%. If a child with the classic syndrome has apparently normal parents, there are two possible explanations: one parent may carry the gene but, because of the effect of other genes, may not have developed the disease; the child may have a new mutation. If some minor features are present in one parent (such as joint laxity and arachnodactyly), this is called 'reduced expression'. It is unusual for carriers of major autosomal dominant disorders to be totally free from clinical disorder (non-penetrance), so if both parents and other family members are normal, the child's disease prob-

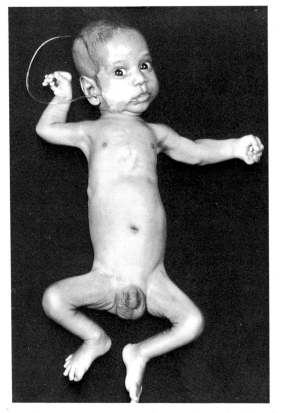

Fig. 2.8 Ellis van Creveld syndrome. Autosomal recessive short rib polydactyly syndrome with common atrium, multiple oral frenulae and natal teeth.

ably results from a new mutation. If a dominant disorder is sufficiently severe to make procreation unlikely, 'genetic fitness' is said to be reduced. The incidence of the disease

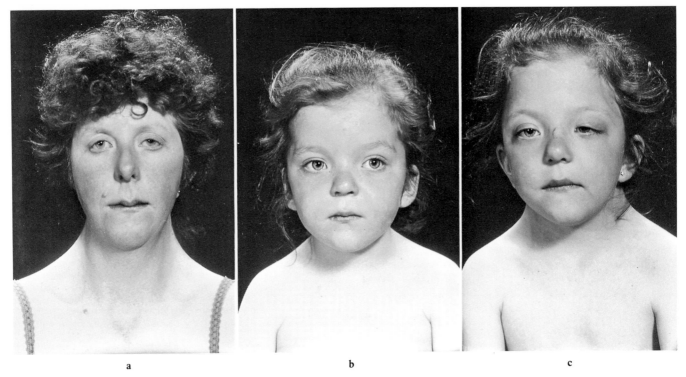

Fig. 2.9 Noonan's syndrome appearing in a mother and her two daughters. (a) The mother has pulmonary stenosis and atrial septal defect, neck webbing, down-slanting eyes and ptosis. She has normal intelligence. (b) The younger daughter has the same heart defect and normal intelligience. (c) The older daughter has a normal heart, but webbed neck, ptosis and moderate mental handicap.

equilibrates where the rate of new mutation equals the loss of defective alleles due to the death of affected individuals.

Noonan's syndrome is an autosomal dominant syndrome involving a high incidence of congenital heart defects (in particular pulmonary stenosis with valve dysplasia, atrial septal defect within the oval fossa and, later, hypertrophic cardiomyopathy). Figure 2.9 shows a mother with the typical facial features of Noonan's syndrome with her two daughters. Mother and the younger daughter are of normal intelligence but required surgical correction of pulmonary stenosis and atrial septal defect. The elder daughter is educationally subnormal, but has a normal heart. Sanchez-Cascos (1983) reviewed 21 children with features of Noonan's syndrome from a series of 2000 children with heart defects. Only one parent had facial features of the syndrome. When dealing with dominant disorders which reduce fertility, it is not uncommon to find a large proportion of affected children who are new mutations and have normal parents. The possibility of heterogeneity must also be considered. Sanchez-Cascos suggested that Noonan's syndrome results from a particular disturbance of development of the sixth branchial arch, and that only a proportion of cases constitute an autosomal dominant single gene defect. In other words, several different aetiological factors may act through a common pathway to produce what appears to be distinct anomaly. This concept is worthy of recall when dealing with non-syndromic heart malformations.

The third form of Mendelian inheritance is X-linked. The male has only one X chromosome in each cell, so any gene locus on the X chromosome has only one allele in male cells. If a boy has a defective allele at an X chromosome locus, a deficiency of gene product must result.

The test of X-linked inheritance is failure of affected males to pass the disease to their sons (a son must receive a Y chromosome from father). If data is limited, transmission through the female line with males suffering a more severe disorder is strongly suggestive.

Duchenne muscular dystrophy is a typical example. Affected patients suffer severe progressive striate muscle degeneration. A cardiomyopathy is evident in many. As has been discussed, the female at an early stage of development has two X chromosomes, one of which is inactivated in each cell. If the chromosome carrying the defective allele is inactivated, the clone derived from that cell will be free from any abnormality. On average, half of the cells in a female will function normally, and half will be defective. The multinuclear muscle cells probably result from fusion of many cells. It is only on rare occasions, therefore, that a female has the misfortune to use only 'defective' cells to make a large proportion of her muscle.

Examples of X-linked genes causing structural heart

defects are rare. One example is the family in which there were 4 males with 'complex dextrocardia', reported by Soltan & Li (1974). They belong to three separate sibships linked by female relatives. A variety of heart defects were associated with their disturbed situs. Monteleone & Fagan (1969) described a family in which all 6 males in three generations had heart defects. Of these, 4 had mitral and aortic incompetence, 1 had mitral stenosis and 1 was not diagnosed. X-linked transmission was probable.

Several hundred syndromes are now recognised on the basis of recognisable patterns of malformation, or pedigree data, or both. Heart defects may occur in a significant proportion. The Appendix (p. 42) contains the more important entities. They are grouped according to the principle extra-cardiac feature. This results in some overlap, but is more useful clinically than alphabetical lists. It is important to remember that this is an area of literature which continues to expand rapidly. If a child has several malformations and normal chromosomes, a syndrome diagnosis should be sought, either by referral or by approaching the literature using the most striking and unusual extracardiac features.

Specific teratogens

The search for specific environmental associations has scored notable successes. This began with the recognition of the congenital rubella syndrome, with its strong association with persistent patency of the arterial duct and peripheral pulmonary stenosis. From 1970–1975 an annual average of 64 cases of congenital rubella were notified in England, Wales and Scotland, of which 39% had multiple malformations. This gave a multiple malformation rate of 3.27/100 000. This is an underestimate of the true incidence, though not all had heart involvement. At this incidence level, recognised congenital rubella contributed just under 0.5% of all heart defects during the early 1970s. The rubella epidemic of 1978–1979 increased briefly the number of malformations caused by rubella in Britain. Since then the first girls to be immunised have reached child-bearing age, so the importance of this teratogen should now recede (National Congenital Rubella Surveillance Programme, 1979).

Table 2.3 lists some other important known teratogenic influences (Nora & Nora, 1983). Diabetes illustrates many important features. There is a clear association between maternal diabetes and congenital heart disease, with the latter forming an important element of a variable malformation complex which is best labelled 'diabetic embryopathy'. The other major feature is 'caudal regression' or sacral agenesis with associated vertebral and lower limb defects. Williamson (1970) reported congenital heart disease in 20% of patients with skeletal features of diabetic embryopathy. A 4% risk of offspring was found by

Table 2.3 Important cardiovascular teratogens (after Nora & Nora, 1983).

Teratogen	Frequency of CV disease	Most common cardiac malformations
Infections		
Rubella	35%	Persistent patency of arterial duct Peripheral pulmonary stenosis Septal defects
Drugs		
Alcohol (high intake)	25–30%	Septal defects
Hydantoin	2–3%	Pulmonary and aortic stenosis Coarctation of aorta Arterial duct
Trimethadione	15–30%	Complete transposition Tetralogy of Fallot Hypoplastic left heart
Thalidomide		Tetralogy of Fallot, septal defects Common arterial trunk
Lithium		Ebstein's anomaly Tricuspid atresia Atrial septal defect
Maternal Disease		
Diabetes (poor control)	3–5%	Complete transposition Ventricular septal defect Coarctation of aorta
Phenylketonuria	25–50%	Tetralogy of Fallot
Systemic lupus erythematosus (Anti-Ro-antibody)	20–40%	Complete heart block

Rowland et al (1973) when the offspring of diabetic mothers were viewed as a whole. Recently it has become increasingly apparent that the quality of diabetic control affects the risk of heart disease. Reviews (Jovanovic et al, 1981; Watkins, 1982) support earlier suggestions that the maintenance of euglycaemia in early pregnancy reduces the risk of malformation to a level little higher than that seen in the general population.

The basis for the ill effect of diabetes is not known. Up to one half of offspring were reported to have significant cardiomegaly, attributed to an anabolic effect of hyperinsulinism. This effect seems distinct from the disturbance of heart morphogenesis. The latter results in an unusual distribution of malformations. Rowland found ventriculo-arterial discordance ('transposition'), ventricular septal defect and aortic coarctation to account for over half of the 19 cases with a heart defect among 470 offspring of diabetic mothers.

With successful treatment for phenylketonuria (dietary modification in childhood), a small but significant number of females have reached child-bearing age with normal intellect. Most relinguish the unpleasant diet in adolescence and may enter pregnancy with high blood levels of phenylalanine. The clinical picture here is different, because the hyperphenylalaninaemia affects the child prenatally only, whereas sufferers from the disease are protected by their healthy mother from high phenylalanine levels until after delivery. Among 524 non-treated phenylketonuria offspring, Lenke & Levey (1980) found microcephaly in two-thirds of cases and congenital heart defects in one-quarter. This was of various types. Often it was severe and led to neonatal death. Even when a phenylalanine-free diet was introduced in the first trimester, 4 of 11 offspring had congenital heart disease. Only preconception dietary modification shows evidence of reducing the teratogenic risk. The occurrence of heart defects in the children of women with a genetic disease illustrates another aspect of the nature/nurture debate. A major element of the 'environment' of an embryo is the mother herself. Variation in the mother, even due to a genetic disease, may contribute to the 'environmental variance' of the embryo.

There is a risk of congenital heart block in the fetus of mothers with systemic lupus erythematosus, probably due to iso-immune damage to the conduction tissues. Circulating anti-Ro antibodies in the mother correlate closely with fetal heart block even if the mother is asymptomatic (Scott et al, 1983). In other maternal diseases it is drug therapy which raises major questions. Among drugs in widespread use, hydantoin and lithium are of particular importance (Table 2.3). Alcohol is attracting increasing attention with the recognition that the fetal alcohol syndrome is not rare (Beattie et al, 1983). Heart defects (particularly septal defects) are common in affected children. It remains to be established whether low levels of intake are damaging.

Teratogens cannot be judged without taking account of genetic variability. As has been discussed, many gene loci are polymorphic; that is, in the population there are several allelic forms – genes may be present at this locus but produce differing polypeptides. The ABO blood group system is a good example. Only 35% of north-west Europeans are A, though this is the commonest ABO blood group in this population. 35% of this population have the rhesus group CCDee. The chance of any individual having both of these common 'phenotypes' is $35/100 \times 35/100$ or about 12%. If this is extended to 10 blood group systems and 12 serum protein polymorphic systems, the chance of any European having in combination even the 22 most common alleles is only 3.1×10^{-5}. In other words, the chance of identifying another European with the same pattern is less than 1 in 30 000. When one considers the large number of gene loci which may be polymorphic, it becomes clear that there are more possible combinations than there are people in the population. With such variability it is likely that teratogens can rarely be considered in isolation from genetic predisposition.

POLYGENIC INHERITANCE AND THE MULTIFACTORIAL MODEL

Polygenic inheritance

The theory of polygenic inheritance works on the principle that a disease is determined by a number of additive genes. In the multifactorial model, additive environmental factors are included. The value of the hypotheses has, in the past, been reduced by applying them to broad diagnostic categories, and by making the term 'multifactorial' synonymous with 'idiopathic'. Figure 2.10 illustrates an imaginary situation which will be used to translate the abstract concepts into practical use. It takes the simplest 'polygenic' situation, with a disease being determined by two additive gene loci, and only two possible alleles at each locus. If this model is examined carefully, it will explain how the rules, or predictions, of the polygenic threshold model are derived. There are six important features.

1. Recurrence risk will depend on the population incidence. The risk to sibs and offspring is approximately the square root of the population incidence.
2. The risk to sibs is comparable to the risk for offspring.
3. The risk is elevated in sibs and offspring, but risk is much less among more distant relatives.
4. The risk is further increased when multiple family members are involved.
5. Recurrence risk may increase when the disorder is more severe.
6. When there is an unequal sex incidence, the risk is greater among relatives of the more rarely affected sex (the Carter effect).

The distinction between a 'genetic' and an 'environmental' disease is arbitary. The term used to describe the proportion of variance due to genetic factors is 'heritability' (symbol h^2). Referring to Figure 2.11, in village 1, heritability was 100%, but in village 2 it was zero. If three additive loci were involved, the smallest category would be 6 minus with a population incidence of $1/4^3$ or 1/64. Again, heritability would be 100% in village 1, even though the recurrence risk in offspring, would be only 1 in 16. Thus a high heritability does not, of necessity, mean a high recurrence risk.

Single gene defects must also be considered. Both autosomal recessive and dominant disorders are known which will cause severe stunting of growth regardless of genetic background. Affected individuals would also fall below the water-level but would be difficult to distinguish in family studies from the polygenic group. For example, if a large number of achondroplastic individuals were present in the population, the effect would be to make the risk to offspring exceed significantly the risk to sibs. Morton et al (1970) have developed a more complex model which takes account of this possibility. It would require a large number of 'single gene' cases to cause a detectable variation from the risks predicted by polygenic inheritance. The

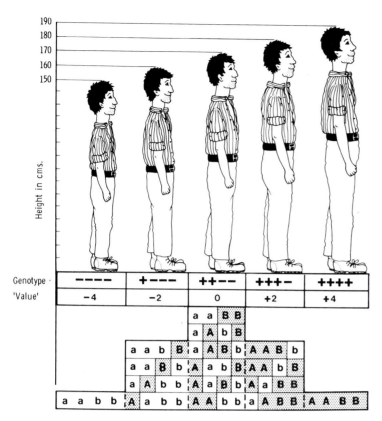

Fig. 2.10 Illustration of the polygenic threshold model. An imaginary population of 18th century Cornishmen had an average height of 170 cm. There was variation between 150 and 190 cm as a result of genetic variation at two gene loci. At the first, there were two alleles A and a, which had an equal frequency in the population as a whole. At the second locus, the alleles were B and b, and again, each made up half of the alleles in the population; a and b had a negative effect on height, one of them reducing adult height by 5 cm. B and A had a positive effect: one positive allele added 5 cm. the histogram shows the 16 possible combinations of A, a, B and b. The mean height of 170 cm, resulted from two negative with two positive alleles, and there were six combinations. One-sixteenth of the population had four negative alleles: aabb. It can be seen that even with two gene loci, the distribution of height falls into five categories whose relative proportion resembles a Gaussian distribution. This is because there is only one way of having four minus alleles, but there are six arrangements of a 2 + 2 combination.

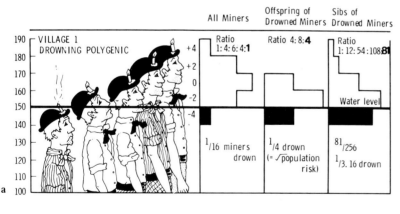

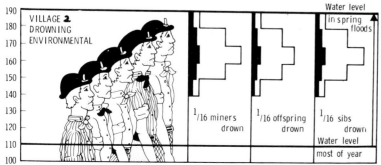

Fig. 2.11 Histograms of height and risks of drowning in imaginary 18th century tin mines.

(a) Tin was discovered! Unfortunately, tin mines in 18th century Cornwall were prone to flooding, and a proportion of the miners drowned. (a) Shows the situation in a mine with a steady water level of 150 cm. This was high enough to embarrass the airway of miners in category −4: aabb. The next histogram shows the height distribution of all prospective miners whose fathers had drowned previously. The offspring of drowned miners had a different height distribution because, with one parent from the aabb group, these individuals had a maximum height of 170 cm – they must have inherited one a and one b from the drowned parent. As the histogram shows, they fell into categories −4, −2 and 0 in a ratio of 4 : 8 : 4, giving a much higher incidence of drowning when they became miners: 1 in 4. This is the square root of the population incidence of 1 in 16, and is a simplified illustration of Edward's observation (1960) that, in the polygenic model, the risk to first degree relatives approximates to the square root of the population incidence.

That it is approximate is shown by the histogram for sibs. Both parents of an aabb child must have had at least one a allele and b allele. Unlike the offspring, it was possible for an aabb miner to have an AABB brother if both parents were AaBb. By adding up the possible combinations it works out that 81/256 (1 in 3.16) sibs were −4 (aabb), while only 1/256 fell in category +4 (AABB). This means that the histogram was skewed towards the lower categories. With more gene loci this difference between the risk to sibs and offspring would become less obvious, illustrating the second rule: in polygenic disorders, the risk to sibs and offspring is approximately the same, due to a shift of their 'curve of liability' towards the threshold.

(b) At a nearby mine, the water level was 110 cm, so no miners drowned, except in early spring when floods raised the level to 185 cm and a whole shift would drown. Again 1 in 16 tin miners drowned each year, but here there was no genetic predisposition, so having a drowned brother or father did not increase a miner's risk of drowning. The lack of familial aggregation and the marked seasonal variation made drowning an environmental trait in village 2.

features which may permit identification of single genes or major environmental factors are listed below.

Effects of major genes
1. Recessive
   a. risk greater for sibs than offspring
   b. the incidence of consanguinity is raised
2. Dominant
   a. risk greater for offspring than sibs
   b. affected members in three generations of a family are more likely.
   c. elevated paternal age

Effects of a major environmental component
1. Disease incidence likely to fluctuate with time and/or season. 'Epidemics' may be seen.
2. Frequent association with specific teratogens.
3. Familial aggregation not marked. Unlikely to involve both sibs and offspring.

Even in the simple model used in Figures 2.10 and 2.11, the collection of possible variables is impressive (the number of loci, the number of alleles at each locus, and the contribution made by spring floods). The water level could vary in all mines, drowning could reduce the number of offspring (reduced genetic fitness), short men could marry short women (assortative mating), and individuals dying in the mines from other causes could be mixed with the study population (clinical heterogeneity). In the face of such complexity, progress seems unlikely. It should, however, be possible to evaluate the contribution of major genes, additive genes and environmental factors using the characteristics listed above.

Sibs and offspring are at greater risk because the death of one family member is evidence of a genetic predisposition. The 'square root' rule is approximate. It is a function of the model used and provides a useful guide. The presence of two or more drowned miners in a family suggests, in retrospect, a predominance of *a* and *b* alleles, so making a further recurrence more likely. Sibships with three affected are possible with polygenic traits. They should be rare in comparison to families with only one affected. As a general rule, three sibs with a rare disorder are strong evidence for a single gene defect causing a recessive disease. Similarly, three consecutive generations of a family with members affected by a rare disorder is suggestive of a single dominant allele causing disease. Consanguinity has a small effect on the incidence of polygenic disorders, but a marked effect on the incidence of autosomal recessive disorders. A recessive contribution is suggested if consanguinity is raised in a population, such as the British Caucasians, where cousin marriage is rare. New mutations for many dominant conditions are more common in the offspring of older fathers, so if the mean age of fathers is greater than normal, this favours the presence of a dominant gene.

Major environmental influences often cause variation with season, social class, or time, and 'epidemics' may occur. If such features are lacking, it implies either that the environment plays a minor role, or that the environmental factor is so widespread as to affect a majority of the population. In the latter situation, genetic predisposition eventually becomes the main deciding factor.

Persistent patency of the arterial duct: practical illustration of multifactorial inheritance

The recognition of a marked increase in the incidence of a patent arterial duct among infants whose mothers were exposed to rubella during the first trimester (Gregg, 1941), provided the first major insight into the aetiology of this condition. It seems likely that the association is the result of direct action by the virus on the developing ductal wall in view of the other cardiovascular effects of the virus, which include a high incidence of peripheral pulmonary artery stenosis and, more rarely, anomalies of other muscular arteries.

Preterm delivery is now the major environmental factor and probably accounts for the increase in population incidence noted recently (Emmanouilides, 1978). It becomes more common with shorter gestation, fluid overload, and associated complications such as respiratory distress syndrome (Siassi et al, 1976). Levin et al (1975) suggested an incidence of 7% among 1150 neonates of less than 2500 grams birth weight, but other studies have suggested that ductal patency may be demonstrated in one-fifth to one-quarter of such infants (Rowe et al, 1981) rising to 35% in those under 1500 grams. Nearly one-tenth of 1081 chidlren with heart defects recorded on the Liverpool malformation registry between 1960 and 1969 had patency of the arterial duct. Just under one-fifth (20/106) had a gestation of less than 38 weeks. Thirty-one (30%) had a birth weight of less than 2.500 kilograms. These figures suggest that the recognised environmental influences should not be held wholly responsible in a large proportion of cases.

Genetic causes are also known, involving chromosomal anomalies such as XXXXY and several single gene defects. The autosomal dominant Treacher-Collins syndrome and the autosomal recessive Carpenter syndrome (craniosynostosis and polysyndactyly) are examples of the latter. Again, the total contribution of these recognised syndromes and genetic disorders to the overall population incidence is small.

Family studies have shown evidence of a polygenic basis in the remaining group. The possibility of a genetic predisposition in isolated persistence of the duct was first raised by the repeated observation of two or more affected individuals in the same family (Carleton, 1958). Systematic analyses based on family studies in the term infant began with Record & McKeown (1953) and Anderson (1954). Their combined data revealed 5, or possibly 6 cases of persistent arterial duct among 269 later born sibs, a recurrence risk of 1 in 50. Anderson further noted that among his uncomplicated cases, only 27% were male. A number of subsequent studies have confirmed that these early estimates were essentially correct (Polani & Campbell, 1960; Wilkins 1969; Ando, 1977; Nora, 1978). One other study stands out for its size, precision and attention to detail. Zetterqvist (1972) examined the records of 479 patients who underwent ligation of the arterial duct in one of three Swedish centres between 1941 and 1965. He selected those born before 1945 who were of Swedish origin, and who had reproduced. He was able to trace 435 of the 479 eligible for study and examine their families. The ratio of males to females was 1 : 3. Among 663 siblings, 17 had congenital heart disease. One had Down's syndrome and an atrioventricular septal defect, and one had preductal aortic coarctation. The rest had persistence of the arterial duct giving a recurrent risk of 15/663 or 2.3% ± 0.6%.

Among 490 offspring, 18 had congenital heart disease; 3 of these did not have a persistently patent duct and were probably random associations. The remaining 15 had persistence of the duct, giving a recurrence risk of 3.7% among offspring. As this is substantially higher than the sib risk, the effect of single dominant genes was considered possible. This was confirmed when Zetterqvist identified two families with a total of 6 children of whom 3 had a duct. All 3 had features of a generalised connective tissue disorder. Excluding these 2 'syndromic' families, 12 offspring out of 484 had ducts. This is 2.5% ± 0.7% – the same risk as was seen in sibs. Zetterqvist looked for evidence of a major environmental contribution, but found none. Birth rank, parental age and seasonal incidence showed no significant associations. Earlier authors had an excess of females in the third quarter of the year. A similar trend was present in the Swedish data but did not reach significant levels. It remains possible that a few cases result from some insult such as fever, cold medications or viral infection affecting women who become pregnant in midwinter. The lack of statistic significance suggests that such an environmental contribution is small.

Zetterqvist's report suggests that persistent patency of the arterial duct is a polygenic threshold trait. The recurrence risk is the same for sibs and offspring. The risk in first degree relatives is the same as the square root of the population incidence. Carlgren (1969) found the incidence of persistent patency of the duct in a comparable group of 116 419 Swedish children to be 6/10 000. The square root of this figure is 2.4%.

Cousins share only one-eighth of their genes in common as opposed to sibs and offspring who share one-half. When a disorder depends on 'negative' alleles being present at several gene loci, it is to be expected that the likelihood of this happening is much smaller in cousins (or third degree relatives) than in first degree relatives. Therefore, the occurrence of a polygenic disorder in one member of a family should be reflected in a high recurrence risk in first, but not in second and third degree relatives. Zetterqvist found only 0.6% of the latter group to be affected.

It was also possible to assess the effect of 'severity' on recurrence risks. At operation, the surgeons measured routinely the widest diameter of the duct. Zetterqvist had 71 probands with a wide duct. They had 7 affected children among a total of 146 (4.8% ± 1.7). The probands in the 'narrow' and 'moderate' categories had 5 affected children among 271 or 1.8% ± 0.9%. This is in keeping with the fifth rule in the list on page 26. Greater severity implies a greater genetic predisposition, which is reflected in the higher risk to relatives. Twenty children were born to probands who themselves had affected sibs. Two of these offspring were affected. This is comparable to the 10% recurrence risk used generally in counselling families with 2 sibs affected by a polygenic trait. The risk of recurrence rises with more affected family members.

The 'Carter effect' (p. 26) states that when there is a sex difference in a polygenic trait the recurrence risk is greater in the relatives of the more rarely affected sex. This is based on the assumption that the more rarely affected sex is, on average, further from the 'threshold' and so requires a greater genetic disadvantage before the 'disease' occurs. The excess of deleterious genes is reflected in a higher incidence of the disorder among close relatives. Since persistence of the arterial duct is 2–3 times as common among females, the recurrence risk should be greater among the relatives of male probands. In the Zetterqvist study, male probands had 100 children of whom 3 had a duct (3.0% ± 1.7%), whereas female probands had 9 affected among 384 offspring (2.3% ± 0.8%). The difference is in the predicted direction, but is not statistically significant.

Persistent patency of the arterial duct provides an excellent example of a multifactorial threshold trait. One environmental insult, rubella, produces persistence of the duct regardless of genetic make-up. With the other important environment factors, (altitude and preterm delivery) there is the possibility that genetic predisposition determines which individuals 'cross the line'. Apart from these categories, there is little evidence of other significant environment 'variance', or contribution to the number of cases born. The family studies, on the other hand, reveal the lesion to comply very well with the six 'polygenic predictions'. The greatest risk would be to the daughter of a man who himself had been found to have a widely patent duct. In Zetterqvist's series there were 16 daughters of such men, of whom 2 were affected.

The animal models of Patterson et al (1971, 1980)

provide biological support for a 'graded character'. In breeding experiments with collies he found some to have an arterial duct and others to have ductal diverticula in which the duct had closed at the extreme pulmonary end, but remained patent over the rest of its length. As in humans, those with a patent duct varied in severity from a narrow channel to a diameter equal to that of the aorta. Crossing an affected dog with an unrelated collie resulted in 22% of offspring crossing the diverticulum threshold and a small number having an open duct. When affected dogs were back-crossed with unaffected first degree relatives there was a much higher incidence of duct anomaly among offspring. This suggests that the population curve for liability was shifted further across the threshold. The worst situation resulted from mating between two affected collies. Only 16% of the offspring had normal closure of the duct. Patterson and his colleagues extended their work to histological examination of abnormal ducts. In cases of ductal diverticulum, they found, instead of the normal muscular media with a few elastic fibres, that the segment of duct adjacent to the aorta had an elastic 'aorta-like' media while normal duct wall was present at the pulmonary end. In cases of persistently patent ducts this 'aortification' extended along the whole length.

The genetic predisposition in humans may be based on a combination of histological abnormality and variation in the speed of maturation. Gittenberger de Groot (1977, 1980 has demonstrated the histological bases of the clinical categories (delayed closure or 'patency' of an otherwise normal duct and 'persistence' of a structurally abnormal duct). The latter results from a primary anatomic defect. An additional subendothelial elastic lamina develops which disrupts normal closure and is the basis for many cases of persistence. The 'aortification' seen in poodles was not seen frequently in human ducts. Also of interest was the recognition that the timing of the maturation process varied so that, for example, one 27-week fetus who died after preterm delivery had a mature duct, whereas another had remained at an early stage throughout much of the third trimester.

Thus, one may deduce that isolated persistent patency of the duct among term infants may be due to a genetically determined abnormality of wall morphology. In some, the change will be such that closure is not possible even with inhibition of prostaglandins. Another genetic factor is exposed with preterm delivery, namely the speed of morphological maturation. As delivery becomes earlier in gestation, an increasing proportion of the population fall over the line dividing closure from patency, so the contribution of genetic predisposition become less visible. Again, attempts to achieve closure by prostaglandin inhibition will depend on maturation. The poorly developed duct is unable to achieve permanent closure. A genetic 'delay' in maturation is likely to be a further factor determining which infants require surgical closure. Delivery at high

altitude will shift the threshold to cover a greater proportion of the population, while the presence of respiratory distress may be seen to be acting as an additive 'environmental variance' in producing scatter. This interpretation may be tested in future by comparing recurrence risks for a child whose duct closed with indomethacin to those needing surgery. One might predict that recurrence will be greater in those families where the child with a persistent duct required surgery.

Zetterqvist reported two families in which an autosomal dominant single gene defect, involving connective tissue structure, seemed to be the cause of patency of the duct. Burman (1961) reported a female infant whose father was affected. Ducts were diagnosed in two of the father's sibs, and their mother died at 48 years from 'dropsy', with features compatible with the diagnosis. A single dominant gene seemed likely in this family. As yet, such families may only be recognised in retrospect, when multiple family members are affected.

EPIDEMIOLOGY, TWIN STUDIES, AND FAMILY STUDIES IN ISOLATED HEART DEFECTS

Epidemiology

Having dealt with chromosome defects, recognised syndromes, known teratogens and persistence of the arterial duct, 75–80% of cardiac malformations remain to be accounted for. Despite frequent assertions in the literature that unrecognised teratogens are at work, the epidemiological evidence provides little support. Though there have been some observations of seasonal variation, the incidence of heart defects has remained remarkably stable in place and time (Taussig, 1982). Most studies give population incidence figures in the range of 6–8/1000 with extremes of 4 and 10/1000. Variations in methods of ascertainment and diagnostic criteria can account for these differences. In the long-term studies in Liverpool, UK (Kenna et al, 1975), and New England, USA (New England Regional Infant Cardiac Programme, 1980), the annual incidence over several years remained almost unchanged. That variation which is noted is more suggestive of genetic variance. For example, the Japanese have a relatively high incidence of ventricular septal defects in the outlet septum with prolapsing aortic cusp, whereas their incidence of muscular ventricular septal defects is lower than that of Caucasians (Takao et al 1980).

Twin studies

If a trait is genetic, monozygotic twins should be concordant; that is, if one of them has the condition the genetically identical co-twin should be affected similarly. Dizygotic or non-identical twins share only half of their genes in common (like ordinary brothers and sisters) so concordance for genetic traits is not as great as the monozygotic group. If a trait is non-genetic, concordance among twins is likely to be less. More important, the difference between monozygotic and dizygotic twins should disappear. This is 'the twin method' of genetic analysis, first proposed by Francis Galton in 1876. The great majority of twin studies carried out over the last twenty-five years have found low concordance rates among monozygotic twins and this has been taken as being strong evidence against a significant genetic contribution. This in turn has led to the assumption that outside environmental agents are pre-eminent. A basic premise of the twin method, however, is that monozygotic twins are comparable to dizygotic twins and singletons in all respects other than their genetic make-up. This is not the case.

McKeown & Record in 1960 commented on the apparent excess of like-sex twins with heart defects. Leck in 1960 and Campbell in 1961 in the same year suggested that the monozygotic twinning process itself might cause a heart defect in one of the pair. A review of subsequent hospital series has shown that the majority have more monozygotic twin pairs than would be expected in the population under study. Furthermore, most population studies have reported an excess of heart defects either among all twins, or among like-sex twins. Unfortunately, the great majority of reports have been open to criticism on one or more of four criteria: namely, proof of zygosity, methods of ascertainment, precision of cardiac diagnosis, and size of sample (Burn & Corney, 1984).

Burn et al (1987) ascertained a consecutive series of 195 twin pairs, in Newcastle and London, where one or both had a heart defect. Exclusion of uncertain diagnoses,

syndromes, conjoined twins and persistence of the arterial duct left 155 pairs. Persistent duct was not included because the tendency of twins to be born 'too small and too soon' makes them particularly prone to this lesion. Zygosity was established in 130, using physical examination and blood group analysis, of which 65 were monozygotic (50%). This represented a significant excess over the expected proportion of monozygotic twins (less than 35% in a British population – Corney et al, 1983). Figure 2.12 shows that the excess remained significant even after allowance was made for the 25 like-sex pairs of uncertain zygosity. Since these were consecutive series, ascertainment bias was avoided. 'Referral bias' remained a possibility with the excess of monozygotic twins being due, perhaps, to such twins finding their way to specialist units more easily.

The second part of the study, based on twin/malformation registers in three British centres (Liverpool, Aberdeen and Birmingham), confirmed that the excess of heart defects in monozygotic twins was a genuine observation. All twins with heart defects were identified in a population of over 20 000 individual twins. Again, only those where diagnosis could be confirmed were included. Thus, in Aberdeen the records of the perinatal malformation survey together with a cross-reference between the twins register and cardiac register revealed 43 children with heart murmurs. After exclusion of uncertain diagnoses and persistent duct, the number fell to 13 twin individuals born between 1968 and 1980 among a total of 1449 (8.97/1000). The incidence of heart defects among singletons in the same area at this time (excluding persistent duct) was just under 6/1000 (A.G.M. Campbell, personal communication). In Liverpool the

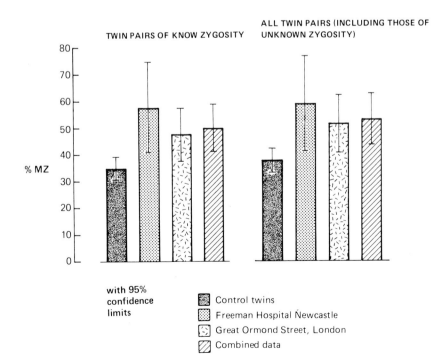

Fig. 2.12 The results of a study of heart defect in twins in two hospitals: monozygotic pairs (one or both affected) as percentage of all twin pairs.

incidence of heart defects in singletons between 1960 and 1969 was also just under 6/1000 (excluding persistent duct; Kenna et al, 1975). Among twins in Liverpool between 1968 and 1980 the incidence of heart malformation was found by Burn et al to be 11.09/1000. In Birmingham the survey of the whole city revealed singleton and twin figures of 3.69 and 5.03/1000 respectively. These are low because only hospital in-patients were included. The excess was confined, however, to like-sex twins, the group which includes the monozygotic twins. Unlike-sex (made up entirely of dizygotic twins) were comparable to singletons.

Taking this as further evidence for an excess of heart malformations confined to monozygotic twins, the incidence of heart defects among Liverpool and Aberdeen twins became more impressive. In order to raise the incidence among all twins to 11.09/1000, the incidence among monozygotic twins would need to be close to 18/1000 (Fig. 2.13).

A second study in Birmingham looked at births in two maternity units between 1960 and 1965 with detailed zygosity analysis. Long-term follow-up review of these data by Burn et al confirmed the presence of heart defects in 13 of the 228 monozygotic twin individuals compared to only 4 among 628 dizygotic twin individuals. When results from this study were pooled with Aberdeen (where zygosity was also established in all available twins) there

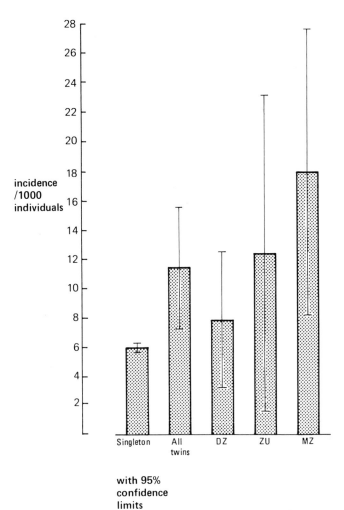

with 95% confidence limits

Fig. 2.14 Heart defects in twins by zygosity. MZ – monozygotic twins; DZ – dizygotic twins; ZU – zygosity uncertain twins.

was, again, a highly significant excess. The incidence of heart defects was 17.2/1000 among monozygotic twin individuals. This is more than double the widely accepted singleton incidence (Fig. 2.14).

These studies gave some support for the concept that haemodynamic disturbance due to twin-twin transfusion could account for the excess of heart defects in monozygotic twins. There was also evidence of disturbance of laterality being an underlying cause of heart defects. The strong association of heart malformation with isomerism and with the genetic defect in the iv/iv mouse supports the belief that the heart is prone to be malformed in the presence of visceral heterotaxy. It has long been recognised that monozygotic twins may, on occasion, show contrasting laterality (or mirror-imagery), though complete mirror-image arrangement is rare. It is now suggested that laterality is determined in the early zygote from a reference point which forms on the extreme left side (Corballis & Morgan, 1978). One piece of evidence in favour of this is that in conjoined twins (which are thought to result from

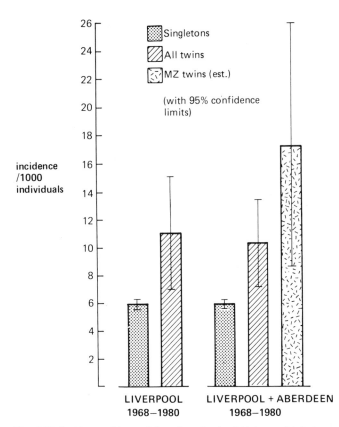

Fig. 2.13 Incidence of heart defects in twins (and higher multiples) compared to singletons.

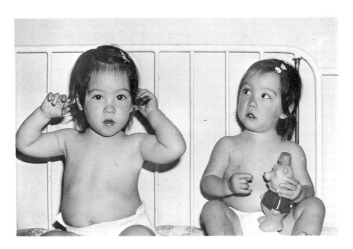

Fig. 2.15 Monoamniotic twins who manifested mirror-imaging for tooth eruption, position of hair whorl and hand preference. The twin on the right has tetralogy of Fallot.

late twinning) it is not uncommon to find the right half of the pair to have a right-sided heart. The twin pair illustrated in Figure 2.15 are monoamniotic twins with interwoven umbilical cords (indicating late twinning). Their mother noted striking mirror-imagery with, for example, the twin on the right having a right-sided hair whorl and eruption of the right teeth, whereas the left twin had the converse. The 'right half' suffered tetralogy of Fallot. This could be explained by suggesting that late twinning caused the right half of the zygote to become separated from its point of reference. This in turn caused a disturbance of laterality in this twin, sufficient to produce mirror-imagery for physical traits and, more important, sufficient to disturb early heart development.

Whatever the explanation for the excess of malformations in monozygotic twins, its existence impairs seriously the use of twin studies to assess genetic contribution. Burn et al found, in round terms, that 8% of monozygotic twin pairs and 4% of dizygotic twins were concordant (i.e. both members of the pair affected). If allowance was made for the excess of monozygotic twins, the concordance figure rose to 16%, four times the figure in dizygotic twins. It was thus possible to construct an estimate of genetic contribution or 'heritability' of 80% rather than 30%. Put another way, an important piece of evidence in favour of environmental insults accounting for the 'unknown' group is invalidated. Nevertheless, the majority of monozygotic twin pairs did have only one affected member. This fact, and the implication of influences such as disturbance of flow or laterality to explain the twin excess, draws attention to a third category of cause – epigenetic factors. These may be defined as variables intrinsic to development but not under direct control. Lenz (1980) reached a similar conclusion. He referred to micro-environmental differences, while Vogel & Motulsky (1979) prefer the term

'random' or 'stochastic' factors. In other words, while genetic predisposition may be essential and external insults overrated, 'chance' events in early development are likely to be a major factor in deciding whether the heart fails to develop normally.

If monozygotic twins have double the incidence of heart malformations, the twinning process is the entire or predominant 'cause' of perhaps 0.5% of all heart defects. If parents have a child with a cardiac malformation who is one of discordant monozygotic twins, their chance of having a further affected child should be less than if the first child was singleton. Burn et al (1987) found none of the 96 sibs of monozygotic twins to have a heart defect indicating a risk close to that of the general population. Two of 85 sibs of dizygotic twins had a heart defect. This figure is in keeping with the 3% quoted for singletons.

Family studies

Attempts to establish precise recurrence risks in sibs and offspring have two purposes. The first is to provide counselling figures. The second is to investigate the existence and nature of genetic contribution.

In 1968 Nora observed that the overall risk of recurrence in sibs was of the order of 3 to 5% for heart defects in general with a comparable risk to offspring. Since these figures were similar to the square root of the population incidence, Nora suggested that the majority of heart defects might be accounted for on the basis of the multifactorial model. While this was a useful advance in understanding, it remains a general observation in need of detailed interpretation. The relative contribution of 'heredity' and 'environment' must be examined. Analysis must be made of whether a majority are cases of environment insult acting on a genetically predisposed fetus, or whether the overall recurrence risks conceal a heterogenous group – some with a single gene basis, some with a purely polygenic basis and others being the primary result of external insult whose effects were determined by timing of the insult and would have been similar in most fetuses. A major criticism of past studies of offspring is that they have largely been confined to those individuals whose heart malformation was relatively mild. The recent report by Whittemore et al (1982) has provided a different perspective. Girls followed through adolescence in the paediatric cardiology clinic were invited to take part in long-term follow-up. In this largely prospective analysis, 60 of 372 offspring (16.1%) had a heart defect. Ascertainment bias through self selection was probably not a major factor. Exclusion of those with dominant syndromes, a positive family history, a history of teratogenic exposure and 12 cases of ventricular septal defect diagnosed clinically which closed spontaneously by 3 years of age, reduces the recurrence risk to 7.9% (Burn, 1983). Nevertheless, this figure is substantially higher than the risk to sibs. It conflicts with earlier suggestions of a multifactorial model with a predominant environmental component.

Where earlier offspring studies selected in favour of probands whose heart defects were relatively mild, the combination of improved surgical techniques and exclusive use of patients retained for follow-up throughout adolescence meant a bias towards the more severe and rare heart malformations in the Whittemore study. Czeizel et al (1982) found an intermediate risk of 5% recurrence in the offspring of patients selected because they had needed corrective surgery but not confined to those in need of prolonged supervision.

The Whittemore study examined the possible effect of maternal cyanosis and poor cardiac output, but found no evidence to suggest more malformations in the 'poor function' group than occurred among those with good haemodynamics. This throws further weight behind the 'genetic' argument. The observation of higher recurrence in the group who, until recently, would not have reproduced, raises the possibility that these probands include a substantial number who represent new mutation autosomal dominant gene defects which were until now 'concealed' by a high mortality.

Further analysis of the overall figures serves little purpose. Instead, attention should be directed towards specific diagnostic categories. Table 2.4 summarises recurrence risks in sibs and offspring for different types of heart defects. In addition to the summary of individual reports, a single estimate is included in bold print to be used in counselling. It should be remembered that parents are often much more reassured by a factual statement such as 'a study of 200 brothers and sisters found a heart defect in only 6' than by being told 'there is a 3% risk'.

In the table, defects which have not been the subject of detailed family study are treated in general terms with a recurrence risk of 3% for another affected sib or, if the parent is affected, a 5% risk of an affected child. If 2 family members are already affected a figure of 10% is appropriate. The specific data are laid out following the sequential classification. This causes the more common lesions to be considered towards the end of the list, but on the other hand, it promotes many of the clinically more severe lesions, which is justified by the greater significance of recurrence for the child and the family. More important, disturbances of atrial arrangement and chamber connexions must pre-date, in embryological development, the majority of other defects. They should therefore be considered as closer to the primary development disturbance. If atrial isomerism is present with a ventricular septal defect, the advice should be based on the isomerism, with the septal defect regarded as a secondary anomaly.

Mirror-image arrangement ('situs inversus')

Complete mirror-image visceral arrangement is associated with a high incidence of affected sibs and a very high consanguinity but rarely with two generation pedigrees. Therefore, a simple autosomal recessive basis has been thought likely (Cockayne, 1938; Torgerson, 1950; Campbell, 1961). The recurrence risk, however, is much less than 1 in 4. In the important category of Kartagener's syndrome (where mirror-imagery is associated with sinusitis and bronchiectasis due to abnormal cilia), there is a 1 in 4 recurrence risk for the cilial anomaly but only a 1 in 8 recurrence risk for the organ arrangement. Moreno & Murphy, (1981) have suggested that this may be explained by random determination of lateralisation in the homozygote. In other words, the affected child has a fundamental defect of the mechanism which decides which side of the embryo will be left and which right. Even with this defect, however, there is a 50% chance of being correct by chance so that only half of those with the gene defect have mirror-image arrangement. This is another example of epigenetic influence. When looking at organ arrangement we are, in the words of Victor McKusick, 'remote from the site of gene action.' In addition to the random distribution of alleles in the egg and sperm there is an additional determinant of expression of the clinical disorder, which is neither 'genetic' nor 'environmental'.

Isomerism sequence

It might be argued that while complete mirror-imagery is not normal, neither is it a malformation in the clinical sense. This is not the case with isomerism sequence. This condition has attracted a plethora of titles. Originally, it was included with 'complete situs inversus' by Cockayne (1938), judging from the list of associated malformations such as absent spleen. 'Incomplete situs inversus', 'complex dextrocardia', 'visceral heterotaxia', 'asplenia polysplenia syndrome', 'Ivemark syndrome', 'bilateral right-sidedness or left-sidedness', and 'situs ambiguus' are among the titles which have enjoyed favour at various times. The term 'isomerism' is preferred because it draws attention to the fundamental anomaly which is that the body has two left sides in left isomerism or two right sides in right isomerism. The various malformations are easily understood as secondary phenomena. Having two right sides typically results in both lungs being trilobed, both bronchi being short and eparterial and both atrial appendages being of right morphology. The spleen, being of left origin, often fails to develop. The pulmonary veins, in the absence of a true left atrium, must always drain anomalously, although sometimes they connect to the heart. The liver and abdominal mesentery tend to remain central and symmetrical, the latter predisposing to malrotation. With left isomerism, bilateral 'left' lungs, bronchi and atrial appendages are typical, while the excess 'leftness' predisposes to the formation of multiple spleens. In this case pulmonary venous connexion is no problem but the upper

Table 2.4 Recurrence risks in sibs and offspring for different types of heart defect.

Cardiovascular malformation	Reference	Number of probands	Number of affected sibs	Total sibs	Percent affected	Counselling figure (%)	Number of affected offspring	Total offspring	Percent affected	Counselling figure (%)	Comments
Disturbance of organ arrangement (mirror image arrangement)	Torgersen, 1950	240	28	1271	2.2	5	–	–	–	1	Torgersen did not examine all sibs. Consanguinity frequent. Evidence points towards a simple autosomal recessive basis with reduced penetrance.
Isomerism sequence	Rose et al, 1975 Burn et al, 1984	60 98	3 2(4)	63 109	4.75 2.0(4.1)	5	–	–	–	1	Frequent cousin marriage and sibships with multiple affected sibs suggests an autosomal recessive basis either as a proportion of cases or in all but with reduced penetrance.
Disturbed atrioventricular connexion Double inlet ventricle ('univentricular heart')	–	–	–	–	–	3	–	–	–	5	
Absent right atrioventricular connexion (tricuspid atresia)	Fuhrmann, 1968 Nora & Nora, 1983	33 52	0(1) 0(1)	92 98	0(0.9) 0(1.0)	1	–	–	–	5	
Absent left atrioventricular connexion (mitral atresia)	Child & Dennis, 1977	–	0(2)	110	0	2	–	–	–	5	No specific study. Figures used are those from 'hypoplastic left heart syndrome'
Disturbed ventriculo-arterial connexion	Nora & Nora, 1983	116	4	229	1.7		–	–	–	5	
Discordant ventriculo-arterial connexion (complete transposition)	Fuhrmann, 1968a Ando et al, 1977 Sanchez-Cascos, 1978	184 153 45	6(22) 3 2	442 171 –	1.4(5.0) 1.8 1.4	2	–	–	–	5	
Single ventriculo-arterial connexion (common arterial trunk)	Nora & Nora, 1983	43	1	86	1.2	1	–	–	–	–	
Pulmonary atresia	Nora & Nora, 1983	36	0(1)	80	1.3	1	–	–	–	5	
Aortic atresia	–	–	–	–	–	–	–	–	–	–	
Associated cardiac anomalies											
Anomalous pulmonary venous connexion	–	–	–	–	–	3	–	–	–	5	No detailed study. A few families show possible dominant transmission with variable penetrance.

Table 2.4 Recurrence risks in sibs and offspring for different types of heart defect (*continued*).

Cardiovascular malformation	Reference	Number of probands	Number of affected sibs	Total sibs	Percent affected	Counselling figure (%)	Number of affected offspring	Total offspring	Percent affected	Counselling figure (%)	Comments
Secundum atrial septal defect	Nora et al, 1967	–	9(10)	279	3.2(3.7)		–	–	–		Literature contains several clearly dominant pedigrees. Prolonged AV conduction is a feature of one dominant form (Bizarro et al, 1970). Williamson recurrence risk excluded one large pedigree with 11 affected members.
	Ando et al, 1977	172	13	1110	1.2		8	252	3.2		
	Nora & Nora, 1983	191	11	380	2.9		5	199	2.5		
	Zetterqvist, 1972		6	645	1.0	3	6	397	1.5	4	
	Sanchez-Cascos, 1978	135	11	335	3.3		4	95	4.2		
	Williamson, 1969	36	7	190	3.7		6	66	9.0		
	Whittemore et al, 1982		–	–	–						
Divided left atrium	–	–	–	–	–	3	–	–	–	5	
Atrioventricular septal defects (includes primum atrial septal defects)	Nora & Nora, 1983	73	4	151	2.6						See text. All Nora's recurrences in single sibship. One large dominant pedigree described. Sanchez-Cascos pooled first degree relatives.
	Emanuel et al, 1968	92	4	229	1.7	2				5–10	
	Ando et al, 1977	80	2	103	1.9						
	Sanchez-Cascos, 1978	51	14		8.7						
	Emanuel et al, 1983						3(2)	52	9.6		
Ebstein's malformation	Nora & Nora, 1983	47	1	105	1	1	–	–	–	5	Associated specifically with maternal lithium ingestion.
Mitral valve prolapse (Barlow syndrome)	Devereux & Brown, 1983						Present in 5% of the population: behaves as variable expression autosomal dominant. Great majority have an affected parent, so risk close to 50% for sibs and offspring. More fully expressed in females and in middle-age. Morbidity and mortality are very low: 1% per year become symptomatic. Major occasional complications are severe mitral regurgitation, bacterial endocarditis, rupture of chordae tendineae, and embolic strokes. Beneficial associations are lower body weight and blood pressure. In four hospital series of selected patients, 62–73% were asymptomatic over 10–24 years follow-up.				
Ventricular septal defect	Campbell, 1965	180	6	359	1.7						Racial variation is evident with Japanese having frequent subaortic defect while caucasions have more muscular defects. Ideally family studies should be subdivided by type of defect but even so, there is likely to be considerable heterogeneity.
	Ando et al, 1977	1241	18	1237	1.5		0	75	0		
	Sanchez-Cascos, 1978	214	12	–	1.7						
	Dennis & Warren, 1981	161	3	345	0.9	3	2	104	1.9	4	
	Nora & Nora, 1983	306	28	672	4.2		7	174	4		
	Czeizel & Meszaras, 1981		2	61	3.3						
	Whittemore et al, 1982	50					17	78	22		
Pulmonary stenosis	Campbell, 1962	125	6	282	2.1		0	15	0		In some families dysplastic pulmonary valve behaves as a simple dominant trait.
	Ando et al, 1977	123	3	99	1.5		4	83	4.6		
	Dennis & Warren, 1981	101	1	208	0.5	2	4	111	3.6	6	
	Nora & Nora, 1983	166	10	375	2.7		7	36	19		
	Whittemore et al, 1982										

Defect	Reference										Comments
Tetralogy of Fallot	Boon et al, 1972	100	4	189	2.1		1	12	8.3		
	Ando et al, 1977	196	6	380	1.6						
	Sanchez-Cascos, 1978	113	4	327	1.2						
	Dennis & Warren, 1981	61	0	100	0		3	118	2.5		
	Nora & Nora, 1983	180	11	366	3.0	**2**	6	141	4.3	**4**	
	Singh et al, 1982						1	30	3.3		
Aortic stenosis	Zoethoet et al, 1964	126	10	246	4.1						Behaves as classic polygenic trait with occasional dominant pedigrees.
	Ando et al, 1977	29	2	41	4.9						
	Nora & Nora, 1983	155	8	361	2.2	**3**	4	103	3.9	**5–10**	
	Whittemore et al, 1982	17					8	27	30		
Coarctation	Campbell & Polani, 1961	109	1	252	0.4		0	45	0		
	Zetterqvist, 1972	94	5	283	1.8		5	191	2.6		
	Boon & Roberts, 1976	100	1	112	0.5		0	8	0		
	Nora & Nora, 1983	131	5	281	1.8	**2**	7	253	2.7	**3**	
	Whittemore et al, 1982	10					4	19	21		
Persistent patency of the arterial duct	Wilkins, 1969	241	3	198	1.5		3	179	1.7		Recurrence risk less if environmental insult such as preterm delivery is identified.
	Zetterqvist, 1972	435	15	663	2.3		12	484	2.5		
	Ando et al, 1977	295	8	408	2.0		0	30	0		
	Whittemore et al, 1982						9	83	10.8		
	Nora & Nora, 1983	220	18	516	3.5	**2.5**	6	139	4.3	**3**	

Figure in bold print is the recommended counselling figure.
Percentage recurrence risk refers to similar defects. The figure in brackets indicates all cardiac defects.

part of the inferior caval vein, in the absence of a right atrium, frequently fails to develop and venous blood instead follows the azygos or hemiazygos path. In aetiological terms then, it is not appropriate to discuss specifically either splenic morphology or bronchial length in isolation, but rather to see these as indicators of the underlying abnormality of laterality.

Wherever a group of malformations are the consequence of another anomaly the term 'sequence' is used. Thus, in the Robin sequence, formerly the 'Pierre Robin syndrome', the micrognathia causes the tongue to be placed posteriorly which in turn prevents normal closure of the palatal shelves. There have been numerous reports of families with two or more sibs with isomerism sequence together with frequent examples of consanguinity.

This led to this disorder being designated autosomal recessive. Among 60 families identified from a necropsy series of asplenia and polysplenia, however, only 3 had two affected children. This gives a recurrence risk of just under 5% (Rose et al, 1975). A recent study based on 109 sibs from 98 cases of documented isomerism (Burn et al, 1984), revealed one sib with right isomerism sequence and two others who died in their first year of life from heart defects. A fourth child, the sister of a girl with right atrial isomerism, had isolated left bronchial isomerism.

If all 4 are taken as recurrences of isomerism sequence the counselling figure becomes 4% or 1 in 25. Two probands of British Caucasian extraction (out of 73 Caucasians) had consanguineous parents (in one case first cousin and in the other second cousin). Given the very low frequency of cousin marriage in Britain this observation adds further weight to the implication of autosomal recessive genes. One possibility is genetic heterogeneity. If one-fifth of cases were recessive and four-fifths non-genetic, the recurrence risk in sibs would be $(1/5 \times 1/4) + (4/5 \times 0)$, or 1 in 20. Alternatively, there may be incomplete penetrance analogous to that seen with Kartagener syndrome. Some of the brothers and sisters may be homozygous for the defective gene and yet develop normally. Layton & Manasek (1980) have studied in detail the iv/iv mouse. When mice are homozygous for the iv gene they have abnormal arrangement of their organs. Half have right-sided hearts. Approximately one-fifth have complex heart defects very similar to those seen in isomerism sequence. The heart defects affect in equal proportions those with left-sided or right-sided hearts. One inference is that organ arrangement is determined in 'pendulum' fashion with one-fifth of homozygotes ending up 'in the middle' with incomplete differentiation of left and right sides and subsequent disturbance of heart development. The distortion of the rightward heart loop seen in the homozygous mice makes it likely that at least some of the heart malformations are secondary to the effect of disturbed laterality on heart looping. This model is numerically attractive because the recurrence of heart malformations in these mice is 1 in 20. If the parents of an iv/iv mouse with a heart defect have another litter, there is a 1 in 4 chance of producing another iv/iv mouse and one-fifth of such mice will have a heart defect – $1/4 \times 1/5 = 1/20$.

The mouse model is not analagous directly to humans because 50% of human sibs do not have right-sided hearts. This mammalian model with incomplete penetrance does, however, serve to illustrate how, thanks to the action of epigenetic influence, an autosomal recessive trait may have low recurrence risk. The clinical significance is that the risks to offspring of affected individuals with isomerism sequence should be small (less than 1%) whereas the polygenic model would have predicted a risk similar to sibs.

Atrioventricular septal defects

In the case of atrioventricular septal defects the converse is true, with recent studies of offspring revealing a much higher incidence of heart malformations in offspring. Emanuel et al (1983) found 5 of 52 offspring to have major heart malformations, a figure which casts further doubt on the relevance of the multifactorial model to this disorder.

Atrioventricular septal defects vary from isolated 'ostium primum atrial septal defects' to those with atrial and ventricular communications and a common valve orifice. The deficiency of the atrioventricular septum itself does not vary, however – only the attachment of the valve apparatus to its margins (see Ch. 24). Thus the different varieties may be analysed as a single pathological entity. This is a good point at which to distinguish more clearly between pathogenesis and aetiology. Aetiology is the study of cause of the lesion whereas pathogenesis refers to the means by which a defect came about. There is considerable debate about the pathogenesis of atrioventricular septal defects. Attention has been directed variously at formation of the atrial septum primum, endocardial cushion growth and adhesion, and the inlet ventricular septum as sites of primary defect (Allwork, 1982). Whichever path or paths prove to be correct, there is evidence of a variety of underlying causes. The strong association with trisomy 21 (such that a quarter to a third of children with atrioventricular septal defects have this chromosome disorder) implies that having an extra copy of a gene or genes on chromosome 21 disturbs the normal septation process.

Isomerism sequence accounts for at least 3% of all heart defects (Deanfield et al, 1980). From the analysis of Van Mierop et al (1972), two-thirds have atrioventricular septal defects (or 2% of the whole). This is analogous to the 2% of the total which have Down's syndrome and atrioventricular septal defects. A large proportion of cases associated with isomerism, however, are also associated with other cardiovascular malformations. These would be classified as 'complex' or 'other' in most studies. Very few isomeric infants have atrioventricular septal defects in isolation. If both groups are taken together, a substantial proportion of infants whose defect includes atrioventricular septal defect have this as a secondary consequence of disturbance of organ arrangement.

In 1968 Yao et al reported 4 siblings suffering from isolated 'ostium primum atrial septal defect' with normal parents. O'Nuallain et al (1977) reported a large pedigree in which this trait behaved as an autosomal dominant. Nora (1971), having found no recurrence in siblings in 70 families, then found 4 siblings with an atrioventricular septal defect in one family. Sanchez-Cascos (1978) found recurrence in 14 of 161 first degree relatives (8.7%). Most recently, Emanuel et al (1983) have found 5 cases of heart malformation among 52 offspring of individuals with atrioventricular septal defect. This 10% recurrence adds further weight to the proposition that in some non-syndromic cases this defect results from a single gene defect, while environmental insults are of little consequence.

One apparent flaw is that, in the Emanuel study, 2 of the 5 recurrences were cases of tetralogy of Fallot. Atrioventricular septal defects and tetralogy would normally be regarded as discordant lesions. Both are associated with malposition of the aorta, however, and this report of occurrences in the same family, on two occasions, would seem to indicate a common aetiology.

Tetralogy of Fallot

When different heart malformations occur within a family it is important not to dismiss these as 'discordant' or chance concurrence. In his study of differing defects in sib pairs Fuhrmann (1968b) observed several examples of tetralogy of Fallot in one and complete transposition in the other. These may be regarded as differing manifestations of a disturbance of connection with double outlet right ventricle as the intermediate form.

In other cases disordered septation may be implicated. Studies in the Keeshond hound suggest this mechanism to account for a form of tetralogy of Fallot. Selective breeding produces a spectrum of malformation which obeys polygenic predictions and which has common arterial trunk as its most extreme manifestation (Patterson et al, 1980). Keeton (personal communication) has seen a Caucasian British family with tetralogy of Fallot in one sib and common arterial trunk in the other. Takao et al (1980) reviewed their observation of a group of patients with 'conotruncal anomalies' with a characteristic facial appearance. None of their 50 cases had relatives with heart defects, though several had a sib or parent with similar facial features. They suggest that this may be a genetic subset among Japanese patients, analagous to the Keeshond model. It is likely that complex lesions such as tetralogy of Fallot represent the 'final common pathway' of a variety

of mechanisms of abnormal development. Such heterogeneity must hinder genetic analysis by family studies alone. Only when a range of polymorphic DNA probes are available (which can act as genetic markers covering the whole genome) might it become possible to characterise genetic subtypes and offer precise counselling to high risk families. In the meantime, advice must be based on empiric risks.

CONCLUSION

Disturbances of genetic control are major causative factors in cardiovascular malformation. In 5% of the total, the malformation is the result of trisomy for chromosome 21 (Down's syndrome). The large range of other chromosomal defects account for at least another 2–3%. With increasing resolution, further cases are likely to be shown to be due to disturbance of genetic control by small deletions and duplications. Single gene defects have been identified mainly on the basis of associated malformations. The role of single gene defects in isolated heart defects has, until recently, been considered small. The high recurrence risk, however, in the offspring of patients with major malformations (who are now surviving to adulthood in increasing numbers) calls this assumption into question. A number of these severe defects may represent autosomal dominant gene defects.

A polygenic predisposition liable to cause malformation (with in some, an additive environmental component – the multifactorial model) is applicable to some cases. Persistent patency of the arterial duct provides a good example. The rising incidence of patent duct in very low birth weight infants, which are surviving more often, is an example of an environmental 'insult' of overriding importance. Rubella infection is another, and for heart defects in general, examples are maternal diabetes and disruption by thalidomide, anticonvulsant drugs and alcohol. The emphasis on 'hidden teratogens' to account for the majority of remaining cases, however, is almost certainly misplaced. In the absence of significant seasonal, social or geographical variation, and in the presence of, at times, a quite high recurrence rate in sibs and offspring, the only support for the 'hidden teratogen' theory has been the low concordance among monozygotic twins. The marked excess of heart malformations in monozygotic twins calls this interpretation into question. It is possible that the twinning process itself causes one twin to suffer a heart defect in about half of monozygotic twin pairs. This observation focuses attention on the role of epigenetic factors such as flow variation and cell interactions in heart formation. It is likely that such random variations within the fetus have a major influence on the expression of genetic predispositions to heart malformations.

REFERENCES

Albright S G, Hook E B 1980 Estimates of the likelihood that a Down's syndrome child of unknown genotype is a consequence of an inherited translocation. Journal of Medical Genetics 17: 273–276

Allwork S P 1982 Anatomical-embryological correlates in atrioventricular septal defect. British Heart Journal 47: 419–429

Anderson R C 1954 Causative factors underlying congenital heart malformations. Paediatrics 14: 143–152

Ando M, Takao A, Mori K 1977 Genetic and environmental factors in congenital heart disease. In: Inouye E, Nishimura H (eds) Gene-environment interaction in common diseases. University Park Press, Baltimore, p 71–88

Beattie J O, Day R, Cockburn F, Garg R A 1983 Alcohol and the fetus in the West of Scotland. British Medical Journal 287: 17–20

Bizarro R O, Callahan J A, Feldt R H, Kurland L T, Gordon H, Brandenburg R O 1970 Familial atrial septal defect with prolonged atrioventricular conduction. Circulation 41: 677–683

Boon A R, Roberts D F 1976 A family study of coarctation of the aorta. Journal of Medical Genetics 13: 420–433

Boon A R, Farmer M B, Roberts D F 1972 A family study of Fallot's tetralogy. Journal of Medical Genetics 9: 179–192

Boue A 1981 European collaborative study on structural chromosome anomalies in prenatal diagnosis. Presented at 6th International Congress of Human Genetics Workshop on collaborative studies in prenatal diagnosis for chromosome disorders, Jerusalem.

Burman D 1961 Familial patent ductus arteriosus. British Heart Journal 23: 603–604

Burn J 1983 Annotation: congenital heart defects – the risks to offspring. Archives of Diseases in Childhood 58: 947–948

Burn J, Corney G 1984 Congenital heart defects and twinning. Acta Geneticae Medicae et Gemellologiae 33: 61–69

Burn J, Baraitser M, Hughes D T, Saldana-Garcia P, Taylor J F N 1984 Absent right atrioventricular connection and double inlet ventricle due to an unbalanced familial 8:13 chromosome translocation: a cautionary tale. Paediatric Cardiology 5: 55–60

Burn J, Coffey R, Allan L D, Pembrey M E, Robinson P, Macartney F J 1985 Isomerism – a family study (abstract). Journal of Medical Genetics 21:301

Burn J, Corney G, Griffiths M, et al 1987 Congenital Heart Defects and twinning. Journal of Medical Genetics (in preparation)

Campbell M 1961 Twins and congenital heart disease. Acta Geneticae Medicae et Gemellologiae 10: 443–455

Campbell M 1962 Factors in the aetiology of pulmonary stenosis. British Heart Journal 24: 625–632

Campbell M 1965 Malformation of the heart. British Medical Journal ii: 895–904

Campbell M, Polani P 1961 The aetiology of coarctation of the aorta. Lancet i: 463–468

Carleton R A, Abelman W H, Hancock E W 1958 Familial occurrence of congenital heart disease: Report of three families and review of the literature. New England Journal of Medicine 26: 1237–1245

Carlgren L E 1969 The incidence of congenital heart disease in Gothenburg Proceedings of the Association of European Paediatric Cardiologists 5: 2–8

Child A H, Dennis N R 1977 The genetics of congenital heart disease. Birth Defects Original Article Series XIII 3A: 85–89

Cockayne E A 1938 The genetics of transposition of the viscera. Quarterly Journal of Medicine 31: 479–493

Corballis M C, Morgan M J 1978 On the biological basis of human laterality. Evidence of a maturational left to right gradient. Behaviour and Brain Science 2: 261–269

Corney G, MacGillivray I, Campbell D M, Thompson B, Little J 1983 Congenital abnormalities in twins in Aberdeen and North East Scotland. Acta Geneticae Medicae et Gemellologiae 32: 31–35

Czeizel A, Meszaros M 1981 Two family studies of children with ventricular septal defect. European Journal of Paediatrics 13: 81–85

Czeizel A, Pornoi A, Peterffy E, Tarcal E 1982 Studies of children of parents operated on for congenital cardio-vascular malformations. British Heart Journal 47: 290–293

David T J 1981 Dermatoglyphics in congenital heart disease. Journal of Medical Genetics 18: 344–349

Deanfield J E, Leanage R, Stroobant J, Chrispin A R, Taylor J F N, Macartney F J 1980 Use of high kilovoltage filtered beam radiographs for detection of bronchial situs in infants and young children. British Heart Journal 44: 577–583

Dennis N R, Warren J 1981 Risks to the offspring of patients with some common congenital heart defects. Journal of Medical Genetics 18: 8–16

Devereux R B, Brown W T 1983 Genetics of mitral valve prolapse. In: Steinberg A G, Bearn A G, Motulsky A G, Childs B (eds) Progress in medical genetics V. Genetics of cardiovascular disease. Saunders, Philadelphia, p 91–137

Down J L H 1866 Observations on an ethnic classification of idiots. Clinical Lecture Reports, London Hospital 3:259

Emanuel R, Nichols J, Anders J M, Moores E C, Somerville J 1968 Atrioventricular defects – a study of 92 families. British Heart Journal 30: 645–653

Emanuel R, Somerville J, Innas A, Withers R 1983 Evidence of congenital heart disease in the offspring of parents with atrioventricular defects. British Heart Journal 49: 144–147

Emmanouilides G C 1978 Incidence, perinatal factors and natural history. In: Heymann M A, Rudolph A M (eds) Report of the seventy-fifth Ross Conference on Paediatric Research. Columbus, Ohio, Ross Laboratories, p 63

Ferguson-Smith M, Yates J 1984 Maternal age specific rates for chromosome and factors influencing them: report of a collaborative European study on 52 965 amniocenteses. Prenatal Diagnosis 4: 5–44

Fricke G R, Mattern H J, Schweikert H U 1981 Mitral valve prolapse in Klinefelter syndrome (letter). Lancet ii:1414

Fuhrmann W 1968a A family study of transposition of the great vessels and in tricuspid atresia. Humangenetik 6: 148–157

Fuhrmann W 1968b Congenital heart disease in sibships ascertained by two affected siblings. Humangenetik 6:1

Gatton F 1876 The history of twins as a criterion of the relative powers of nature and nurture. Journal of the Anthroposophical Institute of Great Britain and Ireland

Gittenberger de Groot A 1977 Persistent ductus arteriosus: most probably a primary congenital malformation. British Heart Journal 39: 610–618

Gittenberger de Groot A C, Ertbruggen I, Moulaert A J M G, Harincke E 1980 The ductus arteriosus in the preterm infant: Histologic and clinical observations. Journal of Paediatrics 96: 88–93

Gregg N M 1942 Congenital cataract following german measles in mother. Transactions of Opthalmological Society Australia (1941) 3: 35–46

Harris D J, Begleiter M L, Chamberlin J, Hankins L, Magenis R E 1982 Parental trisomy 21 mosaicism. American Journal of Human Genetics 34: 125–133

Hook E B, Lindsjo A 1978 Down syndrome in live births by single year maternal age interval in a Swedish study: comparison with results from a New York state study. American Journal of Human Genetics 19–27

Jovanovic L, Druzin M, Peterson C M 1981 Effect of euglycaemia of the outcome of pregnancy in insulin-dependent diabetic women as compared with normal control subjects. American Journal of Medicine 71: 921–927

Kenna A P, Smithells R W, Fielding D W 1975 Congenital heart disease in Liverpool 1960–9. Quarterly Journal of Medicine 44: 17–44

Layton W M, Manasek F J 1980 Cardiac looping in early iv/iv mouse embryos. In: Van Praagh R, Takao A (eds) Etiology and morphogenesis of congenital heart disease. Futura, New York, 8: 109–126

Leck I 1960 Malformations in a population observed for five years after birth. PhD Thesis, University of Birmingham, p 177–9

Lejeune J, Gautier M, Turpin R 1959 Etude des chromosomes somatiques de neuf enfant mongoliens. Compte Rendus de l'Academie des Sciences Paris 248:1721

Lenke R R, Levy H L 1980 Maternal phenylketonuria and hyperphenylalaninemia. An international survey of the outcome of untreated and treated pregnancies. New England Journal of Medicine 1202–1208

Lenz W 1980 Aetiology, incidence and genetics of congenital heart disease. In: Graham G, Rossi E (eds) Heart disease in infants and children. Edward Arnold, London, p 27–35

Levin D L, Stanger P, Kitterman J A, Heymann M A 1975 Congenital heart disease in low birth weight infants. Circulation 52: 500–503

Loonen M C B 1979 The variability of Pompe's disease. MD Thesis, Department Neurology, University of Rotterdam, Netherlands

McKeown T, Record R G 1960 Malformations in a population observed for five years. CIBA Foundation Symposium on Congenital Malformations. Churchill, London 2–21

McKeown T, MacMahon B, Parsons C G 1953 The familial incidence of congenital malformation of the heart. British Heart Journal 15: 273–277

Masterson J G, Law E M, Power M M 1970 Reproduction in two females with Down's syndrome. Annals of Genetics 13: 38–41

Miller M J, Geffner I H, Lippe B M, Itami R M, Kaplan S A, Disessa T G, Isabel-Jones J B, Friedman 1983 Echocardiography reveals a high incidence of bicuspid aortic valve in Turner syndrome. Journal of Paediatrics 102: 47–50

Monteleone P L, Fagan L F 1969 Possible X linked congenital heart disease. Circulation 39: 611–614

Moreno A, Murphy E A 1981 Inheritance of Kartagener syndrome. American Journal of Medical Genetics 8: 305–313

Morton N E, Yee S, Elston R C, Lew R 1970 Discontinuity and quasi-continuity: Alternative hypotheses of multi-factorial inheritance. Clinical Genetics 1: 81–93

Murphy E A 1981 Skepsis dogma and belief: uses and abuses in medicine. Johns Hopkins University Press, Baltimore

National Congenital Rubella Surveillance Progress Report 1979. British Medical Journal 2: 396–397

New England Regional Infant Cardiac Programme Report 1980. Paediatrics (supplement) 65: 377–461

Nora J J 1968 Multifactorial inheritance hypothesis for the etiology of congenital heart disease: the genetic environment interaction. Circulation 38: 604–617

Nora J J 1971 Etiologic factors in congenital heart diseases. Pediatric Clinics of North America 18: 1059–1074

Nora J J, Nora A H 1978 The evolution of specific genetic and environmental counselling in congenital heart diseases. Circulation 57:205

Nora J J, Nora A H 1983 In: Steinberg A G, Bearn A G, Motulsky (eds) Genetic epidemiology of congenital heart diseases. In: Progress in medical genetics V. Genetics of cardiovascular disease. Saunders, Philadelphia, p 91–137

Nora J J, McNamara D G, Clarke Fraser F 1967 Hereditary factors in atrial septal defect. Circulation 35: 448–456

O'Nuallain S, Hall J G, Stamm S J 1977 Autosomal dominant inheritance of endocardial cushion defects. Birth Defects Original Article Series 13(3A): 143–147

Park S C, Mathews R A, Zuberbuhler J R, Rowe R D, Neches W H, Lenox C C 1977 Down's syndrome with congenital heart malformation. American Journal of Diseases in Children 131: 29–33

Patterson D F 1980 Genetic aspects of cardiovascular development in dogs. In: Van Praagh R, Takao A (eds) Etiology and morphogenesis of congenital heart disease. Futura, New York, p 1–20

Patterson D F, Pyle R L, Buchanan J W, Trautveter E, Abt D A 1971 Hereditary patent ductus arteriosus and its sequelae in the dog. Circulation Research 29: 1–13

Polani P E 1982 Pairing of X and Y chromosomes, non-inactivation of X-linked genes, and the maleness factor. Human Genetics 60(3): 207–211

Polani P E, Campbell M 1955 An aetiological study of congenital heart disease. Annals of Human Genetics 19: 209–230

Polani P E, Campbell M 1960 Factors in the causation of persistent ductus arteriosus. Annals of Human Genetics 24: 343–357

Polani P E, Alberman E, Alexander B J, et al 1979 Sixteen years' experience of counselling, diagnosis, and prenatal detection in one genetic centre, progress, results and problems. Journal of Medical Genetics 16: 166–175

Pompe J C 1933 Hypertrophie idiopathique du coeur. Annals d'Anatomie et Pathologie 10: 23–35

Rashkind W J 1972 Historical aspects of congenital heart disease. Birth Defects Original Article Series VIII i: 2–8

Record R G, McKeown T 1953 Observations relating to the aetiology of patent ductus arteriosus. British

Rose V, Izukawa T, Moes C A F 1975 Syndromes of asplenia and polysplenia: A review of cardiac and non-cardiac malformations in 60 cases with special reference to diagnosis and prognosis. British Heart Journal 37: 840–852

Rosenthal A 1972 Cardiovascular malformations in Klinefelter's syndrome: a report of three cases. Journal of Pediatrics 80: 471–473

Rowe R D, Uchida I A 1961 Cardiac malformation in mongolism. A prospective study of 184 mongoloid children. American Medical Journal 31: 726–735

Rowe R D, Freedom R M, Mehrizi A, Bloom K R 1981 Patent ductus arteriosus in the neonate with congenital heart disease. Saunders, Philadelphia, p 271–285

Rowland T W, Hubell J P, Nadas A S 1973 Congenital heart disease in infants of diabetic mothers. Journal of Pediatrics 83: 815–820

Sanchez-Cascos A 1972 Genetics of atrial septal defect. Archives of Diseases in Childhood 47: 581–8

Sanchez-Cascos A 1978 The recurrence risk in congenital heart disease. European Journal of Cardiology 7: 197–210

Sanchez-Cascos A 1983 The Noonan syndrome. European Heart Journal 4: 223–229

Schinzel A A 1983 Cardiovascular defects associated with chromosomal aberrations and malformation syndromes. In: Steinberg A G, Bearn A G, Motulsky A G, Childs B (eds) Progress in Medical Genetics of Cardiovascular Disease. Saunders, Philadelphia, p 303–380

Scott J S, Maddison P J, Taylor P V, Esscher E, Scott O, Skinner R P 1983 Connective-tissue disease, antibodies to ribonucleoprotein and congenital heart block. New England Journal of Medicine 309: 209–212

Siassi B, Blanco C, Cabal L A, Goran A G 1976 Incidence and clinical features of patent ductus arteriosus in low birth weight infants: a prospective analysis of 150 consecutively born infants. Paediatrics 57: 347–351

Simpson J L 1976 Gonadal dysgenesis in disorders of sexual differentiation etiology and clinical delineation. Academic Press, New York

Singh H, Bolton P J, Oakley C M 1982 Pregnancy after surgical correction of tetralogy of Fallot. British Medical Journal 285: 168–170

Soltan H C, Li M D 1974 Hereditary dextrocardia associated with other congenital heart defects: report of a pedigree. Clinical Genetics 5: 51–58

Speed R M, Johnston A W, Evans H J 1976 Chromosome survey of total population of mentally subnormal in North-East Scotland. Journal of Medical Genetics 13: 295–306

Takao A, Ando M, Cho K, Kinouchi A, Murakami Y 1980 Etiologic categorization of common congenital heart disease. In: Van Praagh R, Takao A (eds) Etiology and morphogenesis of congenital heart disease. Futura, New York, p 253–269

Taussig H B 1982 World survey of the common cardiac malformations: developmental error or genetic variant. American Journal of Cardiology 50: 544–559

Torgersen J 1950 Situs inversus, asymmetry and twinning. American Journal of Human Genetics 2: 361–370

Turner H H 1938 A syndrome of infantilism congenital webbed neck and cubitus valgus. Endocrinology 23: 566–574

Ullrich O 1930 Uber typische Kombinationsbilder multipler Abartungen. Zeitschrift Kinderheilkund 49: 271–276

Van Mierop L, Gessner I H, Schiebler G L 1972 Asplenia and polysplenia syndromes. Birth defects original articles series VIII 1: 74–82

Vogel F, Motulsky A G 1979 Human Genetics. Problems and Approaches New York: Springer Verlag 569–577

Warkany J, Passarge E, Smith L B 1966 Congenital malformations in autosomal trisomy syndromes. American Journal of Diseases in Children 112: 502–517

Watkins P J 1982 Congenital malformations and blood glucose control in diabetic pregnancy (editorial). British Medical Journal 1357–1358

Whittemore, R, Hobbins J C, Engle M A 1982 Pregnancy and its outcome in women with and without surgical treatment of congenital heart disease. American Journal of Cardiology 50: 361–370

Wilkins J L 1969 Risks to offspring of patients with patent ductus arteriosus. Journal of Medical Genetics 6: 1–4

Williamson D A J 1970 A syndrome of congenital spinal anomalies in infants of diabetic mothers. Developmental Medicine and Child Neurology 12: 145–152

Williamson E M 1969 A family study of atrial septal defect. Journal of Medical Genetics 6: 255–261

Yao J, Thompson M W, Trusler G A, Trimble A S 1968 Familial atrial septal defect of the primum type: a report of four cases in one sibship. Canadian Medical Association Journal 98: 218–219

Zetterqvist P 1972 A clinical and genetic study of congenital heart defects. University of Uppsala Publication, Sweden, p 1–80

Zoethoet H E, Bonham-Carter R E, Carter C O 1964 A family study of aortic stenosis. Journal of Medical Genetics 1: 2–9

Appendix: Syndromes involving the heart

The word 'syndrome' derives from the Greek 'running together'. When a heart defect is part of the pattern this frequently is the reason for early specialist referral. The problem for the cardiologist is that over a quarter of children with heart defects have abnormalities in other systems, so the question often arises 'Is this a syndrome?' The number of syndromes in the literature continues to expand – now over 1000. Many are rare and some are likely to be merged or erased in time but others are likely to replace them. Even the best reference textbooks have fewer than half of the total. Faced with such complexity there is an urge to dismiss the exercise as pointless, or confine one's attention to the dozen best known disorders. The following tables are an attempt to provide more comprehensive access.

The eleven key tables contain, in alphabetical order, the syndromes which combine the main features, for example, heart defects and polydactyly. Each table is divided into two categories. The first category in each table contains the more common and/or well documented disorders. The second list includes rare or unproven syndromes and those where one or other of the features is 'small-print'.

Table 2A.1 Heart defects and organomegaly.

'Common' syndromes
Aase syndrome
Alagille syndrome
Beckwith-Wiedemann syndrome
Berardinelli syndrome (generalised lipodystrophy)
Glycogen storage disease type IV, Brancher deficiency
Hunter syndrome (mucopolysaccharidosis II)
Hurler syndrome (mucopolysaccharisosis IH)
Maroteaux-Lamy syndrome (mucopolysaccharidosis VI)
Mulibrey Nanism syndrome
Pompe's disease (glycogen storage disease type IIA)
Zewllweger syndrome (cerebrohepatorenal syndrome)

'Rare' syndromes
Fetal cytomegalovirus syndrome
Fetal toxoplasmosis syndrome
Fucosidosis
Geleophysic dysplasia
Klippel-Trenaunay-Weber syndrome
Morquio syndrome (mucopolysaccharidosis IV)
Noonan syndrome
Scheie syndrome (mucopolysaccharidosis IS)

Table 2A.2 Heart defects and mental retardation/abnormal face.

'Common' syndromes
Alagille syndrome (arteriohepatic dysplasia)
Asymmetric crying face syndrome
Beckwith-Wiedemann syndrome (EMG syndrome)
Carpenter syndrome
Campomelic dysplasia
CHARGE syndrome (acronym)
Coffin Siris syndrome
Conotruncal anomaly-face
de Lange syndrome
Ellis-Van Creveld syndrome (chondroectodermal dysplasia)
Fetal alcohol syndrome
Fetal hydantoin syndrome
Goldenhar syndrome
Goltz syndrome
Heart-hand IV
Hunter syndrome (mucopolysaccharidosis II)
Hurler syndrome (mucopolysaccharisosis IH)
Hydrolethalus
LEOPARD syndrome
Manzke syndrome (digitopalatal syndrome)
Maternal phenylketonuria disruption
Meckel syndrome
Miller Dieker syndrome (lissencephaly syndrome)
Mulibrey nanism syndrome
Noonan syndrome
Pompe's disease (glycogen storage disease type IIA)
Pseudo-Hurler polydystrophy (mucolipidosis III)
Rubinstein-Taybi syndrome
Smith-Lemli-Opitz syndrome
Velocardiofacial syndrome (Shprintzen syndrome)
Williams syndrome
Zellweger syndrome (cerebrohepatorenal syndrome)

'Rare' syndromes
Aase Smith syndrome
Acrofacial dysostosis (Miller) syndrome
Allanson syndrome
Antley-Bixler syndrome
Apert syndrome
Andre syndrome
Baetz-Greenwalt syndrome
Baller Gerold syndrome
Barrow syndrome
Behmel syndrome
Beighton type spondyloepimetaphyseal dysplasia
Berardinelli syndrome (generalised lipodystrophy)
Bonneau syndrome
Cerebrocostomandibular syndrome
Char syndrome
Conradi Hunerman syndrome (chondrodysplasia punctata)
Congenital hypothyroidism
Conradi syndrome, chondrodysplasia punctata – rhizomelic type
Cranioectodermal dysplasia
Cutis laxa (recessive form)
C-trigonocephaly syndrome (Opitz C syndrome)

Table 2A.2(*cont'd*)

'*Rare*' *syndromes*
DiGeorge syndrome
Distichiasis – heart defects syndrome (Goldstein syndrome)
Faciocardiomelic syndrome
Faciocardiorenal syndrome
Fanconi syndrome
Femoral hypoplasia – unusual facies syndrome
Fetal aminopterin syndrome
Fetal trimethadione syndrome
Fetal toxoplasmosis syndrome
Fetal warfarin syndrome
Fitch syndrome
FG syndrome (Opitz Kaveggia syndrome)
Fraser syndrome
Fucosidosis
Gastrocutaneous syndrome
Geleophysic dysplasia
Golabi Ito syndrome
Goodman syndrome
Gorlin-Chaudhary-Moss
Grix syndrome
Hallerman-Streiff syndrome
Hay-Wells syndrome
Homocystinuria
Hypertrichosis-osteochondrodysplasia
Jennings syndrome
Johnson syndrome
Kabuki make-up syndrome
Kearns-Sayre syndrome
Klippel-Feil syndrome
Klippel-Trenaunay-Weber syndrome
Lambert syndrome
Larsen syndrome
Lenz microphthalmia syndrome
Laurence–Moon–Biedl syndrome
Limb reduction ichthyosis syndrome
Linear sebaceous naevus syndrome
Lujan syndrome
Majewski syndrome (short rib-polydactyly syndrome II)
Maroteaux-Lamy syndrome (mucopolysaccharidosis VI)
McDonough syndrome
Marden Walker syndrome
Maternal diabetes disruption
Mietens syndrome
Mutchinick syndrome
Morquio syndrome (mucopolysaccharidosis IV)
Mucolipidosis II (I cell disease)
Myotonic dystrophy
Najjar syndrome
Neurofibromatosis
Onat syndrome
Opitz G/BBB syndrome
Osteogenesis imperfecta (four clinical types – ?multiple genetic
    disorders)
Osteogenesis imperfecta-microcephaly-cataracts
Robenhorst syndrome
Robin sequence (Pierre Robin syndrome)
Robinow syndrome
Rogers syndrome (?same as velocardiofacial syndrome)
Rutledge syndrome
Ruvalcaba syndrome
Saethre-Chotzen syndrome
Schinzel-Giedion syndrome
Scheie syndrome (mucopolysaccharidosis IS)
Singleton-Merten syndrome
Steinfeld syndrome
Strong syndrome
Sturge-Weber syndrome
Tamari Goodman syndrome
Thrombocytopenia-absent radius (TAR) syndrome

Table 2A.2 (*cont'd*)

'*Rare*' *syndromes*
Thanatophoric dysplasia syndrome
Treacher Collins syndrome (mandibulofacial dysostosis)
Trigonocephaly C syndrome (Opitz C syndrome)
Tuberous sclerosis
Varadi syndrome
Waardenburg syndrome
Werner syndrome
Woodhouse syndrome

Table 2A.3   Heart defects and eye defects.

'*Common*' *syndromes*
Alagille syndrome (arteriohepatic dysplasia)
CHARGE syndrome
Fraser syndrome
Goldenhar syndrome
Goltz syndrome
Homocystinuria
Hurler syndrome (mucopolysaccharisosis IH)
Laurence-Moon syndrome
Marfan syndrome
Scheie syndrome (mucopolysaccharidosis IS)

'*Rare*' *syndromes*
Acrofacial dysostosis (Miller) syndrome
Alkaptonuria
Beal syndrome
Berardinelli syndrome (generalised lipodystrophy)
Conradi Hunerman syndrome (chondrodysplasia punctata)
Conradi syndrome (chondrodysplasia punctata rhizomelic type)
de Lange syndrome
Distichiasis-heart defects syndrome (Goldstein syndrome)
Fabry's disease
Fanconi syndrome
Fetal cytomegalovirus syndrome
Fetal toxoplasmosis syndrome
Fetal warfarin syndrome
Gastrocutaneous syndrome
Goodman syndrome
Gorlin-Chaudhary-Moss syndrome
Hallerman-Streiff syndrome
Hay-Wells syndrome
Hittner syndrome
Kearns-Sayre syndrome
Klippel-Trenaunay-Weber syndrome
Lenz microphthalmia syndrome
Levin syndrome
Linear sebaceous naevus syndrome
Maroteaux-Lamy syndrome (mucopolysaccharidosis VI)
Maternal phenylketonuria disruption
Meckel syndrome
Mietens syndrome
Morquio syndrome (mucopolysaccharidosis IV)
Mulibrey nanism syndrome
Myotonic dystrophy
Nathalie syndrome
Neurofibromatosis
Osteogenesis imperfecta (four clinical types – ?multiple genetic
    disorders)
Osteogenesis imperfecta-microcephaly-cataracts.
Pseudo-Hurler polydystrophy (mucolipidosis III)
Von Hippel-Lindau syndrome
Waardenburg syndrome
Weill-Marchesani syndrome
Werner syndrome

Table 2A.4 Heart defects and deafness/ear abnormalities.

'Common' syndromes
CHARGE syndrome
Goldenhar syndrome
Jervell-Lange-Nielson syndrome
LEOPARD syndrome
Noonan syndrome

'Rare' syndromes
Acrofacial dysostosis (Miller) syndrome
Apert syndrome
Baller Gerold syndrome
Beckwith-Wiedemann syndrome (EMG syndrome)
Beal syndrome
Cardioauditory syndrome of Sanchez Cascos
Fanconi syndrome
Fetal cytomegalovirus syndrome
Fetal trimethadione syndrome
Forney syndrome
Fraser syndrome
Golabi Ito syndrome
Hittner syndrome
Hunter syndrome (mucopolysaccharidosis II)
Hurler syndrome (mucopolysaccharisosis IH)
Jennings syndrome
Johnson syndrome
Kartagener syndrome
Keutel syndrome
Klippel-Feil syndrome
Lenz microphthalmia syndrome
Lujan syndrome
Maroteaux-Lamy syndrome (mucopolysaccharidosis VI)
McDonough syndrome
Mutchinick syndrome
Morquio syndrome (mucopolysaccharidosis IV)
Nathalie syndrome
Osteogenesis imperfecta (four clinical types – ?multiple genetic disorders)
Osteogenesis imperfecta-microcephaly-cataracts
Roberts syndrome (Pseudothalidomide (SC) syndrome)
Scheie syndrome (mucopolysaccharidosis IS)
Treacher Collins syndrome (mandibulofacial dysostosis)
Velocardiofacial syndrome (Shprintzen syndrome)
Waardenburg syndrome
Woodhouse syndrome

Table 2A.5 Heart defects and limb reduction defects.

'Common' syndromes
Aase syndrome
Coffin Siris syndrome
de Lange syndrome
Fanconi syndrome
Goltz syndrome
Holt-Oram syndrome (heart-hand I)
Maternal diabetes disruption
Thrombocytopenia-absent radius (TAR) syndrome
VACTERL association

'Rare' syndromes
Acrofacial dysostosis (Miller) syndrome
Andre syndrome
Baller Gerold syndrome
Faciocardiomelic syndrome
Fetal alcohol syndrome
Fetal aminopterin syndrome
Fetal hydantoin syndrome
Heart-hand II
Heart-hand III
Hollister syndrome
Keutel syndrome
Limb reduction ichthyosis syndrome
Roberts syndrome (pseudothalidomide (SC) syndrome)
Steinfeld syndrome

Table 2A.6 Heart defects and polydactyly.

'Common' syndromes
Carpenter syndrome
Ellis-van Creveld syndrome (chondroectodermal dysplasia)
Heart-hand IV syndrome
Hydrolethalus syndrome
Meckel syndrome
Saldino Noonan syndrome

'Rare' syndromes
Anocerebrodigital syndromes (CNS hamartoblastoma syndrome)
Andre syndrome
Behmel syndrome
Bonneau syndrome
C-trigonocephaly syndrome (Opitz C syndrome)
Forney syndrome
Ho syndrome
Jeune thoracic dysplasia
Kaufman-McKusick syndrome
Laurence syndrome
Laurence-Moon-Biedl syndrome
Majewski syndrome (short rib-polydactyly syndrome)
Rogers syndrome
Schinzel-Giedion syndrome
Short rib-polydactyly syndrome III
Smith-Lemli-Opitz syndrome
Varadi syndrome

Table 2A.7 Heart defects and other skeletal defects.

'Common' syndromes
Beighton type spondyloepimetaphyseal dysplasia
Campomelic dysplasia
Goldenhar syndrome
Homocystinuria
Manzke syndrome (digitopalatal syndrome)
Marfan syndrome
Maternal diabetes disruption
Mulibrey nanism syndrome
Noonan syndrome
Rubenstein-Taybi syndrome

'Rare' syndromes
Aase Smith syndrome
Alagille syndrome (arteriohepatic dysplasia)
Alkaptonuria syndrome
Allanson syndrome
Antley-Bixler syndrome
Apert syndrome
Asymmetric crying face syndrome
Andre syndrome
Barrow syndrome
Beal syndrome
Behmel syndrome
Cerebrocostomandibular syndrome
Conradi Hunerman syndrome (chondrodysplasia punctata)
Conradi syndrome (chondrodysplasia punctata rhizomelic type)
Cranioectodermal dysplasia
C-trigonocephaly syndrome (Opitz C syndrome)
Distichiasis-heart defects syndrome (Goldstein syndrome)
Femoral hypoplasia – unusual facies syndrome
Fetal warfarin syndrome
Fitch syndrome
Forney syndrome
Fucosidosis syndrome
Gay syndrome
Geleophysic dysplasia
Gorlin-Chaudhary-Moss syndrome
Grix syndrome
Hunter syndrome (mucopolysaccharidosis II)
Hurler syndrome (mucopolysaccharisosis IH)
Hypertrichosis-osteochondrodysplasia syndrome
Jeune thoracic dysplasia
Klippel-Feil syndrome
Klippel-Trenaunay-Weber syndrome
Kozlowski syndrome
Larsen syndrome
Lujan syndrome
Majewski syndrome (short rib-polydactyly syndrome II)
Marfanoid hypermobility syndrome
Martinez syndrome
McDonough syndrome
Marden Walker syndrome
Mietens syndrome
Morquio syndrome (mucopolysaccharidosis IV)
Mucolipidosis II (I cell disease)
Myhre syndrome
Neurofibromatosis
Onat syndrome
Osteogenesis imperfecta (four clinical types – ?multiple genetic
  disorders)
Osteogenesis imperfecta-microcephaly-cataracts
Pseudo-Hurler polydystrophy (mucolipidosis III)
Robinow syndrome
Ruvalcaba syndrome
Saethre-Chotzen syndrome
Schinzel-Giedion syndrome
Scheie syndrome (mucopolysaccharidosis IS)
Short rib-polydactyly syndrome III
Singleton-Merten syndrome
Shwachman syndrome

Table 2A.7 (*cont'd*)

'Rare' syndromes
Tamari Goodman syndrome
Thanatophoric dysplasia syndrome
Weill-Marchesani syndrome
Zellweger syndrome (cerebrohepatorenal syndrome)

Table 2A.8 Heart defects and gastrointestinal/genitourinary anomalies.

'Common' syndromes
Beckwith-Wiedemann syndrome (EMG syndrome)
Campomelic dysplasia syndrome
Isomerism sequence
LEOPARD syndrome (acronym)
Noonan syndrome
VACTERL association

'Rare' syndromes
Allanson syndrome
Anocerebrodigital syndrome (CNS hamartoblastoma syndrome)
Antley-Bixler syndrome
Apert syndrome
Baller Gerold syndrome
Cantrell pentalogy syndrome
CHARGE syndrome (acronym)
de Lange syndrome
Ehlers-Danlos syndrome type IV (arterial or Sack type)
Fabry's disease
Faciocardiorenal syndrome
Fanconi syndrome
Fetal hydantoin syndrome
Fetal trimethadione syndrome
FG syndrome (Opitz Kaveggia syndrome)
Fraser syndrome
Fucosidosis syndrome
Gastrocutaneous syndrome
Gorlin-Chaudhary-Moss syndrome
Harris syndrome
Heart-hand IV syndrome
Hydrolethalus syndrome
Jennings syndrome
Jeune thoracic dysplasia
Johnson syndrome
Kashani syndrome
Kaufman-McKusick syndrome
Klippel-Feil syndrome
Lambert syndrome
Lenz microphthalmia syndrome
Laurence syndrome
Laurence-Moon-Biedl syndrome
Linear sebaceous naevus syndrome
Majewski syndrome (short rib-polydactyly syndrome II)
Marfan syndrome
Maternal diabetes disruption syndrome
Meckel syndrome
Najjar syndrome
Opitz G/BBB syndrome
Robinow syndrome
Rubinstein-Taybi syndrome
Rutledge syndrome
Ruvalcaba syndrome
Sacks syndrome
Schinzel-Giedion syndrome
Shwachman syndrome
Smith Lemli Opitz syndrome
Steinfeld syndrome
Von Hippel-Lindau syndrome
Woodhouse syndrome
Zellweger syndrome (cerebrohepatorenal syndrome)

Table 2A.9   Syndromes involving conduction defects.

'Common' syndromes
Heart-hand III
Jervell-Lange-Nielson syndrome
Kearns-Sayre syndrome
LEOPARD syndrome

'Rare' syndromes
Behmel syndrome
Distichiasis-heart defects syndrome (Goldstein syndrome)
Faciocardiorenal syndrome
Heart-hand II
Hollister syndrome
Holt-Oram syndrome (Heart-hand I syndrome)
Keutel syndrome
Myotonic dystrophy
Nathalie syndrome
Refsum disease (phytanic acid storage disease)
Woodhouse syndrome

Table 2A.10   Syndromes involving cardiomyopathy.

'Common' syndromes
Duchenne muscular dystrophy
Emery Dreifuss muscular dystrophy
Freidrich's ataxia
Glycogen storage disease type IV (Brancher deficiency)
Kearns-Sayre syndrome (mitochondrial cytopathy)
LEOPARD syndrome
Najjar syndrome
Noonan syndrome
Pompe's disease (glycogen storage disease type IIA)
Sacks syndrome

'Rare' syndromes
Berardinelli syndrome (generalised lipodystrophy, Seip syndrome)
Congenital hypothyroidism
Fenichel syndrome
Fetal toxoplasmosis
Fucosidosis
Hurler syndrome (mucopolysaccharisosis IH)
Jeune thoracic dysplasia
Maroteaux-Lamy syndrome (mucopolysaccharidosis VI)
McArdle's disease (glycogen storage disease type V)
Refsum diseases (phytanic acid storage disease)
Spinal muscular atrophy (Kugelberg-Welander disease)
Tuberose sclerosis

Table 2A.11   Syndromes involving vascular defects.

'Common' syndromes
Ehlers-Danlos syndrome type IV (arterial or Sack type)
Fabry's disease
Homocystinuria
Isomerism sequence
Klippel-Trenaunay-Weber syndrome
Marfan syndrome
Osler's hereditary haemorrhagic telangiectasia
Pseudoxanthoma elasticum syndrome
Progeria syndrome (the Hutchinson-Gilford syndrome)
Von Hippel-Lindau syndrome
Williams syndrome

'Rare' syndromes
Alkaptonuria syndrome
Berardinelli syndrome (generalised lipodystrophy, Seip syndrome)
Cutis laxa (recessive form)
Distichiasis-heart defects syndrome (Goldstein syndrome)
Holt-Oram (heart-hand I syndrome)
Hunter syndrome (mucopolysaccharidosis II)
Mucolipidosis II (I cell disease)
Singleton-Merten syndrome
Sturge-Weber syndrome
Werner syndrome

Table 2A.12 Clinical features and aetiology of cardiac syndromes.

Syndrome name	Clinical features	Aetiology	Cardiac defects	Key reference
Aase syndrome	Triphalangeal thumbs, radial hypoplasia, narrow shoulders, late closure fontanelle, hypoplastic anaemia, mild short stature, variable hepatosplenomegaly.	Probable autosomal recessive.	Ventricular septal defect most common anomaly. Common arterial trunk described.	van Weel-Sipman et al, 1977
Aase Smith syndrome	Dandy Walker cerebral malformation, multiple joint contractures, poorly formed flexion creases, cleft palate, ptosis.	Autosomal dominant.	Muscular ventricular septal defects and cardiac hypertrophy reported.	Aase & Smith, 1968
Acrofacial dysostosis (Miller) syndrome	Postaxial reduction defect, dysplastic ears, malar flattening, downslanting palpebral fissures, ectropion, colobomata, cleft palate.	Possible autosomal recessive.	Ventricular septal defect.	Fineman, 1981
Alagille syndrome Arteriohepatic dysplasia	Intrahepatic biliary atresia, embryotoxon of eye (80%), abnormal facies (75%), vertebral anomalies (33%).	At least some cases are autosomal dominant.	Peripheral pulmonary artery stenosis.	Alagille et al, 1975
Alkaptonuria syndrome	Deposition of homogentisic acid, pigmentation sclerae, cartilage, late arthritis.	Probable autosomal recessive.	Accelerated cardiovascular disease, aortic stenosis.	Reginato et al, 1972
Allanson syndrome	Diffuse hypoplasia renal tubules, pulmonary hypoplasia, hypertelorism, fixed flexion knees and hips, lax wrists and ankles.	All cases sporadic to data.	Tetralogy of Fallot.	Allanson et al, 1983
Anocerebrodigital syndrome CNS hamartoblastoma syndrome	Imperforate anus, brain tumours, laryngeal anomaly, postaxial polydactyly, renal agenesis.	All cases sporadic to date.	Pulmonary stenosis.	Hall et al, 1980a
Antley-Bixler syndrome	Coronal, lambdoid suture synostosis, frontal bossing, severe midface hypoplasia, proptosis, choanal stenosis, bowed femora and ulnae, vaginal atresia, renal anomalies.	Probable autosomal recessive.	Oval fossa atrial septal defect.	Schinzel et al, 1983
Andre syndrome	Hypertelorism, downslanting eyes, micrognathia, cleft palate, long bone bowing, fanned toes, occasional polydactyly, kyphoscoliosis.	X-linked recessive.	Occasional ventricular septal defect.	Andre et al, 1981
Apert syndrome	Severe craniosynostosis, flat face, hypertelorism, cleft palate (occ), syndactyly (mitten hands), deafness, occasional retardation, renal anomalies.	Autosomal dominant.	Pulmonary stenosis, ventricular septal defect.	Blank, 1960
Asymmetric crying face syndrome	Hypoplasia or absence of depressor angularis oris on one side.	Sporadic.	Ventricular septal defect.	Levin et al, 1982
Atkin syndrome	Posterior fossa 'Dandy Walker' cyst, microphthalmia, cloudy corneae, cleft lip, malformed ears, webbed neck, cleft hands, renal anomalies, hypospadias.	Single case report.	Atrial septal defect, ventricular septal defect, persistent arterial duct, dysplastic pulmonary valve.	Atkin & Patil, 1984
Baetz-Greenwalt syndrome	Microcephaly (10), micrognathia, cleft palate (2), low set ears (4), arhinencephaly (1).	14 cases in one area, ?seasonal cluster, specific teratogen.	Varying degrees of hypoplastic right ventricle with associated valve defects.	Baetz-Greenwalt et al, 1983
Baller Gerold syndrome	Craniosynostosis, radial aplasia, missing thumbs, short stature, imperforate anus, epicanthic folds, dysplastic ears.	Probable autosomal recessive.	Subaortic valvar hypertrophy, ventricular septal defect.	Pelias et al, 1981

Table 2A.12 Clinical features and aetiology of cardiac syndromes. (*cont'd*)

Syndrome name	Clinical features	Aetiology	Cardiac defects	Key reference
Barrow syndrome	Short-limbed dwarfism (rhizomelic), undescended testes, severe micrognathia, sloping forehead, prominent nasal bridge, facial haemangioma.	Single case.	Double inlet ventricle, common arterial trunk.	Barrow & Fitzsimmons, 1984
Beal syndrome Congenital contractural arachnodactyly	Large joint contractures, arachnodactyly 'crumpled' ear helices. Rarely keratoconus and myopia, kyphoscoliosis.	Autosomal dominant.	Mitral regurgitation, coarctation.	Anderson et al, 1984
Beckwith-Wiedemann syndrome EMG syndrome	Macroglossia, exomphalos, visceromegaly, hypoglycaemia, ear creases, renal anomalies, ?excess insulin-like growth factor.	Some cases duplication 11p. Probable autosomal dominant.	Cardiomegaly, variety of malformations include septal defects, common arterial trunk.	Greenwood et al, 1977
Beemer syndrome	Hydropic, median cleft upper lip, short ribs, short tubular bones, exomphalos.	Probable autosomal recessive.	Complete transposition, ventricular septal defect.	Beemer et al, 1983
Behmel syndrome	General overgrowth, coarse face, postaxial polydactyly, mental retardation, cryptorchidism.	X-linked recessive.	Electrocardiographic abnormality, ventricular septal defect.	Behmel et al, 1984
Beighton type spondylo-epimetaphyseal dysplasia	Short stature, kyphoscoliosis, talipes, joint dislocation, soft skin with hyperelastosis, blue sclerae, prominent eyes, long top lip.	Autosomal recessive.	Mitral incompetence, ventricular septal defect.	Beighton et al, 1984
Berardinelli syndrome (generalised lipodystrophy) Seip syndrome	Lipoatrophy, phallic hypertrophy, hepatomegaly, hyperlipaemia, corneal, opacities, large superficial veins.	Autosomal recessive.	Cardiomegaly.	Berardinelli, 1954
Bonneau syndrome	Polysyndactyly, hypertelorism, telecanthus large nares.	Probable autosomal recessive.	Septal defects, double inlet ventricle, discordant ventriculo-arterial connexion.	Bonneau et al, 1983
Cantrell pentalogy syndrome	Anterior body wall defect; absent diaphragm, short or bifid sternum, gastroschisis.	Sporadic.	A variety of defects including tetralogy of Fallot.	Cantrell et al, 1958
Campomelic dysplasia syndrome	Polyhydramnios, anterior bowed tibiae, hypotonia, small scapulae, males appear female, cleft palate, micrognathia.	Autosomal recessive.	Septal defects, tetralogy of Fallot, aortic stenosis.	Houston et al, 1983
Cardio-auditory syndrome of Sanchez-Cascos	Severe sensorineural deafness. Excess whorls on fingertips.	Autosomal recessive.	Cardiac hypertrophy.	Sanchez Cascos et al, 1969
Carpenter syndrome.	Craniosynostosis (acrocephaly), mental retardation, obesity, polysyndactyly.	Autosomal recessive.	Frequent heart defects include persistent arterial duct, ventricular septal defect, pulmonary stenosis.	Temtamy 1966
Cerebro-costo-mandibular syndrome	Micrognathia, cleft palate, gaps in posterior ribs and fusion of dorsal end to vertebrae, mental retardation.	Autosomal recessive.	Ventricular septal defect.	McNicholl et al, 1970
Char syndrome	Short stature, microcephaly, mental retardation, patchy skin pigmentation, hypertelorism, premature loss of teeth.	Possible autosomal dominant.	Multifocal ventricular ectopic beats.	Char et al, 1975

Table 2A.12 Clinical features and aetiology of cardiac syndromes. (*cont'd*)

Syndrome name	Clinical features	Aetiology	Cardiac defects	Key reference
CHARGE syndrome (acronym)	Colobomaata (iris and/or retina), Heart defects, artresia choanae, Retardation and renal defects, Genitalia small in males, Ears cup-shaped and deaf.	Unknown – all cases sporadic.	Wide variety including ventricular septal defects, atrioventricular septal defects and tetralogy of Fallot.	Pagon et al, 1981
Coffin Siris syndrome	Short stature of prenatal onset, mental retardation, hypotonia, sparse scalp hair, hirsutes, coarse face, deficient terminal phalanges.	Possible autosomal recessive.	Atrial septal defect, partial anomalous pulmonary venous connexion.	Carey & Hall, 1978
Congenital hypothyroidism	Untreated, short stature, coarse facies, mental retardation, hypotonia, constipation, goitre, umbilical hernia.	Autosomal recessive in most cases.	'Cardiac myxoedema' with decreased heart sounds and decreased cardiac output.	Fisher & Klein, 1981
Conotruncal anomaly face syndrome	Small mouth, hypertelorism, nasal voice occcasional cleft palate, mild retardation (1/3), malformed ears.	Sporadic ?branchial arch defect.	Common arterial trunk, complete transposition, tetralogy of Fallot.	Takao et al, 1980
Conradi Hunerman syndrome Chondrodysplasia punctata	Hydramnios and early death in some, punctate epiphyseal calcification, limb asymmetry, scoliosis contractures, flat facies, cataracts (20%), dry skin and alopecia (20%).	Variable autosomal dominant.	Heart defects an occasional feature.	Hyndman et al, 1976
Conradi syndrome Chondrodysplasia punctata rhizomelic type	Short proximal limbs, flat face, lymphoedema of cheeks, cataracts, contractures, stippled epiphyses. Early death, survivors retarded.	Autosomal recessive.	Variety of heart defects described.	Rimoin & Horton, 1978
Cranioectodermal dysplasia syndrome	Dolichocephaly, sparse hair, epicanthic folds, hypodontia, short limbs, brachydactyly, narrow thorax.	Possible autosomal recessive.	Divided left atrium and ventricular septal defects described.	Levin et al, 1977
Cutis laxa syndrome (recessive form)	Lax facial skin, everted lower eyelids, hooked nose, long upper lip, bladder and colonic diverticulae, vaginal and rectal prolapse, hernias.	Autosomal recessive.	Cor pulmonale due to severe emphysema, aortic aneurysm.	Beighton, 1972
C-trigonocephaly syndrome (Opitz C syndrome)	Prominent metopic ridge, microcephaly, upslanting eyes, hypotelorism, telecanthus, characteristic palate, occasional polysyndactyly.	?Heterogeneous – possible autosomal recessive cases.	Persistent arterial duct, septal defects occasionally, 1 case of critical mitral stenosis.	Sargent et al, 1985
de Lange syndrome	Synophrys, thin down-turned upper lip, severe retardation and short stature, malrotation of bowel, micrognathia, severe upper limb reduction defects.	Sporadic.	Most often ventricular septal defects.	Ptacek et al, 1963
DiGeorge syndrome	Congenital hypoparathyroidism, down-slanting eyes, short philtrum, low set ears, micrognathia, thymic hypoplasia (defect in 4th branchial arch).	Sporadic, more in males? Deletion 22 in some.	Outflow defects – interrupted aorta, common arterial trunk, tetralogy of Fallot.	De la Chapelle et al, 1981
Duchenne muscular dystrophy syndrome	Progressive selective wasting of skeletal musculature, worst around pectoral and pelvic girdles, with pseudohypertrophy of calf muscles.	X-linked recessive.	Progressive cardiomyopathy.	Skyring & McKusick, 1961
Distichiasis – heart defects syndrome (Goldstein syndrome)	Extra row of eyelashes, photophobia, squint, vertebral anomalies, oedema, broad neck, small jaw in some.	Autosomal dominant	Ventricular septal defect, persistent arterial duct, varicose veins, bradycardia.	Goldstein et al, 1985

Table 2A.12 Clinical features and aetiology of cardiac syndromes. (*cont'd*)

Syndrome name	Clinical features	Aetiology	Cardiac defects	Key reference
Ehlers-Danlos syndrome type IV (arterial or Sack type)	Most severe form – thin easily bruised skin with prominent veins but only slight increase in stretchability. Tendency to bowel rupture.	Autosomal recessive and dominant forms described.	Spontaneous rupture of large and medium-sized arteries. Mitral valve prolapse. Atrial septal defect.	Pope et al, 1976
Ellis-van Creveld syndrome Chondroectodermal dysplasia	Postaxial polydactyly, rhizomelic limb shortening, short ribs/small chest, oral frenulae, natal teeth, nail dysplasia, sparse hair, thin skin.	Autosomal recessive.	50% have heart defects, typically common atrium, atrioventricular septal defect.	Walls et al, 1959
Emery-Dreifuss muscular dystrophy	Progressive weakness, first in legs, waddling gait, large joint contractures.	X-linked recessive.	Congestive cardiomyopathy.	Emery & Dreifuss, 1966
Fabry's disease	Acroparaesthesiae, corneal opacities, characteristic skin angiomata, abdominal pains, renal failure, aneurysms.	X-linked α-galactosidase A deficiency.	Ventricular hypertrophy, ischaemia, hypertension, cerebral vascular disease.	Wallace, 1973
Faciocardiomelic syndrome	Hypoplastic or absent radius, ulna, tibia and thumb bilaterally, talipes camptodactyly, webbed neck, hypoplastic or absent tongue, hypertelorism.	Autosomal recessive.	Hypoplastic left heart. Common arterial trunk.	Cantu et al, 1975
Facio-cardio-renal syndrome	Prominent and rigid ears, wide nasal bridge, cleft palate, oligodontia, horse-shoe kidneys, absent/hypoplastic nails, big hallux, retardation.	?Autosomal recessive.	Conduction defects, endocardial fibroelastosis.	Eastman & Bixler, 1977.
Fanconi syndrome	Short stature, small eyes and cranium, thumb hypoplasia, pancytopaenia, splenic hypoplasia, brown pigmentation, small genitalia, leukaemia.	Autosomal recessive (chromosome repair defect).	Cardiac defects in 1 in 6 of various types.	Glanz & Clarke Fraser, 1982.
Femoral hypoplasia-unusual faces syndrome	Short bowed femora, long philtrum radio-ulnar synostosis cleft palate.	2/3 sporadic 1/3 maternal diabetes.	Heart defects mainly ventricular septal defects (in maternal diabetic cases only).	Burn et al, 1984
Fenichel syndrome	Slowly progressive humeropelvic weakness, joint contractures in childhood.	Autosomal dominant.	Cardiomyopathy in early adult life.	Fenichel et al, 1982
Fetal alcohol syndrome	Short stature, prenatal onset, short palpebral fissures, hairy forehead, smooth philtrum, thin upper lip, hypoplastic terminal phalanges.	Maternal alcohol disruption	Typically septal defects 1/3 of classic cases.	Jones et al, 1973
Fetal aminopterin syndrome	Growth deficiency, microcephaly, hypoplastic facial bones, broad nasal bridge, upsweep of hair, short forearm, talipes.	Folate antagonist.	Right-sided heart defects in some.	Shaw & Steinback, 1968
Fetal cytomegalovirus syndrome	Hepatosplenomegaly, thrombocytopenia, anaemia, microcephaly, calcification in brain, chorioretinitis, deafness.	Viral disruption.	Occasional mitral or pulmonary valve stenosis, atrial septal defect.	Hanshaw, 1966
Fetal hydantoin syndrome	Growth deficiency, microcephaly, mild retardation, broad depressed nasal bridge, hypoplastic nails.	Drug disruption.	Aortic and pulmonary valve stenosis coarctation, patent arterial duct, septal defects.	Speidel & Meadow, 1972
Fetal rubella syndrome	Sensorineural deafness, growth deficiency, retardation, cataracts.	Viral disruption.	Patent arterial duct, pulmonary stenosis, peripheral arterial stenosis.	Gregg, 1942

Table 2A.12 Clinical features and aetiology of cardiac syndromes. (*cont'd*)

Syndrome name	Clinical features	Aetiology	Cardiac defects	Key reference
Fetal trimethadione syndrome	Developmental delay, speech difficulty, V-shaped eyebrows, epicanthus, low set ears, abnormal palate, irregular teeth, occasional microcephaly, hypospadias, eye defect.	Drug disruption.	Ventricular septal defects, tetralogy of Fallot most common.	Zachai et al, 1975
Fetal toxoplasmosis syndrome	Micro/hydrocephaly, chorioretinitis, hepatosplenomegaly, retardation, thrombocytopenia, jaundice, pneumonitis in newborn period.	Maternal toxoplasmosis in 1st/2nd trimester.	Neonatal carditis.	Desmonts & Couvreur, 1974
Fetal warfarin syndrome	Chondrodysplasia punctata with short limbs and stippled epiphyses. Hypoplastic nasal bridge and/or alae nasae. Occasional eye and cerebral defects.	Drug disruption.	Pulmonary stenosis and persistent arterial duct described.	Hall et al, 1980
FG syndrome (Opitz Kaveggia syndrome)	Postnatal growth failure, hypotonia, severe constipation, anal anomalies, large forehead with developmental delay, agenesis of corpus callosum.	X-linked recessive.	Various ventricular septal defects, pulmonary stenosis; hypoplastic left heart reported.	Burn & Martin, 1983
Fitch syndrome	Microcephaly, abnormal ears, down-slanting eyes, small mouth, cleft palate, flexed overlapping fingers with syndactyly of digits, and polydactyly.	2 half-brothers – ?X-linked, ?variable dominant.	One half-brother had 3/6 murmur, ?ventricular septal defect.	Fitch et al, 1976
Forney syndrome	Proportionate short stature, conductive deafness, vertebral fusion, carpal/tarsal synostosis, skin pigmentation.	Autosomal dominant.	Mitral incompetence.	Forney et al, 1966
Fraser syndrome	Acronym CRASH – Cryptophthalmos, Renal agenesis, Atresia/stenosis larynx and vagina, Syndactyly, Heart defect.	Autosomal recessive.	Variety of defects described.	Burn & Marwood, 1983
Friedreich's ataxia	Progressive cerebellar ataxia, diminished/absent tendon reflexes.	Autosomal recessive.	Hypertrophic cardiomyopathy.	Boyer et al, 1962
Fucosidosis	Coarse face, brachycephaly, hepatomegaly, thick skin, angiokeratomas, CNS deterioration, stiff joints, umbilical hernia.	Autosomal recessive deficiency of α-fucosidase.	Cardiomyopathy.	Kouseff et al, 1973
Gastrocutaneous syndrome	Peptic ulcer/hiatus hernia, lentigines/café au lait patches, hypertelorism, myopia.	Autosomal dominant.	Single pedigree, 10 affected, 1 of whom had mitral valve prolapse, and 1 peripheral pulmonary stenosis.	Halal et al, 1982
Gay syndrome	Laryngeal web, short stature.	Autosomal dominant.	Ventricular septal defect.	Gay et al, 1981
Geleophysic syndrome	Short stature, short broad tubular bones, up-slant of eyes, short nose, thin lip, smooth philtrum (geleo – 'happy' face) hepatosplenomegaly.	Autosomal recessive.	Glycoprotein deposit in all cardiac valves causing stenosis and incompetence. Atrial septal defect.	Spranger et al, 1984
Glycogen storage disease type IV Brancher deficiency	Cirrhosis in infancy, muscular weakness and contractures, storage of abnormal glycogen in liver, heart.	Autosomal recessive.	Cardiomyopathy deficiency of amylo-1,4 to 1,6-trans glucosidase.	Levin et al, 1968
Golabi Ito syndrome	Mental retardation, microcephaly, protruding ears, hypertelorism, brittle dry hair, narrow palate, macrodontia, cutis marmorata.	X-linked recessive.	Atrial septal defect.	Golabi et al, 1984

Table 2A.12 Clinical features and aetiology of cardiac syndromes. (*cont'd*)

Syndrome name	Clinical features	Aetiology	Cardiac defects	Key reference
Goldenhar syndrome	Hemifacial microsomia, epibulbar dermoid, preauricular tags, deafness, colobomata of eyelids, small jaw, cleft palate, vertebral anomalies.	Sporadic, occasional autosomal dominant.	35% of cases, particularly tetralogy of Fallot.	Greenwood et al, 1974
Goltz syndrome	Focal dermal hypoplasia, oligodactyly, irregular small teeth, microphthalmos, alopecia.	Almost all sporadic and female, ?lethal in males.	Pulmonary stenosis and atrial septal defect reported.	Goltz et al, 1970
Goodman syndrome	White forelock, hypertelorism, blue sclerae, epicanthic folds, high palate, prominent philtrum, clinodactyly.	?Autosomal recessive.	Atrial septal defect.	Goodman et al, 1980
Gorlin-Chaudhary-Moss syndrome	Craniofacial dysostosis, hypertrichosis, hypoplasia labia majora, dental defects, small eyes, lid defects, short stature.	?Autosomal recessive.	Persistent arterial duct.	Gorlin et al, 1960
Grix syndrome	Short stature, microcephaly, hirsute, small jaw, cleft palate, long smooth top lip, swollen eyelids, broad first digits, retardation, seizures, spasticity.	?Autosomal dominant.	Ventricular septal defect.	Grix et al, 1975
Hallerman-Streiff syndrome	Microphthalmia, cataract, small jaw, dental anomalies, hypotrichosis, cutaneous atrophy, retardation, short stature.	Almost always sporadic.	Single report of 3 cases, 1 Fallot, 2 pulmonary stenosis and 1 ventricular septal defect.	Dinwiddie et al, 1978
Harris syndrome	Natal teeth, intestinal malrotation, megacolon.	?Autosomal recessive, ?X-linked.	Persistent arterial duct.	Harris et al, 1976
Hay-Wells syndrome	Ankyloblepharon, ectodermal dysplasia, cleft lip and/or palate, hypodontia, dystrophic nails, wiry sparse hair.	Autosomal dominant.	Occasional ventricular septal defect or persistent arterial duct.	Hay & Wells, 1976
Heart-hand II syndrome	Hypoplastic or absent ulna, narrow sloping shoulders, short metacarpals, broad short thumbs.	ECG abnormality.	Atrial fibrillation due to variable heart block.	Temtamy & McKusick, 1978
Heart-hand III syndrome	Brachydactyly, hypoplastic phalanges, extra ossicle in index fingers.	Autosomal dominant.	Intraventricular conduction defect, sick sinus syndrome.	Ruiz de la Fuente & Prieto, 1980
Heart-hand IV syndrome	Proportionate short stature, torticollis, small genitalia, pre- and postaxial polydactyly, synostosis of metacarpals.	Possible autosomal recessive.	Common atrium, pulmonary stenosis, ventricular septal defect, anomalous systemic venous.	Martinezy Martinez et al, 1981
Hittner syndrome	Colobomatous microphthalmia, hearing loss, mental retardation.	Uncertain.	Unspecified congenital heart defects.	Hittner et al, 1979
Ho syndrome	Small jaw, cleft palate, preaxial polydactyly, hip dislocation, hypoplastic/absent tibia, talipes, persistent fontanelle, Wormian bones.	Single case ?due to multiple drug exposures.	Ventricular septal defect, aberrant subclavian artery.	Ho et al, 1975
Hollister syndrome	Brachydactyly with long thumb, narrow shoulders, slight shortness of limbs, stiff joints.	Autosomal dominant	Pulmonary stenosis, ?conduction defect, first-degree heart block.	Hollister & Hollister, 1981
Holt-Oram syndrome Heart-hand I syndrome	Finger-like hypoplastic to absent thumb, variable hypoplasia first metacarpal, radius or whole limb, narrow shoulders.	Autosomal dominant variable expression.	Septal defects usual. Occasional arrhythmia, hypoplastic distal arteries.	Smith et al, 1979

Table 2A.12 Clinical features and aetiology of cardiac syndromes. (*cont'd*)

Syndrome name	Clinical features	Aetiology	Cardiac defects	Key reference
Homocystinuria	Ectopia lentis, mild retardatiaon, Marfanoid habitus, stiff joints, psychiatric disturbance.	Autosomal recessive (cystathionine synthase deficiency).	Vascular thromboses.	Harker et al, 1974
Hunter syndrome (mucopolysaccharidos is II)	Coarse facies, growth deficiency, stiff joints, clear corneas, hepatosplenomegaly, progressive deafness.	X-linked – iduronate sulphatase deficiency.	Valve stenosis and incompetence, coronary artery narrowing due to mucopolysaccharide deposition.	Leroy & Crocker, 1966
Hurler syndrome (mucopolysaccharidosis IH)	Coarse facies, dysostosis multiplex, hepatosplenomegaly, corneal clouding, deafness, mental retardation.	Autosomal recessive – α-iduronidase deficiency.	Cardiomyopathy, valve stenosis and incompetence due to mucopolysaccharide deposition.	Leroy & Crocker, 1966
Hydrolethalus	Hydrocephalus, 'keyhole' foramen magnum, polydactyly, small mandible polyhydramnios, early death, abnormal genitalia.	Autosomal recessive.	Atrioventricular septal defect, others rarely.	Salonen et al, 1981
Hypertrichosis-osteochondrodysplasia	Congenital hypertrichosis, macrosomy, osyteopenia, narrow chest, broad ribs, platyspondyly.	?Autosomal recessive.	All 4 cardiomegaly. 1 had patent arterial duct, 1 had aortic stenosis.	Cantu et al, 1982
Isomerism sequence	Right – typically 2 right atria, bronchi and lungs, absent spleen; left – typically 2 left atria, bronchi and lungs, multiple spleens; both – central liver, malrotation of gut.	Probably hetergeneous – incomplete penetrance, recessive in some	Disturbance of embryonic septation and connexion, worse in right. Venous connection abnormal systemic in left, pulmonary in right.	Burn et al, 1986
Jennings syndrome	Prominent forehead crumpled ears, small palpebral fissures, jaw, and genitalia. Moderate retardation and seizures.	2 brothers. ?X-linked.	Endocardial fibroelastosis.	Jennings et al, 1980
Jervell-Lange-Nielson syndrome	Deafness-sensorineural, occasional hypochromic anaemia.	Autosomal recessive.	Conduction defect, long QT interval.	Jervell et al, 1966
Jeune thoracic dysplasia	Severe rib shortening, short limbs, polydactyly, glomerulonephritis.	Autosomal recessive.	Cardiomyopathy.	Tahernia & Stamps, 1977
Johnson syndrome	Alopecia, anosmia, conductive deafness, microtia and/or atresia of external auditory canal, hypogonadotrophic hypogonadism, occasional retardation, cleft palate.	Autosomal dominant.	Oval fossa atrial septal defect in 1 affected member of pedigree.	Johnson et al, 1983
Kabuki make-up syndrome	Mental retardation, short stature, characteristic face with tented eyebrows and everted lower lips, longer palpebral fissures, prominent ears.	Sporadic.	Ventricular septal defect, double outlet right ventricle and coarctation.	Ohdo et al, 1985
Kartagener syndrome	Cilial dyskinesis due to absent dynein arms, bronchiectasis, conductive deafness.	Autosomal recessive.	Mirror-image arrangement rarely associated with major defects (?overlap with isomerism sequence).	Afzelius, 1976
Kashani syndrome	Obstructive uropathy, ureteral reflux, hydronephrosis.	2 sisters, ?autosomal recessive.	Diffuse hypoplasia of ascending aorta.	Kashani et al, 1984
Kaufman-McKusick syndrome	Postaxial polydactyly, hydrometrocolpos, variable atresia vagina and anus, hydronephrosis.	Autosomal recessive.	Common atrium, ventricular septal defect.	Robinow & Shaw, 1979
Kearns-Sayre syndrome	Mitochondrial cytopathy, muscle weakness, ophthalmoplegia, retinitis pigmentatosa, optic atrophy, endocrine and neurological dysfunction.	Possible mitochondrial inheritance.	Conduction defects.	Egger et al, 1981

Table 2A.12 Clinical features and aetiology of cardiac syndromes. (*cont'd*)

Syndrome name	Clinical features	Aetiology	Cardiac defects	Key reference
Keutel syndrome	Calcification of ear cartilage, neural and conductive deafness, acro-osteolysis (brachytelephalangy), infection-prone.	Autosomal recessive.	Electrocardiographic abnormality, peripheral pulmonary artery stenosis.	Fryn et al, 1984
Klippel-Feil syndrome	Short neck, low hairline, abnormal cervical vertebrae, deafness, Sprengel shoulder, cleft palate, renal agenesis in some.	Most sporadic, may be dominant in some.	Variety of defects, usually ventricular septal defects.	Morrison et al, 1968
Klippel-Trenaunay-Weber syndrome	Asymmetric limb hypertrophy, haemangiomata, visceromegaly, short stature, mild retardation in those with facial involvement, cataracts.	Sporadic.	Arteriovenous fistula, cavernous haemangiomata.	Lindenauer, 1971
Kozlowski syndrome	Talipes equinovarus, coronal clefts of vertebrae, dislocated elbow, bifid distal humerus, rhizomelia upper limbs.	Uncertain – maternal half-sibs affected.	Thickened mitral valve in one, possible ventricular septal defect in other.	Kozlowski et al, 1974
Lambert syndrome	Mild retardation, preauricular tags/pits, dysplastic ears, talipes, macrostomia, hypospadias.	?Autosomal recessive.	Ventricular septal defect.	Lambert et al, 1982
Larsen syndrome	Severe joint laxity, genu recurvatum at birth, flat face, depressed nasal bridge, cleft palate, short stature.	Autosomal dominant.	Aortic root dilatation, aneurysm of arterial duct. Isolated reports of septal defects.	Kiel et al, 1983
Laurence syndrome	Hirschprung's disease, post-axial polydactyly of hands, bifid big toes.	Probable recessive – ?autosomal, ?X-linked.	Ventricular septal defect and mitral stenosis.	Laurence et al, 1975
Laurence-Moon-Biedl syndrome	Mental retardation, ulnar polydactyly and syndactyly, obesity, small genitalia, retinitis pigmentosa, hydronephrosis/renal dysplasia.	Autosomal recessive.	A variety of defects reported. Acquired left ventricular hypertrophy.	Bauman & Hogan, 1973
Lenz microthalmia syndrome	Short, retarded, microphthalmos. Large simple ears, in some facial clefts and genitourinary anomalies.	X-linked recessive.	Unspecified heart defects usually occur.	Baraitser et al, 1982
LEOPARD syndrome (acronym)	Multiple lentigines, ECG anomalies, Ocular hypertelorism, Pulmonary stenosis, Abnormal genitalia, Retardation, Deafness.	Autosomal dominant.	Electrocardiographic anomalies, pulmonary stenosis (?overlap with Noonan).	Gorlin et al, 1969
Levin syndrome	Coloboma of retina, facial weakness (?overlap with CHARGE association)	Both of a pair of monozygotic twins, ?genetic, ?twinning disruption.	Hypoplastic aortic arch.	Levin et al, 1973
Limb reduction ichthyosis syndrome	Acronym CHILD – Cardiac defect, Hemidysplasia, Ichthyosiform erythroderma, Limb defects (severe unilateral reduction defect), mental retardation.	?Autosomal recessive.	2 sisters with partial to complete absence of septation with abnormal valves ± common arterial trunk.	Falek et al, 1968
Linear sebaceous naevus syndrome	Linear pigmented naevus, moderate retardation, hydrocephaly, cloudy cornea, coloboma, renal tumours, seizures.	Sporadic.	Coarctation of aorta, ventricular septal defect. Others less often.	Zaremba, 1978
Lujan Syndrome	Mental retardation, tall slender physique, small mandible, abnormal speech, nasal voice, lax joints, double row of teeth, absent corpus callosum.	X-linked recessive.	Atrial septal defect.	Lujan et al, 1984
Maffuci syndrome	Enchondromatosis, multiple cutaneous haemangiomata.	Sporadic.	Cavernous haemangiomata.	Lewis & Ketcham, 1973

Table 2A.12 Clinical features and aetiology of cardiac syndromes. (*cont'd*)

Syndrome name	Clinical features	Aetiology	Cardiac defects	Key reference
McDonough syndrome	Mental retardation, large nose, bat ears, diastasis recti, kyphoscoliosis, simian crease.	?Autosomal recessive.	Aortic stenosis, pulmonary stenosis, atrial septal defect, ventricular septal defect.	Garcia-Sagredo et al, 1984
Manzke syndrome Digitopalatal syndrome	Micrognathia, cleft palate, accessory second metacarpal.	?X-linked, ?autosomal recessive.	Atrial or ventricular septal defect.	Stevenson et al, 1980
Marden Walker syndrome	Joint contractures, fingers and large joints, small mouth and eye openings, kyphoscoliosis, hypotonia, developmental delay.	Autosomal recessive.	Right-sided heart and anomalous systemic venous connexion.	Jaatoul et al, 1982
Marfan syndrome	Arachnodactyly, lens subluxation, tall and slim with scoliosis, hernia, high palate.	Autosomal dominant collagen defect.	Aortic dilatation, valve incompetence.	Pyeritz & McKusick, 1979
Marfanoid hypermobility syndrome	Disproportionate tall stature, arachnodactyly, joint dislocation, hyperelastosis.	Probable collagen defect, ?autosomal dominant.	Aortic and mitral incompetence.	Walker et al, 1969
Maroteaux-Lamy syndrome Mucopolysaccharidosis VI	Short, coarse face, hepatosplenomegaly, hearing loss, joint contractures, corneal clouding.	Arylsulphatase B deficiency, autosomal recessive.	Valve incompetence, narrow vessels.	Stumph et al, 1973
Martinez syndrome	Camptodactyly, enlarged joints, progressive joint stiffness.	Autosomal recessive.	Pericarditis.	Martinez-Lavin et al, 1983
Maternal diabetes disruption syndrome	Variety of malformations, sacral agenesis (caudal regression), femoral hypoplasia, cleft palate, vertebral anomalies.	(?Poorly treated) maternal diabetes.	Up to 5% – defects include ventricular septal defects and complete transposition.	Rowland et al, 1973
Maternal phenylketonuria disruption syndrome	Microcephaly, retardation, short stature, occasional microphthalmos and cleft palate.	Disruption by high phenylalanine levels in utero.	25% of cases – variety of defects include septal defects and outflow obstruction.	Lenke & Levy, 1980
Meckel syndrome	Encephalocele, polydactyly, cystic renal dysplasia, other neural tube defects, facial clefting, genital anomalies, imperforate anus, coloboma.	Autosomal recessive.	Septal defects, coarctation, aortic stenosis, disturbed organ arrangement, hypoplastic right heart.	Clarke Fraser & Lytwyn, 1981
McArdle's disease Glycogen storage disease type V	Muscle cramping and rapid fatigue, myoglobinuria on exercise.	Autosomal recessive.	Congestive failure due to increased blood flow on exercise and ?involvement of myocardium.	McArdle, 1951
Majewski syndrome Short rib-polydactyly syndrome II	Hydropic at birth, narrow thorax, short limbs, hypoplastic tibiae, pre- and postaxial polydactyly, cleft lip/palate, flat face, genital anomalies, renal cysts.	Autosomal recessive.	A variety of heart defects described.	Spranger et al, 1974
Mietens syndrome	Corneal opacity, nystagmus, flexion contracture at elbows, growth failure, mental retardation, narrow nose.	Autosomal recessive.	Vascular aneurysms.	Mietens & Weber, 1966
Miller Dieker syndrome Lissencephaly syndrome	'Smooth' brain – polymicrogyria, severe retardation, tall furrowed forehead, low-set ears.	Probable autosomal recessive (?chromosomal defect in some).	Wide variety from patent arterial duct through septal defects to left isomerism sequence.	Jones et al, 1980
Mutchinick syndrome	Mental retardation, microcephaly, speech disorders, short stature, ocular hypertelorism, down-slanting eyes, large simple ears, broad straight nose.	?Autosomal recessive.	Atrial septal defect in 1, pulmonary valve stenosis, right bundle branch block in sister.	Mutchinick, 1972

Table 2A.12 Clinical features and aetiology of cardiac syndromes. (*cont'd*)

Syndrome name	Clinical features	Aetiology	Cardiac defects	Key reference
Morquio syndrome Mucopolysaccharidosis IV	Mild coarse face from 3 years on, severe kyphosis, knock knees, platyspondyly, cloudy corneas, hearing loss, hepatomegaly.	Galactosamine-6-sulphate sulphatase deficiency.	Aortic regurgitation.	Di Ferrante et al, 1978
Mucolipidosis II (I cell disease)	Coarse face, thick alveolar ridges, periosteal new bone formation, thick tight skin, psychomotor retardation.	Autosomal recessive – abnormal leak of lysomal enzymes.	Valvar thickening and incompetence. Cavernous haemangiomata.	Leroy et al, 1971
Mulibrey nanism syndrome	Severe short stature, pseudohydrocephalus, strabismus, fibrous dysplasia of bone, e.g. tibia, large hands, flame naevi on face.	Autosomal recessive.	Constrictive pericarditis.	Cumming et al, 1976
Myhre syndrome	Mental retardation, growth deficiency, muscular hypertrophy, joint limitation, short broad digits.	3 sporadic male cases reported.	Atrial septal defect.	Myhre et al, 1981
Myotonic dystrophy syndrome	Myotonia, cataract, ptosis, small testes, frontal balding, muscle weakness.	Autosomal dominant.	Conduction defects, rhabdomyoma.	Harper, 1979
Najjar syndrome	Hypospadias, small penis, mental retardation.	Recessive – 3 brothers, ?autosomal, ?X-linked.	Congestive cardiomyopathy.	Najjar et al, 1973
Nathalie syndrome	Sensorineural deafness, cataract, muscular atrophy, osteochondrosis, growth retardation, hypoplastic breasts.	Autosomal recessive.	Short PR intervals and QRS ventricular extrasystoles.	Cremers et al, 1975
Neurofibromatosis syndrome	Café au lait patches, cutaneous and intracranial tumours, optic glioma, pseudarthrosis, phaeochromocytoma.	Autosomal dominant.	Pulmonary stenosis, neurofibromata of heart.	Feinman & Yakovac, 1970
Noonan syndrome	Short, retarded, down-slanting palpebral fissures, low set ears, short/webbed neck, cryptorchidism, pectus excavatum/carinatum.	Autosomal dominant.	Pulmonary valve stenosis, atrial septal defect, hypertrophic cardiomyopathy.	Duncan et al, 1981
Onat syndrome	Proportionate short stature, upturned nose, anteverted nares, hoarse voice, kyphosis inguinal hernia.	Possible autosomal dominant.	Aortic stenosis.	Onat et al, 1984
Opitz G/BBB syndrome	Hypertelorism, hypospadias, cleft lip and palate, small jaw, laryngotracheal cleft, imperforate anus (occ), (midline defect).	Autosomal dominant (? worse in males).	Anomalous pulmonary venous connexion, central cardiac position.	Funderburk & Stewart, 1978
Osler's hereditary haemorrhagic telangiectasia	Pinpoint spider and nodular telangiectasia, lips, face, mucous membranes and occasionally on viscera.	Variable expression autosomal dominant.	Arteriovenous fistulas, cavernous haemangiomata, cerebral vascular anomalies.	Schaumann & Alter, 1973
Osteogenesis imperfecta (?4 clinical types, multiple genetic disorders)	Multiple fractures, ± blue sclerae, ± abnormal tooth enamel, ± soft deformed cranium, Wormian bones in skull, herniae, deafness. (Collagen defect.)	Types I and IV dominant, II and III mixed.	Mitral valve prolapse, aortic regurgitation.	Sillence et al, 1979
Osteogenesis imperfecta-microcephaly-cataracts	Multiple fractures, broad bones, cataracts, low set ears, microcephaly, cerebral atrophy.	Autosomal recessive.	3 sibs – 1 small left ventricle, 1 ventricular septal defect.	Buyse & Bull, 1978
Pompe's disease Glycogen storage disease type IIA	Severe hypotonia, large tongue, hepatomegaly.	Autosomal recessive acid maltase deficiency.	Progressive cardiac hypertrophy.	Rees et al, 1976
Pseudoxanthoma elasticum syndrome	'Chicken skin' in flexures, lax joints, angioid streaks in retina, chloroidoretinitis.	Dominant and recessive form.	Angina, claudication, hypertension (in dominant type I most often).	Pope, 1974

Table 2A.12 Clinical features and aetiology of cardiac syndromes. (*cont'd*)

Syndrome name	Clinical features	Aetiology	Cardiac defects	Key reference
Progeria syndrome Hutchinson-Gilford syndrome	Premature ageing leading to growth failure, loss of subcutaneous fat, hair and teeth.	Possible autosomal recessive and dominant forms.	Coronary artery disease, general atherosclerosis, congestive heart failure, cerebrovascular accident.	De Busk, 1972
Pseudo-Hurler polydystrophy Mucolipidosis III	Coarse face, corneal opacities, mild retardation, stiff joints, short stature, lysosomal enzymes, high in serum, low in fibroblasts.	Autosomal recessive.	Aortic regurgitation due to valve involvement.	Kelly et al, 1975
Rabenhorst syndrome Cardio-acro-facial syndrome	Narrow face, micrognathia, prominent narrow nasal bridge, small mouth, kyphosis.	Probable autosomal dominant (father and daughter).	Ventricular septal defect, pulmonary stenosis.	Grosse, 1974
Refsum disease Phytonic acid storage disease	Sensorineural deafness, cataract, retinal pigmentation, ataxia, peripheral neuropathy, spontaneous pains, ichthyosis.	Autosomal recessive.	ECG abnormality – ST, T wave changes, congestive cardiomyopathy.	Refsum, 1981
Roberts syndrome Pseudothalidomide (SC) syndrome	Variable reduction defects of all limbs, growth delay, cleft lip/palate, facial flame naevus.	Autosomal recessive.	Atrial septal defect.	Herrman et al, 1969
Robin sequence Pierre Robin syndrome	Micrognathia, posterior horse-shoe-shaped cleft palate, posterior displacement of tongue (small jaw displaces tongue which prevents palate closure).	Most are sporadic.	Heart defects strongly associated, probably where micrognathia due to branchial arch defect.	Hanson & Smith, 1975
Robinow syndrome	Short-limbed dwarfism, 'fetal' face, broad forehead, wide-set, up-turned nose, small midface, thick gums, small penis.	Dominant and recessive forms described.	Heart defects, including Tetralogy of Fallot are described.	Wadlington et al, 1973
Rogers syndrome	Postaxial polydactyly, hypoplasia and fusion vertebral bodies, teeth large, of reduced number with defective enamel, broad toes submucous cleft.	Autosomal recessive.	Right ventricular outflow murmurs in 2, in 1 a common arterial trunk giving rise to 2 pulmonary arteries.	Rogers et al, 1977
Rubinstein-Taybi syndrome	Developmental delay, broad thumbs and great toes, short, small head, down-slanting eyes, beaked nose with downward extension of septum, cryptorchidism.	Sporadic.	33% ventricular septal defect and persistent arterial duct most common.	Simpson & Brissenden, 1973
Rutledge syndrome	Moderate limb-shortening, polydactyly, joint contractures, female external genitalia in males, unilobar lungs, hypoplasia anterior tongue, cleft palate, renal hypoplasia.	Autosomal recessive.	Defects include ventricular septal defects and hypoplastic left ventricle.	Donnai et al, 1986
Ruvalcaba syndrome	Mental retardation, microcephaly, ptosis, small mouth and alae nasi, short fingers, cryptorchidism, craniosynostosis, and elbow limitation in some.	Autosomal dominant.	Cases of atrial septal defect and pulmonary stenosis described.	Hunter et al, 1977
Sacks syndrome	Primary testicular failure, collagenomas of the scalp.	Probable variable.	Congestive cardiomyopathy, mainly right heart with tricuspid incompetence.	Sacks et al, 1980
Saethre-Chotzen syndrome	Asymmetric face, broad forehead, ptosis, squint, beaked nose, broad great toes, skin syndactyly, variable developmental delay, long ear crus.	Variable autosomal dominant.	Occasional heart defect described.	Friedman et al, 1977
Saldino Noonan syndrome Short rib polydactyly I	Short ribs, ulnar polydactyly, short hands and feet, round flattened face, fetal hydrops.	Autosomal recessive.	Variety of heart defects including complete transposition.	Sillence, 1980
Scheie syndrome Mucopolysaccharidosis IS	Broad mouth, full lips, big jaw, cloudy corneas, stiff joints, occasional hepatomegaly and hearing loss.	Autosomal recessive iduronodase deficiency.	Aortic valve defect	Scheie et al, 1962

Table 2A.12 Clinical features and aetiology of cardiac syndromes. (*cont'd*)

Syndrome name	Clinical features	Aetiology	Cardiac defects	Key reference
Schinzel-Geidon syndrome	Short, retarded, severe midface hypoplasia, hydronephrosis, hairy, postaxial polydactyly, wormian bones and sclerosis in skull.	Autosomal recessive.	Atrial septal defect.	Schinzel & Giedion, 1978
Short rib-polydactyly syndrome III	Short stature, short limbs, irregular vertebrae, short ribs, cetabular spurs, hypoplastic ilea and lungs.	Autosomal recessive.	Hypoplastic left heart.	Sillence et al, 1979
Singleton-Merten syndrome	Hypoplastic tooth buds, osteoporosis and widening of metacarpals, carpals and phalanges, osteoporosis of cranial vault.	Sporadic in females to date.	Calcification of aortic arch and aortic valve – high mortality.	Singleton & Merten, 1973
Shwachman syndrome	Pancreatic hypoplasia, short-limbed dwarfism with metaphyseal changes, bone marrow dysfunction – anaemia, neutropenia, thrombocytopenia.	Autosomal recessive.	Endocardial fibrosis.	Shmerling et al, .1969
Smith-Lemli-Opitz syndrome	Mental retardation, microcephaly, ptosis, squint, anteverted nostrils, 2/3 syndactyly of toes, broad alveolar ridges, hypospadias, occasional polydactyly.	Autosomal recessive.	Various cardiac defects reported including atrial and ventricular septal defects and tetralogy of Fallot.	Cherstvoy et al, 1975
Spinal muscular atrophy syndrome Kugelberg-Welander disease	Hypotonia, weakness, depressed reflexes, 'denervation' EMG – anterior horn cell disease.	Autosomal recessive and dominant forms.	Cardiomyopathy leading to cardiac arrhythmia.	Fried & Emery, 1971
Steinfeld syndrome	Holoprosencephaly, hypertelorism, midline cleft upper lip, cleft palate, ectopic and/or dysplastic kidneys, hypoplastic/absent radius, ulnar, thumbs.	Possible autosomal dominant.	Bilobed lungs in proband. Sister died of unspecified heart defect.	Steinfeld, 1982
Strong syndrome	Mental retardation, microcephaly, small mouth, beaked nose, facial asymmetry, down-slanting eyes, large posteriorly rotated ears, dental defects.	Autosomal dominant.	Right-sided aorta, left ventricular hypertrophy.	Strong, 1968
Sturge Weber syndrome	'Port wine' naevus of face, epilepsy, retardation, intracranial calcification.	Sporadic.	Cerebral vascular malformations, coarctation of aorta described.	Chao, 1959
Tamari Goodman syndrome	Short, retarded, microcephaly, wide-set eyes, squint, radio-ulnar synostosis, asymmetry of leg length, 'winging' of scapulae.	Single case.	Atrial septal defect, pulmonary stenosis.	Tamari & Goodman, 1974
Thrombocytopenia-absent radius (TAR) syndrome	Bilateral absent radius, ulnar hypoplasia, thumbs present, occasionally (7%) mentally retarded, squint, small jaw.	Autosomal recessive.	33% have congenital heart defect including tetralogy of Fallot and atrial septal defect.	Hall et al, 1969
Thanatophoric dysplasia syndrome	Severe short-limbed dwarfism, 'telephone handle' femora, flat H-shaped vertebrae, large cranium, depressed nasal bridge.	Most cases sporadic.	Atrial septal defect, persistent ductus arteriosus, 1 case of great artery 'abnormality'.	Harris & Patton, 1971
Treacher Collins syndrome Mandibulofacial dysostosis	Down-slanting eyes, eyelid colobomata, dysplastic ears, small mandible, conductive hearing loss, cleft palate.	Autosomal dominant.	Unspecified heart defects seen on occasion.	Shprintzen et al, 1979
Trigonocephaly C syndrome Opitz C syndrome	Mental retardation, metopic ridge, broad alveolar ridges, up-slanting eyes, telecanthus, capillary haemangiomata.	?Heterogeneous – possible recessive in some cases.	Variety of defects including persistent arterial duct, ventricular septal defect and congenital mitral stenosis.	Sargent et al, 1985

Table 2A.12 Clinical features and aetiology of cardiac syndromes. (*cont'd*)

Syndrome name	Clinical features	Aetiology	Cardiac defects	Key reference
Tuberous sclerosis syndrome	Variable retardation, adenoma sebaceum, seizures, cerebral calcification, renal tumour, depigmented skin patches, periungal fibromata.	Autosomal dominant.	Rhabdomyomata and angiomata of heart may be congenital.	Monaghan et al, 1981
Varadi syndrome	Bifid big toes, ulnar polydactyly, cleft lip/palate, lingual nodules, growth and mental retardation.	Autosomal recessive.	Aortic stenosis described.	Varadi et al, 1980
VACTERL association	Acronym – Vertebral anomalies, Anal atresia, Cardiac defects, Tracheo-Esophageal fistula, Renal anomalies, Limb reduction defects (radial).	Sporadic ?early generally disruption of development	Variety of defects: ventricular septal defects most common.	Temtamy & Miller, 1974
Velo-cardio-facial syndrome Shprintzen syndrome	Cleft palate, nasal voice, square nasal root, mild retardation, short stature, small jaw and head in some, conductive hearing loss.	Probable autosomal dominant.	Ventricular septal defect, right aortic arch, tetralogy of Fallot.	Shprintzen et al, 1981
Von Hippel-Lindau syndrome	Retinal angiomata, hemangioblastoma most often in cerebellum.	Variable autosomal dominant.	Vascular defects, hypertension associated with hypernephroma or phaeochromocytoma.	Horton et al, 1976
Waardenburg syndrome	White forelock, sensorineural deafness, heterochromia of irides, hypertelorism, occasional cleft palate and Hirschsprung's disease.	Autosomal dominant with variable expression.	Occasional heart defect, typically ventricular septal defect.	Hageman & Delleman, 1977
Weil Marchesani syndrome	Short stature, brachycephaly, brachydactyly, myopia, glaucoma, dislocated and/or spherical lenses.	Autosomal recessive.	Cases of infundibular pulmonary stenosis, ventricular septal defect and persistent arterial duct described.	Zabriskie & Reisman, 1958
Werner Syndrome	Arrest of growth at puberty, cataracts, premature greying and balding, muscle wasting, diabetes mellitus, hypogonadism, soft tissue calcification.	Autosomal recessive.	Premature arteriosclerosis leading to congestive heart failure, valvular sclerosis.	Fleischmajer & Nedwich, 1973
Williams syndrome	Mild to moderate mental retardation, medial eyebrow flare, stellate iris, thick lips, zygomatic flattening, infantile hypercalcaemia.	Sporadic, possible new mutation dominant.	Supravalvar aortic stenosis, peripheral valve stenosis.	Williams et al, 1961
Woodhouse syndrome	Hypogonadism, sparse hair and eyebrows, diabetes mellitus, mental retardation, deafness, failure female sexual maturation, moderate retardation.	Autosomal recessive.	Variable ST depression and T wave abnormalities.	Woodhouse & Sakati, 1983
Zellweger syndrome Cerebrohepatorenal syndrome	Profound muscular hypotonia, tall forehead, brachycephaly, up-slanting eyes, epicanthic folds, hepatomegaly, stippled epiphyses.	Autosomal recessive.	Persistent arterial duct, ventricular septal defect.	Smith et al, 1965

APPENDIX REFERENCES

Aase J M, Smith D W 1968 Dysmorphogenesis of joints, brain, and palate: A new dominantly inherited syndrome. Journal of Pediatrics 73: 606–609

Afzelius B A 1976 A human syndrome caused by immotile cilia. Science 193: 317–319

Alagille D, Odievre M, Gautier M, Dommergues J P 1975 Hepatic ductular hypoplasia associated with characteristic facies, vertebral malformations, retarded physical, mental and sexual development and cardiac murmur. Journal of Pediatrics 86: 63–71

Allanson J E, Pantzar J T, MacLeod P M 1983 Possible new autosomal recessive syndrome with unusual renal histopathological changes. American Journal of Medical Genetics 16: 57–60

Anderson R A, Koch S, Camerini-Otero R D 1984 Cardiovascular findings in congenital contractural arachnodactyly: report of an affected kindred. American Journal of Medical Genetics 18: 265–271

Andre M, Vigneron J, Didier F 1981 Abnormal facies, cleft palate and generalised dysostosis: A lethal X-linked syndrome. Pediatrics 98: 747–752

Atkin J F, Patil S 1984 Apparently new oculo-cerebro-acral syndrome. American Journal of Medical Genetics 19: 585–587

Baetz-Greenwalt B, Ratliff N B, Moodie D S 1983 Hypoplastic right-sided heart complex: A cluster of cases with associated congenital birth defects. A new syndrome. Journal of Pediatrics 103: 399–401

Baraitser M, Winter R M, Taylor D S I 1982 Lenz microphthalmia – a case report. Clinical Genetics 22: 99–101

Barrow M, Fitzsimmons J S 1984 A new syndrome: Short limbs, abnormal facial appearance and congenital heart defect. American Journal of Medical Genetics 18: 431–433

Bauman M L, Hogan G R 1973 Laurence-Moon-Biedl syndrome: Review article American Journal of Diseases in Children 126: 119–126

Beemer F A, Langer L O Jr, Klep-de Pater J M, et al 1983 A new short rib syndrome: report of 2 cases. American Journal of Medical Genetics 14: 115–123

Behmel A, Plochl E, Rosenkranz W 1984 A new X-linked dysplasia gigantism syndrome: identical with the Simpson dysplasia syndrome? Human Genetics 67: 409–413

Beighton P 1972 The dominant and recessive forms of cutis laxa. Journal of Medical Genetics 9: 216–221

Beighton P, Gericke G, Kozlowski, Grobler L 1984 The manifestations and natural history of spondylo-epi-metaphyseal dysplasia with joint laxity. Clinical Genetics 26: 308–317

Berardinelli W 1954 An undiagnosed endocrinometabolic syndrome: report of two cases. Journal of Clinical Endocrinology and Metabolism 14: 193–204

Blank C E 1960 Apert's syndrome (a type of acrocephalosyndactyly) observations on a British series of thirty nine cases. Annals of Human Genetics 24: 151–164

Bonneau J C, Moirot H, Bastard C, Petitcolas, Ropartz C 1983 Polysyndactyly, septal defects, double inlet ventricle in 3 sibs. Journal of Human Genetics 31: 93–105

Boyer S H, Chisholm A W, McKusick V A 1962 Cardiac aspects of Friedreich's ataxia. Circulation 25: 493–505

Burn J, Martin N 1983 Two retarded male cousins with odd facies, hypotonia and severe constipation: possible examples of the X linked FG syndrome. Journal of Medical Genetics 20: 97–99

Burn J, Marwood R P 1983 Fraser syndrome presenting as bilateral renal agenesis in three sibs. Journal of Medical Genetics 20: 97–99

Burn J, Winter R M, Baraitser M, Hall C M, Fixsen J 1984 Femoral hypoplasia-unusual facies syndrome. Journal of Medical Genetics 21: 331–340

Burn J, Coffey R, Allan L D, Robinson P, Pembrey M E, Macartney F J 1986 Isomerism: A genetic analysis. In: Doyle, Engle, Gersony, Rashkind, Talner (eds) Pediatric cardiology. (Proceedings of World Congress 1985.) In press

Buyse M, Bull M J 1978 A syndrome of osteogenesis imperfecta, microcephaly and cataracts. Birth Defects XIV(6): 95–98

Cantrell J R, Haller J A, Ravitch M A 1958 Syndrome of congenital defects. Surgery, Gynecology and Obstetrics 107: 602–614

Cantu J M, Hernandez A, Ramifrez J et al 1975 Lethal faciocardiomelic dysplasia: a new autosomal recessive disorder. Birth Defects 11(5): 91–98

Cantu J M, Garcia-Cruz D, Sanchez-Corona J, Hernandez A, Nazara Z 1982 A distinct osteochondrodysplasia with hypertrichosis – individualisation of a probable autosomal recessive entity. Human Genetics 60: 36–41

Carey J C, Hall B D 1978 The Coffin-Siris syndrome. American Journal of Diseases in Children 132: 667–671

Chao D H-C 1959 Congenital neurocutaneous syndrome of childhood III. Sturge-Weber disease. Journal of Pediatrics 55: 635–49

Char F, Douglas J E, Dungan W T 1975 Familial multiforme ventricular extrasystoles with short stature, hyperpigmentation and microcephaly – a new syndrome. Birth Defects 11(5): 63–69

Cherstvoy E D, Lazjuk G I, Lurie I W, Nedzved M K, Usoev S S 1975 The pathological anatomy of the Smith-Lemli-Opitz syndrome. Clinical Genetics 7: 382–387

Clarke Fraser F, Lytwyn A 1981 Spectrum of anomalies in the Meckel syndrome or: 'Maybe there is a malformation syndrome with at least one constant anomaly'. American Journal of Medical Genetics 9: 67–73

Cremers C W R J, Ter Haar B G A, Van Rens T J G 1975 The Nathalie syndrome. A new hereditary syndrome. Clinical Genetics 8: 330–340

Cumming G R, Kerr D, Ferguson C C 1976 Constrictive pericarditis with dwarfism in two siblings (mulibrey nanism). Pediatrics 88: 569–572

De Busk F L 1972 The Hutchinson-Gilford progeria syndrome. Journal of Pediatrics 80: 697–724

De La Chapelle A, Herva R, Koivisto M, Aula P 1981 A deletion in chromosome 22 can cause Digeorge syndrome. Human Genetics 57: 253–256

Desmonts G, Couvreur J 1974 Congenital toxoplasmosis. A prospective study of 378 pregnancies. New England Journal of Medicine 290: 1110–16

Di Ferrante N, Ginsberg L C, Donnelly P V, DiFerrante D T, Caskey C T 1978 Deficiencies of glucosamine-6-sulfate or galactosamine-6-sulfate sulfatases are responsible for different mucopolysaccharidoses. Science 199: 79–81

Dinwiddie R, Gewitz M, Taylor J F N 1978 Cardiac defects in the Hallerman-Streiff syndrome. Journal of Pediatrics 92: 77–79

Donnai D, Young I D, Owen W G, Clark S A, Miller P F W, Knox W F 1986 The lethal multiple congenital anomaly syndrome of polydactyly, sex reversal, renal hypoplasia and unilobular lungs. Journal of Medical Genetics (in press)

Duncan W J, Fowler R S, Farkas L G, Ross R B, Wright A W, Bloom K R et al 1981 A comprehensive scoring system for evaluating Noonans syndrome. American Journal of Medical Genetics 10: 37–50

Eastman J R, Bixler D 1977 Facio-cardio-renal syndrome: A newly delineated recessive disorder. Clinical Genetics 11: 424–430

Egger J, Lake B D, Wilson J 1981 Mitochondrial cytopathy. A multisystem disorder with ragged red fibres on muscle biopsy. Archives of Disease in Childhood 56: 741–752

Emery A E H, Dreifuss F E 1966 Unusual type of benign X-linked muscular dystrophy. Journal of Neurology, Neurosurgery and Psychiatry 29: 338–342

Falek A, Heath C W, Ebbin A J, McLean W R 1968 Unilateral limb and skin deformities with congenital heart disease in twin siblings. A lethal syndrome. Journal of Pediatrics 73: 910–913

Fenichel G M, Chul Sul Y, Kilroy A W, Blouin R 1982 An autosomal-dominant dystrophy with humeropelvic distribution and cardiomyopathy. Neurology 32: 1399–1401

Fienman N L, Yakovac W C 1970 Neurofibromatosis in childhood. Journal of Pediatrics 76: 339–346

Fineman R M 1981 Recurrence of the postaxial acrofacial dysostosis syndrome in a sibship: implications for genetic counseling. Journal of Pediatrics 98: 87–8

Fisher D A, Klein A H 1981 Thyroid development and disorders of thyroid function in the newborn. New England Journal of Medicine 304: 702–712

Fitch N, Jequier S, Papageorgiou A 1976 A familial syndrome of cranial, facial, oral and limb anomalies. Clinical Genetics 10: 226–231

Fleischmajer R, Nedwich A 1973 Werner's syndrome. American Journal of Medicine 54: 111–118

Forney W R, Robinson S J, Pascoe D J 1966 Congenital heart disease, deafness and skeletal malformations: a new syndrome? Journal of Pediatrics 68: 14–26

Fried K, Emery A E H 1971 Spinal muscular atrophy type II. A separate genetic and clinical entity from type I (Werdnif-Hoffman disease) and type III (Kugelberg-Welander disease). Clinical Genetics 2: 203–209

Friedman J M, Hanson J W, Graham C B, Smith D W 1977 Saethre-Chotzen syndrome: A broad and variable pattern of skeletal malformations. Journal of Pediatrics 91: 929–933

Fryn J P, van Fleteren A, Mattelaer P, van der Berghe H 1984 Calcification of cartilages, brachytelephalangy and peripheral pulmonary stenosis. Confirmation of the Keutel syndrome. European Journal of Pediatrics 142: 201–3

Funderburk S J, Stewart R 1978 The G and BBB syndromes: Case presentations, genetics and nosology. American Journal of Medical Genetics 2: 131–144

Garcia-Sagredo J M, Lozano C, Ferrando P, San Roman C 1984 Mentally retarded siblings with congenital heart defect, peculiar facies and cryptorchidism in the male: possible McDonough syndrome with coincidental (X;20) translocation. Clinical Genetics 26: 117–124

Gay I 1981 Laryngeal web, congenital heart disease and low stature. A syndrome? Archives Otolaryngology 107: 510–512

Glanz A, Clarke Fraser F 1982 Spectrum of anomalies in Fanconi anaemia. Journal of Medical Genetics 19: 412–416

Golabi M, Ito M, Hall B D 1984 A new X-linked multiple congenital anomalies/mental retardation syndrome. American Journal of Medical Genetics 27: 367–374

Goldstein S, Qazi Q H, Fitzgerald J, Goldstein J, Friedman A P, Sawyer P 1985 Distichiasis, congenital heart defects and mixed peripheral vascular anomalies. American Journal of Medical Genetics 20: 283–294

Goltz R W, Henderson R R, Hitch J M, Ott J E 1970 Focal dermal hypoplasia syndrome: A review of the literature and report of two cases. Archives of Dermatology 101: 1–11

Goodman R M, Yahav Y, Frand M, Barzilay Z, Nisan E, Hertz M 1980 A new white forelock (poliosis) syndrome with multiple congenital malformations in two sibs. Clinical Genetics 17: 437–442

Gorlin R J, Chaudhary A P, Moss M L 1960 Craniofacial dysostosis, patent ductus arteriosus, hypertrichosis, hypoplasia of labia majora, dental and eye anomalies – a new syndrome? Pediatrics 56: 778–785

Gorlin R J, Anderson R C, Blaw M 1969 Multiple Lentigenes syndrome. American Journal of Diseases in Children 117: 652–662

Greenwood R D, Rosenthal A, Sommer A, Wolff G, Craenen J 1974 Cardiovascular malformations in oculoauriculovertebral dysplasia (Goldenhar syndrome). The Journal of Pediatrics 85: 816–818

Greenwood R D, Somer A, Rosenthal A, Craenen J, Nadas A S 1977 Cardiovascular abnormalities: Beckwith-Wiedemann syndrome. American Journal of Disease in Childhood 131: 293–294

Gregg N McA 1942 Congenital cataract following german measles in the mother. Transactions of the Ophthalmological Society of Australia 3: 35–46

Grix A, Blankenship W, Peterson R 1975 A new familial syndrome with craniofacial abnormalities, osseous defects and mental retardation. Birth Defects: Original Article Series 11: 107–114

Grosse F R 1974 The Rabenhorst syndrome – a cardio-acro-fascial syndrome. Zeitschrift fur Kinderheilkunde 117: 109–114

Hageman M J, Delleman J W 1977 Heterogeneity in Waardenburg syndrome. American Journal of Human Genetics 29: 468–85

Halal F, Gervais M H, Baillargeon J, Lesage R 1982 Gastro-cutaneous syndrome: Peptic ulcer/hiatal hernia, multiple lentigines/café-au-lait spots, hypertelorism and myopia. American Journal of Medical Genetics 11: 161–176

Hall J G, Levin J, Kuhn J P, Ottenheimer E J, van Berkum K A P, McKusick V A 1969 Thrombocytopenia with absent radius (TAR). Medicine 48: 411–439

Hall J G, Pallister P D, Charron S K 1980a Congenital hypothalamic hamartoblastoma, hypopituitarism, imperforate anus and postaxial polydactyly – a new syndrome. Parts I and II. American Journal of Medical Genetics 7: 47–83

Hall J G, Pauli R M, Wilson K M 1980b Maternal and fetal sequelae of anticoagulation during pregnancy. The American Journal of Medicine 68: 122–140

Hanshaw J B 1966 Congenital and acquired cytomegalovirus infection. Pediatric Clinics of North America 13: 279–293

Hanson J W, Smith D W 1975 U-shaped palatal defect in the Robin anomalad: Developmental and clinical relevance. Journal of Pediatrics 87: 30–33

Harker L A, Slighter S J, Scott C R, Ross R 1974 Homocystinuria – Vascular injury and arterial thrombosis. New England Journal of Medicine 291: 537–543

Harper P S 1979 Myotonic dystrophy. Saunders, Philadelphia

Harris D J, Ashcroft K W, Beatty E C, Holder T M, Leonidas J C 1976 Natal teeth, patent ductus arteriosus and intestinal pseudo-obstruction: A lethal syndrome in the newborn. Clinical Genetics 9: 479–482

Harris R, Patton J T 1971 Achondroplasia and thanatophoric dwarfism in the newborn. Clinical Genetics 2: 61–72

Hay R J, Wells R S 1976 The syndrome of ankyloblepharon, ectodermal defects, and cleft lip and palate: an autosomal dominant condition. British Journal of Dermatology 94: 277–289

Herrmann J, Feingold M, Tuffeli G A, Opitz J M 1969 A familial dysmorphogenetic syndrome of limb deformities, characteristic facial appearance and associated anomalies: The 'pseudothalidomide' or 'SC-syndrome'. Birth Defects V(3): 81–89

Hittner H M, Hirsch N J, Kreh G M, Rudolph A J 1979 Colobomatous microphthalmia, heart disease, hearing loss and mental retardation – a syndrome. Journal of Pediatric Ophthalmology and Strabismus 16: 122–128

Ho Chen-Kung, Kaufman R L, McAlister W H 1975 Congenital malformations: Cleft palate, congenital heart disease, absent tibiae and polydactyly. American Journal of Diseases in Children 129: 714–716

Hollister D W, Hollister W G 1981 The 'long thumb' brachydactyly syndrome. American Journal of Medical Genetics 8: 5–16

Horton W A, Wong V, Eldridge A 1976 Von Hippel-Lindau disease. Clinical and pathological manifestations in nine families with 50 affected members. Archives of Internal Medicine 136: 769–777

Houston C S, Opitz J M, Spranger J W, et al 1983 The campomelic syndrome: Review, report of 17 cases, and follow-up on the currently 17-year-old boy first reported by Maroteaux et al in 1971. American Journal of Medical Genetics 15: 3–28

Hunter A G W, McAlpine P J, Rudd N L, Clarke Fraser F 1977 A 'new' syndrome of mental retardation with characteristic facies and brachyphalangy. Journal of Medical Genetics 14: 430–437

Hyndman W B, Alexander D S, Mackie K W 1976 Chondrodystrophia calcificans congenita (the Conradi-Hunermann syndrome). Clinical Pediatrics 15: 317–321

Jaatoul N Y, Haddad N E, Khoury L A, et al 1982 Brief clinical report and review: The Marden-Walker syndrome. American Journal of Medical Genetics 11: 259–271

Jennings M T, Hall J G, Kukolich M 1980 Endocardial fibroelastosis, neurologic dysfunction and unsual facial appearance in two brothers coincidentally associated with dominantly inherited macrocephaly. American Journal of Medical Genetics 5: 271–276

Jervell A, Thingstad R, Endsjo T O 1966 The surdo-cardiac syndrome: three new cases of congenital deafness with syncopal attacks and Q-T prolongation in the electrocardiogram. American Heart Journal 72: 582–593

Johnson V P, McMillin J M, Aceto Jr T, Bruins G 1983 A newly recognised neuroectodermal syndrome of familial alopecia, anosmia, deafness and hypogonadism. American Journal of Medical Genetics 15: 497–506

Jones K L, Gilbert E F, Kaveggia E G, Opitz J M 1980 The Miller-Dieker syndrome. Pediatrics 66: 277–281

Jones K L, Smith D W, Ulleland C N, Streissguth A P 1973 Pattern of malformation in offspring of chronic alcoholic mothers. Lancet 1: 1267–1271

Kashani I A, Strom C M, Utley J E, Marin-Garcia J, Higgins C B 1984 Hypoplastic pulmonary arteries and aorta with obstructive uropathy in 2 siblings. Angiology 35: 252–256

Kelly T E, Thomas G H, Taylor Jr H A, et al 1975 Mucolipidosis III (Pseudo-Hurler polydystrophy): clinical and laboratory studies in a series of 12 patients. Johns Hopkins Medical Bulletin 137: 156–175

Kiel E A, Frias J L, Victoria B E 1983 Cardiovascular manifestations in the Larsen syndrome. Pediatrics 7: 942–946

Kousseff B G, Beratis N G, Danesino C, Hirschhorn K 1973 Genetic heterogeneity in fucosidosis. Lancet 2: 1387–1388

Kozlowski K S, Celermajer J M, Tink A R 1974 Humero-spinal dysostosis with congenital heart disease. American Journal of Diseases in Children 127: 407–410

Lambert J C, Ayraud N, Martin J, Mariani R, Ferrari M, Donzea U M 1982 Familial occurrence of a syndrome with branchial dysplasia, mental deficiency, club feet and inguinal herniae. Journal of Medical Genetics 19: 214–215

Laurence K M, Prosser R, Rocker I, Pearson J F, Richards C 1975 Hirschsprung's disease associated with congenital heart malformation, broad big toes, and ulnar polydactyly in sibs: a case for fetoscopy. Journal of Medical Genetics 12: 334–338

Lenke R R, Levy H L 1980 Maternal phenylketonuria and hyperphenylalaninemia: International survey of treated and untreated pregnancies. New England Journal of Medicine 303: 1202–8

Leroy J G, Crocker A C 1966 Clinical definition of the Hurler-Hunter phenotypes. A review of 50 patients. American Journal of Diseases in Children 112: 518–530

Leroy J G, Spranger J W, Feingold M, Opitz J M, Crocker A C 1971 I-Cell disease, a clinical picture. Journal of Pediatrics 29: 360–365

Levin B, Burgess E A, Mortimer P E 1968 Glycogen storage disease type IV, amylopectinosis. Archives of Diseases in Childhood 43: 548–555

Levin D L, Muster A J, Newfield E A, Paul M H 1973 Concordant aortic arch anomalies in monozygotic twins. Journal of Pediatrics 83: 459–461

Levin L S, Perrin J C S, Ose L, Dorst J P, Miller J D, McKusick V A 1977 A heritable syndrome of craniosynostosis, short thin hair, dental abnormalities, and short limbs: Cranioectodermal dysplasia. Pediatrics 90: 55–61

Levin S E, Silverman N H, Milner S 1982 Hypoplasia or absence of the depressor angularis oris muscle and congenital abnormalities with special reference to the cardiofacial syndrome. South African Medical Journal 61: 227–231

Lewis R J, Ketcham A S 1973 Maffucci's syndrome: functional and neoplastic significance. Journal of Bone and Joint Surgery 55: 1465–1479

Lindenauer S M 1971 Congenital arteriovenous fistula and the Klippel-Trenaunay syndrome. Annals of Surgery 174: 248–263

Lujan J E, Carlin M E, Lubs H A 1984 A form of X-linked mental retardation with marfanoid habitus. American Journal of Medical Genetics 17: 311–322

McArdle B 1951 Myopathy due to a defect in muscle glycogen breakdown. Clinical Science 10: 13–35

McNicholl B, Egan-Mitchell B, Murray J P, Doyle J F, Kennedy J D, Crome L 1970 Cerebro-costo-mandibular syndrome: A new familial developmental disorder. Archives of Disease in Childhood 45: 421–424

Martinez y Martinez R, Corona-Rivera E, Jimenez-Martinez M, Ocampo-Campos R, Garcia-Maravilla S 1981 A new probably autosomal recessive cardiomelic dysplasia with mesoaxial hexadactyly. Journal of Medical Genetics 18: 151–154

Martinez-Lavin M, Buendia A, Delgado E, et al 1983 A familial syndrome of pericarditis, arthritis and camptodactyly. New England Journal of Medicine 309: 224–225

Mietens C, Weber H 1966 A syndrome characterised by corneal opacity, nystagmus, flexion contracture of the elbows, growth failure, and mental retardation. Journal of Pediatrics 69: 624–629

Monaghan H P, Krafchik B R, MacGregor D L, Fitz C R 1981 Tuberous sclerosis complex in children. American Journal of Diseases in Children 135: 912–917

Morrison S G, Perry L W, Scott L P 1968 Congenital brevicollis (Klippel-Feil syndrome) and cardiovascular anomalies. American Journal of Diseases in Children 115: 614–620

Mutchinick O 1972 A syndrome of mental and physical retardation, speech disorders, and peculiar facies in two sisters. Journal of Medical Genetics 9: 60–63

Myhre S A, Ruvalcaba R H A, Graham C B 1981 A new growth deficiency syndrome. Clinical Genetics 20: 1–5

Najjar S S, Der Kaloustian V M, Nassif S I 1973 Genital anomaly, mental retardation and cardiomyopathy: A new syndrome? Journal of Pediatrics 83: 286–288

Ohdo S, Madokoro H, Sonodo T, Nishiguchi T, Kawaguchi K, Hayakawa K 1985 Kabuki make-up syndrome (Niikawa-Kuroki syndrome) associated with congenital heart disease. Journal of Medical Genetics 22: 126–127

Onat A, Onat T, Domanic N 1984 Discrete subaortic stenosis as part of a short stature syndrome. Human Genetics 65: 331–335

Pagon R A, Graham J M, Socana J, Yong S L 1981 Coloboma, congenital heart disease, and choanal atresia with multiple anomalies: CHARGE association. Pediatrics 99: 223–227

Pelias M Z, Superneau D W, Thurmon T F 1981 Brief clinical report: a sixth report (eighth case) of craniosynostosis-radial aplasia (Baller-Gerold) syndrome. American Journal of Medical Genetics 10: 133–139

Pope F M 1974 Autosomal dominant pseudoxanthoma elasticum. Journal of Medical Genetics 11: 152–157

Pope F M, Martin G R, McKusick V A 1976 Inheritance of Ehlers Danlos type IV syndrome. Journal of Medical Genetics 14: 200–4

Ptacek L J, Opitz, J M, Smith D W, Gerritsen T, Waisman H A 1963 The Cornelia de Lange syndrome. Journal of Pediatrics 63: 1000–1020

Pyeritz R E, McKusick V A 1979 The Marfan syndrome: Diagnosis and management. New England Journal of Medicine 300: 772–777

Rees A, Elbl F, Minhas K, Solinger R 1976 Echocardiographic evidence of outflow tract obstruction in Pompe's disease (glycogen storage disease of the heart). The American Journal of Cardiology 37: 1103–1106

Refsum S 1981 Heredopathia atactica polyneuritiformis. Phytanic acid storage disease, Refsum's disease: a biochemically well-defined disease with a specific dietary treatment. Archives of Neurology (Chicago) 38: 605–606

Reginato A, Riera M, Martinez V, Ruiz F 1972 Alkaptonuria, ochronotic arthropathy and aortic stenosis. Rev Med Chile 100: 529–533

Rimoin D L, Horton W A 1978 Short stature. Part II. Journal of Pediatrics 92: 697–704

Robinow M, Shaw A 1979 The McKusick-Kaufman syndrome: Recessively inherited vaginal atresia, hydrometrocolpos, uterovaginal duplications, anorectal anomalies, postaxial polydactyly, and congenital heart disease. Journal of Pediatrics 94: 776–778

Rogers J G, Levin L S, Dorst J P, Temtamy S A 1977 A postaxial polydactyly-dental-vertebral syndrome. Journal of Pediatrics 90: 230–235

Rowland T W, Hubell J P, Nadas A S 1973 Congenital heart disease in infants of diabetic mothers. Journal of Pediatrics 83: 815–820

Ruiz de la Fuente S, Prieto F 1980 Heart-hand syndrome III. Human Genetics 55: 43–47

Sacks H N, Crawley I S, Ward J A, Fine R M 1980 Familial cardiomyopathy, hypogonadism and collagenoma. Annals of Internal Medicine 93: 813–817

Salonen R, Herva R, Norio R 1981 The hydrolethalus syndrome: delineation of a 'new', lethal malformation syndrome based on 28 patients. Clinical Genetics 19: 321–330

Sanchez Cascos A, Sanchez Harguindey L, DeRabago P 1969 Cardioauditory syndromes: cardiac and genetic study of 511 deaf-mute children. British Heart Journal 31: 26–33

Sargent C, Burn J, Baraitser M, Pembrey M E 1985 Trigonocephaly and the Opitz C syndrome. Journal of Medical Genetics 22: 39–45

Schaumann B, Alter M 1973 Cerebrovascular malformations in hereditary hemorrhagic telangiectasia. Minnesota Medicine 56: 951–954

Scheie H G, Hambrick G W Jr, Barnes A 1962 A newly recognised forme fruste of Hurler's disease (gargoylism). American Journal of Ophthalmology 53: 753–769

Schinzel A, Giedion A 1978 A syndrome of severe midface retraction, multiple skull anomalies, club feet, and cardiac and renal malformations in sibs. American Journal of Medical Genetics 1: 361–375

Schinzel A, Savoldelli G, Briner J, Sigg P, Massini C 1983 Antley-Bixler syndrome in sisters: A term newborn and a prenatally diagnosed fetus. American Journal of Medical Genetics 14: 139–147

Shaw E B, Steinback H L 1968 Aminopterin-induced fetal malformation. American Journal of Diseases in Children 115: 477–482

Shmerling D H, Prader A, Hitzig W H 1969 The syndrome of exocrine pancreatic insufficiency, neutropenia, metaphyseal dysostosis and dwarfism. Helvetica Paediatrica Acta 24: 547–575

Shprintzen R J, Croft C, Berkman M D, Rakoff S J 1979 Pharyngeal hypoplasia in Treacher Collins syndrome. Archives of Otolaryngology 105: 127–131

Shprintzen R J, Goldberg R B, Young D, Wolford L 1981 The velo-cardio-facial syndrome: A clinical and genetic analysis. Pediatrics 67: 167–172

Sillence D O 1980 Invited editorial comment: non-Majewski short rib-polydactyly syndrome. American Journal of Medical Genetics 7: 223–229

Sillence D O, Senn A, Danks D M 1979 Genetic heterogeneity in osteogenesis imperfecta. Journal of Medical Genetics 16: 101–116

Simpson N E, Brissenden J E 1973 The Rubinstein-Taybi syndrome: Familial and dermatoglyphic data. American Journal of Human Genetics 25: 225–229

Singleton E B, Merten D F 1973 An unusual syndrome of widened medullary cavities of the metacarpals and phalanges, aortic calcificatioin and abnormal dentition. Pediatric Radiology 1: 2–7

Skyring A P, McKusick V A 1961 Clinical, genetic and

electrocardiographic studies of childhood muscular dystrophy. American Journal of Medical Science 242: 534–547

Smith A T, Sack G H, Taylor G J 1979 Holt-Oram syndrome. Journal of Pediatrics 95: 538–43

Smith D W, Opitz J M, Inhorn S L 1965 A syndrome of multiple developmental defects including polycystic kidneys and intrahepatic biliary dysgenesis in two siblings. Journal of Pediatrics 67: 617–624

Speidel B D and Meadow S R 1972 Maternal epilepsy and abnormalities of the fetus and new born. Lancet 2: 839–843

Spranger J, Grimm B, Weller M, Weissenbacher G, Hermann J, Gilbert E, Krepler R 1974 Short rib polydactyly (SRP) syndromes type Majewski and Saldino-Noonan. Zeitschrift fur Kinderheilkunde 116: 73–94

Spranger J, Gilbert E F, Arya S, Hoganson G M I, Opitz J M 1984 Geleophysic dysplasia. American Journal of Medical Genetics 19: 487–499

Steinfeld H J 1982 Holoprosencephaly and visceral defects with familial limb abnormalities (case report 81). Syndrome Identification VIII: 1–2

Stevenson R E, Taylor H A, Burton O M, Hearn H B 1980 A digitopalatal syndrome with associated anomalies of the heart, face and skeleton. Journal of Medical Genetics 17: 238–241

Strong W B 1968 Familial syndrome of right-sided aortic arch, mental deficiency, and facial dysmorphism. Journal of Pediatrics 73: 882–888

Stumph D A, Austin J H, Crocker A C, LaFrance M 1973 Mucopolysaccharidosis type VI (Maroteaux-Lamy syndrome). I. Sulfatase B deficiency in tissues. American Journal of Diseases in Children 126: 747–755

Tahernia A C, Stamps P 1977 'Jeune syndrome' (asphyxiating thoracic dystrophy). Report of a case, a review of the literature, and an editor's commentary. Clinical Pediatrics 16: 903–908

Takao A, Ando M, Cho K, Kinouchi A, Murakami Y 1980 Etiological categorization of common congenital heart disease. In: Van Praagh R, Takao A (eds) Etiology and morphogenesis of congenital heart disease. Futura, New York, p 253–269

Tamari I, Goodman R M 1974 Upper limb-cardiovascular syndromes: A description of two new disorders with a classification. Chest 65: 632–639

Temtamy S A 1966 Carpenter's syndrome: Acrocephalopolysyndactyly. An autosomal recessive syndrome. Pediatrics 69: 111–119

Temtamy S A, Miller J D 1974 Extending the scope of VATER association. Definition of a VATER syndrome. Journal of Pediatrics 85: 345–349

Temtamy S, McKusick V A 1978 Heart-hand syndrome II (Tabatznik syndrome). Birth Defects XIV(3): 241–4

van Weel-Sipman M, van de Kamp J J P, de Koning J 1977 A female patient with 'Aase syndrome'. Journal of Pediatrics 91: 753–755

Varadi V, Szabo L, Papp Z 1980 Syndrome of polydactyly, cleft lip/palate or lingual lump, and psychomotor retardation in endogamic gypsies. Journal of Medical Genetics 17: 119–112

Wadlington W B, Tucker V L, Schimke R N 1973 Mesomelic dwarfism with hemivertebrae and small genitalia (the Robinow syndrome). American Journal of Disease in Children 126: 202–208

Walker B A, Beighton P H, Murdock J L 1969 The Marfanoid hypermobility syndrome. Annals of Internal Medicine 71: 349–352

Wallace H J 1973 Anderson-Fabry disease. British Journal of Dermatolgoy 88: 1–23

Walls W L, Altman D H, Winslow O P 1959 Chondroectodermal dysplasia (Ellis van Creveld syndrome). Report of a case and review of the literature. American Journal of Diseases in Children 98: 242–8

Williams J C P, Barratt-Boyes B G, Lowe J B 1961 Supravalvular aortic stenosis. Circulation 24: 1311–1318

Woodhouse N J Y, Sakati N A 1983 A syndrome of hypogonadism, alopecia, diabetes mellitus, mental retardation, deafness and ECG abnormalities. Journal of Medical Genetics 20: 216–219

Zabriskie J, Reisman M 1958 Marchesani syndrome. Journal of Pediatrics 52: 158–169

Zachai E H, Mellman W J, Neiderer B, Hanson J W 1975 The fetal trimethadione syndrome. Journal of pediatrics 87: 280–4

Zaremba J 1978 Jadassohn's naevus phakomatosis: A study based on a review of thirty seven cases. Journal of Mental Deficiency Research 22: 103–23

3

Terminology

It is probable that nomenclature and classification are the most contentious topics in paediatric cardiology, with the possible exception of embryology which in itself is responsible for many of the terminological disagreements. Notwithstanding, an unambiguous and simple terminology is essential for successful practice of and communication in paediatric cardiology. Most would now agree that such a system is provided by a sequential segmental approach, but there is no agreement as how best to construct this system (Van Praagh, 1972, 1973, 1977; Van Praagh & Vlad, 1978; Van Praagh et al, 1964a, b, 1971, 1977, 1983; de la Cruz & Nadal-Ginard, 1972; de la Cruz et al, 1967, 1976; Pacifico et al, 1973; Brandt & Calder, 1977; Elliott, 1978). In this book we will use the system we have developed in recent years (Shinebourne et al, 1976; Macartney et al 1976b, 1978; Tynan et al, 1979, 1981; Anderson & Tynan, 1981; Anderson et al, 1981, 1983).

During the evolution of our system, we have realised the need to follow a few simple terminological rules. First and foremost, the system has been based upon observed and observable anatomic facts, and has eschewed all speculative embryological and morphogenetic considerations. Secondly, chamber morphologies, connexions and relations have been recognised as three different facets of the make-up of the heart. Each of the three facets has therefore been differentiated and described using mutually exclusive terms. Morphology has been described using anatomical terms, connexions described using 'connexion terms' (such as concordant, discordant, double inlet, etc.), and relations described using spatial terms (such as right, left, superior, inferior and so on).

If these simple rules are observed, any terminology will be unambiguous. All can then describe the most complex heart in a manner which is readily understandable to all others, providing that one remembers that clarity is more important than brevity.

SEQUENTIAL CHAMBER LOCALISATION – BASIC CONCEPTS

The system we advocate depends firstly upon the establishment of atrial arrangement (situs). Thereafter, the atrioventricular junction is analysed in terms of its connexions (*type* of connexion) and the morphology of the valves which guard it (*mode* of connexion). At the same time, it is necessary to identify the topology of the ventricular mass and the relationships of the ventricular chambers within it. Then the ventriculo-arterial junction is analysed in terms of the type and mode of connexion, at the same time taking cognisance of outflow tract morphology and the relationships of the great arteries. Finally a catalogue is made of all associated cardiac (and, where pertinent, non-cardiac) malformations. Included in this final category are such features as cardiac and visceral positions.

It may seem that use of such a system is like using a sledgehammer to crack a nut, since about nine-tenths of patients with congenital heart disease have simple lesions such as atrial septal defects, an arterial duct or pulmonary stenosis. But a patient cannot be presumed to have a simple lesion such as pulmonary stenosis until it has been demonstrated unequivocally that the cardiac connexions and relations are normal. For example, pulmonary stenosis in the patient with corrected transposition will have very similar symptomatology and haemodynamic findings to pulmonary stenosis in the patient with a normally connected heart, but the prognosis and surgical treatment of the two are poles apart. Sequential segmental analysis imposes a logical approach to the diagnosis of every patient with congenital heart disease. Normal connexions and relations can never be assumed but once established they can be taken as read and will not complicate either the diagnosis or description of the simple lesions. Contrariwise, the use of the sequential segmental approach makes it possible to describe unambiguously the most complicated heart, including hearts which may never have been recognised before, an impossibility using any system based on 'pattern recognition'.

Implicit in the system is the ability to distinguish the morphology of the individual atrial and ventricular chambers and to recognise the types of arterial trunks connected to the ventricles. This is not as straightforward as it may seem, since often in congenitally malformed hearts these chambers do not possess the morphological features which most obviously characterise them in the normal heart. For example, in the normal heart the most obvious feature of the morphologically left atrium is the presence of the pulmonary veins. But in hearts with total anomalous pulmonary venous connexion, these veins connect to a systemic venous site yet still the left atrium is recognisable. Considerations of this type underscore the concept we use for recognition of the cardiac chambers and great arteries. Dubbed by Van Praagh and his colleagues the 'morphological method', and based on the initial work of Lev (1954), it states that structures should be recognised in terms of their own intrinsic morphology, and ideally should not be defined in terms of other structures which are themselves variable.

When this concept is applied to the atrial chambers, then the connexions of the great veins are immediately disqualified as markers of rightness or leftness. Lev (1954) placed great stress on septal morphology as a distinguishing feature. It is certainly true that in the normal heart there are obvious differences between the morphologically right and left sides of the septum. When present, these are very helpful in distinguishing the atria. But septal morphology is of little help when the septum itself is absent, for example in hearts with 'common' atrium. Fortunately there is another component of the atrial chambers which in our experience has been almost universally present and has enabled us to distinguish between morphologically right and left structures. This is the atrial appendage. The morphologically right appendage is characteristically the shape of a blunt triangle with a broad junction to the venous component of the atrium. The junction is marked externally by the terminal sulcus and internally by the terminal crest. The morphologically left appendage is much narrower and crenellated. It has a narrow junction with the venous component which is marked by neither sulcus nor muscular crest (Fig. 3.1).

When considering the ventricular mass, it is first necessary to state that we consider the mass to extend from the atrioventricular to the ventriculo-arterial junctions. In other words, it extends from the fibrous tissue plane between atrial and ventricular muscle masses to the point at which the ventricular musculature changes to the typical structure of the great arteries. This rather obvious definition is needed because recently Van Praagh and his colleagues (Van Praagh & Van Praagh, 1982; Van Praagh et al, 1983) have suggested that there are two additional segments within the heart, namely the atrioventricular canal and the infundibular segment. We consider this an unnecessary complication of a basically simple topic, since within our definitions both of these 'segments' are an integral part of the ventricular mass.

Within the ventricular mass as here defined there are almost always two ventricular chambers. When two ventricles are present, in our experience these have always been of morphologically right and morphologically left type respectively. It is vital to have a uniform means of distinguishing such chambers, no matter how malformed they may be. We have found it helpful in this respect to

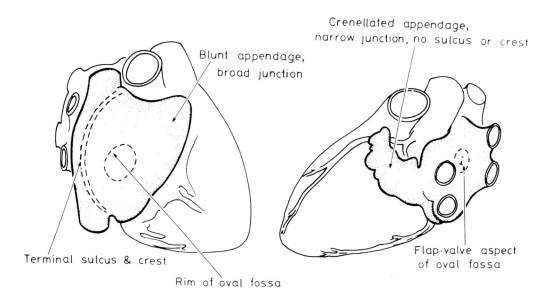

Blunt appendage,
broad junction

Crenellated appendage,
narrow junction, no sulcus or crest

Terminal sulcus & crest

Rim of oval fossa

Flap-valve aspect
of oval fossa

Morphologically Right Atrium   Morphologically Left Atrium

Fig. 3.1 The characteristic morphological features of the right versus the left atrium.

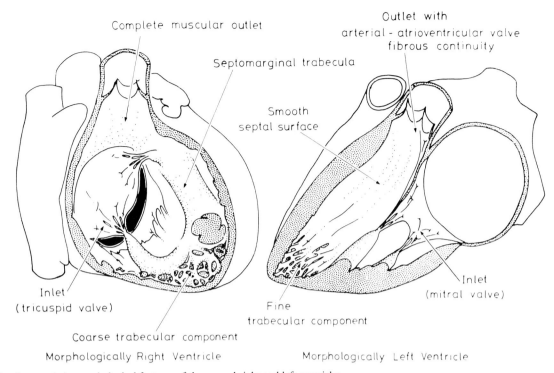

Fig. 3.2 The characteristic morphological features of the normal right and left ventricles.

consider ventricles as possessing three components rather than the traditional sinus and conus. These three components are the inlet, extending from the atrioventricular junction to the distal attachment of the atrioventricular valve tension apparatus, the apical trabecular component and the outlet component which supports the arterial valve (Fig. 3.2). Using the morphological method, it is then self-evident that it is the morphology of the apical trabecular component which must be used to distinguish leftness and rightness. This is because it is the apical trabecular component which is most universally present in malformed ventricles. Fortunately, the apical trabecular component differentiates with great accuracy morphologically right from left ventricles when the two apical components are compared in the same heart (Fig. 3.3). The apical trabecular pattern also permits ventricles to be recognised as left or right ventricles even when the trabecular components exist as isolated pouches without inlet or outlet components (Fig. 3.4). It is then possible to describe simply and accurately all known types of ventricles in hearts with two ventricles on the basis of the way that the inlet and outlet components are shared between the two apical trabecular components (Fig. 3.5). In order fully to describe any ventricle it is then necessary to take cognisance of size. Providing that component make-up, trabecular pattern and size are all described, there can be no room for confusion.

Fig. 3.3 A normal heart dissected in such a way that only the apical trabecular components are visible. It is an easy matter by comparing these to distinguish the morphologically right from the morphologically left ventricle.

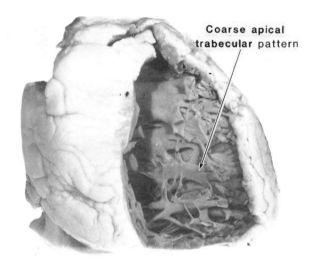

Coarse apical trabecular pattern

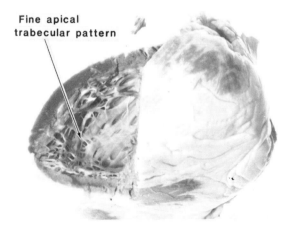

Fine apical trabecular pattern

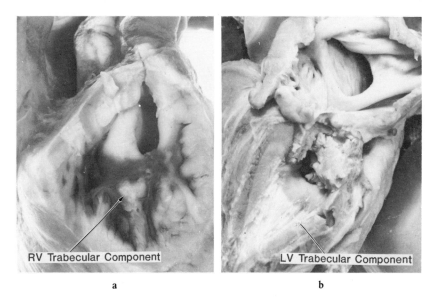

a   b

Fig. 3.4 The ventricles are recognisable as being of right (a) and left (b) morphology even when only represented by their trabecular components. In both of the hearts illustrated there was double inlet and double outlet from the complementary dominant ventricle.

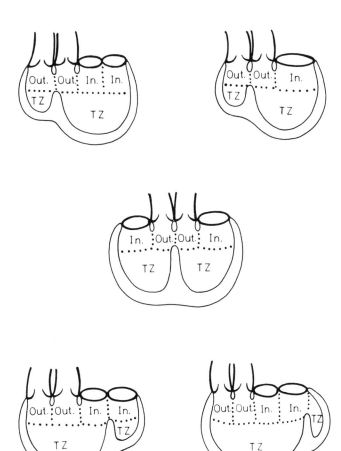

Fig. 3.5 The way in which the ventricular inlet and outlet components can be shared between the apical trabecular components to produce normal, rudimentary or 'super' ventricles. Rudimentary ventricles can also result because of absence of an inlet our outlet component, but only double inlet and double outlet arrangements are illustrated. (Reproduced from Anderson et al, 1983, by kind permission of Castle House Publications Ltd., Tunbridge Wells, UK.)

Rarely hearts will be encountered with a solitary ventricle. Sometimes this may be because a right or left ventricle is present but is so small or rudimentary that it cannot be recognised with usual investigatory techniques. But there is the third pattern of apical ventricular morphology. This is when the apical component is of neither right nor left type but is coarsely trabeculated and crossed by multiple large muscle bundles. This is the third pattern of ventricular morphology, namely the solitary ventricle of indeterminate morphology.

When determining the morphology of the great arteries, unfortunately there are no intrinsic features which enable an aorta to be distinguished from a pulmonary trunk and a common or solitary trunk. To do this we use the branching pattern of the trunks. With rare exceptions, it can be said that the aorta give rise to at least one coronary artery and the bulk of the systemic arteries. The pulmonary trunk gives rise to at least one pulmonary artery. A common trunk gives rise directly to coronary, systemic and pulmonary arteries. A solitary arterial trunk is described in the absence of intrapericardial pulmonary arteries. Even in the rare cases which may transgress one of these rules, by looking at the overall branching pattern it is usually possible to distinguish the nature of the arterial trunk.

ATRIAL ARRANGEMENT

The cornerstone of any sequential system must be accurate establishment of atrial arrangement, since it is not possible to construct a three-storey house based on the atria without having a firm foundation at ground floor level. In some sequential systems, most doubt surrounds atrial arrangement (de la Cruz & Nadal-Ginard, 1972; de la Cruz et al, 1967, 1976; Brandt & Calder, 1977; Stanger et al, 1977;

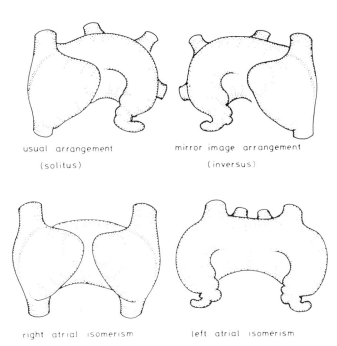

usual arrangement
(solitus)

mirror image arrangement
(inversus)

right atrial isomerism

left atrial isomerism

Fig. 3.6 The four possible arrangements of the atrial chambers based on the morphology of the atrial appendages and their junction with the smooth-walled atrial components.

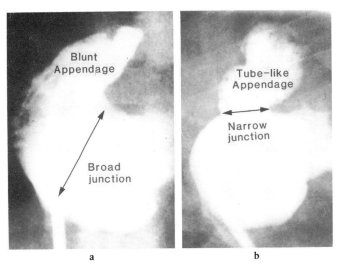

Fig. 3.7 Angiogram illustrating the differences between (a) the morphologically right and (b) the morphologically left atrial appendage. (Reproduced from Anderson et al, 1983, by kind permission of Dr B. Soto and Castle House Publications Ltd., Tunbridge Wells. UK.)

Van Praagh & Vlad, 1978; Van Praagh et al, 1977). This doubt is removed if atrial arrangement is determined from appendage morphology as discussed above (Anderson et al, 1978; de la Cruz et al, 1983), rather than being inferred from other features such as visceral arrangement or else determined from variable features such as the course of the inferior caval vein. Then on the basis of all hearts having two atrial chambers, each of which may be of morphologically right or left type, four types of discrete atrial arrangement (situs) can be recognised (Fig. 3.6). They are, firstly, the usual atrial arrangement (situs solitus) in which the morphologically right atrial appendage is right-sided and the morphologically left atrial appendage is left-sided. The second rare arrangement is the mirror-image of the usual and is generally called situs inversus. These first two atrial arrangements are characterised by lateralisation of the atria, the morphologically right atrium being to one side and the morphologically left atrium to the other. The two remaining atrial arrangements do not show such lateralisation. Instead there is isomerism of atrial morphology. Thus, both the atria have morphological characteristics of either right (right atrial isomerism) or left (left atrial isomerism) type.

Practical recognition of atrial arrangement

These different types of atrial arrangement are readily recognised by direct examination of the atria themselves, and atrial appendage morphology can be recognised by atrial angiography (Fig. 3.7). In expert hands it may also

become possible to identify atrial morphology using cross-sectional echocardiography. But in general clinical practice it is rarely necessary to resort to direct atrial identification. This is because almost always atrial morphology reflects visceral morphology. In patients with lateralised visceral arrangements (usual and mirror-image), it is exceedingly rare for there to be viscero-atrial disharmony. However, when the atria are isomeric, then usually there is visceral heterotaxy, and atrial morphology cannot be determined with any degree of certainty from the abdominal organs (Partridge et al, 1975; Macartney et al, 1978, 1980). But fortunately, even when there is visceral heterotaxy it is rare for there to be disharmony between atrial morphology and *bronchial* morphology (Caruso & Becker, 1979). So, the presence of atrial isomerism can almost always be inferred from the bronchial anatomy (Landing et al, 1971; Partridge et al, 1975; Macartney et al, 1978, 1980; Deanfield et al, 1980). The key is that the morphologically left bronchus is long and branches after the lower lobe pulmonary artery has crossed it (so that the bronchus is hyparterial). In contrast, the morphologically right bronchus is short and is crossed by the lower lobe pulmonary artery after it has branched (eparterial). Four bronchial patterns can then be recognised (usual, mirror-image, right isomerism and left isomerism – Fig. 3.8) which almost invariably will reflect atrial arrangement. These patterns of bronchial anatomy are not always seen in the penetrated chest radiograph, but are readily displayed by so-called 'filter films' (Dunbar, 1970; Macartney et al, 1983). More recently it has been shown that the same information provided by bronchial arrangement can be obtained non-invasively using cross-sectional ultrasonography (Huhta et al, 1982). This is because the abdominal great vessels bear a distinct relation to each other and to the spine according to the atrial

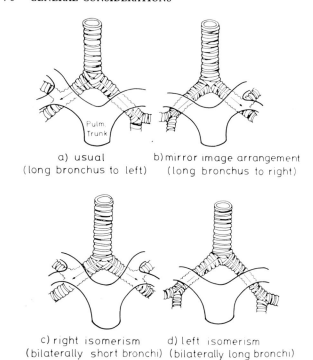

a) usual
(long bronchus to left)

b) mirror image arrangement
(long bronchus to right)

c) right isomerism
(bilaterally short bronchi)

d) left isomerism
(bilaterally long bronchi)

Fig. 3.8 The four patterns of bronchial morphology which, almost without exception, reflect the type of atrial arrangement.

arrangement present (Fig. 3.9) and can be recognised ultrasonically according to their pattern of pulsation. When the atria are lateralised, then the inferior caval vein and aorta lie to opposite sides of the spine, with the caval vein on the side of the morphologically right atrium (see also Ch. 12). When there is atrial isomerism, then almost without exception the great vessels lie to the same side of the spine, with the caval vein in anterior position in right isomerism and posterior (or the azygos vein posterior) in left isomerism.

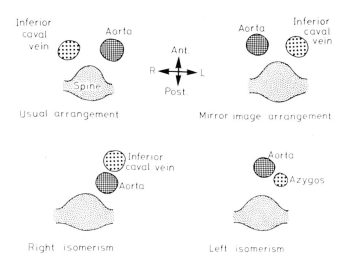

Fig. 3.9 The characteristic arrangements of the abdominal great vessels as seen in the short axis relative to the spine which are excellent indications of the atrial arrangement.

Generally speaking right isomerism is associated with absence of the spleen (asplenia) while left isomerism is associated with multiple spleens (polysplenia). Some authorities use these terms to describe given atrial arrangements (Brandt & Calder, 1977; Stanger et al, 1977), while patients with isomerism are frequently grouped together from the cardiac standpoint under the banner of the 'splenic syndromes'. We find it easier to describe these syndromes in terms of what they are, namely isomeric. This is particularly so because the correlation between right isomerism and asplenia and between left isomerism and polysplenia, though good, is not perfect (Macartney et al, 1980). Right and left atrial isomerism, in contrast, describes what is there and concentrates attention upon the heart.

THE ATRIOVENTRICULAR JUNCTION

In order to analyse accurately the atrioventricular junction, it is self-evidently necessary to know the atrial arrangements. Equally, it is necessary to establish the morphology of the ventricular chambers in order to know which atrium is connected to which ventricle. Then it is possible to define the type of atrioventricular connexion and to determine the morphology of the valves guarding the atrioventricular junction (the mode of connexion). In hearts with complex malformations it is also necessary to check the precise topology of the ventricular mass and to specify the relationships of the ventricular chambers.

Type of atrioventricular connexion

When we use the term 'atrioventricular connexion', we mean simply that atrial myocardium is connected to ventricular myocardium around the atrioventricular junction, the two being separated by the fibrous annulus. The cavities of the atrial chambers are therefore connected to the underlying ventricular mass, the two being in communication via the atrioventricular junction (Fig. 3.10). In every heart, perforce, since there are two atrial chambers there is the possibility for two atrioventricular connexions (Fig. 3.10 – centre). This is irrespective of whether they are guarded by two valves (Fig. 3.10 – top left) or by a common atrioventricular valve (Fig. 3.10 – bottom left). One of the connexions as thus defined may be blocked by an imperforate valve membrane, but this does not alter the fact that there are still two atrioventricular connexions present (Fig. 3.10 – top right). But in some hearts this possibility is not fulfilled because one of the connexions is *absent*. Then the atrial myocardium on that side has no connexion with the underlying ventricular myocardium. Instead it is separated from the ventricular structures by the fibro-fatty tissues of the atrioventricular groove. (Fig. 3.10 – bottom right).

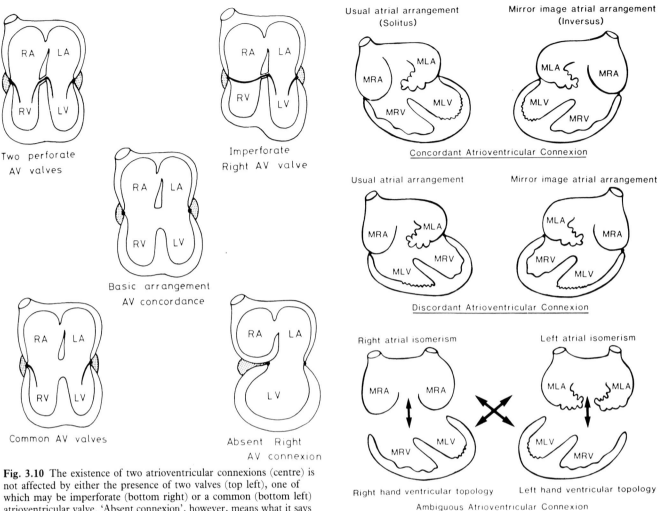

Fig. 3.10 The existence of two atrioventricular connexions (centre) is not affected by either the presence of two valves (top left), one of which may be imperforate (bottom right) or a common (bottom left) atrioventricular valve. 'Absent connexion', however, means what it says (bottom right), namely that only one atrium is connected to the ventricular mass. Although only imperforate right valve or absent right connexion is illustrated, the same morphology can be found on the left side of the heart.

Fig. 3.11 The three different types of biventricular atrioventricular connexion.

When atrioventricular connexions are defined in this fashion, all hearts fit into one of two groups (Anderson, 1983). In the first group, each atrial chamber is connected actually or potentially to its own underlying ventricle. The feature of the second group is that only one of the ventricles (if indeed two are present) is connected to the atria.

There are three possible arrangements in hearts with each of the atria connected to its own ventricle, or in other words three types of biventricular atrioventricular connexion. These depend on the morphology of the chambers connected together (Fig. 3.11). The first is for the morphologically right atrium to be connected to the morphologically right ventricle and the morphologically left atrium to the morphologically left ventricle irrespective of the relationship or architecture of the ventricles or the morphology of the values guarding the junction. This arrangement produces a concordant atrioventricular connexion. The second arrangement is the reverse of the first and is again independent of relationships of valve

morphology. It is a discordant atrioventricular connexion. These first two arrangements are found when the atria are lateralised. The final atrioventricular connexion in which each atrium is connected with its own ventricle is found with isomeric atria, of either right or left morphology. Because of the isomeric atria, this third connexion is neither concordant nor discordant. It is a discrete atrioventricular connexion in its own right, to which we have assigned the term *ambiguous* atrioventricular connexion (Shinebourne et al, 1976). It too is independent of ventricular relationships or topology and atrioventricular valve morphologies.

There are also three possible arrangements which can produce a univentricular atrioventricular connexion (Fig. 3.12). The first is when both atria are connected to the same ventricle – *double inlet* atrioventricular connexion. The other two are found when one atrioventricular connexion is absent. They are *absent right* and *absent left* atrioventricular connexion (Fig. 3.13). The group of

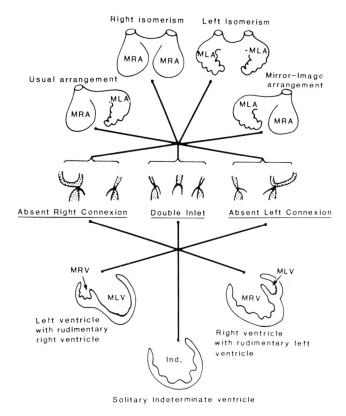

Fig. 3.12 The combinations of atrial arrangement and ventricular morphology which can be found with the three types of univentricular atrioventricular connexion.

univentricular atrioventricular connexions is different from the group of biventricular connexions. Not only is it independent of ventricular relationships and valve morphology, but it is also independent of atrial and ventricular morphologies. Thus hearts with concordant and discordant atrioventricular connexions can only exist when usually arranged or mirror-image atrial chambers are both connected to appropriate ventricles. An ambiguous connexion can only be found with each of two isomeric atrial chambers connected to separate ventricles. In contrast, either double inlet, absent right or absent left atrioventricular connexions can be found with usually arranged, mirror-image or isomeric atria and with these atria connected to a right ventricle, a left ventricle or a morphologically indeterminate ventricle (Fig. 3.12). Ventricular morphology must always, therefore, be described separately in this second group.

Although in these hearts only one ventricle is connected to the atria, in most there is a second ventricle present, albeit rudimentary, which is of complementary trabecular pattern to the dominant ventricle. Most frequently the dominant ventricle will be of left ventricular trabecular pattern and the rudimentary ventricle will be of right ventricular trabecular pattern. More rarely, the dominant ventricle will be a right ventricle and the rudimentary ventricle will be of left ventricular type. Even more rarely, hearts will be found with solitary ventricles. Most frequently these will be of indeterminate morphology. But, at least in clinical practice, it must be expected that solitary left or right ventricles will be encountered with the rudimentary ventricle too small to be demonstrated.

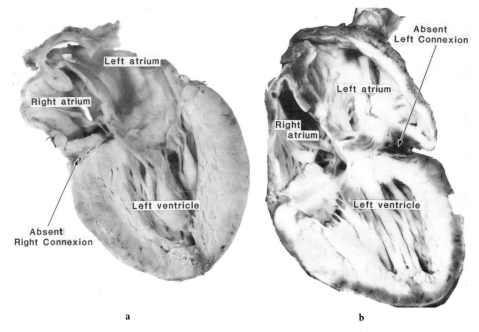

Fig. 3.13 Sections in 'four-chamber' plane illustrating the morphology of absent right (a) and absent left (b) atrioventricular connexion. Both are shown with the other atrium connected to a dominant left ventricle.

Mode of atrioventricular connexion

The type of atrioventricular connexion describes only the way in which the atria are connected to the ventricles. The morphology of the valves guarding the atrioventricular junction is independent of this type of connexion within the constraints imposed by the connexion itself (Fig. 3.10). Thus, when both atria are connected to the ventricular mass, then the two atrioventricular connexions may be guarded by two patent and perforate valves, by one patent valve and one imperforate valve, by a common valve or by straddling and overriding valves (Fig. 3.14). These modes of connexion can be found with concordant, discordant, ambiguous or double inlet types of connexion. When one valve is imperforate, it may be the right or left valve. A common valve guards two atrioventricular connexions irrespective of its morphology. We distinguish between straddling and overriding of an atrioventricular valve by considering the tension apparatus in terms of straddling and the valve annulus in terms of override. Thus, a valve straddles when its tension apparatus is

attached to both sides of a septum within the ventricular mass. It overrides when its annulus is connected to ventricles on both sides of a septal structure. A right valve, a left valve or a common valve can straddle, can override or can straddle and override. Very rarely both right and left valves may straddle or override in the same heart.

When one atrioventricular connexion is absent, then the possible modes of connexion are greatly reduced because there is only one atrioventricular connexion, and hence only one atrioventricular valve is present. The sole valve may be entirely committed to one ventricle, or alternatively it may straddle, override or may straddle and override.

An overriding valve is more than just a mode of connexion, because the degree of commitment of the valve annulus to the ventricles on either side of the septum determines the atrioventricular connexion. Hearts with two valves in which one valve is overriding are anatomically intermediate between hearts with biventricular and univentricular atrioventicular connexions. There are two ways of dealing with such hearts. One way is to consider the hearts as having a special type of atrioventricular connexion (Liberthson et al, 1971; Bharati & Lev, 1979a). The other way is to recognise that hearts with overriding valves are intermediates in a series of anomalies and to split the series depending on whether 50% or more of the valve overrides. For the purpose of categorisation only the two ends of the series are labelled, so that the hearts in the middle are recognised but are then assigned to one or other of the end-point categories (Milo et al, 1979). Our preference is for the second alternative (Fig. 3.15). When most of an overriding valve is connected to a ventricle which already possesses the other atrioventricular connexion, then we designate the connexion as being double inlet. If the overriding valve is connected mostly to a ventricle not itself connected to the other atrium, then each atrium is categorised as though connected to its own ventricle.

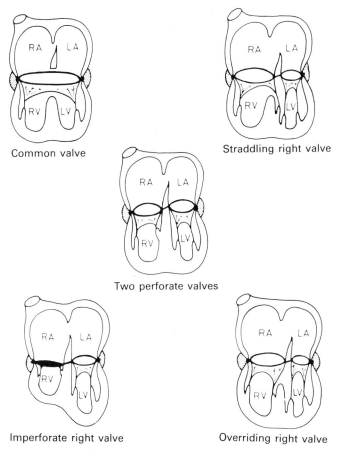

Common valve

Straddling right valve

Two perforate valves

Imperforate right valve

Overriding right valve

Fig. 3.14 The different modes of atrioventricular connexion when two atria connect with the ventricular mass. Although shown affecting a right valve, a left valve can also be imperforate, straddling or overriding.

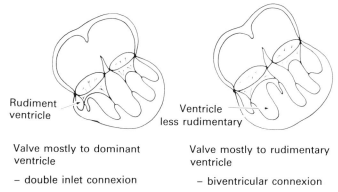

Rudiment ventricle

Ventricle less rudimentary

Valve mostly to dominant ventricle

– double inlet connexion

Valve mostly to rudimentary ventricle

– biventricular connexion

Fig. 3.15 This diagram of two hearts with abnormal right atrioventricular valves which both straddle and override show the two ends of the spectrum of overriding of an atrioventricular valve which results in either a double inlet or a biventricular atrioventricular connexion. We divide this spectrum at its midpoint – the '50%' rule.

Before finishing with atrioventricular valves, it is worthy of emphasis that the terms 'mitral' and 'tricuspid' valve are only appropriate in hearts with biventricular atrioventricular connexions and two valves. In this context, we have never encountered a heart in which the tricuspid valve was other than in the morphologically right ventricle or the mitral valve in the morphologically left ventricle. In hearts with biventricular atrioventricular connexions but with an atrioventricular septal defect, however, it is incorrect to consider the common valve as having 'mitral' and 'tricuspid' components. It has right and left components, but, particularly on the left side, these bear scant resemblance to the normal atrioventricular valves (see Ch. 24). Equally, in hearts with double inlet it is incorrect to consider the two valves as 'mitral' and 'tricuspid'. They are *right* and *left* valves. Similarly, when one connexion is absent, although it is usually possible to deduce the presumed nature of the existing valve from concepts of morphogenesis, this is not always practical or helpful. The valve can always accurately be described as a right or a left valve. For example, possibly contentious arguments are defused when the right or left valve straddles in the absence of the other atrioventricular connexion. Some have suggested that such a valve is a common valve (Van Mierop, 1977). By our definitions, since it drains only one atrium, it can only be a left or right valve.

Ventricular topology and relationships

In the normal heart, the ventricular spatial relationships are complex. The inlet portions are more or less to right and left, with the inlet part of the muscular ventricular septum in an approximately sagittal plane. The outlet portions are more or less anteroposteriorly related, with the outlet muscular septum in an approximately frontal plane. The trabecular portions extend between these two components, with the trabecular muscular septum spiralling between the inlet and outlet septa. Much of the right ventricular trabecular component is inferior to the left ventricular trabecular component. It is understandable that there is a desire to have a 'shorthand' term to describe such a complex spatial arrangement. In normal hearts the term 'normal relations' fulfills this role. The problem with this is that many use 'normal relations' as the point of departure for the construction of complex systems of nomenclature which attempt to combine information concerning both connexions and relationships. Thus 'ventricular inversion' is widely used as a synonym for a discordant atrioventricular connexion, while 'normal relations' is frequently presumed to be the same as a concordant atrioventricular connexion. These systems have at least three major problems. The first is that relationships are usually but not invariably harmonious with atrioventricular connexions. The second is that 'ventricular inversion' is *not* the mirror-image of 'normal relations'. The ventricular septum is usually a relatively straight structure in the presence of 'ventricular inversion'. The third, and perhaps major, problem is that real difficulties arise with these terms in the presence of mirror-image atrial arrangement. Then it may seem that 'normal relations' for the usual situation would be 'inversion' for the mirror-image arrangement. But, as indicated above, 'inversion' is not the isomer of 'normal relations'. Hence the necessity for introduction of the confusing term 'non-inversion' (Espino-Vela et al, 1970; Quero-Jimenez, 1980). This term then means different things to different observers. An alternative to all these terms is to use the ventricular 'loop' to describe atrioventricular relationships (Van Praagh & Vlad, 1978). In this convention, 'd-loop' is frequently considered to be the same as 'normal relations' and 'l-loop' to be the same as 'ventricular inversion'. The same problems then arise as described above when connexions do not harmonise with relationships. Van Praagh and his colleagues now use the 'loop' specifically to describe internal ventricular topology (Van Praagh et al, 1981, 1983). This highlights the need to describe spatial relationships separately from both connexions and morphology, using mutually exclusive terms for these different attributes of the heart. In our view this then allows many if not all the problems of nomenclature to be resolved.

Using this approach, our preference then is to describe ventricular topology in terms of right-hand and left-hand patterns rather than 'd-loop' and 'l-loop'. We then account for ventricular relationships using simple terms. The right-hand and left-hand patterns of ventricular topology describe the way in which, figuratively speaking, the palmar surface of the observer's hands can be placed upon the septal surface of the morphologically right ventricle with the thumb in the inlet, the wrist in the apical trabecular component and the fingers in the outlet. In the person with usual atrial arrangement and a concordant atrioventricular connexion, it is the right hand which can be thus placed (Fig. 3.16 – left). In patients with mirror-image atria and a concordant atrioventricular connexion, it is the left hand which fits the septal surface (Fig. 3.16 – right). In persons with usually arranged atria and a discordant atrioventricular connexion almost always there is a left-hand pattern whereas right-hand topology is found with the combination of mirror-image atria and a discordant atrioventricular connexion. These combinations are almost always present although rare exceptions have been described (Otero Coto et al, 1979; Van Praagh et al, 1981). When describing ventricular relationships, which are independent of the topology, we account for right-left, anterior-posterior and superior-inferior coordinates Where necessary we describe the position of the three ventricular components separately. In most hearts these refinements are unnecessary. Indeed, when the relationships are harmonious with chamber connexions, problems do not arise in any system.

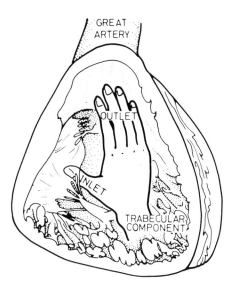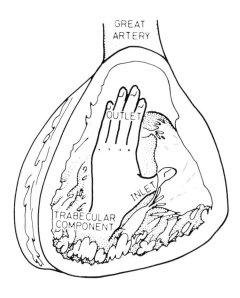

Fig. 3.16 The way in which, figuratively speaking, ventricular topology can be described in terms of the way in which the septal surface of the morphologically right ventricle accepts the palmar surface of the observer's right or left hand.

It is the so-called 'criss-cross' hearts which gave most problems (Anderson et al, 1974; Sato et al, 1978; Freedom et al, 1978; Van Praagh et al, 1980). But the problems were largely in the eyes of the observers. If connexions, relations and ventricular topology are described separately there is no room for confusion (Anderson, 1982). In the typical 'criss-cross' heart with discordant atrioventricular connexion and usual atrial arrangement, the morphologically right ventricular inlet is to the left of the morphologically left ventricular inlet. In these hearts the ventricles are rotated and the morphologically right ventricular trabecular and outlet components are to the right of their morphologically left ventricular counterparts, giving a spurious impression of 'normal relationships'. In the 'criss-cross' hearts seen with usual atrial arrangement and a concordant atrioventricular connexion, the ventricular rotation gives a spurious impression of 'ventricular inversion'. In cases with extreme rotation, the morphologically right ventricular inlet may be right-sided with a discordant atrioventricular connexion (Freedom et al, 1978). 'Criss-cross' hearts are frequently associated with overriding or straddling atrioventricular valves, and can be found with various ventriculo-arterial connexions and relations. Provided relationships are described accurately and separately from either the connexions or the ventricular topology none of these hearts will be difficult either to diagnose or to categorise.

We have indicated above how Van Praagh and his colleagues (1981) now advocate the use of the ventricular loop for description of internal ventricular topology. In most instances separate description of this feature is unnecessary. Apart from rare exceptions, all necessary information is given in the description of atrioventricular connexions and ventricular relationships. But there is one situation where description of internal ventricular topology is essential. That is when there are isomeric atria and an ambiguous atrioventricular connexion. In this arrangement, the same terms would be correctly used to describe the heart in which the left-sided isomeric atrium was connected to a morphologically right ventricle and the heart in which the left-sided atrium was connected to a morphologically left ventricle. It is inadequate to supplement these descriptions with those for ventricular relationships as we suggested before (Shinebourne et al, 1976). This is because the relationships would not convey information concerning ventricular topology when there was any additional ventricular rotation ('criss-cross' heart with ambiguous atrioventricular connexion). The different arrangements are well accounted for simply by describing the ventricular topology. The significance of these patterns in hearts with ambiguous atrioventricular connexion (De Tommasi et al, 1981) is that, as far as we know, they determine the disposition of the atrioventricular conduction tissues (Dickinson et al, 1979).

It is also important to describe the position and relationships of rudimentary ventricles in hearts with univentricular atrioventricular connexions. Here the relationships are largely independent of the connexions and the ventricular morphology. It is known that whilst usually the rudimentary right ventricle is basically anterior and right-sided in classical tricuspid atresia, it can be anterior and left-sided without in any way altering the clinical presentation and haemodynamic findings. Similarly, in hearts with double inlet ventricle the position of the rudimentary ventricle plays only a minor role in determining the clinical presentation (Macartney et al, 1976a). While a case can be made for such hearts with univentricular atrioventricular connexion being developed basically in the setting of 'd-loops' or 'l-loops', there are sufficient exceptions to recommend restriction of this concept to a morphogenetic (but not a descriptive) role. For describing the position of the rudimentary ventricle we simply describe it relative to the dominant ventricle, when necessary describing right-left, anterior-posterior and superior-inferior coordinates. On occasion in may also be necessary to describe separately the position of trabecular and outlet components.

THE VENTRICULO-ARTERIAL JUNCTION

As with problems with other aspects of terminology, most polemics concerning the ventriculo-arterial junction (Van Praagh, 1971; Van Praagh et al, 1971; Van Mierop, 1971) devolve upon the failure to distinguish connexions from relations from infundibular morphology. If we consider the problems concerning 'transposition', it is the prerogative of those who define transposition as an anterior aorta to speak rightly of 'double outlet with transposition', and equally to object to the introduction of the term 'posterior transposition'. Within the system of 'transposition' defined as an anterior aorta, posterior transposition is clearly an impossibility. This is not so when 'transposition' is defined as a ventriculo-arterial connexion. But then, the proponents of the 'connexions definition' must recognise the right of the relationists to their own definition of transposition. However much the historical papers are invoked or however much weight is given to the clinical importance of connexions, there can be no copyright on the definition of 'transposition' The solution to this thorny problem is not to try to define 'transposition' as describing any single facet of the ventriculo-arterial junction, but instead to describe separately connexions, infundibular morphology and relationships (Tynan & Anderson, 1979; Anderson & Tynan, 1981). By this stroke, it is possible at the same time to defuse controversies concerning the role of the 'bilateral conus' in the diagnosis of double outlet right ventricle (Baron, 1971; Anderson & Tynan, 1981). When we describe connexions, infundibular morphology and arterial

relationships independently with mutually exclusive terms (eschewing use of 'transposition'), there can be no room for confusion.

Ventriculo-arterial connexions

As with the atrioventricular junction, it is necessary to account for both the *type* and *mode* of ventriculo-arterial connexion (Tynan et al, 1981; Quero-Jimenez et al, 1981). There are four types of connexion. A concordant ventriculo-arterial connexion exists when the aorta arises from a morphologically left ventricle and the pulmonary trunk from a morphologically right ventricle. The arrangement where the aorta arises from a morphologically right ventricle and the pulmonary trunk from a morphologically left ventricle produces a discordant ventriculo-arterial connexion. Double outlet connexion is found when both arteries are connected to the same ventricle, which may be of right ventricular, left ventricular, or of indeterminate ventricular pattern. As with atrioventricular valves, overriding arterial valves (see below) are assigned to the ventricle connected to their greater parts. The final ventriculo-arterial connexion is single outlet of the heart (Fig. 3.17). This may take one of four forms. A common trunk exists when both ventricles are connected via a common arterial valve to an arterial trunk which gives rise to the coronary arteries, at least one pulmonary artery and the majority of the systemic circulation. A solitary arterial trunk exists when it is not possible to identify any pulmonary arteries (or their remnants) within the pericardial cavity. The other forms of single outlet are single pulmonary trunk with aortic atresia or single aortic trunk with pulmonary atresia. These latter two categories describe only those arrangements in which the atretic arterial trunk has no connexion to a ventricular cavity. If its connexion can be established but is found to be

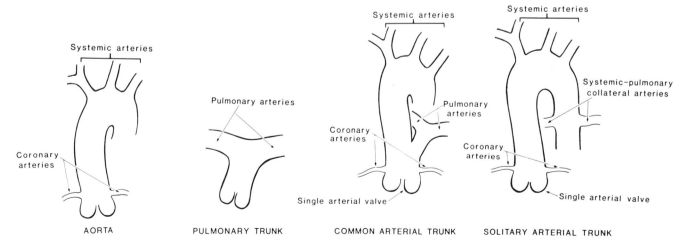

Fig. 3.17 The different patterns of the great arteries which produce single outlet of the heart.

imperforate, then the connexion is described and the imperforate valve categorised as a mode of connexion (see below). In hearts with single outlet, it is also necessary to describe the ventricular connexion of the single trunk. This may be exclusively from a right or left ventricle, but it can override the septum, being connected to both ventricles.

There are fewer *modes* of connexion at the ventriculo-arterial junction than the atrioventricular junction. A common arterial valve is not considered a mode of connexion, because it can only exist with a specific type of single outlet, namely common arterial trunk. Straddling of an arterial valve is impossible because it has no tension apparatus. Thus the possible modes of connexion (Quero-Jimenez et al, 1981) are two perforate valves (one or both of which may override), or one perforate and one imperforate valve. As with overriding atrioventricular valves, the degree of override of an arterial valve determines the ventriculo-arterial connexion present, the overriding valve or valves being assigned to the ventricle conneted to its greater part. For example, if more than half of an overriding pulmonary valve was connected to a right ventricle, the aorta being connected to a left ventricle, we would code a discordant connexion. If more than half the overriding aortic valve was connected to the right ventricle in this situation, we would code a double outlet connexion. In this way, following the precedent of Kirklin et al (1973), we avoid the necessity for intermediate categories, but we

have to describe the degree of override whenever an overriding valve is found. This is done to the best of one's ability, using whichever techniques are available, and recognising the subjective nature of the task.

Infundibular morphology

The infundibular regions are no more and no less than the outlet components of the ventricular mass, but they are the dwelling place of two of the sacred cows of paediatric cardiology. One is the so-called 'bilateral conus', an arbiter of the connexion for some when associated with double outlet right ventricle (Baron, 1971; Sridaromont et al, 1978) but of little import when each great artery is supported by its own ventricle. The other is the enigmatic 'crista', sought here and there as was the Scarlet Pimpernel, and just as elusive. If these structures are recognised for what they are and their morphology described as such then they, too, provide no problems in recognition and description.

The morphology of the ventricular outlet portions is variable for any heart. Potentially each ventricle can possess a complete muscular funnel as its outlet portion, and then each arterial valve can be said to have a complete infundibulum. When considered as a whole, the outlet portions of a ventricular mass exhibiting such a bilateral infundibulum have three discrete parts (Fig. 3.18). Two

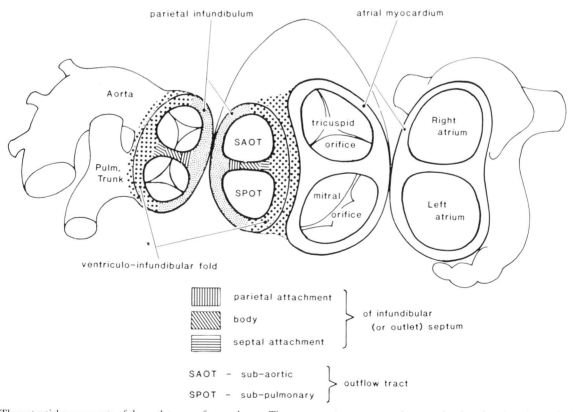

Fig. 3.18 The potential components of the outlet cone of musculature. These are not always present, for example when there is atrioventricular-arterial or intra-arterial valve continuity then some of the components are effaced

of the parts form the anterior and posterior halves of the funnels of muscle supporting the valves. The anterior, parietal part is the free anterior ventricular wall. The posterior part is the inner heart curvature which separates the arterial from the atrioventricular valves, and which we term the 'ventriculo-infundibular fold'). The third part of the outlet portion is the septum separating the two outlets and the two arterial valves, the *infundibular* or *outlet* septum. The dimensions of the outlet septum are independent of the remainder of the infundibular musculature, and it is possible for both arterial valves to be separated from both atrioventricular valves, but for the arterial valves to be in fibrous continuity with one another. Such an occurrence is very rare, but it is usual for some part of the infundibular musculature to be effaced so that valvar fibrous continuity does occur. Most frequently it is the morphologically left ventricular part of the ventriculo-infundibular fold which is attenuated, so that there is fibrous continuity between the mitral valve and the arterial valve of the left ventricle. Whether the arterial valve is aortic or pulmonary will depend on the ventriculo-arterial connexion present. In this usual arrangement the morphologically right ventricular part of the ventricular-infundibular fold persists so that there is tricuspid-arterial valve discontinuity and, depending on the integrity of the outlet septum, usually there is a completely muscular outflow tract or infundibulum in the morphologically right ventricle. When both outlet portions are connected to the morphologically right ventricle, then most frequently the ventriculo-infundibular fold persists in its entirety and there is atrioventricular-arterial valve discontinuity. Hence the suggestion that a bilateral infundibulum should be the criterion of double outlet right ventricle (Baron, 1971; Sridaromont et al, 1978). But many hearts with an unequivocal connexion of double outlet right ventricle have atrioventricular-arterial valve continuity. What are such hearts to be called if not double outlet right ventricle? This is another example of the unnecessary controversy of attempting to determine one feature of cardiac morphology from a second, unrelated, feature. Returning to the basics of outlet morphology, when both outlet portions are connected to the morphologically left ventricle, the tendency is for there to be continuity between both arterial valves and both atrioventricular valves, but the ventriculo-infundibular fold can persist in part or even in its whole. In summary, the state of the ventriculo-infundibular fold determines the infundibular morphology. Ignoring the rare situation of complete absence of the infundibular septum, and considering morphology from the standpoint of the arterial valves, there are then four possible arrangements. There may be a complete subpulmonary infundibulum with aortic-atrioventricular valve continuity. There may be a complete subaortic infundibulum with pulmonary-atrioventricular valve continuity. There may be a bilateral infundibulum without any arterial-atrioventricular valve

continuity. There may be a bilateral infundibulum without any arterial-atrioventricular valve continuity or finally there may be bilaterally deficient infundibula with bilateral arterial-atrioventricular continuity. In themselves, these terms are insufficient. For specificity it is necessary to know which arterial valve is connected to which ventricle. This emphasises the fact that infundibular morphology is independent of the ventriculo-arterial connexion.

The above discussion has been concluded with no mention whatsoever of the enigmatic 'crista'. This is because the term has so many definitions as to become virtually meaningless. Our preference is therefore to reserve the term 'supraventricular crest' for the normal heart or hearts with a normally connected and structured right ventricular outflow tract. Then the 'crest' is the muscular mass in the ventricular roof which separates the tricuspid and pulmonary valves. Dissection easily demonstrates that its greater part is the right ventricular part of the ventriculo-infundibular fold. A small part of its most medial part is the muscular part of the outlet septum. The supraventricular crest of the normal heart is discrete from the extensive muscular trabeculation of the morphologically right ventricle which overlies the muscular septum and which divides into two limbs, these limbs then clasping the body of the supraventricular crest. This extensive morphologically right ventricular trabeculation is the *septomarginal trabecula* (Anderson et al, 1977). Usually these three structures, namely the ventriculo-infundibular fold and outlet septum and the septomarginal trabecula, are so well aligned that it is frequently not possible to say where one starts and the other finishes. But in hearts with ventricular septal defects and/or abnormal ventriculo-arterial connexions, the three parts are frequently widely separated and each can then be clearly recognised in its own right. The problem with the 'crista' is that at some time or in some place each of these three different structures has been nominated as *the* crista, while the left ventricular component of the ventriculo-infundibular fold has been similarly honoured. It is for this reason that we eschew the use of 'crista' except in the normal heart. We describe each muscle bundle in its own right, naming any muscular structure separating the ventricular outflow portions from one another as the 'infundibular' or 'outlet' septum; any muscular structure separating an arterial from an atrioventricular valve as the 'ventriculo-infundibular fold' and naming the extensive septal trabeculation of the morphologically right ventricle as the 'septomarginal trabecula' (Fig. 3.19).

Arterial relationships

The final feature of the ventriculo-arterial junction is the relationships of the great arteries and their valves. Usually relationships are described at valve level, and many systems for nomenclature have been constructed on this basis.

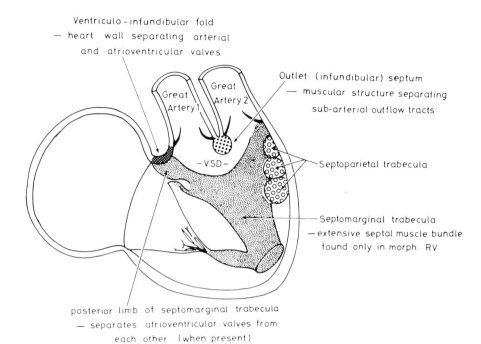

Ventriculo-infundibular fold
— heart wall separating arterial
and atrioventricular valves

Great Artery 1

Great Artery 2

Outlet (infundibular) septum
— muscular structure separating
sub-arterial outflow tracts

— VSD —

Septoparietal trabecula

Septomarginal trabecula
— extensive septal muscle bundle
found only in morph. RV

posterior limb of septomarginal trabecula
— separates atrioventricular valves from
each other (when present)

Fig. 3.19 The definition of the muscular components of the ventricular outlet as often seen in double outlet right ventricle.

Indeed, the concept that the position of the arterial valves reflects the ventricular loop (the 'loop rule' – Van Praagh et al, 1964a, b) has become so entrenched that it is frequent to see 'd-transposition' used as though synonymous with complete transposition (Dillon et al, 1973; Bourlon et al, 1980) and 'l-transposition' as if it were the same as corrected transposition (Ruttenberg, 1977). This is the more surprising since it is well known that arterial valve position is a poor guide to ventricular position, the aortic valve being to the right in only about 60% of the cases of complete transposition with usually arranged atria studied by Carr et al (1968). A further deficiency of describing arterial valve position in terms of leftness and rightness is that the concept takes no cognisance of anteroposterior relationships, an omission no less surprising since we have already indicated how an anterior position of the aorta was for many years the cornerstone for definitions of 'transposition' (Van Mierop, 1971). It is therefore our practice to describe arterial valve relationships in terms of both right-left and anterior-posterior coordinates. Such description can be accomplished with as great a degree of precision as is required, and a system which describes aortic position in degrees of the arc of a circle described around the pulmonary valve (Bargeron, 1981) has much to commend it. Nonetheless, our preference is to describe aortic valve position relative to the pulmonary trunk in terms of eight positions of a 'compass', using the simple terms left, right, anterior, posterior and side-by-side in their various combinations as our adjectives. As long as we then remember that these describe *only* arterial valve relations and convey no information about either connexions or morphology we have no fear of producing confusion.

From the stance of positions of the arterial trunks, the possibilities are either for the pulmonary trunk to spiral round the aorta as it ascends, or else for the two trunks to ascend in parallel fashion (de la Cruz et al, 1976). It is rarely necessary to describe these relationships. Usually, spiralling trunks are associated with concordant ventriculo-arterial connexions, and parallel trunks with discordant or double outlet connexions, but again there is no predictive value in these relationships.

Another relationship of the great arteries which is of significance is that between the aortic arch and the pulmonary arteries. In almost all hearts the aortic arch crosses superiorly to the pulmonary arteries.

Aortic arch malposition is a well-recognised associated anomaly of conditions such as tetralogy of Fallot (see Ch. 32) or common arterial trunk (see Ch. 37). Distinction should be made between the position of the aortic arch and the side of the descending aorta, particularly when describing vascular rings (see Ch. 46). The side of the aortic arch is determined by whether it passes to the right or left of the trachea. This can be easily determined from the plain chest radiograph and corresponds to where the arch crosses the pulmonary artery. The position of the descending aorta is defined relative to the vertebral column.

ASSOCIATED MALFORMATIONS

As we suggested in our introduction, the majority of patients seen with congenital heart disease will have normal chamber connexions, morphology and relations. Then the associated malformation will be *the* anomaly. The body of this book is concerned with describing the specific morphological and clinical features of these anomalies, and they will not be considered further here, except to say that any combination of anomalies which are not mutually exclusive must be anticipated to occur at some time in some heart.

The section on associated malformations cannot, however, be concluded without consideration of the position (within the chest) of the heart itself and of the cardiac apex (or for that matter identification of a heart positioned outside the thoracic cavity – ectopia cordis). Some systems of nomenclature are based primarily upon the cardiac position (Bharati & Lev, 1979b), while complex nosologies have been devised solely to account for the various types of cardiac malposition (reviewed by Wilkinson & Acerete, 1973). We describe an abnormal position of the heart within the chest as an associated malformation, but we do not promote the cardiac malposition as a prime diagnosis. This is not to decry the importance of cardiac malposition (if only to interpret an electrocardiogram), but knowing that the heart is malpositioned gives no information concerning its internal architecture. Full sequential segmental analysis is needed to determine this analysis, and not vice versa.

There are three basic positions for the heart: mostly in the left hemithorax, mostly in the right hemithorax and equally positioned in the mediastinum. There are also three basic positions for the cardiac apex: pointing to the left, to the right, or to the middle. Apical direction is independent of cardiac position and both of these are independent of atrial and visceral arrangement. There is no agreement even amongst ourselves on the most appropriate definitions of dextrocardia, laevocardia, and mesocardia. Some use the terms only to describe cardiac position, taking no cognisance of apical direction (Van Praagh et al, 1977). Others use them to describe a combination of cardiac position with apical direction (Bharati & Lev, 1979b; Calcaterra et al 1979). Since there is no consensus on appropriate usage, it is perhaps less ambiguous although more long-winded to be completely descriptive. Account can then be taken of the cardiac position and the direction of the apex, particularly when the two are not in their anticipated harmony. This is the system we shall use here.

REFERENCES

Anderson R H 1982 Criss-cross hearts revisited. Pediatric Cardiology 3: 305–313

Anderson R H 1983 Weasel words in paediatric cardiology. International Journal of Cardiology 2: 425–429

Anderson R H, Tynan M 1981 Sequential chamber localisation. In: Hamer J, Rowlands D J (eds) Recent advances in cardiology, Vol 8. Churchill Livingstone, Edinburgh, p 265–285

Anderson R H, Shinebourne E A, Gerlis L M 1974 Criss-cross atrioventricular relationships producing paradoxical atrioventricular concordance or discordance: their significance to nomenclature of congenital heart disease. Circulation 50: 176–181

Anderson R H, Becker A E, Van Mierop L H S 1977 What should we call the 'crista'? British Heart Journal 39: 856–859

Anderson R H, Macartney F J, Shinebourne E A, Tynan M J 1978 Definition of cardiac chambers. In: Anderson R H, Shinebourne E A (eds) Definition of cardiac chambers. Churchill Livingstone, Edinburgh, p 5–15

Anderson R H, Becker A E, Freedom R M, et al 1981 Analysis of atrioventricular junction – connexions, relations and ventricular morphology. In: Godman M J (ed) Paediatric cardiology, Vol 4. Churchill Livingstone, Edinburgh, p 169–181

Anderson R H, Becker A E, Lucchese F E, Meier M A, Rigby M L, Soto B 1983 Sequential segmental analysis. In: Morphology of congenital heart disease. Angiocardiographic, echocardiographic and surgical correlates. Castle House, Tunbridge Wells, p 1–22

Bargeron L M Jr 1981 Angiography relevant to complicating features. In: Paediatric Cardiology Volume 3, eds. Becker A E, Losekoot T G, Marcelletti C, Anderson R H (eds) Paediatric cardiology, Vol 3. Churchill Livingstone, Edinburgh, p 33–47

Baron M G 1971 Radiologic notes in cardiology: angiographic differentiation between tetralogy of Fallot and double outlet right ventricle. Circulation 43: 451–455

Bharati S, Lev M 1979a The concept of tricuspid atresia complex as distinct from that of the single ventricle complex. Pediatric Cardiology 1: 57–62

Bharati S, Lev M 1979b Positional variations of the heart and its component chambers. Circulation 59: 886–887

Bourlon F, Fouron J-C, Battle-Diaz J, Ducharme G, Davignon A 1980 Relation between isovolumic relaxation period of left ventricle and pulmonary artery pressure in d-transposition of the great arteries. British Heart Journal 43: 226–231

Brandt P W T, Calder A L 1977 Cardiac connections: the segmental approach to radiologic diagnosis in congenital heart disease. Current Problems in Diagnostic Radiology 7: 1–35

Calcaterra G, Anderson R H, Lau K C, Shinebourne E A 1979 Dextrocardia – value of segmental analysis in its categorization. British Heart Journal 42: 497–507

Carr I, Tynan M J, Aberdeen E, Bonham-Carter R E, Graham G, Waterston D J 1968 Predictive accuracy of the loop rule in 109 children with classical complete transposition of the great arteries (abstract). Circulation 38: V1–52

Caruso G, Becker A E 1979 How to determine atrial situs? Considerations initiated by 3 cases of absent spleen with a discordant anatomy between bronchi and atria. British Heart Journal 41: 559–567

de la Cruz M V, Nadal-Ginard B 1972 Rules for the diagnosis of visceral situs, truncoconal morphologies and ventricular inversions. American Heart Journal 84: 19–32

de la Cruz M V, Espino-Vela J, Attie F, Munoz C L 1967 An embryological theory for the ventricular inversions and their classification. American Heart Journal 73: 777–793

de la Cruz M V, Berrazueta J R, Arteaga M, Attie F, Soni J 1976 Rules for diagnosis of arterioventricular discordances and spatial identification of ventricles. British Heart Journal 38: 341–354

de la Cruz M V, Violini R, Cayre R, Martinez Sanchez A, Arteaga M, Fernandez-Espino R 1983 Caracteristicas anatomicas del corazon normal y del situs visceral en el diagnostico de las cardiopatias congenitas. Revista Latina de Cardiologia 4: 35–42

Deanfield J, Leanage R, Stroobant J, Chrispin A R, Taylor J F N, Macartney F J 1980 Use of high kilovoltage filtered beam radiographs for detection of bronchial situs in infants and young children. British Heart Journal 44: 577–583

De Tommasi S M, Daliento L, Ho S Y, Macartney F J, Anderson R H 1981 Analysis of atrioventricular junction, ventricular mass and ventriculo-arterial junction in 43 specimens with atrial isomerism. British Heart Journal 45: 236–247

Dickinson D F, Wilkinson J L, Anderson K R, Smith A, Ho S Y, Anderson R H 1979 The cardiac conduction system in situs ambiguus. Circulation 59: 879–885

Dillon J C Feigenbaum H, Konecke L L, et al 1973 Echocardiographic manifestations of d-transposition of the great vessels. American Journal of Cardiology 32: 74–78

Dunbar J S 1970 Upper respiratory tract obstruction in infants and children. American Journal of Roentgenology 109: 227–246

Elliott L 1978 An angiocardiographic and plain film approach to complex congenital heart disease: classification and simplified nomenclature. In: Current problems in cardiology. Year Book Medical Publishers, Chicago, p 10–41

Espino-Vela J, de la Cruz M V, Munoz-Castellanos L, Plaza L, Attie F 1970 Ventricular inversion without transposition of the great vessels in situs inversus. British Heart Journal 32: 292–303

Freedom R M, Culham G, Rowe R D 1978 The criss-cross heart and supero-inferior ventricular heart: an angiocardiographic study. American Journal of Cardiology 42: 620–628

Huhta J C, Smallhorn J F, Macartney F J 1982 Two dimensional echocardiographic diagnosis of situs. British Heart Journal 48: 97–108

Kirklin J W, Pacifico A D, Bargeron L M, Soto B 1973 Cardiac repair in anatomically corrected malposition of the great arteries. Circulation 48: 153–159

Landing B H, Tsun-Yee K L, Vaughn C P, Wells T R 1971 Bronchial anatomy in syndromes with abnormal visceral situs, anormal spleen and congenital heart disease. American Journal of Cardiology 28: 456–462

Lev M 1954 Pathologic diagnosis of positional variations in cardiac chambers in congenital heart disease. Laboratory Investigation 3: 71–82

Liberthson R R, Paul M H, Muster A J, Arcilla R A, Eckner F A O, Lev M 1971 Straddling and displaced atrioventricular orifices and valves with primitive ventricles. Circulation 43: 213–226

Macartney F J, Partridge J B, Scott O, Deverall P B 1976a Common or single ventricle. An angiocardiographic and hemodynamic study of 42 patients. Circulation 53: 543–554

Macartney F J, Shinebourne E A, Anderson R H 1976b Connections, relations, discordance and distortions. British Heart Journal 38: 323–326

Macartney F J, Partridge J B, Shinebourne E A, Tynan M J, Anderson R H 1978 In: Anderson R H, Shinebourne E A (eds) identification of atrial situs. Churchill Livingstone, Edinburgh, p 16–26

Macartney F J, Zuberbuhler J R, Anderson R H 1980 Morphological considerations pertaining to recognition of atrial isomerism. Consequences for sequential chamber localisation. British Heart Journal 44: 657–667

Macartney F J, Tynan M, Smallhorn J F, Huhta J C, Deanfield J C, Anderson R H 1983 Clinical recognition of atrial isomerism. In: Anderson R H, Macartney F J, Shinebourne E A, Tynan M (eds) Paediatric cardiology, Vol 5. Churchill Livingstone, Edinburgh, p 205–214

Milo S, Ho S Y, Macartney F J, Wilkinson J L, et al 1979 Straddling and overriding atrioventricular valves morphology and classification. American Journal of Cardiology 44: 1122–1134

Otero Coto E, Wilkinson J L, Dickinson D F, Rufilanchas, J J, Marquez J 1979 Gross distortion of atrioventricular and ventriculo-arterial relations associated with left juxtaposition of atrial appendages – bizarre form of atrioventricular criss-cross. British Heart Journal 41: 486–492

Pacifico A D, Kirklin J W, Bargeron L M Jr 1973 Complex congenital malformations: surgical treatment of double-outlet right ventricle and double-outlet left ventricle. In: Kirklin J W (ed) Advances in cardiovascular surgery. Grune & Stratton, New York, p 57–76

Partridge J B, Scott O, Deverall P B, Macartney F J 1975 Visualization and measurement of the main bronchi by tomography as an objective indicator of thoracic situs in congenital heart disease. Circulation 51: 188–196

Quero-Jimenez M 1980 Inversion ventricular. Concepto, clasificacion y terminologia. Revista Latina de Cardiologia 1: 5–13

Quero-Jimenez M, Anderson R H, Tynan M, et al 1981 Summation of anatomic patterns of atrioventricular and ventriculo-arterial connexions. In: Godman M J (ed) Paediatric cardiology, Vol 4. Churchill Livingstone, Edinburgh, p 211–288

Ruttenberg H D 1977 Corrected transposition (L-transposition) of the great arteries: splenic syndromes (asplenia, polysplenia). Moss A J, Adams F H, Emmanouilides G C (eds) Heart disease in infants,

children and adolescents, 2nd Edn. Williams & Wilkins, Baltimore, p 338–354

Sato K, Ohara S, Tsukaguchi I, et al 1978 A criss-cross heart with concordant atrioventriculo-arterial connections. Circulation 57: 396–400

Shinebourne E A, Macartney F J, Anderson R H 1976 Sequential chamber localization: the logical approach to diagnosis in congenital heart disease. British Heart Journal 38: 327–340

Sridaromont S, Ritter D G, Feldt R H, Davis G D, Edwards J E 1978 Double-outlet right ventricle. Anatomic and angiographic correlations. Mayo Clinic Proceedings 53: 555–577

Stanger P, Rudolph A M, Edwards J E 1977 Cardiac malpositions: an overview based on study of sixty-five necropsy specimens. Circulation 56: 159–172

Tynan M J, Anderson R H 1979 Terminology of transposition of the great arteries. In: Godman M J, Marquis R M (eds) Paediatric cardiology, vol 2. Heart disease in the newborn. Churchill Livingstone, Edinburgh, p 341–349

Tynan M J, Becker A E, Macartney F J, Quero-Jimenez M, Shinebourne E A, Anderson R H 1979 Nomenclature and classification of congenital heart disease. British Heart Journal 41: 544–553

Tynan M, Becker A E, Freedom R M, et al 1981 Analysis of the ventriculo-arterial junction – connexions, infundibulum morphology and arterial relationships. In: Godman M J (ed) Paediatric cardiology, vol 4. Churchill Livingstone, Edinburgh, p 182–190

Van Mierop L H S 1971 Transposition of the great arteries. Clarification or further confusion? Editorial. American Journal of Cardiology 28: 735–738

Van Mierop L H S 1977 Pathology and pathogenesis of endocardial cushion defects. Surgical implications. In: Davila J C (ed) 2nd Henry Ford Hospital international symposium on cardiac surgery. Appleton-Century-Crofts, New York, p 201–207

Van Praagh R 1971 Transposition of the great arteries. II. Transposition clarified. American Journal of Cardiology 28: 739–741

Van Praagh R 1972 The segmental approach to diagnosis in congenital heart disease. Birth Defects 8: 4–23

Van Praagh R 1973 Conotruncal malformations. In: Barratt-Boyes B G, Neutze J M, Harris E A (eds) Heart disease in infancy. Churchill Livingstone, Edinburgh, p 140–188

Van Praagh R 1977 Terminology of congenital heart disease: glossary and commentary. Circulation 56: 139–143

Van Praagh R, Van Praagh S 1982 Embryology and anatomy: keys to the understanding of complex congenital heart disease. Coeur 13: 315–336

Van Praagh R, Vlad P 1978 Dextrocardia, mesocardia and levocardia: the segmental approach to diagnosis in congenital heart disease. In: Keith J D, Rowe R D, Vlad P (eds) Heart disease in infancy and childhood. Macmillan, New York, p 638–695

Van Praagh R, Ongley P A, Swan H J C 1964a Anatomic types of single or common ventricle in man: morphologic and geometric aspects of sixty necropsied cases. American Journal of Cardiology 13: 367–386

Van Praagh R, Van Praagh S, Vlad P, Keith J D 1964b Anatomic types of congenital dextrocardia. Diagnostic and embryologic implications. American Journal of Cardiology 13: 510–531

Van Praagh R, Perez-Trevino C, Lopez-Cuellar M, et al 1971 Transposition of the great arteries with posterior aorta, anterior pulmonary artery, subpulmonary conus and fibrous continuity between aortic and atrioventricular valves. American Journal of Cardiology 28: 621–631

Van Praagh R, Weinberg P H, Van Praagh S 1977 Malposition of the Heart. In: Moss A J, Adams F H, Emmanouilides G C (eds) Heart diseases in infants, children and adolescents. Williams & Wilkins, Baltimore, p 394–416

Van Praagh S, LaCorte M, Fellow K E, et al 1980 Superoinferior ventricles: angiocardiographic findings in ten postmortem cases. In: Van Praagh R, Takao A (eds) Etiology and morphology of congenital heart disease. Futura, New York, p 317–378

Van Praagh R, David I, Gordon D, Wright G B, Van Praagh S 1981 Ventricular diagnosis and designation. In: Godman M J (ed) Paediatric cardiology, vol 4. Churchill Livingstone, Edinburgh, p 153–168

Van Praagh R, Weinberg P M, Matsuoka R, Van Praagh S 1983 In: Adams F A, Emmanouildes G C (eds) Moss' Heart disease in infants and adolescents. Williams & Wilkins, Baltimore, p 422–457

Wilkinson J L, Acerete F 1973 Terminological pitfalls in congenital heart disease. Reappraisal of some confusing terms, with an account of a simplified system of basic nomenclature. British Heart Journal 35: 1166–1177

4

A. C. G. Wenink

Embryology of the heart

From the functional point of view, the heart is simply a specialised part of the vascular system. This is even clearer when regarding the organ from the developmental point of view. The heart forms as a specialised pumping portion of the vascular system, rather than as a pumping organ in itself. The formation of a coelomic cavity around this specialised portion of the vascular network undoubtedly aids its action. In this respect, cardiac development is fully comparable to the development of the digestive system. The primary anlage of the gut is the endodermal tube, whereas the mesoderm of the coelomic wall contributes to its muscular layers. In the case of the heart, the primary structure is formed by a pair of endothelial vessels. Again, the coelomic wall contributes to the muscular portion of the organ (Fig. 4.1).

Although the body of this chapter is devoted to morphogenesis of the heart itself, attention is given to the great veins and arteries as well. Understanding of development of these vessels requires a description of the position of the heart in the embryonic body, and of the processes which lead to the final topography. Therefore, the first section of this chapter concerns the early stages of cardiogenesis.

EARLY CARDIOGENESIS

Development of a vascular system is an early necessity in human embryology. Essentially, three different systems contribute to the vascular network. The yolk sac vessels (which are the first to arise) and the chorionic vessels form the vitelline and umbilical systems respectively. These two are extra-embryonic systems. The third component is completely intra-embryonic and is produced close to the developing central nervous system (Figs. 4.2 & 4.3).

A special site of blood vessel formation is found in the mesoderm at the anterior edge of the embryonic disc. This is the cardiogenic area. Many small vessels unite in this

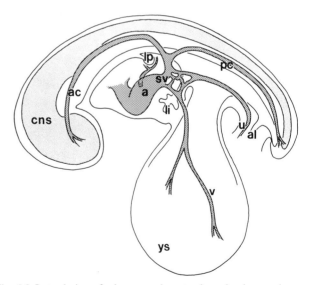

Fig. 4.2 Lateral view of a human embryo to show the three main venous systems draining into the sinus venosus (sv). The anterior (ac) and posterior (pc) cardinal veins develop in close proximity to the central nervous system (cns). Before entering the sinus venosus, the vitelline (v) and umbilical (u) veins have an anastomosing network within the septum transversum, where the liver (li) develops. The vessels surrounding the lung primordium (lp) are connected with the atrium (a) by a single pulmonary vein. ys – yolk sac; al – allantois within connecting stalk. Note that this diagram does not represent one single developmental stage.

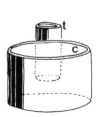 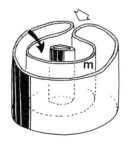

Fig. 4.1 Diagrams to show the principle by which the endocardial heart tube (t) gains an intrapericardial position. Part of the wall of the coelomic cavity (c) becomes the myocardial mantle (m). Initially, the dorsal mesocardium (open arrow) ensures the connection between extracoelomic mesenchyme and the heart tube. The space between heart tube and myocardial mantle (black arrow) is filled with cardiac jelly.

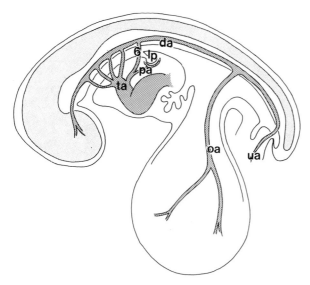

Fig. 4.3 Lateral view of a human embryo to show the main arterial system. The dorsal aorta (da), which is dorsal to the gut, gives rise to omphaloenteric (oa) and umbilical (ua) arteries. The truncus arteriosus (ta) connects with the dorsal aorta by way of branchial arch arteries, which are lateral to the foregut. The proximity of the lung primordium (lp) to the 6th branchial arch artery (6) is compatible with the origin of the pulmonary artery (pa).

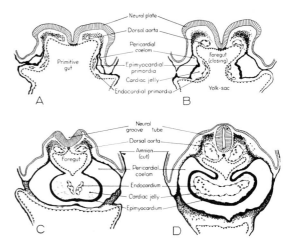

Fig. 4.4 Transverse sections of human embryos to show how the paired heart tubes, which are formed outside the coelomic cavity, fuse to form a single intracoelomic endocardial tube, which is surrounded by the myocardial mantle (here called 'epimyocardium'). (Reproduced with permission from Patten, 1968.)

area to form two distinct heart tubes. These left and right primordia fuse to give rise to a single endocardial heart tube.

Formation of the heart tube takes place in the mesoderm between the yolk sac and the rostral confluence of the left and right coelomic cavities. This rostral cavity will later become the pericardial cavity, but initially the paired heart tubes form outside this cavity. The process of fusion into a single tube is accompanied by invagination into the pericardial cavity. Since this invagination takes place without disruption of the coelomic wall, it provides the heart tube with a second, external layer, the myocardial mantle. At the site of invagination, the mesocardium connects the myocardial mantle with the coelomic wall and partly divides the pericardial cavity into left and right divisions (Fig. 4.4).

The endocardial tube is separated from the myocardial mantle by a space, filled with a loose reticulum – the cardiac jelly.

It has been thought that the external layer of the heart wall, the epicardium, derives from the myocardial mantle in situ, hence the name 'epimyocardium' (Patten, 1968). Evidence now shows, however, that the epicardial cells originate at the venous end of the heart tube, and spread out over the myocardial mantle (Manasek, 1969; Shimada & Ho, 1980; Virágh & Challice, 1981).

The initial site of cardiogenesis is not the most suitable for the heart to receive the veins of all three vascular beds. The heart will acquire this position by development of the head fold. The mesoderm rostral to the cardiogenic area turns ventrally and caudally and is laid down rostral to the

yolk sac and ventral to the foregut which is formed by this same process. This mesodermal mass is the septum transversum. The heart tube itself obtains a similar position ventral to the foregut and its venous end is anchored within the septum transversum. Thus, it is able to receive the vitelline veins, the umbilical veins and the cardinal veins. The first two systems form an anastomosing network.

The septum transversum with this wealth of anastomosing veins, within the area of liver development, is directly caudal to the foregut from which grow the lung buds. These grow out into the mesenchyme of the mediastinum which is continuous with the dorsal mesocardium. Therefore, the presence of the mesocardium is necessary to guarantee the union of the pulmonary venous plexus with the venous end of the heart (Fig. 4.2).

After formation of the head fold, the heart lies ventral to the foregut, whereas the main arteries of the embryo occupy a dorsal position. Communication of the arterial end of the heart with these left and right dorsal aorta can only be effected through the mesenchyme to the left and right sides of the foregut. This is the mesenchyme of the branchial arches, which alternates with the pharyngeal grooves and pouches. The vessels in these arches are the branchial arch arteries (Fig. 4.3).

Since lung development takes place directly caudal to the pharynx, development of the pulmonary arteries from the branchial system is easily understood (see below).

Formation of the cardiac loop

The embryonic heart, which is initially a more or less straight tube, soon acquires several curvatures and becomes an S-shaped organ. This transformation process is called 'looping'. Although it has been thought that the curvatures of the heart are caused by rapid growth of the tube within a much more slowly expanding pericardial cavity (Patten, 1968), transplantation experiments have shown that the heart is capable of looping without its normal arterial and venous attachments (Orts Llorca & Ruano Gil, 1967). Furthermore, exclusion of haemodynamics as a morphogenetic factor by stopping the beating of the heart still does not prevent the looping process (Manasek & Monroe, 1972). These data suggest that the looping process is an intrinsic ability of the heart itself. It has been shown that regional changes in myocardial cell shape and alignment go along with development of the curvatures (Manasek et al, 1972), but the exact cause of the looping process is still considered to be constituted by a number of different factors (Stallsberg, 1970; Manasek, 1981).

Normally, the heart tube curves to the right. Whatever may be the causes of the looping process, they are the expression of the overall left-right asymmetry of the human viscera. This asymmetry is even found at the level of cardiac histology, specifically in the arrangement of the conduction tissues (Anderson et al, 1974a; Gittenberger-de Groot & Wenink, 1978). The intrinsic asymmetry of the heart is even able to overcome temporary changes in the form of the cardiac loop due to experimental manipulation (Steding & Seidl, 1981).

The looping process itself demonstrates that different parts of the heart behave differently. These local differences are already present in the straight heart tube stage, where the myocardial mantle shows several constrictions (Davis, 1927). This means that, before looping, the heart already shows a compartmental organisation. Development of the heart is best described by using a 'segmental' approach,* and this approach is also of paramount importance when describing the mature heart, be it normal or congenitally malformed.

When the segmental approach is used in describing cardiac development, two problems arise. The first problem is that the segmental organisation of the embryonic heart is not as extreme as to enable me to deal with the different segments in a completely separate way. Segmental interactions are so important in development that gradually changing segmental relationships are more essential for the understanding of cardiac morphology than are their individual natural histories.

The second problem inherent to the segmental approach is produced by nomenclature. Many different terms have been used, and still are used, to describe the same part of the embryonic heart. The background of this confusion has

been described (Laane, 1974; Wenink & Gittenberger-de Groot, 1982a) and will not be repeated here. Suffice it to state that, for some structures in the embryonic heart, descriptive rather than nominative terms have been designed (Anderson & Becker, 1980; Wenink & Gittenberger-de Groot, 1982b), and these will be used in this chapter.

Primitive cardiac segments

The heart tube may be divided into five segments because of constrictions in the myocardial mantle (Fig. 4.5). These constrictions play a continuous role in further development. Evidently, they become more pronounced during the looping process, but their morphogenetic interest reaches far beyond the looping stage. Briefly, the events may be summarised as those processes which lead to septation and those which lead to valve formation. On theoretical grounds the two processes are very comparable because in both instances a more or less complete separation of adjacent segments is effected.

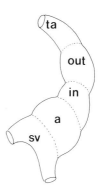

Fig. 4.5 Schematic view of the primitive heart tube, which consists of five individual segments: sinus venosus (sv), atrium (a), inlet (in), outlet (out) and truncus arteriosus (ta).

The junctions of the different segments have important anatomical characteristics. The myocardium at the junctions has been described as sphincters by Benninghoff (1923), who considered these rings to be the phylogenetic and ontogenetic precursors of the conduction system. These rings were described in constant relationships with superficial trabeculations ('Konturfasern', delineating fibres) which in turn indicated the original outline of the lumen of the segments. The 'delineating fibres' were also thought to be involved in the septation processes (Benninghoff, 1923).

On both sides of the myocardial mantle, accumulations of loosely built mesenchyme indicate the junctional zones. Outside the myocardium is found the subepicardial connective tissue ('sulcus tissue') which is a derivative of the epicardium (Virágh & Challice, 1981). Within the heart, the junctional zones are demarcated by 'endocardial

---

* Using the term 'segment' in this respect does not suggest that succeeding parts are identical, but rather that the different segments are separate parts of the initial tube. This usage has a long pedigree in cardiac embryology and morphology, but differs from the common biological usage.

cushions'. The latter are preceded by the 'cardiac jelly' (Davis, 1924, 1927) which is then invaded by cells derived from the endocardium (Markwald et al, 1977).

Intracardiac and extracardiac connective tissues collaborate in the separation of the individual segments. The fibrous atrioventricular rings of the mature heart are the result of this collaboration. For two reasons the separation has to be incomplete. The pumping function requires only cyclic closure of intersegmental junctions, which means valves are produced, not septa. On the other hand, the segments have to remain interconnected for the sake of impulse conduction. Here, the junctional myocardial rings play their role in formation of the conduction system (see below).

Complete septation is only effected within individual segments of the heart so as to separate lung and body circulations. Phylogenetically, valves precede the real septa but in human development valves are only formed after establishment of the segmental septa. Septum formation in the human heart may be effected in several different ways.

At both ends of the heart tube, where it is connected to the mediastinal vessels, the mediastinal mesenchyme plays an important role in septation. The venous sinus septum and the aortopulmonary septum are both of such extracardiac origin.

Within the ventricular part of the heart, two septa develop primarily from myocardium. The *primary septum* (arising between *inlet* and *outlet* – see below) develops as a myocardial fold, whereas the *inlet septum* (belonging to the *inlet* only) originates from coalescence of individual myocardial trabeculations.

Still another mode of septation is seen in the *atrioventricular junction*, where endocardial cushions fuse to separate left and right orifices. This endocardial septum is not important for further development in a material sense, for the cushions do not contribute extensively to any structure in the mature heart. Undoubtedly, however, normal septation will not occur if this endocardial septum fails to form. A similar situation is found in the *outlet* of the heart, where endocardial ridges fuse to form an embryonic *outlet septum*. There is insufficient data presently available on further development of the endocardial outlet septum, but it would not be surprising if it were found to make only a minimal contribution to the mature heart.

Septation may be effected in many different ways, each of which seems to be typical for the cardiac segment concerned. The different segments maintain their individuality throughout development and they are easily recognised in the mature heart.

Before looping, the segments show a caudocranial arrangement (Fig. 4.5). Caudally, the venous segment or *sinus venosus* is anchored within the mesenchyme of the septum transversum. This first segment receives the systemic veins of the embryo. The next segment is the *atrium*. From there, the future *ventricular* part of the heart

is reached, which has two separate divisions. The first division connected to the atrium is the *inlet*, and the next segment is the *outlet*.

As was mentioned above, these latter terms have been introduced recently (Anderson & Becker, 1980) to overcome the extreme terminological confusion which is overshadowing embryological discussions. The advantage of these terms is the fact that they apply to the mature heart as well. As will be shown, the mature ventricles have inlet and outlet portions which derive from the embryonic inlet and outlet respectively.

The final cardiac segment is the arterial segment or *truncus arteriosus* which is anchored in the mediastinal mesenchyme ventral to the foregut and which gives rise to the branchial arch arteries.

The external grooves which indicate the junctions of neighbouring segments are, in the same caudocranial order, the *sinu-atrial groove* between sinus venosus and atrium, the *atrioventricular groove* between atrium and inlet, the *primary groove* between inlet and outlet, and the *arterial groove* between outlet and truncus arteriosus. The latter is never a deep groove, but this junction may be recognised because the wall of the outlet consists of myocardium (myoblastic tissue in these early stages) whereas the truncal wall is made up of compact mesenchyme.

After looping, the grooves are much more pronounced. In particular, the atrioventricular and primary grooves are easily identified. The term 'primary' groove is used to indicate the importance of this junctional area. Earlier, this junction was called 'bulboventricular', in accordance with the fashion of the time (Wenink, 1981a).

DEVELOPMENT OF INDIVIDUAL SEGMENTS

The sinus venosus and the atrium

Development of the sinus venosus is dominated by the changes in the venous system of the embryo. Initially, the sinus venosus has bilaterally symmetrical *left and right sinus horns* which are embedded in the septum transversum. Gradually, the left sinus horn loses its importance because of disappearance of most of the left-sided venous connexions. The last connexion to disappear is that of the left cardinal veins, which leaves the left sinus horn as the exclusive drainage system of the myocardium (±25 mm crown-rump length (CRL), 7th week of development). This asymmetric development is also expressed by a more intimate relationship of the sinus venosus with the right part of the atrium. The sinu-atrial junction is displaced into the atrial cavity and this invagination process leads to valve formation as well as septation. As was suggested above, there is no fundamental difference between these two processes. The invagination process on the left side leads to complete partitioning of the left sinus horn from the left part of the atrium. A 'left sinu-atrial wall' (Los, 1960) is

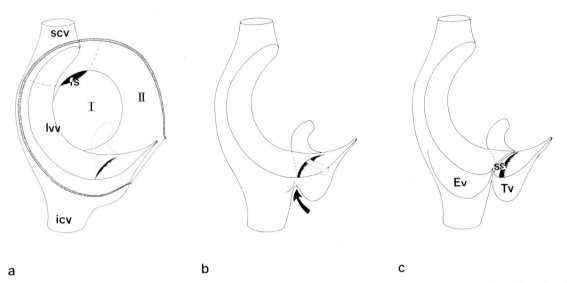

a   b   c

Fig. 4.6 Diagrams to show the incorporation of the sinus venosus into the right part of the atrium. Right lateral views. (a) The right atrium has been opened (cross-hatched sectioning line) and the components of the atrial septum are seen. I – septum primum; II – septum secundum; lvv – left venous valve. The foramen secundum (fs) is shown in black. The superior (scv) and inferior (icv) caval veins both belong to the right sinus horn. The left sinus horn is hidden by the atrial septal components. (b) Isolated illustration of the sinus venosus. Between the left and right sinus horns, the wall of the sinus venosus invaginates (black arrow) and the ostium of the left sinus horn (open arrow) becomes more demarcated. (c) Demarcation of left and right sinus horns is complete, resulting in the sinus septum (ss). By the same process, the right venous valve has been divided into Thebesian (Tv) and Eustachian (Ev) valves.

formed. This wall is a double structure, consisting of the walls of both sinus venosus and atrium, separated by a thin layer of extracardiac connective tissue. Further protrusion of the sinu-atrial junction into the right part of the atrial cavity forms the venous valves (Fig. 4.6).

The fact that the sinus venosus gains an exclusive connection with the right atrium is caused by development of the sinu-atrial septum. This septum is partly represented by the left sinu-atrial wall as mentioned above. The more anterior part of the sinu-atrial septum contributes also to interatrial septation. Before completion of atrial septation, this anterior portion is known as the *left venous valve*. It acquires continuity with the atrioventricular endocardial cushions, which divide the atrioventricular canal, and it extends forwards towards the posterior wall of the arterial pole of the heart. Being an infolding of the cardiac wall, it brings extracardiac connective tissue towards the posterior aortic wall, and it contributes to the fibrous skeleton of the heart (Van Gils, 1981), in particular to the anterior part of the tendon of Todaro (Anderson et al 1977; Wenink et al, 1978) (Fig. 4.7).

In the mature heart, the tendon of Todaro continues between the orifices of the coronary sinus and the inferior caval vein, to extend through the Eustachian valve (i.e. the valve of the inferior caval vein) into the extracardiac connective tissue (Todaro, 1865).

Essentially, the septation processes at the venous and arterial ends of the heart tube are very comparable (Los, 1978). The extracardiac septa may be considered in two different ways. On the one hand, these structures can be looked upon as growing into the heart, where they fuse

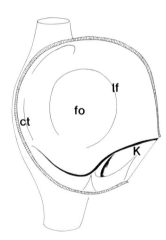

Fig. 4.7 As Figure 4.6a, after completion of atrial septation and formation of the sinus septum. The tendon of Todaro (tendon of the Eustachian valve), is shown in black. It forms the upper border of the triangle of Koch (K). fo – fossa ovalis; lf – limbus fossae ovalis; ct – crista terminalis.

with purely intracardiac septa. Alternatively, the venous and arterial poles may be considered as expanding into the mediastinal mesenchyme, incorporating part of this mesenchyme in the process. The amount of extracardiac connective tissue protruding into the atrial cavity may be considerable. It should not be mistaken for one of the atrioventricular endocardial cushions with which it becomes continuous (Fig. 4.8). Puerto Fonollà & Orts Llorca (1978) described well how the mesenchymal base of the septum primum, which had been called the spina vestibuli by His (1885), had the same appearance as the

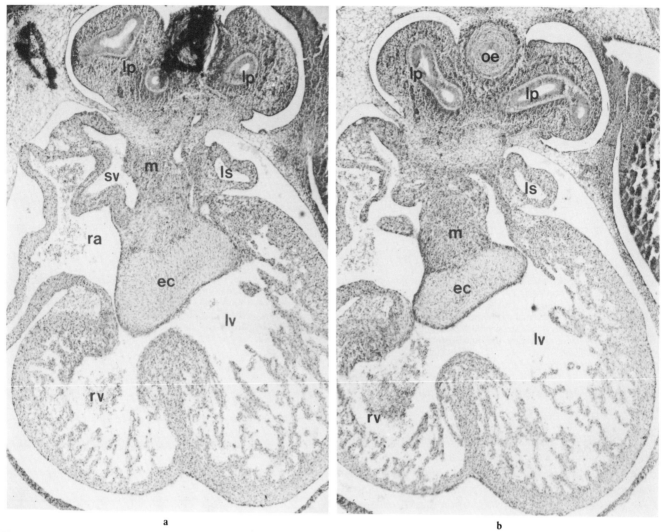

Fig. 4.8 Transverse sections of the heart of a human embryo of 9.5 mm CRL. (a) At the level of the entrance of the sinus venosus (sv) into the right atrium (ra), the mediastinal mesenchyme (m) is contiguous with the inferior endocardial cushion (ec). (b) More cranially, the extracardiac mesenchyme (m) forms a huge mass posterior to the inferior cushion (ec). rv – right ventricle; lv – left ventricle; ls – left sinus horn; lp – lung primordium; oe – oesophagus.

endocardial cushions. They showed its continuity with the mesocardial mesenchyme.

The continuity of extracardiac and intracardiac portions of mesenchyme at the sinu-atrial junction has two implications for further development. As the dorsal mesocardium, this connective tissue mass represents the connection of the dorsal atrial wall with the foregut. It enables the outgrowing pulmonary vein to reach the venous plexus surrounding the developing lungs (Los, 1960). At the same time, the dorsal mesocardium represents a temporary discontinuity in the posterior atrial wall. At this site, myocardial cells may be found in clusters or even seen as individual cells without much contact between them when examined using the light microscope (Fig. 4.9). At this site, and probably from these cells, the primary atrial septum is formed.

A relative lack of cellular coherence in the dorsal atrial myocardium would help to explain further the development of the septum primum. This septum, which develops between the left venous valve and the pulmonary venous orifice (Dalgleish, 1976), has to develop so as also to permit interatrial shunting throughout fetal life. Before closure of the subseptal primary foramen (between the septum primum and the atrioventricular endocardial cushions), the secondary foramen develops by disruption of myocardial continuity within the septum primum. Dalgleish (1976) observed a loose arrangement of the cardiac muscle cells prior to formation of this foramen. Morse (1978) has shown that withdrawal of myocardial cell contacts leaves individual strands of endocardium as the only bridges between the multiple foramina secunda of the chick heart. He subsequently suggested that controlled cell death plays only a minor role in development of these perforations (Morse, 1980).

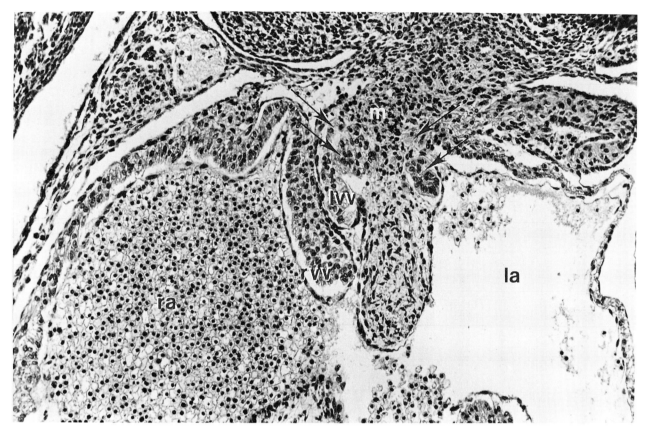

Fig. 4.9 Transverse section of the heart of a human embryo of 9.5 mm CRL (*not* the specimen shown in Fig. 4.8), to show the discontinuity in the dorsal atrial myocardial wall (arrows), which allows the mediastinal mesenchyme (m) to continue into the interior of the atrium. ra – right atrium; la – left atrium; rvv – right venous valve; lvv – left venous valve.

In man, the left venous valve and the septum primum are not the only contributions to the atrial septum. By the time the primary septum fuses with the atrioventricular endocardial cushions (11 mm CRL, 5th week of development) and the secondary foramen has formed, the space between the left venous valve and the septum primum widens. A ridge invaginates within this space, reinforcing the two septa already present. The ridge grows so as to form the septum secundum, which overlaps the flap valve of the septum primum. The space between the flap valve and the ridge is known as the foramen ovale, which only after birth is closed off by apposition of these two structures (Fig. 4.10).

Thus, the definitive atrial septum is a complex structure. At its base, two individual septal structures developed within the segments of the primary heart tube, i.e. the venous sinus septum and the primary atrial septum, the latter being reinforced by the secondary atrial septum, join each other. Between the two, a junctional septum, the sinu-atrial septum, completes partitioning. The free rim of the invaginated secondary septum remains visible as the rim of the oval fossa. The extent to which the right venous valve remains recognisable in the mature heart is variable. In the majority of cases, the Eustachian and Thebesian

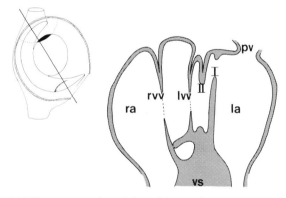

Fig. 4.10 Transverse section of the atrial part of an embryonic heart (about 30 mm CRL). The sectioning plane is indicated in the inset. ra – right atrium; la – left atrium; vs – ventricular septum; rvv – right venous valve; lvv – left venous valve; I – septum primum; II – septum secundum; pv – entrance of pulmonary veins.

valves (Fig. 4.11), together with the terminal crest, represent the embryonic right venous valve. More extensive persistence, may lead to the presence of a valve-like structure to the right of the superior caval vein, similar to and continuous with the Eustachian valve (Fig. 4.12).

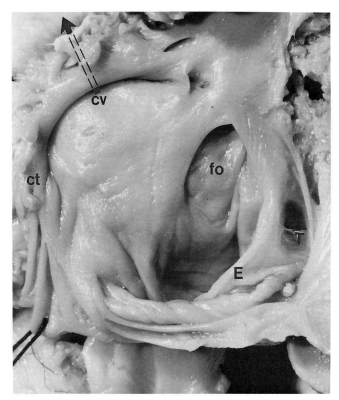

Fig. 4.11 Right atrium of a normal heart. fo – fossa ovalis; ct – crista terminalis; E – Eustachian valve; T – Thebesian valve; cv – superior caval vein.

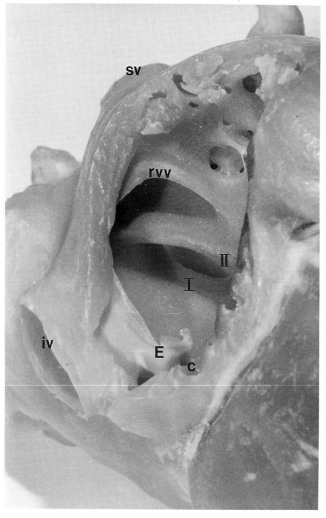

Fig. 4.12 Right atrium of a heart with tricuspid atresia, to show persistence of the cranial part of the right venous valve (rvv), guarding the orifice of the superior caval vein (sv). II – septum secundum; I – septum primum; E – redundant tissue of Eustachian valve; iv – inferior caval vein; c – ostium of coronary sinus.

The atrioventricular canal

In embryonic stages, the junction between the atrium and the inlet of the ventricular loop is indeed a canal with a certain length. It is supplied with a septum of its own, called the 'septum intermedium' by His (1885). However, the septum intermedium which develops by fusion of the upper and lower endocardial cushions (Hay & Low, 1972; Los & Van Eijndthoven, 1973) plays only a temporary role. When formed, it participates in the complex system of structures which divide the embryonic left and right blood streams (Steding & Seidl, 1980). But subsequently, it contributes very little to the mature heart (Van Gils, 1981; Wenink & Gittenberger-deGroot, 1985). Soon after its formation, its destruction by cell death has been observed (Hay, 1978).

The role of the atrioventricular endocardial cushions has probably been overaccentuated because of their visual prominence in embryonic stages. Research has been concentrated on early stages, and developmental studies after completion of septation are scarce. Kramer (1942) stated that, after fusion of the different endocardial swellings, the final fusion site would thin out and become fibrous, to form the membranous septum. I also (Wenink, 1975) described formation of the membranous septum without giving much data on the stages following closure of

the interventricular communication. Hay & Low (1972), describing fusion of the cushions in detail, discussed their work in terms of transformation of cushions into membranous septum. While Shaner (1949) blamed the atrioventricular cushions for having caused many malformations in pig embryo hearts, Doerr (1952) has shown that these cushions have to be considered as forming part of a more important set of ridges which precede development of the septal components. More recently Steding & Seidl (1980) have shown that formation of endocardial swellings is always preceded by changes in the form of the myocardial mantle. This already questions the prime role of the cushions. But, so as to prove the ephemeral significance of the endocardial cushions, it had to be shown that the atrioventricular valves as well as the fibrous skeleton were formed from extracardiac connective tissue (Van Gils, 1979, 1981; Wenink et al, 1985).

In my opinion, the atrioventricular canal should not be dealt with as a separate cardiac segment, such as has been done by Van Praagh (1972). It is a *junctional* structure, which merits discussion where the conducting system is concerned (see below). But apart from that, it is simply the ostium between atrium and inlet and it is best described together with the inlet. Its importance in formation of the atrioventricular valves will be described in a separate paragraph.

The inlet and the outlet

The terminological confusion concerning the ventricular portion of the embryonic heart (Laane, 1974) has made it difficult to use nominative terms, even if properly defined. Careful study of the literature (see Wenink & Gittenberger-de Groot, 1982a) leads to the conclusion that Anderson & Becker (1980) were right in choosing new descriptive terms for the two cardiac segments which contribute to the ventricles. Since recent investigation of development of the ventricles (Wenink, 1981a, b) has shown that, in the human embryonic heart, the two segments which contribute to the ventricles of the mature heart retain their functional status of inlet and outlet throughout development, the descriptive terms 'inlet' and 'outlet' are indeed appropriate. The point to be made is not that the two contributing segments have never been recognised, but that they have been called by the wrong names. The matter is complicated by the fact that more than two segments have been distinguished as contributing to the definitive left and right ventricles. In particular, the work of Pernkopf & Wirtinger (1933) led to a school of embryologists who recognised a proampulla, a metampulla and a bulbus as contributing to the ventricles. Doerr (1980, personal communication) has stated that these terms, which are derived from comparative embryology, probably do not hold for human development. Furthermore, comparative anatomy of the ventricular septum has been shown (Van Mierop & Kutsche, 1981) to accord with the views on human development as presently espoused (Wenink, 1981b). It seems most appropriate, therefore, to ignore these contentious nominative terms and to describe simply the development of the inlet and the outlet, these being the only two cardiac segments which contribute to the mature left and right ventricles.

Three septal components are necessary to divide these two primitive segments. The intimate relationships of inlet and outlet resemble those between sinus venosus and atrium. As was described above, these two segments develop their own individual septa in addition to an intersegmental septum: the sinu-atrial septum. Similarly, expansion of inlet and outlet cavities leads to the formation of a partial septum between the two. This septum can be called the primary ventricular septum. In addition to this intersegmental septum, both the inlet and the outlet are provided with their own intrinsic septa, which can then be called the 'inlet septum' and the 'outlet septum' respectively. The three components of the ventricular septum cannot be formed in one plane. This was recognised by Meredith et al (1979), who described the septum to be formed along a spiral which can be followed from the atrioventricular cushions, along the anterior ventricular wall and into the 'crista supraventricularis'. The incorporation of several different structures in the formation of one ventricular septum may be understood by the notion that functional separation of left and right blood streams has taken place before development of the septum (Steding & Seidl, 1980; McBride et al, 1981), because this means two parallel bloodstreams instead of a single one traversing the serial segments.

Although both segments contributing to the ventricles develop their own septa, the first component of the ventricular septum arises from a fold between the inlet and the outlet. This fold is indicated externally by a groove, the primary groove, and encircles the internal communication between the two segments (Fig. 4.13). The communication is similarly called the 'primary foramen'. Expansion of the cavities of the inlet and outlet takes place predominantly in an anterior and apical direction, causing local elevation of the primary fold. Thus exagerrated, the anterior and apical part of the fold deserves the name of 'primary septum'. It should be noted that this first septum, which will become interventricular, is also intersegmental. It separates the anterior and apical part of the inlet from the anterior and apical part of the outlet. Similarly, the communication above the rim of this septum (the primary foramen) is an intersegmental communication. The adop-

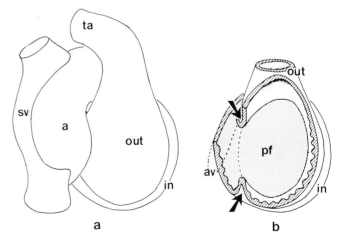

Fig. 4.13 (a) Right lateral views of the segmented heart after looping. sv – sinus venosus; a – atrium; in – inlet; out – outlet; ta – truncus arteriosus. (b) As (a), after removal of sinus venosus, atrium and truncus arteriosus. The remaining inlet (in) and outlet (out) have been opened to show the intervening primary fold (arrows). The primary fold contacts the atrioventricular junction (av) in the inner curvature of the heart (upper arrow). pf – primary foramen. (Reproduced from Wenink & Gittenberger-de Groot, 1982b.)

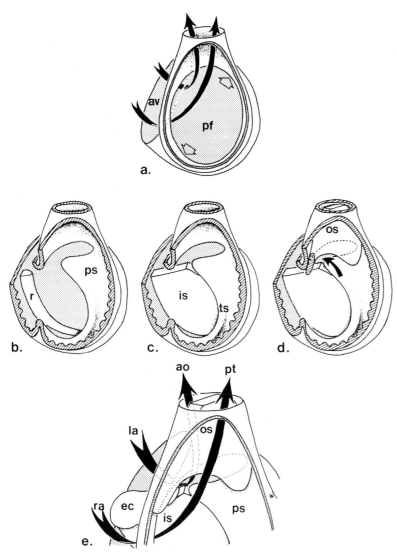

Fig. 4.14 Diagrams to show development of the ventricular septal components. Right lateral views. (a) Before septation. The arrows indicate the left and right blood streams, which have to pass both the atrioventricular (av) and the primary (open arrows) junction. pf – primary foramen. (b) Growth of inlet and outlet segments leads to expansion of the intervening primary fold, resulting in the primary septum (ps). At the same time, inlet trabeculations coalesce to form a muscular ridge (r) on the posterior wall of the inlet. (c) The posterior ridge has grown out to form the inlet septum (is), which has fused with the primary septum. The posterior rim of the latter remains visible as trabecula septomarginalis (ts). (d) Endocardial ridges in the distal part of the outlet have fused to form the outlet septum (os). A small interventricular communication (arrow) is still present. The left part of the primary fold (stippled line) is in the left ventricle, hidden by the outlet septum. (e) As (d), with addition of the fused atrioventricular endocardial cushions (ec), which are present in previous stages, although not depicted. The boundaries of the interventricular communication are: outlet septum (os), primary septum (ps), inlet septum (is) and atrioventricular endocardial cushion (ec). Note that this communication has nothing to do with the primary foramen. The arrows indicate the bloodstreams from right atrium (ra) to pulmonary trunk (pt) (through right part of the primary foramen) and from left atrium (la) to aorta (ao) (through left part of primary foramen). (a) and (e) are reproduced from Wenink & Gittenberger-de Groot, 1982b.

tion of this term 'primary foramen' is an attempt to avoid the possible confusion inherent in the use of the term 'interventricular foramen', which has been described as existing (depending on the developmental stage reached) in two (Van Mierop et al, 1963) or even three different forms (Goor et al, 1970). In contrast, the primary foramen, which connects two serial segments, remains the same throughout development in being traversed by both the left and the right bloodstreams (Fig. 4.14).

The first indication of separation of left and right bloodstreams within the inlet has been observed in an embryo of 3.6 mm CRL (Wenink, 1981a). The myocardial trabeculations, which are particularly numerous on the posterior inlet wall, were seen to have coalesced to form a posterior muscular ridge continuous with the lower atrioventricular cushion. This ridge is the anlage of the inlet septum (Figs. 4.14 & 4.15). On the atrial side it has already been described how the atrial septum primum develops in contiguity with the atrioventricular cushions. Therefore,

the atrial septum primum and the inlet septum develop in the same plane. Completion of septation at this level will make the right atrium communicate with the right part of the inlet and the left atrium with the left part of the inlet. No 'shift' of the atrioventricular canal to the right (de la Cruz & Miller, 1968) is necessary to account for this final arrangement. Similarly, the alternative explanation offered by Dor & Corone (1979), namely that the septum migrates to the left, is unnecessary and takes no account of the fact that the inlet septum is of intrasegmental origin.

Fusion of the inlet septum with the left and posterior side of the primary septum leads to formation of the larger part of the ventricular septum. The multifocal origin of the septum has been denied by Harh & Paul (1975), who described trabecular aggregation as the sole mode of septum formation. As indicated above, my observations show that this is the way in which the inlet septum forms, but it differs from the way in which the primary fold enlarges to form the primary septum. It should also be

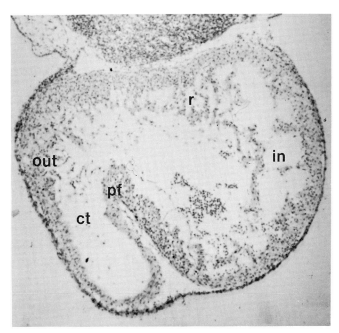

Fig. 4.15 Transverse section of a human embryo of 3.6 mm CRL. The inlet (in) and outlet (out) are partly separated by the anterior primary fold (pf). The posterior wall of the inlet is invested with small trabeculations constituting a loose ridge (r). The distal part of the outlet is filled with endocardial cushion tissue (ct). (Reproduced from Wenink & Gittenberger-de Groot, 1982b.)

stressed that these two septa are not identical to the 'posterior smooth' and 'posterior trabeculated' septa as distinguished by Goor et al (1970). The difference lies in the introduction of 'imaginary lines' by these authors. In fact the demarcation of inlet and primary septa on the right side remains visible throughout development. Because the inlet septum fuses with the posterior and leftward aspects of the primary septum, the posterior and rightward rim of the primary septum remains more or less free. It can be recognised as the septomarginal trabecula of the mature right ventricle. The primary septum is not entirely comparable to the 'trabecular septum' as initially described by Anderson et al (1977), since this septal component was illustrated to be divided by the septomarginal trabecula. In a more recent modification of this concept (Anderson et al, 1981), the septomarginal trabecula was stated to form the posterior border of the 'trabecular septum'. This modification is in keeping with my own concept.*

It is for reasons of clarity that these septal components are described separately (Fig. 4.14). But one must stress that in life they develop as a single unit, no normal developmental stage being known in which the primary septum can be distinguished without there being any indication of the inlet septum.

---

* *Editors' note.* The author is correct in pointing to the early mistake of Anderson et al (1977). We now concur wholeheartedly with his concept as here expressed.

It follows from the discussion thus far that the primary foramen is an intersegmental communication which can never be closed. Both the left and the right bloodstreams (being to the left and right sides of the inlet septum respectively) must traverse the borders of the primary fold so as to reach the outlet. To facilitate this understanding, it is helpful to appreciate that, after formation of the ventricular septum, distinction between left and right ventricles has become possible. The apical component of the inlet, which is to the left of the inlet septum and to the left of the primary septum, has formed the apex of the developing left ventricle. To the right of the inlet and primary septa, the right part of the inlet segment and the apical part of the outlet segment together constitute the developing right ventricle. Thus, the right ventricle too possesses inlet and outlet portions. The boundary between them is indicated by the septomarginal trabecula, which is a derivative of the primary fold. A further derivative of this fold lies in the roof of the right ventricle from whence it passes into the left ventricle. This right-sided portion of the primary fold, which at the same time forms the anterior boundary of the atrioventricular canal, forms part of the crista supraventricularis (Fig. 4.16). Thus, the blood coming from the right atrium has to pass these junctional structures to reach the right ventricular outlet portion. In doing so, it uses the right ventricular part of the primary foramen (Fig. 4.14).

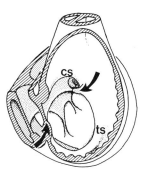

Fig. 4.16 Right lateral view of the mature right ventricle, to show the remnants of the primary fold. The arrows indicate its contribution to the tension apparatus of the tricuspid valve. cs – crista supraventricularis; ts – trabecula septomarginalis. (Reproduced from Wenink & Gittenberger-de Groot, 1982a.)

A similar situation exists in the left ventricle, where the left ventricular part of the primary fold is found as a basal structure, continuing from the crista supraventricularis into the left ventricle where it lies between the atrioventricular canal and the future aortic orifice. Thus the primary fold passes through the roof of the interventricular communication. From its position between atrioventricular and aortic orifices, the fold curves anteriorly. Here, the ring rejoins with the anterior and apical part of the fold which has expanded to form the primary septum. The left part of the fold thus surrounds the outlet portion of the left

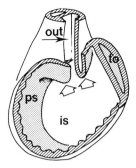

Fig. 4.17 Left lateral view of the left ventricle after completion of septation, but before valve formation. The left ventricular part of the primary fold (open arrows) has been sectioned to show the entrance into the outlet portion of the left ventricle (out). ps – primary septum; is – inlet septum; to – tricuspid orifice. The stippled line indicates the mitral orifice. (Reproduced from Wenink & Gittenberger-de Groot, 1982b.)

with those of McBride et al (1981) insofar as we were unable to demonstrate more than one continuous pair of endocardial outlet ridges. An important factor in this confusion may be the exact site of arterial valve formation, which is discussed below.

Fusion of the endocardial outlet ridges establishes the outlet septum. Before septation is completed, therefore, an interventricular communication is found which has the following boundaries: the outlet septum cranially, the primary ventricular septum anteriorly and caudally, and the inlet septum and the atrioventricular endocardial cushions posteriorly (Fig. 4.14). Here, the primary fold in the roof of the defect is not mentioned as a bordering structure because it is covered by the endocardial cushion tissue of the atrioventricular cushions posteriorly and the outlet septum anteriorly (Fig. 4.18) (Wenink et al, 1985). Ultimate

ventricle. It delimits the left ventricular part of the primary foramen, which is traversed by the blood coming from the left atrium and reaching the left ventricular outlet portion (Fig. 4.17).

It is important to note the difference between the communication that was termed the 'primary foramen' and that which can now justifiably be called the 'interventricular communication'. The primary foramen is a permanent orifice which connects inlet and outlet segments and, after septation, inlet and outlet portions of both ventricles. The very process of septation divides the primary foramen into left and right ventricular parts. The interventricular communication, however, is not intersegmental. It only exists during the process of septation, being closed by the ultimate act of septation. Thus, it may only be recognised from the time at which left and right ventricles are distinguishable, i.e. when the larger part of the ventricular septum is formed. The complete borders of the interventricular communication can only be described when all components of the septum are developed.

It is therefore necessary to account for the third septal component, which has yet to be discussed. It is the intrasegmental septum belonging to the outlet and is called simply the 'outlet septum'. The outlet septum is different from the other two components in that it is not primarily a muscular structure.

In embryos of 6 mm CRL, a pair of endocardial ridges is seen (Los, 1968), having been moulded from the continuous layer of cardiac jelly seen in younger stages. These ridges can be called the 'outlet ridges'. There has been confusion as to the number of outlet ridges. Two pairs of ridges, proximal and distal ones (Van Mierop et al, 1963) were stated to be normal in the chick (Pexieder, 1978). In contrast, de la Cruz & Da Rocha (1956) had distinguished between three sets of ridges: proximal, distal and intermediate ones. The latter were to be found at the level of the arterial valves. The author's findings are in keeping

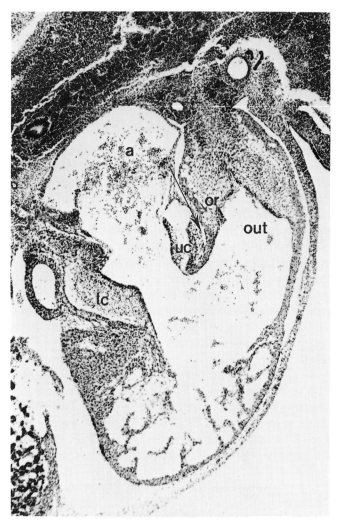

Fig. 4.18 Sagittal section of the heart of a human embryo of 10 mm CRL, to show that primary and atrioventricular grooves coincide in the lesser curvature (arrow). The fold is covered by the upper atrioventricular cushion (uc) and the right posterior outlet ridge (or). lc – lower atrioventricular cushion; a – atrium; out – outlet to pulmonary orifice. (Reproduced from Wenink et al, 1985.)

closure of the interventricular communication (about 16 mm CRL) is effected by fusion of these endocardial structures with each other and with the endocardial ridge on the rim of the primary ventricular septum (Kramer, 1942; Odgers, 1937/1938). The latter is an extension of the left outlet ridge (Wenink, 1971).

Most reports have suggested that the membranous septum is itself formed from these fusing endocardial tissues which surround the interventricular communication. The way in which this fibrous structure is formed has not yet been well established. With respect to the possible role of the outlet septum it has been stated that this endocardial structure leaves no remnants in the mature heart and that it is not muscularised to form an adult outlet septum (Van Mierop, 1977). Okamoto et al (1981), however, have shown cell death foci in the outlet septum which are invaded by myocardial cells. The problem may be solved by further studies in which all structures bordering the interventricular communication are followed into relatively late developmental stages.* It has already been shown that completion of the membranous septum takes place very late (Allwork & Anderson, 1979).

A mechanism which has given problems in understanding is the 'transfer' of the aortic orifice to the left ventricle (Los, 1968). Intricate torsions in the outlet region of the heart have been both described (Pernkopf & Wirtinger, 1933; Asami, 1969) and denied (de la Cruz & Da Rocha, 1956; Pexieder, 1978). Steding & Seidl (1980) have accounted for the final connexion of the aortic orifice to the left ventricle without having any need for recourse to the controversial torsions. The present description of septum formation shows that, simply by the establishment of the outlet septum, the aorta is definitively placed above the left ventricle. The left part of the outlet segment is allotted to the left ventricle by this septation process, in very much the same way as the right part of the inlet was allotted to the right ventricle by formation of an inlet septum.

A further controversial process has been the so-called 'absorption' of part of the outlet, which has been considered necessary to bring the aorta to the left (Goor et al, 1972; Anderson et al, 1974b). de la Cruz & Da Rocha (1956) have denied this 'conus absorption' but they did describe 'disappearance of the conoventricular flange' (this latter structure being the primary fold of this account). Dor & Corone (1973) speak of 'résorption de la chambre conal gauche' (resorption of the left outlet chamber), rather than of resorption of its wall. Such a description would perfectly

fit with my own observations. Indeed, by formation of the outlet septum, the left part of the outlet portion of the heart is *incorporated* into the left ventricle. What, then, happens to the wall of the outlet segment? Does it disappear or can it be distinguished in the mature heart? As will be shown in the paragraph on valve formation, this part of the outlet wall, which is part of the primary fold, does not disappear. It has separated inlet from outlet in early stages, and so it does in the mature heart. It forms the anterior aortic leaflet of the mitral valve. The process by which this valve and its tension apparatus are formed leads to the disappearance of markers on the ventricular septum which might distinguish its three components.

The relative positions of the ascending aorta and the pulmonary trunk are not explained by what happens within the outlet. The spiral course of the arteries is produced at a more distal level, occurring within the arterial segment (truncus arteriosus).

The arterial junction and the truncus arteriosus

It is most practical to define the site of arterial valve formation as the distal end of the outlet, and to consider the truncus arteriosus as part of the arterial system rather than part of the heart itself (Orts Llorca et al, 1982). Prior to formation of the arterial valves, the distinction between these segments is made according to the mesenchymal nature of the truncal wall. Moreover, the myocardial outlet segment is lined internally by endocardial ridges, while the truncus arteriosus is not.

The truncus arteriosus and the sinus venosus are comparable in that they develop intimate relationships with the surrounding mesenchyme (Los, 1978). The way in which their septa develop is an expression of this fact. Furthermore, the sinus venosus exemplifies its relationships with vessels by receiving the cardiac veins, while the truncus arteriosus gives rise to the ostia of the coronary arteries. On the other hand, the two segments differ considerably. The sinus venosus is largely incorporated into the atrium, whilst the truncus arteriosus remains demarcated from the outlet. The way in which the sinu-atrial valves develop is completely different from the mode of arterial valve formation (see below). But this does not mean that the truncus arteriosus is not intimately related to the outlet. The septum of the truncus arteriosus, i.e. the aortopulmonary septum, becomes firmly anchored to the myocardial outlet wall.

Expansion of the truncus arteriosus into the branchial mesenchyme takes place asymmetrically. Less expansion is seen between the origins of the fourth and sixth branchial arch arteries, and branchial mesenchyme between these origins seems to grow inward. This leads to formation of the aortopulmonary septum, which is complete in embryos of 12 mm CRL (Orts Llorca et al, 1982). Los (1978) has shown that this septum is easily identified in

---

* *Author's note*: After completion of this manuscript the studies of Margot M. Bartelings, presently working in our department, have shown that the outlet septum forms as a primarily muscular structure which is only covered by the endocardial outlet ridges. This confirms the statement by Steding & Seidl (1980) that formation of endocardial swellings is preceded by changes in the form of the myocardial mantle.

luminal reconstructions of this region, but not so readily in reconstructions of the solid tissues (i.e. the branchial mesenchyme). This important observation stresses arterial expansion as the primary event. When this is recognised, it becomes clear that any arterial expansion at all will lead to the formation of 'interarterial septa'. A septum defined in these terms is any mesenchymal tissue intervening between arterial lumina. This is exactly what Seidl & Steding (1981) have shown in their scanning electron micrographs of the lumen of the truncus arteriosus and the branchial arch arteries. They have shown that the aorto-pulmonary septum is simply the most prominent of a series of 'interarterial septa'.

Fusion of the aortopulmonary septum with the endo-cardial outlet septum is a complex process. The outlet

ridges have fused at the site of future arterial valve forma-tion before complete fusion with the extracardiac septum takes place (De Vries, 1981). The left and right limbs of the aortopulmonary septum extend towards the endocardial ridges (Seidl & Steding, 1981) and form a sort of root within these ridges (Laane, 1978, 1979; Dor & Corone, 1981) (Figs. 4.19 & 4.20). Laane (1979) has stated that the origin of these roots is not certain. Current investi-gations taking place in the author's department show that the histology of normal human embryos does not always allow full distinction between the endocardial swellings of the outlet segment and the 'roots' of the extracardiac aorto-pulmonary septum (Bartelings, unpublished observations).

More precise knowledge is therefore needed concerning late development and relationships of the aortopulmonary

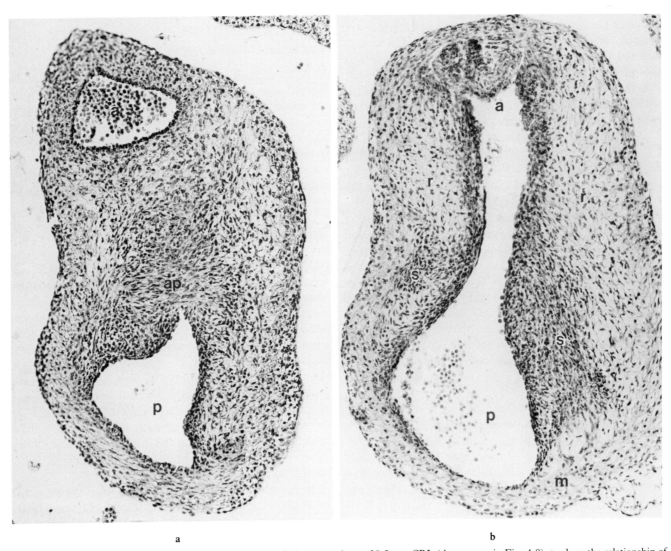

a   b

Fig. 4.19 Transverse sections of the arterial pole of the heart of a human embryo of 9.5 mm CRL (the same as in Fig. 4.8), to show the relationship of extracardiac mesenchyme and endocardial cushion tissue. (a) The aortopulmonary septum (ap) is wedged between the pulmonary orifice (p) and the ascending aorta (a). (b) More apically, the aortopulmonary septum has sent two spurs (s) into the two main endocardial outlet ridges (r). These spurs are contiguous with the myocardial wall (m) of the outlet. At this level, the aortic (a) and pulmonary (p) tracts are not yet fully separated (compare Fig. 4.20).

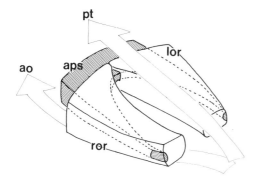

Fig. 4.20 Diagram to show how, in a human embryo of 9.5 mm CRL, the aortopulmonary septum (aps) sends its two spurs into the left (lor) and right (ror) endocardial outlet ridges. These structures are shown in a highly schematic, right lateral view, after removal of the myocardium. The arrows indicate the bloodstreams into the pulmonary trunk (pt) and the aorta (ao). (compare Fig. 4.19). (After a reconstruction by M. Bartelings MD, with her permission.)

septum and the endocardial outlet septum. In this respect, the anomaly of complete transposition has represented a challenge to all cardiac embryologists, and this challenge has lead to a wealth of theories. Only when the exact fate of these embryonic septa in the mature heart is known can the morphogenesis of ventriculo-arterial discordance be clarified. It should be pointed out that the distinction of an outlet septum (or conal or infundibular septum) in malformed hearts is mainly the consequence of definitions. Detailed descriptions of cardiac development are usually concluded at the moment of closure of the interventricular communication, when there is only an endocardial outlet septum. Van Mierop's statement, that this septum has no substantial representation in the mature heart (Van Mierop, 1977), has yet to receive unequivocal confirmation. The exact origin of the muscular septum which separates the subarterial outflow tracts has yet to be established (see footnote to p. 95). Only when it has, might it be clarified whether a discordant ventriculo-arterial connexion is induced below, at, or above the level of arterial valve formation.

VALVE FORMATION

The human heart is provided at several sites with valves. In all instances regurgitation to a proximal segment is prevented. This is the only analogy. Morphogenesis and final anatomy differ from level to level.

The sinu-atrial valves

The valve-like structures at the sinu-atrial junction are most conspicuous during development. The function of their mature remnants seems to be relatively unimportant. From a morphological point of view, however, the developmental histories of the left and right venous valves, i.e.

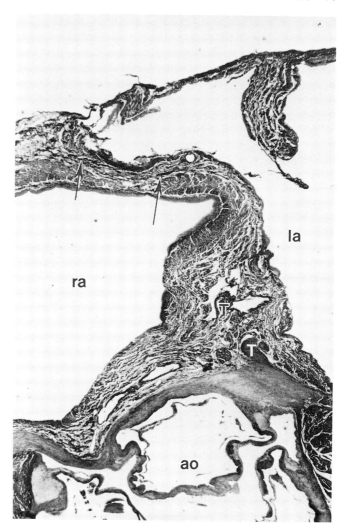

Fig. 4.21 Transverse section of a neonatal heart, showing the complex architecture of the atrial septum. ra – right atrium; la – left atrium; ao – aortic orifice; T – tendon of Todaro. Note also fibrous tissue (arrows) other than Todaro's tendon.

the structures which develop by invagination of the sinus venosus into the right part of the atrium, are very important, particularly because they are different from one another. The left venous or sinu-atrial 'valve' participates in atrial septation, since it reinforces the right side of the primary and secondary atrial septal structures. In the mature heart, no distinct remnant of this 'valve' can be found, unless the very complicated myocardial architecture of the atrial septum (Fig. 4.21) can be taken to indicate its complex developmental background.

The right sinu-atrial valve remains recognisable, albeit in various forms in individual hearts. Here, as in some other regions of the heart, the boundary between normal variation and clear-cut pathology is difficult to establish. In most instances the anterior portion of the right venous valve persists to guard the coronary sinus orifice. It is known as the Thebesian valve and is a thin fibrous structure. The posterior part of the right venous valve usually persists as the Eustachian valve, a similarly fibrous structure which guards the orifice of the inferior caval vein (see Figs. 4.7 & 4.11). The anatomy of this valve may vary considerably. In individual cases it may reach far cranially, so as to provide a valve also for the ostium of the superior caval vein. More usually the Eustachian valve is not so large and most of the right venous valve disappears to leave as its remnant the muscular terminal crest. This internal ridge corresponds with the external terminal sulcus. The terminal crest marks the boundary between the smooth-walled sinus venosus and the trabeculated embryonic atrium.

The right venous valve is a muscular valve-like structure from early stages (6 mm CRL, Los, 1968) and part of it persists as a fibrous flap in the mature heart. As such, it is very different from the other valves in the human heart, which develop in much later stages.

The atrioventricular valves

Initially, the atrioventricular canal is lined by a continuous mass of cardiac jelly (see above) from which develop gradually the superior and inferior atrioventricular endocardial cushions. These cushions undoubtedly have a valve-like function and most investigators (Odgers, 1939; Van Mierop et al, 1962; Ugarte et al, 1976) have described the cushions to be the precursors of the valves. On the other hand, the role of ventricular myocardium in the formation of the tension apparatus has also received attention (Sato, 1914; Van Mierop & Gessner, 1972). More recently the cushions have been described as contributing only minimally to the valves, the major parts of the valve leaflets as well as all of the tendinous chords and papillary muscles being derived from ventricular myocardium (Van Mierop, 1977).

Such contrasting opinions made it necessary to reinvestigate valve development particularly to focus on later stages. Studies in our laboratory have confirmed the role of the endocardial cushions to be temporary and minimal. These observations showed that the atrioventricular valves were formed mainly by invagination of sulcus tissue and by undermining of ventricular myocardium (Van Gils, 1979, Wenink et al, 1985). The process of valve formation is strictly confined to the ventricular inlet segment. The general principle of invagination of the atrioventricular junction concurs with expansion of the inlet, and leads to formation of a three-layered flap hanging down into the inlet. The outer layers of the flap consist of atrial and inlet ventricular myocardium. The middle layer is formed by the ingrowing sulcus tissue. Endocardial cushion tissue is found at the apex of the flap and on its atrial aspect (Fig. 4.22). The initial continuity of atrial and inlet myocardium is disrupted in embryos of 30 mm CRL, in which the extracardiac sulcus tissue is seen to be continuous with the intracardiac cushion tissue (Figs. 4.23 &

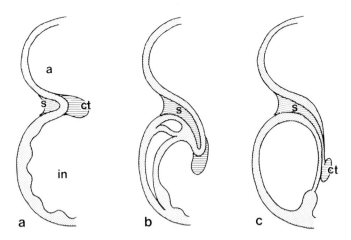

Fig. 4.22 Diagrams to show the processes of invagination of the atrioventricular junction and undermining of inlet myocardium, which lead to formation of the atrioventricular valves. (a) Before valve formation, endocardial cushion tissue (ct) has a valve like function. s – atrioventricular sulcus tissue; a – atrium; in – inlet. (b) Expansion of atrium and inlet leads to invagination of sulcus tissue (s). At the same time, inlet myocardium is undermined to form the tension apparatus. (c) After completion of these processes, valve and papillary muscles are present. Further histogenesis will lead to a fibrous valve leaflet and tendinous chords. The continuity of atrial and ventricular myocardium has been disrupted by sulcus tissue (s). Remnants of cushion tissue (ct) are found on the apical rim of the leaflet. (Reproduced from Wenink et al, 1985.)

4.24). It is important to note that, with this process, the original atrioventricular junction comes to lie near to the apex of the valve leaflet. The invagination of sulcus tissue coincides in time with undermining of the inner layers of the inlet myocardium. The result is production of a complete muscular valve leaflet (albeit with a mesenchymal middle layer) having muscular cords and papillary muscles. Only in fetuses of 3 months is the muscular tissue of the valve leaflets and chords replaced by connective tissue. Not all valve leaflets mature in the same period. Formation of the septal leaflet of the tricuspid valve is completed extremely late. It is the final steps of this undermining process which lead to complete establishment of the membranous septum around the time of birth (Allwork & Anderson, 1979).

The use of the inner layers of the inlet ventricular myocardium to form the valvar tension apparatus has consequences for the anatomy of the endocardial surface of this segment. Before valve formation, the trabeculations in the inlet and the outlet show identical patterns. But the inlet trabeculations are involved in valve formation and at the end of the undermining process a relatively smooth surface with only fine trabeculations is left behind. Therefore, the trabecular pattern of the inlet becomes different from that of the outlet, this latter segment being left undisturbed by valve formation (Wenink & Gittenberger-de Groot, 1982b). The typical differences between left and right ventricular trabecular patterns (Anderson et al, 1978) are caused by the fact that the apex of the left ventricle (its

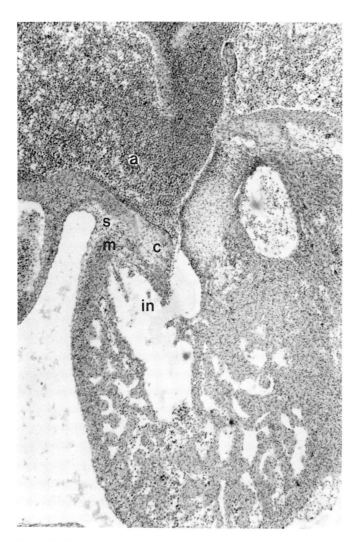

Fig. 4.23 Transverse section of the heart of a human embryo of 18 mm CRL, to show the invaginated atrioventricular junction. a – atrium; in – inlet; s – sulcus tissue; c – cushion tissue; m – myocardium.

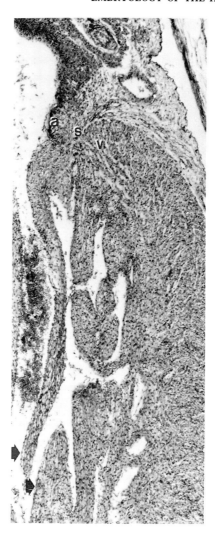

Fig. 4.24 Section of a fetal heart (40 mm CRL), showing an atrioventricular valve leaflet, which still has only muscular tension apparatus (arrows). Further invagination of sulcus tissue (s) has disrupted the continuity of atrial (a) and ventricular (v) myocardium.

'trabecular zone') derives from the inlet, whereas the apex ('trabecular zone') of the right ventricle stems from the outlet. Perhaps it would be more exact (particularly where complex cardiac malformations are concerned) to speak of 'typical inlet and outlet trabecular patterns'.

The topography of atrioventricular valve formation needs further consideration. The walls of the left-sided and right-sided components of the inlet segment (i.e. the inlet portions of the left and right ventricles) are made up of the parietal wall of the inlet, the inlet septum and, of course, the primary fold. In a sense, the looping process which brings the atrioventricular and primary grooves together in the inner curvature of the heart may be considered to be a preliminary to the formation of the anterior leaflets of the atrioventricular valves. The mature anatomy of the tricuspid valve clearly illustrates this. Its anterior leaflet is positioned at the very boundary between inlet and outlet portions of the right ventricle. With its annular attachment

just behind the crista supraventricularis and its anterior papillary muscle originating from the trabecula septomarginalis, this leaflet is completely a junctional structure (see Fig. 4.16). In the left ventricle, the situation is somewhat different. The undermining process which leads to formation of the aortic (anterior) leaflet of the mitral valve completely effaces the boundary between inlet and primary septum. It is because of this that papillary muscles arising from the septum are not found in the mature left ventricle. This means that important changes take place between completion of septation and the final stages of valve development. Initially the left part of the primary fold encircles the entrance into the aortic vestibule. Its position, therefore, marks the junction of the left ventricular inlet and outlet portions. It is directly continuous with the primary septum in the roof of the left ventricle. The left ventricular outlet portion is relatively small. Myocardial undermining then leads to disruption of the continuity be-

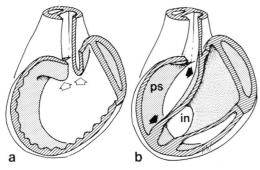

Fig. 4.25 Diagrams to show development of the mitral valve, left lateral views. (a) The same as Figure 4.17, showing the left ventricular part of the primary fold (open arrows). (b) Myocardial undermining removes the attachments to the primary septum (ps), leading to parietal papillary muscles (arrows). In the normal heart, with complete fusion of primary and inlet septa, the undermining process continues posteriorly on the inlet septum (in). (Reproduced from Wenink A C G, Gittenberger-de Groot 1982 British Heart Journal 48: 462–468.)

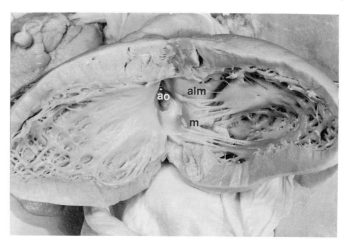

Fig. 4.27 Left ventricle of a normal heart, showing the anterolateral muscle bundle (alm) to wedge into the fibrous continuity between aortic (ao) and mitral (m) valves.

tween fold and septum, the primary fold being completely liberated from the septum. This leads to relative enlargement of the outlet portion (Fig. 4.25) and produces its characteristic posterior diverticulum in the formed heart.

In the mature left ventricle, the embryonic relationship of the aortic leaflet of the mitral valve and the primary septum may still be recognised by the presence of longitudinal trabeculations on the anterior ventricular wall between the septum and the aortic (anterior) mitral leaflet (Fig. 4.26). The anterolateral muscle bundle, which in many normal hearts is found anterolateral to the region of the mitral aortic valve fibrous continuity (Moulaert & Oppenheimer-Dekker, 1976) is probably a muscular remnant of the primary fold (Fig. 4.27).

Not only do the anterior leaflets of the atrioventricular valves develop in different ways, but a further difference

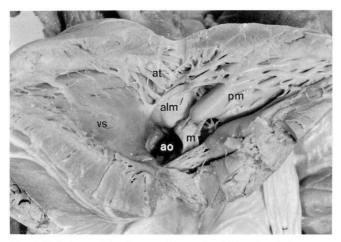

Fig. 4.26 Left ventricle of a normal heart, in which trabeculations on the anterior part of the ventricular septum (vs) and on the anterior ventricular wall (at) form one continuous mass with the anterolateral papillary muscle (pm). An individual anterolateral muscle bundle (alm) may be distinguished as well. ao – aortic orifice; m – mitral valve.

is found in the presence of the septal leaflet of the tricuspid valve which has no counterpart in the normal mitral valve. Undermining of the right side of the inlet septum is a relatively late event which never leads to complete disengagement of the tension apparatus from the septum. The septal leaflet always has 'accessory papillary muscles' on the inlet septum. In the left ventricle, the undermining process which liberates the primary fold continues without interruption onto the inlet septum. Undermining of the left ventricular inlet septal myocardium is more extensive than it is on the right side and formation of the posterior recess behind the aortic leaflet of the mitral valve brings its annular attachment to a somewhat higher level than the attachment of the septal tricuspid leaflet. It is the different planes of mitral and tricuspid annuli which permits the identification of the atrioventricular muscular septum in the normal heart (Allwork, 1982; Wenink et al, 1985) (Fig. 4.28). Because this structure is not an individual entity as the other septal components are, it would perhaps be better to call it the atrioventricular *part* of the septum. This is particularly so since between the annular attachments of mitral and tricuspid valves both the atrial *and* ventricular inlet septum form this atrioventricular part.

The arterial valves

The valves which intervene between the outlet segment and the truncus arteriosus also have their own particular developmental history and are not comparable to the other valves.

At 9 mm CRL, the first anlagen of the arterial valves are formed by the distal extremities of the endocardial outlet ridges (Van Mierop et al, 1963). To these ridges another pair of smaller endocardial swellings is added. The latter have been termed the 'intercalated valve swellings'

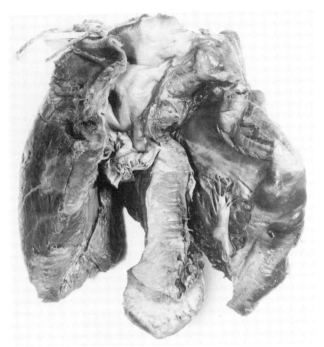
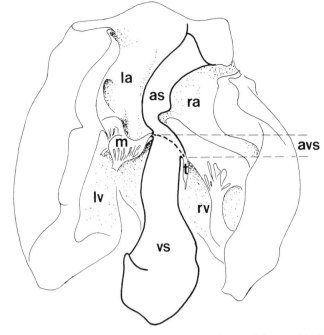

Fig. 4.28 Frontal section of an adult heart, just anterior to the ostium of the coronary sinus, posterior view. The anular attachment of the septal leaflet of the tricuspid valve (t) has a more apical position than that of the mitral valve (m). The intervening atrioventricular septum (avs) is composed of atrial septum (as) as well as ventricular septum (vs). la – left atrium; ra – right atrium; lv – left ventricle; rv – right ventricle. (Reproduced from Wenink et al, 1985.)

(Kramer, 1942). The (major) outlet ridges are divided into aortic and pulmonary halves by the ingrowing aortopulmonary septum (Shaner, 1962). As a result, two separate orifices are formed each of which has its own three leaflet primordia. Excavation of these endocardial masses forms the sinuses of Valsalva and the actual valve leaflets are produced in the 30–40 mm stage (Van Mierop et al, 1963; Maron & Hutchins, 1974). A further developmental phase is that of histological maturation, which is not completed even at birth (Maron & Hutchins, 1974; Hurle, 1979; Hurle et al, 1980).

According to Seidl & Steding (1981), the aortopulmonary septum is just one of a system of interarterial septa which intervene between the different parts of the branchial arch artery system. The work of Shaner (1962) has shown a beautiful correlation between the pattern of branchial arch artery development and formation of the arterial orifices in different animal species (Fig. 4.29). The morphology of the aortopulmonary septum depends very much on this arterial pattern. It is this which determines the way in which the different parts of the endocardial outlet swellings are assigned to individual arterial orifices.

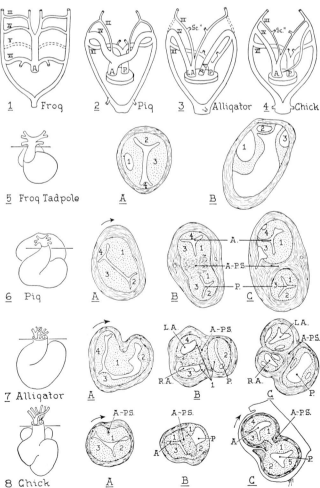

Fig. 4.29 Diagrams to show the different patterns of the branchial arch artery system and the aorticopulmonary septum (A.-P.S.), in relation with the endocardial outlet ridges (1, 2, 3, 4), as seen in different animal species. A – aorta; P – pulmonary trunk; R.A. – right aorta; L.A. – left aorta. (Reproduced with permission from Shaner, 1962.) Anatomical Record 143: 519–529.)

THE CONDUCTION SYSTEM

Histological identification of the embryonic conduction tissues is difficult. In the mature heart they occupy a more or less isolated position because first, they are largely covered by a connective tissue sheath and secondly, their cellular cytoplasm has a more bright appearance because of the relative scarcity of myofibrils. These are only relative differences from the working myocardium.

Early investigations (Mall, 1912; Sanabria, 1936; Walls, 1947) have concentrated upon the developmental stage at which the atrioventricular node and bundle are first distinguishable. In those embryonic hearts in which individual parts of the conduction system are first detectable, however, the myocardium seems to have 'specialised' characteristics at many more, unexpected sites

(Fig. 4.30). I concluded that the mature conduction system developed from four rings of specialised myocardium which intervened between the individual primitive segments of the embryonic heart (Wenink, 1976).

The presence of specialised myocardium at the intersegmental junctions has been given a phylogenetic background by Benninghoff (1923). The sinu-atrial ring bundle is a well-known junctional structure in the rabbit heart (Paes de Carvalho, 1959; Challice, 1966; Tranum-Jensen & Bojsen-Møller, 1973), and the retro-aortic tissue of the guinea-pig (Anderson, 1972) lies at the arterial junction. In the human heart, it is the atrioventricular ring tissue which is most easily identified (Keith & Flack, 1907; Anderson & Taylor, 1972; Anderson et al, 1974a). The ring concept (Wenink, 1976; Anderson et al, 1976) has been further supported by studies on the bird's heart (Kim & Yasuda, 1979, 1980).

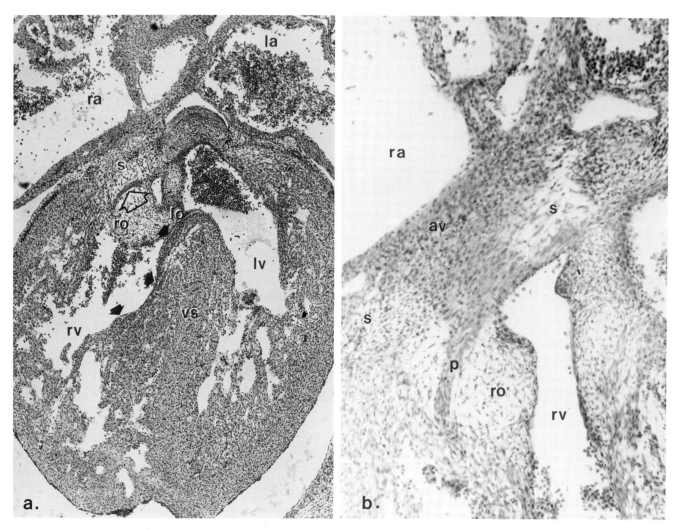

Fig. 4.30 Transverse sections of a human embryo of 17 mm CRL. (a) Low power view to show two portions of the primary ring. On top of the ventricular septum (vs), the ring forms the bundle and its right branch (black arrows). In the inner curvature of the heart, the primary ring (open arrow) does not contribute to the normal conducting system. ra – right atrium; la – left atrium; rv – right ventricle; lv – left ventricle; s – sulcus tissue; ro – right outlet ridge (fused with the left outlet ridge – lo). (b) This section is taken more caudally, and shows the contiguity of primary (p) and atrioventricular (av) ring tissues in the inner curvature. ra – right atrium; rv – right ventricle; s – sulcus tissue; ro – right outlet ridge.

Although Vassall-Adams (1982) has doubted the value of the ring theory, there is little doubt that his illustrations are readily interpreted within this concept.

In man, development of the intersegmental and intra-segmental septa explains the final disposition of those parts of the specialised myocardial rings which contribute to the conduction system (Wenink, 1982). In keeping with the nomenclature of the embryonic cardiac segments, the specialised rings can be termed the sinu-atrial (between sinus venosus and atrium), atrioventricular (between atrium and inlet), primary (between inlet and outlet) and arterial (between outlet and truncus arteriosus) rings (Fig. 4.31).

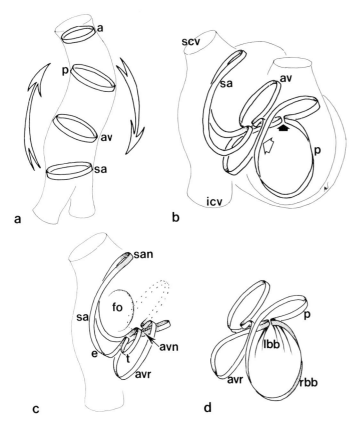

Fig. 4.31 Diagrams to show development of the specialised myocardial rings, right lateral views. (a) Before looping. sa – sinu-atrial ring; av – atrioventricular ring; p – primary ring; a – arterial ring. The arrows indicate the looping process. (b) After looping and septation. The sinu-atrial ring (sa) has been incorporated into the right atrium (compare Fig. 4.6). The atrioventricular ring (av) has developed anterior and posterior invaginations. The posterior ring, which lies on the inlet septum, contacts (black arrow) the primary ring (p) which lies on the primary septum (compare Fig. 4.14). The open arrow indicates the contact of atrioventricular and primary rings in the lesser curvature of the heart (compare Fig. 4.13b). scv – superior caval vein; icv – inferior caval vein. (c) Formation of the sinu-atrial (san) and atrioventricular (avn) nodes, from different portions of the sinu-atrial (sa) and atrioventricular (avr) rings. The sinu-atrial ring passes through the anlagen of the Thebesian (t) and Eustachian (e) valves. fo – fossa ovalis. (d) Contribution of the atrioventricular (avr) and primary (p) rings to the bundle and its branches. The right bundle branch (rbb) develops as part of the primary ring. The left bundle branch (lbb), secondarily, develops from both the atrioventricular and the primary ring. (Reproduced from Wenink, 1982.)

The contribution of the sinu-atrial ring to the sinus node at the junction of superior caval vein and right atrium is self-evident. Formation of the sinu-atrial septum brings part of the sinu-atrial junction into the base of the atrial septum. Here, the sinu-atrial ring contributes to the super-ficial part of the atrioventricular node. In human fetal hearts, further remnants of the sinu-atrial ring have been described (Gittenberger-de Groot & Wenink, 1978). These might be considered in the light of the so-called 'internodal pathways' (Thorel, 1910; James, 1967). In the definitive heart, however, there is no evidence to support the concept of such pathways forming an insulated conduction system (Janse & Anderson, 1974).

The atrioventricular ring is transformed by septation of the atrioventricular canal, or rather, by septation of the atrium and of the inlet. The development of left and right atrioventricular orifices gives the atrioventricular ring the form of a figure of eight. Anterior and posterior inden-tations of the ring meet in the base of the atrial septum. The indentations, together with the basal extension of the sinu-atrial ring mentioned above, form the atrioventricular node. Thus, the node has a complex composition (Wenink, 1976; Anderson et al, 1977). Similar results were described by Marino et al (1979) who delineated the contiguity of a 'left and right nodal primordium' with 'AV bundle cells'. In contrast, Virágh & Challice (1977, 1982) have only distinguished a single nodal primordium, which may be comparable to the 'AV-bundle cells' of Marino et al (1979) or to my 'posterior invagination of the atrioventricular ring' (Wenink, 1976).

This posterior indentation of the atrioventricular ring is found on top of the inlet septum. It not only forms the deep portion of the node but also the proximal part of the penetrating bundle. At the site of fusion of the inlet septum with the primary septum, the atrioventricular ring is contiguous with the primary ring, which lies on the rim of the primary septum. Thus, the distal part of the pen-etrating bundle is derived from the primary ring. The dual origin of the bundle, coinciding with the two underlying septal components, is also found in the mouse heart (Fig. 4.32). Virágh & Challice (1982) have denied this duality in the mouse. More research on the histogenesis of the atrioventricular junction is needed to clarify these different opinions.

The primary ring, which is the junctional myocardium on top of the primary fold, not only contributes to the penetrating bundle, but also forms the right bundle branch. The position of the right bundle branch in the septomarginal trabecula indicates its primary junctional derivation. As Vassall-Adams (1982) has indicated, the development of the left bundle branch is out of harmony with the ring concept. This may well be related to the fact that valve formation in the left and right ventricles differs considerably. In the right ventricle, the original architec-ture is not disturbed and the right part of the primary fold

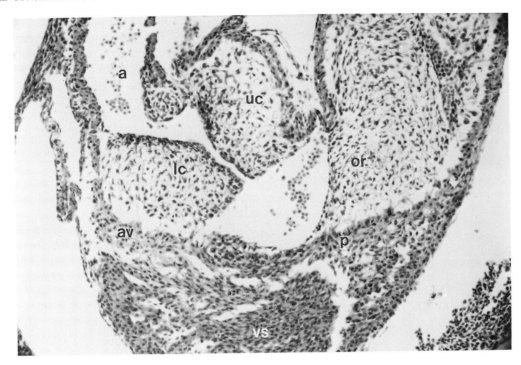

Fig. 4.32 Sagittal section of a mouse embryo heart, showing the atrioventricular (av) and primary (p) rings, contacting each other on top of the ventricular septum (vs). a – atrium; uc – upper atrioventricular cushion; lc – lower atrioventricular cushion; or – outlet ridge.

(septomarginal trabecula and anterior papillary muscle) persists to indicate the junction of inlet and outlet. The right bundle branch is found in this undisturbed landmark. In the left ventricle, however, the tension apparatus of the mitral valve is completely loosened from the septum and no indication of the boundary between inlet septum and primary septum is left. This extensive myocardial transformation may also involve the specialised tissues, which could then explain the fan-like disposition of the left bundle branch. This branch originates from the site of fusion of atrioventricular and primary rings and its dual origin is reflected by its dual blood supply (Frink & James, 1973).

The rim of the ventricular septum is not the only site at which primary and atrioventricular rings meet each other. They are also contiguous in the inner curvature of the heart, where atrioventricular and primary grooves coincide (see above). This contact is found anterior to the right atrioventricular orifice (Fig. 4.31). During normal development this contact disappears and it does not play a role in formation of the mature conduction system. There are, however, many congenital malformations, in which this contact takes over from the usual septal one to establish an anomalous anterior node and bundle (Wenink, 1982).

The fourth, arterial, ring does not seem to be important for the human conduction system, although it does contribute in the bird's heart (Kim & Yasuda, 1980).

Myocardial vascularisation

Because of the typical structure of the myocardium, there is no need for any particular vascular system in early embryonic stages. The myocardium has a spongy structure and is broken up into a mass of individual trabeculations which are lined by endocardium. The intertrabecular spaces, which have been described as reaching the epicardium (Grant, 1926), certainly play a role in the formation of the myocardial vascular bed. According to Virágh & Challice (1981) they are encased within the myocardium by consolidation of the trabeculations.

An extensive description of development of the cardiac vessels has recently been given by Heintzberger (1982). In an embryo of 8 mm CRL, she describes a subepicardial endothelial plexus as the first indication of this vascular system. This network was connected with the left sinus horn. In a later stage, it extended into the myocardium to make continuity with the intertrabecular spaces. Still later (12 mm CRL), continuity was established with endothelial sprouts in the aortic wall. The opinion of Hackensellner (1956) that more than two coronary arterial anlagen arise from both the aortic and the pulmonary truncal walls has been doubted by both Van Mierop (1979) and Heintzberger (1982).

The question as to whether proliferation of the endocardium is the first event (Virágh & Challice, 1981), or whether the myocardial network is primarily formed from the subepicardial network (Heintzberger, 1982), is beyond

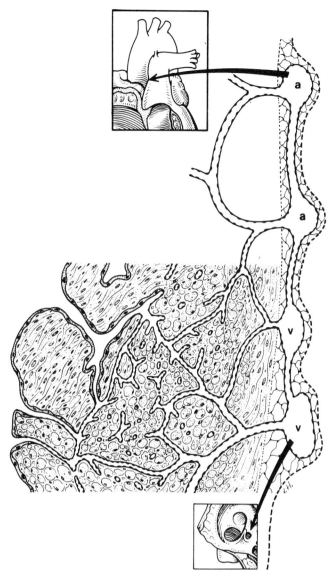

Fig. 4.33 Schematic representation of the dispositions of arterial and venous networks and their interrelations, as well as their connexions with the intertrabecular spaces, the aorta and the coronary sinus in the human heart. a – artery; v – vein. (From Heintzberger, 1982, with her permission.)

the scope of this chapter. An intermediate stage in which a vascular plexus within the myocardium is continuous with the cardiac lumen as well as with the left sinus horn and the ascending aorta explains the mature anatomy (Fig. 4.33). Different types of anastomoses remain in the adult heart (Hadzieselimović & Sećerov, 1979). Before the 15 mm stage, no difference can be seen between arteries and veins and further histogenesis still has to take place. Differentiation of the vessel walls starts at their origin from the aorta and proceeds in an apical direction.

With respect to the subepicardial or intramyocardial position of the main arteries, there appear to be species differences (Heintzberger 1982), although in man the main arterial stems are not exclusively subepicardial (Hadziselimović et al, 1977).

ACKNOWLEDGEMENTS

I am grateful to my Leiden colleagues for their continuous support, to Mr J. Lens for the photography and to Miss M. Stokman for typing of the manuscript.

REFERENCES

Allwork S P 1982 Anatomical–embryological correlates in atrioventricular septal defect. British Heart Journal 47: 419–429
Allwork S P, Anderson R H 1979 Developmental anatomy of the membranous part of the ventricular septum in the human heart. British Heart Journal 41: 275–280
Anderson R H 1972 The disposition, morphology and innervation of cardiac specialized tissue in the guinea pig. Journal of Anatomy 111: 453–468
Anderson R H, Becker A E 1980 Cardiac anatomy. An integrated text and colour atlas. Churchill Livingstone, Edinburgh, 1980
Anderson R H, Taylor I M 1972 Development of atrioventricular specialized tissue in the human heart. British Heart Journal 34: 1205–1214
Anderson R H, Davies M J, Becker A E 1974a Atrioventricular ring specialized tissue in the normal heart. European Journal of Cardiology 2: 219–230
Anderson R H, Wilkinson J L, Arnold R, Lubkiewicz K 1974b Morphogenesis of bulboventricular malformations. I. Consideration of embryogenesis in the normal heart. British Heart Journal 36: 242–255
Anderson R H, Becker A E, Wenink A C G, Janse M J 1976 The development of the cardiac specialized tissue. In: Wellens H J J, Lie K J, Janse M J (eds) The conduction system of the heart: structure, function and clinical implications. Stenfert Kroese, Leiden, p 3–28
Anderson R H, Wenink A C G, Losekoot T G, Becker A E 1977 Congenitally complete heart block. Developmental aspects. Circulation 56: 90–101
Anderson R H, Macartney F J, Shinebourne E A, Tynan M J 1978 Definitions of cardiac chambers. In: Anderson R H, Shinebourne E A (eds) Paediatric cardiology, Vol 1. Churchill Livingstone, Edinburgh, p 5–15
Anderson R H, Ho S Y, Becker A E 1981 The morphology of septal structures in univentricular hearts. In: Wenink A C G, Oppenheimer-Dekker A, Moulaert A J (eds) The ventricular septum of the heart. Leiden University Press, The Hague, p 203–224
Asami I 1969 Beitrag zur Entwicklung des Kammerseptums im menschlichen Herzen mit besonderer Berücksichtigung der sogenannten Bulbusdrehung. Zeitschrift für Anatomie und Entwicklungsgeschichte 128: 1–17
Benninghoff A 1923 Über die Beziehungen des Reizleitungssystems und der Papillarmuskeln zu den Konturfasern des Herzschlauches. Anatomischer Anzeiger, Ergänzungsheft 57: 186–208
Challice C E 1966 Studies on the microstructure of the heart. I. The sino-atrial node and sino-atrial ring bundle. Journal of the Royal Microscopy Society 85–1: 1–21
de la Cruz M V, Da Rocha J P 1956 An ontogenetic theory for the explanation of congenital malformations involving the truncus and conus. American Heart Journal 51: 782–805
de la Cruz M V, Miller B L 1968 Double inlet left ventricle. Two pathological specimens with comments on the embryology and on its relation to single ventricle. Circulation 37: 249–260
Dalgleish A E 1976 The development of the septum primum relative to atrial septation in the mouse heart. Journal of Morphology 149: 369–382
Davis C L 1924 The cardiac jelly of the chick embryo. Anatomical Record 27: 201–202
Davis C L 1927 Development of the human heart from its first appearance to the stage found in embryos of twenty paired somites. Contributions to Embryology 19–107: 247–293
De Vries P A 1981 Evolution of precardiac and splanching mesoderm in relationship to the infundibulum and truncus. In: Pexieder T (ed) Perspectives in cardiovascular research, Vol 5. Mechanisms of cardiac morphogenesis and teratogenesis. Raven Press, New York, p 31–48

Doerr W 1952 Uber ein formales Prinzip der Koppelung von Entwicklungsstörungen der venösen und arteriellen Kammerostien. Zeitschrift für Kreislaufforschung 41: 269–284

Dor X, Corone P 1973 Le rôle du conus dans la morphogenèse cardiaque. Essai d'étude sur l'embryon de poulet. Coeur 4: 207–308

Dor X, Corone P 1979 Experimental creation of univentricular heart in the chick embryo. Herz 4: 91–96

Dor X, Corone P 1981 Cono-truncal torsions and transposition of the great vessels in the chick embryo. In: Pexieder T (ed) Perspectives in cardiovascular research, Vol 5. Mechanisms of cardiac morphogenesis and teratogenesis. Raven Press, New York, p 453–472

Frink R J, James T N 1973 Normal blood supply to the human His bundle and proximal bundle branches. Circulation 49: 8–18

Gittenberger-de Groot A C, Wenink A C G 1978 The specialized myocardium in the fetal heart. In: Van Mierop L H S, Oppenheimer-Dekker A, Bruins C L D C (eds) Embryology and teratology of the heart and the great arteries. Leiden University Press, Leiden, p 15–24

Goor D A, Edwards J E, Lillehei C W 1970 The development of the interventricular septum of the human heart; correlative morphogenetic study. Chest 58: 453–467

Goor D A, Dische R, Lillehei C W 1972 The conotruncus. I. Its normal inversion and conus absorption. Circulation 46: 375–384

Grant R P 1926 Development of the cardiac coronary vessels in the rabbit. Heart 13: 261–271

Hackensellner H A 1956 Akzessorische Kranzgefässanlagen der Arteria pulmonalis unter 63 menschlichen Embryonenseries mit einer grössten Länge von 12 bis 36 mm. Zeitschrift fur mikroskopisch-anatomische Forschung 62: 153–64

Hadziselimović H, Sećerov D 1979 Superficial anastomoses of blood vessels in the human heart. Acta Anatomica 104: 268–278

Hadziselimović H, Sećerov D, Ovćina F 1977 Muscular formations on coronary blood vessels and vascularization of the coronary sinus. Folia Medica XII-1: 35–54

Harh J Y, Paul M H 1975 Experimental cardiac morphogenesis. I. Development of the ventricular septum in the chick. Journal of Embryology and Experimental Morphology 33: 13–28

Hay D A 1978 Development and fusion of the endocardial cushions. Birth Defects Original Article Series XIV-7: 69–90

Hay D A, Low F N 1972 The fusion of dorsal and ventral endocardial cushions in the embryonic chick heart: a study in fine structure. American Journal of Cardiology 133: 1–23

His W 1885 Das Herz. In: W His (ed) Anatomie menschlicher Embryonen. Theil 3: Zur Geschichte der Organe. Vogel, Leipzig, p 129–184

Heintzberger C F M 1982 De relatie van myocardstructuur en vascularisatiepatroon in de ventrikelwand van kip, rat en mens, tijdens de ontwikkeling. Thesis, Amsterdam

Hurle J M 1979 Scanning and light microscope studies of the development of the chick embryo semilunar heart valves. Anatomy and Embryology 157: 69–80

Hurle J M, Colveé E, Blanca A M 1980 Development of mouse semilunar valves. Anatomy and Embryology 160: 83–91

James T N 1967 Anatomy of the cardiac conduction system in the rabbit. Circulation Research 20: 638–648

Janse M J, Anderson R H 1974 Specialized internodal atrial pathways – fact or fiction? European Journal of Cardiology 2: 117–136

Keith A, Flack M 1907 The form and nature of the muscular connections between the primary divisions of the vertebrate heart. Journal of Anatomy and Physiology 41: 172–189

Kim Y, Yasuda M 1979 The cardiac conducting system of the fowl. Zeitblatt für Veterinäre Medizin, Anatomie, Histologie, Embryologie 8: 138–150

Kim Y, Yasuda M 1980 Development of the cardiac conducting system in the chick embryo. Zbl Vet Med C Anat Histol Embryol 9: 7–20

Kramer T C 1942 The partitioning of the truncus and conus and the formation of the membranous portion of the interventricular septum in the human heart. American Journal of Cardiology 71: 343–370

Laane H M 1974 The nomenclature of the arterial pole of the embryonic heart. Acta Morphologica Neerlando-Scandinavica 12: 167–210

Laane H M 1978 The septation of the arterial pole of the heart in the chick embryo. II. Development of the truncus arteriosus of the heart of chick embryos from 4 to 5 days of incubation. Acta Morphologica Neerlando-Scandinavica 16: 29–53

Laane H M 1979 The septation of the arterial pole of the heart in the chick embryo. III. Development of the truncus arteriosus of the heart of chick embryos from 5½ to 7 days of incubation. Acta Morphologica Neerlando-Scandinavica 17: 1–20

Los J A 1960 Die Entwicklung des Septum venosus cordis. Die Herzentwicklung des Menschen, von einer vergessenen Struktur aus untersucht. Zeitschrift für Anatomie und Entwicklungsgeschichte 122: 173–196

Los J A 1968 Embryology. In: Watson H (ed) Pediatric cardiology. Lloyd-Luke, London, p 1–28

Los J A 1978 Cardiac septation and development of the aorta, pulmonary trunk and pulmonary veins: previous work in the light of recent observations. Birth Defects Original Article Series XIV-7: 109–138

Los J A, van Eijndthoven E 1973 The fusion of the endocardial cushions in the heart of the chick embryo. A light-microscopical and electron-microscopical study. Zeitschrift für Anatomie und Entwicklungsgeschichte 141: 55–75

McBride R E, Moore G W, Hutchins G M 1981 Development of the outflow tract and closure of the interventricular septum in the normal human heart. American Journal of Anatomy 100: 309–331

Mall F P 1912 On the development of the human heart. American Journal of Anatomy 13: 249–298

Manasek F J 1969 Embryonic development of the heart. II. Formation of the epicardium. Journal of Embryology and Experimental Morphology 22: 333–348

Manasek F J 1981 Determinants of heartshape in early embryos. Federation Proceedings 40: 2011–2016

Manasek F J, Monroe R G 1972 Early cardiac morphogenesis is independent of function. Developmental Biology 27: 584–588

Manasek F J, Burnside M B, Waterman R E 1972 Myocardial cell shape change as a mechanism of embryonic heart looping. Developmental Biology, 29: 349–371

Marino T A, Truex R C, Marino D R 1979 The development of the atrioventricular node and bundle in the ferret heart. American Journal of Anatomy, 154: 135–150

Markwald R R, Fitzharris T P, Manasek F J 1977 Structural development of endocardial cushions. American Journal of Anatomy 148: 85–120

Maron B J, Hutchins G M 1974 The development of the semilunar valves in the human heart. American Journal of Pathology 74: 331–344

Meredith M A, Hutchins G M, Moore G W 1979 Role of the left interventricular sulcus in formation of the interventricular septum and crista supraventricularis in normal human cardiogenesis. Anatomical Record 194: 417–428

Morse D E 1978 Scanning electron microscopy of the developing septa in the chick heart. Birth Defects Original Article Series XIV-7: 91–107

Morse D E 1980 Formation of foramina secunda in the chick. In: Pexieder T (ed) Perspectives in cardiovascular research, Vol 5: Mechanisms of cardiac morphogenesis and teratogenesis. Raven Press, New York, p 139–149

Moulaert A J, Oppenheimer-Dekker A 1976 Anterolateral muscle bundle of the left ventricle, bulboventricular flange and subaortic stenosis. American Journal Cardiology 37: 78–81

Odgers P N B 1937/1938 The development of the pars membranacea septi in the human heart. Journal of Anatomy 72: 247–259

Odgers P N B 1939 The development of the atrioventricular valves in man. Journal of Anatomy 73: 643–657

Okamoto N, Akimoto N, Satow Y, Hidaka N, Miyabara S 1981 Role of cell death in conal ridges of developing human heart. In: Pexieder T (ed) Perspectives in cardiovascular research, Vol 5: Mechanisms of cardiac morphogenesis and teratogenesis. Raven Press, New York, p 127–137

Orts Llorca F, Ruano Gil D 1967 A causal analysis of the heart curvatures in the chicken embryo. Roux Archiv für Entwicklungsmechanik der Organismen 158: 52–63

Orts Llorca F, Puerta Fonolla J, Sobrado J 1982 The formation, septation and fate of the truncus arteriosus in man. Journal of Anatomy 131: 41–56

Paes de Carvalho A, de Mello W C, Hoffman B F 1959 Electrophysiological evidence for specialized fiber types in rabbit atrium. American Journal of Physiology 196: 483–488

Patten B M 1968 The development of the heart. In: Gould S E (ed) Pathology of the heart and blood vessels, 3rd Edn. Springfield, Illinois, p 20–90

Pernkopf E, Wirtinger W 1933 Die Transposition der Herzostien – ein Versuch der Erklärung dieser Erscheinung. Die Phoronomie der Herzentwicklung als morphogenetische Grundlage der Erklärung. I. Teil. Die Phoronomie der Herzentwicklung. Zeitschrift für Anatomie and Entwicklungsgeschichte 100: 563–711

Pexieder T 1978 Development of the outflow tract of the embryonic heart. Birth Defects Original Article Series 14: 29–68

Puerta Fonollà A J, Orts Llorca F 1978 Origin and development of the septum primum. Acta Anatomica 100: 250–257

Sanabria T 1936 Recherches sur la différenciation du tissu nodal et connecteur du coeur des mammifères Archives de Biologie 47: 1–70

Sato S 1914 Ueber die Entwicklung der Atrioventrikulären Klappen und der pars membranacea unter Berücksichtigung zugehöriger Herzmissbildungen. Anatomische Hefte Abteilung I 50: 195–251

Seidl W, Steding G 1981 Contribution to the development of the heart. Part III: The aortic arch complex. Normal development and morphogenesis of congenital malformation. Thoracic and Cardiovascular Surgeon 29: 359–368

Shaner R F 1949 Malformation of the atrioventricular endocardial cushions of the embryo pig, and its relation to defects of the conus and truncus arteriosus. American Journal of Anatomy 84: 431–456

Shaner R F 1962 Comparative development of the bulbus and ventricles of the vertebrate heart with special reference to Spitzer's theory of heart malformations. Anatomical Record 142: 519–529

Shimada Y, Ho E 1980 Scanning electron microscopy of the embryonic chick heart: Formation of the epicardium and surface structure of the four heterotypic cells that constitute the embryonic heart. In: Van Praagh R, Takao A (eds) Etiology and morphogenesis of congenital heart disease. Futura, New York, p 63–80

Stalsberg H 1970 Mechanism of dextral looping of the embryonic heart. American Journal of Cardiology 25: 265–271

Steding G, Seidl W 1980 Contribution to the development of the heart. Part I: normal development. Thoracic and Cardiovascular Surgeon 28: 386–409

Steding G, Seidl W 1981 Contribution to the development of the heart. Part II: Morphogenesis of congenital heart disease. Thoracic and Cardiovascular Surgeon 29: 1–16

Thorel C 1910 Über die supraventrikulären Abschnitte des sog. Reizleitungs-systems. Zentralblatt fur allgemeine Pathologie und pathologische Anatomie, Erganzungsheft 21: 71–90

Todaro F 1865 Novelle ricerche sopra la struttura muscolare delle orechiette del cuore umano e sopra la valvola d'Eustachio. Stabilimento Civelli, Firenze

Tranum-Jensen J, Bojsen-Møller F 1973 The ultrastructure of the sinuatrial ring bundle and of the caudal extension of the sinus node in the right atrium of the rabbit heart. Zeitschrift für Zellforschung und mikroskopische Anatomie 138: 97–112

Ugarte M, Enriquez de Salamanca F, Quero M 1976 Endocardial cushion defects. An anatomical study of 54 specimens. British Heart Journal 38: 674–682

Van Gils F A W 1979 The development of the human atrioventricular heart valves. Journal of Anatomy 128: 427

Van Gils F A W 1981 The fibrous skeleton in the human heart: embryological and pathogenetic considerations. Virchows Archiv. A. Pathological Anatomy and Histology 393: 61–73

Van Mierop L H S 1977 Pathology and pathogenesis of endocardial cushion defects: surgical implications. In: Davila J C (ed) Second Henry Ford Hospital International Symposium on Cardiac Surgery. Appleton Century Crofts, New York, p 201–207

Van Mierop L H S 1979 Morphological development of the heart. In: Berne R M (ed) Handbook of physiology, Section 2: The cardiovascular system, Vol 1: The heart. Williams & Wilkins, New York, p 1–28

Van Mierop L H S, Gessner I H 1972 Pathogenetic mechanisms in congenital cardiovascular malformations. Progress in Cardiovascular Diseases 15: 67–85

Van Mierop L H S, Kutsche L M 1981 Comparative anatomy of the ventricular septum. In: Wenink A C G, Oppenheimer-Dekker A, Moulaert A J (eds) The ventricular septum of the heart. Leiden University Press, The Hague, p 35–46

Van Mierop L H S, Alley R D, Kausel H W, Stranahan A 1962 The anatomy and embryology of endocardial cushion defects. Journal of Thoracic and Cardiovascular Surgery 43: 71–82

Van Mierop L H S, Alley R D, Kausel H W, Stranahan A 1963 Pathogenesis of transposition complexes. I. Embryology of the ventricles and great arteries. American Journal of Cardiology 12: 216–225

Van Praagh R 1972 The segmental approach to diagnosis in congenital heart disease. Birth Defects Original Article Series 8–5: 4–23

Vassall-Adams P R 1982 The development of the atrioventricular bundle and its branches in the avian heart. Journal of Anatomy 134: 169–183

Virágh S, Challice C E 1977 The development of the conduction system in the mouse embryo heart. II. Histogenesis of the atrioventricular node and bundle. Developmental Biology 56: 397–411

Virágh S, Challice C E 1981 The origin of the epicardium and the embryonic myocardial circulation in the mouse. Anatomical Record 201: 157–168

Virágh S, Challice C E 1982 The development of the conduction system in the mouse embryo heart. IV. Differentiation of the atrioventricular conduction system. Developmental Biology 89: 25–40

Walls E W 1947 The development of the specialized conducting tissue of the human heart. Journal of Anatomy 81: 93–110

Wenink A C G 1971 Some details on the final stages of heart septation in the human embryo. Thesis, Luctor et Emergo, Leiden

Wenink A C G 1975 La formation du septum membranaceum dans le coeur humain. Bulletin de l'Association des Anatomistes 58: 1127–1132

Wenink A C G 1976 Development of the human cardiac conducting system. Journal of Anatomy 121: 617–631

Wenink A C G 1981a Embryology of the ventricular septum. Separate origin of its components. Virchows Archiv. A. Pathological Anatomy and Histology 390: 71–79

Wenink A C G 1981b Development of the ventricular septum. In: Wenink A C G, Oppenheimer A, Moulaert A J (eds) The ventricular septum of the heart. Leiden University Press, The Hague, p 23–34

Wenink A C G 1982 Embryologie des tissus de conduction. Coeur XIII–4: 479–490

Wenink A C G, Gittenberger-de Groot A C 1982a Cloisonnement ventriculaire. Terminologie proposée. Coeur XIII–4: 467–478

Wenink A C G, Gittenberger-de Groot A C 1982b Left and right ventricular trabecular patterns. Consequence of ventricular septation and valve development. British Heart Journal 48: 462–468

Wenink A C G, Gittenberger-de Groot A C 1985 The role of atrioventricular endocardial cushions in the septation of the heart. International Journal of Cardiology 8: 25–44

Wenink A C G, Anderson R H, Thiene G 1978 The conducting system in hearts with atrioventricular canal malformations. In: Van Mierop L H S, Oppenheimer-Dekker A, Bruins C L D C (eds) Embryology and teratology of the heart and the great arteries. Leiden University Press, Leiden p 55–61

Wenink A C G, Van Gils F A W, Gittenberger-de Groot A C, Draulans-Noë HAY, Thiene G, Anderson R H 1985 Developmental aspects of atrioventricular defects. In: Quero Jimenez M (ed) Atrioventricular septal defects (in preparation)

5

Fetal circulation and circulatory changes at birth

Most congenital cardiac anomalies are already present 6 weeks after conception. As a result, congenital heart disease may influence the circulation in the fetus. This applies both to the distribution of the fetal cardiac output and to the relative sizes of the cardiac chambers and great vessels. Of particular note are the relative cross-sectional areas of the aorta and pulmonary trunk. The dimensions of these arteries at birth reflect the proportion of the fetal cardiac output passing through them during fetal development. Not only may the presence of congenital heart disease influence the fetal circulation, but the changes in the circulation normally occurring at birth may also be modified. These in turn may influence the clinical presentation of congenital heart disease in infancy. To provide the basis for understanding these events, we start this chapter with a brief description of the normal fetal circulation.

FETAL CIRCULATION

In the fetus the highest partial pressure of oxygen (P_{O_2} 30–35 mmHg) (Fig. 5.1) is found in blood returning from the placenta (Meschia et al, 1965). This is transported from the placenta through a single umbilical vein which then enters the portal vein. After birth all the portal venous return passes through a venous capillary system in the liver before reaching the inferior caval vein via the hepatic veins. In the fetus, approximately 60% of the umbilical venous return bypasses the liver through the venous duct (ductus venosus) which connects the portal sinus to the junction of the left hepatic and inferior caval veins. In this way, blood with a relatively high oxygen content reaches the inferior caval vein and thence the right atrium. The anatomy of the atrial septum in the fetus is such that there is preferential streaming of the venous return from the inferior caval vein into the left atrium (Fig. 5.2) through the oval foramen (Barclay et al, 1944). As a consequence, about one-third of inferior caval venous return passes across the foramen ovale to the left atrium

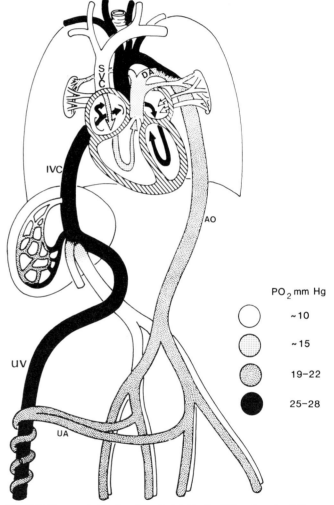

Fig. 5.1 Diagram indicating the arterial P_{O_2} in different parts of the fetal circulation as well as the principle distribution of flow within the heart (shown in more detail in Fig. 5.2). The most highly oxygenated blood (P_{O_2} 25–28) passes from the umbilical vein (UV) through the venous duct (ductus venous) to the inferior caval vein (IVC) and thence preferentially across the oval foramen (foramen ovale) to left atrium, left ventricle and into ascending aorta. Blood from the superior caval vein (SVC) passes preferentially through the tricuspid valve to right ventricle, main pulmonary artery and via the arterial duct (DA) to descending aorta (AO). Paired umbilical arteries (UA) then perfuse the placenta. See text for more detailed discussion.

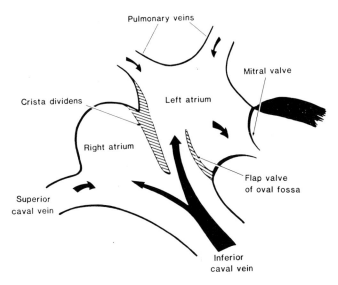

Fig. 5.2 In the fetus most of the blood entering the heart from the inferior caval vein passes preferentially across the oval foramen (foramen ovale) to the left atrium with only a small proportion passing to the right atrium.

while the rest mixes with the superior caval venous return in the right atrium. Blood in the superior caval vein has a P_{O_2} of 12–14 mmHg (Heymann & Rudolph, 1966). Apart from that in the coronary sinus, it is the most desaturated blood in the fetus. This highly desaturated blood passes preferentially from the right atrium through the tricuspid valve to the right ventricle and pulmonary trunk. Not more than 3% of the return from the superior caval vein passes across the oval foramen to the left atrium.

Since the inferior caval vein receives the umbilical venous return, blood entering the left atrium and left ventricle has a higher P_{O_2} (23–25 mmHg) than that in the right ventricle (18–19 mmHg). Blood ejected by the left ventricle passes through the aortic valve to the ascending aorta where it is distributed to the coronary arteries, cerebral circulation, head, neck and upper extremities. Less than 10% of the blood passing from right ventricle to the pulmonary trunk reaches the lungs. Most passes through the widely patent arterial duct (ductus arteriosus) to the descending aorta. In the fetus, gas exchange takes place at the placenta and not in the lungs. The deflated fetal lung has a high pulmonary vascular resistance which is related in part to the relatively low arterial P_{O_2} in the fetus compared with the neonate (see below). A large proportion of the blood entering the descending aorta passes to the very low vascular resistance placenta via paired umbilical arteries arising from the external iliac arteries. The rest supplies the lower body. The organisation of the fetal circulation (Fig. 5.3) thus ensures that the more highly saturated blood returning to the heart passes preferentially to the myocardium and brain. The more desaturated blood is returned to the placenta. This system is facilitated by three channels (the oval foramen

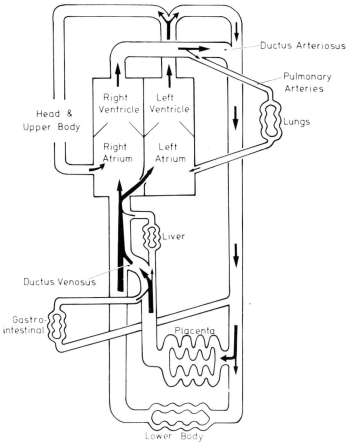

Fig. 5.3 Diagram indicating direction of blood flow within the fetal circulation. See text for fuller discussion.

and the venous and arterial ducts), all of which normally close after birth.

Distribution and control of the fetal circulation

During the latter half of gestation, cardiac output increases in proportion to fetal weight as does umbilical blood flow (Rudolph & Heymann, 1970). As a proportion of total output, however, placental flow falls in late gestation. This implies that placental resistance has risen and/or that the relative vascular resistance of the rest of the fetus has fallen. In the adult, the increased demands of the circulation are met principally by increasing cardiac output. In the fetus, by contrast, higher demands for oxygen and nutrients at different phases of growth are met by a redistribution of flow. Examples of this in the lamb are the increase in pulmonary flow at about 120 days (term = 150 days). These correspond to the development of significant amounts of surfactant in the lung (Howatt et al, 1965) and possibly the increase in flow to the gut at around 110 days gestation. The increase in flow in both these situations is fairly abrupt and would appear to be due to local vasodilation perhaps, dependent on local metabolites. In contrast, the gradual increase in cerebral blood flow occurring throughout gestation could be explained by enlargement of the vascular bed from the production of new capillary networks.

RELATIONSHIP OF FETAL BLOOD FLOW TO NEONATAL AORTIC AND PULMONARY ANATOMY: THE NORMAL CHILD

There is an intimate relationship between the course of the circulation through the heart, patterns of flow in the major blood vessels of the fetus, and the anatomy of the great vessels at birth. The angiographic appearances of the neonatal human aorta, pulmonary arteries and (when patent) the arterial duct reflect the distribution and pattern of flow in the fetus. During intrauterine life, the right ventricle ejects approximately two-thirds of the combined fetal cardiac output (data extrapolated from fetal lambs – Rudolph, 1974). As both ventricles eject blood against a similar vascular resistance, there is little difference in thickness between their free walls (St John Sutton et al, 1985). This is reflected by the relative right ventricular dominance present in the normal neonatal electrocardiogram. The dimensions of the great arteries reflect flow through them. Approximately one-third of the total fetal cardiac output enters the ascending aorta, 4% going to the coronary arteries and 20% to the head and neck arteries. This leaves about 10% to traverse the aortic isthmus. Two-thirds of the combined fetal cardiac output passes to the pulmonary trunk. Because of the high fetal pulmonary vascular resistance, only 8% (of the combined fetal cardiac output) reaches the lungs. The rest passes via the arterial duct to the descending aorta. The cross-sectional area of the isthmus is consequently considerably smaller than that of the descending aorta (Fig. 5.4). In clinical practice it is important not to consider the normal neonatal isthmus as

representing a 'hypoplastic' segment of the aorta or aortic coarctation. As the fetal pulmonary trunk is perfused at the same pressure as the ascending aorta, the two vessels at birth have similar histological characteristics (Heath et al, 1959). The pulmonary arterial wall then becomes relatively thinner with fewer elastic lamellae over the first year. With not more than 8% of the combined fetal cardiac output going to the lungs, the right and left pulmonary arteries are small during intra-uterine life. In contrast, the arterial duct is a wide channel connecting the pulmonary trunk to the descending aorta – a pattern well-demonstrated in infants with a patent arterial duct. The difference in diameters of the pulmonary arteries and the arterial duct are not perhaps as great as might be expected from the proportions of right ventricular output they are purported to carry. Nonetheless, even after closure of the arterial duct, its previous importance as the channel which carried most of the right ventricular output may be reflected by the size of the ductal diverticulum seen in some normal neonatal pulmonary arteriograms (Fig. 5.5). The presence of a 5–8 mmHg pressure gradient between the main and peripheral pulmonary arteries in young human infants up to the age of 4 months also reflects the disparity between pulmonary flow in the fetus and newborn. The right and left pulmonary arteries, unaccustomed to a high flow, initially arise at an acute angle from the pulmonary trunk and are of disproportionately small size compared to those of a 1-year-old (Danilowicz et al, 1965).

AORTIC AND PULMONARY ARTERIAL ANATOMY IN THE CHILD WITH CONGENITAL HEART DISEASE

When pulmonary atresia is present from early fetal life, the whole of the fetal cardiac output leaves the heart via the

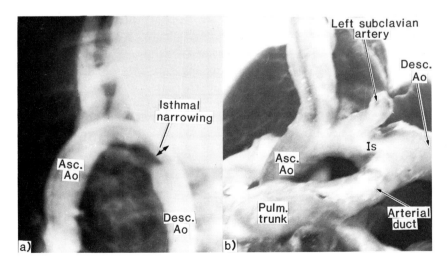

Fig. 5.4 (a) Lateral projection of aortogram in a neonate. The isthmus is narrower than both ascending (Asc Ao) and descending aorta (Desc Ao). An arterial duct is also shown. (b) Anatomical specimen of normal neonatal aorta and pulmonary trunk. The arterial duct is demonstrated as a continuation of the pulmonary trunk. The aortic isthmus (Is) is seen to be narrower than both ascending and descending aorta.

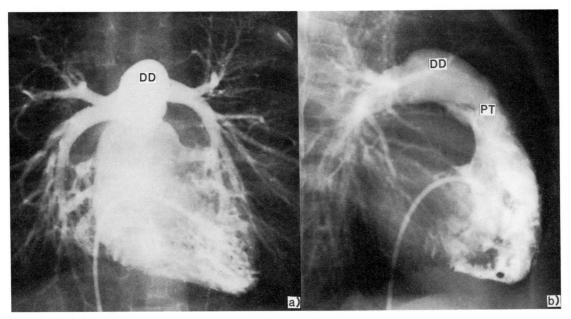

Fig. 5.5 Right ventriculogram in frontal (a) and lateral (b) projections. A ductal diverticulum (DD) is seen. Also demonstrated is the relatively small calibre of the right and left pulmonary arteries compared with the pulmonary trunk (PT).

ascending aorta irrespective of other associated intracardiac anomalies. The ascending aorta is usually of greater cross-sectional area than in the normal child. Flow through the arterial duct will be from left to right (that is from aorta to pulmonary trunk, the converse of that in the normal fetus). As a consequence, the neonate with pulmonary atresia lacks the usual narrowing of the aortic isthmus, while the arterial duct has a different angle of insertion

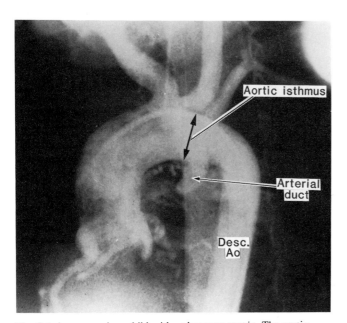

Fig. 5.6 Aortogram in a child with pulmonary atresia. The aortic isthmus is wider than the descending aorta while the abnormal angle of insertion of the arterial duct with aorta contrasts with that found in the normal neonate (Fig. 5.4).

(Fig. 5.6) to the descending aorta compared with the normal (Fig. 5.4) (Santos et al, 1980). Coarctation of the aorta never occurs (or, at least, is extremely rare) in neonates with severe pulmonary outflow tract obstruction (Shinebourne & El Seed, 1974). This is because the distribution of flow in the fetus results in an abnormal increase in cross-sectional area of the aortic isthmus which mitigates against coarctation. Alternatively it could be argued that if pre-ductal coarctation of the aorta was present alongside pulmonary atresia, descending aortic and hence placental flow would be inadequate to sustain fetal life. To take this one stage further, if isthmal narrowing were found in conjunction with pulmonary atresia or critical stenosis at birth (Wilson et al, 1987), it could imply that the atresia was acquired later in fetal development, or at least late enough not to distort the normal aortic arch anatomy.

Conversely, any intracardiac anomaly that results in reduced aortic and excessive pulmonary blood flow in the fetus will be associated with exaggeration of the normal neonatal isthmal narrowing to produce so-called 'pre-ductal coarctation' (Rudolph et al, 1972). Perhaps the most striking example is the association of interruption of the aortic arch with a ventricular septal defect (Van Praagh et al, 1971). The subaortic stenosis is typically due to leftwards deviation of the outlet septal (Moulaert et al, 1976; see Ch. 45). In this and other comparable situations, such as double outlet right ventricle with subpulmonary ventricular septal defect and a restrictive subaortic infundibulum (Fig. 5.7), preferential flow to the pulmonary trunk results in a small ascending aorta. After the blood entering the aorta has supplied the head and neck vessels, little flow is left to perfuse the aortic isthmus, which is consequently

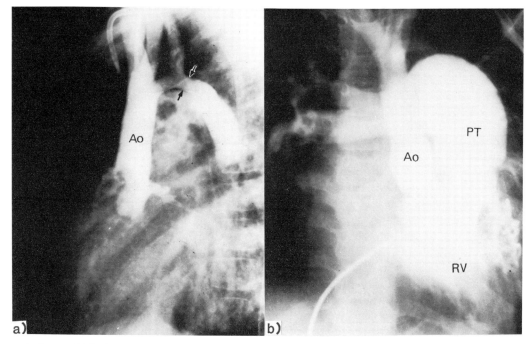

Fig. 5.7 Right ventriculogram (b) in frontal projection in a child with double outlet right ventricle. Preferential flow to pulmonary trunk has resulted in a small ascending aorta. (a) Lateral projection of aortogram. As the head and neck vessels arise, so further narrowing of the aorta results in isthmal hypoplasia. A persistent arterial duct is present.

narrow. A further example is provided by the frequent association of aortic coarctation in univentricular atrioventricular connexion to a left ventricle in presence of a discordant ventriculo-arterial connexion but not with a concordant ventriculo-arterial connexion. Since the ventricular septal defect is often restrictive, it results effectively in subaortic stenosis. Antegrate aortic flow is reduced in this setting, while in the situation with a concordant ventriculo-arterial connexion, aortic flow may be increased as pulmonary flow is frequently reduced.

BLOOD PRESSURE, CARDIAC OUTPUT AND MYOCARDIAL FUNCTION IN THE FETUS

Since the fetus is surrounded by amniotic fluid, fetal vascular pressures are recorded in relation to the pressure in the amniotic cavity. The fetal blood pressure is low throughout most of gestation despite a high cardiac output. This is accounted for principally by the very low resistance of the placental vascular bed. Fetal lambs of 90 days have a systolic pressure of about 40 mmHg, rising to 65–70 mmHg at term (150 days) (Rudolph, 1979). The rise in pressure with gestation age depends on complex alterations in the resistance of each organ. It is most probably dominated by the increase in placental vascular resistance with maturation. As the arterial duct is widely patent, both ventricles eject against the same vascular resistance. The pressures in the aorta and pulmonary trunk are therefore equal at 65–70/30–35 mmHg. In late gestation, pulmonary arterial and right ventricular systolic pressures may be 5–8 mmHg higher than those in the aorta and left ventricle, probably because of mild constriction of the arterial duct.

The term 'cardiac output' has different connotations in the fetus and neonate. After birth, the pulmonary and systemic circulations are in series whereas in the fetus this is not so. Comparison of fetal and neonatal cardiac output is therefore not straightforward. Nonetheless, since umbilical flow roughly equates with half the combined fetal ventricular output and left ventricular output equates with cardiac output in the infant or adult, these may be used for comparison.

The most important single fact about cardiac output in the fetus and newborn is that it is greater per kg body weight than in the adult (Dawes, 1968). In the sheep, measurements of umbilical flow range from 140–180 ml/kg/min (Dawes et al, 1954) in anaesthetised fetuses near term, to 240 ml/kg/min in anaesthetised fetuses in utero (Rudolph & Heymann, 1970). In the first 10 days following delivery, the output rises to 450 ml/kg/min (Stahlman et al, 1967), falling to 325 ml/kg/min between 20 and 60 days (Cross et al, 1959) and to 115–120 ml/kg/min in the adult (Metcalfe & Parer, 1966). Human infants similarly have resting cardiac outputs (180–240 ml/kg/min) which are 2–3 times in excess of adult values.

In the fetus the low resistance placental circuit is

thought to facilitate a high cardiac output. The higher cardiac output in the newborn may reflect a higher oxygen consumption (metabolic rate) (up to 7 ml O_2/kg/min at 10 days) than in the adult (3.9 ml O_2/kg/min). This is probably related to temperature homeostasis (Dawes, 1968). Small animals have a greater surface area in relation to body mass than large animals and therefore lose heat more readily.

As there is limited ability of the fetal heart to alter stroke volume, cardiac output is closely related to heart rate. Thus an increase in heart rate in lambs from 160–240/min (Rudolph, 1977) causes a 15% increase in stroke volume. A fall to 120/min decreases cardiac output by about one-quarter. There is less ability of isolated strips of fetal lamb myocardium to generate tension than an equivalent mass of adult lamb myocardium (Friedman, 1973). Similarly, stroke volume in fetal lambs studied in utero falls more than in adult animals subsequent to surgical constriction of the pulmonary trunk or aorta. The fetal heart increases its output less when given a rapid volume load by intravenous infusion than does the adult animal given a comparable load.

There is evidence that myocardial performance improves with gestational age, but it is not known when precisely after birth function approaches that of the adult myocardium. Morphological characteristics of fetal compared with mature myocardium account for some of the differences in function. Fetal myocardium has a higher water content and fewer contractile elements than adult muscle and there may be differences in metabolism (Friedman, 1973).

Another factor that may influence fetal or neonatal ventricular function is the relative lack of sympathetic innervation. For normal responses to sympathetic control, there must be an adequately functional nerve supply with an intact reflex arc. The myocardial cells must have the capacity to respond to the neurohumoral transmitter, which in turn must be synthesised and produced in adequate amounts. There are marked species differences in this respect. Man is somewhere between rats (largely postnatal development) and guinea-pigs (remarkably well innervated during fetal life). The newborn human infant does have a well-developed cardiac sympathetic innervation but this is not as extensive as in the adult. There is, therefore, considerable postnatal development.

The differences between fetal and adult myocardium may partially explain why the preterm infant tolerates volume loads poorly and why congestive cardiac failure rapidly ensues in the presence of a large arterial duct. Similarly, preterm and young neonates may not tolerate surgery (particularly cardiopulmonary bypass surgery) as well as older children. This is not only due to technical considerations related to size. If the myocardium already has a high water content, there may be poor tolerance of further increases that may occur due to increased capillary permeability following cardiopulmonary bypass with or without hypothermia.

THE CHANGE FROM FETAL TO NEONATAL CIRCULATION

At birth the course of the circulation changes abruptly. The placenta is withdrawn from the circulation and gas transfer now takes place at the lungs. Withdrawal of the low resistance placental vascular bed (accompanied by constriction of the umbilical arteries) causes an increase in the systemic vascular resistance. As is discussed in more detail later, mechanical expansion of the lungs (and a rise in alveolar and arterial Po_2) initiates dilation of the pulmonary vascular bed. The pulmonary vascular resistance then falls and pulmonary blood flow increases. Also, in response to the increase in arterial Po_2, the arterial duct constricts (see below). It is functionally closed in the normal baby within 48 hours. With removal of the placenta from the circulation there is a reduction in umbilical venous return to the portal vein, venous duct and right atrium. At the same time, the increase in pulmonary blood flow augments pulmonary venous return to the left atrium. Although in the fetus the right atrial pressure was marginally higher than that in the left atrium, this situation becomes reversed after birth with functional (but not anatomical) closure of the oval foramen. This occurs by apposition of the flap valve with the rest of the atrial septum.

The pulmonary and systemic circulations are now essentially in series, although the oval foramen and arterial duct remain possible sites for left-to-right or right-to-left shunting for some days or even weeks after birth. There is evidence in normal neonates that small left-to-right shunts may be found at both atrial and ductal levels in the first 48 hours after birth. More important is the continuing potential for right-to-left shunting at either site, should the pulmonary vascular resistance rise or remain high for any reason. This may occur with respiratory infections, hyaline membrane disease or in particular with the condition termed 'persistent fetal circulation' (Gersony et al, 1969), or better, 'transitional circulation' (Brown & Pickering, 1974). The umbilical circulation in man is usually arrested by tying the cord, although umbilical arteries constrict in response to an increased oxygen tension as well as to mechanical and probably hormonal stimuli. How long after birth the cord should be tied remains debatable. The longer it is left, the greater the time for placental transfusion. A maximum of 30 ml/kg (Yao & Lind, 1974) is available. Maximum transfer does, however, confer the hazard of neonatal polycythaemia (Saigal & Usher, 1977). As half this transfusion occurs during the first 30–45 seconds (Yao et al, 1968), this may be taken as an appropriate time.

Closure of the venous duct is principally passive (Meyer & Lind, 1966) rather than as a result of constriction of a sphincter (Chacko & Reynolds, 1953) as was once thought. After birth, flow through the duct continues for some hours or days, the duct becoming smaller as the portal sinus itself becomes smaller as a consequence of the reduction of umbilical venous return. Contraction of the smooth muscle cells in the wall may also play some part in its closure. Whether it constricts or dilates in response to certain prostaglandins or to changes in Po_2 as yet has not been established. Organic closure of the venous duct usually takes place between the 15th and 20th days of life (Meyer & Lind, 1966).

The major importance of the venous duct in congenital heart disease is in the setting of infradiaphragmatic total anomalous pulmonary venous connexion to the portal vein. In this condition, severe pulmonary venous obstruction and oedema develop when the duct closes. The pulmonary venous return, inconveniently, must then have to pass through the portal and hepatic vascular capillary beds before returning to the heart. Of interest is the potential for demonstration of this type of anomalous pulmonary venous connexion by injection of radio-opaque contrast medium via a catheter introduced into the umbilical vein and passed to the portal vein (Tynan et al, 1974).

The mechanism of closure of the arterial duct and the postnatal changes in the pulmonary circulation will be described later (see below and Ch. 38).

The arterial duct (ductus arteriosus)

The arterial duct develops from the distal portion of the left 6th aortic arch and connects the pulmonary trunk to the aorta just distal to the left subclavian artery. While almost always left-sided, a right-sided duct may be found with a right aortic arch (Knight & Edwards, 1974). Rarely the arterial duct may persist as a bilateral structure. By the 6th week of life, the arterial duct carries over 90% of the right ventricular output. It therefore diverts blood to the descending aorta and thence to the low resistance placental circuit.

Anatomy

This is dealt with in detail in Chapter 38. It is of note that the histological, but not the gross morphological structure of the duct, contrasts with that of the surrounding vessels (Ho, 1977). Whereas the media of the pulmonary trunk and aorta are composed mainly of circumferentially arranged layers of elastic fibres, the media of the arterial duct consists largely of smooth muscle fibres arranged spirally. The ductal intima consists of an endothelial cell lining with subendothelial avascular connective tissue separated from the media by an internal elastic lamina (Ho & Anderson, 1979).

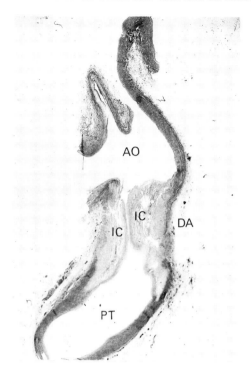

Fig. 5.8 Histological section through the pulmonary trunk (PT), arterial duct (DA) and aorta (AO). Mounds or cushions (IC) of intimal and medial tissue encroach upon the ductal lumen which is almost completely obliterated.

No close correlation exists between gestational age and ductal maturity (Gittenberger-de Groot et al, 1980b). In general, the more mature duct shows development of mounds or cushions of medial and intimal tissue which encroach on the ductal lumen (Fig. 5.8). After closure, spaces filled with mucoid tissue develop in the media with fragmentation of the internal elastic membrane and cytolytic necrosis. Closure is produced initially by muscular contraction which both narrows and shortens the duct.

Of note is the finding of a thick, wavy, unfragmented elastic lamina in a persistent patent duct in a term or older child. This suggests strongly that true persistence of the duct is a primary congenital malformation (Gittenberger-de Groot, 1977) which can be distinguished histologically from prolonged patency of an immature duct. One exception to this is the persistently patent duct found in cases of congenital rubella. This has been shown to reflect arrested development rather than a specific anatomical abnormality (Gittenberger-de Groot et al, 1980a).

Why the arterial duct remains widely patent during fetal life is not fully known. The concept has developed that patency is actively maintained in response to certain prostaglandins produced in the ductal wall (Coceani & Olley, 1980). The intramural mechanism may be reinforced by circulating prostaglandins produced elsewhere. Prostaglandins are oxygenated derivatives of polyunsaturated fatty acids. The most abundant mammalian precursor is arachidonic acid, which is esterified to phospholipids in cell membranes (Moncada & Vane, 1979). Arachidonic acid is released by a phospholipase and can then be metabolised by lipoxygenase or cyclo-oxygenase enzymes to a prostaglandin endoperoxide such as PGH_2. This in turn may be converted to a stable vasoactive prostaglandin such as PGE_2. The arterial duct contains a cyclo-oxygenase and possibly a lipoxygenase (Olley & Coceani, 1981). It has the capacity to synthesise prostaglandins. Certain anti-inflammatory compounds such as indomethacin which inhibit cyclo-oxygenases (prostaglandin synthetase) constrict the fetal duct both in vitro and in vivo in doses below the range for most non-specific actions. Other cyclo-oxygenase inhibitors such as aspirin also induce ductal constriction. The effect correlates closely with their relative potencies as cyclo-oxygenase inhibitors. The constricting effect of the agents is more marked in immature than in mature fetuses.

Of many prostaglandins tested on isolated ductal strips from the fetal lamb, PGE_2 is the most potent relaxant (Coceani et al, 1978a & b) with only PGE_1 being comparable. This effect was noted at all stages of gestation. The constrictor effect of indomethacin is completely reversed by PGE_1 or PGE_2. Although other prostaglandins may play a role in influencing ductal tone, evidence at present strongly supports the notion that murally produced PGE_2 is the prime mediator of ductal patency.

Closure of the arterial duct

Whether specific prostaglandins cause ductal closure remains uncertain. One hypothesis (Starling & Elliot, 1974) is that oxygen promotes production from arachidonic acid of PGE_2 which is known to constrict the duct. Indomethacin, however, still causes ductal constriction in high oxygen concentrations, thus making this an unlikely explanation. Another possibility is that thromboxane A2 (a powerful constrictor of other vessels) may play a part (Friedman, 1978). Against this is the lack of effect of thromboxane A2 in vitro (Coceani et al, 1978a) and its short half-life in blood.

The alternative and more attractive hypothesis is that ductal closure occurs due to the withdrawal of the relaxant effect of PGE_2. This is supported first by the findings that PGE_2 is less effective postnatally than prenatally (Coceani et al, 1975). Further evidence comes from the known decline in prostaglandin activity in the last trimester of pregnancy (Clyman et al, 1978), and the rapid fall in prostaglandin levels after birth (Challiss et al, 1976).

Contraction of the smooth muscle wall of the arterial duct in the full-term neonate results in functional closure within 10–15 hours of birth (Moss et al, 1963; Rudolph et al, 1961). This is related to the rise in arterial P_{O_2} with respiration which in some way modifies synthesis of local prostaglandins.

Studies in fetal lambs have shown that constriction of the arterial duct during the last trimester is stimulated by increasing arterial and venous P_{O_2} (McMurphy et al, 1972). With advancing gestational age the amount of constriction in response to an increasing P_{O_2} is greater and the level of P_{O_2} required to initiate a response falls (McMurphy et al, 1972). It is, therefore, not surprising to find the relatively high incidence of persistent patency of the arterial duct in preterm infants.

Failure of ductal closure at birth may lead to cardiac failure in early life or pulmonary vascular occlusive disease in later life. In infants with certain types of congenital heart disease, however, residual patency of the duct may be life-saving. This occurs when pulmonary blood flow is maintained by left-to-right shunting through the duct (pulmonary atresia for example) and when aortic obstruction is bypassed by right-to-left shunting from pulmonary trunk to the descending aorta (as in interrupted aortic arch).

The magnitude of left-to-right shunting through an arterial duct is governed by its diameter, the pressure difference between its aortic and pulmonary ends and the difference between the systemic and pulmonary vascular resistances. As already discussed, animal studies have shown that ductal constriction can be produced by inhibition of prostaglandin synthesis (Heymann & Rudolph, 1976; Sharpe et al, 1974). Successful closure or reduction in size of a persistent arterial duct has been reported using aspirin or indomethacin, potent inhibitors of prostaglandin synthetase (Friedman et al, 1976; Rudolph, 1977). This is discussed in more detail in Chapter 38.

The pulmonary circulation

Pulmonary arterial and aortic pressures are equal in the normal fetus (Lewis et al, 1976). As a result of the extremely high fetal pulmonary vascular resistance, pulmonary blood flow is low. More than 90% of the right ventricular output is diverted away from the lungs via the arterial duct. Why is the pulmonary resistance so high? Although tortuosity and kinking of small pulmonary vessels has been suggested (Reynolds, 1956), a more probable explanation is the low P_{O_2} to which the small muscular pulmonary arteries are exposed during fetal life. Changes in gas composition of blood perfusing unventilated fetal lung or of the gas mixture used for ventilation (Cassin et al, 1964; Cook et al, 1963) produce large alterations in pulmonary vascular resistance. Gaseous expansion alone also causes pulmonary vasodilation irrespective of changes in arterial blood gases (Cassin et al, 1964; Lauer et al, 1965). Nonetheless, the effects of ventilation with air- or oxygen-enriched mixtures are far greater than those of nitrogen (Dawes et al, 1953). Changes in alveolar P_{O_2} without gaseous distension of the lungs (and without appreciable changes in arterial P_{O_2}) also result in pulmonary vasodilation in the mature fetal limb. This is shown by the response to expanding the lungs with dextran-saline solution of high O_2 content (Lauer et al, 1965). Whether arterial or alveolar P_{CO_2} influence the fetal or newborn pulmonary vascular resistance remains debatable. Cassin et al (1964) found in their experiments with mature fetal lambs that, over the range of P_{O_2} 16–34 mmHg and P_{CO_2} 25–42 mmHg, either a 10 mmHg rise in P_{O_2} or a 10 mmHg fall in P_{CO_2} caused the same degree of pulmonary vasodilation. In contrast, Rudolph & Yuan (1966), working with newborn calves, found no relation between P_{CO_2} and pulmonary vascular resistance. Be that as it may, hypoventilation with a raised P_{CO_2} in clinical practice causes profound pulmonary vasoconstriction even with minimal change in pH. All workers agree that a fall in pH causes pulmonary vasoconstriction in the newborn.

Reflecting the high vasoconstrictor tone, the small pulmonary arteries in the fetus are more muscular than in the adult. Wall thickness for the same sized external diameter vessel is approximately double in the fetus (Hislop & Reid, 1981). The notion that there is a progressive increase in the ratio of the area of the media to the area of the intima in small pulmonary arteries under 50 μm diameter (i.e. an increase in the amount of smooth muscle in their walls – Naeye, 1961), is a simplification (see Ch. 6). At all fetal ages, partially muscular and non-muscular arteries are found in the same size-range vessels as the adult (Elliott, 1964). All vessels below 35 μm diameter, however, are non-muscular. The diameters of the most proximal muscular arteries in the fetus are less than those in the adult. The main resistance to pulmonary flow is probably situated at the fifth and sixth generation vessels.

All the factors mentioned previously operate at birth to lower pulmonary vascular resistance and increase pulmonary blood flow. The introduction of air into the alveoli with the first breath produces a gas-fluid interface. Surface forces tending to collapse alveoli may exert some distending force on the small vessels in the interalveolar spaces by holding them open (Macklin, 1946; Rudolph, 1970). At first sight it is not apparent how changes in alveolar gases should influence the precapillary pulmonary vessels which constitute the major site of pulmonary vascular resistance. Using a rapid freezing technique, however, Staub (1963) showed that oxygen could diffuse from alveoli directly into the small pulmonary arteries, so influencing them in this way. Another fascinating question is why does oxygen cause dilation of pulmonary vessels while causing constriction of all other vascular smooth muscle (including the arterial duct)? Lloyd (1968) suggested this was related to a substance produced by lung parenchyma: isolated carotid and pulmonary artery strips

suspended in a bath failed to constrict in response to hypoxia, though both vessels constricted when surrounded by a cuff of lung tissue. Bradykinin is a potent vasodilator of fetal pulmonary blood vessels (Campbell et al, 1968). It has also been thought to play an important part in events at birth (Melmon et al, 1968). Left atrial blood samples showed a fall in levels of kininogen, a bradykinin precursor, when fetal lambs were ventilated with oxygen but not with nitrogen, suggesting that bradykinin is formed in the lungs (Heymann et al, 1969). Similarly, when the fetal P_{O_2} was raised by placing the ewe in a hyperbaric oxygen chamber, there was enhanced bradykinin formation.

More recently the role of prostaglandins in influencing pulmonary vascular resistance has been appreciated. As previously discussed (when considering the arterial duct) arachidonic acid, which is widely distributed in fetal and neonatal vessel walls, is one of the principal precursors of prostaglandins. Prostacyclin, PGI_2, has been shown to be the major product of arachidonic acid metabolism in neonatal pulmonary vessel walls (Pace-Asciak & Rangaraj, 1978). It is an extremely powerful pulmonary vasodilator. The dilator effect of PGI_2 on pulmonary vessels is strikingly more consistent and profound than that of PGE_1 or PGE_2, although E series prostaglandins (the most powerful known relaxants of the arterial duct) also cause pulmonary vasodilation (Lock et al, 1980a). Significantly, even in hypoxic lambs, PGI_2 has a far more potent pulmonary vasodilator action than PGE_1 or PGE_2. This fact is made the more significant by the finding of minimal one-pass clearance or deactivation by the pulmonary vascular bed of PGI_2 (Dusting et al, 1978) in contrast to other prostaglandins.

Further to support the notion that prostaglandins regulate fetal and neonatal pulmonary vascular resistance is the finding that indomethacin, a prostaglandin synthetase inhibitor, induces pulmonary vasoconstriction in newborn dogs (Kadowitz et al, 1975) or goats (Leffler et al, 1978). Chronic therapy, however, did not affect baseline pulmonary vascular tone. Responses to hypoxia or other agents such as acetylcholine or histamine, suggest that other mechanisms also regulate fetal or neonatal pulmonary vascular tone (Lock et al, 1980a).

Other prostaglandins may also be important. Thus, Lock et al (1980b) demonstrated marked vasoconstrictor effects of PGD_2 and PGF_2 in newborn lambs. The response was diminished by alveolar hypoxia in contrast to the dilator effect of PGI_2 which was enhanced. This group has suggested that the principal mediator of pulmonary vascular tone is continuous local production of prostaglandin which actively maintains the neonatal pulmonary vessels in a relaxed state. Developing this further, it could be that certain neonatal conditions resulting in an elevated pulmonary vascular resistance (such as persistent fetal or transitional circulation – Gersony et al, 1969; Brown & Pickering, 1974) are caused by abnormalities of prostaglandin synthesis. Such abnormalities may also explain a further phenomenon. Most infants with large ventricular septal defects exhibit a fall in pulmonary vascular resistance 2–3 months after birth. A small group, however, with similar intracardiac anatomy do not show such a fall. They present with irreversible pulmonary vascular disease in early childhood (Hislop et al, 1975). Perhaps abnormalities in PGI_2 production explain the latter. The reactivity of the pulmonary vasculature decreases with age and shows marked species differences. The small pulmonary vessels of newborn animals have thick muscular walls and their pulmonary arterial pressure is at systemic levels. In the newborn infant, following ductal closure, pulmonary arterial pressure falls to adult levels in about 2 weeks (James & Rowe, 1957), most of the change taking place in the first 2–3 days. The initial fall is due to release of pulmonary vasoconstrictor tone with later thinning of the medial muscle layer in the vessel wall (Naeye, 1966). Newborn puppies (Phillips et al, 1960) show a similar pattern to man, but calves at sea level may take 4–5 weeks before their pulmonary artery pressure reaches adult levels (Reeves & Leathers, 1964). Small pulmonary vessels in these animals have extremely thick muscular walls. This feature is also thought to account for the greater reactivity of the newborn calf to a fall in PO_2 or pH (Rudolph & Yuan, 1966). Similarly, the pulmonary vasculature of the newborn human infant reacts more briskly (pulmonary artery pressure rises) to falls in alveolar or arterial PO_2 than does that of an older child or adult (Emmanouilides et al, 1964; James & Rowe, 1957; Rudolph et al, 1961).

After the first 2–3 weeks of life, mean pulmonary arterial pressure in man remains constant at around 15 ($\pm$5) mmHg. Systolic pressure varies from 15–30 mmHg and diastolic pressure from 5–10 mmHg. With growth, more blood passes through the lungs but the pressure drop across them remains constant. In the lungs the ratio of pressure drop (mmHg) to flow (litres/min) is loosely termed 'resistance' (PVR). If flow is normalised for body surface area and expressed as cardiac index (i.e. litres/min/m^2), pulmonary vascular resistance remains constant from the age of 1 month to late adulthood. (If resistance is expressed simply as litres/min/mmHg, resistance is higher in the first year of life.) As resistance remains constant with age but the pulmonary vessels increase in length, either resistance vessels must dilate or the number of vessels must increase. As the vessels still retain some capacity for dilation, the former is unlikely. It is now known (Hislop, 1971) that the number of small pulmonary arteries (acinar vessels) increase markedly during postnatal growth. Should this normal proliferation of vessels not occur, pulmonary hypertension would be expected.

Influence of congenital heart disease on changes in the pulmonary circulation at birth

The normal postnatal fall in pulmonary vascular resistance may be influenced by the presence of certain congenital cardiac anomalies. Particularly significant are those where there is a large communication between the pulmonary and systemic circulations. A further influence is hypoxia from any cause such as a respiratory tract infection or hyaline membrane disease.

Infants who are hypoxic from lung disease, or who exhibit persistent hypoventilation from cerebral causes for prolonged periods after birth show a slower rate of fall of pulmonary vascular resistance (Naeye & Letts, 1962). Similarly, infants born at high altitude show a delayed fall of resistance compared to those born at sea level. They have more muscle in the walls of small pulmonary arteries (Arias-Stella & Saldana, 1962). The higher pulmonary pressures and resistance may persist into adult life (Penaloza et al, 1963; Sime et al, 1963). The retention of smooth muscle in the media of the pulmonary vessels is associated with enhanced responsiveness to vasoactive stimuli (Grover et al, 1963).

Many congenital cardiac anomalies are characterised by free communication at ventricular or great arterial level between the pulmonary and systemic circulations. In the absence of pulmonary outflow tract obstruction, many will have excessive pulmonary blood flow due to a left-to-right shunt. The magnitude of shunting then depends on the ratio of pulmonary to systemic vascular resistance – a so-called 'dependent' shunt (Rudolph, 1977).

Patients with a large ventricular septal defect or widely patent arterial duct might be expected to go into cardiac failure in the first week of life. This is unusual and symptoms of left ventricular failure seldom occur before 3–12 weeks (Hoffman & Rudolph, 1965). The explanation is a delay in fall of pulmonary vascular resistance accompanied by persistence of the fetal amount of muscle in the media (Wagenvoort, 1962). It is not known why subjection of the pulmonary artery to systemic pressures should cause a delayed fall in resistance. The delayed fall in pulmonary vascular resistance limits the left-to-right shunt in term babies and accounts for the time of onset of symptoms. In premature babies with a dependent shunt, however, cardiac failure may appear in the first week of life. This had previously been thought due to the more rapid fall in pulmonary vascular resistance in the preterm group, as some studies had shown less muscle in the media of the small pulmonary arteries (Wagenvoort, 1962). The assumption had been that, in this group, a high pulmonary vascular resistance could not be maintained in the face of systemic pressures. More recently, other workers have indicated that there is no change in the amount of pulmonary vascular smooth muscle during the latter half of gestation, which would make it unlikely that this factor is important (Levin et al, 1976). Alternative factors are that sympathetic innervation of the left ventricle is incomplete (Friedman et al, 1968; Lebowitz et al 1972) and that Starling's law is less applicable to the preterm myocardium (Friedman, 1973). Furthermore, the relatively high resting cardiac output of preterm compared with term infants allows them little or no capacity to increase stroke volume or heart rate in response to an increased pulmonary venous return (Rudolph, 1977).

Paradoxically, the hypoxia and acidosis of respiratory infections may limit the magnitude of dependent left-to-right shunts and prevent heart failure (Vogel et al, 1967). In the same way, a higher resistance at altitude limits dependent left-to-right shunts. Infants with ventricular septal defects in Denver (at the moderate altitude of 5280 ft) have lower pulmonary blood flows and a lower incidence of heart failure than infants with similar defects at sea level (Rudolph, 1977).

The concept of dependent versus obligatory shunting is also helpful in planning management of certain patients with cardiac anomalies (Rudolph, 1970). In obligatory shunt situations (perhaps typified by some atrioventricular septal defects with a left ventricular to right atrial communication, or sinus of Valsalva fistula from aortic root to right atrium), there is a shunt of blood from a high pressure ventricle or great artery to a low pressure atrium. This left-to-right shunt may occur irrespective of the ratio of pulmonary to systemic vascular resistance. Hence, in this group, banding of the pulmonary trunk as palliation may be contraindicated. This is in contrast to the dependent shunt group where banding may be appropriate (e.g. hearts with univentricular atrioventricular connexions and grossly excessive pulmonary flow). Care must be taken, however, not to apply this principle too rigidly in the setting of atrioventricular septal defects where there may be dependent as well as obligatory shunting. The presence of regurgitation through an atrioventricular valve has also to be considered in this situation (see Ch. 24).

REFERENCES

Arias-Stella J, Saldana M 1962 The muscular pulmonary arteries in people native to high altitude. Med. Thorac. 19: 484–493

Barclay A E, Franklin K J, Prichard M M L 1944 The foetal circulation and cardiovascular system and the changes that they undergo at birth. Blackwell Scientific, Oxford

Brown R, Pickering D 1974 Persistent transitional circulation. Archives of Disease in Childhood 49: 883–885

Campbell A G M, Dawes G S, Fishman A P, Hyman A I, Perks A M 1968 The release of a Bradykinin-like pulmonary vasodilator substance in foetal and newborn lambs. Journal of Physiology 195: 83–96

Cassin S, Dawes G S, Mott J C, Ross B B, Strang L B 1964 The vascular resistance of the foetal and newly ventilated lung of the lamb. Journal of Physiology 171: 61–79

Chacko A W, Reynolds S R M 1953 Embryonic development in the human of the "sphincter" of the ductus venosus. Anatomical Record 115: 151–163

Challis J R G, Dilley S R, Robinson J S 1976 Prostaglandins in the circulation of the fetal lamb. Prostaglandins 11: 1041–1052

Clyman R I, Mauray F, Heymann M A 1978 Ductus arteriosus: developmental response to oxygen and indomethacin. Prostaglandins 15: 933–998

Coceani F, Olley P M 1980 Role of prostaglandins, prostacyclin and thromboxanes in the control of prenatal patency and postnatal closure of the ductus arteriosus. Seminars in Perinatology 4: 109–113

Coceani F, Olley P M, Bodach E 1975 Lamb ductus arteriosus: effect of prostaglandin synthesis inhibitors on the muscle tone and the response to prostaglandin E2. Prostaglandins 9: 299–308

Coceani F, Bishai I, White E, Bodach E, Olley P M 1978a Action of prostaglandins, endoperoxides, and thromboxanes on the lamb ductus arteriosus. American Journal of Physiology 234: H 117–122

Coceani F, Bodach E, White E, Bishai I, Olley P M 1978b Prostaglandin I2 is less relaxant than prostaglandin E2 on the lamb ductus arteriosus. Prostaglandins 15: 551–556

Cook C D, Drinker P A, Jacobson H N, Levison M, Strang L B 1963 Control of pulmonary blood flow in the foetal and newly born lamb. Journal of Physiology 169: 10–29

Cross K W, Dawes G S and Mott J C 1959 Anoxia, oxygen consumption and cardiac output in newborn lambs and adult sheep. Journal of Physiology 146: 316–43.

Danilowicz D, Rudolph A M and Hoffman J I E 1965 Vascular resistance in the large pulmonary arteries in infancy. Circulation Suppl II 32: (abstr) p. 74

Dawes G S 1968 Foetal and neonatal physiology. Year Book, Chicago, p 141–159, 32–37

Dawes G S, Mott J C, Widdicombe J G, Wyatt D G 1953 Changes in the lungs of the newborn lamb. Journal of Physiology 121: 141–162

Dawes G S, Mott J C, Widdicombe J G 1954 The foetal circulation in the lamb. Journal of Physiology 126: 563–587

Dusting G J, Moncada J S, Vane J R 1978 Recirculation of prostacyclin (PGI2) in the dog. British Journal of Pharmacology 64: 315–320

Elliott F M 1964 The pulmonary artery system in normal and diseased lungs – structure in relation to pattern of branching. PhD Thesis, University of London

Emmanouilides G C, Moss A J, Duffie E R Jr, Adams F H 1964 Pulmonary arterial pressure changes in human newborn infants from birth to 3 days of age. Journal of Pediatrics 65: 327–333

Friedman W F 1973 The intrinsic physiologic properties of the developing heart. In: Friedman W F, Lesch M, Sonnenblick E M (eds) Neonatal heart disease. Grune & Stratton, New York, p 21–49

Friedman W F 1978 Studies of responses of the ductus arteriosus in intact animals. In: Heymann M A, Rudolph A M (eds) The ductus arteriosus. The 75th Ross Conference on Pediatric Research. Ross Laboratories, Columbus, Ohio, p 35–43

Friedman W F, Pool P E, Jacobowitz D, Seagren S C, Braunwald E 1968 Sympathetic innervation of the developing rabbit heart. Biochemical and histochemical comparisons of fetal, neonatal and adult myocardium. Circulation Research 23: 25–32

Friedman W F, Hirschklau M J, Printz M P, Pitlick P T, Kirkpatrick S E 1976 Pharmacologic closure of patent ductus arteriosus in the premature infant. New England Journal of Medicine 295: 526–529

Gersony W M, Duc G V, Sinclair J C 1969 'PFC' syndrome (persistence of the fetal circulation). Circulation 40: 111–115

Gittenberger-de Groot A C 1977 Persistent ductus arteriosus: most probably a primary congenital malformation. British Heart Journal 39: 610–618

Gittenberger-de Groot A C, Moulaert A J M, Hitchcock J F 1980a Histology of the persistent ductus arteriosus in cases of congenital rubella. Circulation 62: 183–186

Gittenberger-de Groot A C, Van Ertbruggen I, Moulaert A J M G, Harinck E 1980b The ductus arteriosus in the preterm infant: histologic and clinical observations. Journal of Pediatrics 96: 88–93

Grover R F, Reeves J T, Will D H, Blunt S G Jr 1963 Pulmonary vasoconstriction in steers at high altitude. Journal of Applied Physiology 18: 567–574

Heath D, Du Shane J W, Wood E H, Edwards J E 1959 The structure of the pulmonary trunk at different ages and in cases of pulmonary hypertension and pulmonary stenosis. Journal of Pathology and Bacteriology 77: 443–456

Heymann M A, Rudolph A M 1966 Physiological observations of the normal fetus in utero. Journal of Pediatrics 69:967 (Abstract)

Heymann M A, Rudolph A M 1976 Effects of acetylsalicyclic acid on the ductus arteriosus and circulation in fetal lambs in utero. Circulation Research 38: 418–422

Heymann M A, Rudolph A M, Nies A S, Melmon K L 1969 Bradykinin production associated with oxygenation of the fetal lamb. Circulation Research 25: 521–534

Hislop A 1971 The fetal and childhood development of the pulmonary circulation and its disturbance in certain types of congenital heart disease. PhD Thesis, University of London

Hislop A, Reid L 1981 Growth and development of the respiratory system. In: Davis J A, Dobbing J (eds) Scientific foundations of paediatrics, 2nd Edn. Heinemann, London

Hislop A, Haworth S G, Shinebourne E A, Reid L 1975 Quantitative structural analysis of pulmonary vessels in isolated ventricular septal defects in infancy. British Heart Journal 37: 1014–1021

Ho S Y 1977 The ductus arteriosus and its relationship to tubular hypoplasia and coarctation. M Phil Thesis

Ho S Y, Anderson R H 1979 Coarctation, tubular hypoplasia and the ductus arteriosus: a histological study of 35 specimens. British Heart Journal 41: 268–274

Hoffman J I E, Rudolph A M 1965 The natural history of ventricular septal defects in infancy. American Journal of Cardiology 16: 634–653

Howatt W F, Avery M E, Humphreys P W, Normand I C S, Reid L, Strang L B 1965 Factors affecting pulmonary surface properties in the foetal lamb. Clinical Science 29: 238–248

James L S, Rowe R D 1957 The pattern of response of pulmonary and systemic arterial pressures in newborn and older infants to short periods of hypoxia. Journal of Pediatrics 51: 5–11

Kadowitz P J, Chapnick B M, Joiner P D, Hyman A L 1975 Influence of inhibitors of prostaglandin synthesis on the canine pulmonary vascular bed. American Journal of Physiology 229: 941–946

Knight L, Edwards J E 1974 Right aortic arch: types and associated cardiac anomalies. Circulation 50: 1047–1051

Lauer R M, Evans J A, Aoki M, Kittle C F 1965 Factors controlling pulmonary vascular resistance in fetal lambs. Journal of Pediatrics 67: 568–577

Lebowitz E A, Novick J S, Rudolph A M 1972 Development of myocardial sympathetic innervation in the fetal lamb. Pediatric Research 6: 887–893

Leffler C W, Tyler T L, Cassin S 1978 Effect of indomethacin on pulmonary vascular response to ventilation of fetal goats. American Journal of Physiology 234 (Heart Circ Physiol 3): H 346–351

Levin D L, Rudolph A M, Heymann M A, Phibbs R H 1976 Morphological development of the pulmonary vascular bed in fetal lambs. Circulation 53: 144–151

Lewis A B, Heymann M A, Rudolph A M 1976 Gestational changes in pulmonary vascular responses in fetal lambs in utero. Circulation Research 39: 536–541

Lloyd T C 1968 Hypoxic pulmonary vasoconstriction: role of perivascular tissue. Journal of Applied Physiology 25: 560–565

Lock J E, Olley P M, Coceani F 1980a Direct pulmonary vascular responses to prostaglandins in the conscious newborn lamb. American Journal of Physiology 238 ii: H631–H638

Lock J E, Olley P M, Soldin S, Coceani F 1980b Indomethacin-induced pulmonary vasoconstriction in the conscious newborn lamb. American Journal of Physiology 238 ii: H639–H651

McMurphy D M, Heymann M A, Rudolph A M, Melmon K L 1972 Developmental change in constriction of the ductus arteriosus: response to oxygen and vasoactive substances in the isolated ductus arteriosus of the fetal lamb. Pediatric Research 6: 231–238

Macklin C C 1946 Evidences of increase in the capacity of the pulmonary arteries and veins of dogs, cats and rabbits during inflation of the freshly excised lung. Revue Canadienne de Biologie 5: 199–232

Melmon K L, Cline M J, Hughes T, Nies A S 1968 Kinins: possible mediation of neonatal circulatory changes in man. Journal of Clinical Investigation 47: 1295–1302

Meschia G, Cotter J R, Breathnach C S, Barron D H 1965 The hemoglobin, oxygen, carbon dioxide and hydrogen ion concentrations in the umbilical bloods of sheep and goats as sampled via indwelling plastic catheters. Quarterly Journal of Experimental Physiology 50: 185–195

Metcalfe J, Parer J T 1966 Cardiovascular changes during pregnancy in ewes. American Journal of Physiology 210: 821–825

Meyer W W, Lind J 1966 The ductus venosus and the mechanism of its closure. Archives of Disease in Childhood 41: 597–612

Moncada S, Vane J R 1979 Pharmacology and endogenous roles of prostaglandin and endoperoxides, thromboxane A2, and prostacyclin. Pharmacological Reviews, 30: 293–330

Moss A J, Emmanouilides G C, Duffie E R Jr 1963 Closure of the ductus arteriosus. Lancet i: 703–704

Moulaert A J, Bruins C C, Oppenheimer Dekker A 1976 Anomalies of the aortic arch and ventricular septal defects. Circulation 53: 1011–1015

Naeye R L 1961 Arterial changes during the perinatal period. Archives of Pathology 71: 121–128

Naeye R L 1966 Development of systemic and pulmonary arteries from birth through early childhood. Biology of the Neonate 10: 8–16

Naeye R L, Letts H W 1962 The effects of prolonged neonatal hypoxaemia on the pulmonary vascular bed and heart. Pediatrics 30: 902–908

Olley P M, Coceani F 1981 Prostaglandins and the ductus arteriosus. Annual Review of Medicine 32: 375–385

Pace-Asciak C R, Rangaraj G 1978 Prostaglandin biosynthesis and catabolism in the lamb ductus arteriosus, aorta and pulmonary artery. Biochimica et Biophysica Acta 529: 13–29

Penaloza D, Sime F, Banchero N, Gamboa R 1963 Pulmonary hypertension in healthy man born and living at high altitudes. In: Normal and abnormal pulmonary circulation. Fifth Annual Conference on Research in Emphysema. Aspen, Colorado. Karger, New York, p 257

Phillips C E Jr, De Weese J A, Manning J A, Mahoney E B 1960 Maturation of small pulmonary arteries in puppies. Circulation Research 8: 1268–1273

Reeves J T, Leathers J E 1964 Circulatory changes following birth of the calf and the effect of hypoxia. Circulation Research 15: 345–354

Reynolds S R M 1956 Fetal and neonatal pulmonary vasculature in guinea-pig in relation to hemodynamic changes at birth. American Journal of Anatomy 98: 97–123

Rudolph A M 1970 The changes in the circulation after birth: their importance in congenital heart disease. Circulation 41: 343–359

Rudolph A M 1974 Congenital diseases of the heart. Year Book, Chicago, p 1–48

Rudolph A M 1977 The ductus arteriosus. In: Anderson R H, Shinebourne E A (eds) Paediatric cardiology. Churchill Livingstone, Edinburgh, p 406–414

Rudolph A M 1979 Fetal and neonatal pulmonary circulation. Annual Review of Physiology 41: 383–395

Rudolph A M, Heymann M A 1970 Circulatory changes during growth in the fetal lamb. Circulation Research 26: 289–299

Rudolph A M, Yuan S 1966 Response of the pulmonary vasculature to hypoxia and H+ ion concentration changes. Journal of Clinical Investigation 45: 399–411

Rudolph A M, Drorbaugh J E, Auld P A M, et al 1961 Studies on the circulation in the neonatal period. The circulation in the respiratory distress syndrome. Pediatrics 27: 551–566

Rudolph A M, Heymann M A, Spitznas U 1972 Hemodynamic considerations in the development of narrowing of the aorta. American Journal of Cardiology 30: 514–525

Saigal S, Usher R H 1977 Symptomatic neonatal plethora. Biology of the Neonate 32: 62–72

St John Sutton M G, Raichlen J S, Reichek N, Huff D S 1984 Quantitative assessment of right and left ventricular growth in the human fetal heart: pathoanatomic study. Circulation 70: 935–941

Santos M A, Moll J N, Drummond C, Araujo W B, Romao N, Reis N B 1980 Development of the ductus arteriosus in right ventricular outflow tract obstruction. Circulation 62: 818–822

Sharpe G L, Thalme B, Sune Larsson K 1974 Studies on closure of the ductus arteriosus. XI. Ductal closure in utero by a prostaglandin synthetase inhibitor. Prostaglandins 8: 363–368

Shinebourne E A, Elseed A M 1974 Relation between fetal flow patterns, coarctation of the aorta and pulmonary blood flow. British Heart Journal 36: 492–498

Sime F, Banchero N, Penaloza D, Gamboa R, Cruz J, Marticorena E 1963 Pulmonary hypertension in children born and living at high altitudes. American Journal of Cardiology 11: 143–149

Stahlman M, Gray J, Young W C, Shepard F M 1967 Cardiovascular response of the neonatal lamb to hypoxia and hypercapnia. American Journal of Physiology 213: 899–904

Starling M B, Elliot R B 1974 The effects of prostaglandins, prostaglandin inhibitors and oxygen on the closure of the ductus arteriosus, pulmonary arteries and umbilical vessels in vitro. Prostaglandins 8: 187–203

Staub N C 1963 Site of action of hypoxia on the pulmonary vasculature. Federation Proceedings 22:453 (Abstract)

Tynan M, Behrendt D, Urquhart W, Graham G R 1974 Portal vein catheterisation and selective angiography in diagnosis of total anomalous pulmonary venous connexion. British Heart Journal 36: 1155–1159

Van Praagh R, Bernhard W P, Rosenthal A, Parisi L F, Fyler D C 1971 Interrupted aortic arch: surgical treatment. American Journal of Cardiology 27: 200–211

Vogel J H K, McNamara D G, Blount S G Jr 1967 Role of hypoxia in determining pulmonary vascular resistance in infants with ventricular septal defects. American Journal of Cardiology 20: 346–349

Wagenvoort C A 1962 The pulmonary arteries in infants with ventricular septal defect. Med. Thorac. 19: 354–361

Wilson N, Fonseka S, Walker D 1987 Severe pulmonary stenosis and duct dependent coarctation in a neonate. International Journal of Cardiology (in press)

Yao A C, Lind J 1974 Blood flow in the umbilical vessels during the third stage of labor. Biology of the Neonate of 25: 186–193

Yao A C, Hirvensalo M, Lind J 1968 Placental transfusion rate and uterine contraction. Lancet i: 380–383

Pulmonary vasculature

Clinical practice has changed in paediatric cardiology during the past 10 years. With improvements in surgical technique and in the management of cardiopulmonary bypass and cardioplegia many children now undergo surgery during the first months of life. Not surprisingly, the structural changes in the lungs of very young infants with heart disease are unlike those seen in older patients. The pulmonary circulation is normally remodelled after birth. Thus, the emphasis has shifted from descriptive pathology of established disease to studying the effect of abnormalities of pulmonary arterial pressure and flow on the growth and development of the pulmonary vasculature.

Haemodynamic abnormalities frequently prevent the pulmonary circulation from developing normally. When the structural abnormalities in the vessels are severe they may progress despite surgical repair of the cardiac abnormality which caused them. Occasionally, the progression of hypertensive pulmonary vascular disease may even accelerate following surgical repair. The optimal time for surgical intervention increasingly becomes a compromise between the surgical problems of operating on a small sick infant with little pulmonary vascular change and the risk of operating on an older, larger patient with more advanced vascular change. When the risk of an intracardiac repair is unacceptably high, abnormalities in pulmonary arterial pressure and flow can be corrected by palliative surgery. This encourages the pulmonary circulation to grow and develop normally, making a later intracardiac repair possible.

In children with pulmonary vascular abnormalities we ought to be able to predict not only the immediate outcome of an operation, but also the reversibility of the pulmonary vascular changes present at the time of surgery, and the potential for further normal growth. Unfortunately, the natural history of pulmonary vascular change and the effect of surgical intervention in the different types of congenital heart disease is still not completely understood.

NORMAL ANATOMY OF THE PULMONARY CIRCULATION

The functional unit of the lung is the acinus. An acinus is all the lung tissue supplied by a terminal bronchiolus. In the mature lung it includes up to eight generations of respiratory bronchioles, alveolar ducts and the alveoli beyond (Fig. 6.1). It is the respiratory unit of the lung. At the end of any airway, 3–5 acini are grouped to form a lobule. Each small airway is accompanied by a branch of the pulmonary artery until the arteries finally enter the capillary network of the alveolar walls. The acini and lobules with their accompanying arteries are the last part of the lung to appear before birth. It is these structures which are remodelled in the normal lung with growth and which change most readily in disease.

The bronchopulmonary segment is the basic topographical unit of the lung. It is a wedge of lung tissue supplied by a principal branch of a lobar bronchus and its accompanying pulmonary artery (Figs. 6.1, 6.2). The pulmonary veins and lymphatics lie in the intersegmental plane and receive tributaries from adjacent segments. The bronchopulmonary segment is the surgical unit of lung tissue, since a segment can be resected along its intersegmental boundaries. Familiarity with normal bronchopulmonary segmental anatomy is needed by the cardiologist. On pulmonary angiography, he must ensure that all the bronchopulmonary segments are normally connected to the central pulmonary arteries (Fig. 6.3a). Segments which are not perfused by a normal pulmonary arterial supply must be identified and their source of systemic blood supply sought (Figs. 6.3b, c). In patients with congenital heart disease the lobar and segmental arteries are sometimes dilated, displaced, stenosed, extremely small or are connected to a large collateral artery (Fig. 6.3b). The interpretation of the abnormal angiographic findings depends on systematic definition of the blood supply of each bronchopulmonary segment. Large collateral systemic arteries arising from the aorta (major aortopulmonary collateral arteries) are distinguished angiographically from

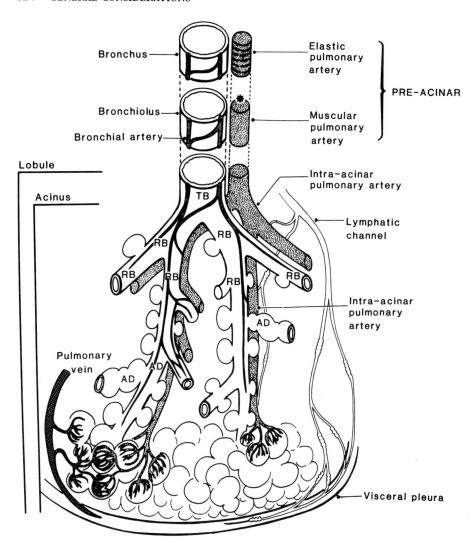

Fig. 6.1 Diagram of the airway and arterial pathway, showing an elastic artery which accompanies cartilaginous lobar, segmental and subsegmental bronchi. The pulmonary artery becomes muscularised at the 7–9th division from the segmental hilum, as indicated by * in this figure and in Figure 6.2. TB = terminal bronchiolus; RB = respiratory bronchiolus; AD = alveolar duct.

large bronchial arteries by their origin, distribution and proximal connexions with the hilar, lobar or segmental arteries (Figs. 6.3c, d). The final destination of bronchial arteries is not seen angiographically, since the majority of them connect with the intra-acinar pulmonary arteries.

The bronchial circulation

In children with congenital heart disease, the bronchial circulation may provide an alternative source of blood supply to the pulmonary capillaries when there is little or no flow of blood down the lobar or segmental arteries. In the presence of obstruction to or absence of the pulmonary veins, the bronchial veins drain oxygenated blood from the lung into the systemic venous system.

The main bronchial arterial supply usually arises from the aorta either directly or from an intermediary intercosto-bronchial artery. The number of arteries arising from the aorta to supply each lung varies in the normal. The commonest anatomical patterns seen in the series of Liebow (1965) included two posterior bronchial arteries supplying each lung in 30% of cases, with two arteries supplying the left and one the right lung in 20%. This last relationship was seen in mirror-image pattern in 16% and a single trunk supplied each bronchus in a further 10% of cases. The successive branches of each bronchial artery are described as superior, middle, and inferior with reference to their relative levels of aortic origin and not to their ultimate level of distribution within the lung. Additional 'accessory' bronchial arteries may arise from the subclavian, brachiocephalic, or internal mammary arteries. When the bronchial arterial circulation is expanded to provide an alternative source of pulmonary blood supply, these and other vessels enlarge. They then distribute blood through the bronchial arteries via the pulmonary ligaments and retroperitoneal tissues. Blood is also distributed from the pericardiophrenic, oesophageal and other mediastinal vessels and occasionally from a coronary artery. Each lobar and segmental bronchus within the lung is accompanied by two large bronchial arteries which anastomose frequently around the bronchus.

The bronchial arteries are readily distinguishable micro-

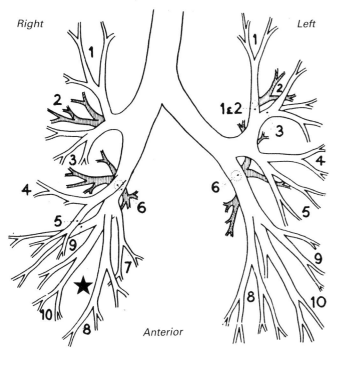

Right   *Left*

UPPER LOBE
1. Apical bronchus
2. Posterior bronchus
3. Anterior bronchus

Right	*Left*
MIDDLE LOBE	LINGULA
4. Lateral bronchus	4. Superior bronchus
5. Medial bronchus	5. Inferior bronchus

LOWER LOBE

6. Apical bronchus	6. Apical bronchus
7. Medial basal (cardiac)	8. Anterior basal bronchus
8. Anterior basal bronchus	9. Lateral basal bronchus
9. Lateral basal bronchus	10. Posterior basal bronchus
10. Posterior basal bronchus	

Fig. 6.2 Diagram showing the bronchopulmonary nomenclature. In the anterior basal bronchus of the right lower lobe the point at which the artery accompanying the bronchus changes from an elastic to a muscular wall structure is indicated *. Note that not all the divisions of the segmental bronchi are shown. (Reproduced by kind permission of Butterworths.)

scopically from the pulmonary arteries by their position in the lung and by their wall structure. They accompany the bronchi to supply the bronchial adventitia and mucosa together with the walls of large pulmonary arteries. They lie next to the bronchial veins and the nerves which supply the large airways. Like other systemic arteries, the media is thick and muscular, the internal elastic lamina is well defined and the external elastic lamina is interrupted or absent. The structure of bronchial arteries frequently changes with age in the normal lung. Longitudinal muscle bundles develop within the walls which may even occlude the lumen. The mechanism for this change is not understood.

There are two types of bronchial vein. These are the deep and the superficial (or pleurohilar) veins. Both types communicate freely with the pulmonary veins (Miller, 1947; Marchand et al, 1950). The deep veins originate in the walls of the terminal bronchioli and eventually drain into the left atrium directly or via the pulmonary veins. The pleurohilar veins from the right lung drain into the azygos vein. Those from the left lung drain into the hemiazygos, superior intercostal or left brachiocephalic veins. A bronchial vein has a thinner wall than a pulmonary vein for a given diameter. Unlike pulmonary veins, bronchial veins contain delicate bicuspid valves which are more commonly seen in the immature than in the mature lung.

Anastomoses between pulmonary and bronchial circulations

The presence of anastomoses between the pulmonary and bronchial arteries was first postulated by Virchow in 1854 because 'blocking' a pulmonary artery in the dog did not affect the nutrition of the lung. Zuckerkandl (1883) then demonstrated 'deep' anastomoses in the bronchial wall and 'superficial' ones in the pleura. Most of the proximal connexions between the pulmonary and bronchial arteries in the normal adult which accompany the same airway occur at the level of non-cartilaginous bronchioli (Tobin, 1952). More peripherally, the small bronchial arteries become indistinguishable as they anastomose with small pulmonary arteries around the necks of respiratory and terminal bronchioli. In addition, branches of the bronchial arteries which accompany large and small airways anastomose in the surrounding lung tissue with adjacent thin-walled pulmonary arteries. These connexions are called bronchopulmonary arteries (Wagenvoort & Wagenvoort, 1967). Subepithelial bronchial arteries also anastomose with small pre-capillary pulmonary arteries.

Wagenvoort & Wagenvoort (1967) found more bronchopulmonary anastomoses in the normal fetal and newborn lung than in the older lung. They therefore suggested that such connexions are normally more important before birth when pulmonary blood flow is low. Branches arising from small pulmonary arteries to supply the walls of the bronchi (called pulmobronchial arteries) are also more common in the immature than in the mature lung. A greater number of anastomoses would predispose to the more rapid enlargement of the bronchial circulation and hence to the greater adaptability of the newborn than the adult lung.

In the venous circulation, there are many connexions between bronchial and pulmonary veins. These enlarge in the presence of pulmonary venous hypertension (Marchand et al, 1950; Wagenvoort et al, 1972). Blood may then flow from the pulmonary veins indirectly to the right atrium.

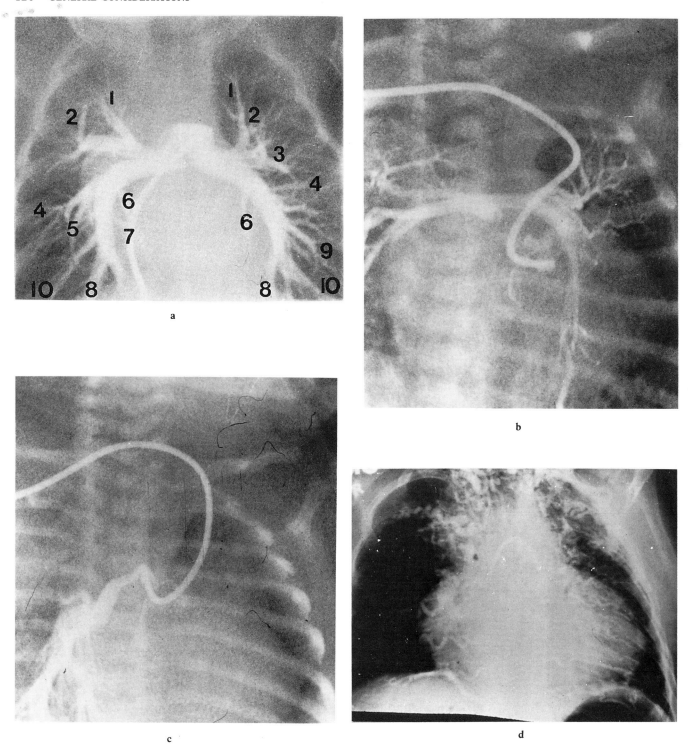

a

b

c

d

Fig. 6.3 (a) Normal pulmonary angiogram. The figures refer to the segmental pulmonary arteries indicated in Figure 6.2, identified by inspection of anteroposterior and lateral projections. The intrapulmonary arteries are closely related to the bronchi. In the left upper lobe there may be 2–7 segmental arteries in contrast to the 3 segmental bronchi, which are anatomically constant. (b) Angiogram from a case of pulmonary atresia with ventricular septal defect and major aortopulmonary collateral arteries in which the collateral artery supplying the left pulmonary artery was injected. The central pulmonary arteries are not connected to all the segmental arteries in either lung. (c) Angiogram from the case illustrated in Figure 6.3b, showing an injection into the collateral artery which anastomoses with the medial and anterior basal segmental arteries of the right lower lobe. The collateral arteries injected in Figures 6.3b and c arose from the descending thoracic aorta, behind the origin of the left main bronchus. (d) Angiogram from a case of acquired pulmonary atresia, showing innumerable small bronchial and other systemic arteries which supplied the pulmonary circulation. (Reproduced by kind permission of Dr Jane Somerville.)

Arterio-venous connexions

These are not found in the normal lung.

Pulmonary lymphatics

The superficial lymphatic network lies in the pleura while the deep network lies in the interstitium. The two networks anastomose around the hilum and drain to the hilar and tracheobronchial lymph nodes. Lymphatics are present in the pleura, connective tissue septa around the pulmonary arteries and veins and in the bronchial wall (including the mucosa). Small lymphatics consist of endothelial cells lying on a basement membrane. In the large channels the walls are strengthened by the addition of collagen and elastic fibres and an occasional muscle cell. The lymphatics contain delicate bicuspid valves. When pulmonary venous return is obstructed (either at the mitral valve or within the pulmonary veins themselves) the lymphatics become dilated. In the presence of longstanding obstruction (as in children with rheumatic heart disease and mitral stenosis), the walls of the lymphatics may be thickened by an increase in the amount of smooth muscle.

METHODS OF STUDYING PULMONARY VASCULAR PATHOLOGY

Biopsying the lung

For many years, the assessment of hypertensive pulmonary vascular disease by lung biopsy in young children with congenital heart disease proved to be a disappointing exercise. Biopsies were generally taken only from the most severely ill children in whom the structural changes of severe obstructive pulmonary vascular disease tended to confirm the clinical impression of inoperability. Interest was renewed, however, once it became apparent that the influence of pulmonary hypertension on the growth and development of the pulmonary circulation could be assessed in terms of size, number and muscularity of the pulmonary arteries (Haworth & Hislop, 1983).

The problems associated with biopsying the lung are first the state of preservation of the lung tissue. Equally significant is whether the structural changes in the biopsy are representative of those in the entire pulmonary circulation. Alveolar collapse does not occur when the biopsy is taken from the inflated lung fixed so that the airways are distended. Structures can then be identified easily (Fig. 6.4a). The distribution of pulmonary vascular change can vary throughout the lung in adults, the lower lobes generally being more severely affected (Harrison, 1958). In young children, however, extensive post-mortem studies have not demonstrated regional differences in pulmonary vascular structure. One study designed to detect regional difference in arterial muscularity, size and number demon-

strated none (Haworth & Reid, 1978). Nonetheless, when taking a lung biopsy the lingula is best avoided. Even in the normal lung, the intra-acinar pulmonary arteries in the lingula tend to have a thicker muscle coat than those in other parts of the lung (Heath & Best, 1958).

Analysis of pulmonary vascular change using frozen lung biopsy material has been advocated in children in whom there are clinical and haemodynamic doubts about operability. This is particularly so when the pulmonary arterial pressure was not measured at the cardiac catheterisation study (Rabinovitch et al, 1981). In deciding the feasibility of doing a corrective procedure, it is generally preferable to take an open lung biopsy and stain it appropriately. The structural, clinical and haemodynamic findings should then be re-discussed before making a final decision. More recent studies in lungs from children with various congenital cardiac malformations have confirmed the role of taking a lung biopsy and have endorsed its value providing the sample taken is of reasonable depth (Haworth, 1984).

Autopsy studies

In studying a post-mortem lung specimen, the technique used to prepare the specimen depends on the questions to be answered. The best results are often achieved by using a combination of techniques. These include injection of the pulmonary arterial or venous circulation with a radio-opaque contrast medium, radiographic examination, dissection of the fixed specimen and histological examination, including serial reconstruction of the arterial pathways.

For precise measurement of vessel size, wall thickness and number, the system must be distended before fixation. Injection of one system ensures easy identification of both arteries and veins.

Injection of the pulmonary arterial (or venous) system with a warm radio-opaque barium-sulphate gelatin mixture permits both arteriographic study and histological examination. The injection mixture solidifies at room temperature thus allowing the material to be cut for histological preparation (Elliott & Reid, 1965; Davies & Reid, 1970). The lung is fixed by injecting the airways under pressure with buffered formol saline. Alternatively, the pulmonary arteries and the airways can be injected with a fixative such as glutaraldehyde in cacodylate or phosphate buffer. This gives better preservation of cellular detail, but less satisfactory vascular distension for accurate quantitative morphometry (Gil & Weibel, 1969; Meyrick & Reid, 1979). The latter injection technique is more suitable for experimental studies when electron microscopic examination is the most important objective. Corrosion casts may be helpful in studying the relation between two or more vascular systems, particularly when seeking anastomoses

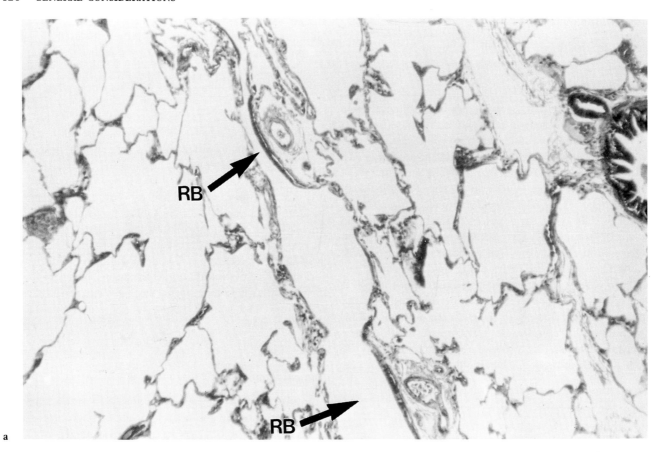

a

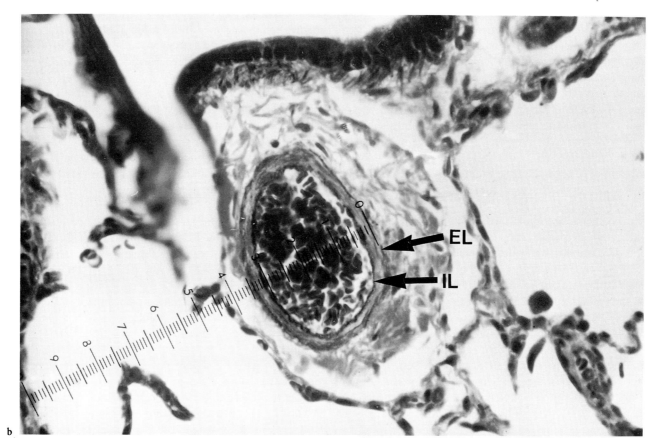

b

between the pulmonary and bronchial arterial circulations (Liebow et al, 1947; Liebow et al, 1950). The combination of arteriography and serial reconstruction, however, is generally the most satisfactory approach. Changes in wall structure are usually of concern. When using a corrosion technique, the evidence is dissolved during the preparation of the cast!

Identification of the intrapulmonary arteries

In the normal child the lung is remodelled with growth. The size, number and composition of different structures in the lung changes with age (Hislop & Reid, 1972, 1973a, b). In the abnormal lung, therefore, each structural feature must be compared with that of age-matched controls in tissue prepared and analysed in the same manner. The intrapulmonary arteries must be identified in order to make a comparison. They cannot be identified according to their size, because size in the normal lung changes with age and may also change in disease. In an autopsy specimen the elastic and large muscular arteries are identified by counting the number of generations which separate them from the segmental hilum, the segmental artery being counted as the first generation. Their wall structure is determined by their position in the lung (Hayward & Reid, 1952; Elliott & Reid, 1965; Hislop & Reid, 1973b). Arteries continue to branch with the airways within the acinus. On microscopic examination (of both biopsy and autopsy tissue), the arteries are identified according to the type of airway they accompany (terminal or respiratory bronchioli or alveolar ducts). They may also lie within the alveolar walls (Fig. 6.4a). The term 'arteriole' is best avoided. It is open to different interpretations which may be based on size, structure or function or on a combination of these attributes.

Techniques of morphological analysis

The same techniques of morphometric analysis are used to study biopsy and either injected or uninjected autopsy material. Quantitative studies include the determination of the amount of pulmonary arterial or venous muscularity, vessel size and number. In making a qualitative analysis, the appearance of the pre-acinar arteries and of each type of intra-acinar artery is described. Combining the different techniques provides a comprehensive assessment of pulmonary vascular structure and a means of cross-checking the validity and relevance of each individual assessment.

Fig. 6.4 (a) Photomicrograph of a lung biopsy showing respiratory bronchioli (RB), each accompanied by a pulmonary artery. (× 152) (b) Photomicrograph of a lung biopsy with a graticule superimposed to measure the external diameter, the distance between the external elastic laminae (EL), and the medial thickness, and the distance between internal (IL) and external elastic laminae. (× 620)

Assessment of pulmonary arterial muscularity

Several techniques are available. In a large and unselected population of arteries, the mean percentage medial thickness can be calculated from measurements of medial thickness and external diameter (Fig. 6.4b) (Davies & Reid, 1970). Other assessments include the mean arterial lumen : wall ratio, the area of muscle present, and an index of medial muscle tissue present in the lung (Dammann & Ferencz, 1956; Könn & Storb, 1960; Wagenvoort, 1960; Naeye, 1961a). Population counts reveal the relationship between wall structure and size. The muscularity of the intra-acinar arteries is also studied by determining the proportion of arteries accompanying the terminal bronchioli, respiratory bronchioli, alveolar ducts and alveolar walls which have a muscular, partially muscular or non-muscular structure. Arterial muscularity is usually assessed by determination of percentage medial thickness and by finding the extent to which muscle has differentiated along the arterial pathway as judged both by the size and the position of the arterial pathway in the lung field.

Assessment of arterial number

The number of arteries per unit area or volume of lung can be determined. The ratio of alveoli to arteries is then calculated to overcome any difference in the degree of inflation in different lungs (Dunnill, 1962). The effect of hypoperfusion on lung growth can be studied in autopsy specimens by determining the number and size of the alveoli.

Assessment of the pulmonary veins

Wall thickness is measured from the internal elastic lamina to the outer edge of the most peripheral muscle cells or an elastic lamina. The percentage of vein wall thickness is then calculated as for the arteries. Like the arteries, the number of veins per unit area of lung and the ratio of alveoli to veins can be determined.

Assessment of right ventricular hypertrophy

The amount of muscle increases in the pulmonary vascular bed in patients having pulmonary hypertension. It also increases in the systemic venous ventricle, normally the morphologically right ventricle. In the normal heart the septum is usually considered as part of the left ventricle. Hypertrophy of the right ventricle is therefore indicated by a decrease in the ratio:

$$\frac{\text{weight of the left ventricle + septum}}{\text{weight of the right ventricle}}$$

(Fulton et al, 1952). The right ventricle during fetal life forms a greater proportion of the total ventricular weight than it does in the child or adult. At sea level the 'adult' heart weight ratio of 2.3 : 1–3.3 : 1 is normally achieved by 4 months of age (Recavarren & Arias-Stella, 1964).

NORMAL DEVELOPMENT OF THE PULMONARY CIRCULATION

Prenatal development

Early fetal development

The heart tube is formed by the end of the 3rd week of gestation (see Ch. 4). About 5 days later, the lung bud develops at the caudal end of the laryngotracheal sulcus. The lung bud expands laterally and divides into two lung sacs. Each sac elongates and divides first into lobes and then into bronchopulmonary segments. The lobar bronchi to each lung are present by 5 weeks (8 mm stage) and all sub-segmental bronchi are present by 6 weeks (13.4 mm) (Wells & Boyden, 1954). As the lung buds push out from the laryngeal floor they become invested by the surrounding mesenchyme of the splanchic mesoderm of the ventral surface of the foregut. From this mesenchyme develop the pulmonary blood vessels and lymphatics. The vascular plexus within each lung bud comes to be supplied by paired segmental arteries which arise from the dorsal aorta cranial to the coeliac arteries.

At about 32 days of gestation (5 mm stage), the 6th branchial arches appear. These supply branches to the lungs, namely the pulmonary arteries (Congdon, 1922). The segmental arteries subsequently cease to supply the lung, but for several days the lungs are probably connected to both segmental and pulmonary arteries. The adult pattern of blood supply is achieved by 50 days after ovulation (18 mm stage). All the bronchopulmonary segments are then connected exclusively to the central pulmonary arteries (derived from the 6th branchial arches). These arteries thus provide the intrapulmonary arteries with their only source of blood supply. One or more of the early segmental arteries occasionally persists, permanently capturing a lobe or segment of lung (Hessel et al, 1970).

The intrapulmonary veins (like the arteries) are derived from the splanchnic plexus associated with the lung buds. Initially, they drain into the systemic venous system. The proximal pulmonary vein develops as an outgrowth from the left atrium and becomes connected with the intrapulmonary veins by the 28–30th day of gestation. Following this, pulmonary venous blood drains into the left atrium. In the human some connexions remain between oesophageal and pulmonary veins at the hilum of the lung (Butler, 1952). These connexions offer an alternative pathway for pulmonary venous outflow and may assume considerable importance in babies born either with absent extrapulmonary veins or obstructed pulmonary venous return.

The bronchial arteries appear relatively late in fetal life.

They arise between the 9th and 12th week of gestation from the aorta itself or from the right or left posterior intercostal branches of the aorta (Boyden, 1970). They are implanted as a secondary arterial system on the walls of the bronchi and large pulmonary vessels, extending down the bronchial tree as the cartilage develops.

Branching pattern of arteries and veins

The arteries and airways develop together. The pre-acinar arteries and airways are those structures extending down to (but not including) the respiratory or acinar region of the lung (see Fig. 6.1). They are formed during a relatively short period of time (Bucher & Reid, 1961; Hislop & Reid, 1972). About three-quarters of the branches present at birth are formed between the 10th and 14th weeks of gestation. The longer segments of lung continue developing until the 16th week. By this time, pre-acinar airway and arterial branching is complete (Fig. 6.5a). In contrast, the intra-acinar arteries develop relatively late in fetal life and continue to form after birth as the alveolar ducts and alveoli develop (Fig. 6.5b, c). The pre- and postnatal development of the intrapulmonary veins parallels that of the arteries. The branching pattern of the pre-acinar veins is complete by 20 weeks of gestation (Hislop & Reid, 1973a). New veins develop after birth in the intra-acinar region of the lung.

Arterial wall structure

The proximal half of the pre-acinar arterial pathway down to the 7th generation in the adult lung has an elastic wall structure and beyond this it is muscular (Reid, 1968). This adult distribution of elastic structure is achieved in fetal life by the 19th week of gestation (Hislop & Reid, 1972). Wall structure in the smaller pre-acinar and intra-acinar arteries is related to the diameter of the artery. The muscular segment gives way to a partially muscular and thence to a non-muscular structure at the same diameter in the fetus as in the adult lung, but these changes occur at a more proximal level along the arterial pathway (Fig. 6.6). At birth, therefore, relatively few intra-acinar arteries contain muscle. Muscle cells gradually differentiate in progressively more peripheral arteries as the child grows.

During fetal life the wall thickness of the muscular and partially muscular pulmonary arteries is high (Civin & Edwards, 1951; Naeye, 1961a) (Fig. 6.7). As new arteries are formed, they acquire a muscle coat whose thickness is commensurate with their size (Hislop & Reid, 1972). Thus, as gestation advances, the number of muscularised arteries increases. The thickness of the muscle coat of each individual artery does not.

The wall structure of the pulmonary circulation reflects the high pulmonary vascular resistance and low blood flow characteristic of fetal life. The pulmonary trunk is exposed

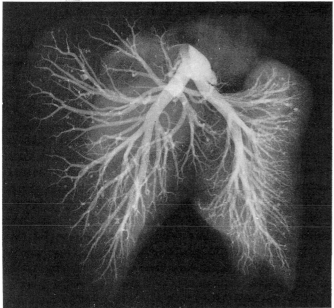

a

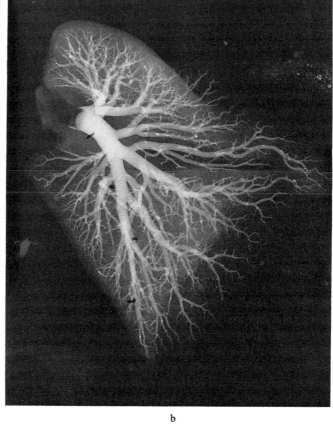

b

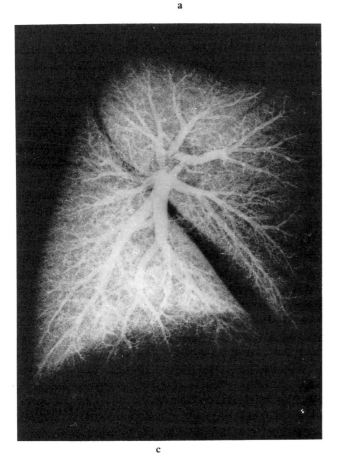

c

to the same pressure as the aorta. It has a similar wall thickness and is composed of parallel elastic fibres of uniform thickness arranged in a compact fashion (Heath et al, 1959). The muscular, partially muscular and non-muscular arteries all have a low lumen-to-wall ratio and appear to offer a high resistance to blood flow.

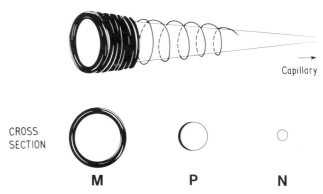

Fig. 6.5 (a) Post-mortem arteriogram of a normal fetus of 19 weeks gestation. The pre-acinar arteries are all present. (× 2.5) (Reproduced by kind permission of Dr A. Hislop.) (b) Post-mortem arteriogram of a normal fetus of 40 weeks gestation. (× 0.95) (Reproduced by kind permission of Heinemann Medical Books Ltd.) (c) Post-mortem arteriogram of a normal 18 month old child. A dense background haze has appeared since birth, due to filling of newly formed intra-acinar arteries. (× 0.5) (Reproduced by kind permission of Dr A. Hislop.)

Fig. 6.6 Diagram of the terminal part of each arterial pathway as the muscular vessel (M) becomes partially (P) and then non-muscularised (N). (Reproduced by kind permission of Heinemann Medical Books Ltd.)

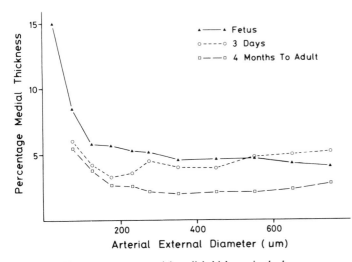

Fig. 6.7 Mean percentage arterial medial thickness in the human related to external diameter (μm) in the normal fetus, at 3 days and at 4 months to adult life. (Reproduced by kind permission of Heinemann Medical Books Ltd.)

Vein wall structure

The vein wall is thin throughout fetal and postnatal life. Muscle cells are rarely found in the wall before 28 weeks of gestation (Hislop & Reid, 1973a).

Adaptation to extra-uterine life

At birth the lung suddenly becomes responsible for the oxygenation of the newborn baby. It must, therefore, adapt rapidly to extra-uterine life. The blood-gas barrier is extremely thin before and at birth, measuring only 200 nm in its thinnest region. The wall structure of the pulmonary arteries, however, changes from the pulmonary valve to the precapillary bed during the first weeks of life. The most important change is the dilation of the non-muscular and small partially muscular arteries in the pre-capillary region. This occurs immediately after birth and lowers the pulmonary vascular resistance (Civin & Edwards, 1951; Naeye, 1961a; Parmentier, 1962; Hislop & Reid, 1973b). In the normal human lung the relative pulmonary arterial medial thickness decreases rapidly during the first days of life, particularly in arteries < 250 μm in diameter. It reaches a mature adult level in all arteries during the first 3 months of life (Hislop & Reid, 1973b; Haworth & Hislop, 1983) (Fig. 6.7). Studies on the normal pig lung have shown that the pulmonary arteries adapt to extrauterine life not by reducing the amount of muscle present but by reorganising the components of the arterial wall, thus reducing wall thickness and increasing lumen diameter. During fetal life, there is considerable overlap between endothelial cells and between smooth muscle cells in the peripheral pulmonary arteries. The lumen of many small vessels is occluded by interdigitating endothelial cells. Adaptation to extrauterine life can be divided into overlapping stages. The first stage extends from birth to 4 days. Immediately after birth, adaptation begins with a reduction in cell/cell overlap, all the cells becoming significantly thinner. Endothelial cells show a reduction in depth and complexity of interdigitating contacts. The peripheral arteries of the newborn lung contain only a small amount of relatively unyielding, stable connective tissue. They do not have a well-defined external elastic lamina which could limit expansion. The second stage is one of structural stabilisation and extends from 4 days to 3 weeks. A rapid phase of adaptation is followed by a period of stabilisation during which the smooth muscle cells, having taken up a more definitive position within the vessel wall lay down connective tissue around themselves to stabilise the newly organised wall structure. The third stage, that of growth, takes place from 3 weeks to 6 months. Wall thickness increases as lumen diameter increases and the vessels grow. Endothelial and smooth muscle cells which are relatively immature at birth become more fully differentiated.

The increase in luminal cross-sectional area and the reduction in medial thickness reduces the resistance to blood flow. In the pig the pulmonary-systemic resistance ratio decreases from 0.8 to 0.18 between 24 hours and 2 weeks. The period of time during which blood flows forward into the pulmonary vascular bed during each cardiac cycle increases rapidly. In the fetal lamb, blood flows forward in the pulmonary arteries only during early systole when velocity is high. This is presumably because of the high resistance maintained by thick walled peripheral pulmonary arteries (Rudolph et al, 1977). Administration of acetyl choline lowers resistance and extends forward flow throughout systole as occurs in the normal lamb after birth. The adaptational changes also reduce the lability of the pulmonary circulation and reduce the brisk fetal response to vasoconstrictor agents.

Because of the dramatic changes which occur in the peripheral pulmonary arteries at birth, changes in the proximal arteries are frequently ignored. Considerable amounts of collagen and elastin are deposited in the elastic and large pulmonary arteries of the pig lung in the neonatal period. These structural changes are associated with an increase in the structural stiffness of the vessel wall (Greenwald et al, 1982). The pressure decreases from about 6.0 kPa at birth to 1.3 kPa by 2 weeks of age. The greater distensibility at high pressures is then no longer necessary.

During fetal life the pulmonary trunk continues as the arterial duct into the descending thoracic aorta. The right and left pulmonary arteries have a smaller diameter than the pulmonary trunk and arise from the trunk at a more acute angle than is seen in post-natal life (Fig. 6.8). This appearance can persist for several weeks after birth and accounts for a small pressure gradient of 5–8 mm between the trunk and the right and left pulmonary arteries (Danilowicz et al, 1965).

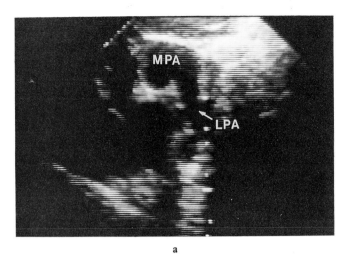

a

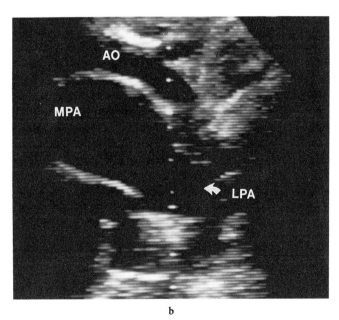

b

Fig. 6.8 Cross-sectional echocardiograms showing a suprasternal cut in (a) a neonate, where the left pulmonary artery (LPA) forms an acute angle with the pulmonary trunk (MPA), and in (b) an older child with complete transposition, hence the anterior aorta. The left pulmonary arises from the pulmonary trunk at a more acute angle in the younger child. (Reproduced by kind permission of Dr Jeffrey Smallhorn).

At birth, adaptive changes in the pulmonary circulation are accompanied by adaptive changes in the heart. The ability to increase cardiac output by increasing stroke volume improves, the myocardium develops greater active tension with age, and at molecular level, the ratio of the different cardiac myosin isoenzymes alters (Rudolph, 1974; Lompre et al, 1981). The cardiopulmonary system adapts rapidly to extrauterine life so that it may function efficiently as an integrated whole.

Postnatal development

The progressive growth and remodelling of the pulmonary vascular bed ensures that, as the cardiac output increases with growth, pulmonary vascular resistance does not rise. Proximal to the arterial pathways of the microcirculation, resistance is mainly determined by lumen diameter. Total pulmonary vascular resistance is determined by the number of resistance pathways arranged in parallel. Not only does arterial size increase with growth, but the number of peripheral arterial pathways also increases (Haworth & Hislop, 1983). This ensures a progressive rise in capacity of the peripheral pulmonary vascular bed during childhood. The multiplication of intra-acinar arteries keeps pace with alveolar multiplication (Hislop & Reid, 1973b).

Muscle continues to differentiate throughout childhood in the intra-acinar arteries. The intra-acinar arterial bed is less muscular in childhood than in adult life. This structural difference has important practical implications for the cardiologist. In a lung biopsy, the presence of muscle in more peripheral arteries than those in which it is normally seen at that age is an important early indication of the structural response of the pulmonary circulation to pulmonary hypertension.

The structure of the pulmonary trunk changes more gradually. The ratio of the thickness of the media to that of the aorta decreases from 1 to a mean value of 0.6 at about 8 months of age. This ratio is then maintained throughout life (Heath et al, 1959). The elastic fibres of the pulmonary trunk become fragmented and consist of short thick rods, some with clubbed ends. The trunk has an adult appearance by the end of the 2nd year of life.

Hypoperfusion in children with congenital heart disease may lead to one or both lungs being small with respect to age and height. A radiological comparison with the normal is possible. The overall growth of the normal lung in childhood has been assessed by measuring the lung on serial radiographs of normal children who were contacts of tuberculous patients (Simon et al, 1972). Centile standards for the length, width and area of the lung and for heart diameter were compiled, together with mean velocity growth curves.

THE PULMONARY CIRCULATION IN CONGENITAL HEART DISEASE

In children with congenital heart disease the pulmonary circulation may fail to develop normally even before birth.

Abnormal prenatal development

Abnormalities of pulmonary vascular development which arise during fetal life may be divided into primary developmental abnormalities (those occurring during the first 16 weeks of gestation) and secondary abnormalities which are probably due to haemodynamic changes caused by the presence of congenital heart disease. The latter therefore develop later in fetal life. Primary abnormalities may include an absent right or left pulmonary artery, failure of some or all of the intrapulmonary arteries to connect exclusively with the central intrapericardial pulmonary arteries, a reduction in the number of generations of intra-pulmonary arteries, and stenoses of the pulmonary arteries. These abnormalities may occur in children with a normal heart. They are then usually associated with disordered airway development. A persistent systemic arterial supply is a feature of a sequestrated segment or malformed hypo-plastic lung. A reduction in the pulmonary arterial branching pattern is seen in the hypoplastic lung of renal agenesis and dysplasia, congenital diaphragmatic hernia and rhesus iso-immunisation (Kitagawa et al, 1971; Cham-berlain et al, 1977; Hislop et al, 1979). Pulmonary arterial stenoses occur in the rubella syndrome with or without an associated intracardiac abnormality (Rowe, 1963; Wasserman et al, 1968).

Absent pulmonary artery

Absence of a central pulmonary artery can occur in patients with and without intracardiac anomalies. It can occur in the presence of patent pulmonary trunk when the pulmonary artery at the hilum is connected to an artery arising from the ascending aorta or aortic arch. This is sometimes known as a 'distal ductal origin' of a pulmonary artery (Sotomora & Edwards, 1978). Patients with an absent pulmonary artery on angiography can be divided into 2 groups, those with and those without an intrapericardial pulmonary artery. Typically, in those without an intrapericardial vessel the absent pulmonary artery is on the side opposite the aortic ach, and there is angiographic evidence of an arterial duct coming from the brachiocephalic artery on the side of the interruption. At operation there is a large gap between the pulmonary trunk and the hilar vessel which may require insertion of a conduit to achieve continuity. By contrast, patients with an intrapericardial pulmonary artery have an occluded pulmonary artery in continuity with the hilar vessel on the left side, the interruption is on the same side as the aortic arch and is associated with a left-sided arterial duct which descends vertically from underneath the aortic arch in patients with severe or complete right ventricular outflow tract obstruction. In these cases the occluded gap is relatively short and continuity is more readily established than in patients without an intrapericardial vessel. In both groups serial angiography occasionally demonstrates the acquired nature of the lesion, showing that interruption may be associated with closure of the arterial duct. Histologically, serial reconstructions show ductal tissue extending from the duct into the pulmonary artery, producing a coarctation of the pulmonary artery at the site of insertion of a vertical duct which carries blood from the aorta to the pulmonary artery in duct-dependent lesions. The picture is reminiscent of coarctation of the aorta

associated with insertion of a normal horizontal duct which carries blood from the pulmonary trunk to the descending aorta in fetal life. Stenosis at the origin of the left pulmonary artery is a recognised complication of tetralogy of Fallot and may represent the incompletely developed picture of interrupted, angiographically absent, pulmonary artery.

Where no large systemic artery anastomoses with the hilar pulmonary artery, the pulmonary blood supply is derived from an expanded bronchial circulation. When the central pulmonary artery is absent or interrupted, the pulmonary artery is usually patent at the hilum although it is frequently small. All such patients should thus be regarded as potential candidates for correction by insertion of a prosthesis between the pulmonary trunk (or right ventricle) and the hilar pulmonary artery.

Failure of all intrapulmonary arteries to connect exclusively with the central pulmonary arteries

In the majority of patients with pulmonary atresia and ventricular septal defect, the lungs are perfused by large arteries which arise from the aorta. These are the major aortopulmonary collateral arteries (Fig. 6.9). Airway development is normal. The central pulmonary arteries are usually present, although they may be extremely small or even incompletely canalised. Major aortopulmonary collateral arteries are not to be confused with the enlarged

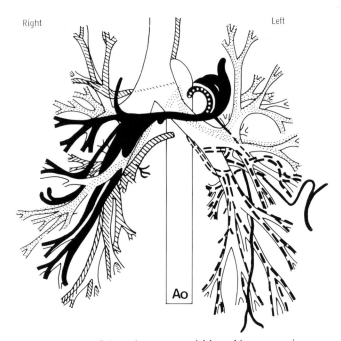

Fig. 6.9 Diagram of the pulmonary arterial branching pattern in a case of pulmonary atresia with ventricular septal defect and major aortopulmonary collateral arteries. The solid lines indicate the central pulmonary arteries and their branches, and the cross-hatched, stippled, interrupted and dotted lines, the collateral arteries and the intrapulmonary arteries with which they connect. Ao = aorta. (Reproduced by kind permission of the Editors of the *British Heart Journal*.)

bronchial arteries seen after birth in several types of congenital heart disease characterised by presence of a low pulmonary blood flow (see Fig. 6.3d).

The source of blood supply to the lungs in the presence of collateral arteries is frequently complex and varies in different patients (Haworth & Macartney, 1980). Collateral arteries are thought to be persistent segmental arteries which have retained their early fetal connexion with the intrapulmonary arteries (Hessel et al, 1970). The complexity of their connexions with the intrapulmonary arteries and with each other is not, therefore, surprising. A collateral artery in children with pulmonary atresia and a ventricular septal defect may connect with the pulmonary artery at the hilum and, if the central pulmonary arteries are patent, so perfuse both lungs (see Fig. 6.3b). Alternatively, a collateral artery may anastomose end-to-end with a lobar or segmental pulmonary artery and have no connexion with the central pulmonary artery at the hilum or with its branches within the lung. More than one collateral artery may perfuse the same intrapulmonary artery at the hilum. The pulmonary artery is then said to have a duplicate blood supply (Fäller et al, 1981).

Collateral arteries which do not connect with a central or hilar pulmonary artery run to the hilum of the lung and then accompany a lobar bronchus until they anastomose with an intrapulmonary artery. A vessel which has the basic structure of a muscular systemic artery then becomes a vessel with the structure of an elastic pulmonary artery (Haworth, 1980). The pulmonary artery subsequently branches with the airways in a normal manner to perfuse the capillary bed.

Different bronchopulmonary segments within a lobe may be connected to several different vessels, some segments being connected to a central pulmonary artery and others only to collateral arteries. Because of this, several arteries may accompany the main and lobar bronchi. The orderly appearance of one pulmonary artery accompanying each bronchus as seen on angiography is lost. The only method of ensuring that the anatomy is understood in each patient is to account for the blood supply of each bronchopulmonary segment on the anteroposterior and lateral projections of the cineangiograms. In addition, sources of a duplicate supply to each segment are sought together with connexions between different collateral arteries.

The collateral arteries commonly arise from the descending thoracic aorta behind the origin of the left main bronchus in the presence of a left aortic arch. They tend to arise almost in the midline when the arch is on the right. They may also arise from beneath the aortic arch and less commonly from the supracoeliac aorta below the diaphragm. They frequently divide near their aortic origin.

Collateral arteries are commonly stenosed where they anastomose with a hilar or intrapulmonary artery. In postnatal life, a degree of stenosis is desirable since it reduces the systemic arterial pressure to a level more suited to the pulmonary circulation (Haworth, 1980). Collateral arteries may, however, be severely stenosed either at their origin from the aorta or, more commonly, in the mid-portion of the vessel between aorta and lung. Here the lumen may even be occluded by large mounds of proliferating intimal tissue. It is not uncommon for children to become increasingly cyanosed during the first months of life. This is probably due to progressive intimal proliferation in the collateral arteries. Children are occasionally born with minute central and intrapulmonary arteries and small or occluded collateral arteries. Multiple aortopulmonary collateral arteries seen in infancy are best regarded as precarious fetal connexions.

In pulmonary atresia with ventricular septal defect, the lungs may also be perfused by persistent branchial arch structures other than the normal 6th arch. It is the arterial duct which usually persists after birth. More rarely it is the 5th aortic arch (Macartney et al, 1974). When the lungs are perfused by an arterial duct, all the intrapulmonary arteries are usually connected at the hilum. A duct may, however, connect with a hilar pulmonary artery to perfuse some bronchopulmonary segments while major aortopulmonary collateral arteries provide the only blood supply to other segments. Bilateral ducts also occur.

The development of the pre and intra-acinar arteries within the lung before and after birth depends on the lumen diameter of the perfusing vessels. The lungs are usually hypoperfused.

Developmental abnormalities of the intrapulmonary arteries

The various types of congenital heart disease may be regarded as vicarious experiments in which to study the relationship between structural development and changes in pulmonary arterial pressure and flow. Children in whom the aortic valve is atretic or severely stenosed and those with pulmonary atresia and an intact ventricular septum are born with structural abnormalities of the intra-acinar arteries. These two types of cardiac anomaly produce a different and almost diametrically opposite structural effect on the lung (Haworth & Reid, 1977a, b).

In atresia or critical stenosis of the aortic valve, the entire cardiac output is ejected into the pulmonary trunk and the body is perfused via the arterial duct. During fetal life there is an increase in thickness of the medial coat in arteries which are normally muscularised. Muscle is then present in smaller and more peripheral arteries than is normal (Naeye, 1962; Haworth & Reid, 1977a). In some patients the number of intra-acinar arteries per unit area of lung is also increased and these vessels also are heavily muscularised. The veins are abnormally thick-walled. The increase in the amount of vascular smooth muscle suggests an increase in pulmonary vascular resistance to ensure adequate perfusion of the systemic circulation. At birth patients with aortic atresia or critical stenosis have severe pulmonary hypertension and the majority die within the first few days of life. Those in whom the aortic valve is stenosed, and in whom the left ventricle is relatively well developed, may undergo aortic valvotomy or palliative surgery as an emergency procedure. In such children the increased muscularity of the arterial pathway increases the tendency to react to vasoconstricting agents such as acidosis and hypoxia.

By contrast, children with pulmonary atresia (in whom the arterial duct is the only source of blood supply to the lung) are born with abnormally small pre- and intra-acinar arteries and may have a reduction in the number of intra-acinar arteries (Haworth & Reid, 1977b). The muscle coat is abnormally thin although the distribution of muscle along the arterial pathway is normal (Naeye, 1961b; Haworth & Reid, 1977b). When the arterial duct is relatively large, pulmonary arterial muscularity develops normally and intra-acinar arterial multiplication is almost normal.

In pulmonary atresia, the pulmonary vessels are probably exposed before birth to a lower than normal pressure and flow. The pressure generated by the left ventricle is probably not transmitted to the pulmonary circulation across the rather small, abnormally angulated arterial duct found in these patients. A low pulmonary arterial pressure may help explain the reduced arterial muscularity. The low wall thickness might also be due to an increase in the oxygen tension of blood perfusing the lung. This is because, in pulmonary atresia, oxygenated placental blood mixes with deoxygenated blood in the left ventricle. The oxygen tension of the perfusing blood, however, may also be greater than normal in aortic atresia due to mixing in the right ventricle. In this abnormality, the muscularity is increased.

A reduction in arterial number implies a reduction in capacity of the pulmonary circulation. In the normal lung, recruitment of additional channels is said to be more important than distension of channels already perfused in accommodating an increase in blood volume (Maseri et al, 1972). A reduction in both number and size of intra-acinar arteries might help explain why some newborn infants with pulmonary atresia develop pulmonary oedema following an aortopulmonary anastomosis.

Babies with total anomalous pulmonary venous connexion who present with obstructed venous return during the 1st week of life may show a marked increase in muscularity of both intrapulmonary arteries and veins (Haworth & Reid, 1977c; Haworth, 1982). The findings are consistent with prenatal obstruction to pulmonary venous return. The majority of patients dying during the first days of life have the infradiaphragmatic type of anomaly. The descending vein can be narrowed or even occluded by fibrous tissue. The extrapulmonary veins may also be smaller than normal and show intimal proliferation. Within the lungs the increased muscularity is potentially reversible. In the extrapulmonary veins, however, prenatal obstruction may instigate intimal proliferation and fibrosis. This can progress despite a technically successful operation which relieves the obstruction by anastomosing the common pulmonary vein to the left atrium. There are several reports of postoperative stenosis developing in the extrapulmonary veins at some distance from the suture lines (see Ch. 21). Patients with the infradiaphragmatic type of anomalous connexion are probably particularly vulnerable.

These findings in the pulmonary circulation of patients with aortic atresia or stenosis, pulmonary atresia and total anomalous pulmonary venous connexion illustrate the susceptibility of the developing pulmonary circulation to changes in pressure and flow during fetal life. They show how prenatal structural changes in the lung can prejudice survival.

PULMONARY HYPERTENSION IN CHILDHOOD

In congenital heart disease the variability of the structural response to an increase in pulmonary arterial pressure and flow is not understood. Some disorders are almost always associated with rapidly progressive pulmonary vascular disease, the best example being complete transposition with ventricular septal defect. Other abnormalities are usually associated with pulmonary vascular disease, as in a large ventricular septal defect. In yet other abnormalities pulmonary vascular disease either never develops or does so later in adult life, as in the 'secundum' atrial septal defect. 'Individual susceptibility' is said to explain the variable response seen in many types of congenital heart disease. This term implies a variety of functional and structural differences in susceptible individuals. The list of possibilities is long, including an excessive amount of pulmonary vascular smooth muscle present from birth; an excessive tendency to vasoconstrict and a reduction in size and number of intra-acinar arteries. Variation in animals in the propensity to vasoconstrict has been related to genetically determined differences in the medial thickness of the muscular pulmonary arteries (Grover et al, 1963).

In general, patients with post-tricuspid shunts such as a ventricular septal defect, a large arterial duct, an atrio-ventricular septal defect, aortopulmonary window or common arterial trunk are more likely to develop pulmonary hypertension and severe pulmonary vascular disease than those with a pre-tricuspid shunt, such as an atrial septal defect. Patients with a 'secundum' atrial septal defect do not usually develop severe pulmonary hypertension before the 3rd decade, although there are exceptions (Haworth, 1983).

Recent refinements in surgical techniques have encouraged studies of pulmonary vascular pathology in very young patients. Abnormalities in arterial remodelling and growth have been detected using the quantitative morphometric techniques described earlier in this chapter from the newborn period in children with pulmonary hypertension. Even when the pulmonary circulation is probably structurally normal at birth, the presence of pulmonary hypertension soon influences pre- and intra-acinar wall structure together with the number and size of intra-acinar arteries. Pulmonary arterial medial thickness is relatively normal in patients with complete transposition who have an intact ventricular septum and normal pulmonary arterial pressure. In those with a ventricular septal defect and pulmonary hypertension, however, it is significantly increased by 2 months of age. Furthermore, a reduction in the number of patent intra-acinar arteries has been reported in various cardiac anomalies. Occluded arteries within the alveolar walls can be seen with the electron microscope in patients having an increase in both pre- and intra-acinar arterial muscularity (Fig. 6.10). Such changes precede many of the abnormalities of arterial wall structure described in the classical studies of Heath & Edwards (1958). Heath & Edwards studied pulmonary vascular structure in older patients with pulmonary hypertension. At that time, they excluded from study infants in whom the pulmonary arterial pressure was higher than

expected for the severity of the structural change. The more recent quantitative studies on pulmonary vascular structure help explain why this is so. They also help explain why, after corrective surgery, some children show progression of pulmonary vascular disease, or have an inappropriate increase in pulmonary arterial pressure on exercise, despite their young age and the absence of severe obliterative disease at the time of surgery (Hallidie-Smith et al, 1969; Friedli et al, 1974).

Since many cardiac anomalies can now be repaired in early infancy the emphasis must be on the detection of early pulmonary vascular disease and the prevention of established, 'fixed' obstructive disease.

Heath and Edwards classification (1958)

Heath & Edwards (1958) described the appearance of the pulmonary arteries in patients with pulmonary hypertension. They classified pulmonary vascular change into 6 grades arranged in order of increasing vascular damage. The structural features of each grade were related to measurements of pulmonary arterial pressure, resistance and flow, and to the outcome of surgery.

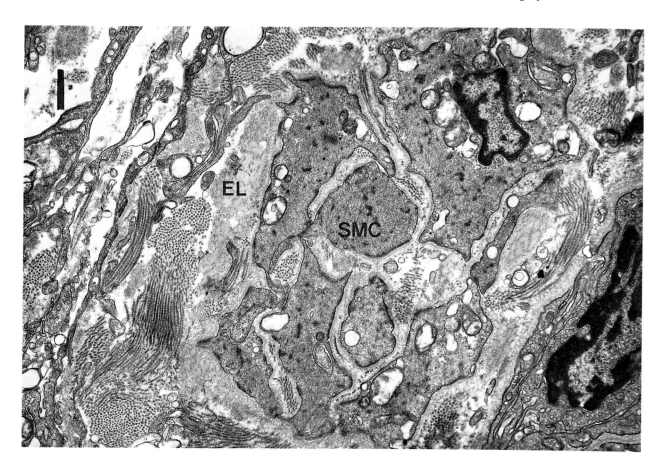

Fig. 6.10 Electromicrograph of occluded alveolar wall artery, from a lung biopsy specimen of a 7-month-old child with double inlet ventricle. Mature smooth muscle cells (SMC) are seen within internal elastic lamina (EEL), without in this instance, any endothelial cells. Bar represents 1 μm.

Grade I	– Medial hypertrophy
Grade II	– Medial hypertrophy with cellular intimal proliferation
Grade III	– Progressive fibrous occlusion
Grade IV	– Progressive generalised arterial dilation with the formation of complex dilation lesions
Grade V	– Chronic dilation with numerous dilation vessels throughout the lung and pulmonary haemosiderosis
Grade VI	– Fibrinoid necrosis of the media.

Grades I–III indicate a 'high resistance, high reserve', pulmonary vascular bed which is still labile (Edwards, 1957). The pulmonary arterial pressure is high, the pulmonary blood flow is high and the direction of the shunt is left to right. Grades V–VI indicate a 'high resistance, low reserve' pulmonary vascular bed which is no longer labile because the lumen of many of the arteries is occluded. Pulmonary arterial pressure is higher than in patients with grades I–III pulmonary vascular disease. Flow is low and the direction of the shunt is predominantly right to left. Grade IV represents a transitional stage. Although grades I–III reflect a succession of structural changes, grades IV–VI probably do not. Wagenvoort & Wagenvoort (1977) believe that necrotising arteritis can precede the development of plexiform lesions. Many changes such as necrotising arteritis, plexiform lesions or dilation lesions may certainly be seen alone or in combination with other changes. Wagenvoort & Wagenvoort (1977) found that none of these lesions carried a more severe prognosis than the others save for the plexiform lesion.

A classification system is useful in describing the principal structural abnormalities in a group of patients, particularly when relating structural to functional change. Using a classification system to evaluate and give a prognosis on an individual lung biopsy is, however, fraught with difficulties, particularly in childhood. The relationship between structure and function is too poorly understood. We do not know how changes in pulmonary arterial size, number and wall structure are inter-related.

Structure of the muscular pulmonary arteries

Medial hypertrophy

The media is composed of a dense layer of circumferentially arranged smooth muscle cells interspersed with thin elastic fibres (Fig. 6.11). Longitudinal muscle bundles may develop in contact with the external elastic lamina. Less commonly such bundles may be found internal to the internal elastic lamina. The internal elastic lamina is thickened and in uninjected tissue is often crenellated. The adventitial coat appears more dense than normal and is composed largely of thick collagen fibres. Because these

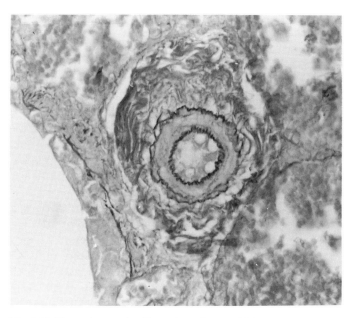

Fig. 6.11 Photomicrograph of lung tissue from a child aged 3 months who died with complete transposition showing severe medial hypertrophy in a respiratory bronchiolar artery. (× 620) (Reproduced by kind permission of Springer-Verlag.)

vessels are often tortuous, multiple cross-sections of the same vessel may be seen on microscopic examination.

Cellular intimal proliferation

Cellular intimal proliferation is usually concentric in pulmonary hypertensive congenital heart disease (Fig. 6.12). Initially the cells are loosely arranged perpendicular to the intima. Gradually the cell layer becomes more compact. The term 'intimal proliferation' implies that the cells originate in the intima. In fact, they are derived from the media. Cells with the ultrastructural features of smooth muscle cells can be seen penetrating the internal elastic lamina. Electron microscopy shows that the proliferating cells in the intima have the characteristics of smooth muscle cells. Mucopolysaccharides are occasionally deposited in this layer.

Intimal fibrosis

Collagen fibres and then elastic fibres are gradually deposited in the cellular intimal layer (Fig. 6.13). The extent to which elastin is deposited varies, and is age-related. Intimal fibrosis has a compact, lamellar appearance, and may completely occlude the arterial lumen.

Generalised arterial dilation and the formation of dilation lesions

Chronic pulmonary hypertension leads to thinning and atrophy of the media (Compare Figs. 6.11, 6.13). Atrophy

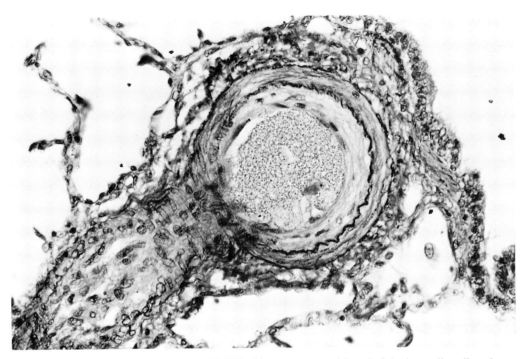

Fig. 6.12 Photomicrograph of lung tissue from an 11-month-old child with a common arterial trunk. Injection medium distends an artery showing medial hypertrophy with circumferential intimal proliferation. (× 460)

and dilation is associated with (and probably the result of) narrowing or obliteration of the parent artery by intimal fibrosis.

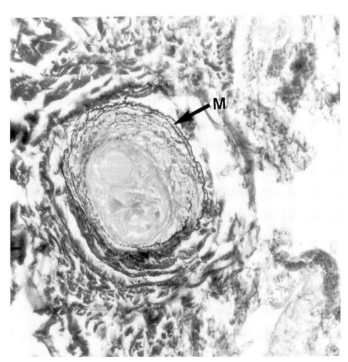

Fig. 6.13 Photomicrograph of lung tissue from an Indian child with severe rheumatic mitral stenosis, who died at 9 years of age, showing a small pre-acinar artery with atrophy of the media (M), and circumferential intimal proliferation. (× 380) (Reproduced by kind permission of Springer-Verlag.)

Haemosiderosis

Haemosiderin is produced by disintegrated erythrocytes after rupture of small blood vessels or diapedesis. It accumulates in macrophages, which are then called 'siderophages', and is deposited in the vessel wall and connective tissue of the lung. It is most pronounced in cases of long-standing pulmonary hypertension.

Fibrinoid necrosis of the media

Fibrinoid necrosis is found in the muscular pre-acinar and intra-acinar arteries. A part of the arterial wall becomes necrotic in severe pulmonary hypertension. The nuclei of the smooth muscle cells then disappear and fibrin is deposited in the necrotic area. The affected part of the wall has an acellular, homogenous, opaque appearance which is eosinophilic and stains bright pink with haematoxylin. The media is swollen and the internal and external elastic laminae tend to bulge. Fibrinoid necrosis may excite an inflammatory response with infiltration by polymorphonuclear leucocytes. The inflammatory response often extends into the adventitia and surrounding alveolar tissue. The entire circumference of the vessel may be affected, generally over a short segment of the arterial pathway. When the entire circumference of the artery is involved a fibrin clot is usually present.

Plexiform lesions

Plexiform lesions are complex lesions found in patients

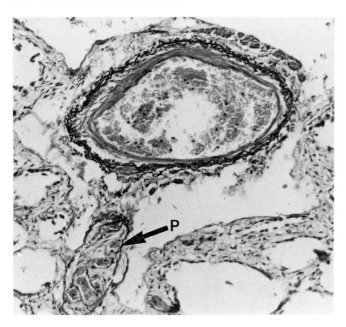

Fig. 6.14 Photomicrograph of lung tissue showing a respiratory bronchiolar artery with medial atrophy, intimal fibrosis and a branch containing a plexiform lesion (P). (× 380) (Reproduced by kind permission of Springer-Verlag.)

with severe pulmonary hypertension. The incidence of the lesion varies considerably in different cases. The lesion arises from an artery showing medial hypertrophy, often with concentric lamellar fibrosis. The branch is dilated, parts of the wall are necrotic and the large lumen is filled with strands of proliferating intimal cells separated by a plexus of narrow channels (Fig. 6.14). The arteries arising from a plexiform lesion are thin-walled distally. The plexiform lesion is thought to be located between a high pressure vessel and those arteries in the alveolar wall in which the pressure is not elevated. Plexiform lesions are not anastomotic channels, nor are they multiple angiomas or congenital malformations of the pulmonary arteries (Wagenvoort, 1973). Mature plexiform lesions are rare in infancy, but arteries showing the early features of the lesion have been reported in infants between 3 weeks and 4 months of age (Hruban & Humphreys, 1960; Kanjuh et al, 1964).

Compression of the airways

Dilated pulmonary arteries frequently compress the main and lobar bronchi in children with a high pulmonary blood flow with and without pulmonary hypertension. In infants with severe pulmonary hypertension, this leads to the familiar clinical problem of recurrent collapse of different lobes or segments of lung. Not infrequently the respiratory complications of congenital heart disease constitute an indication for corrective surgery in infancy. The deformity of the bronchi may persist after operation for some time.

In some patients prolonged compression appears to be associated with bronchomalacia.

Structure of the pulmonary trunk

In the presence of severe pulmonary hypertension, the luminal diameter of the pulmonary trunk is frequently larger than that of the aorta. When pulmonary hypertension is present from birth, the relative wall thickness remains similar to that of the aorta. The elastic laminae then tend to remain long and continuous, as in fetal life. The pulmonary trunk retains its 'aortic configuration' in most (but not all) patients (Heath et al, 1959). Aneurysmal dilation is not uncommon in children with severe pulmonary hypertension and is sometimes associated with bacterial endocarditis. Yellow streaks of patches of atheroma may be found in the extrapulmonary and elastic intrapulmonary arteries. It is particularly common in the presence of a large arterial duct.

Application of quantitative morphometric techniques to the study of pulmonary vascular disease

Quantitative morphometric analysis of lung biopsies taken from 95 patients with congenital heart disease and pulmonary hypertension showed that the abnormalities in pulmonary arterial growth and development could be related to the level of pulmonary arterial pressure and resistance (Rabinovitch et al, 1978a). Grouping the patients with different types of cardiac anomalies together, the structural changes fell into 3 patterns. Of the 95 patients, 21 (22%) showed only abnormal extension of muscle into peripheral intra-acinar arteries, and this type of structural change was found in patients who had only an increase in pulmonary blood flow. In a second group, 59 of the 95 patients (62%) had an increase in percentage medial thickness in normally muscularised arteries in addition to abnormal extension of the muscle. Of these 59 patients, percentage medial thickness was greater than twice the normal value in 32 and the arteries were smaller than normal for age. Patients with the early manifestations of a slight increase in percentage wall thickness had an increase in pulmonary blood flow, but little if any increase in pressure. In those showing the later manifestations, pulmonary arterial pressure was moderately to severely elevated. The level of pulmonary arterial pressure correlated with the percentage arterial medial thickness (r = 0.74; p < 0.005). The third group of 15 patients (16%), had a reduction in arterial number in addition to the increased muscularity and a reduction in arterial size as seen in the more advanced cases in the second group. In those patients pulmonary vascular resistance was generally greater than 3.5 units/m². For the entire group of 95 patients the number of intra-acinar arteries, expressed as the alveolar : arterial ratio, was significantly related to pulmonary vascular resist-

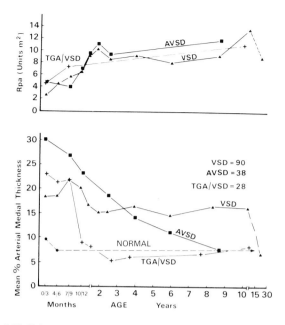

Fig. 6.15 Pulmonary arteriolar resistance (Rpa) and mean percentage arterial medial thickness related to age in cases of isolated ventricular septal defect (VSD) atrioventricular septal defect (AVSD) and complete transposition with ventricular septal defect (TGA/VSD).

The effect of pulmonary hypertension on the development of pulmonary vasculature in different types of congenital cardiac anomalies

The natural history of pulmonary vascular disease differs according to the type of cardiac abnormality.

A high level of resistance in older patients with ventricular septal defect is caused by obliterative changes in small muscular pulmonary arteries which gradually reduce the cross-sectional area of the pulmonary vascular bed. During the first few years of life, however, obliterative changes of this kind rarely occur. This suggests that, at this young age, a different mechanism is associated with a high pulmonary arterial pressure and, in some cases with an elevated resistance. Quantitative morphometric techniques applied to the analysis of structural change in the lungs of 10 children dying between the ages of 3 months and 10 years showed that the presence of pulmonary hypertension interfered with the growth and development of the pulmonary circulation (Haworth et al, 1977). Most of these children had had a high pulmonary blood flow and had been in congestive cardiac failure. At autopsy the pre-acinar arteries showed little (if any) dilation but an increase in medial thickness (Fig. 6.16). Arterial muscularity was increased within the acinus (as judged by an increase in percentage medial thickness of normally muscularised arteries and by the presence of muscle in smaller and more peripheral arteries than normal). Vein wall muscularity was also increased and the small veins were 'arterialised' (Wagenvoort, 1970). The intra-acinar arteries were abnormally small, generally being similar to the normal at birth (Fig. 6.17). Post-mortem arteriography showed a reduction in the density of the background haze, suggesting a reduc-

ance (r = 0.77; p < 0.005), and the correlation was greater in children over the age of 1 year (r = 0.84). Of the patients with a reduction in arterial number, 33% also had severe structural change within the arterial walls, described as being at least of grade III pulmonary vascular disease (Heath & Edwards, 1958).

Recent studies in which pulmonary vascular structure has been analysed separately in cases of ventricular septal defect, atrioventricular septal defect and complete transposition with ventricular septal defect have shown that the percentage medial thickness becomes reduced as intimal proliferation develops in small pre-acinar, terminal and respiratory bronchiolar arteries (Fig. 6.15). With time, intra-acinar arterial muscularity becomes inversely related to the pulmonary arterial pressure and resistance. This occurs before medial atrophy and the classical changes of grade IV disease are evident. In the presence of severe pulmonary hypertension, determination of intra-acinar arterial muscularity helps assess the severity of intimal obstruction in more proximal arteries.

In assessing a lung biopsy specimen, quantitation of arterial muscularity, size and number is accompanied by a description of the appearance of the vessel wall at each level along the arterial pathway. In the normal lung the structure of the pre-acinar arteries is unlike that of the more distal intra-acinar arteries. The appearance of arteries at each level along the arterial pathway will, therefore, differ also in disease. No pathologic finding should be considered in isolation, but should be related to, and explained by, other findings observed in the biopsy specimen.

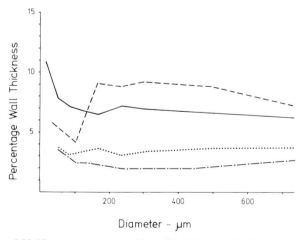

Fig. 6.16 Mean percentage arterial medial thickness related to external diameter (µm) in patients with ventricular septal defect, showing in all cases medial hypertrophy and in infancy the presence of muscle in smaller arteries than is normal. ——— = infants less than 1 year; ----- = children aged 3 and 4 years; ...... = child aged 3 months; -.-.-.- = normal. (Reproduced with permission from the *American Journal of Cardiology*.)

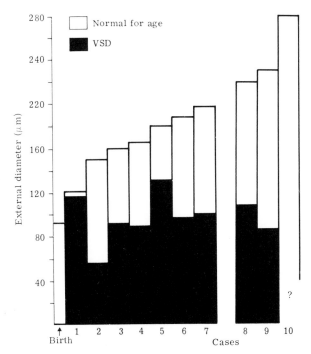

Fig. 6.17 Mean external diameter (μm) of arteries accompanying respiratory bronchioli in the normal infant at birth, in 9 children with a ventricular septal defect together with the normal of the same age, showing growth failure of the intra-acinar arteries. Case 10 died aged 10 years with obliterative pulmonary vascular disease and destruction of the intra-acinar vessels made accurate quantitation impossible. (Reproduced with permission from the *American Journal of Cardiology.*)

tion of the number of intra-acinar arteries (Fig. 6.18). This was confirmed by counting microscopically the number of arteries per unit area of lung tissue. Occluded alveolar wall arteries are seen on electron microscopic examination (see Fig. 6.10). Occlusion is probably secondary to the hypertrophy and hyperplasia of the differentiating smooth muscle cells seen in this normally thin-walled precapillary segment of the arterial pathway (Fig. 6.19). This is the clinical and pathological picture seen in many young children who die with a large hypertensive ventricular septal defect. A minority appear never to have been in congestive heart failure and to have had a high pulmonary vascular resistance from birth. Post-mortem arteriography in such children shows a reduction in the lumen diameter of the axial arteries from the hilum to the pleural surface. The changes in pulmonary arterial muscularity, size and number are similar to those in patients with a higher pulmonary blood flow (Hislop et al, 1975).

Recent studies on lung biopsy specimens from 90 children with a large isolated ventricular septal defect have shown that pulmonary arterial muscularity is increased from 3 weeks until 10–15 years of age (Fig. 6.15). Muscularity is greatest at 7–9 months of age, and does not change significantly with age thereafter until 10–15 years. Mild non-occlusive cellular proliferation is first seen at 7–9 months and fibrosis is relatively common between 2 and 4 years of age. A

progressive increase in fibrotic luminal obstruction by 10–15 years of age is associated with a marked reduction in muscularity in intra-acinar arteries lying distal to the obstructed vessels and to the subsequent development of grade IV changes. A graded assessment of arterial wall damage correlated with age (r = 0.4; p < 0.0003), mean pulmonary artery pressure (r = 0.6; p < 0.0003), and resistance (r = 0.6; p < 0.0003). Mean percentage arterial medial thickness was not significantly related to age, pulmonary arterial pressure, or vascular resistance. Factors that appeared to predispose individual children to more severe disease than others of similar age included patency of the arterial duct or coarctation, even when these lesions had previously been repaired. Thus, in young children, a ventricular septal defect with pulmonary hypertension appears to be associated with severe muscularisation of the intra-acinar arteries which may be accompanied by a reduction in size and number of intra-acinar arteries, abnormalities which must prevent the pulmonary vasculature from growing and developing normally. The intimal changes characteristic of obstructed pulmonary vascular disease are superimposed on an imperfectly developed pulmonary vascular bed if the pulmonary arterial bed is allowed to remain elevated.

In cases of atrioventricular septal defect, cellular intimal proliferation is more severe in infancy and early childhood than in children with an isolated ventricular septal defect. The more severe luminal obstruction is associated with a reduction in muscularity with age (r = −0.5; p < 0.001), pulmonary arterial pressure (r = −0.6; p < 0.001), and resistance (r = −0.4; p < 0.001) (Fig. 6.15).

In children with complete transposition and ventricular septal defect, obstructive cellular intimal proliferation develops earlier than in the previous two anomalies (by 4–6 months of age) and is associated with a rapid reduction in intra-acinar pulmonary arterial muscularity by 10–12 months of age (Fig. 6.15). Mean percentage arterial medial thickness is inversely related to mean pulmonary arterial pressure (r = −0.6; p < 0.001). Serial reconstructions of the arterial pathways in autopsy specimens showed that, by 6 months of age, an increase in pulmonary vascular resistance was due to the development of severe medial hypertrophy and cellular intimal proliferation at the end of the arterial pathways just proximal to and within the acinus (Fig. 6.20) (Haworth, 1984). The structural abnormalities are strategically placed to obstruct the flow of blood into the acinus and their development precedes the classical changes of advanced pulmonary vascular obliterative disease. Generalised arterial dilation begins to appear during the first year of life before the marked intimal fibrosis characteristic of late grade III or IV disease has had time to develop. In a series of 200 lungs biopsy specimens from children with complete transposition, Newfeld et al (1974) showed that, in the presence of a ventricular septal defect, two-fifths of cases had more than grade II pulmonary

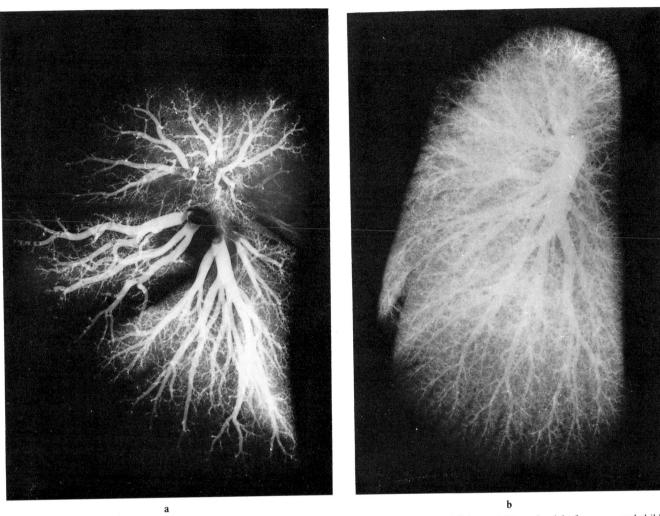

a   b

Fig. 6.18 Post-mortem arteriograms, (a) on the left from a 9-month-old child with a ventricular septal defect and (b) on the right from a normal child of the same age. (× 1) (Reproduced with permission from the *American Journal of Cardiology*.)

vascular disease. Of those aged 1 year or more, three-quarters had grade IV disease. By contrast, of those with an intact ventricular septum, only 8.4% had more than grade II pulmonary vascular disease.

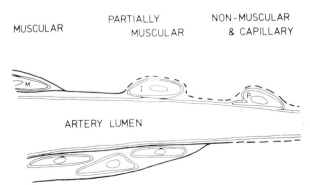

Fig. 6.19 Diagram of the precapillary region of rat pulmonary artery. M = smooth muscle cell; I = intermediate cell; P = pericyte. (Reproduced by kind permission of the Wistar Institute Press.)

Pulmonary vascular disease is uncommon in children with complete transposition and an intact ventricular septum except in the presence of a large arterial duct. If the duct is not closed, severe obliterative pulmonary vascular disease develops rapidly during the first year of life. In the absence of a large arterial duct, the development of pulmonary vascular disease is difficult to explain in the few cases in which it occurs. A high haematocrit causing multiple small pulmonary thromboses is a possible initiating factor. More recently, the bronchial arterial circulation has been incriminated. Angiographic studies indicate that the bronchial circulation is more prominent in children with complete transposition than in the normal child, particularly in those with an intact septum. Aziz et al (1977) suggested that the low arterial oxygen tension of the systemic arterial blood flowing into the pulmonary vascular bed (and also into the vessels supplying the arteries themselves) encouraged vasoconstriction and thus medial hypertropy. Equally, an enlarged bronchial arterial circulation may be harmful by

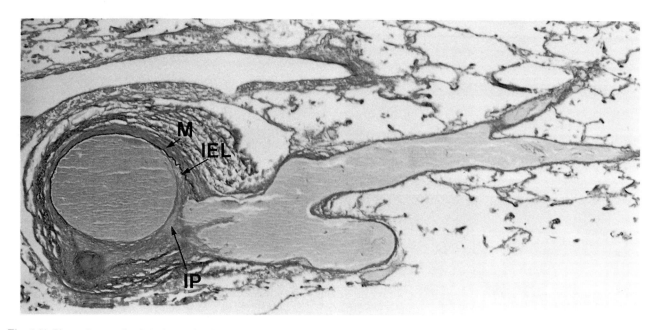

Fig. 6.20 Photomicrograph of the lung of a 5-month-old infant with transposition of the great arteries and ventricular septal defect showing a terminal bronchilar artery distended by injection medium having a thick media (M). Intimal proliferation (IP) surrounds the origin of the thin-walled branches. IEL = internal elastic lumina. (× 200)

increasing the pressure and flow of blood entering the intra-acinar arteries.

Thus, each of the common types of congenital cardiac anomalies elicits a different structural response from the pulmonary circulation. In ventricular septal defect, a marked increased in muscularity is sustained with relatively little trauma to the intima – unlike atrioventricular septal defect with common orifice and particularly unlike complete transposition with ventricular septal defect, where the intima is severely damaged during the first months of life. A similar increase in pulmonary arterial pressure and vascular resistance in children of the same age may imply a different pathological picture in different conditions.

Pathogenesis of pulmonary vascular disease

In patients with an increase in pulmonary blood flow but little or no increase in pressure, pericytes and intermediate cells differentiate into mature smooth muscle cells in the normally thin-walled precapillary vessels (Fig. 6.19). In the presence of pulmonary hypertension this change is more pronounced and is accompanied by medial hypertrophy in more proximal arteries. There may be an early reduction in number of patent and newly muscularised alveolar wall arteries. If the pulmonary hypertension is not relieved, intimal proliferation develops in more proximal small pre-acinar, terminal and respiratory bronchiolar arteries. Increased muscularity is a response to increased isometric or isotonic work but intimal proliferation suggests intimal damage. Summarising current theory, blood flow velocity is

increased in conditions such as complete transposition with ventricular septal defect, double inlet ventricle and isolated ventricular septal defect where pulmonary blood flow is increased without a concomitant increase in vessel size and with, in some cases, a reduction in peripheral arterial number. The resulting high shearing forces damage the endothelial cells, particularly at arterial bifurcations (Fry, 1968). Migration and proliferation of smooth muscle cells derived from the media is stimulated (Ross et al, 1984).

A mitogen is produced by platelets which become activated when they adhere to the damaged endothelium (Ross et al, 1974). In addition, endothelial cells and macrophages produce mitogens in vitro, but their contribution to mitogenesis in vivo remains to be elucidated (Gajdusek et al, 1980; Bitterman et al, 1982). An endothelial-derived mitogen can, in the test tube cause quiescent smooth muscle cells to proliferate under hypoxic stress. A macrophage-derived mitogen could be important in stimulating the connective tissue synthesis associated with pulmonary arterial medial hypertrophy. The damaged endothelial, adherent degranulated platelets and leukocytes release arachadonic acid metabolites which influence vascular wall function and the balance between thrombogenesis and thrombolysis. In the simplest terms, platelet derived thromboxane A_2 encourages vasoconstriction and platelet aggregation while PGI_2 relaxes the vessel wall and prevents platelet aggregation. Experimental studies suggest that regeneration of endothelium or the formation of a neointimal surface by smooth muscle cells leads to restoration of PGI_2 production (Eldor et al, 1981).

The pulmonary endothelial cell obviously plays a central role in the pathogenesis of pulmonary vascular disease, which is as yet incompletely defined. The presence of endothelial cells is essential for acetyl choline-dependent contraction of underlying smooth muscle cells (Furchgott & Sawadki, 1980). Endothelial cells process prostaglandins, biogenic amines, steroids, chylomicrons and haemostatic factors, while angiotensin converting enzymes and other peptidase enzymes are situated on the luminal surface (Ryan & Ryan, 1984). Like the smooth muscle cells, they synthesise and export extracellular materials such as fibronectin, collagen and elastin (Birdwell et al, 1978; Mecham et al, 1983; Sage et al, 1979). Damage to endothelial cells in pulmonary vascular disease could be associated with release into the circulation of abnormal amounts of a normal cell product or release of an abnormal metabolite.

Exciting advances in cell biology encourage parallel investigations into the physical properties of the hypertensive pulmonary circulation. Attention is traditionally focused on the peripheral pulmonary arteries, but pulmonary hypertension also elicits a structural response from the proximal intrapulmonary arteries. The medial thickness of the large muscular and elastic arteries increases and this increases wall stiffness, which may increase the transmission of pulsatile pressure and flow to the peripheral vessels, encouraging further damage to the walls of the peripheral vessels (Berry et al, 1981).

Pulmonary hypertension and the effect of palliative surgery on the lung

In patients with pulmonary hypoperfusion, insertion of a systemic-pulmonary shunt may lead to pulmonary hypertension, while in patients with congenital heart disease associated with pulmonary hypertension, banding the pulmonary trunk may fail to reduce the pulmonary arterial pressure and flow adequately. For many years a less than perfect result has not impaired the outcome of intracardiac repair in the majority of patients. Now, however, the introduction of the Fontan procedure, cardiac transplantation and other types of operation has emphasised the need to achieve a structurally normal pulmonary vascular bed.

The perfect shunt produces symptomatic relief. It ensures that the lungs are equally well perfused and that the central and intrapulmonary arteries grow normally (see below). It must be sufficiently large to prevent the occurrence of the thromboemboli associated with a low pulmonary blood flow and polycythaemia and sufficiently small to avoid the development of pulmonary vascular disease. The type of shunt can influence the outcome. In a Waterston anastomosis, kinking of the right pulmonary artery may be attributable either to technical difficulties or to rapid growth and realignment of the aorta and pulmonary trunk (Rao et al, 1978). The incidence of pulmonary hypertension is higher in

patients who have had a Waterston shunt than in those who have had a Blalock-Taussig shunt. In the minority of patients, the pulmonary blood flow is excessive following a shunt operation. Uncommonly patients die in severe cardiac failure during the first week after operation with distended vessels and capillaries and thickened alveolar walls (Ferencz, 1960a). If a child dies 2 or 3 weeks after the operation, then medial hypertrophy of the muscular pulmonary arteries with extension of muscle into smaller arteries than normal can be demonstrated. The lungs of patients who survive longer with pulmonary hypertension due to an aortopulmonary anastomosis show the structural changes associated with cardiac defects and pulmonary hypertension. Even in the absence of significant pulmonary hypertension, however, the muscularity of the pulmonary arteries on the same side as the shunt is frequently greater than in the contralateral lung. It may be greater than normal even when the pressure is not elevated. Radionuclide studies after corrective surgery have shown relative hypoperfusion of the lung which had received the shunt, resulting in ventilation-perfusion imbalance (Alderson et al, 1976).

The pulmonary trunk is banded to reduce pulmonary blood flow in babies in cardiac failure and to prevent the development of pulmonary vascular disease. The success of the operation is related to age and to the type of intracardiac anomaly present. In conditions associated with the rapid development of pulmonary vascular disease the pulmonary trunk should be banded by 4–6 months of age. Early rebanding should be considered if a satisfactory result is not obtained, particularly in patients destined for a Fontan type of procedure.

The criteria for an ideal shunt and for an ideal pulmonary arterial band are related to the type of intracardiac repair for which the patient is destined. A moderate increase in pulmonary arterial medial thickness can prejudice the outcome of a Fontan operation by increasing right atrial afterload. Such changes may have little or no effect on the outcome of repair of tetralogy of Fallot or atrioventricular septal defect. In patients in whom the pulmonary trunk has been banded, it can be particularly difficult to predict the pulmonary vascular structure and 'operability' from the haemodynamic findings. Pulmonary vascular smooth muscle can be increased in such patients even when the criteria for a Fontan operation have been largely fulfilled.

In recent operations to palliate children with the hypoplastic left heart syndrome, the pulmonary trunk has been connected to the aortic arch, after first disconnecting the central pulmonary arteries which are then perfused by a systemic-pulmonary shunt (Norwood et al, 1983). I have been personally informed by Professor Thomas Graham of Nashville, Tennessee, that the lungs occasionally remain persistently hypoperfused. This is probably due to the marked increase in pulmonary arterial muscularity which develops in the lungs of these children during fetal life. Such an increase in pulmonary vascular smooth muscle offers a greater resistance to blood flow than is usually seen in shunted patients, the majority of whom have a hypoperfused pulmonary circulation with abnormally thin-walled arteries.

Cardiac transplantation demands that the pulmonary circulation should be structurally normal or show only minimal abnormalities. In congenital heart disease (and in cor pulmonale) an increase in pulmonary arterial smooth muscle is associated with hypertrophy of the pulmonary ventricle. Following cardiac transplantation, a normal right ventricle may fail in the presence of only a moderate increase in pulmonary arterial muscularity.

Preoperative assessment of pulmonary vascular disease

The cardiologist is constantly trying to predict the structural changes present in the lungs from the clinical, radiological and haemodynamic findings without having to resort to biopsy of the lung. Prediction is frequently difficult.

The chest radiograph is reassuringly plethoric when the resistance is sufficiently low to permit a high blood flow. It is depressingly evident when pulmonary vascular disease is advanced. The development of severe obstructive disease in the muscular pulmonary arteries leads to peripheral pruning and a hypertranslucent appearance in association with dilation of the hilar and proximal vessels. Wedge angiography is not widely used. This is because although it is helpful in demonstrating advanced pulmonary vascular obstructive disease, it does not discriminate between less severe degrees of pulmonary vascular disease when the patient may still be potentially operable. The abnormal pulmonary wedge angiogram is characterised by decreased arborisation, reduced background opacification, and delayed venous filling. The arteries may appear tortuous and have segments of dilation or constriction with marginal defects suggestive of obliterative disease.

The technique of wedge angiography has been revived recently in an attempt to improve the correlation between structural and functional change in the pulmonary vascular bed by measuring the rate of tapering of a subsegmental branch of the right posterobasal artery in patients with pulmonary hypertension (Rabinovitch et al, 1978b). In the normal lung the pulmonary arteries taper towards the periphery, but the vessels narrow over a shorter distance in the presence of an elevated pulmonary vascular resistance. In a group of patients with pulmonary hypertension, the rate of tapering corresponded both with the measurements of pulmonary arterial pressure and vascular resistance made at cardiac catheterisation and with the structural changes found at lung biopsy. Three groups of patients could be identified. Those with gradual tapering had a high pulmonary blood flow and an increased extension of muscle into the arteries. Those with an intermediate degree of tapering had some elevation in pulmonary arterial pressure, but the resistance was generally less than 3.5 units/m², and there was an increase in the percentage wall thickness. Those with abrupt tapering had a resistance greater than 3.5 units/m², and showed a reduced number of arteries or more advanced structural change characteristic of at least grade III pulmonary vascular disease (Heath & Edwards, 1958).

Attempts at the time of cardiac catheterisation to assess the potential reversibility of pulmonary vascular disease clinically are based on the premise that, if the only structural change in the pulmonary vascular bed is an increase in muscularity, then the circulation will respond to vasodilator substances such as oxygen and tolazoline. The release of vasoconstrictor tone will lower pulmonary vascular resistance, increase the magnitude of the left-to-right shunt and may lower the pulmonary arterial pressure. Failure to achieve this response implies fixed, organic obstruction of the pulmonary circulation. In practice, however, it is often difficult to predict pulmonary vascular structure in this manner, particularly after the 1st year of life. Children with Down's syndrome are particularly difficult to assess because they often suffer from upper airways obstruction which may contribute to the increased pulmonary vascular resistance determined at cardiac catheterisation. The pathologist will then find less pulmonary vascular damage in a lung biopsy than expected for the increase in pulmonary arterial pressure and resistance.

Non-invasive methods of estimating the level of pulmonary arterial pressure and vascular resistance in patients at risk of developing pulmonary vascular disease are not yet sufficiently reliable for routine clinical use. The pulmonary arterial systolic pressure can be related, using phonocardiography or Doppler ultrasound to detect valve movement, to the duration of the interval between pulmonary valve closure and tricuspid opening (Burstin, 1967; Hätle et al, 1981). The mean pulmonary arterial pressure, diastolic pressure and vascular resistance are related to the right ventricular systolic time intervals measured from the M-mode echocardiographic tracing from the pulmonary valve. The relationship is not sufficiently precise to avoid cardiac catheterisation in patients at risk from developing pulmonary vascular disease (Hirschfeld et al, 1975; Silverman et al, 1980). An open lung biopsy is taken when the prognosis remains uncertain after assessment of the clinical and haemodynamic data.

Survival after intracardiac repair

In patients with pulmonary hypertension the outcome of a satisfactory intra-cardiac repair is determined by the state of the pulmonary vascular bed at the time of repair. Survival after leaving hospital depends on the potential reversibility of the different types of pathological abnormalities present in the lung. Patients who have potentially reversible pathological lesions occasionally die at (or soon after) operation because the "mild" abnormalities prevent the pulmonary circulation from functioning normally in the perioperative period. Potential reversibility of pulmonary vascular disease is not synonymous with operability.

Cardiopulmonary bypass damages the lung. The effect is most traumatic in patients who have preoperative abnormalities of pulmonary vascular structure (Ratliffe et al, 1973). Recent studies suggest that the foreign substances encountered by the blood during cardiopulmonary bypass lead to compliment activation. Such compliment activation, together with generation of anaphylatoxins C3a and C5a and other products leads to a wholebody inflammatory reaction (Kirklin et al, 1983). Polymorphonuclear leukocytes and monocytes have membrane binding sites for C5a. C5a release results in altered mobility of these cells and their sequestration in lung capillaries (Hammerschmidt et al, 1981). Studies in the test tube have shown that damage to the endothelium (endothelial abnormalities precede intimal proliferation in pulmonary vascular disease) can increase adherence of granulocytes to the endothelial surface and enhance granulocyte-mediated endothelial injury, resulting in a vicious circle which leads to increase microvascular permeability (Brigham and Merrick, 1984; Flick et al, 1981). The endothelial cells have receptors for some compliment components and latent receptors for others (Ryan and Ryan, 1984). Evidence suggests that the pulmonary endothelial cell is both a target of the inflammatory response and an active participant. The integrity of the pulmonary endothelium at the onset of bypass is probably crucial in avoiding the "post-perfusion" lung.

The postoperative management of patients with long-standing pulmonary hypertension is often difficult and prolonged artificial ventilation may be required. Even in young infants who do not suffer from advanced obliterative pulmonary vascular disease, the postoperative course may be complicated by sudden, apparently unprovoked increases in pulmonary arterial pressure which are usually followed by a fall in cardiac output. Such episodic pulmonary hypertension may respond to the administration of a pulmonary vasodilator drug such as tolazoline (Jones et al, 1981). In young infants with a marked increase in pulmonary vascular smooth muscle, the capacity of the pulmonary circulation to vasoconstrict is considerable and the child may die despite the absence of severe obliterative pulmonary vascular disease. In patients at risk, the pulmonary arterial pressure should be monitored postoperatively.

The structural effect of lowering the pulmonary arterial pressure in children with congenital heart disease is rarely seen because the lung is rarely biopsied after an intracardiac repair. After banding the pulmonary trunk to reduce the pulmonary arterial pressure and flow, however, medial hypertrophy regressed and cellular intimal proliferation generally showed deposition of collagen-rich fibrous tissue which retracted towards the media and increased the luminal diameter (Dammann et al, 1961; Wagenvoort, 1974). Cases showing obstruction of the arterial lumen in the first biopsy showed similar changes in the second. In the presence of more advanced arterial lesions, clinically the prognosis is less optimistic but the fate of the lesions themselves is unknown (Wagenvoort & Wagenvoort, 1974). Medial atrophy and dilation is associated with, and probably the result of, narrowing or obliteration of the lumen of the parent artery by intimal proliferation and, more usually, with fibrosis. Such changes are probably not reversible. Recent experimental studies also suggest that, although a reduction in pulmonary arterial pressure is associated with regression of muscularity, there may be a permanent increase in the amount of connective tissue in the subendothelial layer, media and adentitia of the arteries and a permanent reduction in intra-acinar number (Meyrick & Reid, 1980a).

In a recent study, the pulmonary vascular abnormalities present at the time of intracardiac repair were correlated with the haemodynamic findings one day, and one year after repair (Rabinovitch et al, 1984). During the first day after operation, the mean pulmonary arterial pressure was commonly elevated in patients with severe medial hypertrophy with or without intimal proliferation, and was invariably increased in those with Grade III pulmonary vascular disease or more. One year after repair, the pulmonary arterial pressure and resistance were normal in all patients who underwent intracardiac repair before 9 months of age irrespective of the severity of the pulmonary vascular lesions present at the time of repair. Pressure and resistance were also normal in older patients who at the time of repair had a lung biopsy specimen showing Grade A or B morphometric findings (Rabinovitch et al, 1978) with any Heath and Edwards grade or with Grade B morphometric findings and Heath and Edwards Grade I change. Pressure and resistance were increased in half of the patients with Grade B and Heath and Edwards Grade II disease or with Grade C and Heath and Edwards Grade I or II changes. Pulmonary arterial pressure and resistance were increased in all patients who had an intracardiac repair after 2 years of age and who had Grade C morphometric findings. Morphometry and assessment of intimal damage are helpful in predicting post operative pulmonary hypertension and in selecting those patients whose pulmonary arterial pressure and resistance will eventually return to normal after intracardiac repair.

The prognosis must therefore depend on a combination of factors. These include the luminal diameter of pre- and intra-acinar arteries, the number of patent intra-acinar arteries, and the thickness and composition of the arterial walls from the pulmonary trunk to the capillary bed. The relationship between these factors is not understood. We do not know, for example, to what extent a reduction in arterial size and number can lead to further structural damage to the arterial wall. Understanding the cell biology of pulmonary vascular disease is only now beginning.

Emphasis in clinical management must be on the prevention of pulmonary vascular disease. When the natural history of the cardiac abnormality is that of rapidly progressive pulmonary vascular disease, as in complete transposition with ventricular septal defect, or double inlet ventricle without pulmonary outflow tract obstruction, then the child should either undergo corrective surgery or banding of the pulmonary trunk during the first 6 months of life. Where the natural history of pulmonary vascular disease is less aggressive, as in a ventricular septal defect, the abnormality should be corrected before 1 year of age if the pulmonary arterial pressure remains high.

PULMONARY HYPOPERFUSION IN CHILDHOOD

Effect of hypoperfusion on lung development

The effects of hypoperfusion on the developing pulmonary circulation may be as deleterious as those of hyperperfusion and pulmonary hypertension. The proximal elastic arteries may develop less elastin than normal, while the intra-acinar arteries are usually smaller and have a thinner muscle coat. Pulmonary arterial thromboses can occur and account for eccentric areas of intimal fibrosis. Enlargement of the bronchial arterial circulation supplements (or even replaces) a normal pulmonary arterial blood supply in many forms of cyanotic congenital heart disease, including tetralogy of Fallot and pulmonary atresia. When the lung is severely hypoperfused the development of the alveoli can also be impaired.

Fortunately, the full impact of pulmonary hypoperfusion on the developing lung is rarely seen nowadays since the pulmonary blood flow can be increased as early as is necessary by medical or surgical treatment. Neonates, in whom the pulmonary blood flow depends on the continued patency of the arterial duct, may present as emergencies when the duct begins to close after birth. In pulmonary atresia with an intact ventricular septum, for example, ductal patency is maintained by treatment with prostaglandin E_1 or E_2. Neither of these potent drugs is without side-effects and prolonged administration of prostaglandin E_1 can damage the intrapulmonary arteries (Haworth et al, 1980). Irrespective of age, however, the pulmonary blood flow in the majority of patients is increased surgically by a palliative aortopulmonary shunt or by a 'corrective' operation.

Even in those patients with an adequate pulmonary blood flow who thrive in early childhood without palliation, there may be abnormalities of lung development. This applies to many children with tetralogy of Fallot. For the majority of patients with tetralogy of Fallot the prognosis is good. The 5-year survival of patients having had a Blalock-Taussig anastomosis followed by 'corrective' surgery is 85%. Many children undergo elective repair without

having needed palliative surgery (Macartney et al, 1980). In such children, the extrapulmonary arteries may be of normal size and the intrapulmonary pre-acinar arteries may even be large for age (Johnson & Haworth, 1982). By contrast, the intra-acinar arteries are significantly smaller than normal. In both pre- and intra-acinar muscular arteries the media is abnormally thin, although muscle is normally distributed along the arterial pathway. Eccentric areas of intimal fibrosis are usually small and uncommon. The bronchial arteries may be more prominent than usual both macroscopically and microscopically, but no abnormal bronchopulmonary connexions occur. Thus, even those patients with the most favourable clinical picture of tetralogy of Fallot have abnormalities of pulmonary vascular development.

Several studies describe atrophy of the media in patients with tetralogy of Fallot. Atrophy, however, implies a secondary reduction in muscularity, and muscularity is probably never normal in postnatal life in these patients. Indeed, babies with pulmonary atresia and intact ventricular septum are born with abnormally thin-walled arteries (Haworth & Reid, 1977b). Despite the media being thin, it hypertrophies in response to an increase in pressure or flow. This response is seen either following a Waterston-Cooley anastomosis or in the presence of a residual post-operative ventricular septal defect. Recent experimental studies have shown that in pulmonary hypertension smooth muscle cells increase in size rather than in number (Meyrick & Reid, 1980b). The ability of the medial coat to hypertrophy in tetralogy of Fallot suggests that the children are probably born with a normal number of abnormally small medial smooth muscle cells. Supporting this hypothesis is the observation that, in these children, the muscle cells extend as far down the arterial pathway as in the normal child.

Pulmonary atresia with ventricular septal defect and multiple aortopulmonary collateral arteries can be regarded as a vicarious experiment in which the size of the intrapulmonary arteries is determined by the size of the collateral arteries or arterial duct which perfuses them (see Fig. 6.9). Although perfusion by a large collateral artery can lead to pulmonary hypertensive vascular disease, in the majority of patients the problem is hypoperfusion. Stenoses of the collateral arteries occurred in 58.8% of collaterals in one pathological study and 42% of vessels in a radiological study (McGoon et al, 1977; Haworth & Macartney, 1980). Unfortunately, although stenoses 'protect' the pulmonary vascular bed from developing pulmonary vascular disease, they may also prevent the lung from being adequately perfused. This then prevents the pulmonary vessels from developing normally. Thus, the pre-acinar arteries, both those connected to collateral arteries and those connected to central pulmonary arteries, are generally smaller than normal. This is in both absolute terms and in relation to the size of the accompanying airway. The pre-acinar arteries may also show saccular dilatation at lobar or segmental level, stenoses of the lobar arteries and smaller lateral branches than normal. Quantitative morphometric analysis shows that the intra-acinar arteries frequently have a reduced external diameter and that the percentage arterial medial thickness is normal or reduced.

Several studies have reported a reduction in postmortem lung volume in children dying with tetralogy of Fallot (Hislop & Reid, 1973c; Johnson & Haworth, 1982). A group of adults who in life had undergone a successful repair had a reduction in thoracic gas volume to 75% of the predicted value. The findings were similar in those with and without initial palliative surgery (Bjarke, 1974). The magnitude of the reduction in thoracic gas volume in the in vivo series was similar to the magnitude of the reduction in lung volume in an autopsy study. Postoperative lung function studies have also demonstrated only a restrictive defect, there being no evidence of obstruction to air flow. The alveoli and airways appear normal, both macroscopically and microscopically.

The reduction in lung volume is largely due to a reduction in total alveolar number. The reduction in number is not as great as the reduction in volume because the number of alveoli per unit volume of lung tissue is greater than normal. In young animals, a reduction in blood flow is associated with a small lung composed of many small alveoli (Haworth et al, 1981). These observations are encouraging because, after corrective surgery, the lung probably has a better chance of achieving normal alveolar development if an increase of size of existing alveoli is required rather than the formation of new alveoli. A corrective operation performed before the critical growth period of the lung is over will presumably encourage normal alveolar development. An early repair also permits greater physical activity. Physical training in normal children increases both total lung volume and vital capacity (Ekblom, 1969). In the lung function study mentioned previously, the mean age at repair was 19 years. The relative reduction in thoracic gas volume in these patients was probably similar to what it had been in childhood.

Pulmonary arterial thromboses

Pulmonary arterial thromboses with intimal proliferation were previously an important feature of the pulmonary vascular bed in tetralogy of Fallot. The absence of postoperative pulmonary hypertension was attributed to the reserve capacity of the pulmonary vascular bed being sufficient to compensate for the reduction in cross-sectional area. Such severe change is unusual nowadays with earlier palliative and corrective surgery.

The aetiology and incidence of thrombotic lesions is uncertain. Best & Heath (1958) related the presence of thromboses to a pulmonary blood flow of <2.5 l/min:m^{-2}. They did not find thrombi when the pulmonary blood flow

was normal or increased. By contrast, Newfeld et al (1977) found that, of 73 patients with tetralogy who had a patent systemic pulmonary anastomosis, pulmonary arterial thromboses were present in 70%. In many, thromboses were present when the pulmonary blood flow was sufficient to achieve a systemic arterial oxygen saturation greater than 90%. The presence of thromboses is also related to the degree of polycythaemia (Best & Heath, 1958). The age at which thromboses appear is controversial. Naeye (1963) described thrombi in the newborn lung, and Ferencz (1960a) suggested that they appear as frequently in children as in adults in cases of tetralogy of Fallot. Best & Heath (1958), however, found them more commonly in patients above 10 years of age.

Thromboses in the presence of a low pulmonary blood flow are characterised by a peculiar form of recanalisation in which strands of fibrous tissue of varying thickness divide the arterial lumen into several channels (Rich, 1948; Wagenvoort et al, 1964). A similar appearance is found in the lungs of children with hypertensive obliterative pulmonary vascular disease. Whatever their aetiology, in patients with a typical and favourable clinical picture of tetralogy, pulmonary vascular thromboses do not cause postoperative pulmonary hypertension.

Growth potential of hypoplastic central pulmonary arteries

In patients with pulmonary atresia and ventricular septal defect, and in those with tetralogy who have severe right ventricular outflow tract obstruction, the central pulmonary arteries may be hypoplastic. We recently observed that the central pulmonary arteries were hypoplastic in all cases studied with multiple aortopulmonary collateral arteries. In only 2 of 11 cases, however, would the central vessels have been too small to take a prosthetic shunt (Haworth & Macartney, 1980). It is difficult in life to assess the adequacy of central pulmonary arteries for insertion either of a prosthetic shunt or valve-bearing conduit. One radiological study considered the vessels to be hypoplastic in almost half the cases in relation to the size of the aortic root and vertebral bodies (McGoon et al, 1977). Even when the central pulmonary arteries are severely hypoplastic, the hilar pulmonary arteries are usually sufficiently large to accommodate an aortopulmonary anastomosis.

Growth of small right and left pulmonary arteries is encouraged by increasing the flow of blood through them for some time before performing the definitive repair. Kirklin et al (1977) increased flow either by creation of a systemic-pulmonary anastomosis or by patch enlargement of the right ventricular outflow tract in 4 patients (in 3 of whom the pulmonary valve was atretic). 2–4 years later the vessels were sufficiently large to permit complete repair. Alfieri et al (1978) reported an increase in size of the pulmonary trunk and its right and left branches after a

Waterston anastomosis, the increase in diameter of the pulmonary arteries to that of the aorta being 0.38 and 0.2 respectively. This reflects an increase in size of 50% in the trunk and 30% in the right and left pulmonary arteries. More recently, Lincoln et al (1980) increased pulmonary arterial size in 10 patients by either patch enlargement of the right ventricular outflow tract, insertion of a valved homograft conduit or by infundibulectomy. All had the basic morphology of tetralogy of Fallot and in 3 the pulmonary outflow tract was atretic.

The growth potential of the pulmonary arteries is uncertain. Increased distensibility of a vessel consequent upon an increase in flow must be distinguished from growth. The magnitude of the response and the relatively long time interval between operation and restudy in the cited investigations suggests that growth has indeed occurred. We do not know, however, whether or not these vessels will grow sufficiently to achieve a size commensurate with the size of the lung and that of the child. The abnormal wall structure of the extrapulmonary vessels when pulmonary blood flow is low points to an abnormal growth potential. The elastic fibrils of the media are thin and sparse, or are clumped together in irregular masses, separated by collagen and scanty muscle fibres. Such changes will also change the static and functional mechanical properties of the vessel wall and hence its physical response to an increase in blood flow.

Bronchial arterial circulation

An enlarged bronchial arterial circulation is rarely found in newborn infants with an abnormally low pulmonary blood flow. Infants with pulmonary atresia and intact ventricular septum, for example, die when the arterial duct closes because at that time the bronchial arterial circulation is not sufficiently enlarged. Ferencz (1960b) reported 2 cases of tetralogy of Fallot with enlarged bronchial arteries who died at 17 and 21 days of age. In 5 older patients aged 11 months to 13 years dying with tetralogy of Fallot, Hales & Liebow (1948) using Vinylite corrosion casts demonstrated an increase in bronchial arterial circulation and pre-capillary bronchopulmonary anastomoses. In older patients with pulmonary atresia and a ventricular septal defect, the enlarged bronchial arterial circulation can frequently be demonstrated angiographically as numerous small systemic arteries (Jefferson et al, 1972). Serial cardiac catheterisation studies in such patients frequently show progressive enlargement of the bronchial arterial circulation.

In interruption of a pulmonary artery, the extent to which the bronchial arteries enlarge depends on whether or not the pulmonary artery distal to the interruption is adequately perfused by an arterial duct or by a major aortopulmonary collateral artery.

The frequency with which anastomoses occur between the bronchial and pulmonary arterial circulations explains why accidental surgical interruption of a pulmonary artery (or ligation of a collateral artery providing the only source of blood supply to a region of lung) does not usually lead to infarction of the lung. By contrast, experimental stripping of the bronchial arteries at the hilum leads to perihilar necrosis of the bronchial wall (Ellis et al, 1951).

Summary

In children with a reduction in pulmonary blood flow, the pulmonary arterial circulation and the alveoli may fail to develop normally. This should ideally influence the age at which the abnormality is corrected since the potential for growth decreases with age. The alveoli in the normal lung are formed most rapidly during the first 3 years of life. Subsequent growth is by increase in size rather than number. The ability to produce elastin in the pulmonary circulation decreases with increasing age. The elastin also becomes more stable, suggesting a reduction in the remodelling capacity as haemodynamic conditions change (Farrar et al, 1965). The extent to which the intra-acinar arteries can grow and catch up to achieve a normal size is not known. The thin-walled muscular arteries probably achieve a normal wall thickness since they have the capacity to develop medial hypertrophy in the presence of too large an aortopulmonary shunt.

Growth and remodelling in the normal lung occurs most rapidly during the first 2 years of life. Pulmonary blood flow should ideally be restored to normal during this time.

ACQUIRED HEART DISEASE

Pulmonary hypertension in rheumatic heart disease

In developing countries rheumatic heart disease is a common cause of severe pulmonary hypertension in childhood. In a study of 100 Indian patients with mitral stenosis, 42 patients were less than 20 years of age (Tandon & Kasturi, 1975). The more severe structural changes in the lungs were seen in the younger patients. As in adult patients with mitral stenosis, the structural changes consist chiefly of medial hypertrophy of the pulmonary arteries, the development of muscle in smaller arteries than normal; intimal thickening of peripheral pulmonary arteries and capillaries, thickening of the walls of lymphatics, hypertrophy of the pulmonary veins, and 'arterialisation' of the small veins (Wagenvoort, 1970). Generalised thickening and fibrosis of the alveolar walls is often particularly severe in children with mitral stenosis. The more advanced changes of obliterative pulmonary vascular disease are uncommon.

Following mitral valvotomy, the pulmonary arterial pressure usually falls as judged clinically. Many children, however, suffer repeated attacks of carditis and can develop severe pulmonary vascular disease.

PULMONARY HYPERTENSION OF VARIABLE AETIOLOGY

Effect of altitude on adaptation to extra-uterine life

The weight of the morphologically right ventricle and the muscularity of the pulmonary arterial circulation in babies born at altitude is similar at birth to that found in babies born at sea level (Arias-Stella & Recavarren, 1962). After birth, however, pulmonary arterial muscularity does not decrease at the same rate nor reach the same low level as in infants born at sea level (Arias-Stella & Saldana, 1962; Naeye, 1965). From the age of 1 month, the peripheral pulmonary arteries show medial hypertrophy as compared with normal at sea level. This difference represents an adaptive phenomenon and not disease. There is evidence, however, to suggest that the incidence of 'primary' pulmonary hypertension in childhood is greater at altitude than at sea level (Berthong & Cochran, 1955; Khoury & Hawes, 1963).

Persistent pulmonary hypertension

Excluding children in whom the fetal pattern of blood flow persists due to an anatomical abnormality in the heart, persistence of the fetal circulation implies a primary failure of the pulmonary circulation to adapt normally to extra-uterine life. Pulmonary vascular resistance remains elevated and right-to-left shunting persists across the arterial duct and or the foramen ovale. The heart is anatomically normal. Since its initial description, persistent fetal circulation has been recognised with increasing frequency as a cause of neonatal cyanosis (Gersony et al, 1969; Siassi et al, 1971; Brown & Pickering, 1974).

Persistent fetal circulation is associated with perinatal hypoxia in 80% of cases. It is seen less frequently in term babies following a normal delivery when it is termed 'idiopathic persistence of the fetal circulation' because no 'trigger' factor can be identified (Gersony, 1973). The clinical course is variable. Most infants improve gradually during the 1st week of life, but there may be little or no response to pulmonary vasodilator drugs such as tolazoline. In several series, however, up to one-third of infants have died (Gersony et al, 1969; Brown & Pickering, 1974; Levin et al, 1976). Persistent pulmonary hypertension is occasionally seen in babies born to mothers taking prostaglandin synthetase inhibitors (Manchester et al, 1975). It is postulated that prostaglandin synthetase inhibitors such as aspirin and indomethacin can cause constriction or premature closure of the arterial duct and thus produce severe prenatal pulmonary hypertension. In two

studies of babies born of mothers taking indomethacin, 10 out of a total of 39 babies had persistence of the fetal circulation and 2 died (Csaba et al, 1978; Rubatelli et al, 1979). The offspring of sheep and rats given indomethacin show constriction of the arterial duct together with structural changes in the lungs similar to those in babies with persistent fetal circulation (Levin et al, 1978; Harker et al, 1981).

In young infants who die with idiopathic persistent pulmonary hypertension, the application of quantitative morphometric techniques to the injected and uninjected pulmonary arterial circulation of post-mortem lung specimens shows an increase in peripheral arterial muscularity (Wagenvoort & Wagenvoort, 1970; Haworth & Reid, 1976; McKenzie & Haworth, 1981). Mature smooth muscle cells are present in smaller and more peripheral intra-acinar arteries than normal. Arteries which in the normal lung are non-muscular or only partially muscularised are surrounded by a thick coat of muscle cells. The larger arteries with an external diameter greater than 150 μm generally show an increase in the amount of muscle present but the response is variable, probably due to differences in the duration of pulmonary hypertension. Serial sections of the arterial pathways show progressive encroachment on the lumen by smooth muscle cells and enlarged swollen endothelial cells. In the small pre-capillary arteries the lumen is occluded. Whether or not some of these vessels are occluded from birth (and thus are never recruited into the pulmonary circulation) is not clear. If this does happen, then it probably induces a secondary increase in intra-acinar arterial muscle.

Relation between persistent pulmonary hypertension and 'primary' pulmonary hypertension in children and adults

Wagenvoort & Wagenvoort (1970) described 110 cases of pulmonary hypertension of unknown aetiology which they called 'vasoconstrictive' because of the type of morphological change in the lungs. 39 of the patients were less than 15 years old, the youngest being 4 days. The structural changes were age-related. In infants and young children the small pulmonary arteries showed only medial hypertrophy. With increase in age, the percentage arterial medial thickness decreased as the media atrophied and the percentage intimal thickness increased. Intimal proliferation and lamellar concentric fibrosis, dilation lesions and plexiform lesions appeared in older patients. Because medial hypertrophy was the only early lesion found, a vasoconstrictive mechanism was proposed, the inference being that the pulmonary circulation was affected at or soon after birth. More recent studies on normal adaptation of the pulmonary arterial circulation to extra-uterine life (and on the lungs of babies dying in the first months of life with persistent pulmonary hypertension) supports this hypothesis. We do not know, however, whether vasoconstriction is the first abnormality or is a response to an elevated pulmonary arterial pressure. If the latter, it is perhaps caused by failure of dilation or recruitment of intra-acinar arteries at birth.

If pulmonary hypertension is present from birth, the media of the pulmonary trunk retains the aortic configuration of elastic fibres normally present at birth (Heath et al, 1959). In some adult patients with 'primary' pulmonary hypertension the pulmonary trunk has an aortic configuration. In most it does not, suggesting that pulmonary hypertension is usually not present from birth (Wagenvoort & Wagenvoort, 1977). This does not imply that the pulmonary arterial circulation necessarily adapts to extra-uterine life and grows normally in all patients. The pulmonary vascular reserve is large and the pulmonary arterial pressure may have fallen despite a persistent reduction in capacity of the intra-acinar pulmonary arterial circulation.

Primary pulmonary hypertension in older patients is almost certainly multifactorial, the clinical and structural changes representing the final common pathway. Post-mortem arteriography shows narrowing of the pre-acinar arteries and a loss of background haze. In adults as well as children this appearance can be associated with an increase in muscularity and occlusion of intra-acinar pulmonary arteries without the more advanced changes of concentric lamellar intimal fibrosis and plexiform lesions (Anderson et al, 1973).

In children the sex ratio in primary pulmonary hypertension is equal, while in adults, females predominate. Familial pulmonary hypertension is well described. It is generally a spontaneous occurrence but sometimes can be an autosomal dominant inheritance of a single genetic trait. It may present in childhood (Thompson & McRae, 1970).

Indian children suffer from a particularly vicious form of primary pulmonary hypertension. Children of other nationalities are also affected, but less commonly. The clinical picture is distinctive. The majority of patients present in late adolescence, although they can present as early as 4 years of age. Many patients die within 2 years of diagnosis, a few surviving as long as 10 years. Pulmonary vascular change is described as grade IV–VI, using the Heath & Edwards classification (Heath & Edwards, 1958; Subramanian et al, 1974). In patients from Sri Lanka, the picture may be one of plexogenic pulmonary arteriopathy (Wagenvoort & Wagenvoort, 1977). There is generally no familial incidence and no evidence of collagen disorder, coagulation defect, eosinophila or thromboembolism.

Pulmonary hypertension in lung disease

Chronic lung disease can lead to sustained pulmonary hypertension particularly when associated with hypoxia.

Structural changes develop in the intrapulmonary arteries and the right ventricle hypertrophies. 'Hypertrophy of the right ventricle resulting from diseases affecting the function and/or structure of the lung, except when these pulmonary alterations are the result of diseases that primarily affect the left side of the heart or of congenital heart disease', is how a World Health Organisation Committee (1961) defined cor pulmonale. This definition is unsatisfactory. To the purist, only the pathologist can diagnose right ventricular hypertrophy. Nonetheless, a clinical assessment of right ventricular hypertrophy may be at least as accurate as a pathologist's assessment. Moreover, 'cor pulmonale' to the clinician describes a clinical entity. The term is best avoided.

Chronic lung disease in childhood damages the airways and alveoli during their development and may affect the structural development of the accompanying arteries. Thus, lung disease in childhood may have a longstanding effect on the pulmonary circulation. The commonest causative disease in Europe and the United States is probably cystic fibrosis. Heart failure may also complicate scoliosis in childhood. Extensive small airway and alveolar disease occurring in bronchiolitis, fibrosing alveolitis and the collagen vascular disorders can lead to pulmonary vascular change and hypertension, but this is not common in childhood. Chronic upper airways obstruction due to large tonsils and adenoids is a well recognised cause of pulmonary hypertension and right heart failure in children. In these cases there is rapid improvement following surgery and no evidence of permanent pulmonary vascular damage. Pulmonary hypertension and right heart failure are an important feature of the disease in a minority of patients with cystic fibrosis. Right axis deviation on the electrocardiogram usually indicates an abnormally heavy right ventricle at autopsy, but absence of electrocardiographic changes does not preclude the presence of right ventricular hypertrophy (Ryland & Reid, 1975). These authors studied the hearts and lungs of 36 children aged between 5 years and 12 years who died with cystic fibrosis. Intimal change was patchy, developed in the most severely diseased parts of the lung, and was most common in patients with right ventricular hypertrophy. The most marked pulmonary arterial changes occurred in the most diseased parts of the lungs which were presumably the most hypoxic. All cases showed extension of muscle into smaller arteries than normal and an increase in wall thickness of normally muscularised arteries. These features are common to almost all types of pulmonary hypertension irrespective of aetiology. The differentiation of smooth muscle cells in the non-muscular arteries of the precapillary bed is, however, one of the earliest structural changes seen in experimental hypoxia. The first change to occur in experimental animals exposed to hypoxia is swelling of the endothelial cells which occlude the lumen (Meyrick & Reid, 1980a). The reduction in number of intra-acinar arteries in children with cystic fibrosis is probably due to loss of arteries during acute infective hypoxic episodes. This causes further damage to parts of the lung which are already diseased.

As in cystic fibrosis, in the majority of children with scoliosis the lung is probably normal at birth. With progressive spinal deformity the space available for lung growth diminishes. Repeated respiratory tract infections further compromise lung growth. When scoliosis is severe, signs of pulmonary hypertension and right ventricular hypertrophy frequently develop. Cardiac failure may then supervene. Morphological studies on the lungs of patients dying with scoliosis show a reduction in the number of alveoli. Some alveoli are emphysematous and others atrophied. The changes distributed irregularly throughout the lung according to the distortion of the thoracic cage (Davies & Reid, 1971). The size of the pre-acinar arteries in the pulmonary circulation is appropriate to the volume of the lung. Hence these vessels are small for age. There are many reports of an increase in peripheral arterial muscularity (Bergofsky et al, 1959; Naeye, 1961; Davies & Reid, 1971). The surface area available for gas exchange decreases in scoliosis, thereby causing extensive areas of lung to be poorly ventilated. As in cystic fibrosis, hypoxia probably explains the increased pulmonary arterial muscularity in these patients.

Thromboembolic pulmonary hypertension

Thromboembolic hypertension in children is usually iatrogenic or due to schistosomiasis (see Ch. 56). It is a complication of intravenous hyperalimentation, catheterisation of the umbilical vein in the newborn and of ventriculovenous shunts for hydrocephalus (Emery & Hilton, 1961; Emery, 1962; Noonan & Ehmke, 1963; Firor, 1972). Showers of emboli are discharged from the tip of the catheter and become lodged in elastic or muscular pulmonary arteries. They can gradually occlude a large proportion of the pulmonary vascular bed. Pulmonary hypertension in schistosomiasis is probably caused by embolic obstruction by ova, an allergic response to the ova and vasoconstriction followed by plexogenic pulmonary arteriopathy (Shaw & Ghareeb, 1938). The pulmonary vascular morphology is well reviewed by Wagenvoort & Wagenvoort (1977).

EXPERIMENTAL MODELS

Animal models have been designed to study the effect on pulmonary vascular structure of an increase or decrease in pulmonary blood flow and an increase in pressure. An increase flow has been produced either by creating an aortopulmonary anastomosis or by pneumonectomy in both adult and immature animals (Levy & Blalock, 1939; Rudolph et al, 1961; Dammann et al, 1978; Rendas et al, 1979). The increase in flow and pressure is usually suffi-

cient to produce medial hypertrophy but not to produce severe pulmonary vascular obliterative disease. Creation of an aortopulmonary anastomosis in immature pigs leads to a reduction in intra-acinar arterial size in addition to medial hypertrophy (Rendas et al, 1979). Creating an aortic coarctation in fetal lambs causes arterial medial hypertrophy and a reduction in peripheral arterial size and number (Levin et al, 1978). The pulmonary blood flow can be reduced by banding one pulmonary artery. In the immature pig, pre- and intra-acinar arterial size and muscularity is reduced (Haworth et al, 1981). Animal models are thus useful in studying the effect of haemodynamic abnormalities on lung growth and development. They are less successful in studying the evolution of severe hypertensive pulmonary vascular obliterative disease.

Chronic hypoxia has been used to study the evolution and reversibility of structural change in pulmonary hypertension. The early extension of muscle into smaller and more peripheral arteries than normal (Hislop & Reid, 1976) is explained by the differentiation of muscle cells (Fig. 6.19) from precursor cells (the intermediate cell and pericyte) which are normally present in the partially muscular and non-muscular arteries of the precapillary bed (Meyrick & Reid, 1978, 1979). Hypoxia also produces a reduction in intra-acinar arterial size and number. The pulmonary arterial pressure following recovery from hypoxia returns to normal in adult rats. In the immature animals, however, the pressure remains elevated and there is a persistent reduction in number of intra-acinar arteries. Hypoxia-induced pulmonary hypertension is also associated with an increase in perivascular connective tissue. This does not regress on recovery from hypoxia (Meyrick & Reid, 1980b).

CONCLUSION

The growth and development of the pulmonary circulation may be severely impaired in children with congenital heart disease. This may prejudice or prevent repair of the intracardiac abnormality. Given our present state of knowledge, the pulmonary arterial pressure and flow should be made as normal as possible at the earliest possible age. If necessary this should be done by palliative surgery in order to encourage normal pulmonary vascular development.

The aim of future studies in children with pulmonary hypertension will include first, a greater understanding of the cellular and molecular basis of pulmonary vascular disease. A second aim is the improved understanding of the physical properties of the diseased pulmonary circulation and the relation between structural and functional changes. Thirdly, the potential reversibility of the different ultrastructural abnormalities present and how changes in arterial wall structure relate to the size and number of patent arteries deserve attention. A vasodilator drug acting selectively on the pulmonary arteries is urgently needed to improve the pre- and postoperative management of children with pulmonary hypertension. Lastly, there is a need to study the growth potential of the pulmonary circulation with respect to age, and the structural and functional nature of the pulmonary vascular reserve.

REFERENCES

Alderson P O, Boonvisut S, McKnight R C, Hartmann A F 1976 Pulmonary perfusion abnormalities and ventilation-perfusion imbalance in children after total repair of tetralogy of Fallot. Circulation 53: 332–337

Alfieri O, Blackstone E H, Kirklin J W, Pacifico A D, Bargeron L M 1978 Surgical treatment of tetralogy of Fallot with pulmonary atresia. Journal of Thoracic and Cardiovascular Surgery 76: 321–335

Anderson E G, Simon G, Reid L 1973 Primary and thrombo-embolic pulmonary hypertension. A quantitative pathological study. Journal of Pathology 110: 273–293

Arias-Stella J, Recavarren S 1962 Right ventricular hypertrophy in native children living at high altitude. American Journal of Pathology 41: 55–64

Arias-Stella J, Saldaña M 1962 The muscular pulmonary arteries in people native to high altitude. Medicina Thoracis 19: 484–493

Aziz K U, Paul M H, Rowe R D 1977 Bronchopulmonary circulation in d-transposition of the great arteries: a possible role in the genesis of accelerated pulmonary vascular disease. American Journal of Cardiology 39: 432–438

Bergofsky E H, Turino G M, Fishman A P 1959 Cardiorespiratory failure in kyphoscoliosis. Medicine 38: 263–317

Berry C L, Greenwald S E, Haworth S G 1981. Mechanical properties of the pulmonary vessels in the normal and in congenital heart disease. In: Godman M J (ed) Paediatric cardiology Vol 4. Churchill Livingstone, Edinburgh, p 64–70.

Berthrong M, Cochran T H 1955 Pathological findings in nine children with 'primary' pulmonary hypertension. Bulletin of Johns Hopkins Hospital 97: 69–111

Best P V, Heath D 1958 Pulmonary thrombosis in cyanotic congenital heart disease without pulmonary hypertension. Journal of Pathology and Bacteriology 75: 281–291

Birdwell C R, Gospodarowicz D, Nicholson G L 1978. Identification localization and role of fibronectin in cultured bovine endothelial cells. Proceedings of the National Academy of Science. USA 75: 3273–3277

Bitterman P B, Rennard S I, Hunninghake G W, Crystal R G 1982. Human alveolar macrophage growth factor for fibroblasts. Journal of Clinical Investigation 70: 806–822

Bjarke B 1974 Spirometric data, pulmonary ventilation and gas exchange at rest and during exercise in adult patients with tetralogy of Fallot. Scandinavian Journal of Respiratory Diseases 55: 47–61

Boyden E A 1970 The developing bronchial arteries in a fetus of the twelfth week. American Journal of Anatomy 129: 357–368

Brigham K L, Meyrick B 1984 Granulocyte-dependent injury of pulmonary endothelium: A case of miscommunication? Tissue and Cell 16: 137–155

Brown R, Pickering D 1974 Persistent transitional circulation. Archives of Disease in Childhood 49: 883–885

Bucher U, Reid L 1961 Development of the intrasegmental bronchial tree: the pattern of branching and development of cartilage at the various stages of intra-uterine life. Thorax 16: 207–218

Burstin L 1967 Determination of pressure in the pulmonary artery by external graphic recordings. British Heart Journal 29: 396–404

Butler H 1952 Some derivatives of the foregut venous plexus of the albino rat, with reference to man. Journal of Anatomy (London) 86: 95–109

Chamberlain D, Hislop A, Hey E, Reid L 1977 Pulmonary hypoplasia in babies with severe rhesus isoimmunisation: a quantitative study. Journal of Pathology 122: 43–52

Civin W H, Edwards J E 1951 The postnatal structural changes in the intrapulmonary arteries and arterioles. Archives of Pathology 51: 192–200

Congdon E D 1922 Transformation of the aortic arch system during the development of the human embryo. Contributions to embryology, Carnegie Institute 14: 47–110

Csaba I P, Sulyok E, Ertle T 1978 Relationship of maternal treatment with indomethacin to persistent fetal circulation syndrome. Journal of Pediatrics 92:484

Dammann J F Jr, Ferencz C 1956 The significance of the pulmonary vascular bed in congenital heart disease. I. Normal lungs. II. Malformations of the heart in which there is pulmonary stenosis. American Heart Journal 52: 7–17

Dammann J F Jr, McEachen J A, Thompson W H Jr, Smith R, Muller W H 1961 The regression of pulmonary vascular disease after the creation of pulmonary stenosis. Journal of Thoracic and Cardiovascular Surgery 42: 722–734

Dammann J F Jr, Baker J P, Muller W H Jr 1959 Pulmonary vascular change induced by experimentally produced pulmonary hypertension. Surgery, Gynecology and Obstetrics 105: 16–26

Danilowicz D, Rudolph A M, Hoffman J I E 1965. Vascular resistance in the large pulmonary arteries in infancy. Circulation 32 (Suppl II): 74

Davies G, Reid L 1970 Growth of the alveoli and pulmonary arteries in childhood. Thorax 25: 669–681

Davies G, Reid L 1971 Effect of scoliosis on growth of alveoli and pulmonary arteries and on right ventricle. Archives of Disease in Childhood 46: 623–632

Dunnill M S 1962 Quantitative methods in the study of pulmonary pathology. Thorax 17: 320–328

Edwards J E 1957 Functional pathology of the pulmonary vascular tree in congenital cardiac disease. Circulation 15: 164–196

Ekblom B 1969 Effect of physical training in adolescent boys. Journal of Applied Physiology 27: 350–355

Eldor A, Falcone D J, Hajjar D P, Minick C R, Weksler B B 1981 Recovery of prostacyclin production of deendothelialized rabbit aorta. Critical role of neointimal smooth muscle cells. Journal of Clinical Investigation 67: 735–741

Elliott F M, Reid L 1965 Some new facts about the pulmonary artery and its branching pattern. Clinical Radiology 16: 193–198

Ellis F H, Grindlay J H, Edwards J E 1951 The bronchial arteries. I. Experimental occlusion. Surgery 30: 810–826

Emery J L 1962 Pulmonary embolism in children. Archives of Disease in Childhood 37: 591–595

Emery J L, Hilton H B 1961 Lung and heart complications of the treatment of hydrocephalus by ventriculo-auriculostomy. Surgery 50: 309–314

Fäller K, Haworth S G, Taylor J F N, Macartney F J 1981 Duplicate sources of pulmonary blood supply in pulmonary atresia with ventricular septal defect. British Heart Journal 46: 263–268

Farrar J F, Blomfield J, Reye R D K 1965 The structure and composition of the maturing pulmonary circulation. Journal of Pathology and Bacteriology 90: 83–96

Ferencz C 1960a The pulmonary vascular bed in tetralogy of Fallot. II. Changes following a systemic-pulmonary arterial anastomosis. Bulletin of Johns Hopkins Hospital 106: 100–118

Ferencz C 1960b The pulmonary vascular bed in tetralogy of Fallot. I. Changes associated with pulmonic stenosis. Bulletin of Johns Hopkins Hospital 106: 81–99

Firor H V 1972 Pulmonary embolization complicating total intravenous alimentation. Journal of Pediatric Surgery 7:81

Flick M R, Perel A, Staub N C 1981 Leukocytes are required for increased lung microvascular permeability after micro-embolization in sheep. Circulation Research 58: 344–351

Friedli B, Kidd B S L, Mustard W T, Keith J D 1974 Ventricular septal defect with increased pulmonary vascular resistance. Late results of surgical closure. American Journal of Cardiology 33: 403–409

Fry D L 1968 Aortic vascular endothelial changes associated with increased blood velocity gradients. Circulation Research 22: 165–197

Fulton R M, Hutchinson E C, Jones A M 1952 Ventricular weight in cardiac hypertrophy. British Heart Journal 14: 413–420

Furchgott R F, Zawadzki J V 1980 The obligatory role of endothelial cells in the relaxation of arterial smooth muscle by acetycholine. Nature 288: 373–376

Gajdusek C, Dicorleto P, Ross R, Schwartz S M 1980 An endothelial cell-derived growth factor. Journal of Cell Biology 85: 467–472

Gersony W M 1973 Persistence of the fetal circulation. A commentary. Journal of Pediatrics 82: 1103–1106

Gersony W M, Duc G V, Sinclair J C 1969 'PFC' syndrome (persistence of the fetal circulation) (Abstract). Circulation 40 (Suppl III):87

Gil J, Weibel E R 1969 Improvements in demonstration of lining layer of lung alveoli by electron microscopy. Respiration Physiology 8: 13–36

Greenwald S E, Berry C L, Haworth 1982 Changes in the distensibility of the intrapulmonary arteries in the normal newborn and growing pig. Cardiovascular Research 16: 716–725

Grover R F, Vogel J H K, Averill K H, Blount S G 1963 Pulmonary hypertension. Individual and species variation relative to vascular reactivity. American Heart Journal 66: 1–3

Hales M R, Liebow A A 1948 Collateral circulation to the lungs in congenital pulmonic stenosis. Bulletin of the International Association of Medical Museums 28: 1–22

Hallidie-Smith K A, Hollman A, Cleland W P, Bentall H H, Goodwin J F 1969 Effects of surgical closure of ventricular septal defects upon pulmonary vascular disease. British Heart Journal 31: 246–260

Hammerschmidt D E, Stroncek D F, Bowers T K, et al 1981 Complement activation and neutropenia occurring during cardiopulmonary bypass. Journal of Thoracic and Cardiovascular Surgery 81: 370–377

Harker L C, Kirkpatrick S E, Friedman W F, Bloor C M 1981 Effects of indomethacin on fetal rat lungs; a possible cause of persistent fetal circulation (PFC). Pediatric Research 15: 147–151

Harrison C V 1958 The pathology of the pulmonary vessels in pulmonary hypertension. British Journal of Radiology 31: 217–226

Hätle L, Angelsen B A J, Tromsdal A 1981 Non-invasive estimation of pulmonary artery systolic pressure with Doppler ultrasound. British Heart Journal 45: 157–165

Haworth S G 1980 Collateral arteries in pulmonary atresia with ventricular septal defect. A precarious blood supply. British Heart Journal 44: 5–13

Haworth S G 1982 Total anomalous pulmonary venous return. Prenatal damage to pulmonary vascular bed and extrapulmonary veins. British Heart Journal 48: 513–524

Haworth S G 1983 Pulmonary vascular disease in secundum atrial septal defect in childhood. American Journal of Cardiology 51: 265–272

Haworth S G 1984 Pulmonary vascular disease in different types of congenital heart disease: implications for interpretation of lung biopsy findings in early childhood. British Heart Journal 52: 557–571

Haworth S G, Hislop A 1981 Adaptation of the pulmonary circulation to extrauterine life in the pig and its relevance to the human infant. Cardiovascular Research 15: 108–119

Haworth S G, Hislop A A 1983 Pulmonary vascular development: Normal values of peripheral vascular structure. American Journal of Cardiology 52: 578–583

Haworth S G, Macartney F J 1980 Growth and development of pulmonary circulation in pulmonary atresia with ventricular septal defect and major aortopulmonary collateral arteries. British Heart Journal 44: 14–24

Haworth S G, Reid L 1976 Persistent fetal circulation: newly recognised structural features. Journal of Pediatrics 88: 614–620

Haworth S G, Reid L 1977a A quantitative structural study of the pulmonary circulation in the newborn with aortic atresia, stenosis or coarctation. Thorax 32: 121–128

Haworth S G, Reid L 1977b Quantitative structural study of the pulmonary circulation in the newborn with pulmonary atresia. Thorax 32: 129–133

Haworth S G, Reid L 1977c Structural study of pulmonary circulation and of heart in total anomalous pulmonary venous return in early infancy. British Heart Journal 39: 80–92

Haworth S G, Reid L 1978 A morphometric study of regional variation in lung structure in infants with pulmonary hypertension and congenital cardiac defect: a justification of lung biopsy. British Heart Journal 40: 825–831

Haworth S G, Sauer U, Bühlmeyer K, Reid L 1977 Development of

the pulmonary circulation in ventricular septal defect: a quantitative structural study. American Journal of Cardiology 40: 781–788

Haworth S G, Sauer U, Bühlmeyer K 1980 The effect of prostaglandin E₁ on the pulmonary circulation in pulmonary atresia: a quantitative morphometric study. British Heart Journal 43: 306–314

Haworth S G, de Leval M, Macartney F J 1981 Hypoperfusion and hyperperfusion in the immature lung. Pulmonary arterial development after ligation of left pulmonary artery in newborn newborn pig. Journal of Thoracic and Cardiovascular Surgery 82: 281–292

Haworth S G, McKenzie S A, Fitzpatrick M L 1981 Alveolar development following ligation of left pulmonary arter in newborn pig: clinical relevance to unilateral pulmonary artery. Thorax 36: 938–943

Hayward J, Reid L 1952 Observations on the anatomy of the intrasegmental bronchial tree. Thorax 7: 89–97

Heath D, Best P V 1958 The tunica media of the arteries in pulmonary hypertension. Journal of Pathology and Bacteriology 76: 165–174

Heath D, Edwards J E 1958 The pathology of hypertensive pulmonary vascular disease. A description of six grades of structural changes in the pulmonary artery with special reference to congenital cardiac septal defect. Circulation 18: 533–547

Heath D, Wood E H, DuShane J W, Edwards J E 1959 The structure of the pulmonary trunk at different ages and in cases of pulmonary hypertension and pulmonary stenosis. Journal of Pathology and Bacteriology 77: 443–456

Hessel E A, Boyden E A, Stamm S J, Sauvage L R 1970 High systemic origin of the sole artery to the basal segments of the left lung: findings, surgical treatment and embryologic interpretation. Surgery 67: 624–632

Hirschfeld S, Meyer R, Schwartz D C, Korfhagen J, Kaplan S 1975 The echocardiographic assessment of pulmonary artery pressure and pulmonary vascular resistance. Circulation 52: 642–650

Hislop A, Reid L 1972 Intrapulmonary arterial development during fetal life – branching pattern and structure. Journal of Anatomy 113: 35–48

Hislop A, Reid L 1973a Fetal and childhood development of the intrapulmonary veins in man-branching pattern and structure. Thorax 28: 313–319

Hislop A, Reid L 1973b Pulmonary arterial development during childhood – branching pattern and structure. Thorax 28: 129–135

Hislop A, Reid L 1973c Structural changes in the pulmonary arteries and veins in tetralogy of Fallot. British Heart Journal 35: 1178–1183

Hislop A, Reid L 1976 New findings in pulmonary arteries of rats with hypoxia-induced pulmonary hypertension. British Journal of Experimental Pathology 57: 542–554

Hislop A, Haworth S G, Shinebourne E A, Reid L 1975 Structural changes in the pulmonary circulation in isolated ventricular septal defect in infancy. British Heart Journal 37: 1014–1021

Hislop A, Hey E, Reid L 1979 The lungs in congenital bilateral renal agenesis and dysplasia. Archives of Disease in Childhood 54: 32–38

Hruban Z, Humphreys E M 1960 Congenital anomalies associated with pulmonary hypertension in an infant. Archives of Pathology 70:766

Jefferson K, Rees S, Somerville J 1972 Systemic arterial supply to the lungs in pulmonary atresia and its relation to pulmonary artery development. British Heart Journal 34: 418–427

Johnson R J, Haworth S G 1982 Pulmonary vascular and alveolar development in tetralogy of Fallot: a recommendation for early correction. Thorax 37: 893–901

Jones O D H, Shore D F, Rigby M L, et al 1981 The use of tolazoline hydrochloride as a pulmonary vasodilator in potentially fatal episodes of pulmonary vasoconstriction after cardiac surgery in children. Circulation 64(Suppl III): 134–139

Kanjuh V I, Sellers R D, Edwards J E 1964 Pulmonary vascular plexiform lesion Archives of Pathology 78:513

Khoury G H, Hawes C R 1963 Primary pulmonary hypertension in children living at high altitude. Journal of Pediatrics 62: 177–185

Kirklin J W, Bargeron L M, Pacifico A D 1977 The enlargement of small pulmonary arteries by preliminary palliative operations. Circulation 56: 612–617

Kirklin J K, Westaby S, Blackstone E H, Kirklin J W, Chenoweth D E, Pacifico A D 1983. Complement and the damaging effects of cardiopulmonary bypass. Journal of Thoracic and Cardiovascular Surgery 86: 845–857

Kitagawa M, Hislop A, Boyden E A, Reid L 1971 Lung hypoplasia in congenital diaphragmatic hernia. A quantitative study of airway, artery and alveolar development. British Journal of Surgery 58: 342–346

Könn G, Storb R 1960 Über den Formandel der kleinen Lungenarterien des Menschen nach der Geburt. Beitraege zur Pathologie und Anatomie 123:212

Levin D L, Heymann M A, Kitterman J A, Gregory G A, Phibbs R H, Rudolph A M 1976 Persistent pulmonary hypertension. Journal of Pediatrics 89: 626–630

Levin D L, Fixler D E, Moriss F C, Tyson J 1978 Morphologic analysis of the pulmonary vascular bed in infants exposed in utero to prostaglandin synthetase inhibitors. Journal of Pediatrics 92: 478–483

Levy S E, Blalock A 1939 Experimental observations on connecting by suture the left main pulmonary artery to the systemic circulation. Journal of Thoracic Surgery 8:525

Liebow A A 1965 Patterns of origin and distribution of the major bronchial arteries in man. American Journal of Anatomy 117: 19–32

Liebow A A, Hales M R, Lindskog G E, Bloomer W E 1947 Plastic demonstrations of pulmonary pathology. Journal of Technical Methods 27: 116–129

Liebow A A, Hales M R, Bloomer W E, Harrison W, Lindskog G E 1950 Studies on the lung after ligation of the pulmonary artery. II Anatomical change. American Journal of Pathology 26: 177–195

Lincoln C, Shinebourne E, Treasure T, Leijala M, Lane I 1980 Direct surgical management of right ventricular outflow tract obstruction in children with diminitive pulmonary arteries. In: Stone S (ed) World Congress of Paediatric Cardiology Abstracts. Ciba-Geigy, Sussex, p. 42

Lompre A M, Mercadier J J, Wisnewsky C, et al 1981 Species and age-dependant changes in the relative amounts of cardiac myosin isoenzymes in mammals. Developmental Biology 84: 286–290

Macartney F J, Scott O, Deverall P B 1974 Haemodynamic and anatomical characteristics of pulmonary blood supply in pulmonary atresia with ventricular septal defect – including a case of persistent fifth arch. British Heart Journal 36: 1049–1060

Macartney F J, Taylor J F N, Graham G R, de Leval M, Stark J 1980 The fate of survivors of cardiac surgery in infancy. Circulation 62: 80–91

McGoon M D, Fulton R E, Davis G D, Ritter D G, Neill C A, White R J Jr 1977 Systemic collateral and pulmonary artery stenosis in patients with congenital pulmonary valve atresia and ventricular septal defect. Circulation 56: 473–479

McKenzie S, Haworth S G 1981 Occlusion of peripheral pulmonary vascular bed in a baby with idiopathic persistent fetal circulation. British Heart Journal 46: 675–678

Manchester D, Margolis H S, Sheldon R E 1975 Possible association between maternal indomethacin therapy and primary pulmonary hypertension of the newborn. American Journal of Obstetrics and Gynecology 126: 467–469

Marchand P, Gilroy J C, Wilson V H 1950 An anatomical study of the bronchial vascular system and its variation in disease. Thorax 5: 207–221

Maseri A, Caldini P, Harward P, Joshi R C, Permutt S, Zierler K L 1972 Determinants of pulmonary vascular volume. Recruitment versus distensibility. Circulation Research 31: 218–228

Mecham R P, Madaras J, Bogar L, McDonald J A, Ryan U S 1983 Elastin production by cultured calf pulmonary artery endothelial cells. Journal of Cellular Physiology 116: 282–288

Meyrick B, Reid L 1978 The effect of continued hypoxia on rat pulmonary arterial circulation. Laboratory Investigation 38: 188–200

Meyrick B, Reid L 1979 Ultrastructural features of the distended pulmonary arteries of the normal rat. Anatomical Record 193: 71–98

Meyrick B, Reid L 1980a Endothelial and subintimal changes in rat hilar pulmonary artery during recovery from hypoxia. A quantitative ultrastructural study. Laboratory Investigation 42: 603–615

Meyrick B, Reid L 1980b Hypoxia-induced structural changes in the media and adventitia of the rat hilar pulmonary artery and their regression. American Journal of Pathology 100: 151–169

Miller W S 1947 The lung. Thomas Springfield, Illinois

Naeye R L 1961a Arterial changes during the perinatal period. Archives of Pathology 71: 121–128

Naeye R L 1961b Perinatal changes in the pulmonary vascular bed with stenosis and atresia of the pulmonic valve. American Heart Journal 61: 586–592

Naeye R L 1962 Perinatal vascular changes associated with underdevelopment of the left heart. American Journal of Pathology 41: 287–293

Naeye R L 1963 Arteriosclerosis in congenital heart disease. Archives of Pathology 75: 162–170

Naeye R L 1965 Children at high altitude: pulmonary and renal abnormalities. Circulation Research 16: 33–38

Newfeld E A, Paul M H, Muster A J, Idriss F S 1974 Pulmonary vascular disease and complete transposition of the great arteries. A study of 200 patients. American Journal of Cardiology 34: 75–82

Newfeld E A, Waldman J D, Paul M H, et al 1977 Pulmonary vascular disease after systemic–pulmonary arterial shunt operation. American Journal of Cardiology 39: 715–726

Noonan J A, Ehmke D A 1963 Complications of ventriculovenous shunts for control of hydrocephalus. New England Journal of Medicine 269: 70–77

Norwood W I, Lang P, Hansen D 1983 Physiologic repair of aortic atresia – hypoplastic left heart. New England Journal of Medicine 308: 23–26

Parmentier R 1962 L'aeration neonatale du poumon. Contribution experimentale et anatomo-clinique. Revue Belge de Pathologie 29: 123–244

Rabinovitch M, Haworth S G, Castaneda A R, Nadas A S, Reid L M 1978a Lung biopsy in congenital heart disease: a morphometric approach to pulmonary vascular disease. Circulation 58: 1107–1122

Rabinovitch M, Keane J F, Murray K, et al 1978b Quantitative pulmonary wedge angiography (QPWA) in assessing pulmonary vascular disease (PVD) in congenital heart defects (CHD). Circulation 58: 11–68

Rabinovitch M, Castaneda A R, Reid L 1981 Lung biopsy with frozen section as a diagnostic aid in patients with congenital heart defects. American Journal of Cardiology 47: 77–84

Rabinovitch M, Keane J F, Norwood W I, Castaneda A R, Reid L 1984 Vascular structure in lung tissue obtained at biopsy correlated with pulmonary hemodynamic findings after repair of congenital heart defects. Circulation 69: 655–667

Rao P S, Ellison R G 1978 The cause of kinking of the right pulmonary artery in the Waterston anastomosis. Journal of Thoracic and Cardiovascular Surgery 76: 126–129

Ratliff N B, Young W G Jr, Hackel D B, Mikat E, Wilson J W 1973 Pulmonary injury secondary to extracorporeal circulation. Journal of Thoracic and Cardiovascular Surgery 65: 425–432

Recavarren S, Arias-Stella J 1964 Growth and development of the ventricular myocardium from birth to adult life. British Heart Journal 26: 187–192

Reid L 1968 Structural and functional reappraisal of the pulmonary artery system. In: The scientific basis of medicine annual reviews. The Athlone Press, London, p. 289–307

Rendas A, Lennox S, Reid L 1979 Aorta-pulmonary shunts in growing pigs. Journal of Thoracic and Cardiovascular Surgery 77: 109–118

Rich A R 1948 A hitherto unrecognized tendency to the development of widespread pulmonary vascular obstruction in patients with congenital pulmonic stenosis (tetralogy of Fallot) Bulletin of Johns Hopkins Hospital 82:389

Ross R, Glomset J, Kariya B, Harker L 1974 A platelet-dependent serum factor that stimulates the proliferation of arterial smooth muscle cells in vitro. Proceedings of National Academy of Science, USA 71: 1207–1210

Ross R, Faggiotto A, Bowen-Pope D, Raines E 1984 The role of endothelial injury and platelet and macrophage interactions in atherosclerosis. Circulation 70 (Suppl III): 77–82

Rowe R D 1963 Maternal rubella and pulmonary artery stenosis. Report of eleven cases. Pediatrics 32: 180–185

Rubatelli F F, Chiazza M L, Zanardon V, Cantarutti F 1979 Effect on neonate of maternal treatment with indomethacin (letter). Journal of Pediatrics 94:161

Rudolph A M 1974 Congenital diseases of the heart. Year Book Medical Publishers, Chicago, p 10

Rudolph A M, Neuhauser E D B, Golinko R J, Auld P A M 1961 Effects of pneumonectomy on pulmonary circulation in adult and young animals. Circulation Research 9: 856–861

Rudolph A M, Heymann M A, Lewis A B 1977 Fetal and neonatal pulmonary circulation. In: Hudson W A (ed) Development of the lung. Marcel Dekker, New York, p. 503–505

Ryan U S, Ryan J W 1984 Cell biology of pulmonary endothelium. Circulation 70 (Suppl III): 46–62

Ryland D, Reid L 1975 The pulmonary circulation in cystic fibrosis. Thorax 30: 285–292

Sage H, Crouch E, Bornstein P 1979 Collagen synthesis by bovine aortic endothelial cells in culture. Biochemistry 18: 5433–5441

Shaw A F B, Ghareeb A A 1938 The pathogenesis of pulmonary schistosomiasis in Egypt with special reference to Ayerza's disease. Journal of Pathology and Bacteriology 46: 401–424

Siassi B, Goldberg S J, Emmanouilides G C, Higoshino S M, Lewis E 1971 Persistent pulmonary vascular obstruction in newborn infants. Journal of Pediatrics 78: 610–615

Silverman N H, Snider A R, Rudolph A M 1980 Evaluation of pulmonary hypertension by M-mode echocardiography in children with ventricular septal defect. Circulation 61: 1125–1132

Simon G, Reid L, Tanner J M, Goldstein H, Benjamin B 1972 Growth of radiologically determined heart diameter, lung width, and lung length from 5–19 years, with standards for clinical use. Archives of Disease in Childhood 47: 373–381

Sotomora R F, Edwards J E 1978 Anatomic identification of so-called absent pulmonary artery. Circulation 57: 624–633

Subramanian N, Bakthaviziam A, Sukamar I P, Krishnaswami S, Cherian G 1974 Primary pulmonary hypertension. A clinocopathological study of 11 cases. Indian Heart Journal 26: 171–178

Tandon H D, Kasturi J 1975 Pulmonary vascular changes associated with isolated mitral stenosis in India. British Heart Journal 37: 26–36

Thompson, McRae 1970 Familial pulmonary hypertension. Evidence of autosomal dominant inheritance. British Heart Journal 32: 758–760

Tobin C E 1952 The bronchial arteries and their connections with other vessels in the human lung. Surgery, Gynecology and Obstetrics 95:741

Virchow R L K 1854 'Zur Geschichte der Lehre von der Arterienverstopfung'. Archiv für pathologische Anatomie und Physiologie und für klinishe Medicin 6: 583–584

Wagenvoort C A 1960 Vasoconstriction and medial hypertrophy in pulmonary hypertension. Circulation 22: 535–546

Wagenvoort C A 1970 Morphologic changes in intrapulmonary veins. Human Pathology 1: 205–213

Wagenvoort C A 1973 Hypertensive pulmonary vascular disease complicating congenital heart disease: A review. Cardiovascular Clinics 5: 43–60

Wagenvoort C A 1974 Classification of pulmonary vascular lesions in congenital and acquired heart disease. Advances in Cardiology 11: 48–55

Wagenvoort C A, Wagenvoort N 1967 Arterial anastomoses, bronchopulmonary arteries and pulmobronchial arteries in perinatal lungs. Laboratory Investigation 16: 13–24

Wagenvoort C A, Wagenvoort N 1970 Primary pulmonary hypertension: a pathologic study of the lung vessels in 156 clinically diagnosed cases. Circulation 42: 1163–1184

Wagenvoort C A, Wagenvoort N 1974 Pathology of the Eisenmenger syndrome and primary pulmonary hypertension. Advances in Cardiology 11: 123–130

Wagenvoort C A, Wagenvoort N 1977 Pathology of pulmonary hypertension. Wiley, New York p. 48

Wagenvoort C A, Heath D, Edwards J E 1964 The pathology of the pulmonary vasculature. Thomas. Springfield, Illinois

Wagenvoort C A, Wagenvoort N, Becker A E 1972 The effect of obstructed venous blood flow on the development of alternative pathways in the lung. Journal of Pathology 107: 21–25

Wasserman M P, Varghese P J, Rowe R D 1968 The evolution of pulmonary arterial stenosis associated with congenital rubella. American Heart Journal 76: 638–644

Wells L J, Boyden E A 1954 The development of the bronchopulmonary segments in human embryos of Horizon XVII to XIX. American Journal of Anatomy 95: 163–201

World Health Organisation 1961 Chronic cor pulmonale. Technical Report Series No. 212, WHO, Geneva, p. 6

Zuckerkandl E 1883 'Uber die Verbindungen Zwischen den Arteriellen Gefässen der Menschlichen Lunge'. Sitzungsberichte der Kaiserlichen Akademie der Wissenschafte A. Mathematisch-Naturwissenschaftliche Classe, Wein 87: 171–186

Ventricular function

Ventricular function is more complex to study in patients with congenital than acquired heart disease. The reason for this is obvious. There may be developmental abnormalities of the ventricles themselves, leading to structural distortion and mutual interaction. The range of variation in volume and pressure loading is large, and present at a period of life when growth is rapid and when fundamental adaptations to the circulation occur. The functions of the ventricles themselves may be reversed. Chronic arterial hypoxia can be more severe and prolonged than in patients with acquired heart disease and there may be primary metabolic abnormalities of the myocardium itself. Superimposed on this complex base are the effects of growth, homeostasis, fibrosis and other degenerative processes, as well as the results of palliative or definitive surgery (Somerville, 1979). The relatively narrow range of ideas derived from acquired disturbances of ventricular function forms a restricted basis for the discussion of those seen in congenital heart disease, and a wider view will be needed. Ideally, a return should be made to basic principles, but it is by no means clear what these 'basic principles' should be. The approach used here will therefore be descriptive, recognising that many different types of ventricular disease may exist, which can be present singly or in combination in any given patient. As the heart disease evolves, so different facets may become more or less significant at different times. Finally, the properties of the two circulations must be considered. These can profoundly affect the way in which blood flows through them and thus the function of the ventricles themselves. The present discussion will therefore review different approaches to the study of the functions of the ventricles, with emphasis more on the nature of the measurements made than in enumerating abnormalities in single diseases. An attempt will be made to combine these different entities into a coherent picture based on the belief that fundamentally left ventricular disease has a physical basis, so that it is worthwhile defining its components unambiguously in physical terms.

NORMAL MYOCARDIAL ANATOMY

Myocardial fibre architecture in the normal ventricle is complex and highly organised (Streeter & Hanna 1973a, b; Greenbaum et al, 1981). Fibre orientation on the epicardial aspect can be examined by simple inspection and is strikingly non-uniform. It is longitudinal over the acute margin of the heart and oblique on the anterior surface between the vortex and the anterior interventricular groove. The fibres of the diaphragmatic and obtuse marginal surfaces are more circumferentially arranged. Microscopic examination combined with detailed morphometric analysis of fibre angle shows them to be continuous with the deeper circumferential layer. The superficial fibres at the vortices are directly continuous with the subendocardial fibres (and thus with the trabeculations and papillary muscles) which run longitudinally

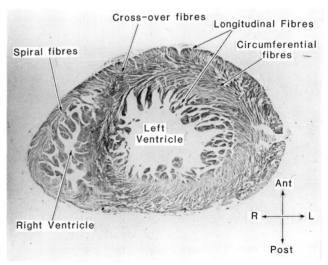

Fig. 7.1 Normal ventricular fibre architecture in man. Tranverse section of normal ventricular mass showing circumferential fibres in the mid-portion of the left ventricular wall, with longitudinally directed subendocardial and subepicardial fibres. The right ventricular wall is formed of spirally arranged fibres, with cross-over fibres in the region of the anterior interventricular sulcus. (Reproduced from Greenbaum et al, 1981, by permission of the Editor of the *British Heart Journal*.)

upwards from the apex, becoming more circumferential as they approach the base (Fig. 7.1). Between these two, a thick circumferential layer of myocardium encircles both inlet and outlet portions of the left ventricle. The bulk of the septum consists of circumferential fibres but it also contains subendocardial components from the right and left ventricles. The circumferential layer is less well developed in the right ventricle. The infundibulum is formed of longitudinally directed superficial fibres, which interdigitate with 'cross-over' fibres from the left ventricle.

There is surprisingly little information available about abnormalities of ventricular structure occurring in patients with congenital heart disease. In general, muscle fibre structure adjusts itself to the functional anomaly. For example, the normal region of fibre crossover between the two outflow tracts is absent when there is a common arterial trunk. The degree of dominance of one or other ventricle is a major factor with respect to the final arrangement of fibres (Fig. 7.2). When right ventricular hypertrophy develops, the amount of muscle of right ventricular origin encircling the apex of the left ventricle is increased and modulates the normal pattern of fibre orientation in this region. It may also be associated with a change in the geometry of the interventricular septum (Becker & Caruso, 1981).

The functional significance of this complex arrangement has been little explored, although it is likely to shed light on the nature of the relationship between 'pump' and 'muscle' aspects of left ventricular performance. Significant implications can be identified. Normal sarcomeres shorten by approximately 10% in normal beats and up to 15% in postectopic beats (Sonnenblick et al, 1967). The normal reduction in the minor axis of the left ventricle is

25–40% under resting conditions and may be very much greater when the resistance to ejection is reduced. It can reach 80% or more in patients with complete transposition after a Mustard operation when the left ventricle ejects into a normal pulmonary circulation. Changes in minor axis are thus much greater than those of normal sarcomere shortening. This discrepancy can be explained from the observation that minor axis shortening is due as much to wall thickening as to inward movement of epicardium. The extent of this thickening is too great to be explained on the basis of shortening of circumferentially arranged fibres. It is necessary to invoke the effects of shortening and hence fattening of longitudinally directed ones (Dumesnil et al, 1979). If a spherical ventricle is constructed of normal myocardium arranged circumferentially, and normal sarcomere shortening is allowed to take place, then the resulting ejection fraction is only of the order of 30–33%. A normal ejection fraction can be achieved only when the cavity shape departs from spherical and fibres are arranged obliquely around it. These relationships have been studied in detail by Sallin (1969).

CAVITY SIZE AND SHAPE

A number of methods are available to study cavity size and shape. Historically, most information is available from angiography. More recently M-mode and cross-sectional echocardiography and radionuclide angiography have been used. Methods for deriving ventircular volume from angiograms have been reviwed in detail (Sandler & Alderman, 1974). The left ventricle has usually been assumed to be an ellipsoid of revolution and the area-length method used to calculate major and minor axes. If biplane angiograms are available, then two separate minor axes can be calculated. The method has been calibrated against a series of casts and regression equations which are used to correct observed values (Dodge et al, 1966). Angiography was used to measure left ventricular volume in a series of patients aged from one day to 16 years by Graham et al (1968, 1971). They demonstrated that a separate regression equation was required for end-diastolic volume in patients less than two years old, while end-systolic volume behaved uniformly throughout the age-range studied. Right ventricular volume can be measured in a similar way. Its shape departs even more significantly from that of the left from any simple ellipsoid so a number of alternative approaches have also been used. They include one based on Simpson's rule and a two chamber model in which the outflow tract is considered separately (Graham et al, 1973). Somewhat surprisingly, all three methods gave similar values. Correlation with ventricular casts shows no significant difference between them. Measurement of right ventricular cavity volume presents a number of difficulties not apparent for that of the left. Its shape is irregular and its trabeculation

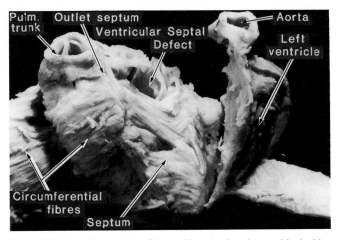

Fig. 7.2 Abnormal ventricular fibre architecture in a heart with double outlet right ventricle. The aorta, which overrode the ventricular septal defect, has been reflected laterally with the left ventricle to show the outlet septum between subaortic and subpulmonary outflow tracts. Note the circumferential fibres round the right ventricle and note also that the ventricular septum is of right ventricular origin. (Reproduced with permission from Becker & Caruso, 1981).

heavy (causing an irregular cavity outline). The normal interventricular septum bulges into the left ventricle in a manner that cannot easily be detected on standard orthogonal views. Together, these factors lead to overestimation of cavity volume. More complex methods of reconstruction of ventricular shape can be used based on three-dimensional reconstruction from biplane angiograms (Heintzen et al, 1974). These do not depend on assuming any idealised geometry and are capable of demonstrating distorted and abnormal cavity shape. In addition, volume estimates derived from them appear appreciably more accurate than those based on a simple ellipsoid.

Angiographic determinations have their limitations although they are still used as the standard of comparison against which other methods are judged. Of these, the major one is lack of certainty of the relation between the position of endocardium and that of the outer border of opacified dye, particularly at end-systole and early diastole. At these times in the cardiac cycle, metal markers on the endocardium in experimental animals may become widely separated from the outer border of the cavity as outlined by contrast (Mitchell et al, 1969). Wall thickness is overestimated and end-systolic volume is probably too low, causing an apparent increase in ventricular mass during systole. In addition, the outline of the cavity is frequently invaginated and complex, bearing no clear relation to any simple geometrical figure. It may also be difficult to reconstruct the ventricle when the cavity is not ellipsoidal unless more complex methods are used. In particular, the direction of curvature is frequently reversed along the inferior wall as seen in the right anterior oblique projection (Grant, 1953; Greenbaum & Gibson, 1981) and around the insertion of the papillary muscles. The advantages of angiography should also be recapitulated in the light of the development of newer imaging techniques. In contrast with echocardiography, the physical basis of image generation by angiography is well understood. Its resolution is unrivalled by any other available method. By demonstrating a profile, the problem of oblique cuts across the ventricle does not arise although the axis may be foreshortened with respect to the X-ray beam. A clear boundary is demonstrated at a rate of at least 50 frames per second, a rate that can be doubled if this is thought to be desirable. The method can easily be quantified by the simple manoeuvre of exposing a grid at mid-chest level. It does not require to be gated as do magnetic resonance imaging or computerised tomography. Although it is invasive, angiograms are widely performed for diagnostic purposes and are thus available for physiological studies. Finally, the development of digital techniques for image storage greatly increases the versatility of the method, allowing manipulations to be performed automatically rather than by time-consuming manual methods.

A number of the difficulties associated with angiography can be circumvented by using echocardiography. M-mode echocardiography can be used to measure the transverse dimension of the left ventricle at the level of the aortic leaflet of the mitral valve, and correlation with angiography has been reported. Particular advantages of the method include its rapid repetition rate (1000/s), and its ability to display the position of endocardium throughout the cardiac cycle. For these reasons, discrepancies in comparison with angiography are as likely to be due to the limitations described above as to any inadequacy of echocardiography. The method can also be used in truly normal subjects. Measurements should be made following the recommendations of the American Society of Echocardiography (Sahn et al, 1978) or the European Society of Cardiology (Roelandt & Gibson, 1980). Its main disadvantage is that a single ventricular dimension is measured rather than a ventricular volume. The dimension can be used to give a good impression of cavity size of the left ventricle (and even a semi-quantitative estimate of volume) provided that cavity size is normal (Kaye et al, 1975). Precise quantification of left ventricular volume from M-mode echocardiography is not possible and such calculations should now be regarded as obsolete. Right ventricular dimension as measured by standard parasternal M-mode echocardiography passes through the lower portion of the outflow tract and thus gives little useful information about volume. When right ventricular dimension is measured from the subcostal approach, however, a very much more satisfactory idea of cavity size can be gained (Saito et al, 1981).

As cross-sectional echocardiography has become more generally available, so its use in measuring cavity size has been explored. Two general methods have been used, either a combination of a single apical four-chamber view with two or more parasternal minor axis views or two orthogonal views (Silverman et al, 1980; Mercier et al, 1982). These allow three-dimensional reconstruction of the left ventricle to be undertaken (Fig. 7.3). Endocardium is outlined in end-diastolic and end-systolic views with a light pen and volume thus calculated. Similar results for the right ventricle have also been reported (Yagihara et al, 1981). Cross-sectional echocardiography appears to be a good predictor of angiographic ventricular volume, although estimates have been consistently lower. The technique has a number of problems. The apparent apex of the heart determined by palpation is not the anatomical one but represents a point approximately one-third of the way up the free wall of the left ventricle. For the greater part of the cavity outline, endocardium is approximately parallel rather than perpendicular to the ultrasound beam and is thus not well demonstrated. An injection of contrast medium shows the apparent position of left ventricular endocardium to be outside the outer border of the cavity accessible to the bubbles. This poor definition of endocardium may also be associated with areas of drop-out where endocardium is not demonstrated at all. A considerable

END-DIASTOLIC FRAMES

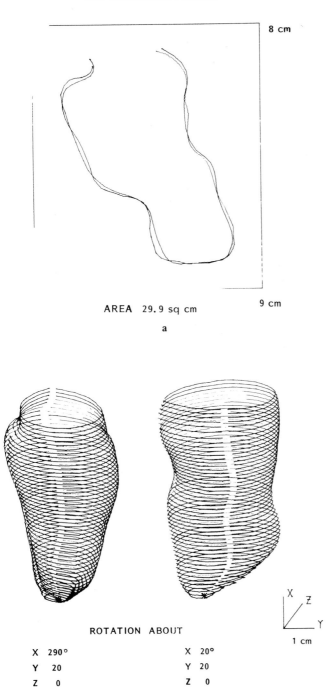

AREA 29.9 sq cm

Fig. 7.3 (a) Digitised outline of left ventricular cavity in a patient with left ventricular hypertrophy derived from the apical four-chamber view. Two outlines are superimposed to assess reproducibility. (b) Three-dimensional reconstruction at end-diastole of left ventricular cavity from apical four- and two-chamber views from the patient shown in (a). The three-dimensional orientation of the structure is indicated in terms of x, y, and z coordinates. The discontinuities in the rings of the reconstruction represent the orientations of the outlines from which it is derived. In the left hand reconstruction, the apical two-chamber outline is in profile, and on the right, the apical four-chamber view.

subjective element is thus often present when the cavity is outlined on such images. This has led to poor reproducibility between duplicate determinations on the same patient. In addition, the repetition rate of cross-sectional echocardiography is very considerably less than that of M-mode, being 30/s, or even less if the path-length is long. Automatic boundary detection is still at an early stage of development and not yet suitable for routine clinical practice (Logan Sinclair et al, 1983).

Radionuclide angiography

Ventricular volumes can readily be measured using radionuclides which bind to blood elements – either plasma proteins or red cells. Two approaches have been used (see also Ch. 10). In the first-pass technique, a single bolus of tracer is followed through the heart from a peripheral venous injection. The right and left ventricular cavities are successively outlined for a few beats each (so that their ejection fraction can be calculated) and circulation time measured (Burger & Zaret, 1981). The alternative approach is to allow the tracer to equilibrate with the blood pool and to count over the precordium for a time interval corresponding to 100–200 beats. Counts are gated with respect to the electrocardiogram (and the cardiac cycle divided into approximately 30 ms intervals) so that a single time-activity curve can be generated (Kurtz et al, 1976). All nuclear techniques have the disadvantage that radionuclides must be administered, which is undesirable in infants and children. The gated blood pool method also has the disadvantage that, in order to avoid counts from the two ventricles being superimposed, the left anterior oblique projection must be used. Nuclear methods also have definite advantages: unlike angiography or cross-sectional echocardiography (where a projection or a section is studied), the number of counts recorded is proportional to the volume itself. Nuclear methods can be used satisfactorily during exercise and it is possible that the response of the ejection fraction to exercise may be more sensitive than resting values in detecting the presence, though not necessarily the nature, of ventricular disease. Information about counts is automatically digitised, so that boundary detection is possible, although the necessary criteria for the boundary itself must first be enunciated, which may introduce a subjective component. It is thus possible to study regional wall motion, and, in particular, to look for regional abnormalities in the timing as well as in the amplitude of motion (Botvinick et al, 1982).

EFFECTS OF GROWTH

If the effects of disease on ventricular size are to be studied, those of growth must first be allowed for. The aspect of body size most commonly used is surface area.

This is difficult to measure directly, so that weight, height, or age have also been used. The normal response to growth has been studied by M-mode echocardiography, allowing truly normal subjects to be used. Disregarding early reports in which standard deviations were incorrectly determined, simple 95% confidence limits are now available for all measurements of ventricular cavity size and wall thickness (Rogé et al, 1978; Henry et al, 1978). All dimensions increase with growth and all correlate with height, weight, age, and body surface area (which are themselves closely correlated with one another during childhood and adolescence). The range of normality is wide. When considering left ventricular end-diastolic dimension in a child of 10 years, the mean value is 38 mm and the 95% confidence limits ±10 mm. Ratios such as ejection fraction or shortening fraction remain constant with age, although angiographically determined ejection fraction is rather higher in infants (68 ± 5%) than in children (63 ± 5%). The 95% confidence limits about both echocardiographic and angiographic estimates are equally wide, an observation that should be borne in mind if abnormal cavity size alone is to be used as evidence of ventricular disease.

SIGNIFICANCE OF CAVITY SIZE AND EJECTION FRACTION

The size of the ventricles during growth is closely related to the functions that they are called upon to perform. End-diastolic volume represents the sum of stroke volume and end-systolic volume. Stroke volume at rest is related to heart rate and oxygen uptake. Although both the latter increase very substantially on exercise, stroke volume changes little. Stroke volume forms a substantial part of end-diastolic volume; this ratio, SV/EDV or ejection fraction, has proved an easily measured quantity of remarkable clinical utility in detecting the presence of certain types of left ventricular disease. Normal left ventricular ejection fraction (Graham et al, 1973) differs little from that of the right. Apart from a minor reduction in left ventricular ejection fraction until the age of two, neither change significantly with growth. When stroke volume is increased by a shunt or valvar regurgitation, ejection fraction is maintained by a corresponding increase in end-diastolic volume. Reduction in resting ejection fraction is strong evidence of ventricular disease. In addition, ejection fraction is sensitive to preload and resistance to ejection (Krayenbuhl et al, 1968). It normally increases with exercise. Throughout the fields of paediatric and adult cardiology, reduction in ejection fraction represents a major manifestation of chronic ventricular disease and an important determinant of long-term prognosis (Field et al, 1973). The basis of its physiological significance is still not clear. For reasons discussed above, it is not a measure of contractility but may represent an index of the integrity of myocardial fibre organisation.

WALL THICKNESS AND VENTRICULAR MASS

Estimates of ventricular wall thickness are necessary for the diagnosis of hypertrophy and for the estimation of ventricular mass. Those of the left ventricle have received particular attention in the literature. Free wall thickness can be measured from the left ventriculogram as seen in postero-anterior projection as the distance between the outer border of the opacified cavity and the cardiac outline (Rackley et al, 1964; Eber, 1969). It may also be measured along the inferior border on the lateral view. It is essential at both sites that no portion of the right ventricle is interposed between these two landmarks. Such estimates include pericardial thickness as well as that of any fat or fluid that may be present. Measurements can only be made satisfactorily at end-diastole due to difficulties in the identification of endocardium later in systole. Angiography cannot therefore be used satisfactorily to follow changes in wall thickness during the cardiac cycle.

Alternatively, M-mode echocardiography can be used. An instrument of adequate dynamic range can demonstrate the pericardial space and distinguish fibrous pericardium from epicardium (Sjogren et al, 1970; Troy et al, 1972). By custom, the thickness of the latter is included with that of the myocardium. Since endocardium can be followed throughout the cardiac cycle, wall thickness can be measured continuously. Septal thickness can be determined in the same way. For both methods, it is desirable that the site of measurement be localised from a cross-sectional display and the orientation of the myocardium with respect to the ultrasound beam checked. Errors may occur if the angle between the two departs significantly from perpendicular. These estimates have been validated against angiography, by direct determination at postmortem study and at operation. Those of the posterior wall seem well established but the reliability of those of the septum has proved questionable. Right ventricular wall thickness can be measured from either the parasternal or from the subcostal approach provided that adequate demonstration of epi- and endocardium can be achieved. These estimates correlate well with postmortem determinations in the adult (Prakash, 1978).

If estimates of thickness are combined with those of cavity volume, the mass of a shell of myocardium surrounding the cavity can be calculated whose thickness is that of the ventricular free wall (Rackley et al, 1964). Both angiographic and echocardiographic measurements have been used for such determinations, which are referred to as 'ventricular mass'. As with cavity volume, so regression equations have been derived from postmortem specimens and used to correct estimates made during life.

These estimates are obviously dependent on the original data and do not allow for variation in wall thickness in different parts of either right or left ventricular cavities; neither do they take account of the papillary muscles or trabeculations. There is probably little to be gained by increasing their precision until imaging systems are developed which are more capable of taking account of the complex regional differences in ventricular structure.

Wall stress

A major function of the ventricles is to develop stress in their walls during systole. A stress is a force per unit area and so has the same physical dimensions as pressure. A force not only has magnitude but also direction so that the net force at any point within the wall of the myocardium may be considered as the result of a number of forces acting in different directions. These forces in the ventricle are usually resolved into components passing longitudinally, circumferentially, and perpendicular to the myocardium. Shear stresses may also be present. These are tangential components between neighbouring elements within the wall. Wall stress is not usually measured directly in man but is calculated from the cavity pressure and the dimensions of the ventricle (Yin, 1981). The simple formation used is referred to as the 'Laplace relation':

$$F = Pr/t$$

where F = wall stress, P = cavity pressure, r = cavity radius and t = wall thickness. A very significant limitation of this approach is that the relation properly applies only when the wall is 'thin'. In the physical science this is usually taken as being less than one-tenth of the local radius of curvature. Unfortunately this does not apply to the left ventricle and barely to the right, particularly at end-systole. A more rewarding technique for calculation of wall stress is to use the finite element method. This has been developed by engineers for use with structures of irregular shape and non-uniform composition (Janz & Grimm, 1972). It allows for stresses to be calculated within the wall and possible effects of localised irregularities to be investigated. Elaborate computing facilities are required, however, making it a technique of research but not of clinical application.

Myocardial stress development

In spite of its well-recognised inadequacies, use of Laplace's law allows a number of semiquantitative deductions to be made about stress development in the myocardium (Fig. 7.4). Peak wall stress is normally of the order of 150–250 g/cm² and is reached early in systole (Hood et al, 1968; Falsetti et al, 1970). Wall stress falls as ejection proceeds because left ventricular cavity dimension falls and

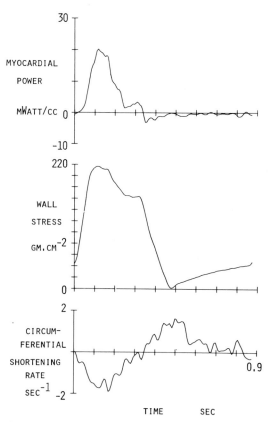

Fig. 7.4 Normal myocardial mid-wall stress derived from simultaneous M-mode echocardiogram and high fidelity pressure. Pressure, wall stress and shortening rate are shown. Peak wall stress is reached early in systole, and then falls off as ejection proceeds.

the wall becomes thicker. When the cavity is enlarged, peak systolic wall stress is increased unless there has been compensatory hypertrophy. When ejection fraction is reduced the percentage reduction in cavity dimension and increase in wall thickness during systole are both low. The myocardium must therefore generate high values of stress throughout ejection. A low end-systolic volume and a high ejection fraction thus have the considerable functional advantage of reducing myocardial oxygen consumption which depends not only on peak wall stress but also on the time over which stress is maintained.

Significance of wall thickness measurements

As might be expected, wall thickness increases with age. During the whole period of growth, however, its relation to cavity size remains virtually constant. Indeed, a similar relation applies throughout a very wide range of mammalian hearts (Ford, 1976). This results in the ratio of wall thickness to cavity radius (t/r) being virtually constant over the range of cardiac size studied. Laplace's law demonstrates that wall stress is directly proportional to cavity pressure, the constant of proportionality being t/r. The relative constancy of this ratio can thus be seen as reflecting the corresponding constancy of peak systolic wall stress regardless of cavity size. This relation can be used to assess ventricular hypertrophy. Left ventricular systolic pressure may be considerably increased in the presence of outflow tract obstruction. If wall stress is to remain constant, there must be a concomitant increase in wall thickness (Gaasch, 1979). Assumed constancy of left ventricular wall stress has been made the basis of a method for estimating peak systolic pressure. Valve gradients have thus been calculated in patients with aortic stenosis by measuring cavity size and wall thickness (Bennett et al, 1975). Unfortunately, wall stress does not always remain constant. When it does, one can speak of left ventricular hypertrophy as being 'appropriate' in that compensation has occurred. If wall thickness fails to increase, wall stress must rise. Failure of appropriate hypertrophy to occur is most commonly seen when the increase in wall stress is associated with cavity dilation, such as occurs in congestive cardiomyopahty. In such cases, the cavity radius increases so that that ratio t/r falls even though ventricular muscle mass may actually increase. Conversely, when hypertrophy occurs with normal cavity pressure (as with hypertrophic non-obstructive cardiomyopathy), wall stress falls. The hypertrophy can be recognised as occurring in the absence of adequate stimulus. The t/r ratio has also proved of value in analysing the ventricular response to a volume load, due, for example, to valvar regurgitation. Failure of appropriate increase in t/r ratio to occur in such patients has a negative effect on survival independent of a low ejection fraction.

VENTRICULAR SYSTOLIC FUNCTION

Measurements of ventricular function made during systole differ fundamentally from those described above, since they are frequently related to the velocity of contraction. This represents a major change in emphasis from the largely anatomical features described above. The former are time-related and the latter are not.

One approach to assessing systolic function which has received great prominence in the literature is to assume that changes in ventricular performance occurring in the intact heart are identical to those seen acutely in isolated papillary muscle. The velocity of shortening of a papillary muscle following stimulation depends on both afterload and preload (Fig. 7.5). Afterload represents the force against which active contraction occurs. There is an inverse and curvilinear relation between contraction velocity and afterload (termed a 'force-velocity' relation) such that the greater the afterload, the lower the velocity of contraction. Preload represents the force extending the muscle in its relaxed state at the onset of contraction. If preload is increased, the muscle will be stretched to an extent determined by its passive length-tension relation.

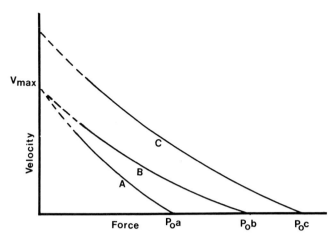

Fig. 7.5 Idealised relation between the rate of shortening and the force developed by an isolated myocardial fibre. Curves A and B were recorded at the same inotropic state, but preload was greater for curve B. Curve C was recorded at the same preload as B, but in the presence of a positive inotropic stimulus. As force (afterload) falls, shortening velocity of the muscle increases with all three, reaching a maximum (V_{max}) when afterload is zero. For each curve, P_o represents peak force achieved in the absence of shortening, i.e. an isometric contraction. At constant isotropic state, an increase in preload (curve B) increases P_o but not V_{max}. A positive inotropic stimulus increases V_{max} and P_o (curve C).

The force of muscular contraction depends (within fixed limits) on resting length and thus on preload (Braunwald et al, 1967). It was suggested that a series of force-velocity curves, arising from different levels of preload and extrapolated back to zero afterload, all met at a single point, which corresponded to the maximum velocity of contraction termed V_{max} (Sonnenblick, 1965). V_{max} derived in this way is independent of preload and afterload. It thus fulfils the criteria for a quantity termed 'contractility', this being a measure of the intrinsic ability of the muscle to contract independent of its external loading conditions. A drug or other manoeuvre with an inotropic action moves the force-velocity curve in its entirety, so that contraction velocity is altered at fixed preload and afterload. If velocity is increased, the stimulus is referred to as a 'positive inotropic effect'. If velocity is reduced, it is considered a negative inotropic effect. Drugs such as isoprenaline or adrenaline (and manoeuvres such as postectopic potentiation or stimulation of the sympathetic nervous system) have a positive inotropic action. Depressant drugs such as disopyramide have a negative inotropic effect. Beta-blocking drugs have an overall negative inotropic effect due almost entirely to competitive blockade of endogenous sympathetic activity rather than to any direct effect at therapeutic doses. When extended from a single muscle to the whole heart, these results have given rise to a framework of ideas which are still in widespread current use for assessing ventricular function. Preload in the papillary muscle has been equated with end-diastolic pressure or volume in the whole heart, so that its effect on contraction velocity has been presumed to correspond almost exactly with that of Starling's law (Patterson et al, 1914). Afterload has been variously identified with systolic pressure, resistance or impedance to ejection, and peak systolic wall stress. Of particular significance has been the theoretical basis given by the model for distinguishing the effects of a change in contractility from those of a change in preload. If these ideas are to be applied to chronic left ventricular disease, rather than simply documenting the effects of pharmacological or other manoeuvres, it must be assumed that disturbances of function seen in patients with chronic ventricular disease have their exact counterpart in acute alterations of inotropic state. It has thus become widely accepted that ventricular function depends only on preload, afterload, and contractility. Once the effects of the two former variables have been allowed for, any departure from normal must be due to some defect in contractility.

This 'contractility' theory of left ventricular disease makes a number of fundamental assumptions that must be examined in detail before it can be accepted into clinical practice (Noble 1972). Its theoretical basis (that preload, afterload, and contractile state are separable in the isolated papillary muscle) has repeatedly been challenged and is no longer tenable (Pollack, 1970). Indeed, non-uniformity of contraction can be demonstrated even within isolated papillary muscle preparations (Vassallo & Pollack, 1982). These fundamental limitations apart, there are major difficulties in accepting the hypothesis. The assumption that disturbances occurring in chronic left ventricular disease can be explained in the same terms as acute alterations in the function of a papillary muscle will be examined in a later section. The failure of sarcomere shortening to explain the observed extent of reduction in left ventricular minor axis demonstrates the fundamental inadequacy of this extrapolation even in normal subjects at rest, and there is no reason to suppose that it should be any more reliable in disease. The highly organised ventricular architecture necessary to explain this relation might itself be abnormal, fundamentally altering observations made in disease. It must be assumed that ventricular function is uniform if an index based on a single measurement of velocity is to provide a description of the function of the whole. Since many types of ventricular disease seen in clinical practice manifest themselves with regional rather than generalised abnormalities of function, this assumption must also be questioned. Also unsatisfactory has been the way in which pre- and afterload have been identified with various measurements made in the intact circulation. For example, if 'preload' can be equated with either a pressure or a volume, it is inadequately defined and is not a physical entity in the usual sense of the term. The same applies to the various measurements of 'afterload' in the intact circulation. This approach is limited to an examination of systolic function, and can take no account of disturbances

of diastole. These reasons seem enough to justify abandoning it as unsuitable for describing the disturbances of ventricular function seen in clinical practice, particularly since it has proved unreliable in identifying patients with advanced ventricular disease. Instead, a multifactorial approach will be examined, in which a variety of different disturbances can be identified. These may occur independently and manifest themselves at any time throughout the cardiac cycle.

PHASES OF THE CARDIAC CYCLE

In order to describe and analyse ventricular function in the beating heart from this point of view, it is first necessary to define the phases of the cardiac cycle at which measurements are being made. To do this unambiguously, the system established by Wiggers (1921) is usually used. The start of the cardiac cycle is taken as the onset of the Q wave of the electrocardiogram. The first manifestation of mechanical activity of the ventricles is the onset of pressure rise within the cavity, or, for the left ventricle, the onset of the upstroke of the apex cardiogram (which is synchronous with it). The interval between the start of electrical and mechanical activity is referred to as the 'activation time'. When activation is normal, the onset of pressure rise in the right ventricle precedes that in the left. The time interval from the onset of pressure rise to the onset of opening of the appropriate arterial valve is termed 'isovolumic contraction time'. Isovolumic contraction time depends on the rate of rise of ventricular pressure, and the difference between end-diastolic pressures in the ventricle and great artery. No isovolumic contraction occurs in the presence of atrioventricular valve regurgitation or a ventricular septal defect. Ejection time is taken from opening to closing of the arterial valve, although at the end of this period, ventricular relaxation may already have started. This earliest period of relaxation is termed 'proto-diastole'. The closure of the arterial valve marks the onset of isovolumic relaxation which ends as the atrioventricular valve opens. Again it may be absent when there is aortic or pulmonary regurgitation or a ventricular septal defect. Finally, ventricular filling is characteristically divided into the phases of rapid filling, diastasis during mid-diastole, and atrial systole.

Isovolumic contraction

The normal duration of isovolumic contraction of the left ventricle shows considerable variation, ranging from 15–55 ms, while that of the right is 20–60 ms. An increase in isovolumic contraction time on the right side of the heart has been used to detect pulmonary hypertension. The peak rate of rise of left ventricular pressure during isovolumic contraction can be determined by differentiating the signal from a micromanometer, the frequency response of a fluid-filled catheter system being inadequate for this purpose. This quantity (peak dP/dt) normally has a resting value of approximately 1500–2000 mmHg/s. It is increased by positive inotropic stimuli such as isoprenaline administration, circulating catecholamines during anaesthesia or with postectopic potentiation (Gleason & Braunwald, 1962). It is reduced in left ventricular disease but is an unsatisfactory measure of resting left ventricular function, since it is also sensitive to end-diastolic cavity size and to resistance to ejection. Thus, it is low in mitral or aortic regurgitation and increased in aortic stenosis. If peak rates of ventricular pressure increase are to be used to assess myocardial function, therefore, it would seem reasonable to relate the rate of rise to the instantaneous pressure. This approach was investigated by Mason (1969) who suggested that it was possible to measure V_{max} directly from the ventricular pressure pulse. This approach is theoretically attractive but has been found to have considerable disadvantages in practice. It is invalidated by any change in cavity shape during isovolumic contraction, be this due to a shunt, valvar regurgitation or incoordinate onset of tension development. There has also been doubt as to the correct zero for pressure measurement. For example, sternal angle, mid-thoracic, and atmospheric values all give different values of V_{max} for the same beat. An alternative suggestion has been to use 'developed' pressure, in other words, the pressure above end-diastolic. End-diastolic pressure, however, may depend on the connective tissue within the wall or even the pericardial pressure and so have no relation to systolic function. In addition, the range of normality is very wide as measured by this technique. In a group of patients with obvious and advanced left ventricular disease (defined in terms of reduced ejection fraction, raised end-diastolic pressure and regional abnormalities of contraction), determination of V_{max} proved very insensitive in separating normal from abnormal (Peterson et al, 1973).

Pre-ejection period

A much simpler approach to the assessment of ventricular function during early systole has been to measure the pre-ejection period. This represents the time interval between the onset of activation and the opening of the arterial valve. Left ventricular pre-ejection period, in particular, has been examined very extensively (Lewis et al, 1977). It can most conveniently be determined from simultaneous recording of the electrocardiogram, phonocardiogram and the indirect carotid pulse as QA2 interval minus the ejection time (Fig. 7.6). In the absence of activation abnormalities such as left bundle branch block, pre-ejection period (like isovolumic contraction time) depends on the difference between the end-diastolic pressures in the aorta and left ventricle and the rate of rise of pressure. All these

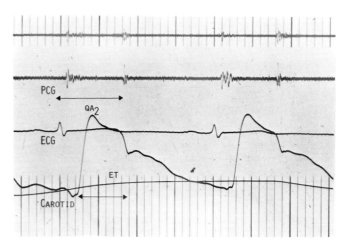

Fig. 7.6 Measurement of pre-ejection period from simultaneous ECG, phonocardiogram (PCG), and indirect carotid pulse. ET – ejection time.

variables are important. In complete transposition, when pulmonary vascular resistance is normal, left ventricular pre-ejection period is very short. It is prolonged in patients with aortic stenosis, even though the rate of rise of pressure is normal. The pre-ejection period is shortened by positive inotropic stimuli and it is lengthened by negative ones. It is also increased in patients with chronic left ventricular disease. In severely ill patients, however, this latter effect may be reversed by the action of endogenous sympathetic stimulation. The pre-ejection period is virtually unaffected by heart rate. Due to its multifactorial basis, pre-ejection period has proved relatively insensitive as an index of chronic left ventricular disease, although it has been used to separate congestive cardiomyopathy from constrictive pericarditis. Its main value lies in detecting acute changes of function brought about by drug administration or other relatively simple manoeuvres.

Ventricular ejection

Events during ventricular ejection have been studied in great detail, and there are many measurements that can be made.

Stroke volume. One of the simplest measurements is to determine stroke volume, either as cardiac output divided by heart rate, or as the difference between end-diastolic and end-systolic volumes if valvar regurgitation or a shunt is present. Stroke volume is related to body surface area and may be maintained in spite of severe ventricular disease. This is particularly so if resistance to ejection is low as in mitral regurgitation. Stroke work is derived as the product of stroke volume and mean arterial pressure. Values of stroke work can be used to analyse ventricular function on the basis of Starling's law of the heart. This 'law' states that the mechanical energy set free with each contraction depends on the end-diastolic fibre

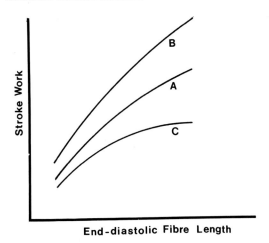

Fig. 7.7 Idealised normal relationship between stroke work and end-diastolic myocardial fibre length – 'Starling's law' (curve A). A positive inotropic stimulus (B) displaces the curve to the left, and a negative inotropic stimulus (C) has the reverse effect.

length (Patterson et al, 1914). In practice, a ventricular function curve is usually constructed by plotting stroke work against end-diastolic pressure, the latter being taken as an index of end-diastolic fibre length (Fig. 7.7). A positive inotropic intervention increases stroke work at constant end-diastolic fibre length. A negative action, such as ventricular disease has the reverse effect. This method has been widely used to assess cardiac function by assuming that ventricular disease has the same effect as a positive inotropic stimulus. End-diastolic pressure can be varied by alteration of plasma volume, transient obstruction of venous flow, or by atrial pacing. The resulting changes in stroke work can then be measured. This approach has the advantage that measurements are relatively easy to make and that both stroke work and end-diastolic pressure have clinical as well as physiological significance. There are difficulties, however, attending its use in defining chronic left ventricular disease. These are related in part to problems in the interpretation of end-diastolic pressure described in a later section. Stroke work is also sensitive to the nature of aortic or pulmonary impedance. In patients with intact reflexes, the manoeuvres used to alter end-diastolic pressure may alter endogenous sympathetic activity. These then have secondary effects on the isotropic state of the myocardium superimposed on those of Starling's law. End-diastolic pressure itself relates poorly to end-diastolic volume in chronic ventricular disease (Rackley et al, 1970). Cavity dilation in ventricular disease is often explained on the basis of Starling's law, the suggestion being made that end-diastolic fibre length has increased to 'compensate' for a reduction in ventricular contractility. There is little evidence to suggest, however, that a large cavity is simply a small one stretched. In particular, histological studies have shown that the Z-band to Z-band distance in such ventricles is normal, indicating

that enlargement has been on the basis of rearrangement or 'slippage' of fibres rather than simple elongation (Linzbach, 1960).

Ventricular ejection time. Ventricular ejection time is measured either from direct observation of the appropriate arterial valve leaflets by echocardiography or from a direct or indirect trace of the pressure in the great artery (Weissler et al, 1963). As with other systolic time intervals, a great deal more information has been published about events on the left side of the heart than the right. Though ejection time is relatively easy to measure, it is affected by many factors. Heart rate is a major determinant, ejection time falling as rate rises. A number of regresssion equations have been proposed to allow for this effect although the relations derived from spontaneous variation in heart rate, exercise, and atrial pacing are all different from one another. Left ventricular ejection time is proportional to stroke volume and is independently shortened by a positive inotropic effect. The effects of ventricular disease are usually small and unpredictable. This is because ejection time is reduced by a low stroke volume, increased by contraction abnormalities and is also affected by the added changes in the function of the autonomic nervous system present in severe heart disease. When ejection time measurements are combined with those of pre-ejection period (by using the ratio of pre-ejection period of left ventricular ejection time), some increase in sensitivity is obtained in detecting ventricular disease.

Velocity of ejection. The velocity of ejection of blood into the great arteries may be reduced in ventricular disease. Mean systolic ejection rate is determined as (stroke volume)/(ejection time). It is a simple and satisfactory means of documenting inotropic effects of drugs (Ross et al, 1965). Alternatively, peak blood flow velocity can be measured, either with a catheter tip electromagnetic flow meter or non-invasively (using the Doppler technique). Flow velocity in the aorta reaches its peak during the first third of systole. It declines thereafter, often with a short period of backward flow just before closure of the aortic valve, which corresponds to protodiastole. Normal peak flow velocity in the ascending aorta is in the range 55–85 cm/s. The rate of change of velocity (that is, acceleration) at the start of ejection is in the range 1500–2500 cm/s^2. Both these values are very sensitive to acute inotropic interventions, while aortic acceleration has been found to be virtually insensitive to changes in end-diastolic cavity size. Transcutaneous Doppler measurements of the velocity and acceleration of blood flow in the descending thoracic aorta have therefore been made as an index of acute changes in left ventricular function. It is thus disappointing that measurement of aortic blood velocity and initial acceleration have both proved to be insensitive measures of chronic ventricular disease. The same applies to determinations of peak ejection rate, expressed in cm^3/s, derived from angiograms (Hammermeister et al, 1974), where there is very considerable overlap between values from normal and abnormal ventricles.

Pressure-flow relations in the great arteries

An important aspect of ventricular function can be examined by assessing pressure-flow relations in the great arteries. Blood flow velocity in the great artery is measured as described in the previous section and pressure is determined with a micromanometer. Instantaneous relations between the two can therefore be studied. Blood enters a great artery as the result of work done on it by the ventricle. The rate at which this work is done (that is, the power of the ventricle) may give information about its function. At any instant during ejection, ventricular power is given by the product of pressure (a force per unit area) and flow (ml/s). This can be referred to as 'hydraulic power' since it is measured from bulk movement of blood rather than from ventricular wall motion. The total work done on the blood can be derived by integrating the power output over the period of ejection. Pressure-flow relations in the great arteries are complex. Paradoxically, aortic pressure is slightly higher than that in the left ventricle for the greater part of ejection. The blood enters the aorta not because of a pressure gradient but as a result of inertia imparted to it early in systole by the initial ventricular impulse (Spencer & Greiss, 1962). Inertia causes peak pressure to precede peak flow rather than to occur simultaneously with it as would be the case for a system showing resistance only. Capacitance has the reverse effect, with peak flow preceding peak pressure. This is seen, for example, when blood enters a compliant vascular bed. Both these effects are taken into account when aortic impedance rather than simple resistance is calculated. The magnitude of inertial and capacitive effects depends on the exact contour of the wave forms, with components at different frequencies varying independently of one another. In order to calculate total power, therefore, it is necessary to sum these frequency components. The greatest contribution to total power comes from the lowest frequencies, but significant energy is present up to frequencies of 10 Hz. Though complex, this method has the potential advantage of allowing the effects of afterload (interpreted as the impedance of the peripheral vascular bed) to be separated from the characteristics of ventricular ejection. It is likely to prove particularly valuable in analysing the effects of pulmonary vascular disease on right-sided events.

Left ventricular wall motion during ejection

The characteristics of wall motion during ejection have been widely used as a measure of function. Motion of the minor axis of the left ventricle has been studied in particular detail. This quantity is frequently referred to as the mean velocity of circumferential fibre shortening (VCF), and is calculated as:

$$(Dd-Ds)/Dd.ET$$

where Dd and Ds are end-diastolic and end-systolic dimensions respectively, and ET is left ventricular ejection time measured from an indirect carotid pulse or aortic valve echogram (Karliner et al, 1971; Paraskos et al, 1971). It has the units s^{-1}. The normal range is $0.8-1.2$ s^{-1}. Low values are seen in patients in whom the cavity is dilated and ejection fraction reduced. It has been shown to correlate well with other manifestations of left ventricular disease, particularly with a reduced ejection fraction. A low value of peak VCF might therefore be taken as evidence that contraction velocity is reduced in these patients. This is not necessarily the case. Mean VCF merely represents (shortening fraction)/(ejection time). Since ejection time is either normal or short in left ventricular disease, mean VCF must be low if shortening fraction is low. The two variables thus measure virtually the same aspect of ventricular function and both therefore reflect ejection fraction. The same applies to peak VCF, which can be measured from digitised echocardiograms or angiograms. Normal values lie between 1.8 and 2.5 s^{-1}. These are again inversely proportional to ventricular cavity size at constant ejection rate. If slow contraction is to be documented as a manifestation of ventricular disease (which would be the case if contractility were indeed depressed), it must be demonstrated in patients in whom cavity size is normal. Such patients are uncommon, although such slow contraction has been found in those with certain types of muscular dystrophy (Venco et al, 1978) or myocardial infiltration. It is possible that slow contraction will be documented more frequently in patients of the paediatric age-group, particularly in those with inherited disorders of myocardial or skeletal muscle.

Pressure-volume relations

Pressure-volume relations of the ventricles (particularly the left) are also informative. Volume has usually been measured angiographically and the results presented as a pressure-volume loop. The area of such a loop represents stroke work. This technique is of particular value in assessing the disturbance caused by valvar heart disease which causes volume overload (Dodge et al, 1966).

Pressure-volume relations can be used to assess a further aspect of systolic left ventricular function (Sagawa, 1981). The end-systolic tension of isolated cardiac muscle depends only on end-systolic length and contractile state. It is virtually independent both of end-diastolic length and mode of contraction, whether isometric or isotonic. When extrapolated to the whole heart, this finding forms the basis of a method potentially able to assess contractile

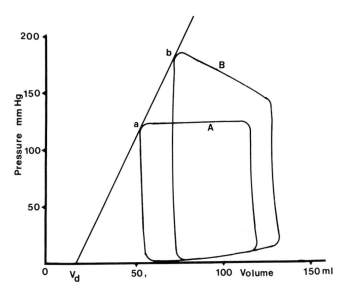

Fig. 7.8 Left ventricular pressure-volume loops, under control conditions (A) and after administration of a pressor agent (B). The end-systolic points, a and b, respectively lie on the same straight line, which has the intercept Vd on the X-axis. The slope of this line represents E_{max}. A positive inotropic stimulus is associated with an increase in E_{max}.

state. The method takes account of afterload yet is independent of preload. End-systole in the intact heart can be defined from the pressure-volume loop as the time of onset of rapid pressure drop. At any time during systole, left ventricular elasticity, E, can be defined as $P/(V-Vd)$, where P and V are instantaneous values of pressure and volume and Vd an intercept representing ventricular volume at zero pressure (Fig. 7.8). As ejection proceeds, E increases, reaching a maximum value, E_{max}, approximately at end-systole. If arterial pressure is raised by methoxamine administration, a series of pressure-volume loops can be constructed whose end-systolic points are found to lie on a straight line. The slope of this line is equivalent to E_{max}, and its intercept on the volume axis is Vd. The slope is independent of end-diastolic pressure or volume but is increased by positive inotropic stimuli. It has thus been identified with contractility.

These observations have been repeated in intact man, with pressure measured by a micromanometer, and volume by angiography. The end-systolic pressure-volume line has proved to be approximately linear over the relatively narrow range in which it can be studied clinically. Its slope is increased by extrasystolic potentiation (Mehmel et al, 1981). In patients with normal ventricular function, the slope has a value of 4–6 mmHg/ml, while values of 1 mmHg/ml or even less are seen in those in whom the left ventricular cavity is dilated. Values of the intercept (Vd)

range from small and positive to large and negative so that their physical significance is not clear.

It is laborious to determine two or more sets of pressure-volume relations in this way, so alternative approaches have been sought. The technique can be greatly simplified if ventricular volume is measured by gated blood pool scintigraphy which allows multiple determinations to be made (McKay et al, 1984). A totally non-invasive method is to substitute end-systolic cavity dimension measured by M-mode echocardiography for volume and to combine it with end-ejection pressure determined from a calibrated indirect carotid pulse tracing. End-systolic pressure-dimension relations are also linear (Marsh et al, 1979) with a normal slope of 78 ± 26 mmHg/mm. This slope is increased both in post-extrasystolic beats and with dobutamine infusion (Colan et al, 1982). Normal values of slope have been recorded in patients who have undergone anatomical correction of complete transposition (Borow et al, 1984). They are reduced in children with transfusion-dependent thalassaemia major over the age of 13 (Borow et al, 1982).

Measurement of end-systolic pressure-volume or pressure-dimension relations thus gives useful information about left ventricular systolic function. Like other measurements of contractility, the implicit assumption is made that ventricular function is uniformly depressed in patients with disease. Little is known of the performance of these indices in patients in whom regional abnormalities are present. In addition, concomitant appearance of a positive inotropic stimulus such as increased sympathetic activity may prevent the detection of left ventricular disease, since its effect on the index is exactly opposite. A similar state of affairs is seen after acute myocardial infarction in adults where measures of overall function such as ejection fraction or pre-ejection period can be entirely within normal limits in spite of severe regional disease. Values of slope are also likely to be related to those of ejection fraction for purely computational reasons, since both contain end-systolic volume in their derivation. Mehmel et al (1981) showed such correlation to exist not only when ejection fraction was depressed but to an even greater extent when it was normal. Some depression of any sensitive index of contractility might be expected in a minority of patients in whom ejection fraction is normal by virtue of its identifying those who have disease too subtle to be detected by other methods. Even closer correlation between slope and the largely random variation in ejection fraction seen in the normal range is not at all compatible with this idea. Rather, it would seem to suggest that end-systolic volume is the main factor determining both. Definite evidence that these new methods are able to detect subclinical left ventricular disease in man as distinct from acute changes in inotropic state caused by drugs or other manoeuvres must be awaited.

INCOORDINATE CONTRACTION

Quite apart from the generalised disturbances described above, regional abnormalities may also interfere with ventricular function. These require an imaging system for their identification and display. So far, the most substantial body of work has been based on angiography, but an increasing contribution is coming from cross-sectional echocardiography or blood pool scanning. Any regional difference in function is frequently taken as evidence of disease. But this assumes that normal ventricular function is uniform. This assumption is unjustified. A series of echocardiographic observations have shown regional differences in the velocity and extent of endocardial motion and, more significant, in myocardial thickening in different parts of the left ventricle (Shapiro, 1982; Haendchen et al, 1983). The significance of these differences is not clear, although they may relate to the efficient bulk movement of blood, particularly in early diastole.

Regional wall motion may be studied in a number of ways. Perhaps the least satisfactory is simply to view a film or videotape in real time and then make subjective judgements. This method has been used widely to compare angiography with cross-sectional echocardiography. Although gross disturbances can be detected in this way, it is unsuitable for detailed analysis or quantification. A second approach has been to use a 'two-frame' display. Here, end-diastolic and end-systolic cavity outlines are superimposed on one another. The method has again been used very extensively and is the basis of the current classification of regional wall motion. Three types of abnormality are recognised: hypokinesis (a reduction in the amplitude of wall motion), akinesis (its absence) and dyskinesis (its reversal, with outward displacement throughout systole) (Herman & Gorlin, 1967). In some patients, however, particularly those with abnormalities in the timing of wall motion, its use can lead to very misleading results (Marier & Gibson, 1980). These arise from lack of definition of the timing of end-systole in patients with incoordinate contraction, since it ends at different times in different parts of the same ventricle. The apparent pattern of regional wall motion displayed is thus influenced critically by the exact timing of the frame taken as end-systolic.

Inco-ordinate wall motion has additional significance in reducing the mechanical efficiency of energy transfer from the myocardium to the circulation. When present during isovolumic contraction, it may cause a reduction in the peak rate of rise of left ventricular pressure (dP/dt). It follows, therefore, that peak values of dP/dt (and thus of variables derived from it such as V_{max}) in patients with left ventricular disease cannot be ascribed to slow contraction (that is, reduced contractility) unless incoordinate contraction has been positively excluded. There do not appear to be any studies in the literature in which this has been done.

SUMMARY OF SYSTOLIC FUNCTION

There have been many approaches to the study of systolic function, which might seem to have little in common with one another. Nevertheless, a number of general principles do become apparent. The first is the overriding physiological significance of normal cavity architecture and end-diastolic cavity size. Normal myocardial architecture is indispensible for the maintenance of normal ejection fraction. With fibres arranged circumferentially around a spherical ventricle, normal sarcomere shortening will lead to an ejection fraction of approximately 30%. The physiological effects of a large cavity and low ejection fraction include an increase in peak wall stress, with loss of the normal fall as ejection proceeds and so to increased myocardial oxygen requirements. At constant ejection rate, peak rates of dimension change fall as the square of cavity dimension. Power transfer from the myocardium to the circulation occurs in unfavourable circumstances. Finally, end-systolic cavity pressure-volume relations may be abnormal, in spite of stress-strain relations of the myocardium being unimpaired. Unless these effects of cavity size are allowed for, normal myocardium is at a considerable mechanical disadvantage if it is abnormally arranged around a ventricular cavity that is too large and its function becomes modified in a way that might suggest impaired 'contractility'. Whatever its pathological basis, anatomical studies have made it clear that a dilated cavity is not simply a small one stretched but that rearrangement of muscle fibres has occurred. A reduced ejection fraction in a patient with chronic ventricular disease thus has nothing in common with acute changes brought about by Starling's law.

A second process, quite separate from enlargement of cavity size is incoordinate contraction. Its presence implies a heterogeneity of function which may manifest itself at any time during the cardiac cycle. It reduces the peak rate of rise of ventricular pressure (and hence in values of V_{max} derived from it) and prolongs pre-ejection period. It makes the process of energy transfer from the myocardium to the circulation mechanically inefficient. Incoordinate relaxation interferes with the early diastolic fall in pressure and may well impair rapid filling and diastolic pressure-volume relations.

When the effects of these two important mechanisms are taken into account, there is little evidence for the third possibility, namely that the equivalent of an acute depression of inotropic state may have its counterpart as a mechanism of chronic ventricular disease. In order to document this, slow contraction must be demonstrated in a patient with normal cavity size and systolic wall stress.

This combination is very uncommon. When present it does not usually lead to clinical manifestations characteristic of ventricular disease. The existence of isolated slow contraction even as a significant – let alone dominant – mechanism of clinical left ventricular disease remains unproven.

DIASTOLIC FUNCTION

Diastolic is as important as systolic ventricular function. When heart rate is increased, the time available during each beat for filling is significantly less than that for ejection. Complex mechanisms are hence likely to be present which allow rapid inflow of blood into the ventricle in the absence of measureable pressure elevation. Right-sided diastolic events, in particular, have been little studied, so that the greater part of what follows will be concerned with the left ventricle. It is likely, however, that major insight into right ventricular function will come from analysis of disturbances seen in patients with congenital heart disease.

Isovolumic relaxation

Isovolumic relaxation is the time interval between closure of the arterial and opening of the atrioventricular valve. For the left ventricle, aortic valve closure is timed from the phonocardiogram as the onset of the first high frequency vibration of the aortic component of the second sound. This should routinely be identified from a simultaneous aortic echogram. Mitral valve opening is timed from the M-mode echocardiogram as the time of initial separation of the two leaflets. It is essential that the recording be made exactly at the level in the ventricle at which this occurs. Alternatively, isovolumic relaxation has been measured from dual echograms of aortic and mitral valves (Sahn et al, 1978). The duration of isovolumic relaxation time is of physiological significance. The normal range in adults is 60 ± 10 ms (Chen & Gibson, 1979). It is rather less in children (Sahn, 1977). As might be expected, it depends on the end-diastolic pressures in the aorta and left ventricle together with the rate of fall of ventricular pressure. It is little affected by variation of aortic end-diastolic pressure within the normal range. Isovolumic relaxation time on the right side of the heart, cannot be measured as simply as on the left, because pulmonary valve closure and P_2 are delayed with respect to the fall in right ventricular pressure. This phenomenon is termed 'hangout' (Curtiss et al, 1975). It is due to the low impedance of the normal pulmonary vascular bed and is lost if severe pulmonary vascular disease is present. The interval from P_2 to opening of the tricuspid valve is thus normally very short or may even be negative. A similar finding has been recorded on the left side of the heart in patients with complete transposition after Mustard's operation. In these patients, the left ventricle ejects into a normal pulmonary circulation (Bourlon et al, 1980). Isovolumic relation time on the left side of the heart may also be very short or even negative in the normal circulation when left ventricular end-diastolic pressure is raised, frequently being zero at 30 mmHg or above. A short isovolumic relaxation time may also be recorded in certain patients with hypertrophic cardiomyopathy in whom the aortic valve is isolated from the left ventricle by severe outflow tract obstruction (Gamble et al, 1983). By contrast, isovolumic relaxation time is prolonged in patients with left ventricular disease (particularly hypertrophy), provided that end-diastolic (pre-a) pressure is normal.

Rate of fall of left ventricular pressure

Ventricular pressure begins to fall before the end of left ventricular ejection, its onset marking the start of the period of 'protodiastole'. Peak rate of fall (or peak negative dP/dt) occurs just after A_2. It is measured by differentiation of the signal from a micromanometer. In general its magnitude is greatest when systolic pressure is high. The rate of fall is reduced in adults in the presence of acute ischaemia, but normal values are usually recorded in patients with left ventricular hypertrophy. An alternative approach to the quantification of the ventricular pressure pulse during isovolumic relaxation has been to assume its fall is exponential and to measure a time constant (T). This method has been investigated in detail by Weiss et al (1976). Values of T are relatively insensitive to heart rate, end-systolic volume and the height from which the pressure falls, but are prolonged in ischaemia and left ventricular hypertrophy. The technique has the drawbacks of any method dependent on fitting simple geometrical curves to biological traces. If deductions are to be made which depend on the curve being specifically exponential (such as deriving a time constant – a property not shown by other monotonically decreasing functions such as a parabola or a hyperbola), then the identity must be rigorously demonstrated. It is not enough to superimpose the exponential of best fit; this can be performed for almost any arbitrary curve. The hypothesis can be tested by using the convenient relation that the first differential of an exponential is itself an exponential. By this test, significant departures can be demonstrated in traces recorded in man (Thompson et al, 1983a). A second problem is that an exponential is defined not only by a time constant but also by the zero level to which the left ventricular pressure is tending. This pressure is undefined but is frequently taken as atmospheric, or the pressure at the mid-chest or sternal angle. Use of all these values, however, give different values for the calculated time constant. Better fits are frequently obtained when sub-zero pressures are taken (Thompson et al, 1983b). The time constant also changes if pericardial pressure is raised.

Of greater significance in patients with congenital heart disease is the asynchrony that may occur between pressure fall in the two ventricles, even when peak values are identical due to a septal defect. Thus, in Fallot's tetralogy, the right ventricular pressure follows the left. During this period, therefore, there is a net right-to-left shunt. During isovolumic contraction, left ventricular pressure rise precedes that in the right, with a dominant left-to-right shunt. The same applies in patients with a ventricular septal defect and high right ventricular pressures (Levin et al, 1966, 1970).

VENTRICULAR FILLING

Ventricular filling starts with opening of the atrioventricular valve. This can be timed from the appropriate echogram. The pattern of inflow is very characteristic. Filling is rapid in both ventricles in early diastole for a period of 120–200 ms (Hammermeister & Warbasse, 1974). The peak rate of inflow into the left ventricle during this time is of the order of 500–1000 ml/s. This may be considerably exceeded in patients with mitral regurgitation or a large ventricular septal defect (Fig. 7.9). Volume changes little during mid-diastole, a period termed 'diastasis'. There is a further increase (amounting to approximately one-third of the total inflow) during atrial systole. This pattern of filling is best demonstrated at rest. Diastole shortens with exercise so that diastasis is lost and early diastolic rapid filling becomes continuous with atrial systole.

Left ventricular filling time

The overall time available for left ventricular filling can readily be measured from the mitral valve echogram. Filling time is long in normal subjects at rest, being 500 ms or more depending on RR interval. During exercise, however, it shortens strikingly. At heart rates of 140/min or more it has dropped to 100 ms (Oldershaw et al, 1983). Since normal stroke volume is of the order of 100 ml during moderate exercise, this implies a mean filling rate of approximatley 1000 ml/s. The duration of filling time during exercise is less than half that of ejection time. It is not surprising, therefore, that this ability to fill the ventricle rapidly during exercise, without a measurable pressure gradient between atrium and ventricle, presupposes complex physiological mechanisms. It is not the behaviour that would be expected if the diastolic left ventricle were simply a passively filling sac.

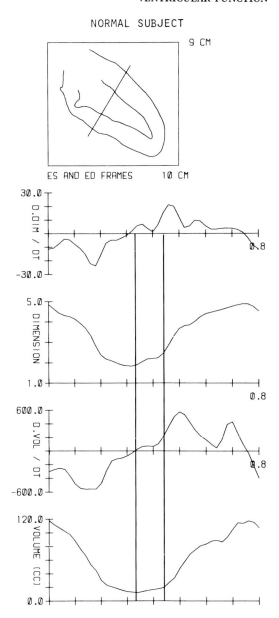

Fig. 7.9 Normal left ventricular volume changes, determined by angiography. The traces show, from below, cavity volume, rate of change of volume, changes in transverse dimension and rate of change of dimension, and (top) superimposed end-diastolic and end-systolic cavity outlines, indicating the position of the dimension measured. The two vertical lines represent the timing of aortic valve closure and mitral valve opening. Note that the period of rapid filling is reflected in the dimension trace, but not the volume increase during atrial systole.

End-diastolic pressure

Ventricular end-diastolic pressure is widely used as a measure of left ventricular function (Rahimtoola, 1973). It has been held to be synonymous with an increased end-diastolic volume. Similarly, an elevated end-diastolic pressure has been taken to indicate a state of cardiac compensation in which output is maintained only at the expense of cavity dilatation. This view is no longer tenable. Correlation between end-diastolic pressure and volume in chronic heart disease is poor (Rackley et al, 1970). In particular, end-diastolic pressure may be high when cavity size is normal but the walls stiff due to increased fibrosis. This is frequently seen in patients with left ventricular outflow tract obstruction. End-diastolic pressure is also independent of left ventricular mass, stroke volume, peak systolic pressure and ejection fraction (Braunwald & Ross, 1963). Even in an individual patient, end-diastolic pressure can be changed without any significant alteration in end-diastolic volume, for example by administration of drugs such as propranolol or nitrates. End-diastolic pressure in one ventricle may be elevated as the result of changes in the size or shape of the other (Ludbrook et al, 1979; Becker & Caruso, 1981). There is also much evidence to suggest that the pressure in the pericardial space may itself be raised when ventricular size increases (Smiseth et al, 1985). If this occurs, pressures measured relative to some external reference point (such as mid-thoracic or atmospheric pressure) cannot reflect the transmural pressure difference (Fig. 7.10). It seems very likely that dilation of one or other ventricle (particularly if this occurs relatively acutely) is restricted by the pericardium. These limitations must be borne in mind when considering the significance of measurements of end-diastolic pressure (or their changes with disease or interventions). Although a

raised end-diastolic pressure may indicate some abnormality, it should not be assumed to indicate an increase in end-diastolic transmural pressure gradient, volume or fibre length. Other information must be taken into account before its significance can be interpreted.

Left ventricular pressure-volume relations

Pressure falls as volume increases during the period of rapid filling. Minimum pressure occurs approximately 150 ms after mitral valve opening and 50 ms after the time of peak rate of volume increase. This anomalous relationship between pressure and volume probably reflects the effects of forces restoring the ventricle towards its end-diastolic cavity shape. Their exact nature is still not clear, but they appear to arise from energy stored in the myocardium during the previous systole. The onset of passive diastole can be taken as occurring at minimum pressure. It continues until the onset of the succeeding atrial systole. Pressure and volume increase together during this time so that the ventricle exhibits elastic behaviour (Grossman & McLaurin, 1976; Mirsky, 1976). The normal pressure-volume relation at this time is curvilinear. At any point during diastole, the slope of this line gives the ventricular compliance, defined as

$$(\text{delta volume})/(\text{delta pressure})$$

Compliance is thus a property of the cavity as a whole (Fig. 7.11). It varies during diastole, becoming lower as filling proceeds, indicating that the cavity has become stiffer. Diastolic pressure-volume curves, being non-linear, are usually assumed to be exponential and to show behav-

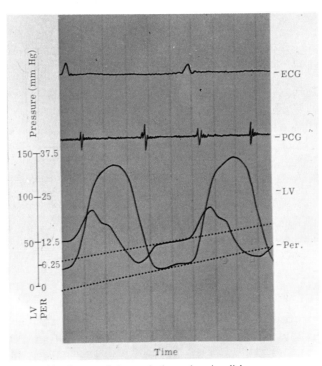

Fig. 7.10 Simultaneous left ventricular and pericardial pressures measured in a postoperative patient. Note that during diastole there is a progressive increase in both so that left ventricular diastolic pressure does not represent true transmural pressure. LV – left ventricular pressure; Per – pericardial pressure; PCG – phonocardiogram.

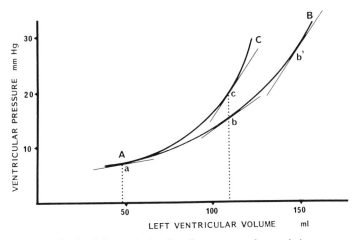

Fig. 7.11 Passive left ventricular diastolic pressure volume relations. AB represents a normal curve. The stiffness at a, b, and b' are given by the tangents to the curve at these points. These show a progressive increase as the ventricle fills. AC represents the pressure volume curve of a less compliant ventricle. Note that at point a, its stiffness is the same as that of the normal ventricle. At the volume corresponding to b and c, its stiffness is increased. However, a further increase in the volume of the normal ventricle to the value corresponding to b' leads to a similar increase in stiffness.

iour characteristic of Lagrangian stress. If pressure is plotted logarithmically and volume linearly, then the curve of ventricular pressure against volume is approximately linear. It is thus possible to calculate its slope and intercept. Ventricular compliance is reduced in patients with ventricular hypertrophy and also in those in whom the cavity is dilated (Fester & Samet, 1976).

Analysis along these lines makes a number of assumptions. If terms such as 'compliance' are used, it is tacitly assumed that the walls of the ventricle are passive and that measurements are made under equilibrium conditions. Both these assumptions can be questioned, even during the period of passive diastole. Equilibrium conditions are not attained, since measurements of pressure and volume have to be made as the ventricle fills. Additional dynamic components due to the filling process itself must therefore be considered. Of these, the most significant is viscosity. Viscous forces are proportional to the rate of filling and cause the ventricle to appear stiffer than at equilibrium. Their presence has been demonstrated experimentally in isolated papillary muscles which have been stretched at rates greater than approximately 2 s^{-1} (Noble, 1977). There is evidence to suggest that they may also be clinically significant in patients with left ventricular hypertrophy (Gaasch et al, 1975). Viscous forces were detected in these studies simply from discrepancies between observed behaviour and an assumed exponential. The possibility was not considered that other factors might be involved, such as the effect of right ventricular filling or pericardial constraint (Pouleur et al, 1979). Inertia is a second dynamic component that must be considered. It is the result of outward acceleration of the walls and causes cavity pressure to be lower at the same cavity size compared with the equilibrium state. Inertial forces are small, however, and even when wall motion is rapid, they seldom result in discrepancies of more than 0.1 mmHg.

Compliance describes a property of the cavity as a whole. An alternative approach has been to consider the stress-strain relations of the myocardium itself (Mirsky & Parmley, 1973). A stress is a force per unit area. A strain is a deformation produced by a stress and, when fibres are considered, it refers to the increase in length. A strain is measured as the increase in length normalised to unit initial length, rather than simply the increase in length. Elasticity at any fibre length represents the ratio of stress to strain, that is, to the slope of the stress-strain relation. Myocardial elasticity, measured in this way, is found to be raised when the cavity is dilated and ejection fraction low, but it is frequently normal or only slightly raised in the presence of ventricular hypertrophy.

Ventricular hypertrophy

Major abnormalities of diastolic function occur in ventricular hypertrophy. As with other diastolic abnormalities, the right side of the heart has been little studied, so that this discussion will be confined to the left ventricle. It seems highly desirable, nonetheless, that diastolic events should be studied in greater detail in patients with right ventricular hypertrophy.

All stages of diastole are involved in patients with left ventricular hypertrophy, whether primary (as occurs in hypertrophic cardiomyopathy) or secondary to increased pressure load. Changes are most marked in patients in whom cavity size is normal and wall thickness increased. Isovolumic contraction time at rest is greatly prolonged, from normal values of around 60 ms up to 150 ms or more (Chen & Gibson, 1979). Once the mitral valve opens, peak filling rate is frequently reduced, particularly in patients with secondary left ventricular hypertrophy. This change in overall left ventricular function is best demonstrated by contrast or radionuclide angiography (Hammermeister & Warbasse, 1974). Regional wall motion can be studied by angiography. Only in occasional cases is the rate of outward wall motion uniformly reduced. Striking regional differences are seen much more commonly with asynchrony in the timing of outward motion, so that peak local values may be within the normal range. The anatomical basis of these regional differences is not clear, although loss of normal ventricular architecture and its replacement by fibre disarray seems a possibility. Further information about filling can be gained from M-mode echocardiography, particularly when used in association with a cross-sectional display. The peak rate of dimension increase is greatly reduced and the early diastolic filling period prolonged (Gibson et al, 1979). This reduced rate of outward motion of endocardium is due to a corresponding reduction in the rate of posterior wall thinning, which may be reduced to as low as 3–4 cm/s from a normal of 15–20 cm/s in children.

These changes in diastolic function may also occur in other conditions such as myotonic muscular dystrophy, diabetes associated with microangiopathy (Shapiro, 1982) and Friedreich's ataxia. They should probably be regarded as non-specific markers of disease. Their exact relation to limitation of exercise tolerance remains to be determined in children. In adults at least, their presence at rest is associated with loss of the normal adaptation of diastolic events associated with an increase in heart rate (Oldershaw et al, 1984).

Incoordinate relaxation

Incoordinate relaxation results from regional variation in the timing of the termination of systole in different parts of the ventricle. Tension persisting in affected areas leads to premature outward motion elsewhere, thus causing changes in cavity shape during the period of isovolumic relaxation. Although the velocity of outward motion may be normal in all regions of the cavity, this movement is not synchronous, so that overall filling rate may be reduced. Incoordinate wall motion is common in patients with ventricular disease, including severe left ventricular hypertrophy, coronary arteriovenous fistula, and tricuspid atresia. It may result in these conditions from abnormal myocardial architecture or ventricular damage due possibly to ischaemia or prolonged hypoxia (Becker & Caruso, 1981). It is also the rule postoperatively, either as the result of myocardial damage during surgery or as a temporary phenomenon as the ventricle adapts to correction of a pressure or a volume load.

SUMMARY OF DIASTOLIC DISTURBANCES

Left ventricular relaxation and filling are complex. A number of different processes can be distinguished, which should be described separately, even though more than one may be present in an individual patient. Relaxation occurs within the myocardium as a result of metabolic activity. It is a time-related process, and can be regarded as a rate of change of wall stress. Although it is associated with a fall in pressure in the cavity, neither the time relations nor the constant of proportionality between the two is fixed. Incoordinate relaxation will not only prolong the duration of pressure fall but also, by causing a change in cavity shape at a time when volume is constant, will alter their relation. Quite separate from the changes in myocardial properties associated with relaxation are the effects of restoring forces. They can be thought of as storing potential energy within the myocardium from the preceding systole. Their dissipation may well contribute to negative pressures recorded in the ventricle early in diastole, as well as to the rapid phase of ventricular filling. Until recently, even their existence has been questioned. Even now their exact nature remains in doubt as does their involvement in disease. Abnormalities of ventricular filling are well documented, however, which may be assessed as a reduction in the peak rate of volume increase. A reduction in the peak rate of dimension increase is a related disturbance. The two are not identical. At constant rate of volume change, the corresponding rate of dimension change is inversely proportional to the square of transverse dimension. A large ventricle may thus have a reduced rate of dimension increase although its filling rate is entirely normal. In addition, dimension changes may occur in the absence of volume change before mitral valve opening if wall movement is incoordinate during the period of isovolumic relaxation. Rates of increase of transverse dimension should not therefore be referred to as 'filling' rates, still less as 'relaxation' rates. Viscous and inertial forces depend on filling rate. They must be taken into account when the diastolic properties of the ventricle are studied in the beating heart and not under equilibrium conditions. Quite separate from these disturbances are alterations in cavity compliance and myocardial elasticity. Neither of these are time-related and so are potentially independent of abnormalities in the rate of dimension change. It is frequently implied that there is a direct relation between cavity compliance and filling rate, such that a stiff ventricle invariably fills slowly. There is no evidence whatever to support this contention. The least compliant ventricles are those in which end-diastolic volume is increased and ejection fraction low and whose filling rate is within the normal range (Hammermeister & Warbasse, 1974). In addition, peak filling rate is registered at a time when ventricular pressure is falling rather than rising, so that it is not possible to speak of the ventricle having elastic properties at this time in the cardiac cycle. Finally, both ventricles are subject to external influences. Of these, the most important are the parietal pericardium and the other ventricle, the latter possibly mediated by abnormal septal position or movement. These disturbances must be identified in individual patients, and their effects separated from those of altered blood flow and viscosity, and from congenital abnormalities of structure of the heart itself.

ASSESSMENT OF VENTRICULAR FUNCTION IN CLINICAL PRACTICE

The very size of the literature on left ventricular function, and the multiplicity of 'indices' that have been described may make it difficult to decide how to investigate an individual case. It is essential to determine ventricular volumes at end-diastole and end-systole (and hence ejection fraction). This can be done by any of a number of imaging techniques, including contrast or nuclear ventriculography, echocardiography, recently introduced methods such as computerised tomographic scanning or magnetic resonance imaging. In spite of its physiological importance, cavity shape is less commonly assessed. Indeed, it is often simply assumed to be ellipsoidal. The relation between volume and surface area, however, is fundamental to understanding the interrelations between muscle and pump function. It would seem to deserve more study, particularly in view of the range of abnormalities seen in patients with congenital heart disease.

A striking feature of the normal ventricle is its coordinate motion. This aspect has been stressed since loss of coordination can mimic other types of systolic and diastolic disease. It is probably in this area that the most satisfactory definition of normality is currently to be found. The regional non-uniformity present in normal ventricles is characteristic, while the effects of pathological disorganisation cannot be counteracted by compensatory mechanisms such as increased sympathetic stimulation or other inotropic stimuli. Again, appropriate information can be obtained using contrast or nuclear angiography or echocardiography.

Some aspect of the velocity of contraction should also be measured in any patient in whom ventricular function is being assessed. The velocity of circumferential fibre shortening is simple to measure, but both it, and the peak fibre shortening are almost completely dependent on left ventricular cavity size. Alternatively, peak left ventricular ejection rate can be measured. This can be done either from the rate of fall of left ventricular volume, or from peak aortic blood flow velocity and cross-sectional area. Measurements of peak left ventricular dP/dt (or derived estimates of V_{max}) are now seldom undertaken. Loading conditions must be determined in detail if these measures of the velocity of contraction are to be used to give information about the behaviour of the myocardium itself. In addition, it is desirable to stress the response of the ventricle to a physiological stress such as exercise. Measurements of flow (such as stroke volume or cardiac output) are of little discriminating value taken on their own, but an attempt should be made to assess the intensity of the homeostatic mechanisms by which they are maintained. The end-systolic pressure-volume slope is theoretically unaffected by loading conditions. Its dependence on end-systolic volume, however, and the unknown effects of incoordination may make its interpretation difficult in patients with congenital heart disease.

Diastolic performance must also be assessed. This is particularly the case in ventricular hypertorphy, where it may become impaired at a time when systolic function is still intact. The process of relaxation can be assessed from determination of the time constant of pressure fall. A less satisfactory method is to determine the magnitude of peak negative dP/dt, provided that the volume of the ventricle remains constant at the time that the measurement is made. This assumption does not necessarily apply in the presence of a shunt or valvar regurgitation. The duration of isovolumic relaxation time depends not only on the properties of the myocardium itself but is also very sensitive to loading conditions, particularly end-diastolic pressure. These are relatively simple to determine, so that if end-diastolic aortic and left ventricular pressures are known, prolongation of isovolumic relaxation time may give useful information about early diastolic function. During rapid filling, one should determine peak filling rate, the duration of the rapid filling period and preferably investigate also the presence or absence of regional abnormalities of wall movement. Rapid filling is of considerable physiological significance when heart rate is high and so may potentially be a factor limiting exercise tolerance. The later mid-diastolic period of passive filling is studied at rest when the heart rate is low. Here the aim is to determine cavity stiffness and myocardial stress-strain relations along with the possible effects of filling of the opposite ventricle and of pericardial constraint. These can be supplemented from observation of pressure and volume during atrial systole.

It will not be necessary to collect all this information routinely, but long-term follow-up of increasing numbers of patients who have undergone anatomical 'correction' suggests that survival is frequently limited by ventricular disease. Such disease often becomes clinically apparent only in its late stages when no more than ineffective pharmacological palliation is available. If, as seems likely, impaired function is due to progressive loss of organisation rather than to some specific, acquired abnormality, it will be irreversible. In this case, it cannot be 'cured' but only prevented. Prevention presupposes a clear understanding of the genesis and natural history of ventricular disease. This in turn can only come from careful documentation of its appearance at the earliest possible stage, analysis of its nature in individual patients and follow-up over many years using methods with a clearly defined physical basis.

REFERENCES

Becker A E, Caruso G 1981 Congenital heart disease – a morphologist's view on myocardial dysfunction. In: Becker A E, Losekoot T G, Marcelletti C, Anderson R H (eds) Paediatric Cardiology, Vol 3. Churchill Livingstone, London, p 307–323

Bennett D H, Evans D W, Raj M V J 1975 Echocardiographic left ventricular dimensions in pressure and volume overload: their use in assessing aortic stenosis. British Heart Journal 37: 971–977

Borow K M, Propper R, Bierman F Z, Grady S, Inati A 1982 The left ventricular end-systolic pressure-dimension relation in patients with thalassemia major. Circulation 66: 980–985

Borow K M, Arensman F W, Webb C, Radley-Smith R, Yacoub M H 1982 Assessment of left ventricular contractile state after anatomic correction of transposition of the great arteries. Circulation 69: 106–112

Botvinick E, Dunn R, Frais M, et al 1982 The phase image: its relationship to patterns of contraction and conduction. Circulation 65: 551–560

Bourlon F, Fouron J-C, Battle-Diaz J, Ducharme G, Davignon A 1980 Relation between isovolumic relaxation period of left ventricle and pulmonary artery pressure in d-transposition of the great arteries. British Heart Journal 43: 226–231

Braunwald E, Ross J Jr 1963 The ventricular end-diastolic pressure: appraisal of its value in the recognition of ventricular failure in man. American Journal of Medicine 34:147

Braunwald E, Ross J Jr, Sonnenblick E H 1967 Mechanisms of contraction in the normal and failing heart. New England Journal of Medicine 277:1012

Burger H J, Zaret B L 1981 Nuclear cardiology. New England Journal of Medicine 305: 855–865

Chen W, Gibson D G 1979 Relation of isovolumic relaxation to left ventricular wall movement in man. British Heart Journal 42: 51–56

Colan S D, Borow K M, Gamble W J, Sanders S P 1983 Effects of enhanced afterload (methoxamine) and contractile state (dobutamine) on left ventricular late-systolic wall stress-dimension ratio. American Journal of Cardiology 52: 1304–1309

Curtiss E I, Matthews R G, Shaver J A 1975 Mechanism of normal splitting of the second heart sound. Circulation 51: 157–164

Dodge H T, Sandler H, Baxley W A, Hawley R R 1966 Usefulness and limitations of radiographic methods for determining left ventricular volume. American Journal of Cardiology 18: 10–24

Dumesnil J G, Shoucri R M, Laurenceau J-L, Turcot J 1979 A mathematical model of the dynamic geometry of the intact left ventricle and its application to clinical data. Circulation 59: 1024–1034

Eber L M, Greenberg H M, Cooke J M, Gorlin R 1969 Dynamic changes in left ventricular free wall thickness in the human heart. Circulation 39: 455–466

Falsetti H L, Mates R E, Grant C, Greene D G, Bunnell I L 1970 Left ventricular wall stress calculated from one-plane cineangiography. An approach to force-velocity analysis in man. Circulation Research 26: 71–83

Fester A, Samet P 1974 Passive elasticity of the human left ventricle. The 'parallel elastic element'. Circulation 50: 609–618

Field B J, Baxley W A, Russel R O, et al 1973 Left ventricular function and hypertrophy in cardiomyopathy with depressed ejection fraction. Circulation 47: 1022–1030

Ford L E 1976 Heart size. Circulation Research 39: 297–303

Gaasch W H 1979 Left ventricular wall thickness ratio. American Journal of Cardiology 43: 1189–1193

Gaasch W H, Cole J S, Quinones M A, Alexander J K 1975 Dynamic determinants of left ventricular pressure-volume relations in man. Circulation 51: 317–323

Gamble W H, Shaver J A, Alvares R F, Salerni R, Reddy P S 1983 A critical appraisal of diastolic time intervals as a measure of relaxation in left ventricular hypertrophy. Circulation 68: 76–87

Gibson D G, Traill T A, Hall R J C, Brown D J 1979 Echocardiographic features of secondary left ventricular hypertrophy. British Heart Journal 41: 54–59

Gleason W L, Braunwald E 1962 Studies on the first derivative of the ventricular pressure pulse in man. Journal of Clinical Investigation 41: 80–96

Graham T P, Jarmanaki M M, Canent R V Jr, Capp M P, Spach M S 1968 Characterization of left heart volumes and mass in normal children and in infants with intrinsic myocardial disease. Circulation 38: 826–837

Graham T P, Jarmanaki J J M, Canent R V Jr, Morrow M N 1971 Left heart volume estimation in infancy and childhood. Circulation 43: 895–904

Graham T P, Jarmakani J M, Atwood G F, Canent R V Jr 1973 Right ventricular volume determinations in children. Normal values and observations with volume or pressure overload. Circulation 47: 144–153

Grant R P 1953 Architectonics of the heart. American Heart Journal 46: 405–431

Greenbaum R A, Gibson D G 1981 Regional non-uniformity of left ventricular wall movement in man. British Heart Journal 45: 29–34

Greenbaum R A, Ho S Y, Gibson D G, Becker A E, Anderson R H 1981 Left ventricular fibre architecture in man. British Heart Journal 45: 248–263

Grossman W, McLaurin L P 1976 Diastolic properties of the left ventricle. Annals of Internal Medicine 84: 316–326

Grossman W, Stefadouros M A, McLaurin L P, Rolett E L, Young D T 1973 Quantitative assessment of left ventricular stiffness in man. Circulation 37: 567–574

Haendchen R V, Wyatt H L, Maurer G, et al 1983 Quantitation of regional cardiac function by two dimensional echocardiography. I. Contraction patterns in the normal ventricle. Circulation 67: 1234–1245

Hammermeister K E, Brooks R C, Warbasse J R 1974 The rate of change of left ventricular volume in man. I. Validation and peak systolic ejection rate in health and disease. Circulation Research 49: 729–738

Hammermeister K E, Warbasse J R 1974 The rate of change of left ventricular volume in man. II. Diastolic events in health and disease. Circulation 49: 739–747

Heintzen P H, Moldenhauer K, Lange P E 1974 Three-dimensional computerized contraction pattern analysis. European Journal of Cardiology 1: 229–239

Henry W L, Ware J, Gardin J M, Hepner S I, McKay J, Weiner M 1978 Echocardiographic measurements in normal subjects. Growth related changes that occur between infancy and early adulthood. Circulation 57: 278–285

Herman M V, Gorlin R 1969 Implications of left ventricular asynergy. American Journal of Cardiology 23: 538–547

Hood W P, Rackley C E, Rolett E L 1968 Wall stress in the normal and hypertrophied human left ventricle. American Journal of Cardiology 22: 550–558

Janz R F, Grimm A F 1972 Finite element model for the mechanical behavior of the left ventricle. Prediction of deformation in the potassium-arrested rat heart. Circulation Research 30: 244–252

Karliner J S, Gault J H, Eckberg D, Mullins C B, Ross Jr J 1971 Mean velocity of fiber shortening. A simplified measure of left ventricular myocardial contractility. Circulation 44: 323–333

Kaye H H, Tynan M, Hunter S 1975 Validity of echocardiographic estimates of left ventricular size and performance in children. British Heart Journal 37: 371–375

Krayenbuhl H P, Bussman W D, Turina M, Luthy E 1968 Is ejection fraction an index of myocardial contractility? Cardiology 53: 1–12

Kurtz D, Ahnberg D S, Freed M, LaFarge C G, Trevers S 1976 Quantitative radionuclide angiocardiography. Determination of left ventricular ejection fraction in children. British Heart Journal 38: 966–973

Levin A R, Boineau J P, Spach M S, Canent R V, Capp M P, Anderson P A W 1966 Ventricular pressure-flow dynamics in tetralogy of Fallot. Circulation 34: 4–13

Levin A R, Spach M S, Canent R V, Boineau J P 1970 Dynamics of interatrial shunting in children with obstruction of tricuspid and pulmonary valves. Circulation 41: 503–512

Lewis R P, Boudalas H, Forester W F, Weissler A M 1977 A critical review of systolic time intervals. Circulation 56: 146–158

Linzbach A J 1960 Heart failure from the point of view of quantitative anatomy. American Journal of Cardiology 5: 370–382

Logan Sinclair R B, Oldershaw P J, Gibson D G 1983 Computing in Echocardiography. Progress in Cardiovascular diseases 25: 465–486

Ludbrook P A, Byrne J D, McKnight R C 1979 Influence of right ventricular hemodynamics on left ventricular diastolic pressure-volume relations in man. Circulation 59: 21–31

McKay R G, Aroesty J M, Heller G V, et al 1984 Left ventricular pressure-volume diagrams and end-systolic pressure-volume relations in human beings. Journal of the American College of Cardiology 3: 301–312

Marier D L, Gibson D G 1980 Limitations of two frame method for displaying regional left ventricular wall motion in man. British Heart Journal 44: 555–559

Marsh J D, Green L H, Wynne J, Cohn P F, Grossman W 1979 Left ventricular end-systolic pressure-dimension and stress-length relations in normal human subjects. American Journal of Cardiology 44: 1311–1317

Mason D T 1969 Usefulness and limitations of the rate of rise of intraventricular pressure (dp/dt) in the evaluation of myocardial contractility. American Journal of Cardiology 25: 516–527

Mehmel H C, Stockins B, Ruffmann K, von Olshausen K, Schuler G, Kubler W 1981 The linearity of the end-systolic pressure-volume relationship in man and its sensitivity for assessment of left ventricular function. Circulation 63: 1216–1222

Mercier J C, DiSessa T G, Jarmanaki J M, et al 1982 Two-dimensional echocardiographic assessment of left ventricular volumes and ejection fraction in children. Circulation 65: 962–969

Mirsky I 1976 Assessment of passive elastic stiffness of cardiac muscle: Mathematical concepts, physiologic and clinical considerations, direction of future research. Progress in Cardiovascular Diseases 18: 277–308

Mirsky I, Parmley W W 1973 Assessment of passive elastic stiffness for isolated heart muscle and the intact heart. Circulation Research 33: 233–243

Mitchell J H, Wildenthal K, Mullins C B 1969 Geometrical studies of the left ventricle utilizing biplane cinefluorography. Federation Proceedings 28: 1334–1338

Noble M I M 1972 Editorial: problems concerning the application of muscle mechanics to the determination of the contractile state of the heart. Circulation 45: 252–254

Noble M I M 1977 The diastolic viscous properties of cat papillary muscle. Circulation Research 40: 288–292

Oldershaw P J, Dawkins K D, Ward D E, Gibson D G 1983 Effect of exercise on left ventricular filling in left ventricular hypertrophy. British Heart Journal 49: 568–573

Paraskos J A, Grossman W, Soltz S, Dalen J E, Dexter L 1971 A noninvasive technique for the determination of the velocity of circumferential fiber shortening in man. Circulation Research 29: 610–618

Patterson S W, Piper H, Starling E H 1914 The regulation of the heart beat. Journal of Physiology 48: 465–573

Pollack G H 1970 Maximum velocity as an index of contractility in cardiac muscle. A critical evaluation. Circulation Research 26: 111–127

Pouleur H, Karliner J S, LeWinter M, Covell J 1979 Diastolic viscous properties of the left ventricle. Circulation Research 45: 410–419

Prakash R 1978 Determination of right ventricular wall thickness in systole and diastole. Echocardiographic and necropsy correlations in 32 patients. British Heart Journal 40: 1257–1261

Rackley C E, Dodge H T, Coble Y D, Hay R E 1964 A method for determining left ventricular mass in man. Circulation 29: 666–679

Rackley C E, Hood Jr W P, Rolett E L, Young D T 1970 Left ventricular end-diastolic pressure in chronic heart disease. American Journal of Medicine 48: 6–14

Rahimtoola S H 1973 Left ventricular end-diastolic and filling pressures in assessment of left ventricular function. Chest 63: 858–862

Roelandt J, Gibson D G 1980 Recommendations for standardization of measurements from M-mode echocardiograms. European Heart Journal 1: 375–378

Rogé C L L, Silverman N H, Hart P A, Ray R M 1978 Cardiac structure growth pattern determined by echocardiography. Circulation 57: 285–290

Ross Jr J, Linhart J W, Braunwald E 1965 Effects of changing heart rate in man by electrical stimulation of the right atrium. Circulation 32: 549–558

Sagawa K 1981 Editorial: The end-systolic pressure-volume relation of the ventricle: definition, modifications and clinical use. Circulation 63: 1223–1227

Sahn D J 1977 A dual M-mode system for simultaneous time-motion analyses of cardiac structure and evaluation of cardiac function. In: Bom N (ed) Echocardiology. Martinus Nijhoff, The Hague, p 83–93

Sahn D J, DeMaria A, Kisslo J, Weyman A 1978 Recommendations regarding quantitation in M-mode echocardiography. Results of a survey of echocardiographic measurements. Circulation 58: 1072–1083

Saito A, Ueda K, Nakano K 1981 Right ventricular volume determination by two dimensional echocardiography. Journal of Cardiography 11: 1159–1168

Sallin E A 1969 Fiber orientation and ejection fraction in the human left ventricle. Biophysics Journal 9: 954–964

Sandler H, Alderman E 1974 Determination of left ventricular size and shape. Circulation Research 34: 1–8

Shapiro E, Marier D L, St John Sutton M G, Gibson D G 1980 Regional non-uniformity of wall dynamics in the normal left ventricle. British Heart Journal 45: 1264–270

Shapiro L M 1982 Echocardiographic features of impaired ventricular function in diabetes. British Heart Journal 47: 439–444

Silverman N H, Ports T A, Snider A R, Schiller N B, Carlsson E, Heilbron D C 1980 Determination of left ventricular volume in children: echocardiographic and angiographic comparisons. Circulation 62: 548–557

Sjogren A L, Hytonen I, Frick M H 1970 Ultrasonic measurement of left ventricular wall thickness. Chest 57: 37–43

Smiseth O A, Frais M A, Kingma I, Smith E R, Tyberg J V 1985 Assessment of pericardial constraint in dogs. Circulation 71: 158–164

Somerville J 1979 Congenital heart disease – changes in form and function. British Heart Journal 41: 1–22

Sonnenblick E H, Braunwald E, Morrow A G 1965 Instantaneous force-velocity determinants in the contraction of heart muscle. Circulation Research 16: 441–453

Spencer M P, Greiss F C 1962 Dynamics of ventricular ejection. Circulation Research 10: 274–279

Streeter D D, Hanna W T 1973a Engineering mechanics for successive states in canine left ventricular myocardium. Circulation Research 33: 639–655

Streeter D D, Hanna W T 1973b Engineering mechanics for successive states in canine left ventricular myocardium. II. Fiber angle and sarcomere length. Circulation Research 33: 656–664

Thompson D S, Waldron C B, Coltart D J, Jenkins B S, Webb-Peploe M M 1983a Estimation of time constant of left ventricular relaxation. British Heart Journal 49: 250–258

Thompson D S, Wilmshurst P, Juul S M, Jenkins B S, Coltart D J, Webb-Peploe M M 1983b Pressure-derived indices of left ventricular isovolumic relaxation in patients with hypertrophic cardiomyopathy. British Heart Journal 49: 259–267

Troy B L, Pombo J, Rackley C E 1972 Measurement of left ventricular wall thickness by echocardiography. Circulation 45: 602–611

Vassallo D V, Pollack G H 1982 The force-velocity relation and stepwise shortening in cardiac muscle. Circulation Research 51: 37–42

Venco A, Saviotti M, Besana D, Finardi G, Lanzi G 1978 Noninvasive assessment of left ventricular function in myotonic muscular dystrophy. British Heart Journal 40: 1262–1266

Weiss J L, Fredericksen J W, Weisfeldt M L 1976 Hemodynamic determinants of the time-course of fall in canine left ventricular pressure. Journal of Clinical Investigation 58: 751–760

Weissler A M, Harris L C, White G D 1963 Left ventricular ejection time index in man. Journal of Applied Physiology 18: 919–931

Wiggers C J 1921 Studies on the duration of the consecutive phases of the cardiac cycle. I. The duration of the consecutive phases of the cardiac cycle and criteria for their precise determination. American Journal of Physiology 56: 415–438

Yagihara T, Kitamura S, Nakano et al 1981 Determination of right ventricular volume by sub-xiphoid two dimensional echocardiography. Journal of Cardiography 11: 1263–1272

Yin F C P 1981 Ventricular wall stress. Circulation Research 49: 829–842

General Clinical Topics

8

History and physical examination

Nowadays early detection of congenital heart disease is the rule. A definitive diagnosis is arrived at by one month of age in 70% of patients (Hoffman & Christianson, 1978). Indeed, this stage is reached in nearly half the patients by the age of one week. Thus, in many instances it is the medical and paramedical support personnel who notice something amiss, rather than the parents seeking medical advice for problems they have encountered. This means that the burden of recognition of affected infants is squarely on the shoulders of the professionals. The signs which direct attention towards the heart include tachypnoea, dyspnoea, poor feeding, abnormalities of weight gain and cyanosis. Although all of these can be manifestations of diseases other than those of the cardiovascular system, the possibility of heart disease must always be entertained. Whilst signs noted by professionals are of great importance, complaints by the parents of poor feeding, cyanosis or 'funny turns' must never be ignored.

HISTORY

In many instances, the advice of the paediatric cardiologist is sought because a murmur has been detected at a routine medical examination. Here the history serves to assist in the assessment of the significance of the murmur to the presence of structural or functional heart disease (see Ch. 41), in ascertaining the functional status of the patient who has heart disease, in the uncovering of any aetiological factors and in establishing any genetic predisposition that might influence counselling and management.

Since many children have few (if any) symptoms, history-taking in the paediatric cardiology clinic frequently comes to resemble an interrogation rather than a medical interview. This must be guarded against. Parents and children must be given time and encouraged to ask questions and voice their concerns no matter how distant they may appear from the purely technical decisions that have to be made. Parents need time and 'space'. This is emphasised

by the observations that, with increasing familiarity with both the cardiac unit and the child's disease, parents ask more questions and obtain longer interviews (Silverman, 1983; Silverman et al, 1984). Thus, whilst a check list of questions has to be worked through, this must be done with sympathy and interested attention on the part of the physician.

Specific questions must include the ability of a baby to take feeds. A good guide is the length of time taken over a feed. A normal baby takes most feeds in 10–20 minutes. Poor feeding with accompanying breathlessness is frequently seen in patients with large left-to-right shunts. Together with direct questioning about feeding, parents must be asked about the rate of respiration and any apparent difficulty with breathing. It is foolhardy to ignore the parents' report of rapid breathing – and more so the report of difficult breathing – yet this is often done.

Whilst breathlessness or tachypnoea are important, tiredness is rarely a symptom of heart disease. Rather it indicates anxiety on the part of the child. This, of course, may be related to his response to the management of his heart condition.

Cyanosis must also be asked about. Parents frequently do not notice mild cyanosis if it is present continuously. It is important to direct their attention to this possibility. It must then be remembered that many normal children are noted to have blue lips or hands and feet on occasions, particularly in the bath or swimming pool. Such episodic peripheral cyanosis is rarely, if ever, of cardiac significance.

Syncope, although rarely of cardiac origin, must be asked about, particularly when assessing the functional state of patients with aortic stenosis, hypertrophic cardiomyopathy, pulmonary stenosis or arrhythmias. The fact that a child has fainted does not indicate a high likelihood of the presence of congenital heart disease. A child with congenital heart disease who faints, however, may be at risk of developing severe if not fatal consequences. Details of this type of 'spell' are important so as to differentiate syncope from epilepsy. In the case of tetralogy of Fallot they must be distinguished from 'cyanotic spells' as an indication for surgery.

Always remember that the history may be in error. For example, parents of children with a simple atrial septal defect having no preoperative symptoms frequently report a great improvement after surgery. Enquiries related to aetiology must include details of untoward events during pregnancy. The taking of drugs or excess alcohol or the occurrence of infections in the early months are particularly important. A complete family history must be taken to provide adequate genetic counselling (see Ch. 2). Although in many cases the history is entirely negative, failure to take it in a complete manner significantly limits the standard of care given to the child and its family.

PHYSICAL EXAMINATION

As far as possible, the physical examination should be carried out in a warm, quiet and congenial environment. The temptation immediately to reach for the stethoscope must be resisted. Inspection, particularly in the case of young infants and newborns, is of paramount importance for diagnosis. Infants are usually examined as they lie flat whilst older children should be sitting at 45 degrees. This is to facilitate inspection of the jugular venous pressure and pulse.

Inspection

An overall impression of the general health of the child is obtained. Is the state of nutrition good? The presence or absence of cyanosis, often best assessed by examining the finger- and toenail beds, is ascertained. At the same time, finger and toe clubbing is looked for. Tachypnoea and dyspnoea, although obvious, must consciously be sought since they are often missed or more probably disregarded. Subcostal, intercostal and supraclavicular recession are present with dyspnoea. The accessory muscles of respiration may be in use. Harrison's sulcus (observed by a general practitioner, Edward Harrison, from the English county of Lincolnshire) is a transverse depression passing laterally from the xiphisternum to the mid-axillary lines. Initially discerned following rickets, it is now more frequently seen in patients with chronic dyspnoea.

Apart from features bearing directly on the cardiovascular system, attention must be given to appearances which indicate recognisable syndromes of malformation known to be associated with cardiac lesions. In many instances it will be recognition of such a syndrome that has brought the heart into question. Thus, chromosomal anomalies like Down's syndrome, or those genetically determined like the Ulrich-Noonan syndrome, will be obvious. It is always important, however, to ascertain

personally that the patient's appearance is normal. If this is not done, entities such as William's syndrome and the asymmetric cry or cardiofacial syndromes may be missed.

Inspection of the jugular venous pulse is rarely of value in infants since, with their short necks, little of value can be seen. It should not be ignored, however, since marked venous and arterial pulsations in the neck may provide the only evidence for an intracranial arterio-venous malformation (given that such a lesion were large enough to cause congestive cardiac failure). In older children, examination of the neck normally reveals three segments to each pulse, the 'a', the 'c' and the 'v' waves. The 'a' wave coincides with atrial systole, the 'v' wave with atrial filling during the latter part of the ventricular systole, whilst the 'c' wave is transmitted arterial pulsation during ventricular systole. The 'a' wave is followed by the 'x' descent which continues after the 'c' wave. The 'v' wave is followed by the 'y' descent as the atrioventricular valves open with the onset of ventricular diastole. The 'a' wave is accentuated in the presence of severe right ventricular hypertrophy or right atrial hypertrophy with tricuspid atresia. In the presence of severe right atrioventricular valve regurgitation, a systolic wave incorporating the 'v' wave will be easily seen. With heart block, intermittent 'cannon waves' will be seen when the right atrium contracts against a closed right atrioventricular valve. With congestive cardiac failure the overall jugular venous pressure will be elevated, whilst restricted filling of the heart (as in constrictive pericarditis) and overall high venous pressure are accompanied by deep and jerky 'x' and 'y' descents. Cardiac tamponade is evidenced by increasing venous pressure on inspiration (Kussmaul sign). Hepatojugular reflux is of little significance except where caval vein obstruction is suspected, for example after venous redirection operations for complete transposition (see Ch. 34). Here presence of the hepatojugular reflux is reassuring.

Palpation

Although the information obtained from palpation (or auscultation) must be systematised and complete, the approach to the child and strategies used to achieve this information are varied. They depend both on the personality of the child (and the family) and that of the clinician. The experienced paediatric cardiologist may at times be able to examine the child while talking to its parents. This can be almost before the child has realised he is being examined. To this end distraction is always better than coercion. In all patients the pulses should be examined in both upper and lower limbs. The carotids or superficial temporals should also be palpated. Important signs include absent or weak femoral pulses with normal or increased upper limb pulses. These indicate coarctation of the aorta. If, in addition to absent lower limb pulses, the left or right arm pulses are weak or absent, the most likely reason is anomalous origin of the corresponding subclavian artery. But interruption of the aortic arch, particularly in young infants, must be excluded. The combination of increased carotid or temporal artery pulsations with absent limb pulsations is uncommon but may be found. It occurs either with large cerebral arterio-venous fistulae; a left aortic arch interrupted distal to the left common carotid artery in presence of an anomalous right subclavian artery; or with an interrupted right arch distal to the right subclavian co-existing with an anomalous left subclavian artery (Sharratt et al, 1979).

Qualitative abnormalities in the pulses are more difficult to assess. High volume pulses are found with persistent patency of the arterial duct. In the premature baby they are the major diagnostic sign of this condition. Pulses of similar character even amounting to collapsing pulses are seen with other causes of rapid aortic run-off, for example aortic regurgitation or ruptured aneurysm of the sinus of Valsalva. As the arterial duct closes, weak pulses become evident in newborns with aortic atresia. In infants with severe aortic stenosis, weak or absent pulses, rather than the classical slow rising pulse, are of diagnostic importance. Palpation of the carotid pulse (and also the suprasternal notch) will reveal a systolic thrill with aortic stenosis or with bicuspid aortic valve. In the latter case the thrill is very delicate and can be obliterated by finger pressure. Irregularities of the pulse will be noticed during arrhythmias. The analysis of the arterial and venous pulses can give assistance in their elucidation. Electrocardiographic analysis, however, is better.

The apex beat should be localised on palpation of the precordium. It is defined as the further and lowest point at which the cardiac impulse moves the examining finger. Its recognition provides a clinical impression of cardiac size, although this is more reliably determined from the chest radiograph. The character of the cardiac impulse gives further information. A parasternal heave indicates right ventricular hypertrophy. Especially in infants such palpation is superior to the radiograph in differentiating between left, right, and combined ventricular hypertrophy. Thrills during the cardiac cycle are detected by palpation with the flat hand using the metacarpal heads as low frequency sensors. Accurate timing should be by the apex beat and is rarely a problem. Further information includes palpation of a loud (pulmonary component) to the second heart sound in the presence of severe pulmonary vascular disease. A palpable second heart sound (aortic) may also be found in any malformation with an anteriorly placed aorta.

Measurements of the blood pressure should be part of the physical examination of patients of all ages. Technical difficulties in performing this test have been largely overcome by the introduction of Doppler shift detection of either arterial flow or wall motion. In this simplest form, an ultrasound Doppler probe is placed over the radial or posterior tibial artery whilst a cuff of appropriate size is deflated. The onset of detection of arterial blood flow indicates accurately the systolic blood pressure (Elseed et al, 1973). This simple and relatively cheap technique supersedes the palpation and the flush methods. The later technical advances which employ Doppler detection of arterial wall motion are equally accurate and have the advantage of also giving a diastolic blood pressure (Savage et al, 1979), although the accuracy of the latter has previously been doubted (Whyte et al, 1975). It must then be remembered that, in young infants, the blood pressure may be 10–20 mmHg higher in the upper limbs (de Swiet et al, 1974). This is presumed to be related to the relatively narrow aortic isthmus in the neonate and young infant. Further information concerning the measurement and significance of blood pressure is given in Chapter 55.

Auscultation

This must be carried out in a quiet warm room with a warm stethoscope of a size appropriate to the child. Because of the small radius of curvature of the infant chest, a stethoscope with a small diaphragm is essential to ensure even application. The bell size is less critical. Low pitched sounds are best heard with the lightly applied bell whilst high pitched sounds are ideally auscultated with the diaphragm. An early diastolic murmur may only be audible with the diaphragm. The best overall performance, if a compromise is necessary, is obtained using the bell and varying the pressure of application. Such a compromise may be needed with a restless or uncooperative child when auscultation is needed urgently. If a child is uncooperative, it is best not to fight, but perhaps to accept only a limited examination to gain his confidence. In certain circumstances, particularly if the electrocardiogram and chest radiograph are normal, a return visit at a later date may be the only answer.

Auscultation must be performed systematically. The whole precordium and the lung fields must be listened to. In addition, auscultation of the neck should be performed, though bruits in the neck are so common in small children that they must be interpreted with extreme caution. Over the precordium both the bell and the diaphragm must be used in all areas. The key to successful auscultation is the identification of systole and diastole. Usually systole is audibly shorter than diastole. Thus the interval between the first and second heart sounds is shorter than that following the second sound up to the first sound again. Furthermore, splitting of the second heart sound is more easily appreciated than that of the first sound and, when present, helps to define the phases of the cardiac cycle.

The sequence in which the areas of precordium are examined is a matter of personal preference. We ourselves begin in the second left intercostal space and progress along the left sternal edge and define the phases of cardiac cycle as discussed above. Then, in order, the apex, the second right intercostal space and the neck are examined. Finally, the lung fields are examined using the bell of the stethoscope. In each site the first and second heart sounds are evaluated for intensity and splitting, and systole and diastole are listened to for additional heart sounds and for murmurs.

When examining children unable to stand and sit it is important to place them in different postures. When they can sit, it is often easier to identify splitting of the second heart sound with the child sitting on the examining couch. One diagnostic criterion for judging a murmur to be normal is the extent of its variation in intensity with change of position. Since the clinical features are the most important diagnostic criteria for the judgement of cardiac normality or abnormality (Newburger et al, 1983), auscultation must be carried out through several respiratory cycles before judgement is passed.

Heart sounds

The normal heart sounds are associated with atrioventricular and arterial valve closure. This is shown by simultaneous recording of the phonocardiogram, the electrocardiogram and the echocardiogram. The exact mechanism of their production is not definitely known (see Zuberbuhler, 1981, for review). The greater the energy being applied to close the valves, however, the louder are the sounds. Thus aortic closure is normally louder than pulmonary closure, and mitral louder than tricuspid closure.

The first heart sound

This is usually heard as a single sound. It is heard over the whole precordium but is loudest at the apex. Variations in its intensity are related to the energy of closure. Thus, in mitral stenosis when left atrial pressure is high, the mitral valve does not close until the left ventricular pressure has risen significantly. Closure is then late and loud. When left ventricular contractility is high, as in anxious patients or with exercise, the sound will again be loud. Conversely, when left ventricular contractility is low (as in congestive cardiomyopathy) the first sound is soft. If the valve leaflets are partially closed before the onset of ventricular systole, the sound is soft. This is the case in severe aortic regurgitation when the regurgitant jet is tending to close the valve. Similarly when the PR interval is long and atrial systole is completed early, the valve leaflets will have drifted towards the closed position before the left ventricular pressure rises. The first sound will then be soft. Conversely when the PR interval is short, atrial systole tends to keep the valve leaflets open until well into the rapid rise of left ventricular pressure, and the first sound is loud. A soft first heart sound is heard in the

presence of left bundle branch block because this is associated with a slow rise of left ventricular pressure (Thompson et al, 1975). Alternating loud and soft first heart sounds are heard with 'pulsus alternans' (Sakamoto et al, 1966). Variable intensity of the first heart sound is found with complete atrioventricular block, reflecting a variable PR interval.

Splitting of the first heart sound is rarely heard in normal children but may on rare occasions be heard in the presence of right bundle branch block. Loud and delayed closure of the tricuspid valve is associated with the heart sound heard in Ebstein's anomaly (Fontana & Wooley, 1972). It is related to sudden arrest of the excessive motion of the anterior leaflet of the deformed valve (see Ch. 30).

On occasions it is the tricuspid component which is the dominant sound in a single first heart sound. This is the case in complete transposition and in some cases of atrial septal defect. It will always be tricuspid or right atrioventricular valve closure which is heard in cases with 'mitral' atresia. In all these latter conditions, other features will point to the diagnosis and the tricuspid origin of the first heart sound will be inferred after the diagnosis is known.

The second heart sound

In the normal subject it is more correct to speak of the second heart *sounds*. They coincide with arterial valve closure. Aortic closure is louder than pulmonary closure and is usually earlier. This is particularly so during inspiration. In expiration the two closure sounds are usually so close in timing that only one sound is heard. This sequence of increased temporal separation (splitting) of the two closure sounds with inspiration is in small part due to earlier aortic closure but in the main is due to delayed pulmonary closure. The accepted explanation of this respiratory variation in splitting of the second heart sound is as follows. During inspiration negative intrathoracic pressure augments systemic venous return to the right heart with consequent prolongation of right ventricular systole and delay of pulmonary valve closure. At the same time increased lung volume slightly slows pulmonary venous return to the left atrium so that aortic closure occurs a little earlier. During expiration, right-sided venous return is diminished whilst pulmonary venous return is augmented. The ejection times of both ventricles become similar and the valves close more synchronously. The maximal splitting of the second heart sound is of the order of 20–30 milliseconds in inspiration. The normal second heart sound thus exhibits variable splitting. Absence of this implies that the second heart sound is abnormal. Time and again in a teaching session one is told that the second sound is normal. But, to the question, 'Can you split the second heart sound?' the answer is negative. If the second heart sound is split, it must be possible to ascertain whether the first or second component is louder.

Wide splitting with normal respiratory variation is heard in pulmonary stenosis and with right bundle branch block. Fixed splitting is heard in atrial septal defect. This describes the lack of temporal variation of the aortic and pulmonary sounds to each other during the respiratory cycle. During expiration the wide split is maintained by prolongation of right ventricular systole because of the left-to-right shunt. During inspiration the increased systemic venous return maintains the prolonged right ventricular systole and is associated with the decrease of blood flow from left to right atrium. The net result is absence of the normal respiratory variation, although the times between the first heart sound and the two components of the second sound do vary with respiration (Leatham, 1954).

Paradoxical splitting (greater separation of the two heart sounds in expiration than in inspiration) usually results from prolongation of left ventricular systole to such an extent that aortic closure is later than pulmonary closure during expiration. Increase in duration of right ventricular systole during inspiration delays pulmonary closure so that the temporal separation of the components is lessened or abolished. This is a rare physical sign and is heard occasionally with left bundle branch block, sometimes when left ventricular function is poor, but more frequently with aortic stenosis, when it indicates that the stenosis is very severe. Exceedingly rarely, paradoxical splitting of the second heart sound is due to early closure of the pulmonary valve as may occur with the Wolff-Parkinson-White syndrome (Zuberbuhler & Bauersfeld, 1965).

This simple approach to splitting of the second heart sound and its variations is adequate for a working understanding. Explaining variations in the timing of closure of the arterial valves in terms of variations in the duration of ventricular systole, themselves due to variations in stroke volume or in ventricular electrical activation, may be too simple. The timing of arterial valve closure is also affected by the impedance in the vascular bed distal to the valve. When impedance is high the dichrotic notch of the arterial pressure is almost superimposed on the descending limb of the ventricular pressure. If impedance is low then the dichrotic notch is later than the corresponding point on the descending ventricular pressure curve (Shaver et al, 1975). This delay has the endearing name 'hang out'. 'Hang out' of pulmonary closure is increased when the pulmonary trunk is dilated with resulting wide splitting of the second heart sound. Conditions associated with wide splitting include mild pulmonary stenosis and atrial septal defect. In both these conditions the pulmonary trunk is frequently dilated. This concept may explain why pulmonary closure is delayed in mild pulmonary stenosis when the mechanical duration of systole would not of itself be a sufficient explanation.

A further observation confirming the role of impedance in the timing of valve closure has been made in the case of pulmonary vascular disease. Here dilation of the pulmonary trunk accompanies high impedance in the pulmonary circuit. This is associated with little pulmonary 'hang out'. Delay in pulmonary closure only occurs when right ventricular systole is prolonged due to right dysfunction. In this case wide splitting of the second heart sound is a bad prognostic sign. A single second heart sound is also heard when there is only one functioning arterial valve, although some cases of common arterial trunk are said to have split second sounds. One explanation for this may be that the sounds heard are in part related to rapid deceleration of two columns of blood returning back from the pulmonary and systemic circulations when the truncal valve moves back to close. This finding, if true, gives some credence to the view that the heart sounds originate from rapid deceleration of blood, rather than from closure of the valves themselves. A single sound may also exist when one component is so soft as to be inaudible. It is usually the pulmonary component which is diminished in intensity as in severe pulmonary stenosis. Only one sound will be appreciated when closure of one valve is very loud and closure of the other is soft. Thus in any heart when the aorta is anterior to the pulmonary trunk (as in complete transposition) the close proximity of aortic closure renders it very loud, even palpable, whilst the posterior position of the softer pulmonary component renders it inaudible. A single second sound will also be heard when both aortic and pulmonary components coincide, as may rarely be the case in the presence of pulmonary vascular disease.

The loudness of the components of the second heart sound depends on their proximity to the stethoscope and to the energy of closure. As stated, a loud aortic component is heard when the aorta is anterior, and in systemic hypertension. This concept can also be used in the evaluation of the pulmonary component of the second heart sound. Splitting is normally heard at the left sternal edge because the pulmonary valve is closer to the stethoscope than is the normally situated aortic valve. In contrast, when listening at the apex the two valves are approximately equidistant from the stethoscope. Thus pulmonary closure of normal intensity will usually not be heard. When splitting of the second heart sound is heard at the apex, it is suggestive of a loud pulmonary component. The latter event occurs only when diastolic pressure is elevated as in pulmonary vascular disease.

The third heart sound

This is heard in early diastole. It is due to rapid filling of the ventricle and is usually heard best at the apex when the sound originates in the left ventricle. It is a normal finding in children. When it is associated with congestive cardiac failure the usual coexistent tachycardia renders the term 'gallop rhythm' appropriate. A third heart sound originating in the left ventricle does not vary with respiration. When it originates in the right ventricle, it may increase in intensity during inspiration. The differentiation of right from left ventricular gallop rhythms may be important in the clinical evaluation of older children with rheumatic mitral valve disease (see Ch. 50). In this situation a left ventricular gallop rhythm suggests predominant mitral regurgitation whilst a right ventricular gallop rhythm is heard in mitral stenosis with pulmonary hypertension. By itself a third heart sound does not indicate heart disease in childhood.

The fourth heart sound

This sound is heard in late systole. It is related to ventricular filling in atrial systole and implies a stiff ventricle, usually the left ventricle. It is never heard in normal children. Indeed, it is rarely heard in children at all. When it is, it is usually in the setting of hypertrophic cardiomyopathy.

Additional heart sounds

Ejection clicks

High pitched sharp sounds, known as 'ejection clicks', are heard in early systole with abnormal arterial valves, usually stenotic ones. In pulmonary valve stenosis the click is best heard in the second or third left intercostal space at the left sternal edge and may increase in intensity on expiration. In aortic valve stenosis, particularly with bicuspid aortic valve, the ejection click is heard best at the apex and the lower left sternal edge. Clicks can also be heard when either arterial trunk is dilated even though its valve is not stenosed. Such sounds originate from the aorta in pulmonary atresia, from the dilated pulmonary trunk in some patients with pulmonary vascular disease and from a common arterial trunk. A mid-systolic click is heard at the lower left sternal edge and at the apex when there is prolapse of the mitral valve during systole. It is usually accompanied by a late systolic murmur. The click appears to be generated by the billowing leaflet of the mitral valve (Barlow et al, 1963).

Additional diastolic sounds

Apart from third and fourth heart sounds the only diastolic additional sounds are opening snaps originating from a stenosed mitral or, more rarely, tricuspid valve. The mitral opening snap is high pitched and heard best at the apex. The closer it is to the second heart sound, the more severe the stenosis. An opening snap indicates significant stenosis but with a mobile valve. In Ebstein's anomaly, opening sounds may originate from the flail-like abnormal anterosuperior leaflet. These may be heard maximally at the lower sternal border or at the apex.

Murmurs

The precise mechanisms which result in a cardiac murmur are a matter of debate. Whether they are due to turbulence or vortex shedding, they occur when flow is disordered. Zuberbuhler (1981) has suggested for simplicity's sake that this disordered flow be called 'turbulence'. This is how the term is used in this chapter.

Turbulence of sufficient degree to be audible depends in part on the velocity of blood flow and on the geometry of the lumen through which it is flowing. Gradients of pressure are detected across lumens where turbulence becomes audible. These gradients may be obvious such as those seen with arterial valve stenosis. Small instantaneous pressure gradients have been demonstrated across normal aortic and pulmonary valves in the normal heart (Murgo et al, 1975). These early systolic gradients are more pronounced in the pulmonary trunk than the aorta. Increased velocity of flow occurs with exercise, fever, anxiety, and so on. Thus the innocent systolic murmur may well be due to accentuation of the normal early systolic gradient across the pulmonary valve (see Ch. 41). Description of murmurs is best systematised under the headings of loudness, timing and character, location and radiation, and, finally, variation with change in position or with respiration.

Loudness. This is conventionally divided into six grades. Grade I is a murmur so soft that it is only heard with concentration. Such murmurs are frequently not heard by inexperienced and non-specialised examiners. Grade II is soft, but immediately audible. Grade III is a loud murmur without a thrill. Grade IV is a loud murmur with a thrill. Grade V is a murmur audible with the stethoscope tilted so that only part of its circumference is in contact with the chest. Grade VI is the loudest and can be heard with the stethoscope held just above the chest but not in contact with it. Loudness is conventionally noted as, for example, grade IV/VI.

Timing and character. Timing is described according to the phase of the cardiac cycle. Basically murmurs are systolic, diastolic or continuous. The latter is defined as a murmur starting in systole then continuing through the second heart sound. It does not have to be heard throughout the whole of systole and diastole (see Ch. 41). Systolic and diastolic murmurs when of brief duration may be identified as early, mid or late in that phase of the cycle.

Systolic murmurs are basically of two types: ejection and pan-systolic. With the ejection murmur there is audible variation of loudness giving a crescendo-diminuendo pattern. The pan-systolic murmur, in contrast, starts with the first heart sound and by definition occupies the whole of systole with no audible variation in its loudness. The systolic murmur of some small ventricular septal defects starts with the first sound but finishes before the second sound. This is neither ejection nor truly pan-systolic, and is best described fully. Ejection murmurs generally originate in the ventricular outflow tracts, the arterial valves or the main arterial trunks. For example, an ejection systolic murmur is typical of subvalvar, valvar and of supravalvar aortic stenosis (see Ch. 40). Pan-systolic murmurs are heard with ventricular septal defect and atrioventricular valve regurgitation. Mid to late systolic murmurs, maximal at the apex, often with a mid-systolic click, indicate regurgitation through a prolapsed mitral leaflet. Occasionally the term 'holosystolic' is used to describe a murmur. This indicates indecision on the part of the physician, rather as the term 'bass-baritone' often indicates indecision in the description of a singer.

Diastolic murmurs, when early, usually diminish in intensity after the second sound. Early diastolic murmurs are due to arterial valve regurgitation. Mid-diastolic murmurs are usually crescendo-diminuendo in character. They are due either to high flow across the mitral or tricuspid valve or to stenosis of either or both of these valves. When the mitral valve is the origin of the murmur, it is best heard at the apex, often with the patient tilted to the left side. Tricuspid origin is indicated by the parasternal site of the murmur. The mid-diastolic murmur as heard with mitral stenosis during sinus rhythm may exhibit presystolic accentuation and crescendos up to the first heart sound.

A continuous murmur is classically maximal in intensity at about the time of second heart sound and has minimum intensity at around the first sound. When heard under the left clavicle it usually indicates persistent patency of the arterial duct. When heard over the lung fields, it may be due to systemic-to-pulmonary collateral arteries, to pulmonary arterio-venous malformation or to multiple peripheral pulmonary stenoses. When heard over the precordium, a coronary arterio-venous malformation must be considered. These murmurs must be differentiated from the innocent venous hum. This is done by moving the head of the patient from left to right and by assessing the extreme variation in loudness with changing position. The venous hum is the one murmur usually best heard with the patient standing up. Murmurs due to the collateral circulation in coarctation of the aorta are also continuous run-off from the arterial to the venous circuits. They are usually limited to the scapular area (see Ch. 45).

The character of the murmur includes variations in its loudness and sometimes an estimation of its pitch, which should be limited to differentiating high from low. In general, describing the pitch is of limited value in the diagnosis of the cause of the murmur. In the case of continuous murmurs, that originating from the arterial duct tends to be of lower pitch than those with other origins.

Location. The location of maximal intensity is described by reference to the sternum, the left and right sternal borders, the rib spaces and by proximity to the apex of the heart. In shorthand terms, the left second interspace at the sternal edge is known as the 'pulmonary area' and the second interspace at the right sternal edge is called the 'aortic area'. The use of such terms is to be discouraged, as false inferences are all too easily drawn, especially with complex congenital heart disease. We do not make reference to mitral or tricuspid areas. The location of murmurs heard in other areas (such as the subclavicular murmur of the arterial duct) are described in detail. Radiation of a murmur is usually to the lung fields, to the neck or to the axilla.

Aortic systolic murmurs are generally best heard in the second right intercostal space and radiate to the neck. Pulmonary systolic murmurs are maximal in the second left intercostal space and radiate to the lung fields. At the left sternal edge are heard the murmurs of a ventricular septal defect, the early diastolic murmur of arterial valve regurgitation and murmurs originating from the tricuspid valve. Mitral murmurs are heard at the apex, that of mitral regurgitation generally radiating to the axilla.

Variation in intensity with changing position has been discussed in relation to innocent murmurs. The murmur of aortic regurgitation may only be heard when the patient is sitting up and leaning forward with the breath held in expiration. Similarly, the murmur of mitral stenosis may only be heard with the patient supine and tilted to the left. Variation in intensity of a murmur during the respiratory cycle is said to differentiate pulmonary from aortic regurgitation. Such a respiratory variation is rarely detected in childhood. Additional noises with respiratory variation which are difficult to time tend to be extracardiac sounds such as a pericardiac friction rub or the clicking noises heard with a pneumopericardium.

The systematic examination of the cardiovascular system together with careful history-taking will frequently lead to the correct diagnosis. It is certainly the most important aspect of the differentiation of innocent from pathological murmurs. At the very least such a careful approach will make the choice of investigations logical and economic. But attention must not be focused solely on the heart. Careful enquiry and examination should be made to exclude associated congenital malformations. When appropriate, the signs of intercurrent illness (such as pneumonia, urinary tract infection or infective endocarditis) must be sought. Systemic diseases with cardiac involvement must all be borne in mind. These aspects are beyond the scope of this chapter and will be dealt with elsewhere (see Ch. 53).

REFERENCES

Barlow J B, Pocock W A, Marchand P, Denny M 1963 The significance of late systolic murmur. American Heart Journal 66: 443–452
de Swiet M, Peto J, Shinebourne E A 1974 Difference between upper and lower limb blood pressure in normal neonates using Doppler technique. Archives of Diseases in Childhood 49: 734–735

Elseed A M, Shinebourne E A, Joseph M C 1973 Assessment of techniques for measurement of blood pressure in infants and children. Archives of Diseases in Childhood 48: 932–936

Fontana M E, Wooley C F 1972 Sail-sound in Ebstein's anomaly. Circulation 46: 155–164

Hoffman J I E, Christianson R 1978 Congenital heart disease in a cohort of 19 502 births with long-term follow-up. American Journal of Cardiology 42: 641–647

Leatham A 1954 Splitting of the first and second heart sounds. Lancet 2: 607–613

Murgo J P, Altobelli S A, Dorethy J F, Logsdon J R, McGranahan G M 1975 Normal ventricular ejection dynamics in man during rest and exercise. Physiologic principles of heart sounds and murmurs. American Heart Association Monograph No. 46. American Heart Association, New York, p 92–101

Newburger J W, Rosenthal A, Williams R G, Fellows K, Miettinen O S 1983 Noninvasive tests in the initial evaluation of heart murmurs in children. New England Journal of Medicine 308: 61–64

Sakamoto T, Kusukawa R, MacCanon D M, Luisada A A 1966 First heart sound amplitude in experimentally induced alternans. Diseases of the Chest 50: 470–475

Savage J M, Dillon M J, Taylor J F N 1979 Clinical evaluation and comparison of the Infrasonde, Arteriosonde and mercury sphygmomanometer in measurement of blood pressure in children. Archives of Diseases in Childhood 54: 184–189

Sharratt G P, Leanage R, Monro J O, Shinebourne E A 1979 Aortic arch interruption presenting with absence of all limb pulses. Archives of Diseases in Childhood 54: 49–53

Shaver J A, O'Toole J D, Curtiss E I, Thompson M E, Reddy P S, Leon D F 1975 Second heart sound: the role of altered greater and lesser circulation. Physiologic principles of heart sounds and murmurs. American Heart Association Monograph No. 46. American Heart Association, New York, p 58–73

Silverman D 1983 Family adaptation to congenital heart disease: adjusting to physical and moral realities. In: Anderson R M, Macartney F J, Shinebourne E A, Tynan M (eds) Paediatric cardiology, Vol 5. Churchill Livingstone, Edinburgh p 317–327

Silverman D, Hilliard R, Baruch G, Shinebourne E A 1984 Factors influencing parenteral participation in a paediatric cardiology outpatient clinic. International Journal of Cardiology 6: 689–695

Thompson M E, Shaver J A, Leon D F, Reddy P S, Leonard J J 1975 Pathodynamics of the first heart sound. Physiologic principles of heart sounds and murmurs. American Heart Association Monograph No. 46. American Heart Association, New York, p 8–18

Whyte R K, Elseed A M, Fraser C B, Shinebourne E A, de Swiet M 1975 Assessment of Doppler ultrasound to measure systolic blood pressure in infants and young children. Archives of Diseases in Childhood 50: 542–544

Zuberbuhler J R, Bauersfeld S R 1965 Paradoxical splitting of the second heart sound in the Wolff-Parkinson-White syndrome. American Heart Journal 70: 595–602

9

Clinical presentation of heart disease in infants and children

How or why does the child with congenital heart disease present to those responsible for primary medical care? It is to this question that this chapter is addressed. In addition, the basic steps necessary to place a cardiac anomaly into a diagnostic group will be considered. Later sections of the book cover the detailed findings in individual anomalies. In practice some of the detailed findings may be easier to elicit when the diagnosis is already known! Furthermore, few abnormal physical findings are found only in one condition. Hence a full and unequivocal segmental diagnosis can rarely be made on clinical examination alone. This is especially so in infancy. It is important for paediatricians to know which babies should be referred to a paediatric cardiological unit and the urgency with which that referral should be made. Despite the large number of congenital cardiac defects that exist alone or in combination, there are a limited number of physiological disturbances produced. By these, anatomical entities are recognised.

Congenital heart disease usually presents in infancy as cyanosis, heart failure or a combination of both. These modes of presentation will therefore first be considered in detail. In the latter part of the chapter we discuss other ways in which the infant or child with suspected congenital heart disease presents to the paediatrician.

CYANOSIS IN CONGENITAL HEART DISEASE

Since cyanosis is due to the presence of more than 5 g/dl circulating reduced haemoglobin, clinical detection depends both on the proportion of haemoglobin in arterial blood that is desaturated and on the total haemoglobin concentration. Thus when there is an arterial oxygen saturation of 60%, cyanosis will be detectable in a child with a haemoglobin concentration of more than 12.5 g/dl, but not if the haemoglobin concentration is below 10 g/dl. In the former case 40% of reduced haemoglobin would amount to at least 5.0 g/dl whereas in the latter 4.0 g/dl reduced haemoglobin is insufficient to be clinically detectable with certainty. Clinical assessment of cyanosis (or more specifi-

cally of arterial desaturation) is therefore inaccurate.

Many forms of cyanotic heart disease with a right-to-left shunt, but increased pulmonary blood flow (e.g. hearts with univentricular atrioventricular connexion or common arterial trunk) may achieve oxygen saturations at which cyanosis is undetectable. Furthermore, infants with 'acyanotic' cardiac anomalies may become cyanosed when heart failure or a chest infection is present. Similarly, primary lung disease may mimic cyanotic congenital heart disease, especially in the neonatal period when pulmonary vascular resistance is labile and right-to-left shunting may occur at ductal or foramen ovale level. Children with polycythaemia may appear cyanosed and reduced respiratory drive due to central nervous system depression may also result in cyanosis. Signification methaemoglobinaemia will also simulate cyanosis.

To resolve the question as to whether or not a patient has cyanotic congenital heart disease, 100% oxygen shoud be administered to the infant for 5–10 minutes. If (right) radial arterial blood samples are taken whilst oxygen administration continues, a P_{O_2} value of more than 250 mmHg effectively excludes cyanotic heart disease. Values of more than 160 mmHg make it unlikely (Jones et al, 1976). Failure of P_{O_2} to rise to this level is strongly suggestive of cyanotic heart disease, though it can also occur in severe lung disease, particularly respiratory distress syndrome, and in 'transitional circulation' (persistent fetal circulation).

As a single discriminant, radial artery blood gas sampling (when the patient's inspired oxygen concentration is high – $FiO_2 > 80\%$), is more useful than the electrocardiogram or chest X-ray in deciding if an infant has cyanotic rather than acyanotic congenital heart disease or lung disease (Warburton et al, 1981).

In the newborn, the arterial duct may persist or be potentially patent. If the pulmonary vascular resistance is elevated, for instance due to lung disease, there may be a right-to-left shunt through the duct resulting in lower body arterial desaturation. A low P_{O_2} in femoral arterial blood may thus reflect lung disease rather than cyanotic heart disease. For this reason, a radial artery sample is used. The right radial artery is preferred as its origin is normally furthest removed from the duct.

The majority of patients with lung parenchymal disease who remain desaturated despite high inspired oxygen concentrations will have obvious pulmonary abnormalities on the chest radiograph, such as the ground appearance of the lungs in hyaline membrane disease. A raised P_{CO_2} may be further evidence of primary lung disease. In this group a history of birth asphyxia, aspiration pneumonia, or for that matter prematurity may further suggest lung disease as a cause for cyanosis.

The lungs may appear normal in transitional circulation. This condition occurs in particular after perinatal asphyxia and/or when the patient is polycythaemic or the mother is diabetic. There is persistent pulmonary vascular vasoconstriction similar to that present in the fetus. If the arterial duct remains patent, blood shunts right-to-left through it. In addition, desaturated blood entering the right atrium from the inferior caval vein streams preferentially across the oval foramen to left atrium as occurs in the fetus. There is thus no sampling point for systemic arterial blood proximal to a right-to-left shunt despite the fact that the heart is structurally normal. The hyperoxia test will therefore fail to exclude 'cyanotic heart disease'.

Right-to-left shunting across an oval foramen in the absence of a structural cardiac abnormality may also follow transient myocardial ischaemia principally affecting the right ventricle. This produces functional tricuspid or even pulmonary incompetence (Rowe & Hoffman, 1972). Echocardiography can play a major part in assessing myocardial function in this situation. It also confirms normal intra-cardiac anatomy when cyanosis results from lung disease or from transitional (persistent fetal) circulation (see Ch. 5). Nonetheless, even in the best run centres, there may be a small number of blue neonates where non-invasive techniques fail to exclude with certainty a diagnosis of cyanotic heart disease. Cardiac catheterisation will then be necessary.

The term 'cyanotic congenital heart disease' is in our view most sensibly applied to those cardiac anomalies in which, because of the anatomy of the heart, some of the systemic venous return will inevitably reach the systemic circulation without passage through the lungs. Having stated this, however, cyanosis is produced in different ways in different groups of anomalies.

As always with congenital heart disease, different anomalies can coexist and complicate the haemodynamic disturbances produced by any single anomaly. Nonetheless cyanosis occurs principally under three major circumstances. The first is when obstructive lesions cause right-to-left shunting and reduce pulmonary blood flow. The second is in the presence of discordant ventriculo-arterial connexions (complete transposition) (or the very rare isolated discordant atrioventricular connexion). The final possibility is a common mixing situation.

In the case of the overtly cyanosed patient or of the infant who has (in our units' parlance) failed his nitrogen wash-out test (Jones et al, 1976), careful clinical examination must be the primary step in diagnosis. Nonetheless, the first major step in allocating patients to a particular diagnostic group is probably to decide on the basis of the chest radiograph whether they have reduced pulmonary vascular markings (pulmonary oligaemia) or normal to increased pulmonary vascular markings (pulmonary plethora).

Cyanotic heart disease presenting with radiographic evidence of pulmonary oligaemia

These patients will be blue because part or all of the systemic venous return is frustrated in its attempt directly to reach the lungs. Instead, it is shunted from the right side of the heart to the left, or at least away from the pulmonary circulation. For this to occur, in addition to obstruction to pulmonary blood flow, there must be a defect through which the right-to-left shunt can occur or alternatively a common chamber in which the systemic and pulmonary venous returns mix. The obstruction may be at right atrial outlet (tricuspid), infundibular or pulmonary valve level. More rarely, it may be within the body of the right ventricle or at peripheral pulmonary artery level. A very high pulmonary vascular resistance due to obstruction in the small pulmonary arterioles may also cause a reduction in pulmonary flow. Strictly speaking, however, any coexistent right-to-left shunting and cyanosis would then be due to pulmonary vascular disease rather than to the primary cardiac anomaly. The defect may be in the atrial septum, the ventricular septum or between the great arteries. Any obstructive right-sided lesion may produce cyanosis in the neonate since a patent oval foramen provides a route for right-to-left shunting.

Clinical differential diagnosis

If right ventricular outflow tract obstruction is complete (pulmonary atresia), pulmonary blood flow will be via a persistent arterial duct or by systemic-pulmonary collateral arteries. More specifically when a continuous murmur is maximal under the left clavicle on the same side as the aortic arch (demonstrated by the chest radiograph), a duct is the usual cause. If the continuous murmur is maximal in other sites, then systemic-pulmonary collateral arteries are the more likely finding, especially when loud and heard by all auscultators. Pulmonary atresia (with or without a ventricular septal defect) may be found with no murmurs (especially in the deeply cyanosed patient), both when pulmonary flow is markedly reduced and when there is polycythaemia and a high blood viscosity. An ejection systolic murmur maximal at the second left intercostal space is heard with mild or moderate pulmonary stenosis, but this disappears with increasing pulmonary outflow tract obstruction. This is particularly so when associated with a large ventricular septal defect or double inlet ventricle. In tetralogy of Fallot, where the obstruction to pulmonary flow is at infundibular level, the usual systolic murmur disappears during hypercyanotic spells due to infundibular spasm.

The presence of a pulmonary ejection click suggests that the ventricular septum is intact. By inference, right-to-left shunting can be presumed to occur at atrial level, although care must be taken to distinguish this from the aortic ejection click which may accompany tetralogy or pulmonary atresia with ventricular septal defect.

Pulmonary closure is not audible with severe stenosis or complete pulmonary outflow tract obstruction. The second sound is then single. Ebstein's or Uhl's anomaly, congenital tricuspid incompetence or a hypoplastic right ventricle should all be considered when the second sound is normal but there are cyanosis and decreased pulmonary vascular markings (Haworth et al, 1975).

A right aortic arch, especially if associated with a pulmonary artery bay (concave upper left cardiac border) and/or an enlarged ascending aorta, strongly suggests tetralogy of Fallot or pulmonary atresia with ventricular septal defect (see Ch. 32). If the pulmonary trunk is dilated in association with reduced pulmonary vascular markings, valvar pulmonary stenosis with right-to-left shunting at atrial level is probable (see Ch. 39). Auscultation will then be required to confirm that the findings are not those of severe pulmonary vascular disease. The pulmonary component of the second sound would be very loud in the latter situation.

In this group of patients with cyanotic heart disease and reduced pulmonary vascular markings, the electrocardiogram adds important diagnostic information. Evidence of right ventricular hypertrophy or dominance is found in the majority. Consequently the presence of left ventricular dominance is a particularly useful indicator of the probable diagnosis. Usually the right ventricle will be rudimentary (univentricular connexion to a left ventricle), absent (univentricular hearts of indeterminate type), or very small, e.g. pulmonary atresia with intact septum. In this group with cyanosis and left ventricular dominance a superior mean frontal QRS axis between 0° and −90° favours a univentricular atrioventricular connexion to a morphologically left ventricle. Perhaps the most distinctive electrocardiogram of all is that of classical tricuspid atresia where the combination of right atrial hypertrophy, left ventricular dominance (in particular a deep S wave in the right praecordial leads), and a superior mean frontal QRS axis is almost diagnostic (Neill & Brink, 1955). Even if

criteria for left ventricular hypertrophy are not present, similar inferences can be drawn from the findings of an adult R/S progression across the chest leads (i.e. dominant S V1 and dominant R V6) in a cyanosed patient.

As previously mentioned, left ventricular dominance on the electrocardiogram is also a feature of pulmonary atresia with intact septum (or for that matter critical pulmonary stenosis in the neonate; Miller et al, 1973). In these conditions the mean frontal QRS axis is usually inferior.

Once these patients have been referred from the paediatric unit to a specialised paediatric cardiology centre, cross-sectional echocardiography allows differentiation.

Cyanotic heart disease presenting with radiographic evidence of normal or increased pulmonary vascular markings

The entities in this group are complete transposition of the great arteries (the commonest causes of cyanotic heart disease in the newborn period) and common mixing situations. A 'common' mixing situation is that in which there is obligatory mixing of the pulmonary and systemic venous returns. The admixed blood is then distributed to both pulmonary and systemic arteries. Such mixing can occur at atrial, ventricular or great arterial level. Examples of the former are total anomalous pulmonary venous connexion and common atrium. In hearts with univentricular atrioventricular connexion or double outlet ventricles, mixing occurs at ventricular level, and in common arterial trunk, at arterial level. Although pulmonary plethora characterises the majority of common mixing situations, coexistent obstruction to pulmonary blood flow would produce oligaemic lung fields. Thus in double outlet right ventricle with pulmonary stenosis, oligaemia will be present despite the 'common' mixing situation.

Patients with 'common mixing' and increased pulmonary blood flow will tend to present with both cyanosis and heart failure, as will those with complete transposition complicated by a large ventricular septal defect or persistent arterial duct. Aortic atresia (hypoplastic left heart syndrome) is another example of a common mixing situation (see Ch. 31). In this group of conditions the clinical picture is dominated by a low cardiac output with pallor, systemic hypotension and metabolic acidosis.

Clinical differential diagnosis

Clinical differentiation is not always possible although the added use of cross-sectional echocardiography has considerably enhanced pre-catheter diagnosis. Complete transposition of the great arteries is the probable diagnosis if cyanosis is severe ($Po_2 < 30$mmHg in 100% oxygen). This anomaly alone is unlikely if the Po_2 rises above

50 mmHg (Jones et al, 1976). Extreme tachypnoea is a feature of pulmonary venous obstruction as in obstructed total anomalous pulmonary venous connexion or the hypoplastic left heart syndrome. Peripheral pulses are increased in the presence of a common arterial trunk, reduced in aortic atresia and are usually normal in the rest. Since many of the anomalies in this group will result in a split second heart sound with an accentuated pulmonary component, as well as a systolic murmur, auscultation is not particularly helpful in differential diagnosis. A continuous murmur, however, is occasionally heard in mitral atresia, being generated at a restrictive interatrial communication. It may also occasionally be heard with total anomalous pulmonary venous connexion, originating at a site of pressure drop within the anomalous channel. Incompetence of a common arterial valve (in common trunk) may produce systolic and early diastolic murmurs that merge to become continuous. A prominent ejection click is also the rule in this condition.

Cyanosis with increased pulmonary vascular markings on chest X-ray and *no* heart murmurs is most common in complete transposition. It is sometimes found with total anomalous pulmonary venous connexion. The 'characteristic' chest radiograph of complete transposition with its narrow pedicle and 'egg-shaped' heart is useful if present. Unfortunately it is not seen in the majority of patients (Counahan et al, 1973). A right aortic arch suggests a common arterial trunk but tetralogy of Fallot with pulmonary atresia and excessive pulmonary blood flow via systemic-pulmonary collateral arteries must also be considered. In the latter condition widespread continuous murmurs are usual and an abnormal vascular pattern may be seen on the chest radiograph (see Ch. 33). Pulmonary oedema (or at least upper lobe blood diversion) suggests obstructed total anomalous pulmonary venous connexion, especially if heart size is normal.

From the stance of the electrocardiogram, total anomalous pulmonary venous connexion tends to have the most marked right ventricular forces. Hearts with univentricular atrioventricular connexion to a left ventricle will have dominant left or posterior forces (plus or minus a superior mean frontal QRS axis). Plethora in the latter group would reflect absence of significant associated pulmonary stenosis. Most other anomalies in this group with cyanosis and radiographic evidence of pulmonary plethora tend to have biventricular or some degree of right ventricular hypertrophy.

HEART FAILURE

Heart failure most commonly presents as tachypnoea or dyspnoea at rest or on exercise. For a baby, this means on feeding. The mother may also notice subcostal recession, tachycardia or excessive sweating, especially if she has had a previous normal baby. Poor feeding in general and failure to thrive are also manifestations of chronic heart failure. Again the experienced mother will detect symptoms earlier than parents with their first child. Other frequent consequences of heart failure with pulmonary venous congestion and/or excessive pulmonary flow are recurrent chest infections. Respiratory infections in otherwise normal children are common, but evidence of underlying heart defects should be sought with recurrent or persistent infections. The radiological appearance of 'infection' may be pulmonary oedema! A chest infection may also give rise to cyanosis due to areas of lung being perfused with blood but not ventilated. Hence, in cyanosed children with suspected congenital heart disease, lung disease is the major differential diagnosis. Less frequent causes of tachypnoea are cerebral abnormalities and acidosis resulting from renal failure or other metabolic disorders.

Signs

Tachypnoea, tachycardia and hepatomegaly are the commonest signs of heart failure in infancy and childhood. Subcostal and even intercostal recession accompany tachypnoea, particularly in infants. This reflects reduced lung compliance (Fisk & Deal, 1970; Griffin et al, 1972; Phelan et al, 1972; Howlett, 1972). On inspiration, the soft tissues are sucked inwards rather than air passing easily into the lungs when a negative intrathoracic pressure is generated. Since the bronchial tree is of small calibre, further narrowing of the lumen by venous congestion of the mucosa or as a result of an increase in peribronchial fluid may lead to airways obstruction, diminished alveolar ventilation, and trapping of secretions. Expiratory or even inspiratory wheezing is therefore common and CO_2 retention may result (Talner et al, 1965). Similarly, bronchopneumonia and recurrent chest infections are common in infants with heart failure, as is difficulty in feeding due to breathlessness. Tachycardia with weak pulses, cold extremities, pallor and sweating reflect increased sympathetic activity, itself a consequence of a low or reduced cardiac output. Profound pallor can be particularly noticeable in long-standing left ventricular inflow or outflow tract obstruction. Fluid retention in infants and children usually expresses itself as hepatomegaly as well as an abnormal increase in weight. Peripheral oedema is the exception. Swollen ankles are more likely to suggest lymphoedema (as in Turner's syndrome) than heart failure. Occasionally peri-orbital oedema is seen in babies.

Acyanotic heart disease presenting with heart failure

In acyanotic congenital heart disease, three main groups of lesion are responsible. The first are obstructive 'left-sided lesions' which impede forward flow of blood into the systemic circuit. The second group consists of large communications between the systemic and pulmonary circulation resulting in left-to-right shunts and excessive pulmonary blood flow. The final group is constituted by intrinsic or extrinsic myocardial disease.

Other causes of heart failure to be considered in acyanotic infants are mitral or aortic incompetence, paroxysmal supraventriuclar tachycardia, arterio-venous fistulas, anaemia (haemolytic disease of the newborn), septicaemia and over-transfusion. Cyanotic congenital heart disease may also be accompanied by heart failure (see above). This can be excluded by arterial blood gas sampling in 100% oxygen (see p. 191).

The commonest cause of heart failure in acyanotic infants in the first week of life is aortic coarctation. Primary myocardial disease and aortic stenosis are less frequent causes in this period. Left ventricular dysfunction, however, may occur secondary to these obstructive left-sided lesions.

Patients with *dependent* left-to-right shunts (see p. 119), even with large defects and potentially large shunts, tend to present in heart failure after the first two weeks of life and up to the second month (Rudolph, 1965). Those with obligatory shunts may present earlier.

Clinical differential diagnosis

The diagnosis can be established clinically in many of these lesions. Thus, aortic coarctation is diagnosed from the discrepancy between upper and lower limb pulses or blood pressure. Palpation of femoral pulses is mandatory in the evaluation of all infants or children (especially of neonates in heart failure). Pressures should be measured if possible in both an upper and a lower limb using an ultrasonic Doppler technique. Decreased pulses can generally be seen in advanced heart failure of any aetiology. They are more characteristic of aortic stenosis and, to a lesser degree, of myocardial disease. Increased pulses in the acyanotic infant are most commonly due to persistent patency of the arterial duct. Except in the premature infant, this entity rarely causes heart failure during the first month. Very early heart failure with full pulses should therefore suggest a systemic arterio-venous fistula such as is associated with an aneurysm of the vein of Galen (see Ch. 41). In this condition the neck veins may be quite dilated. A pulsatile fontanelle and rapidly growing head circumference are other clues. Although discussed here as an acyanotic anomaly, an intra-cranial or arterio-venous fistula may cause cyanosis. This is because part of the huge systemic venous return crosses the oval foramen as right ventricular failure becomes worse (Rowe & Mehrizi, 1968).

After a month of age the most common cause of heart failure is increased pulmonary blood flow. This is usually the result of left-to-right shunting at ventricular (ventricular septal defect) or great artery level (persistent arterial duct, aortopulmonary window). The characteristic murmurs are discussed elsewhere (see Ch. 41). Shunting occurs at both atrial and ventricular levels with an atrioventricular septal defect and common atrioventricular valve orifice. Heart failure may then be aggravated by regurgitation through the common valve.

In infants with heart failure the chest radiograph typically shows cardiomegaly and often increased pulmonary vascular markings. Notable exceptions in the acyanotic group are mitral stenosis and supraventricular tachycardia. In each the chest radiograph may show pulmonary oedema in the absence of cardiomegaly. The pulmonary oedema of supraventricular tachycardia is probably due to impedance to left atrial emptying, induced by the *very* short diastolic filling period. Poor ventricular filling may be aggravated in the neonate by a high haemoglobin level and a consequent increase in blood viscosity. Conversely, heart failure from any cause may be exacerbated by anaemia.

In these acyanotic lesions, the electrocardiogram can be most helpful in differential diagnosis. Primary myocardial disease must always be considered if left sided T waves (V6, V7) are inverted. If the R waves in the same leads are very tall (>30 mm) then endocardial fibroelastosis (or more rarely hypertrophic cardiomyopathy) should be considered. Very low voltages suggest myocarditis.

A rare cardiac anomaly which produces heart failure in infancy is glycogen storage disease of the heart (Pompe's disease). The electrocardiogram typically shows a short PR interval and left ventricular hypertrophy with or without 'strain'. (Caddell & Whitemore, 1962; Gillette et al, 1974). Anomalous origin of the left coronary artery (see Ch. 44) is usually first suspected when an infarction pattern is seen on the electrocardiogram of an infant in heart failure. It should also be considered in an infant with otherwise unexplained heart failure who has left ventricular hypertrophy on the electrocardiogram.

A superior mean frontal QRS axis in an acyanotic infant with heart failure often indicates an atrioventricular septal defect. A common valve is usually present if there is marked right ventricular hypertrophy, while evidence of right ventricular hypertrophy is less when there are separate valve orifices. Other electrocardiographic findings are not so characteristic and will be dealt with under specific conditions.

PRESENTATION BECAUSE OF A HEART MURMUR

In older children, but also in many infants, congenital heart disease presents as a heart murmur detected on routine or incidental examination in an otherwise asymptomatic child (see Ch. 18). The differential diagnosis of heart murmurs in general and of continuous murmurs in particular are dealt with in Chapter 8 and Chapter 41 respectively. Not only may heart murmurs cause the child to be referred to a paediatric cardiologist but abnormal heart sounds or added sounds are sometimes the reason for referral. Perhaps the most dramatic is the very loud pulmonary component of the second sound in patients with a high pulmonary artery diastolic pressure. When pulmonary vascular disease is the cause, the second sound may be so accentuated as to be palpable while cyanosis may be additionally present. Isolated ejection clicks may be produced by a bicuspid aortic valve, idiopathic dilation of the pulmonary artery, or dilation of ascending aorta as in coarctation. Mid-systolic clicks from prolapsing mitral valves have been a cause of referral to our unit, as have the abnormal scratchy mid-systolic sounds produced by the tricuspid valve in Ebstein's anomaly.

PRESENTATION BECAUSE OF SHOCK

Cardiac malformations resulting in a hypoplastic ascending aorta, most commonly aortic atresia associated with the hypoplastic left heart syndrome (see Ch. 31), result in a low cardiac output. In this group survival is dependent on the arterial duct remaining widely open. The child deteriorates rapidly when the duct constricts, and dies when it finally closes. These patients therefore present as extremely ill, semi-comatose, shocked neonates. They are ashen grey in colour with peripheral cyanosis and cold extremities. Other consequences of the low cardiac output are oliguria or anuria and a profound metabolic acidosis.

PRESENTATION BECAUSE OF DEFICIENT PULSES

Absent or reduced femoral pulses detected on routine examination may be the first evidence of aortic coarctation (see Ch. 45). The child may be asymptomatic but, particularly in the neonatal period, breathlessness may be present due to heart failure. Urgent action may be needed in the symptomatic infant (see Ch. 45) to prevent further deterioration. Again this is because of possible dependence of lower body blood flow on ductal patency.

Reduced pulse volumes in all limbs may be a feature of severe aortic stenosis in the neonate. In this respect, the symptoms of critical aortic stenosis merge with those of the hypoplastic left heart syndrome. More commonly, reduced pulses are a non-specific feature of an ill infant whatever the cause, while very fast heart rates (greater than 250/min plus or minus breathlessness) suggest the possibility of paroxysmal supraventricular tachycardia.

PRESENTATION WITH UPPER OR LOWER AIRWAYS OBSTRUCTION

Other less common modes of presentation in infancy are inspiratory and expiratory stridor or rarely difficulty in swallowing ('dysphagia lusoria'). These symptoms may be caused by compression of the trachea or bronchi by vascular rings (see Ch. 46), anomalous origin of the aortic arch vessels, or rarely by a pulmonary vascular sling (see Ch. 46). Bronchi may also be partially or completely obstructed by compression from dilated pulmonary arteries in patients with excessive pulmonary blood flow (Stanger et al, 1969). This is especially produced by the grossly dilated proximal pulmonary arteries found in the absent pulmonary valve syndrome (see Ch. 32). Segmental or lobar collapse may occur. More dramatically, lobar emphysema may develop due to a ball valve effect where air passes into the bronchus during inspiration but is trapped when the bronchial cross-sectional area decreases during expiration. Most commonly the left upper lobe is affected due to compression of the hyparterial left upper lobe bronchus by the left pulmonary artery. Next in frequency is compression of the right-sided intermediate bronchus by the right pulmonary artery, Any bronchus may be involved at different times in the same patient.

FITS, FAINTS AND FUNNY TURNS

Episodic loss of consciousness in otherwise asymptomatic infants is one of the modes of presentation of tetralogy of Fallot in infancy (Shinebourne et al, 1975) (see Ch. 32). In the typical hypercyanotic attack or spell caused by infundibular shut-down (Wood, 1958) the patient is overtly blue, has other signs of cyanotic congenital heart disease such as clubbing, and often a well-documented history of increasing exercise intolerance. In infancy, however, whether or not a murmur has been previously documented, the parents, or for that matter their medical attendants, may not associate the heart with the loss of consciousness or fit. We have seen several patients extensively investigated for epilepsy and thought also to have a small ventricular septal defect who were examples of children with 'acyanotic' tetralogy undergoing episodes of acute severe infundibular spasm.

The relationship between cerebral events and cardiac arrhythmias is slowly being further understood. In reflex anoxic (or perhaps better described 'reflex asystolic') seizures (Stephenson, 1978), the fit or loss of consciousness is associated with transient asystole. The heart and its conduction system are normal, being affected as the end organ of a cerebral discharge mediated through the autonomic nervous system.

Transient loss of consciousness may be associated with

ventricular or supraventricular tachycardia or fibrillation. This would be an unusual mode of presentation for re-entry tachycardias associated with the Wolff- Parkinson White, Lown-Ganong-Levine or other pre-excitation syndromes. The long QT syndrome, however, may well present in this way as a consequence of ventricular fibrillation, torsade de pointes or ventricular tachycardia.

Syncope on exercise is a classical feature of severe aortic stenosis or any severe left ventricular outflow tract obstruction (or for that matter of any severe left ventricular muscle disease such as hypertrophic cardiomyopathy, whether or not it is obstructive). Again this symptom may not be mentioned by parents if their child is referred to a paediatric cardiologist. The loss of consciousness may not be connected to the heart murmur for which they may have been referred.

Palpitations are an unusual presenting symptom in young children. Older children, however, may volunteer the information that their heart 'misses a beat'. Much more common is a syncopal episode. Many children will have an episode of fainting at some time, especially in hot, stuffy, poorly ventilated surroundings. These events tend to occur in stressful or potentially stressful situations such as standing in a school assembly, attending a church service, or (more challenging to the body than soul) awaiting dental treatment or an injection. Older children and adolescents are the usual age-groups affected. If 24-hour tape recordings are performed it is important to realise that approximately half of all normal children will have episodes of junctional rhythm (Southall et al, 1981). Nine-tenths will have episodes of varying degrees of sinuatrial block (or at least an electrocardiographic pattern indistinguishable from sinuatrial block) (Southall et al, 1981; Dickinson & Scott, 1984). These normal findings are not directly associated with a vasovagal episode, nor are they an indication for a pacemaker!

CHEST PAIN

Episodes of screaming, pallor and sweating in neonates or young infants may be due to myocardial ischaemia when there is anomalous origin of a left coronary artery or severe aortic stenosis. The symptoms are analogous to angina pectoris. Classical angina pectoris – i.e. central chest pain on effort, perhaps radiating to the jaw or left arm, which disappears in about a minute on cessation of exercise – is extremely uncommon in paediatric practice. Both severe aortic stenosis (or, for that matter, severe pulmonary stenosis) may uncommonly present in this way.

Chest pain on inspiration nearly always has a respiratory cause (such as bronchitis or pleurisy) but can indicate pericarditis. The majority of other non-specific chest pains are non-cardiac.

ABNORMAL CHEST RADIOGRAPH IN AN ASYMPTOMATIC CHILD

Infants or older children may have a chest radiograph for many reasons not necessarily related directly to the heart. Examples would be because of a cough or chest infection, as part of routine screening at school entrance, as part of assessment after an accident and so on. This may then bring to light isolated cardiomegaly, or an abnormal 'cardiac contour'. In our experience many children referred in this way will have normal hearts, the apparent cardiomegaly being spurious and related to poor inspiration, a large thymus or both. It is not so easy to obtain films on full inspiration in young children, so that allowance must always be made for this. Optimally the anterior aspect of six ribs and the posterior aspect of ten should be seen above the diaphragm. If this is not so, the diaphragm appears to compress the heart from below. The transverse diameter of the heart is then increased. Pectus excavatum and other skeletal abnormalities will also do this, although scoliosis does not affect apparent heart size on a chest radiograph. The very best inspiratory films, however, with small narrow hearts, may result from air trapping and should suggest a diagnosis of asthma! The cardiac silhouette is enlarged on the chest radiograph in presence of a pericardial effusion, although the heart itself may well be of normal size. Other causes of isolated cardiomegaly include Ebstein's malformation of the tricuspid valve or giant right atrium. Congenital absence of the pericardium is rare (Southworth & Stevenson, 1938). In most congenital pericardial defects, only the left side is affected. If there is total absence of the left side of the pericardium, the heart is displaced to the left as well as being enlarged (Nasser, 1970). Cardiomyopathies may give rise to isolated cardiomegaly, although usually only enlargement of the ventricular shadow results. Pompe's disease (type II glycogen storage disease) is the exception, where massive cardiomegaly may result from accumulation of glycogen within heart muscle cells (Ehlers et al, 1962).

An abnormal cardiac contour apart from isolated cardiomegaly is an uncommon mode of presentation for haemodynamically important cardiac anomalies. Nonetheless, if seen, it may result from a wide variety of lesions. This is dealt with in more detail in Chapter 10, but in a paediatric practice the following are some of the possibilities.

The upper right cardiac border may have a bulge due to anomalous connexion of pulmonary veins, either total or partial, or to an azygos continuation of the inferior caval vein. A right aortic arch (or for that matter a double aortic arch or other vascular ring) may present in the same way either by displacing the right superior caval vein laterally, or by giving rise to an abnormal shadow itself. Right juxtaposition of atrial appendages can also cause an abnormal contour to the right upper or middle cardiac border. Dilation of the right atrium causing bulging of the right lower cardiac border may be a consequence of Ebstein's anomaly, of other congenital tricuspid valve anomalies, or of a giant right atrium. Cardiac tumours or pericardial cysts can cause a bulge or abnormal appearance of virtually any part of the cardiac shadow. They affect the left side more than the right. A dilated ascending aorta due to aneurysm or medial necrosis of the ascending aorta may cause an abnormal right-sided cardiac shadow, as would dilation of the aorta in previously undetected isolated aortic incompetence.

An abnormal appearance of the left upper cardiac border may result from a left superior caval vein, left juxtaposition of atrial appendages, total anomalous pulmonary venous connexion, or hemiazygos continuation of an inferior caval vein. Coarctation of the aorta can produce a so-called 'E sign'. The upper convexity represents a dilated aortic knob and left subclavian artery, and the lower convexity reflects post-stenotic dilatation (Figley, 1954). More frequently the aortic knob is obscured (Baron, 1971). Aortic aneurysms are very rare in children but cause a dilated aortic arch and knuckle. Pseudocoarctation of the aorta, with a dilated unfolded aorta common in atherosclerotic adults, can also be found in infants. This is possibly related to abnormal vascular architecture.

Dilation of the pulmonary trunk may represent idiopathic dilation but can also reflect increased pulmonary flow in an asymptomatic child with a previously unsuspected atrial septal defect. A murmur would usually have been previously detected in post-stenotic dilation of the pulmonary trunk accompanying pulmonary stenosis. Some patients referred with radiographic cardiomegaly may also turn out to have an atrial septal defect. Dilated proximal pulmonary arteries may reflect unsuspected pulmonary vascular disease or primary pulmonary hypertension.

As previously mentioned, a cardiomyopathy may cause generalised cardiomegaly. It may also cause left ventricular dilation with an abnormal bulging of the left lower cardiac border. When left ventricular dilation is due to conditions such as endocardial fibroelastosis there will usually be accompanying symptoms of tiredness and breathlessness on exertion. Abnormal left mid or lower cardiac border shadows can be found in asymptomatic patients with a cardiac tumour (such as a fibroma). They may also be produced by left ventricular diverticulum, hypertrophic cardiomyopathy, or pericardial defects or cysts.

Apart from an abnormal cardiac shadow, there are other abnormalities which may be detected on a chest radiograph in an asymptomatic child. These include rib notching due to aortic coarctation (see Ch. 45), isolated circular opacities suggesting pulmonary arteriovenous fistulas and abnormal vascular shadows in patients with pulmonary atresia, a ventricular septal defect and large abnormal systemic-pulmonary collaterals (Ch. 33).

The above account of clinical presentation is pertinent to the general paediatrician who has to decide which infant or child to refer to a paediatric cardiology unit. Once referred, however, specific anatomical diagnosis of the cardiac anomaly is relatively simple. In most patients, cross-sectional echocardiography will allow precise diagnosis non-invasively. The next few years will show the extent to which this and other non-invasive techniques (for example magnetic resonance) will negate the need for cardiac catheterisation and angiography and hence further reduce the risks involved in management of congenital heart disease.

REFERENCES

Baron M G 1971 Obscuration of the aortic knob in coarctation of the aorta. Circulation 43: 311–316

Caddell J L, Whitemore R 1962 Observations on generalized glycogenosis with emphasis on electrocardiographic changes. Pediatrics 29: 743–763

Counahan R, Simon G, Joseph M C 1973 The plain chest radiograph in d-transposition of the great arteries in the first month of life. Pediatric Radiology 1: 217–223

Dickinson D F, Scott O 1984 Ambulatory electrocardiographic monitoring in 100 healthy teenage boys. British Heart Journal 51: 179–183

Ehlers K H, Hagstrom J W C, Lukas D A, Redo S F, Engle M A 1962 Glycogen storage disease of the myocardium with obstruction to left ventricular outflow. Circulation 25: 96–109

Figley M M 1954 Accessory roentgen signs of coarctation of the aorta. Radiology 62: 671–686

Fisk G C, Deal C W 1970 Volume pressure relations of the lungs of children measured during thoracotomy. Australian Paediatric Journal 6: 203–212

Gillette P C, Nihill M R, Singer D B 1974 Electrophysiological mechanism of the short PR interval in Pompe disease. American Journal of Diseases of Children 128: 622–626

Griffin A J, Ferrara J D, Lax J C, Cassells D E 1972 Pulmonary compliance. An index of cardiovascular status in infancy. American Journal of Diseases of Children 123: 89–95

Haworth S G, Shinebourne E A, Miller G A H 1975 Right-to-left interatrial shunting with normal right ventricular pressure. A puzzling haemodynamic picture associated with some rare congenital malformations of the right ventricle and tricuspid valve. British Heart Journal 37: 386–391

Howlett G 1972 Lung mechanics in normal infants and infants with congenital heart disease. Archives of Disease in Childhood 47: 707–715

Jones R W A, Baumer J H, Joseph M C, Shinebourne E A 1976 Arterial oxygen tension and response to oxygen breathing in differential diagnosis of congenital heart disease in infancy. Archives of Disease in Childhood 51: 667–673

Miller G A H, Restifo M, Shinebourne E A, et al 1973 Pulmonary atresia with intact ventricular septum and critical pulmonary stenosis presenting in first month of life. Investigation and surgical results. British Heart Journal 35: 9–16

Nasser W K 1970 Congenital absence of the left pericardium. American Journal of Cardiology 26: 466–470

Neill C A, Brink A J 1955 Left axis deviation in tricuspid atresia and single ventricle: the electrocardiogram in 36 autopsied cases. Circulation 12: 612–619

Phelan P D, Gillam G L, Menahem S A, Coombs E, Venables A W 1972 Respiratory function in infants with a ventricular septal defect. Australian Paediatric Journal 8: 79–85

Rowe R D, Hoffman T 1972 Transient myocardial ischemia of the newborn infant: a form of severe cardiorespiratory distress in full-term infants. Journal of Pediatrics 81: 243–250

Rowe R, Mehrizi A 1968 The neonate with congenital heart disease. Saunders, Philadelphia, p 374

Rudolph A M 1965 The effects of postnatal circulatory adjustments in congenital heart disease. E. Mead Johnson Award Address, October 1964. Pediatrics 36: 763–772

Shinebourne E A, Anderson R H, Bowyer J J 1975 Variations in clinical presentation of Fallot's tetralogy in infancy. Angiographic and pathogenic implications. British Heart Journal 37: 946–955

Southall D P, Johnston F, Shinebourne E A, Johnston P G B 1981 24 hour electrocardiographic study of heart rate and rhythm patterns in population of healthy children. British Heart Journal 45: 281–291

Southworth H, Stevenson C S 1938 Congenital defects of pericardium. Archives of Internal Medicine (Chicago) 61: 223–240

Stanger P, Lucas Jr R V, Edwards J E 1969 Anatomic factors causing respiratory distress in acyanotic congenital heart disease: special reference to bronchial obstruction. Pediatrics 43: 760–769

Stephenson J P B 1978 Reflex anoxic seizures ('white breath-holding'): nonepileptic vagal attacks. Archives of Disease in Childhood 53: 193–200

Talner N S, Sanyal S K, Halloran K H, Gardner T H, Ordway N K 1965 Congestive heart failure in infancy. I. Anomalies in blood gases and acid-base equilibrium. Pediatrics 35: 20–26

Warburton D, Rehan M, Shinebourne E A 1981 Selective criteria for differential diagnosis of infants with symptoms of congenital heart disease. Archives of Disease in Childhood 56: 94–100

Wood P 1958 Attacks of deeper cyanosis and loss of consciousness (syncope) in Fallot's tetralogy. British Heart Journal 20: 282–285

Imaging the heart and chest

1. The chest radiograph
   A. Chrispin

2. Cardiac aspects of computerised tomographic scanning
   A. Chrispin

3. Paediatric nuclear cardiology
   E. J. Baker

4. Magnetic resonance imaging
   A. Chrispin

It was in 1895 that Roentgen discovered the medical application of X-rays and within a year the first untoward side-effects upon the skin had been observed. Since then more well known side-effects of radiation usage have been recognised. In 1973 the imaging potential of nuclear magnetic resonance became apparent with the pioneer work of Mansfield and Grannel in Britain and Lauterbur in North America. After being brought into use, and after many thousands of studies, it may be said that the technique of magnetic resonance imaging seems to be virtually devoid of hazard (Lancet, 1985). This chapter begins with the chest radiograph and concludes with magnetic resonance imaging and so covers the earliest and the latest of non-invasive investigations for heart disease in infants and children. Between lie certain cardiac aspects of computerised scanning and cardiac nuclear medicine.

1. THE CHEST RADIOGRAPH

The chest radiograph of patients who may have heart disease continues to be important because of the speed with which it can be taken and because of the information it may yield. Nevertheless, the findings on a chest radiograph must be set in the context of the clinical findings together with the information accruing from the electrocardiogram and echocardiography. With the advent of ultrasound studies, the value of the chest radiograph has increased rather than diminished. It is with this range of studies – the clinical evaluation, the chest radiograph, the electrocardiogram and echocardiographic examination – that increasing numbers of infants and children go forward to cardiac surgery. The invasive procedures of cardiac catheterisation and selective angiocardiography maintain their position in patients who may have a complicated type of cardiac defect. These major invasive diagnostic procedures are likely to decline further as the role of digital vascular imaging develops and clinical confidence is sustained. Injections of contrast medium show not only morphological abnormality but also altered patterns of blood flow within the heart and pulmonary circulation. Yet another imaging modality, nuclear magnetic resonance, has now appeared. The fact that it employs neither ionising radiation nor invasion should accelerate its development. The first part of this chapter, however, is primarily concerned with the plain chest radiograph, whose importance seems likely to endure (Kurlander et al, 1968; Elliot & Schiebler, 1979; Swischuk, 1979).

At the first examination an anteroposterior radiograph usually suffices. A lateral projection may also be important when stridor is present. It is on the latter view that the trachea is visible throughout its intrathoracic course and narrowing caused by a vascular ring may be detected. Oblique projections cannot be standardised in infants or children and are best avoided. If an oblique view is thought desirable, it is wise to undertake fluoroscopy, whereby the full range of oblique projections can be rapidly obtained. In this way the problem of possible pericardial effusion, disorders of left ventricular movement and postoperative aneurysms can be studied rapidly. In general, cardiac chamber size can be evaluated on the anteroposterior chest projection by inference from the cardiac contour. Left atrial size, bronchial arrangement (situs) and the size of the azygos vein (in either a congenital anomaly or when obstructed after intra-atrial repair for complete transposition) can all be evaluated on a high kilovoltage filtered beam radiograph (Deanfield et al, 1980). For this type of radiograph, as well as for the orthodox anteroposterior radiograph, a film exposed during a good inspiratory breath is essential.

Table 10.1 Features to be be determined.

Heart
Heart size
Heart configuration

Pulmonary features
Narrow pulmonary vessels
Large pulmonary vessels
Pulmonary vessels of intermediate size
Pulmonary venous hypertension ('upper zone diversion')
Pulmonary oedema
Miscellaneous

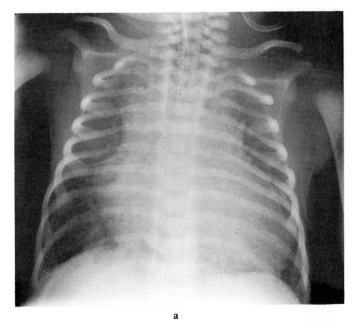

a

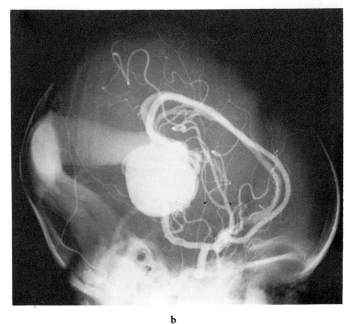

b

Fig. 10.1 This radiograph (a) illustrates cardiac failure due to high output caused by aneurysm of the vein of Galen (b). There is generalised cardiac enlargement affecting all chambers. The pulmonary vessels are not narrow. The horizontal fissure is prominent, there are perihilar line shadows and a little mottled shadowing caused by pulmonary oedema. The aneurysm of the vein of Galen which caused the high cardiac output is shown by angiography (see also Ch. 41).

In many texts, findings from the plain film are described under definitive diagnoses. Informative as this approach may be, when put to practical use, one simple fact soon becomes apparent. It is that patients very often do not have a definitive diagnosis at the time of radiography. What follows is an attempt to analyse the film evidence and deduce from it what is reasonable. It is imperative to avoid making too much of, or inferring too little from, what is seen. The features are considered in the sequence shown in Table 10.1 and summarised in further tables.

Heart size

Most people who pick up the chest radiograph of an infant or child suspected of having heart disease begin by looking at the overall heart size in relationship to the thorax. The transverse diameter of the heart of a normal young patient tends to be slightly in excess of half of the greatest transverse diameter of the chest as seen on an anteroposterior radiograph. If the chest is radiographed during the expiratory phase of respiration, then even a normal heart will have a diameter well in excess of half that of the chest. It follows that radiographs of the chest in full, or reasonably full, inspiration are required for assessment of heart size. Either for technical or clinical reasons, it is not always possible to obtain such inspiratory radiographs. The times when an adequate radiograph is not available, however, should be few. By using fluoroscopy, the heart size can be related to chest size during the various phases of respiration and any doubts about heart size resolved in this way.

When there is clinical evidence of a heart lesion and the heart is not large, it is likely that either the heart lesion is minor or the predominant problem is one of the heart working at increased pressure (especially increased right heart pressure, as in isolated pulmonary valve stenosis). Additionally, and especially in young infants with complete transposition, there may be very serious circulatory problems without much increase in heart size in the first day or two of life. Increases in heart size are a feature of either increased blood flow (Fig. 10.1) or heart failure, particularly left heart failure (Fig. 10.2). An increment in blood flow arises in a variety of ways. There may be a shunt from the physiologically left side of the heart to the

right side, as in persistent patency of the arterial duct, ventricular or atrial septal defect, or arteriovenous fistula (Hellenbrand et al, 1977). Incompetence of one or more valves leads to an increase of 'flow work' in the heart, because blood expelled from one chamber of the heart during systole returns to that chamber during its diastolic phase. For example, when the aortic valve is incompetent,

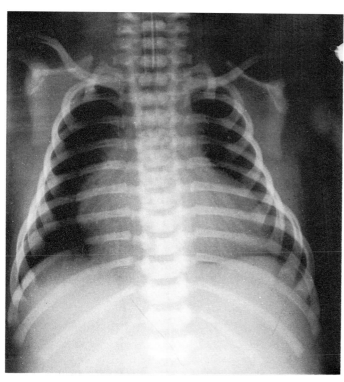

Fig. 10.2 Cardiac failure following circulatory collapse at birth. There is generalised cardiac enlargement affecting all chambers. The pulmonary vessels are narrow because of low output. There had been assisted ventilation via an endotracheal tube.

blood expelled into the aorta returns to the left ventricle during diastole and so left ventricular size increases. Further, if the tricuspid valve is incompetent, the right ventricle expels its content not only into a great artery but also through the incompetent tricuspid valve. Both the right ventricle and the right atrium increase in size because of the to-and-fro movement of blood through the incompetent tricuspid valve.

Heart failure affecting the left side of the heart generally produces an increase in heart size because of an increase in ventricular size. In lesions associated with obstruction of left ventricular output (such as aortic stenosis or coarctation in infants), there may also be a considerable degree of ventricular hypertrophy as well as an increase in ventricular size. Both these contribute to the increase in heart size as the ventricle fails. When the muscle of the ventricle is damaged by, say, endocardial fibroelastosis, viral myocarditis, subacute bacterial endocarditis, or rheumatic heart disease, then the ventricular size increases because of increased end-diastolic volume. In such disorders there is often a concomitant valve incompetence which adds to the problems of the heart and increases its size. A variety of the cardiomyopathies produce an increase in heart size. Two important types of ischaemia of the myocardium are associated with characteristic electrocardiographic patterns. One is caused by precipitate delivery and an ensuing shock

state. The other is due to anomalous coronary arterial supply (Askenazi & Nadas, 1975). In both instances the heart is large, often grossly so.

Increases in 'heart size' may also be apparent on chest radiographs when there is a pericardial effusion (either serous or purulent). Tamponade frequently develops in these circumstances as the heart increases in size. At fluoroscopy the cardiac movement is diminished by the effusion and there may be a differential density (Tehranzadeh & Kelly, 1979). Patients who have advanced constrictive pericarditis often have cardiac enlargement because of the myocardial damage which is also sustained. The major causes of increased heart size are summarised in Table 10.2.

Table 10.2 Summary of changes in heart size.

Heart minimally increased in size
— Pressure work heart as in pulmonary valve stenosis and hypertrophic cardiomyopathy
— Minor lesion which is haemodynamically insignificant
— Complete transposition in first days of life

Major increase in heart size
— Left-to-right shunt at atrial, ventricular or ductal level and any arteriovenous fistula – natural or man-made such as in Blalock shunt
— Valve incompetence – either atrioventricular or arterial because of to-and-fro blood movement
— Left ventricular failure as in coarctation in infancy, aortic valve stenosis, bacterial endocarditis, endocardial fibroelastosis, rheumatic fever and renovascular hypertension
— Pericardial effusion, be it serous, purulent or due to acid-fast bacillus infection in acute stage or in late stage constrictive pericarditis
— Miscellaneous cardiomyopathies, such as Friedreich's ataxia and Kawasaki's disease

Heart configuration

It is wise to be circumspect about information derived from study of the cardiac configuration on a plain chest radiograph. One reason for this attitude is that the cardiac borders in the infant and young child are partly obscured by the thymus. Indeed, it can be impossible to define the base of the heart and the position of the aorta in relationship to the trachea. Another reason is that, in congenital heart disease, a multiplicity of individual cardiac lesions often make up a definitive complex. Yet, at the moment in time when the plain radiograph is important, the knowledge and discrete evaluation of these individual lesions has to be obtained. Evaluating the configuration of the heart is a subjective exercise. Nevertheless, skill in this field increases quite rapidly when findings from angiocardiography and its definitive diagnosis are correlated with the preceding chest radiograph. What follows is a series of guidelines and no more. It is important not to speculate unduly and to avoid too much inference from uncertain features.

Ventricular enlargement

The apex lies to the left in the chest when the heart is normally located. Right ventricular enlargement results in the movement of the apex of the heart across the antero-posterior radiograph towards the lateral part of the chest. The degree to which the anterior margin lies in apposition to the sternum on the lateral chest radiograph is generally of little help in this assessment. This is because the thymus lies between the heart and the sternum.

When the left ventricle enlarges, the apex of the heart moves downwards and, to a lesser degree, also moves laterally across the chest. For this reason, when there is only right ventricular enlargement, the apex of the heart lies clear of the diaphragm. When there is solely left ventricular enlargement, the apex lies below or very close to the diaphragamatic contour (Fig. 10.3).

Changes in convexity of the contour around the cardiac apex are implicit as the position of the apex changes. In many common congenital heart lesions, such as ventricular septal defect, there is an increase in size of both ventricles. Displacement of the apex is then both lateral and downward as the heart increases in size.

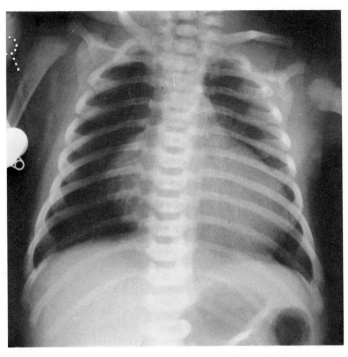

Fig. 10.4 Cardiac failure 12 h after birth due to isolated pulmonary valve stenosis with a closed arterial duct. The heart is large. The right atrial margin lying to the right of the spine is unduly prominent and convex because of right atrial enlargement. The apex of the heart is well clear of the diaphragm on this film taken in deep inspiration. The pulmonary vessels are narrow.

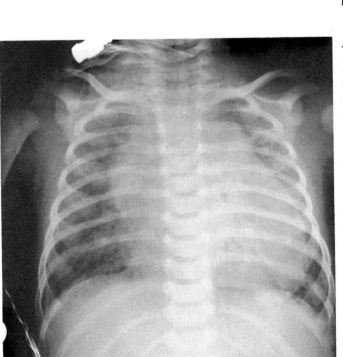

Fig. 10.3 Cardiac failure 1 week after birth due to coarctation of the aorta. The apex of the large heart is low and there is no prominence of the right atrial contour. The pulmonary vessels cannot be identified in the right perihilar region because of pulmonary oedema which highlights the air content seen end-on in three bronchi. The periphery of the lungs is clear and the diaphragmatic and cardiac contours are easily defined.

Atrial enlargement

Right atrial enlargement (Fig. 10.4) is assessed by looking for an increase in the convexity of the margin of the heart lying to the right of the sternum. As this chamber enlarges, so the distance between the most lateral part of the cardiac contour and the midline increases. The margin of the left atrium can sometimes be identified on the anteroposterior chest radiograph as a second shadow lying within the margin of the right atrium. Indeed, the margin of a normal left atrium can often be identified on radiographs of asthmatic children. Left atrial enlargement characteristically opens up the carinal angle by elevating the left main bronchus. Rarely the left atrium enlarges to such a degree and at such a pressure (as in endocardial fibroelastosis) that the left main bronchus is narrowed. Air is then trapped inside, or else there is some collapse of, the left lung. The posterior margin of the left atrium can be identified as an impression on the barium-filled oeso-phagus. In practice, it is rarely necessary to carry out a barium swallow with a lateral projection. Should it be necessary, it is important to remember that the left atrial impression is often quite prominent in normal young children and infants. Massive left atrial enlargement, as, for example, in serious lesions of the mitral valve, may displace the oesophagus not only posteriorly but also laterally.

Pulmonary infundibulum

The subpulmonary infundibulum may enlarge in pulmonary valve stenosis when there is post-stenotic dilatation and when there is a large pulmonary blood flow as in an atrial septal defect. When the pulmonary trunk lies behind the ascending aorta, the shadow of the base of the heart is narrow. This occurs in simple complete transposition to produce the classic (but relatively uncommon) 'egg on the side' cardiac silhouette.

Aortic arch

It may not be possible to see on which side of the trachea the aortic arch lies. A right-sided aortic arch may occur in an otherwise normal patient but also in the tetralogy of Fallot and in common arterial trunk (Daves, 1968; Calder et al, 1976). The ascending aorta lies to the right in the upper mediastinum. In aortic valve stenosis, the post-stenotic dilation in the older child may produce an accentuated convexity above that of the right atrium. Much of the description relating to coarctation is no longer relevant. With present methods of management, signs in the vicinity of the coarctation site (Figley, 1954) are as uncommon as rib notching. The cardiac contour immediately below the point where the descending aorta crosses the left cardiac margin may have a curious added convexity in an older child. This feature, almost never identified in infants, suggests the presence of a pericardial defect (Nasser, 1970). Abnormalities of the descending aorta are rarely seen in children.

Discordance between cardiac position and atrial and visceral arrangement

So far it is assumed that the apex of the heart can be identified with certainty as lying in the left side of the chest. A check to see that the fundus of the stomach is beneath the left dome of the diaphragm and that the liver is beneath the right dome of the diaphragm must be made. When this has been done, it may be concluded that all the abdominal organs are normally located.

When the heart is normally located but the fundus of the stomach lies under the right dome of the diaphragm and the liver principally under the left dome of the diaphragm, then, for practical purposes, it may be presumed at this stage of evaluation that the patient has a degree of mirror-imagery of the organs and an abnormal heart ('isolated laevocardia'), 'Isolated dextrocardia' is seen when the abdominal organs are normally located, but the apex of the heart appears to lie in the right hemithorax. Rarely patients who have such discordance in visceral and cardiac positions may have normal hearts. More commonly they have complex congenital heart defects with abnormal atrioventricular and ventriculo-arterial connexions (Stanger

et al, 1977). Often in these circumstances the precise arrangement of the organs cannot be identified with certainty (Van Mierop et al, 1970). An assessment of lung and bronchial arrangement can then be made on a filter film (Deanfield et al, 1980). In brief, the origin of the upper lobe bronchus lies at a considerable distance from the carina when the bronchial tree has left morphology (Fig. 10.5). When the lung has right morphology, the upper lobe bronchus lies nearer to the carina. Using this information, it may be inferred that the right hemithorax contains a lung with a left type of structure and so on. Abnormalities of bronchial arrangement may then be used as a predictor of atrial arrangement. When the two lungs have identical structure, then either right or left bronchial isomerism is present. Left isomerism is most frequently associated with interruption of the inferior caval vein (see Ch. 19) and this has implications for attempts at catheterisation from the leg. Right isomerism has an almost complete association with total anomalous pulmonary venous connexion. To a considerable measure, however, these interesting evaluations have been superceded by echocardiographic studies of the heart and the great vessels connected to it. The causes of alterations in cardiac configuration are summarised in Table 10.3.

Table 10.3 Summary of changes in cardiac configuration.

— Position of apex — right ventricular enlargement alone shifts apex across chest and clear of diaphragm
— left ventricular enlargement alone shifts apex downward and outward with apex at or below diaphragm
— biventricular enlargement combines the above features.

— Right atrial enlargement increases convexity of right cardiac border and its lateral margin moves more laterally

— Left atrial enlargement opens the carinal angle and may elevate the left main bronchus. The contour of the left atrium may be identified on a filter film

— Posterior margin of large left atrium accentuates the impression on the oesophagus

— Upper mediastinal content in infants and young children (e.g. aortic arch or azygos vein) may be difficult to identify without either filter film or echocardiographic study

Pulmonary features

When assessing the lung fields it is important to make a decisive evaluation of pulmonary vessel size (Simon 1968; Coussement & Gooding, 1973). Identification of definitive features is more valuable in the initial survey than is speculation on the basis of doubtful entities. The features in infants and children suffering from heart disease are generally clear-cut. If the features are not identifiable as such, then usually it is most helpful to consider them as being 'within normal limits'. After lung assessment it is

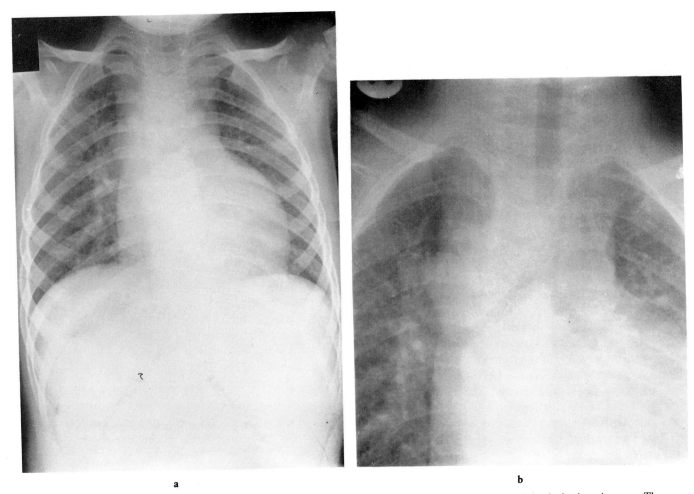

a   b

Fig. 10.5 This radiograph (a) in a young child shows the liver lying under the left dome of the diaphragm — abdominal mirror-imagery. The heart and its apex lie in the left side of the chest (so-called 'isolated levocardia'). Aortic arch position is indeterminate on this radiograph and the mediastinal content cannot be analysed except on the filter film (b). The filter film shows a large azygos vein carrying blood from the abdomen as a continuation of the inferior caval vein. Slightly above and medially the aortic arch lies to the right of the trachea, creating an impression on its right lateral margin. There is a long main stem bronchus to the right lung — 'left bronchial morphology'. The bronchus to the left lung is only slightly shorter and also shows left bronchial morphology. The inference to be made is that the patient has left atrial isomerism and, most probably, complex intracardiac malformations.

possible to integrate radiological findings of the heart size and configuration. A further step in an initial survey is to synthesise radiological observations with clinical, electrocardiographic and echocardiographic findings. This synthesis generally leads to a diagnosis without invasive investigations, at least in terms of categorising a paediatric cardiological problem. It is on this basis that decisions about the next step in management are made.

In looking at the radiological features in the lungs of children with a cardiological problem, the greater the experience of the observer, the more valuable is his interpretation. Experience is acquired not only by studying chest radiographs of children with heart disease, but also by studying carefully the radiographs of children without heart disease. In this way the observer builds a knowledge of what is normal so that he can recognise the abnormal.

There are five general types of finding in the lung in patients with heart disease.

Narrow pulmonary vessels

Presence of narrow pulmonary vessels reflects, in general, an obstruction to filling of the pulmonary circulation. For example, in isolated and clinically significant pulmonary valve stenosis the infundibular region along the left heart border may be prominent, but the pulmonary vessels in the lung are narrow (Fig. 10.6). If the obstruction is below the pulmonary valve (as in infundibular stenosis) then the subpulmonary infundibulum itself is not prominent. This appearance is exemplified by tetralogy of Fallot (Fig. 10.7). Experience in assessing pulmonary vasculature is invaluable. In this respect, there are two

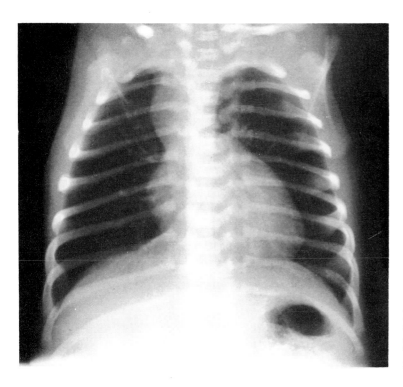

Fig. 10.6 The anteroposterior radiograph of an infant aged 2 days with narrow pulmonary vessels due to pulmonary valve stenosis. The heart is not large but the apex is not low. There is a right aortic arch and the pulmonary infundibulum in this instance is not prominent.

Fig. 10.7 Anteroposterior radiographs in patients with tetralogy of Fallot. (a) Narrow pulmonary vessels in the left lung. There is extensive bronchopneumonic consolidation in the right lung. The circular translucency over the liver and right costophrenic angle is caused by the incubator construction. The heart is not increased in size but the apex is high and extends transversely, reflecting right ventricular hypertrophy. (b) A 'classic' appearance, showing narrow pulmonary vessels, especially notable in the periphery of the lung. The heart is not increased in size. The apex of the heart is blunted and 'double' as a consequence of severe right ventricular hypertrophy. The aortic arch is on the right and the pulmonary infundibulum is not prominent. This is reflected in the concave left cardiac margin beneath the left hilum.

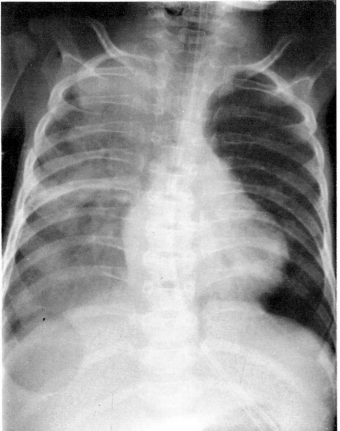

a

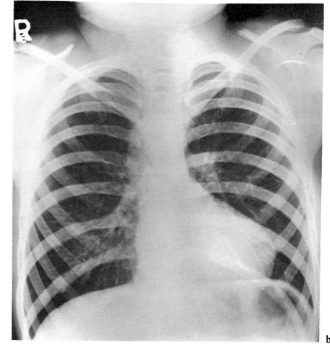

b

collateral points to be made. First, when the pulmonary vessels are narrow, it is also generally true that it is less easy to define the vessels in the periphery of the lung field in the anteroposterior chest radiograph. The second point is that it is usually possible to make an assessment of calibre of the lumen of the right lower lobe bronchus and compare it with the calibre of the artery to the right lower (and middle) lobe in the hilum. Normally these are roughly of equal calibre. Narrow pulmonary vessels are usually associated with a relative diminution of calibre of the right lower lobe artery. Obstructions to filling of the pulmonary circulation are very commonly associated with right ventricular hypertrophy. This affects the position of the cardiac apex (Figs. 10.6, 10.7).

Large pulmonary vessels

Large pulmonary vessels are generally an indication of an increase in pulmonary blood flow. Two sets of circumstances can give rise to this phenomenon. The first is the presence of a left-to-right shunt. This can be caused, for example, by an atrial septal defect (Fig. 10.8), a ven-

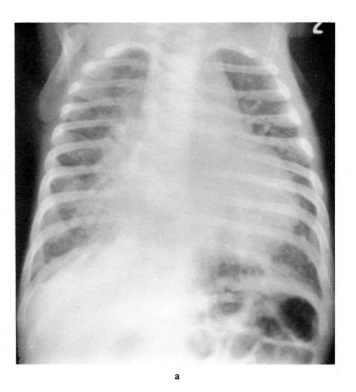

a

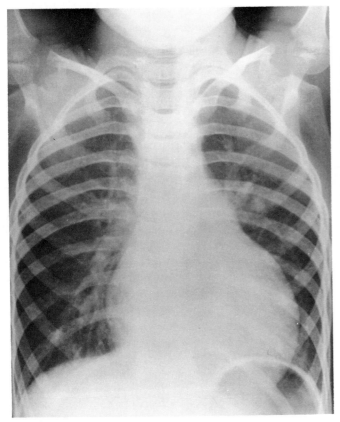

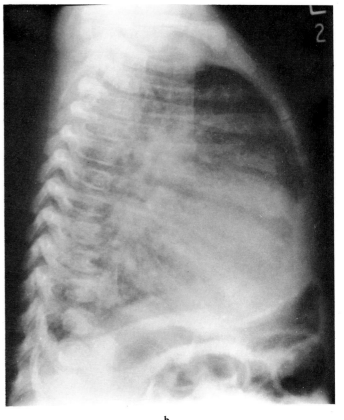

b

Fig. 10.8 The frontal radiograph in a child with atrial septal defect and increased pulmonary vessel size. The transverse diameter of the heart is increased with a prominent right atrial convexity lying on the right cardiac margin and reflecting right atrial enlargement. The rounded apex is displaced across the chest due to right ventricular enlargement. A large pulmonary infundibulum is seen below the left aortic arch along the left cardiac margin.

Fig. 10.9 Anteroposterior (a) and lateral (b) radiographs in a child with ventricular septal defect at 2 months of age with very large pulmonary blood flow and large pulmonary vessels. The lung compliance is reduced ('stiff lungs') and the diaphragm is low and flat. Increase in heart size is present with a cardiac apex which is neither elevated nor depressed, reflecting biventricular enlargement.

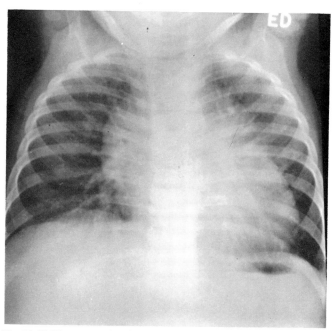

Fig. 10.10 The anteroposterior radiograph of an infant at 9 months of age with persistent patency of the arterial duct. The pulmonary vessels are large. The large heart has a low apex associated with left ventricular enlargement due to increase in flow through the left ventricle.

tricular septal defect (Fig. 10.9), persistent patency of the arterial duct (Fig. 10.10), common arterial trunk (Fig. 10.11), total anomalous pulmonary venous connexion (Fig. 10.12) or a large arteriovenous fistula. The second circumstance is produced by complete transposition (Fig. 10.13) in which the pulmonary and systemic circuits are in parallel, giving limited opportunities for mixing of blood between the two. Patients with left-to-right shunts seldom have systemic arterial desaturation. In contrast, patients with complete transposition characteristically have systemic arterial desaturation and cyanosis.

When pulmonary blood flow is increased, the pulmonary vessels are large and identifiable well out into the periphery of the lung field on the anteroposterior chest radiograph. In these circumstances the pulmonary artery to the right lower lobe is large. An increase in pulmonary vessel size is often well seen on the lateral chest radiograph (Fig. 10.9b). The potential for an increase in pulmonary blood flow develops as the neonate grows during the first few months of life (Collins et al, 1972). Infants whose pulmonary blood flow increases may have incipient heart

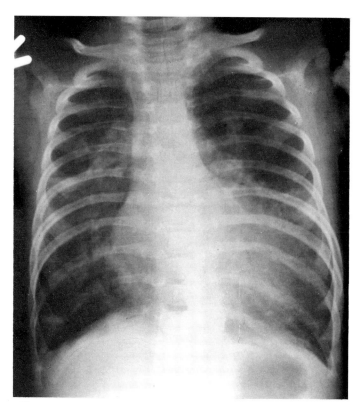

Fig. 10.11 The anteroposterior radiograph in a child with common arterial trunk with increased pulmonary blood flow and large pulmonary vessels. The ill-defined cardiac apex is low. There is a narrow cardiac base because the pulmonary trunk is absent and large pulmonary arteries originate directly from the common trunk. Lung volume is increased, and the diaphragm is flat. Some bronchopneumonic change is present in the lingula segment of the left upper lobe which obscures the cardiac apex.

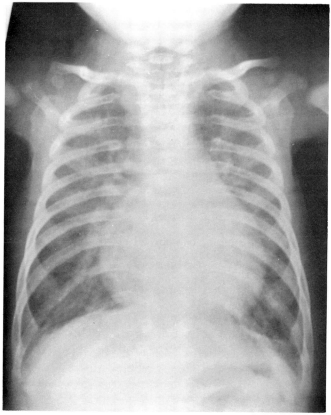

Fig. 10.12 The anteroposterior radiograph in an infant at 4 months of age with total anomalous pulmonary venous connexion to coronary sinus. The pulmonary vessels are large and the cardiac configuration is rather similar to the atrial septal defect shown in Figure 10.8. The upper mediastinum is not wide. Even with total anomalous connexion to left innominate vein the 'cottage-loaf' or 'snowman' configuration is seldom discernible in infancy as separate from other vascular or thymic shadows.

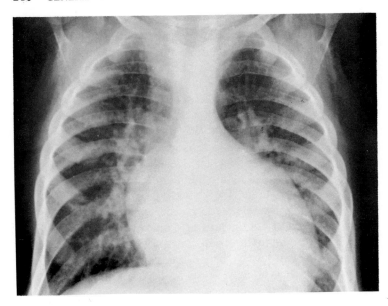

Fig. 10.13 The anteroposterior radiograph in a young child with complete transposition with large pulmonary vessels. Since the pulmonary trunk lies behind the anteriorly placed aorta, there is narrowing of the base of the heart with production of the classic 'egg-on-side' configuration.

failure or they may develop frank heart failure. Such increases in pulmonary blood flow are associated with diminished lung compliance and tachypnoea. Radiologically (and best observed on the lateral chest radiograph), the diaphragm flattens and the sternum bows forward as lung volume increases.

If untreated, some patients with an initially high pulmonary blood flow develop increasing pulmonary vascular disease and pulmonary hypertension with a diminishing blood flow. Such a sequence is faster in young children with complete transposition and slower in children with supratricuspid shunts. The heart tends to become smaller in size as vascular disease starts and progresses. This is as it converts from a 'flow work pattern' to a 'pressure work pattern'. Valve incompetence may mitigate against this transition to a smaller heart. The central pulmonary arteries remain large as the haemodynamic change occurs, or even increase in size. In contrast, children who present with primary pulmonary hypertension may have a pulmonary vessel pattern and heart size indistinguishable from normal throughout life.

Pulmonary vessels of intermediate size

The cardiac abnormality may be a minor one, such as a small ventricular septal defect in patients who have pulmonary vessels of normal calibre. Alternatively, there may be a combination of defects in the heart which produce small deviations in systemic and pulmonary blood flow. The lesions which balance each other in this way include a ventricular or atrial septal defect balanced by pulmonary valvar or subvalvar stenosis or simple complete transposition in the first day of life (Fig. 10.14). Furthermore, in very young infants, the pulmonary vascular resistance may be sufficient to give vascularity within normal limits. When banding of the pulmonary trunk was a popular measure to reduce flow, then the common sequel was pulmonary vessels of normal size. A variety of cardiac problems in the field of acquired and congenital disease may not have any impact on the pulmonary circulation during childhood. Among these conditions may be included rheumatic carditis and aortic stenosis. Neither is a minimal lesion.

Pulmonary venous hypertension: vascular pattern giving the 'upper zone diversion phenomenon'

It has been known for decades that adults who have mitral valve disease and pulmonary venous hypertension have pulmonary vessels in the upper zones which are widened relative to the narrower vessels in the lower zones of the lung. A similar appearance can be seen in older infants and children (Chrispin, 1973) who have pulmonary venous hypertension associated with variants of divided left atrium (cor triatriatum) and mitral valve disease, whether the lesion is of a congenital (Fig. 10.15) or acquired type. Such findings on the chest radiograph are, nevertheless, rather uncommon. Upper zone pulmonary oedema may also occur when upper zone diversion is present.

Pulmonary oedema

Pulmonary oedema is one of the most important diagnoses to make on a chest radiograph of an infant or child. The reason is simply that it indicates a very serious threat to life. Furthermore, specific clinical signs of pulmonary oedema are generally not present in the paediatric age-group and so radiography is the only method of diagnosis. Young patients who have pulmonary oedema have chest radiographs in which the pulmonary vessels in the hilar

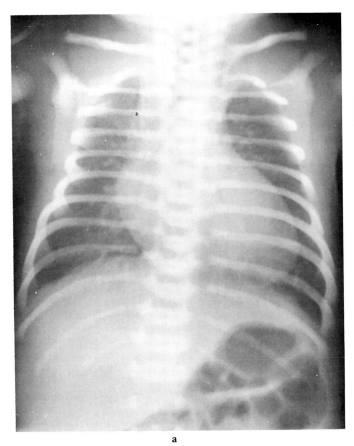

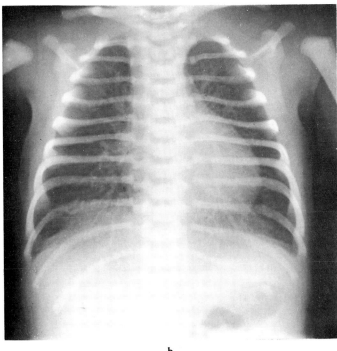

a   b

Fig. 10.14 These radiographs are from patients with simple complete transposition on the first day of life. In Figure 10.14a, the pulmonary vessels are neither large nor small, but are of intermediate size. A classic 'egg-on-side' configuration is visible prior to balloon atrial septostomy. This configuration (see Fig. 10.13) is uncommonly seen at this age. The more usual pattern is seen in Figure 10.14b, again taken prior to balloon atrial septostomy. The pulmonary vessels are also of intermediate size but the cardiac configuration in unremarkable. This appearance is much commoner than the supposed classic 'egg-on-side' (Fig. 10.14a).

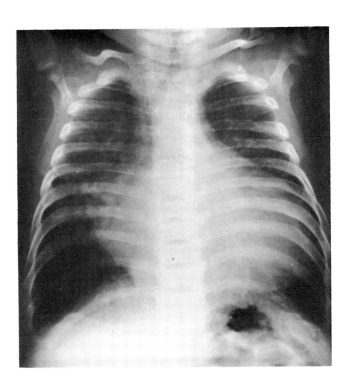

regions of the lung cannot be clearly identified. This is because the oedema produces additional shadowing which obscures the vascular detail in the hilar region. The large bronchi in the hilar region tend to be seen exceptionally clearly since the air within their lumens is surrounded by the bronchial wall and its lymphatics and lung containing oedema. A centrally located hilar and perihilar 'air bronchogram' may thus be evident.

The periphery of the lung appears clear beyond the perihilar shadowing except for septal line shadows. In most infants these can best be seen in the retrosternal area on the lateral chest radiograph and in the costophrenic angles on the anteroposterior chest radiograph in most children.

Fig. 10.15 The anteroposterior radiograph from a child aged 8 months with congenital mitral stenosis and pulmonary venous hypertension. The pulmonary vessels in the lung bases are narrow, giving increased basal transradiancy. The upper zone vessels are increased in size ('upper zone diversion'). The heart is increased in size with a very large left atrium forming the right cardiac margin. The hypertrophied right ventricle is associated with a cardiac apex which is displaced transversely.

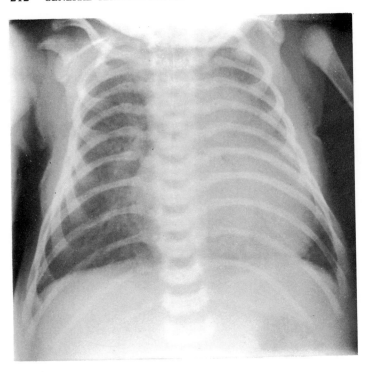

Fig. 10.16 The anteroposterior radiograph in a patient with coarctation of the aorta and pulmonary oedema. Pulmonary vessels in the hilar and perihilar regions cannot be clearly identified because of infiltrated oedema. The periphery of the lungs is clear. An increase in heart size is present due to left ventricular enlargement with a low cardiac apex.

The accentuated lines of the fissures between the lobes of the lung are easily seen on the lateral radiograph. The right horizontal and the lower end of the left oblique fissures are commonly definable on the anteroposterior radiograph. The reason why, even in a small patient, the fissure lines are so easily seen is probably because of pleural oedema and the presence of a trace of fluid in the pleural cavities. Sizeable pleural effusions, however, are exceptionally rare in association with pulmonary oedema due to heart disease in infants or children. Renal failure is often the cause when large effusions are present together with pulmonary oedema. The lungs have diminished compliance in the infant with pulmonary oedema and there is clinical tachypnoea. The diaphragm is low and flattened on radiographs and the sternum is bowed forward. Among the foremost causes of pulmonary oedema in infants with congenital heart disease must be aortic coarctation and total anomalous pulmonary venous connexion with obstruction of the common pulmonary vein. Coarctation of the aorta (Fig. 10.16) is diagnosed on clinical grounds while the chest radiograph indicates the severity of the lesion. The infant is in heart failure when pulmonary oedema is present. The left side of the heart is affected and so the heart is large with the apex low in relationship to the diaphragm. In obstructed pulmonary venous connexion (Fig. 10.17) the left ventricle is not large and the main impact falls upon the right ventricle. The infant who has this defect does not have a large heart. A divided left atrium ('cor triatriatum') is a rare lesion and, when found in symptomatic infants, it is associated characteristically with pulmonary oedema. Among the acquired heart

lesions which have accompanying pulmonary oedema are those in which there is a myocardial problem (as in endocardial fibroelastosis or viral myocarditis). In such circumstances the heart tends to be enlarged and it may be grossly enlarged.

The radiologic features of pulmonary oedema in the young infant have to be differentiated from those of other conditions. There is a range of radiological features in the respiratory distress syndrome which can be staged according to radiological criteria of severity. Patients with respiratory distress syndrome of intermediate severity have a widespread granularity which extends throughout all lung areas and into the periphery of the lung. The margins of the diaphragm and heart are consequently obscured. In moderate or severe respiratory distress syndrome, there is a localised increase in shadowing in the perihilar regions which produces the appearance of an air bronchogram. The condition has a deleterious effect on gaseous interchange. Persistent patency of the arterial duct may then add to systemic arterial desaturation (Higgins et al, 1977). The patency of the duct with respiratory distress syndrome, however, is seldom associated with the type of cardiac enlargement seen when the duct is the primary heart lesion. Furthermore, respiratory distress syndrome is very much associated with low birth weight and prematurity. There is a relatively uncommon type of pulmonary oedema in some infants with obstructed total anomalous pulmonary venous connexion in which the lungs have a mottled appearance. This phenomenon must be differentiated from the miliary shadowing encountered in miliary tuberculosis or neonatal haematogenous bacterial infection

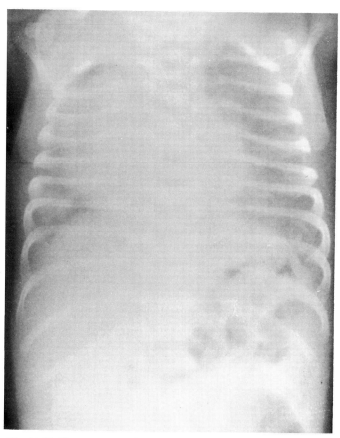

Fig. 10.17 The anteroposterior radiograph in a patient with obstructed total anomalous pulmonary venous connexion to the hepatic portal vein. The liver is large. The pulmonary vessels in the left lung hilum are not definable because of pulmonary oedema. The transverse diameter of the heart is not increased. Much of the right hemithorax is occupied by the thymic shadow on this film, which was taken with the infant supine.

of the lung. None of these conditions have the distinctive perihilar features of pulmonary oedema nor are the septal lines visible in the retrosternal area or costophrenic angles. Clinical and laboratory findings as part of an 'infection screening' can be decisive in showing that infection is the cause of the lung problem.

Pneumonia due to *Pneumocystis carini* occurs as an opportunist infection in premature infants and those with immune deficiency. This clinical context is important, but radiological differentiation from pulmonary oedema is also possible. There is perihilar shadowing in the early stages of pneumocystis infection, producing an air bronchogram and obscuring the detail of pulmonary vessels in the hilum. Nevertheless, the periphery of the lung is clear at this stage. In advanced infection, the lungs have a diffusely granular shadowing or may show severe uniformly diminished transradiancy. Simple bronchopneumonia can be differentiated from pulmonary oedema. The changes associated with bronchopneumonia are mottled shadowing localised to one or two lung lobes and extending to the periphery. They are very often associated with degrees of lung deflation and collapse. Bronchopneumonia is a fairly frequent complication for infants who have heart disease.

Pulmonary oedema in infancy has a symmetrical distribution. In older children, however, this is often not so. One lung in a child may be more affected than the other and there is often more oedema posteriorly than anteriorly. These features are particularly evident in older children with pulmonary oedema of recent onset. Awareness of this should avoid diagnostic error.

Summation of radiologic findings relative to heart and lungs

A systematic evaluation is invaluable when looking at the chest radiograph of an infant or child with congenital or acquired heart disease. Further aid comes from putting the evaluation into the interrogative (Table 10.4). Is this a good inspiratory film? Is the diaphragm unduly flat? Is the heart large? Where is the apex? Which cardiac chamber is large? What about the mediastinum, and is a filter film necessary to define where the aortic arch lies? And so the process continues. In this way the appropriate conclusions are drawn. All this may seem trite, but it is the way to avoid mistakes. After evaluating the chest radiograph in this way the conclusions drawn can be set alongside those deriving from other non-invasive studies. All should fit together in a congruous way like pieces of a jigsaw puzzle.

Table 10.4 Overall findings.

HEART SIZE
Large or not large?

CARDIAC CONFIGURATION
Position of apex?
Which chamber is large?

LUNGS
Pulmonary vessels small?
— as in pulmonary stenosis or pulmonary atresia

Pulmonary vessels large?
— as in atrial or ventricular septal defect, arterial duct, common, arterial trunk or total anomalous pulmonary venous connexion
— as in arterio-venous 'fistula', or
— as in complete transposition

Pulmonary vessels of intermediate size?
— as in defects balancing each other such as ventricular septal defect with pulmonary stenosis
— as in minor lesions or lesions such as aortic stenosis when not decompensated
— as in complete transposition in the first hours of life

Pulmonary vessels large at the apices and narrower at the bases?
— as in pulmonary venous hypertension due to mitral valve disease

Pulmonary oedema present?
— as in coarctation, aortic valve disease, obstructed total anomalous pulmonary venous connexion or divided left atrium in an infant

Miscellaneous features

There are still a number of varied and often apparently unrelated features to be considered in the context of the chest radiograph. They have one common factor – heart disease.

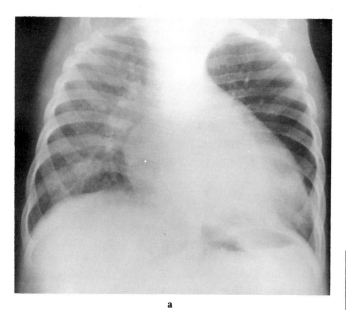

a

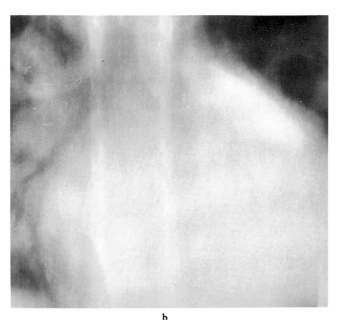

b

Fig. 10.18 This patient has endocardial fibroelastosis with a large left ventricle. The anteroposterior radiograph (a) reveals increased transradiancy of the left lung and diminution in pulmonary vascularity. This is the 'left heart-left lung' syndrome. The tomographic cut (b) shows the large left atrium associated with narrowing of the larger left main bronchus and an increase in the carinal angle. Note the air bronchogram with peribronchial cuffing due to perihilar oedema at the right hilum.

The thorax

Ordinarily the lungs in heart disease have comparable characteristics. There are exceptions to this generalisation. If one lung has not grown, instead remaining hypoplastic, then the mediastinum and heart are displaced to the side of the smaller lung. Such a displacement to the right can given the impression of so-called 'isolated dextrocardia'. It is usually possible to identify the cardiac apex, however, and the smaller lung usually has narrower pulmonary vessels. A barium swallow will exclude an oesophageal bronchus coexisiting with a small lung. Ventilation in the small lung may be studied during the fluoroscopic procedure which this examination entails. There is often deflation or collapse of the left lower lobe when the heart is normally located but grossly enlarged. Alternatively, the left lung may have its bronchus narrowed by a large left atrium and then it will show signs of air-trapping (Fig. 10.18). A very small number of patients may have overdistension of the right middle lobe and they may have congenital heart disease, often with a considerable right-to-left shunt. Although many of these patients do not fall into

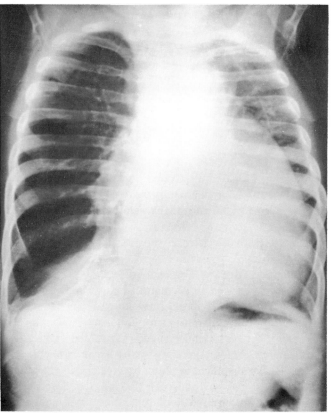

Fig. 10.19 Anteroposterior radiograph in a patient with coarctation of the aorta. The cardiac configuration is typical. There is also some mediastinal shift to the left. There is diaphragmatic flattening and there is emphysema of the middle lobe of the right lung resulting in deflation of the lower right lobe. The pulmonary vessels are crowded in this area.

the category of having true congenital lobar emphysema, some do (Fig. 10.19). Quite a lot of patients with congenital heart disease and severe pulmonary hypertension may have increased transradiancy in the left upper lobe. This is due to vascular occlusion, as shown at angiography.

When the whole of one lung shows increased transradiancy and its overall volume is much as would be expected normally, then the possibility of absence of a central pulmonary artery should be entertained. The peripheral pulmonary vessels are narrow in such circumstances and the central hilar vessels are clearly abnormal. Unilateral lung plethora is often a feature of a pulmonary artery connected to the systemic circulation. Rarely this

may be a natural occurrence but more commonly it is due to a Blalock-Taussig, Waterston or similar shunt (Litwin & Fellows, 1973).

Thromboembolic disease associated with a central indwelling catheter or an intracranial ventricular drain to the right side of the heart may produce localised areas of increased transradiancy where local arterial occlusion has occurred. Septic emboli are uncommon but important. Their origin may be in the abdominal organs, such as the kidney with a renal abcess. Bacterial endocarditis may develop when the heart is damaged by, for example, rheumatic carditis or a congenital anomaly. Bacterial endocarditis with a left-to-right shunt may be associated with septic embolisation and infarction of lung (Fig. 10.20).

Rib anomalies (Fig. 10.20) are quite commonly seen in patients with congenital heart disease. Rib notching occurs either in aortic coarctation (Fig. 10.21) or as a late sequel to the Blalock-Taussig shunt, but is uncommon (Boone et al, 1964). Abnormal segmentation of vertebral bodies in the thoracic spine may be observed in the chest radiograph. An angular spinal curve, which is often stable, may be associated with such vertebral anomalies. In contrast, idiopathic scoliosis may occur in conjunction with congenital heart disease (Luke & McDonnel, 1968). Scoliosis may be detected early on the chest radiograph and it may progress rapidly. This adds to the hazards of the cardiac problem because lung ventilation becomes unequal and lung growth is handicapped.

When the dorsal spine of a child lacks its normal kyphosis (Twigg et al, 1967) and the manubriosternal junction is rather flat, the upper mediastinal shadow appears wide, although the mediastinal content is normal.

The idea that congenital heart disease is a congenitally isolated defect (a clean lesion) is not true. For example, a multiplicity of renal abnormalities may occur in conjunction. There is a spectrum of recognised syndromes of which congenital heart disease is a component, and these are discussed elsewhere. Not all entities and constellations,

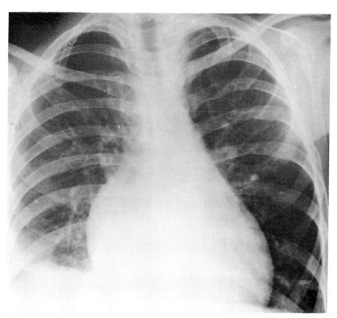

Fig. 10.20 This patient had a ventricular septal defect of small size but with cardiac enlargement due to bacterial endocarditis. There is a wedge shadow in the costophrenic angle of the base of the right lung which results from a septic pulmonary infarction. Note the minor first right rib anomaly.

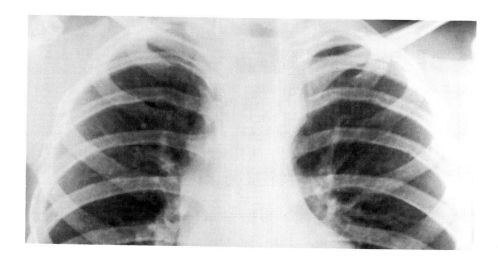

Fig. 10.21 Detail of the top half of the anteroposterior radiograph in an 8-year-old with aortic coarctation found to be hypertensive with absent femoral pulses on routine childhood medical assessment. There is notching of the fourth and fifth ribs posteriorly but the mediastinal configuration is unremarkable.

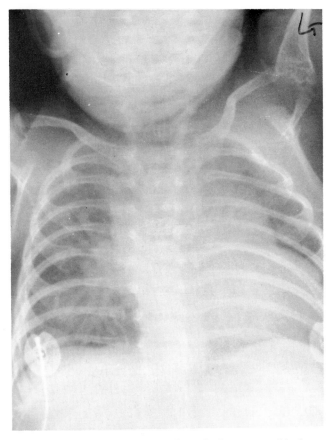

Fig. 10.22 In this anteroposterior radiograph of a neonate with absent pulmonary valve syndrome, the right main pulmonary artery is very large and is seen as a rounded shadow in the right hilum. As yet, compression of the main airways by the pulmonary arteries has not supervened so the aeration of the lungs is normal and there is neither air-trapping nor collapse. The costochondral junctions are broad, however, and there is clear-cut evidence of metaphysical chondrodysplasia in the proximal end of the humerus.

however, are fully described. Occasionally they may be suspected on the chest radiograph (Fig. 10.22).

The trachea

The trachea, as seen on the anteroposterior chest radiograph of a normal infant, often deviates acutely to the right before descending into the thorax. On the lateral chest radiograph, the trachea can be seen above the thoracic inlet and throughout its length in the thorax. Narrowing of the tracheal lumen on this projection is seen in infants who have vascular rings or slings (Stewart et al, 1964; Roesler et al, 1983). Such infants may also have an additional congenital heart defect, but the vascular ring may be an isolated finding. Symptoms are usually due to recurrent infections affecting the respiratory tract, or more commonly there is stridor. Sometimes there are difficulties on swallowing. The diagnosis is confirmed by a barium swallow taken in the true lateral and anteroposterior projections. In the presence of a vascular ring, the lateral view

shows the posterior aspect of the barium-filled oesophagus to be sharply indented at the site of the tracheal narrowing. There is no separation of the oesophagus from the trachea (Fig. 10.23). When a vascular sling is present, the aberrant left pulmonary artery runs to the left lung between the trachea and the oesophagus and thus separates these structures (Fig. 10.24). The common types of vascular ring have a right aortic arch component which comprises part of the ring. The arch gives a high impression on the right of the oesophagus on the anteroposterior projection (Fig. 10.23b). If this feature cannot be identified on the oesophogram, it will be shown by either an ultrasonographic study or a filter film. When the right aortic arch component is absent, thought must be given to the possibility of a left arch with a right arterial duct or ligament. Only in this circumstance will an angiogram be needed (Fig. 10.25). At that time, the anatomy can be discerned further with the aid of a radio-opaque catheter placed in the oesophagus. These investigations permit the patient to have the appropriate thoracotomy instead of the classic and commoner left thoracotomy.

Slings (Berdon et al, 1984) and rings compress and narrow the trachea from behind. They are also associated with a widening of the carinal angle (Fig. 10.26). There are two additional lesions which compress the trachea from the front. The first is the grossly dilated pulmonary arteries which are found with absent leaflets of the pulmonary valve. The second is the compression seen nearer the thoracic inlet and higher in the chest when where is a late origin of the brachiocephalic artery from a left aortic arch. Stridor is a feature of this last entity. In the absent pulmonary valve syndrome, however, the trachea is compressed in the vicinity of the carina while the left and right pulmonary arteries may compress the main bronchi in the hilar regions. Whatever the mechanism, the lungs may show symmetry of air-trapping of life-threatening degree, or there may be varied patterns of air-trapping and lung collapse.

The liver

The liver enlarges clinically in patients with heart failure and this can be seen on radiographs. The liver is especially large in young infants who have an infradiaphragmatic total anomalous pulmonary connexion which terminates in the portal venous system. Gross liver enlargement is seen in older children who have severe tricuspid incompetence or constrictive pericarditis. The pericardium may be calcified in the latter. The liver may also enlarge grossly in patients with thalassaemia and other blood dyscrasias which have a haematological and cardiovascular impact. It may herniate when there is an anterior defect in the diaphragm and produce a concatenation shadow composed of the liver and heart, thereby giving a false impression of cardiac enlargement. The radiological clue which is diag-

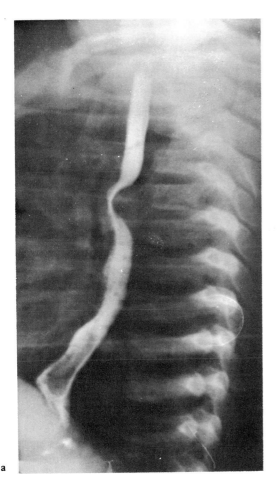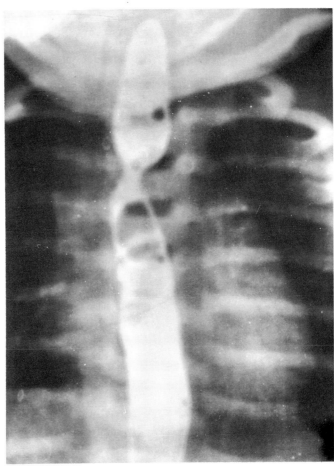

a   b

Fig. 10.23 Vascular rings are well demonstrated by the barium swallow. (a) A barium swallow in lateral projection. The ring encircles both the trachea and the oesophagus and indents the posterior aspect of the oesophagus. The tracheal lumen is narrowed anterior to the oesophagus and is displaced forward at the level of the ring. (b) An anteroposterior projection in a different patient. There is an indentation due to the dominant right arch component on the right aspect of the oesophagus. The smaller left arch produces an impression on the left aspect at a slightly lower level. Appearance of compression of trachea and oesophagus are usually more impressive on the lateral projection.

nostic in this situation is that the left lobe of the liver does not occupy its customary infradiaphragmatic position. Echocardiograms are conclusive.

The gut

Young infants who have severe heart failure and are in a state of shock cease to suck and instead they swallow air. Bowel sounds are clinically in abeyance. Gas may be seen in the stomach in such circumstances and the duodenum and upper jejunum are visible as loops of gut filled with air. When this radiological finding is present, it is important to avoid making a diagnosis of obstruction within the small intestine. This can be done in the clinical context because the gas-containing gut is not distended and contains gas in continuity. Although this consideration is strictly outside the chest, the upper abdomen is invariably included on the chest radiograph. Free air seen under the dome of the diaphragm in an infant with congenital heart

disease who has necrotising enterocolitis indicates that gut perforation has occurred.

2.   CERTAIN CARDIAC ASPECTS OF COMPUTERISED TOMOGRAPHIC SCANNING

Among the more modern methods of investigation, conventional computerised tomographic scanners have never really found a place in the evaluation of heart disease in infants and children. The exposure time is too long for paediatric cardiac imaging. Short exposures of the order of 240 ms, however, are obtained with the multislice real time scanner developed in California in conjunction with the University of California School of Medicine, San Francisco. In this machine, an electron gun produces a beam which is focused on to tungsten target rings, each ring producing a fan beam of radiation which is rotated through the patient. To investigate the interior of the heart,

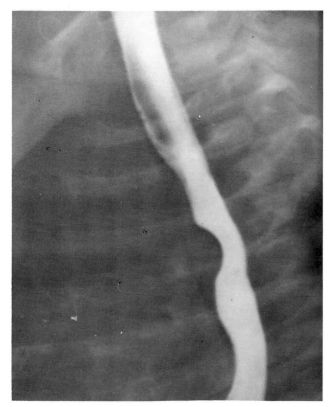

Fig. 10.24 This is a barium swallow from patient with a vascular sling. The left pulmonary artery originates from the pulmonary trunk to the right of the trachea and then passes to the left lung between the trachea and the oesophagus. The barium in the oesophagus shows an anterior impression. The trachea is narrow anterior to the left pulmonary artery.

substantial amounts of radiographic contrast agent are given by bolus injection. Movies permit the evaluation of cardiac anatomical detail. Ventricular volumes can be calculated, as can myocardial wall thickness and perfusion. Time-density curve analysis may be employed to estimate blood flow and cardiac output. For its successful use in cardiac work, the multislice/millisecond scanner utilises both incising radiation and radiographic contrast agents in quantity. It has been used for the study of congenital heart disease with success. Computerised tomography as a method has shown itself capable of development and refinement. It is rather early, therefore, to define the future role of the multislice/millisecond scanner in the study of heart disease in infants and children.

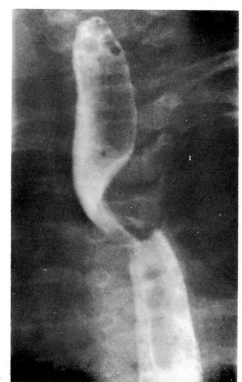

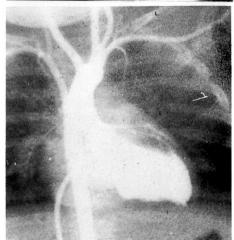

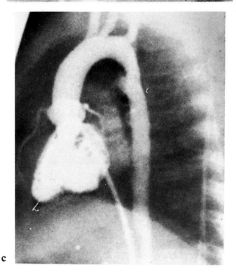

Fig. 10.25 The barium swallow (a) in this patient with a vascular ring shows a very deep impression on the left aspect of the oesophagus – compare with (b). One may infer that the right arch is not dominant. The left ventricular angiogram seen in anteroposterior (b) and lateral (c) projections shows a single left aortic arch matching the oesophageal impression on the anteroposterior projection chest radiograph (a). The lateral angiogram (c) shows some catheter-induced mitral incompetence and an arterial duct which is broad at its base but which tapers towards its entry into the right pulmonary artery.

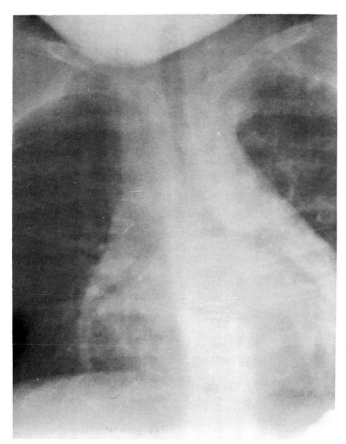

Fig. 10.26 This filter film from a patient with a vascular ring shows the wide carinal angle.

3. PAEDIATRIC NUCLEAR CARDIOLOGY

Radionuclide imaging has been established for many years as a non-invasive technique for the investigation of congenital heart disease. The earliest applications were limited to making structural diagnoses by following the sequence of chamber-filling during a first pass radionuclide angiogram. For such a study, a bolus of a radionuclide is injected into a peripheral vein and images are acquired with a gamma camera as the radioactive material passes through the central circulation. This has proved to be a sensitive method for the detection of intracardiac shunt, but the images are of poor resolution. This limits the structural detail that can be identified. Digitisation of the data from the first pass angiogram and computer analysis of the passing of the radionuclide through the heart and lungs has now, however, greatly increased the functional information that can be obtained. The magnitude of simple left-to-right shunts can be measured with great precision (Treves, 1980), right-to-left shunts can be detected and quantified (Peter et al, 1981), and both right and left ventricular function can be measured (Steele et al, 1976). A second form of radionuclide angiography has also been developed in which red blood cells are selectively labelled with techne-

tium-99m so that an image of the 'equilibrium cardiac blood pool' can be acquired (Strauss et al, 1971). If the acquisition is gated to the electrocardiogram, a cardiac blood pool angiogram can be accumulated over several minutes with sufficient counts for functional data to be obtained.

Radionuclide angiography

If a first pass radionuclide angiogram is acquired in the anterior projection in a patient without a shunt, the radionuclide bolus will be clearly seen to pass in sequence through the right heart, the lungs and the left heart (Fig. 10.27). Recirculation of the radionuclide through a left-to-right shunt will cause persistence in the lungs with

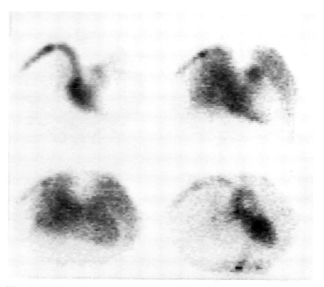

Fig. 10.27 Four frames from a first pass radionuclide angiogram in a patient with no intracardiac shunts, anterior projection.

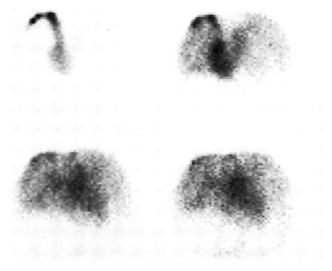

Fig. 10.28 Four frames from a first pass angiogram in a patient with a left-to-right shunt. The lungs do not clear at the end of the study because of recirculation through the shunt.

poor definition of the left heart phase of the angiogram (Fig. 10.28). Such inspection of the first pass angiogram is a sensitive method of detecting left-to-right shunts. With computer analysis, a histogram of counts from the lungs can be drawn against time. In the normal case (Fig. 10.29), there is a single peak as the radionuclide passes through the lungs and then the counts return to a background level. There is a late, broad peak due to systemic recirculation. Where there is a left-to-right shunt (Fig. 10.30), the peak of the first pass is interrupted by an early recirculation peak and then by further multiple peaks which merge into one another due to repeated recirculation. The total pulmonary flow is proportional to the area under the first pass peak, while the shunt is proportional to the area under the first recirculation peak. These areas can be estimated by fitting computer-derived curves to the original pulmonary time-activity curve. A curve with area A1 is fitted to the first pass peak and then this is subtracted from the pulmonary time-activity curve so that only the recirculation peaks remain. A second curve, area A2, is then fitted to the first recirculation peak. The left-to-right shunt is therefore A2/A1. If there is no significant right-to-left shunt, the pulmonary-to-systemic flow ratio can then be calculated (Fig. 10.31) as

$$Qp/Qs = \frac{A1}{A1 - A2}$$

If this measurement is to be accurate, it is essential to give a discrete and rapid bolus of radionuclide. It must therefore be administered via a proximal peripheral vein through as large an intravenous cannula as possible. The quality of the bolus can be assessed by creating a time-activity curve from the superior caval vein (Fig. 10.32). Studies in which the bolus is unduly prolonged or multiple will not give accurate results.

This radionuclide technique correlates well with oximetric measurements in large groups of patients with simple left-to-right shunts (Maltz & Treves, 1973; McIlveen et al, 1981). Indeed, the radionuclide measurement is more accurate than the one normally obtained with oximetry, especially in patients with shunts at atrial level (Baker et

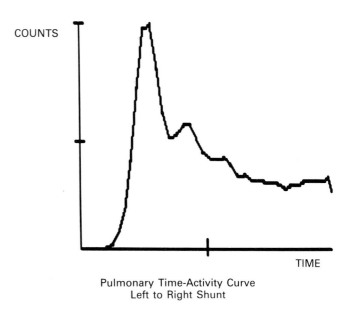

Pulmonary Time-Activity Curve
Left to Right Shunt

Fig. 10.30 A pulmonary time-activity curve in a patient with a left-to-right shunt.

al, 1985). Nonetheless, when interpreting first pass time-activity curves it is important to be aware of the limitations of the method. It is potentially inaccurate when the pulmonary transit time is prolonged, as may be seen in severe pulmonary or mitral regurgitation or very poor cardiac performance. Where the shunt is not symmetrical in the two lungs, as may occur with persistence of the arterial duct (Fig. 10.33), an overall measurement of the pulmonary-to-systemic flow cannot be made. Limitations of the curve-fitting technique and normal bronchial blood flow can lead to measured pulmonary-to-systemic flows of up to 1.2 : 1 in normal patients. Increased collateral flow within the chest in patients with aortic coarctation may lead to an erroneous shunt measurement even greater than this.

Right-to-left shunts

Right-to-left shunts are detected from the first pass radionuclide angiogram by early appearance of the radionuclide in the left heart or aorta (Fig. 10.34). In a normal study, counts are not acquired from the aorta until after the pulmonary phase. In contrast, when there is a right-to-left shunt, the first peak of activity in the aorta is simultaneous with the first pulmonary peak (Fig. 10.35). Analysis of the time-activity curve from the aorta (by using a method originally described for the analysis of dye-dilution curves) can give an estimate of the magnitude of the right-to-left shunt (Peter et al, 1981). Right-to-left shunts can also be measured from the trapping in precapillary arterioles of radionuclide-labelled particles previously injected into a peripheral vein (Gates et al, 1971). Either human albumin

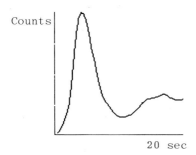

Counts

20 sec

Fig. 10.29 A normal first pass pulmonary time-activity curve.

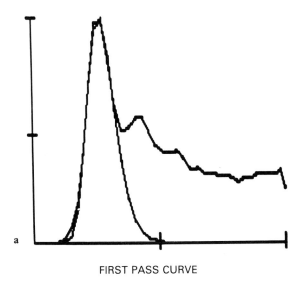

a

FIRST PASS CURVE

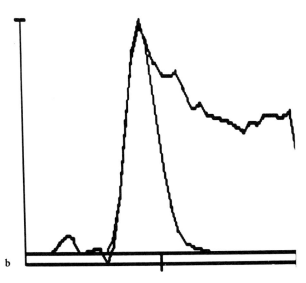

b

RECIRCULATION CURVE

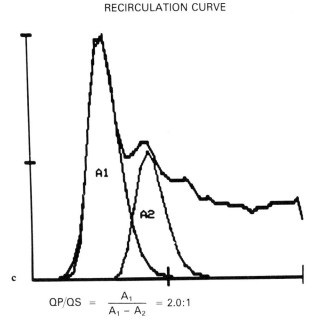

c

$$QP/QS = \frac{A_1}{A_1 - A_2} = 2.0:1$$

Fig. 10.31 (a) Computer fit to the first peak of the pulmonary curve, area A1. (b) Computer fit to the first recirculation curve, area A2. (c) The two fitted curves with the original pulmonary time-activity curve. Qp/Qs is calculated from the areas of the curves fitted by the computer.

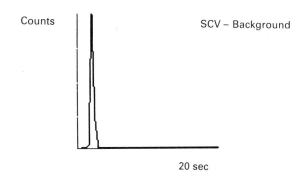

Fig. 10.32 The time-activity curve from the superior caval vein (SCV) corrected for background showing that a satisfactory bolus of radionuclide has been administered.

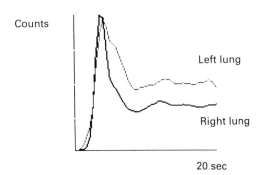

Fig. 10.33 Right and left pulmonary time-activity curve in a patient with persistence of the arterial duct. The first recirculation peak (and therefore the shunt) is larger in the left lung.

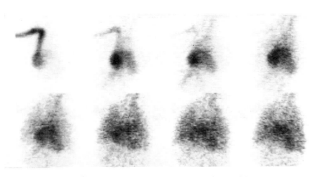

Fig. 10.34 Eight frames from the first pass radionuclide angiogram in a patient with tricuspid atresia. There is bidirectional shunting. Note the appearance of radionuclide in the carotid arteries before the lungs and the persistence of activity in the lungs at the end of the study.

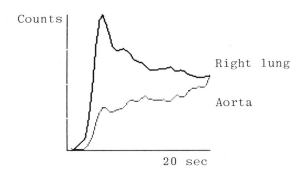

Fig. 10.35 Time-activity curve from a patient with bidirectional shunting. There is a simultaneous peak in the aorta and right lung, indicating a right-to-left shunt. Early recirculation in the lung indicates that there is also left-to-right shunting.

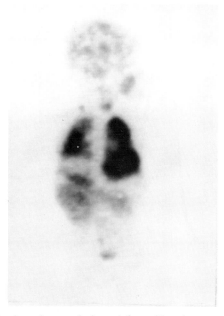

Fig. 10.36 A microsphere study in an infant with pulmonary atresia. The radionuclide was given via a peripheral vein. From distribution of microspheres, the pulmonary to systemic flow can be estimated. Anterior projection.

microspheres or macro-aggregated albumin may be given safely in the presence of right-to-left shunting. Whole body imaging is performed once the radionuclide has been given to estimate the counts in the systemic and pulmonary circulations.

Isolated measurements of right-to-left shunts are of little clinical value. In most patients with bidirectional shunting, measurement with radionuclide techniques of the pulmonary-to-systemic flow ratio (which would be valuable) is not possible. In the special case when there is total mixing of the systemic and pulmonary venous blood within the heart (such as in pulmonary atresia) the pulmonary-to-systemic flow ratio can be calculated from studies with radionuclide-labelled particles. A typical dose of technetium-99m-labelled microspheres is 30 000 per square metre of body surface area. Anterior and posterior whole body images are acquired immediately after administration of the microspheres (Fig. 10.36). The geometric means of the counts from the two views are determined for the whole body and for the lungs. It is then possible to calculate the right-to-left shunt as

$$\frac{\text{whole body counts} - \text{pulmonary counts}}{\text{whole body counts}}$$

and pulmonary-to-systemic flow as

$$\frac{\text{pulmonary counts}}{\text{whole body counts} - \text{pulmonary counts}}$$

Pulmonary perfusion studies

Injection of radionuclide particles may also be used for imaging of the distribution of pulmonary perfusion. If injected into a peripheral vein it is possible to obtain an image of the total pulmonary perfusion. Such studies are especially useful for demonstrating the distribution of perfusion following the creation of surgical shunts (Haroutanian et al, 1969; Gates et al, 1974). In congenital heart malformations with multifocal pulmonary perfusion,

microspheres may be given selectively through a cardiac catheter placed in the pulmonary and the collateral arteries (Baker et al, 1984). Separate perfusion images can be acquired for several sources of pulmonary perfusion using microspheres labelled with different radionuclides or by using image subtraction techniques (Fig. 10.37).

Measurement of left ventricular function

The left ventricular ejection fraction can be measured from both the first pass (Kurtz et al, 1979) and the equilibrium-gated angiogram (Parrish et al, 1982). The first pass study is acquired in either right anterior oblique or anterior projections. It is analysed at a fast frame rate and a time-activity curve is created for the left ventricle (Fig. 10.38). The left ventricular count rate is assumed to be proportional to its volume. Once background counts have been subtracted, the ejection fraction can be calculated from the peaks and troughs of the time-activity curve. The equilibrium-gated study can be acquired in several projections. The images (approximately 20 frames) are viewed in a continuous cine format which enables the operator to detect regional wall motion abnormalities and abnormal chamber enlargement. The left anterior oblique projection is used for calculation of the left ventricular ejection fraction in the structurally normal heart. Slight caudal angulation of the camera (or the use of a 30 degree slant-hole collimator) will improve the separation of the left ventricular cavity from the remainder of the heart (Fig. 10.39). This view will have to be adjusted in patients with abnormal anatomy to provide optimal imaging of the left

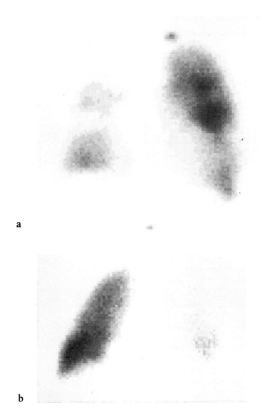

Fig. 10.37 A patient with pulmonary atresia was given an injection of microspheres into a Blalock-Taussig shunt via a cardiac catheter (a). This anterior image shows the distribution of blood flow from the main pulmonary artery. A second injection of microspheres (b) was given into a major aortopulmonary collateral artery arising from the descending aorta. By digital subtraction this image of the distribution of blood flow from the collateral was obtained.

ventricle. Accurate measurement of the ejection fraction is not possible if the separation of the left ventricle is inadequate. A time-activity curve of left ventricular counts throughout the study, corrected for background activity, is a representative volume curve from which ejection fraction can be calculated (Fig. 10.40).

Each of these two methods has advantages and disadvantages. The equilibrium angiogram provides better

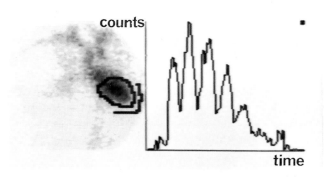

Fig. 10.38 The background corrected left ventricular time-activity curve from a first pass radionuclide angiogram. The frame rate is 32 frames per second. The ejection fraction can be calculated from the peaks and troughs of the curve. Here it is 67%.

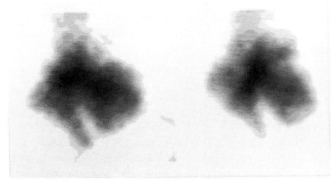

Fig. 10.39 (Left) Diastolic frame. (Right) Systolic frame from an equilibrium gated radionuclide angiogram in the left anterior oblique projection. The ejection fraction is 43%.

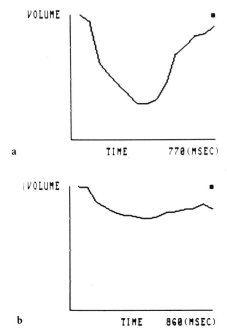

Fig. 10.40 (a) A left ventricular volume curve from an equilibrium radionuclide angiogram. The left ventricular function is normal, ejection fraction 68%. (b) The volume curve from a patient with global left ventricular dysfunction, ejection 24%.

counting statistics than the first pass study and so is to be preferred for study of regional wall motion abnormalities. Repeated views can be obtained without further doses of the radionuclide. The angiogram, however, takes several minutes to acquire, perhaps longer in young children. Motion artefacts can therefore be a problem, especially during exercise studies. The first pass angiogram can be acquired much more rapidly and so is suited to studies for assessing the effects of stress or exercise on left ventricular function. Technetium-99m with a half-life of 6 h is commonly used for these studies, but short half-life radionuclides (such as gold-195 m; half-life 30 s) are ideal. This is because the angiogram can be repeated several times during one investigation (Fazio et al, 1984). One major drawback is that first pass measurements of left ventricular performance are not possible in patients with intracardiac shunts.

Measurement of right ventricular function

It is not possible in the equilibrium angiogram completely to separate the right ventricle from the other chambers of the heart. A valid measurement of the right ventricular ejection fraction cannot, therefore, be made by this technique. While some workers have reported results that correlate remarkably well with cineangiography, the measurement in children with congenital heart malformations is not sufficiently accurate or reproducible to be recommended. The first pass measurement of right ventricular ejection fraction is, however, valid in this group of patients provided there is not an intracardiac right-to-left shunt. The measurement can be made in the same way as described for the left ventricle or by averaging the counts from several individual heart beats from the first pass study to create a single representative right ventricular volume curve (Berger et al, 1979).

Measurement of valve incompetence

Significant volume overload of either ventricle, if present, is usually apparent on viewing the equilibrium angiogram. Relative right or left ventricular volume overload can be quantitated by comparing the stroke counts (and therefore stroke volumes) of the left and right ventricles. Such a measurement is of use in the assessment of the severity of valve incompetence in patients without shunts. Good correlation with cineangiographic estimates of left-sided valve incompetence and stroke volume measurements has been reported (Rigo et al, 1979). The problems of defining the right ventricle in equilibrium angiograms limit the accuracy of this measurement, and the normal range for the radionuclide stroke volume ratio is wide. It is, nonetheless, a valuable non-invasive, semi-quantitative index of valve incompetence.

Phase imaging

Fourier analysis of the time-activity curve for each pixel of the equilibrium angiogram can be performed to generate an image of the timing of contraction within the heart. Such images can sensitively detect abnormally contracting areas within the myocardium (Dae & Botvinick, 1984). Intracardiac conduction defects may be demonstrated by this form of analysis (Underwood et al, 1984). In conditions with right ventricular volume overload, right ventricular contraction may be seen to be delayed in the absence of a conduction defect. This is found even when the right ventricular ejection fraction is normal.

Myocardial scintigraphy

Thallium-201 is taken up by the myocardium in a manner analogous to potassium (Lebowitz et al, 1975). Its use is well established as a myocardial perfusion imaging agent but it is not widely employed in children. Abnormalities of myocardial perfusion have been identified using this technique, however, in transient myocardial ischaemia of the newborn (Finley et al, 1979), cardiomyopathies (Dunn et al, 1982) and in presence of anomalies of the coronary arteries (Gilday, 1981). But the resolution obtainable with thallium imaging is poor and so images from small children are difficult to interpret. The sensitivity of the technique may be improved in older children by giving the thallium during maximal exercise and comparing images acquired immediately with those obtained after a delay of several hours (Fig. 10.41). There is no established clinical role for thallium imaging in childhood. Detailed studies of myocardial perfusion in congenital heart disease studied in this age-group will not be possible until improved imaging techniques are available.

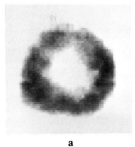 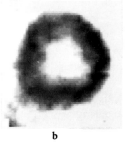

a   b

Fig. 10.41 Thallium myocardial perfusion images. Tomographic reconstructions of a short axis section through the left ventricle in a 13-year-old boy with a fistula between the left coronary artery and the coronary sinus. (a) After maximal bicycle exercise. There is perfusion defect in the anterior wall (top of figure). (b) After 4 h the defect has partially reperfused.

The role of radionuclide imaging

Radionuclide studies are a powerful non-invasive investigative tool in congenital heart disease. They can be used in all age-groups with no risk. The radiation dose from these investigations is small. Preoperatively they can be used for the detection and measurement of intracardiac shunts, the assessment of right and left ventricular performance and the severity of valve incompetence. Radionuclide studies are also valuable in the study of pulmonary perfusion abnormalities. Radionuclide investigations are also ideal for the non-invasive postoperative assessment of long-term surgical results. Residual shunts and valve incompetence can be detected and ventricular performance can be measured at rest and during exercise. Published studies have shown that these investigations can identify abnormalities of cardiac function in asymptomatic patients who have had correction of congenital defect (Reduto et al, 1980; Hurwitz et al, 1982; Ramsay et al, 1984).

4. MAGNETIC RESONANCE IMAGING

In principle, the heart and great veins leading into it and the great arteries leading from it are particularly appropriate for study by magnetic resonance imaging. There is a natural resonance contrast both between the lungs containing air and their blood vessels and also in the heart between its associated vascular structures. The pattern of periodic blood flow within the chambers of the heart and great vessels adds to the scope for this type of imaging. Stationary blood at the moment of image-acquisition returns a high signal and so appears bright in the picture. Blood moving out of the plane of imaging returns little signal and so appears black. Patterns of blood flow can be studied in a qualitative way and there are opportunities to employ formulas which permit quantitation of blood flow in blood vessels. Thus, it is possible, for example, to quantitate shunt size.

Two types of machine have been employed to study congenital heart diasese. One is the conventional commercially available unit. The other is the echoplanar imaging machine. Orthodox commercial resonance imaging machines acquire data for transectional images over a long period of time, usually between 2 and 8 min. There are many heart beats during this period. The cardiac movement associated with these normal events of the cardiac cycle produces artefact which obscures cardiac detail. By using electrocardiographically triggered gating techniques, however, any phase of the cardiac cycle may be studied with diminished cardiac motion artefact. Additionally, a multislice technique may be employed which presents images of contiguous slices acquired at the same time. The images may be viewed in sequence when data-acquisition is complete, thus presenting a 'pseudo real time' image sequence rather like a cineangiocardiogram. As with cineangiocardiographic studies, the human eye perceives more detail when moving structures (black through shades of grey to white) are viewed in the dark or with low levels of light intensity in the room. There is yet a further problem with conventional machines which relates to respiratory movement. As the chest wall and diaphragm move during respiration, so the heart moves. Cardiac function and rhythm may further vary with respiration. To ameliorate those potential problems, acquisition must be additionally gated either to the inspiratory or expiratory phase of respiration. When such gating methods are employed, cardiac image acquisition is a lengthy procedure. There are additional fundamental physical limits which are imposed by the conventional imaging technique. Taken together, this means that, for a three-

dimensional matrix (which is essential for cardiac study), the imaging time may be from 30–90 min.

In contrast, echoplanar magnetic resonance imaging employs a method in which the image acquisition time is 65 ms or less. Data are acquired which yield transectional images. The images may be viewed as they are acquired in real time and are free of motion artefact. No cardiac or respiratory gating is required, Transectional image sequences may be electrocardiographically triggered and related to the events of the cardiac cycle. Movie loops of the cardiac cycle are created in the transection sequence. As with transections, constructions in the sagittal, coronal or any other plane may be viewed as a still picture. Constructions may also be linked so that the events of the cardiac cycle may be viewed as movies. The total time period for an echoplanar image study of the heart has been less than 4 min. Even shorter times are in prospect, as is the employment of a multislice facility. Whereas sedation of young patients seems to be needed for studies using a conventional commercial magnetic resonance machine, the fast image acquisition which characterises the echoplanar method minimises the need for sedation. Indeed, in many cases, sedation may not be needed at all.

Thus, both echoplanar and conventional magnetic resonance methods yield data which may be used to create transections of the heart and thorax. Sagittal and coronal images may be produced and images may be displayed in any other plane. The images may be viewed as still snapshots or as movie loops. Since the heart is located anteriorly and superficially in the chest, the use of surface coils gives a prospect of even greater resolution using either technique. With its short acquisition time, the echoplanar method produces images with true resolution of structures within the limits of the equipment. Because of the size of the installation, however, neither the conventional nor the echoplanar machines will ever be able to be used in the way echocardiography is currently used for the examination of the infant in the incubator or cot or the outpatient in the clinic. Furthermore, as with a gamma camera machine or a computed tomographic scanner, the equipment is enormously expensive when compared with a cross-sectional echocardiographic machine.

Parameters of cardiac function measured by magnetic resonance

Ventricular volume and cardiac output

When the cardiac septum is intact at both atrial and ventricular levels, the output from each ventricle may be measured by several methods. First, the volume of each ventricle can be assessed at end-systole and end-diastole, permitting the stroke volume and ejection fraction to be determined separately for each ventricle. The ventricles are imaged in transection. Data on contiguous slices may be summed, with the area of the ventricular cavity on each transection being multiplied by slice thickness to give volume. Secondly, the formulas used in orthodox angiocardiography can be employed by assessing the area and length of the ventricular cavity. Thirdly, the volume of blood flowing through a vessel such as the aorta or pulmonary trunk during one cardiac cycle may be measured. Given the appropriate software, such a calculation leads to the assessment of systemic and pulmonary blood flow. If no shunt is present, the output from each ventricle may be quantified. Fourthly, the advent of contrast agents for resonance imaging should give the opportunity for quantitation as with other indicator dilution techniques.

Valve incompetence and shunt size

The functional impact on the heart of valve incompetence may be derived and quantified, given that the septal structures are intact, by using any of the four methods given above. The size of a shunt (left-to-right or right-to-left) may be calculated using the ventricular volume or area/length methods if the ventricular septum is intact or by using the other methods when there is a defect in the ventricular septum. All these methods depend on the development and application of appropriate software. As inspection of the echoplanar images will show, however, magnetic resonance does give the prospect of assessing the right ventricle in a better way than other imaging methods. The extent to which such assessments are relevant to management in infancy and childhood is open to question. For example, a little experience with something as simple as a chest radiograph will enable an informed observer to estimate the size of the shunt in terms of the flow ratio being less than 1.5 or greater than 2.5. Furthermore, experience with standard echocardiographic techniques tell us that estimation of valve incompetence and ventricular volumes taken in conjunction with a chest radiograph gives a very good idea of the cardiac status.

Myocardial assessments

Myocardial assessment in terms of wall movement is not difficult using the echoplanar imaging method. Wall movement in the ventricle during systole produces blood movement. This blood movement during ventricular systole normally results in the ventricular cavity appearing black in the image. Abnormalities of wall movement can be observed directly in the myocardium, as may the consequences of that muscle abnormality when it results in no (or limited) blood movement. This is because the blood, which is stationary (or nearly so) returns a high signal and appears white instead of black. Magnetic resonance spectroscopy permits the evaluation of muscle metabolism by identifying resonance peaks corresponding to levels of inorganic phosphate, creatine phosphate and

high energy phosphate within tissue. Perhaps more important in the paediatric field is the study of wall thickness and ventricular size in the various cardiomyopathies. It is also possible to envisage the study of myocardial perfusion when contrast agents are used in combination with magnetic resonance.

Diagnosis of the morphological abnormality in congenital heart disease

In assessing the structural defects of congenital heart disease there are four requirements: the sequential localisation of chambers and vessels; the identification of their connexions (normal or abnormal); the detail of the relationships of the various structures to each other; and the particular abnormality of each structure identified. The echoplanar imaging technique gives information about most of these four requirements. The images are 'still' snapshot pictures which are analogous to the individual frame of an angiocardiogram. The angiocardiogram, however, yields projections of structures opacified by contrast medium, whereas magnetic resonance methods give transections or constructions in the short axis, sagittal or coronal planes. A systematic analysis of the representation of the heart is essential. When this is carried out the pictures are not difficult to interpret. All the cases to be illustrated were correctly analysed with regard to diagnosis without information being available from the other imaging modalities such as the chest radiograph, echocardiography or angiocardiography.

I have found it useful in systematic analysis to develop a style of notation for description of the cardiac segmental connexions from the venous to the arterial end of the heart. Thus, in the normal heart the systemic veins (SV) connect with the right atrium (RA) and thence through the right ventricle (RV) to the pulmonary trunk (PT). On the left side, the pulmonary veins (PV) connect with the left atrium (LA) and then through the left ventricle (LV) to the aorta (AO). The septal structures are continuous and intact, and can be represented by a solid line in the sequential notation which reads

$$\frac{SV - RA - RV - PT}{PV - LA - LV - AO}$$

The echoplanar pictures give a unique sense of the cardiac structure in the context of the normal heart (Figs. 10.42, 10.43). It is in the abnormal heart, however, that the echoplanar transections relate to the decades of transectional postmortem studies in a way which perhaps approach. I have also found it helpful to keep in mind the essentials of embryological development (see Ch. 4). It is in such studies of malformed hearts that the validation of the echoplanar method is to be found (Chrispin et al, 1986a). Recollections of angiocardiographic studies are

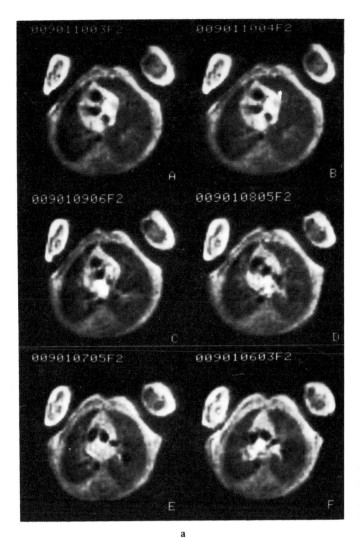

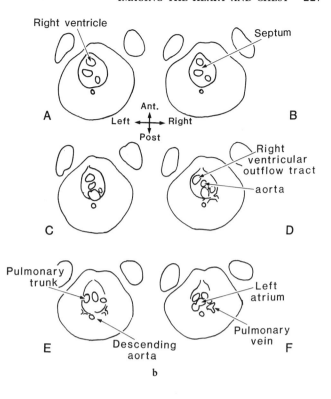

Fig. 10.42 Short axis echoplanar constructions progressing from caudal (A) to cephalad (F) in a patient with cystic fibrosis who has an anatomically normal heart. The drawings illustrate the salient landmarks and the 'compass' shows the orientation. See text for discussion. (Fig. 10.42a is reproduced by permission of Springer-Verlag from Chrispin et al, 1986a.)

helpful when viewing echoplanar constructions in the coronal or sagittal planes, but study of contiguous constructions is essential (Chrispin et al, 1986b). Just as with all magnetic resonance methods applied to other systems, the yield of cardiac information is very large.

The normal heart

Echoplanar transections of the heart are most easily analysed by starting with the transection just below the diaphragm and then progressing in a cephalad direction.

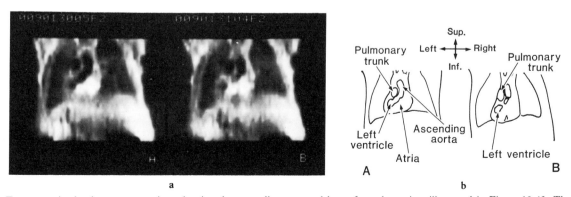

Fig. 10.43 Two coronal echoplanar constructions showing the normally connected heart form the patient illustrated in Figure 10.43. The 'compass' shows the orientation.

Slices of 7.3 mm thickness are shown in Figure 10.43, the interval between each being 3 mm to 7 mm. In viewing the transections the observer should imagine he is looking down from above. The cardiac apex then lies to the observer's left. The most caudal section illustrated (Fig. 10.42 – A) is at midventricular level. Thereafter, the sequence progresses cephalad from A to F to show the remainder of the ventricles and the great arteries. The right ventricle is seen to lie anteriorly to the left ventricle (Fig. 10.42 – A). At midventricular level the septum in this patient makes an angle of 90° to the sagittal plane, although in transections more caudal (not illustrated) the septum makes an angle of 50° to the sagittal plane. Rotation of the septum increases in cephalad direction (Fig. 10.42 – C), continuing to show separation of the right ventricular outflow tract from the aorta until the pulmonary trunk is separated from the aorta. Thus, at ventricular and great arterial level there is a separation of the flow of blood as rotation of septation through a total of about 130° occurs. Two contiguous coronal constructions are shown in Figure 10.43. The heart is viewed, as it were, from the back of the patient. The left ventricle connects to the aorta. The right ventricular outflow tract and pulmonary trunk are seen lying adjacent to the aorta and left ventricle. Thus, in this normal heart the connexions from the right ventricle to the pulmonary trunk and the left ventricle to the aorta are clearly defined together with their relationships. It is worth noting that the heart lies at some distance from the anterior chest wall. This infant had cystic fibrosis with an increase in lung volume. This increase makes the heart particularly difficult to assess by echocardiography, rather as occurs in adults with chronic bronchitis and emphysema.

Complete transposition

The cardiac connexions in complete transposition with intact ventricular septum following balloon atrial septostomy may be represented in my simple notation as

$$\frac{SV - RA - RV - AO}{PV - LA - LV - PT}$$

The break in the continuity of the line between the atrial chambers represents the defect in the interatrial septum. The discordant ventriculo-arterial connexion is shown, since the right ventricle connects to the aorta and the left ventricle connects to the pulmonary trunk. Echoplanar transections from a 3-month-old infant with complete transposition after balloon atrial septostomy are shown in Figure 10.44. Short axis sections are shown in Figures 10.44 (A & B).

The right ventricle at midventricular level is anterior to the septum and the left ventricle is posterior (Fig. 10.44 – A). The aorta also lies anteriorly while the bifurcation

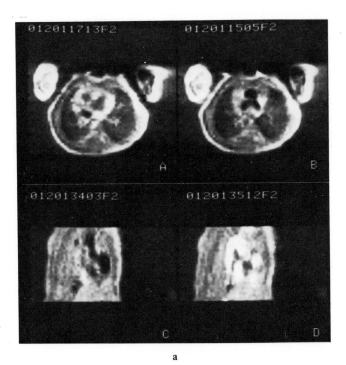

a

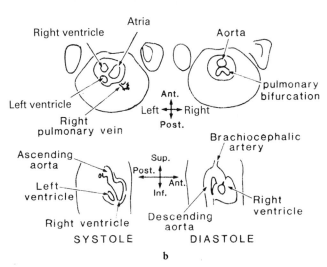

b

Fig. 10.44 Short axis (A & B) and sagittal (C & D) echoplanar transections from 3-month-old patient with complete transposition and intact ventricular septum who had undergone balloon atrial septostomy. The diagrams show the orientation and important structures.
(Fig. 10.44A & B is reproduced by permission of Springer-Verlag from Chrispin et al, 1986a.)

of the pulmonary trunk (seagull sign) lies posteriorly (Fig. 10.44 – B). There is virtually no rotation in septation at ventricular or great arterial level. Note also that there is no evidence of the atrial septum. This is the case through much of the cardiac cycle because of almost continuous mixing of the blood at atrial level. The right pulmonary vein can be seen as a white structure connecting to the left atrium during a period of slow venous blood flow (Fig. 10.44 – B). Sagittal constructions are shown in Figures 10.44 – C, D. During ventricular systole (Fig. 10.44 – C) the right ventricle and ascending aorta are seen as black structures because of blood movement. During ventricular diastole the right ventricle becomes white (Fig. 10.44 – D). Arterial branches from the aortic arch extend towards the thoracic inlet to supply the head and neck. These vessels have an internal calibre of the order of 3 mm at this age. This was the limit of true resolution in the echoplanar equipment at this time. Forward flow is visible during ventricular systole, analysis of sagittal sections showing the aortic arch and descending aorta. With the onset of diastole, flow first ceases at the aortic valve and at the level of the arterial ligament. Flow continues down the descending aorta and from the aortic arch to the vessels supplying the head and neck. Thus, there is a 'watershed' in flow pattern at the junction of the posterior end of the aortic arch and the descending aorta (at the level of the arterial ligament), with this site having the longest period without blood flow.

Tetralogy of Fallot

The essence of tetralogy of Fallot is a ventricular septal defect with overriding of the aorta and, usually, reduced calibre of the pulmonary arteries. Using the conventional notation, this is represented as

$$\frac{SV - RA - RV - pt}{PV - LA - LV - AO}$$

The gap in continuity of the line represents the ventricular septal defect while the 'pt' (in lower case) represents the reduced calibre of the pulmonary trunk. This arrangement as seen using echoplanar transections in an infant is shown in Figure 10.45. In pictures acquired during atrial systole the right atrium is visible (Fig. 10.45) while the left atrium is seen in a more cephalad transection (Fig. 10.45 – B). The right ventricle is anterior to the septum and the left ventricle. A more cephalad transection (Fig. 10.45 – C) shows the infundibular narrowing anteriorly and, posteriorly, the left ventricular outflow tract. The septal defect is seen between the ventricular outlets. The large aortic root and the narrow subpulmonary infundibulum and pulmonary trunk are seen (Figs. 10.45 – D, E). The aorta is large, right-sided and unduly anterior, producing the typical override. These transections highlight the

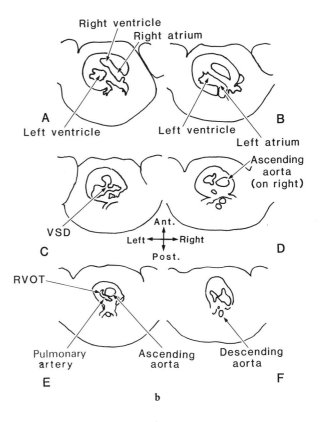

Fig. 10.45 Short axis (A–F) echoplanar transections in a patient with severe tetralogy of Fallot. See text for discussion. (Fig. 10.45a is reproduced by permission of Springer-Verlag from Chrispin et al, 1986a.)

notion that the cardinal problem in severe tetralogy is abnormal septation at great arterial level, with discontinuity of septation at ventricular level to create the ventricular septal defect.

Common arterial trunk

The circulation and connexions in common arterial trunk may be represented notationally as

$$\frac{SV - RA - RV}{PV - LA - LV}TRUNK$$

Here the cessation of continuity of the line represents the subtruncal ventricular septal defect. In lieu of pulmonary trunk and aorta leaving the heart, there is the single great artery, the common trunk. Thus, there is a complete defect of septation beginning at ventricular level and continuing through the great arteries. The pictures in Figures 10.46 and 10.47 show the arrangement in the first infant with this lesion which we studied using this method. Short axis transections during ventricular systole are shown in Figure 10.46. The apex of the large left ventricle is seen in Figure 10.46 – A with the interventricular septum seen in Figure 10.46 – B. Rotation of the interventricular septum is very limited, as seen in Figures 10.46 – A, B & C. Figure 10.46 – D shows the subtruncal defect. One of the sagittal constructions is shown in Figure 10.47. During ventricular systole the large left ventricular cavity is shown and lies posterior to the septum. Anterior to the septum lies the smaller right ventricle. Moving blood is seen as black in the ventricles. In the most caudal part of

the right ventricle there is stationary blood returning a bright signal. Although not quantified, the inference is that, since this was a continuing feature of the right ventricular cavity, ventricular function is abnormal. Even though the right ventricle is small, its contribution to cardiac output is disproportionately small. In movie loops of the echoplanar images, the difference between the nature of the left and right ventricular contraction and emptying is uniquely demonstrated in the normal and abnormal heart. Progressing cephalad in this sagittal construction, the subtruncal ventricular septal defect is shown, as is the truncal valve (seen as a white line at the origin of the common trunk). Valves are visible during systole because, even with the resolution depicted in these pictures, there is blood around the surfaces of the valves which is either moving very slowly or is stationary and so returns a high signal.

Right heart hypoplasia

The connexions and circulation in this entity may be represented notationally as

$$\frac{SV - RA \star rv \star pt}{PV - LA - LV - AO}$$

The defect in continuity of the line represents the defect in atrial septation. The asterisks represent the stenosed diminutive tricuspid and pulmonary valves respectively while the symbols in lower case letters (rv, pt) represent the small right ventricle and pulmonary trunk. In a patient we studied with this lesion (Fig. 10.48), the left ventricle

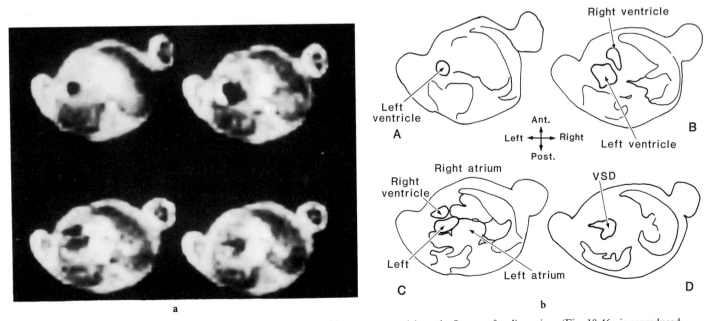

Fig. 10.46 Short axis (A–D) echoplanar transections in a patient with common arterial trunk. See text for discussion. (Fig. 10.46a is reproduced by permission of Springer-Verlag from Chrispin et al, 1986a.)

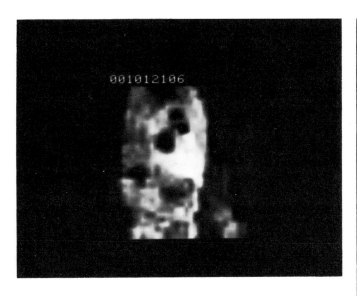

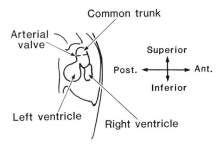

Fig. 10.47 A sagittal echoplanar transection in the patient shown in Figure 10.46 with common arterial trunk. (Fig. 10.47 is reproduced by permission of Springer-Verlag from Chrispin et al, 1986a.)

was shown to be very large by comparison with the diminutive right ventricle. In sagittal constructions the diminutive right ventricle is seen anteriorly and is dark and round (Fig. 10.48 – top). It is also seen as a triangular dark image (Fig. 10.48 – bottom). The very large aorta is seen ascending into the thorax from the left ventricular outflow tract (partly visible – Fig. 10.48 – top). A considerable deformity of the chest with prominent sternal bowing is associated with the cardiac lesion. The echoplanar study gives a good representation of the altered thoracic configuration and also the lack of subcutaneous fat when the infant is ill. The small amount of fat covering these patients is well shown.

Comments and perspectives

This is not the place to discuss the technology of either radiology or magnetic resonance imaging. The development of magnetic resonance technology may be studied in the works of Mansfield & Grannell (1973), Mansfield (1977) and Mansfield & Morris (1982). Reports by Jacobstein et al (1984a, b) and by McNamara & Higgins (1984) give a very clear idea of the potential for gated cardiac imaging using magnetic resonance in congenital heart

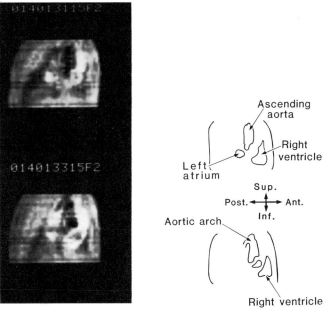

Fig. 10.48 Two sagittal echoplanar constructions in a patient with pulmonary atresia, intact ventricular septum and hypoplastic right ventricle.

disease. Early reports by Rzedzian et al (1983, 1984) and by Chrispin and colleagues (1986a, b) describe the initial echoplanar imaging work in infants with congenital heart disease. The Lancet (1984) observed that the projections for annual sales of magnetic resonance scanners will reach a value of $2500 million worldwide in 1988. The conclusion reached was that 'If manufacturers are correct in their estimates, sales of NMR imagers will have expanded at a rate too quick for any realistic assessment of the true place of these devices'. In short, magnetic resonance scanners will be acquired even though their clinical relevance and worth has not been proved. Costs per patient study when using a conventional magnetic resonance unit are inevitably high. The studies take a long time and so patient throughput on the machine is low. Time is very much shorter with echoplanar imaging. With the additonal use of a multislice technique it will become shorter still, say 1 or 2 min. A high patient throughput on an echoplanar machine is possible. As a result, the costs will be very much lower per patient study. The costs of echoplanar studies might well compete with the costs of radiographs and echocardiograms combined. Echoplanar imaging studies show overall heart size, chamber size and myocardial function. They also show cardiovascular connexions and cardiac defect. Already there is the qualitative assessment of blood flow and quantitation of blood flow in prospect. It is conceivable that such studies could provide all the essential information prior to paediatric cardiac surgery. Nevertheless, all magnetic resonance machines are fixed installations. In contrast, both echocardiographic and radiographic machines are mobile and consequently are available at the place of need. Additionally, the ability to place and angle the transducer of an echocardiographic unit in an almost infinitely variable way will mean that, for example, echocardiograhic studies will continue for demonstration of the detail of a 'cleft' and incompetent left atrioventricular valve in an atrioven-

tricular septal defect. It is a tenable viewpoint that no paediatric cardiologist or paediatric surgeon should feel that there is a compelling need to acquire conventional magnetic resonance equipment before 1989 in addition to that equipment already available. By 1990 high speed magnetic resonance imaging should have come of age.

REFERENCES

Askenazi J, Nadas A S 1975 Anomalous left coronary artery originating from the pulmonary artery. Circulation 51: 976–987

Baker E J, Malamitsi J, Jones O D H, Maisey M N, Tynan M J 1984 Use of radionuclide labelled microspheres to show the distribution of the pulmonary perfusion with multifocal pulmonary blood supply. British Heart Journal 52: 72–76

Baker E J, Ellam S V, Lorber A, Jones O D H, Tynan M J, Maisey M N 1985 Superiority of radionuclide over oximetry measurement of left to right shunts. British Heart Journal 53: 535–540

Berdon W E, Baker D H, Wung J T, et al 1984 Complete cartilage-ring tracheal stenosis associated with anomalous left pulmonary artery: the ring-sling complex. Radiology 152: 57–64

Berger H J, Matthay R A, Pytlik L M, Gottschalk A, Zaret B L 1979 First pass radionuclide assessment of right and left ventricular performance in patients with cardiac and pulmonary disease. Seminars in Nuclear Medicine 9: 275–295

Boone M L, Swenson B E, Felson B 1964 Rib notching: its many causes. American Journal of Roentgenology 91: 1075–1088

Calder L, Van Praagh R, Van Praagh S, et al 1976 Truncus arteriosus communis. Clinical, angiographic, and pathologic findings in 100 patients. American Heart Journal 92: 23–38

Chrispin A 1973 The lung in mitral valve disease. Annales de Radiologie 26:259

Chrispin A, Small P, Rutter N, et al 1986a Transectional echo planar imaging of the heart in cyanotic congenital heart disease. Pediatric Radiology 16: 293–297

Chrispin A, Small P, Rutter N, et al 1986b Echo planar imaging of normal and abnormal connections of the heart and great arteries. Pediatric Radiology 16: 289–292

Collins G, Calder L, Rose V, Kidd L, Keith J 1972 Ventricular septal defect: clinical and haemodynamic changes in the first five years of life. American Heart Journal 84: 695–705

Coussement A M, Gooding C A 1973 Objective radiographic assessment of pulmonary vascularity in children. Radiology 109: 649–654

Dae M W, Botvinick E H 1984 Characterisation of conduction and contraction abnormalities by scintigraphic phase analysis. International Journal of Cardiology 5: 244–253

Daves M L 1968 Roentgenology of tetralogy of Fallot. Seminars in Roentgenology 3:377

Deanfield J, Leanage R, Stroobant J, Chrispin A R, Taylor J F N, Macartney F J 1980 Use of high kilovoltage filtered beam radiographs for detection of bronchial situs in infants and young children. British Heart Journal 44: 577–583

Dunn R F, Uren R F, Sadich N, et al 1982 Comparison of thallium-201 scanning in idiopathic dilated cardiomyopathy and severe coronary artery disease. Circulation 66: 804–810

Elliot L P, Schiebler G L 1979 The X-Ray diagnosis of congenital heart disease in infants, children and adults. Charles C. Thomas, Springfield, p 296–341

Fazio F, Gerundini P, Margonato A, et al 1984 Quantitative radionuclide angiocardiography using gold-195m. American Journal of Cardiology 53: 1442–1446

Figley M M 1954 Accessory roentgen signs of coarctation of the aorta. Radiology 62: 671–686

Finley J P, Howman-Giles R B, Gilday D L, Rowe R D 1979 Transient myocardial ischaemia of the newborn infant demonstrated by thallium myocardial imaging. Journal of Pediatrics 94: 263–270

Gates G F, Orme H W, Dore E K 1971 Measurement of cardiac shunting with technetium labelled albumin aggregates. Journal of Nuclear Medicine 12: 746–749

Gates G F, Orme H W, Dore E K 1974 Cardiac shunt assessment in children with macroaggregated albumin technetium-99m. Radiology 112: 649–653

Gilday D L 1981 Radionuclides in paediatric cardiology. In: Friedman L M, Weissman H S (eds) Nuclear medicine annual. Raven Press, New York, p 251–273

Haroutanian L M, Neill C A, Wagner H N 1969 Radioisotope scanning of the lung in cyanotic congenital heart disease. American Journal of Cardiology 23: 387–395

Hellenbrand W E, Kelley M J, Berman M A 1977 Heart failure and cyanosis in a newborn. Cerebral arteriovenous malformation involving the vein of Galen. Chest 72: 225–227

Higgins C B, Rausch J, Friedman W F, et al 1977 Patent ductus in preterm infants with idiopathic respiratory distress syndrome. Radiographic and echocardiographic evaluation. Radiology 124: 189–195

Hurwitz R A, Papanicolaou N, Treves S, Keane J F, Castaneda A D 1982 Radionuclide angiocardiography in evaluation of patients after repair of transposition of the great arteries. American Journal of Cardiology 49: 761–765

Jacobstein M D, Fletcher B D, Nelson A D, Clampitt R T, Alfidi R J, Riemenschneider T A 1984a Magnetic resonance imaging: evaluation of palliative systemic-pulmonary shunts. Circulation 70: 650–656

Jacobstein M D, Fletcher B D, Nelson A D, Goldstein S, Alfidi R J, Riemenchneider T A 1984b ECG-gated nuclear magnetic resonance imaging: appearance of congenitally malformed heart. American Heart Journal 107: 1014–1020

Kurlander G J, Petry E L, Girod D A 1968 Plain film diagnosis of congenital heart disease in the new born period. American Journal of Roentgenology 103: 66–77

Kurtz D, Ahnberg D S, Freed M, LaFarge C G, Treves S 1979 Quantitative radionuclide angiocardiography. Determination of left ventricular ejection fraction in children. British Heart Journal 38: 966–973

Lancet 1984 The big business of NMR scanners. Lancet 2:1169

Lancet 1985 Editorial. Safety of NMR. Lancet 1: 913–914

Lauterbur P 1973 Image formations by induced local interactions: examples employing nuclear magnetic resonance. Nature 242: 190–191

Lebowitz E, Green M W, Fairchild R, et al 1975 Thallium-201 for medical use. I. Journal of Nuclear Medicine 16: 151–155

Litwin S B, Fellows K 1973 Systemic to pulmonary arterial shunts for patients with cyanotic congenital heart disease. Pediatric Radiology 1: 41–46

Luke M J, McDonnel E J 1968 Congenital heart disease and scoliosis Journal of Pediatrics 73: 725–733

McIlveen B M, Murray I P C, Giles R W, Molk G H, Scarf C M, McCredie R M 1981 Clinical applications of radionuclide quantitation of left to right shunts in children. American Journal of Cardiology 47: 1273–1278

McNamara M T, Higgins C B 1984 Cardiovascular applications of magnetic resonance imaging. Magnetic Resonance Imaging 2: 167–186

Maltz D L, Treves S 1973 Quantitative radionuclide angiography:

determination of Qp : Qs in children. Circulation 47: 1049–1056

Mansfield P 1977 Multi-planar image formation using NMR spin echoes. Journal of Physics C. Solid State Physics 10:L55

Mansfield P, Grannell P K 1973 NMR diffraction in solids. Journal of Physics C. Solid State Physics 6:L422

Mansfield P, Morris P G 1982 Echo planar imaging in NMR imaging in biomedicine. Academic Press, New York, p 143–154

Nasser W K 1970 Congenital absence of the left pericardium. American Journal of Cardiology 26: 466–470

Parrish M D, Graham J P Jr, Born M L, Jones J 1982 Radionuclide evaluation of right and left ventricular function in children: validation of methodology. American Journal of Cardiology 49: 1241–1247

Peter C A, Armstrong B E, Jones R H 1981 Radionuclide quantitation of right-to-left intracardiac shunts in children. Circulation 64: 572–577

Ramsay J M, Venables A W, Kelly M J, Kalff V 1984 Right and left ventricular function at rest and with exercise after the Mustard operation for transposition of the great arteries. British Heart Journal 51: 364–370

Reduto L A, Berger H J, Johnstone D E, et al 1980 Radionuclide assessment of right and left ventricular exercise reserve after total correction of tetralogy of Fallot. American Journal of Cardiology 45: 1013–1018

Rigo P, Alderson P O, Robertson R M, Becker L C, Wagner H N Jr 1979 Measurement of aortic and mitral regurgitation by gated cardiac blood pool scans. Circulation 60: 306–312

Roesler M, de Leval M, Chrispin A, Stark J 1983 Surgical management of vascular ring. Annals of Surgery 197: 139–146

Röntgen W C 1975 In: Encyclopaedia Britannica – Macropaedia Vol 15. Encyclopaedia Britannica Inc, London, p 383

Rzedzian R, Doyle M, Mansfield P, et al 1983 Real-time NMR clinical imaging in paediatrics. Lancet 2: 1281–1282

Rzedzian R, Doyle M, Mansfield P, et al 1984 Echo planar imaging in Paediatrics: real-time-nuclear magnetic resonance. Annales de Radiologie 27: 182–186

Simon M 1968 The pulmonary vasculature in congenital heart disease. Radiologic Clinics of North America 6: 303–317

Stanger P, Rudolph A M, Edwards J E 1977 Cardiac malpositions. Circulation 56: 159–172

Steele P, Kirch D, LeFree M, Battock D 1976 Measurement of right and left ventricular ejection fractions by radionuclide angiocardiography in coronary artery disease. Chest 70: 51–56

Stewart J R, Kincaid O W, Edwards J E 1964 Atlas of vascular rings and related malformations of the aortic arch system. Charles C. Thomas, Springfield, Illinois

Strauss H W, Zaret B L, Hurley P J, Natarajan T K, Pitt B 1971 A scintiphotographic method for measuring left ventricular ejection fraction in man without cardiac catheterisation. American Journal of Cardiology 28: 575–580

Swischuk L E 1979 Plain film interpretation in congenital heart disease. Williams & Wilkins, Baltimore

Tehranzadeh J, Kelly M J 1979 The differential density sign of pericardial effusion. Radiology 133: 23–30

Treves S 1980 Detection and quantitation of cardiovascular shunts with commonly available radionuclides. Seminars in Nuclear Medicine 10: 16–25

Twigg H L, deLeon A C, Perloff J K, Majid M 1967 The straight back syndrome: Radiographic manifestations. Radiology 88: 274–277

Underwood S R, Walton S, Laming P L, Ell P J, Emanuel R W, Swanton R H 1984 Patterns of ventricular contraction in patients with conduction abnormality studied by radionuclide angiocardiography. British Heart Journal 51: 568–574

Van Mierop L H S, Eisen S, Schiebler G L 1970 The radiographic appearance of the tracheobronchial tree as an indicator of visceral situs. American Journal of Cardiology 26: 432–435

11

A. Garson

Electrocardiography

'There are comparatively few people who are not in greater danger of having their peace and happiness destroyed by an erroneous diagnosis of cardiac abnormality based on a faulty interpretation of an electrocardiogram than of being injured or killed by an atomic bomb'. Thus began Frank Wilson's introduction to Lepeschkin's *Modern electrocardiography*, over 30 years ago (1951). The same holds true today. Because it is so important to understand the basis and range of the normal, we will devote the first half of this chapter to the normal electrocardiogram, its electrophysiologic principles, the summation of cellular events on the body surface, the definition and proper measurement of the electrocardiographic waveforms, and finally the variations produced by malposition of the heart within the thorax. In the second half of the chapter, we will consider the abnormal electrocardiogram. Since electrocardiography provides both complementary and supplementary information to echocardiography and nuclear imaging in terms of cardiac chamber enlargement and hypertrophy, we will consider the continuing contribution of the electrocardiogram in this area. The specific morphology of ventricular depolarisation and repolarisation will be shown to provide information on conduction disturbance, myocardial ischaemia, injury and infarction. The effect of systemic alterations on the electrocardiogram will be discussed: electrolyte abnormality, drug effects, and the effect of diseases in other parts of the body on the heart. Finally, a systematic approach to the recognition of artifacts will be presented in the hope that the patient with a normal heart will not become an 'electrocardiographic casualty' (Surawicz, 1966) due to an erroneous interpretation of what is truly sinus rhythm.

ANATOMY OF THE CONDUCTION SYSTEM

The cardiac conduction system extends from the sinus node to the atrial and ventricular myocardium. The sinus node is a fusiform structure, 10–20 mm long in the adult, which lies in the terminal groove slightly lateral to the junction of the right atrial appendage and the superior caval vein (Lev & Bharati, 1977). It is usually located immediately below the epicardium and extends transmurally close to the endocardium (Fig. 11.1). The sinus node surrounds the largest atrial artery, the sinus node artery. In 55–65% of cases it is a branch of the right coronary artery, being a branch of the left circumflex coronary artery in the remainder (Kulbertus & Demoulin, 1975).

The cellular constituents of the sinus node are supported by a collagen framework which increases in density with age. The primary cells are the nodal cells. These are round, pale staining cells which occur in clusters close to the central artery (James, 1977). These are thought to be the true pacemaking cells. The nodal cells are connected either to other nodal cells or to transitional cells. These are small fusiform cells. They have some of the characteristics of nodal cells combined with those of atrial muscle cells. Transitional cells completely surround the borders of the sinus node and are thought to be the site of sinu-atrial entrance and exit block (Kugler, 1981). Parasympathetic ganglia border the anterior and posterior portions of the sinus node.

The mode of conduction of impulses within the atria has been the subject of much controversy. The major question concerns the existence of the internodal tracts. Does conduction proceed preferentially through the atria via specialised pathways? Certain facts can be brought to bear. Electrophysiologically, the conduction velocity has been shown to be increased in three areas of the right atrium. The 'anterior internodal pathway' extends from the sinus node, runs anteriorly to the superior caval vein, through the anterior part of the atrial septum and to the superior part of the atrioventricular node. The 'middle internodal pathway' proceeds posterior to the superior caval vein and then to the rim of the oval fossa where it joins the anterior pathway. The 'posterior internodal pathway' (Thorel, 1910) runs in the terminal crest to the inferior atrial septum adjacent to the inferior caval vein. It then travels superior to the orifice of the coronary sinus and terminates in the posterior part of the atrioventricular node. The 'anterior

235

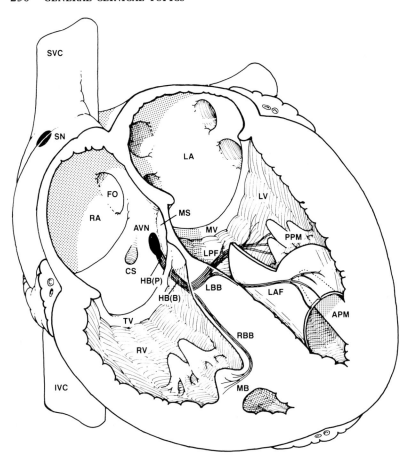

Fig. 11.1 Anatomy of the conduction system. Abbreviations: APM – anterior papillary muscle; AVN – AV node; CS – coronary sinus; FO – oral foramen; HB (P) – conduction axis, penetrating portion; HB(B) – conduction axis, branching portion; IVC – inferior caval vein; LA – left atrium; LAF – left anterior fascicle; LBB – left bundle branch; LV – left ventricle; LPF – left posterior fascicle; MB – moderator band; MS – membranous septum; MV – mitral valve; PPM – posterior papillary muscle; RA – right atrium; RV – right ventricle; SVC – superior caval vein.

intra-atrial tract' (Bachmann, 1916) is a thick band of muscle that courses from the anterior part of the sinus node anteriorly to the superior caval vein and thence through the atrial septum to the left atrial musculature.

In these areas of more rapid conduction, the atrial muscle cells are oriented in a parallel fashion (Spach & Barr, 1976). These pathways are not, however, isolated from the rest of the atrium by connective tissue (Lev & Bharati, 1977). These facts have been interpreted by James (1963), Waldo et al (1971), Merideth & Titus (1968) and Liebman & Plonsey (1978) as indicating the presence of true specialised conduction. On the other hand, the view that these pathways are the shortest anatomic distance between the sinus and atrioventricular nodes and that conduction may be facilitated only by the parallel fiber orientation (rather than the existence of true tracts) is held by Spach & Barr (1976), Lev & Bharati (1977), Durrer et al (1970) and Janse & Anderson (1974). The finding by Gillette et al (1974b) that, after the Mustard operation for complete transposition, the internodal conduction time from the high right atrium to low septal right atrium is normal, supports the view that there are no true internodal tracts. If there were, these tracts should have been injured by atriotomy, suturing of the baffle or coronary sinus cutback, and the conduction time should have been prolonged, which it was not. Our view is that conduction

spreads radially and syncytially from the sinus node to the atrioventricular node by the fastest possible route. The concept of 'specialised tracts' should be reserved for intraventricular conduction via the bundle branches and does not apply to intra-atrial conduction.

The specialised atrioventricular conduction axis is the only normal conduction pathway from atria to ventricles. The nodal component of the axis is located in the right atrium on the right side of the central fibrous body. It is located within the triangle of Koch between the mouth of the coronary sinus and the annulus of the septal leaflet of the tricuspid valve (Ho & Anderson, 1985; Fig. 11.1). The left surface of the node rests on the mitral annulus. The blood supply to the node is via the artery of Haas (1911). This arises from the dominant coronary artery, which is the right in 90% of cases. The compact node is composed of nodal cells with small transitional cells interweaving with collagen in all different directions in the upper and middle portions of the node. In the anterior and inferior part of the node, the fibres begin to orient longitudinally to form the penetrating atrioventricular bundle. Parasympathetic ganglia and sympathetic nerve endings are located posteriorly to the compact node.

When the axis has penetrated the central fibrous body, it is designated the 'penetrating bundle' (or 'bundle of His'). This proceeds anteriorly and medially through the central fibrous body and emerges inferiorly to become the non-branching bundle along the rim of the membranous ventricular septum immediately below the non-coronary leaflet of the aortic valve. In approximately 75% of human hearts, the non-branching bundle runs along the left side of the crest of the muscular ventricular septum. In the remainder, it courses along the right side. It is made up of small oval cells which are longitudinally oriented. There are fibrous collagen septa in this portion of the bundle, which divide the fibres 'predestined' for one of the bundle branches even at this proximal level. A fibrotic lesion in part of the penetrating bundle may, therefore, simulate a more distal lesion in the bundle branches.

The branching portion of the conduction axis begins as fibres forming the left bundle branch cascade down the septal surface from the main bundle. This occurs at the level of the commissure formed by the right and non-coronary cusps. The origin of the left bundle branch is quite variable. All of the fibres may fan out together, or they may be given off in separate fascicles (Rosenbaum et al, 1970; Kulbertus & Demoulin, 1976). The fascicles are composed of cells which are minimally larger than ordinary myocardial cells. Each fascicle is surrounded by a connective tissue sheath and therefore makes no contact with the ventricular muscle for approximately 20 mm. Then, multiple 'Purkinje' fibres branch throughout the endocardium of the left ventricle. The posterobasal left ventricle is virtually devoid of rapidly conducting fibres. This area of the left ventricle is therefore the last part to be activated.

After the last fibres of the left bundle branch are given off from the branching bundle, the axis continues as the right bundle branch. The right bundle branch proceeds subendocardially or intramyocardially within the septo-marginal trabecula (septal band), running immediately inferior to the medial papillary muscle (muscle of Lancisi or papillary muscle of the conus) until the bundle runs through the moderator band. The entire right bundle branch is insulated throughout its non-branching course. When it reaches the anterior papillary muscle of the right ventricle, it separates into numerous Purkinje fibres which ramify throughout the endocardium. The right ventricular infundibulum is virtually devoid of Purkinje tissue. This, added to the normally delayed right ventricular activation due to the insulated right bundle branch, makes the infundibulum the last part of the heart to be activated.

DEPOLARISATION AND REPOLARISATION: CELLULAR ELECTROPHYSIOLOGY

The single cell: cardiac action potential

It is important to begin the consideration of depolarisation and repolarisation with the action potential of the single cell. This is not only because the surface electrocardiogram is a summation of cellular potentials, but also because the effects on the electrocardiogram of alterations in the cardiac milieu (for example by drugs or ischaemia) are more easily understood at the cellular level and then applied to the intact heart. The cardiac action potential is the net result of a sequence of changes in the ionic permeabilities of the cell membrane with different ions carrying charges into and out of the cell. In the normal heart, two different types of action potentials are generated, depending upon the type of cell. These action potentials are named by the rapidity of their upstroke in the initial part of depolarisation: the 'fast response' and the 'slow response' (Reder & Rosen, 1981).

Fast response action potential

Atrial and ventricular myocardial cells and ventricular conduction cells normally have fast response action potentials. The resting cell membrane is permeable to potassium but relatively impermeable to sodium ions. If a microelectrode is passed inside such a cell, the inside is negatively charged with respect to the outside, the magnitude being approximately –90 mV (Fig. 11.2). This is the 'resting membrane potential'. When a cell is stimulated, sodium

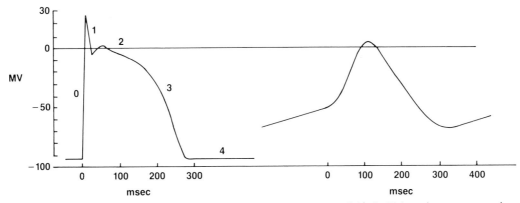

Fig. 11.2 Left – fast response action potential similar to that found in a ventricular myocardial cell. Right – slow response action potential similar to that found in a sinus node P cell.

permeability increases markedly. There is a rapid inflow of sodium causing a rapid depolarisation such that the inside of the cell is positive with respect to the outside (Cooksey et al, 1977). This is the most rapid phase of the action potential (phase 0) and is completed within several milliseconds. The rapidity with which phase 0 occurs is defined as the change in voltage with respect to time and is called V_{max}. This correlates with the conduction velocity in a single cell. Phase 1 of 'early rapid repolarisation' is primarily due to an outward repolarising chloride current. At the same time as the chloride current occurs, the inward sodium current is decreasing and the outward potassium current beginning. During phase 2, the plateau, there is a balance of currents. Slow inward currents are caused by calcium and sodium, and outward currents are caused by chloride and potassium. During repolarisation (phase 3), the balance changes such that the inward currents decrease and the outward potassium current predominates.

It becomes possible to stimulate the cell to depolarise again during phase 3. The ability to re-excite a cell depends on both the time elapsed since the last depolarisation (phase 0) and the absolute voltage that the membrane has reattained during repolarisation. A normal Purkinje cell cannot be re-excited unless approximately 200 ms has passed since the last depolarisation, or unless the membrane potential has returned to –55 to –60 mV. In cellular electrophysiology, the time period when the cell is inexcitable is called the 'absolute refractory period'. In the cardiac electrophysiology catheterisation laboratory this generally corresponds to the effective refractory period. In general, a shorter action potential duration is associated with a shorter effective refractory period. In the 'relative refractory period', the cell is not fully excitable but has repolarised sufficiently to generate an action potential. The resultant action potential from stimulation during the relative refractory period may be distorted with a less rapid rate of rise of phase 0 and therefore a slower conduction velocity within the cell. In some cells, rapid repolarisation (phase 3) overshoots and the membrane potential hyperpolarises (becomes more negative than the resting membrane potential). If the cell is stimulated during this period, V_{max} during phase 0 of the resultant action potential may be increased over that of the normal action potential resulting in more rapid conduction. For this reason, this has been called the 'supernormal period' (Fig. 11.3; Watanabe & Dreifus, 1977).

When repolarisation is complete, phase 4 begins. In atrial and ventricular myocardial cells, there is no net movement of charge during phase 4. Rather there is a balance between slow inward sodium current and an outward potassium current. In Purkinje cells, however, there may be spontaneous diastolic depolarisation. The membrane potential during phase 4 gradually decays to less negative values because of reduction in the outward potas-

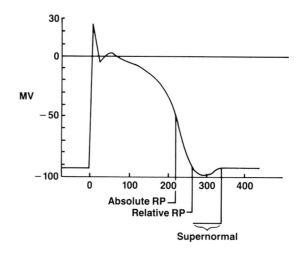

Fig. 11.3 Absolute refractory period, relative refractory period and 'supernormal period' of the ventricular muscle action potential.

sium current, leaving the inward (depolarising) sodium current. This spontaneous depolarisation during phase 4 is termed 'automaticity'. Automatic cells in the specialised conduction axis are normally suppressed by the sinus node. Should the sinus node fail to depolarise, these cells will take over the pacemaker activity of the heart. The rate of diastolic depolarisation in cells of the atria are faster than those of the ventricles. The level of membrane potential at which an action potential is initiated is called the 'threshold potential'. The threshold can be reached by spontaneous diastolic depolarisation of a single cell, by spread of a depolarising wave-front from adjacent cells, or by injection of a depolarising current from an electrode.

Slow response action potential

A second type of action potential occurs in cells of the normal sinus node, the atrioventricular node, coronary sinus and in some cells of the atrioventricular valves (Cranefield, 1975). Other cardiac cells may display action potentials of this type when they are injured (Ten Eick & Singer, 1979). Compared to the 'fast' type there is a lower (i.e. closer to zero) maximum diastolic potential of –50 to –65 mV in the 'slow' action potential. The upstroke (V_{max} of phase 0) is much slower and the conduction velocity much slower. Depolarisation of these cells is dependent upon a slow inward current of calcium and sodium as opposed to the more rapid inward sodium current in the 'fast' action potential (Fig. 11.2). The majority of cells with slow action potentials display automaticity with spontaneous diastolic depolarisation during phase 4. Such phase 4 depolarisation may be due to a slow inward calcium current rather than the loss of outward potassium current found in Purkinje cells. The sinus nodal cells have this type of action potential and normally have the most rapid diastolic depolarisation resulting in the most rapid automatic rate in the heart. It is a property of cardiac cells that stimulation from an external source suppresses their inherent automaticity (Boineau et al, 1980). Therefore, the sinus node is not only dominant because it has the fastest inherent rate, but also because the conduction of the sinus impulses to other cells naturally suppresses them. In addition, there may be selective vagal inhibition of other potentially automatic cells throughout the atrium (Kang et al, 1981). Normally, cells in other parts of the heart with slow response action potentials do not have an opportunity to become the pacemaker of the heart. In diseased states, however, these cells may be responsible for abnormal rhythms.

Current flow within a cell: the dipole concept

A dipole consists of a single pair of positive and negative charges lying in close proximity to each other. The cardiac cell membrane at rest can be represented as a capacitor, with negative charges on the inside and positive on the outside. Current flow is prevented by the high resistance cell membrane. If an excitatory stimulus is applied to the cell surface, the resistance of the membrane is lowered and positive charge (sodium) rushes in. The flow of current also stimulates adjacent resting membrane of the same cell. In so doing, it lowers the electrical resistance of the adjacent resting membrane. As a consequence, a new membrane current appears which initiates discharge of the next point along the cell surface (Cooksey et al, 1977).

Membrane current flows *out* of the cell ahead of the depolarisation wave-front and back into the cell behind it (Fig. 11.4). The greatest amount of current flow causing a positive potential exists immediately in front of the

depolarisation wave-front. The greatest amount of negative potential is immediately behind the wave-front. Depolarisation is, therefore, an advancing wave-front of positive charge that extends in a plane perpendicular to the direction of propagation.

As the movement of the dipole occurs in a single cell, the potential variations at several fixed points surrounding the cell can be recorded with a galvanometer. In the 'unipolar' recording configuration, one lead is close to the muscle cell while the other lead, the 'indifferent lead', is at a relatively large distance. The indifferent lead remains at zero potential, and the active lead records all local events. In Figure 11.5A, three unipolar exploring electrodes are shown surrounding a single muscle cell. These electrodes are similar to those of the chest leads in the electrocardiograph. The potential variations of the cell are recorded by the galvanometer as deflections in a moving baseline. The wave-forms represent voltage plotted against time (paper speed). The size of the deflection measured from the isoelectric baseline is determined by the magnitude of the voltage. The direction of deflection is shown by the voltage sign. Positive voltage is recorded when the wave of depolarisation is moving toward the electrode. It causes an up-swing of the baseline. A negative voltage causes a down-swing. If the muscle cell is stimulated at its left end, electrode A (Fig. 5A – top diagram), facing the stimulated end of the cell, is in closer proximity to the negative charge of the dipole than at any time subsequently. Therefore, electrode A is at maximum negative potential. This is evidenced graphically by a sharp downward deflection. The other two electrodes lie in the positive field of the dipole. Since electrode B, overlying the centre of the cell, is closer to the positive dipole charge than is electrode C, electrode B shows a greater positive deflection. As depolarisation continues, and the equivalent dipole moves further away from electrode A, the negative potential at A diminishes and the positive potential at B and C increases. The maximum positive voltage for electrode B is reached just before the dipole passes under electrode B. At the instant the dipole moves under B, the electrode is equidistant from positive and negative charges. B is therefore at zero potential with the voltage on the isoelectric, or zero line (Fig. 11.5A – second diagram). As the dipole continues to the right (Fig. 11.5A – third diagram), the potential at electrode B falls to a maximum negative potential because of the close proximity to the negative charge of the dipole. During the remainder of depolarisation, the dipole moves steadily away from electrodes A and B (which record progressively smaller negative potentials) and approaches electrode C. The increase in positive potential at electrode C reaches its peak just before the completion of depolarisation. When the fibre is completely depolarised, the dipole is extinguished and the voltage curve for each electrode returns to the isoelectric line (Fig. 11.5A – bottom diagram).

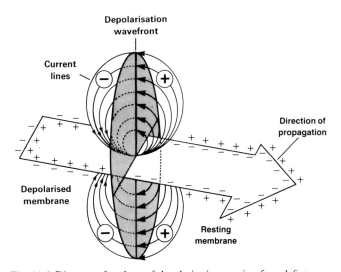

Fig. 11.4 Diagram of a plane of depolarisation moving from left to right along the surface of a membrane. The outside of the membrane is positively charged in front of the plane and negatively charged behind the plane. The plane represents a 'wall' of positive charge moving from left to right.

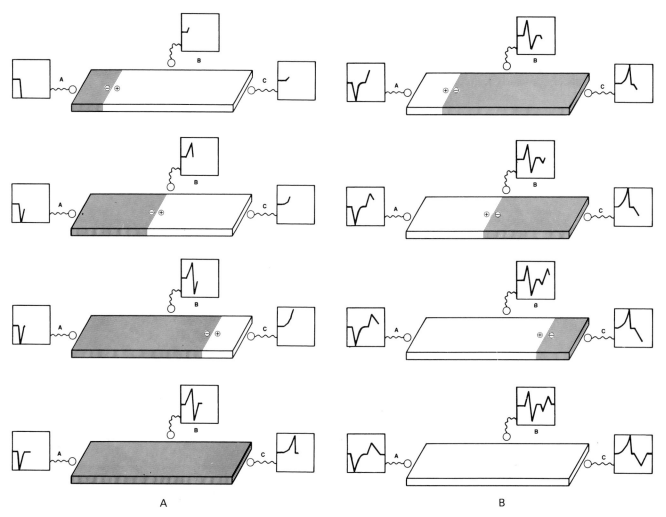

Fig. 11.5 (A) Depolarisation sequence in a hypothetical cardiac cell. Unipolar electrodes surround the cell. The potential found at these electrodes is shown in the accompanying graphs (see text). (B) Sequence of repolarisation in a hypothetical cardiac cell.

Repolarisation (Fig. 11.5B) begins at the left end of the cell and proceeds in the same direction as depolarisation. The potential changes are similar, but are of opposite polarity. Because of the long plateau of the action potential, the processes of repolarisation take much longer than depolarisation. In Figure 11.5B, at electrodes A and C, the different polarities can be seen. At electrode B, the deflection of repolarisation is biphasic just like depolarisation. But, in repolarisation, the downward deflection is written before the upward deflection because the negative part of the dipole is the leading edge.

The 'dipole vector' is a straight line running from the negative to the positive charges of the dipole. In depolarisation, the dipole vector parallels the direction of physiologic activity. In repolarisation, the negative charge of the dipole precedes the positive charge. The repolarisation dipole, therefore, is oriented opposite to the depolarisation dipole since reversed electrical processes are occurring (Fig. 11.6).

From the cell to the body surface

The events of depolarisation and repolarisation that have been described in a single cell must be transmitted from cell to cell. The membrane surrounding each cardiac cell has a high resistance. At the ends of each cardiac cell, the opposing cellular membranes form into intercalated discs. The intercalated discs are thought to be the sites of low resistance such that current flow can be readily transferred from cell to cell (Weidman, 1965). Conduction between cells is considerably slower in a lateral direction (perpendicular to the long axis of a cell). Orientation of fibre bundles would therefore be expected to contribute to the overall conduction velocity and sequence of electrical activity (Spach et al, 1980).

During activation of the atria and ventricles, depolarisation spreads such that there is great cancellation of electrical force. The electrical field generated at the body surface is an 'equivalent dipole' which represents the

DEPOLARISATION

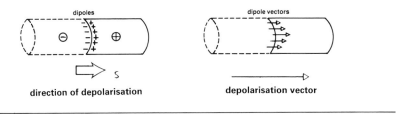

REPOLARISATION

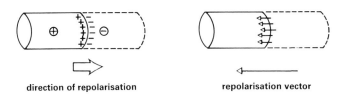

Fig. 11.6 Dipole vectors. The dipole vector in depolarisation parallels the direction of depolarisation; the repolarisation vectors occurs in the opposite direction to the direction of repolarisation.

uncancelled elements. At any instant other than during the isoelectric period between ventricular repolarisation and atrial depolarisation, an electrical potential exists at every point on the body surface. This can be described as the summation of forces, or a vector with magnitude and direction. The magnitude is inversely proportional to the cube of the distance between the dipole and the electrode lead on the body surface. One would therefore expect a greater voltage in leads recorded from the chest wall than from leads recorded on the extremities. The electrocardiogram calculates the projection of the mean instantaneous vector on its lead axis by the electronic equivalent of vector addition. The changing projections of these vectors on a given lead axis, plotted against time, produce the P, QRS and T waves.

RECORDING THE SEQUENCE OF CARDIAC ACTIVITY

Electrocardiographic standardisation and measurement

The electrocardiogram is recorded on standardised paper, with the light lines separated by 1 mm and the heavy lines separated by 5 mm (Fig. 11.7). The voltage is standardised such that 1.0 mV equals 10 mm of deflection. For large amplitude complexes, the calibration can be changed such that 1.0 mV equals either 2.5 mm or 5 mm; for small signals, the calibration can be changed such that 1.0 mV equals 20 mm. A calibration spike should be recorded on the electrocardiogram each time the calibration is changed (Fig. 11.8). The normal paper speed is 25 mm/s. At this speed, the light lines are separated by 0.04 s (40 ms) and

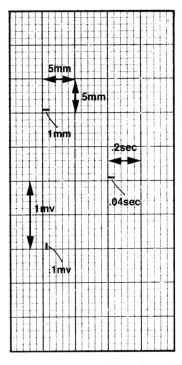

Fig. 11.7 Electrocardiographic paper with usual standardisation (1.0 mV equals 10 mm) and usual timing (the 0.2 s equals 5 mm).

the heavy lines are separated by 0.20 s (200 ms) (see Fig. 11.9). In order to time events more precisely, or in order to examine the electrocardiographic morphology during a rapid heart rate, the paper speed can be increased to 50 mm/s. If a rapid paper speed is used, this should be indicated on the margin of the electrocardiogram for the

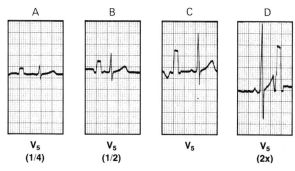

A	B	C	D
V₅ (1/4)	V₅ (1/2)	V₅	V₅ (2x)

Fig. 11.8 Calibration of the electrocardiogram. (A) Lead V₅ at one-quarter standardisation (1.0 mV equals 2.5 mm). Since the electrocardiograph standardisation output is always 1.0 mV, the height of the spike is 2.5 mm with the calibration spike at one-quarter standardisation. (B) Lead V₅ at one-half standardisation (1.0 mV equals 5 mm). (C) Lead V₅ at full (normal) standardisation (1.0 mV equals 10 mm). (D) Lead V₅ at double standardisation (1.0 mV equals 20 mm). For the remainder of the figures, standardisation will be labelled as in this diagram. Unless the standardisation is different from normal calibration, the standardisation will not be specifically indicated.

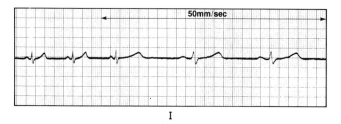

I

Fig. 11.9 Paper speed. The normal paper speed is 25 mm/s. On the right side of this electrocardiographic tracing, the speed has been increased to 50 mm/s and this is marked on the tracing. All other electrocardiograms in the figures are recorded at 25 mm/s.

period of 50 mm/s recording. Since the electrocardiographic tracing drawn by the stylus has a width of its own, measurements should be taken consistently from the same side of the line. For example, in determining amplitude, measurements should be taken from the bottom of one line to the bottom of the other line; and in determining intervals, measurements should be taken from the left side of one line to the left side of the other line.

Computer analysis of the electrocardiogram

In the data by Davignon et al (1979) which are included in this chapter as our normal values, the electrocardiograms were analysed primarily by computer. The electrocardiograms were recorded using a conventional electrocardiograph with a stylus, but in addition, the output was coupled to an FM tape recorder. These 'analog' signals were sampled 333 times/s (every 3 ms) for deflection from the baseline and the measured deflection was stored in a computer in 'digital' (Fig. 11.10). The analysis of these electrocardiograms using the Mayo Clinic program has

been described in detail elsewhere (Davignon et al, 1979; Smith & Hyde, 1969).

Electrocardiographic waves and intervals

Cardiac activation begins in the sinus node. The sinus node, however, has no expression on the surface electrocardiogram (Fig. 11.11). Atrial activation causes the P wave on the electrocardiogram. The atria begin to be activated from the high right atrium at the beginning of the P wave, and the distal parts of the left atrium are depolarised approximately 60 ms (1½ small boxes on the electrocardiogram) after the onset of the P wave (Fig. 11.12A). Therefore, the normal *P wave duration* is about 60 ms measured from the onset to the termination of the P wave. P waves are generally small (less than 2.5 mm tall), 'bullet-shaped' waves.

It takes approximately 40 ms for the impulse to travel from the high right atrium to the low septal right atrium in the region of the atrioventricular node. Thus the node may be activated before the end of the P wave. Depolarisation of the node and the atrioventricular conduction axis do not produce visible deflections on the routine surface electrocardiogram.

The *PR interval* is caused by a relatively major delay in the atrioventricular node and usually a relatively minor delay in conduction through the specialised axis to the ventricular myocardium. The PR interval is measured from the onset of the P wave to the onset of the QRS complex. The normal PR interval varies with age, but is approximately 0.12 s in children. The PR segment is the period between the end of the P wave and the beginning of the QRS complex. The duration of the PR segment is generally not measured. The Ta wave, caused by atrial repolarisation, begins during the PR segment and may extend through the ST segment. In general, the Ta wave is not observed since it is obscured by other waves.

The *QRS complex* is caused by ventricular depolarisation. This is usually the tallest, most rapid deflection on the electrocardiogram. If the QRS complex begins with a negative deflection, this negative deflection is called a Q wave. A Q wave is not seen in all leads. The first positive deflection is the R wave. The second negative deflection is the S wave. If there is only one large negative deflection, this is called a QS wave (Fig. 11.12B). If there is a second R wave, this is called an R′, and the negative deflection which follows an R′ is labelled the S′ (Fig. 11.12C). The QRS duration is measured from the beginning of the Q wave to the end of the QRS complex, whether the last wave is an RSR′ or S′. The normal QRS duration varies with age but is approximately 0.08 s. The *J point* occurs at the juction at the end of the QRS complex with the ST segment.

The *ST segment* extends from the end of the QRS complex to the beginning of the T wave. If there are

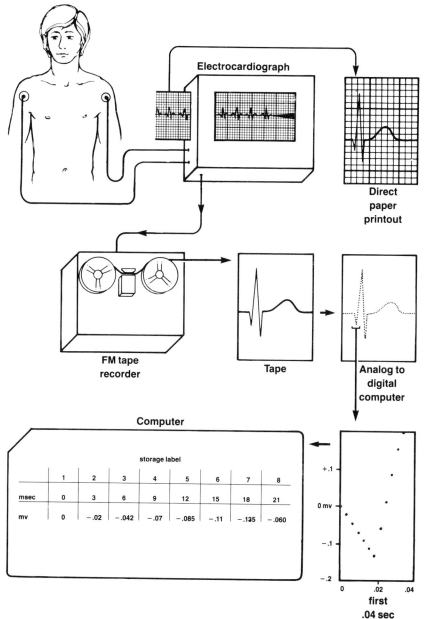

Fig. 11.10 Computer analysis of the electrocardiogram. From the electrocardiograph, the signal is transferred to a tape recorder and then to an analog to digital converter. In the diagram below, the first 0.04 s of the electrocardiographic tracing are shown. The electrocardiogram is sampled every 3 ms and the voltages of the first 0.04 s of the electrocardiogram are shown as they would appear in the storage registers of a computer. The storage label corresponds to the number of the sample point. For example, the seventh sample point is at the deepest point of the Q wave, 18 ms into the QRS complex, and this measures −0.135 mV below the baseline.

abnormalities of ventricular repolarisation, they may be marked by elevation or depression of the ST segment from the baseline. Repolarisation of ventricular myocardium generates the T wave. The T wave is usually rounded with a shallow upstroke and a more rapid downstroke. The *QT interval* is measured from the beginning of the QRS complex to the end of the T wave. It indicates the total duration for electrical depolarisation and repolarisation of ventricular muscle. The QT interval varies with heart rate but is usually about half the interval between QRS complexes. The *Q-OT interval* is measured from the beginning of the QRS complex to the beginning of the T wave. This measures the time to the onset of repolarisation. The Q-OT is not generaly measured but may be prolonged or shortened by abnormalities of serum calcium. In some leads, a *U wave* may be visible. This is thought to be due to ventricular Purkinje cell repolarisation. Normally, the U wave has a lower amplitude than the T wave with an even shallower upstroke and downstroke than the T wave. The *T-P interval* (or U-P interval if there is a U wave) is the true isoelectric baseline and measurements of amplitude are usually made relative to the T-P interval.

Electrocardiographic leads

The electrocardiograph calculates and displays the projection of the three-dimensional vector onto any single lead axis. Examination of a single bipolar lead provides much

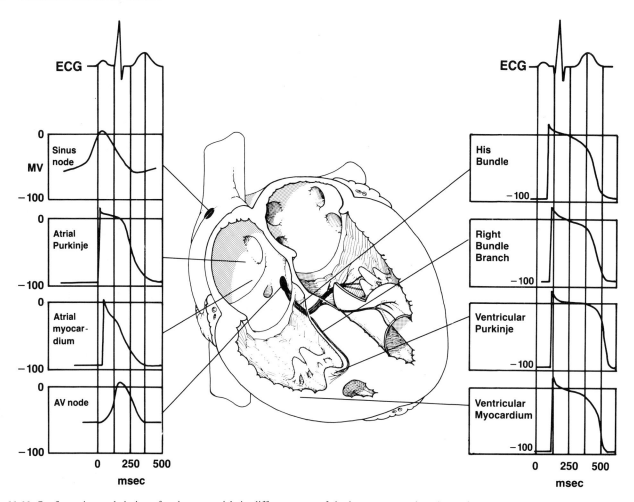

Fig. 11.11 Configuration and timing of action potentials in different parts of the heart compared to the surface electrocardiogram. Activation begins in the sinus node with a 'slow' action potential. This occurs before the P wave on the surface electrocardiogram. The physiologically specialised atrial and working atrial myocardial action potentials occur during the P wave. These are relatively short 'fast' action potentials. Activation of the atrioventricular (AV) node occurs during the PR segment. The AV node has a 'slow' action potential without diastolic depolarisation. The remainder of the action potentials are 'fast'. Activation of the AV bundle, right bundle branch and ventricular conduction cells occur within the PR segment. At the onset of depolarisation of ventricular myocardium, the QRS complex begins.

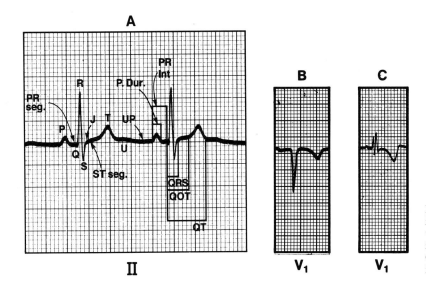

Fig. 11.12 (A) Normal electrocardiographic waves and intervals, lead II. P, Q, R, S, T, U refer to their respective waves. Abbreviations: P Dur – P duration; PR Int – PR interval; PR Seg – PR segment; QRS – QRS duration; QOT – QOT interval; QT – QT interval; UP – UP interval. (B) QS pattern. (C) RSR′ pattern.

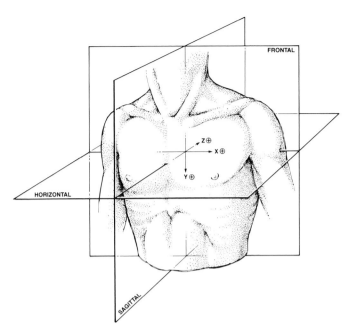

Fig. 11.13 Demonstration of the frontal, horizontal and saggital planes.

information about the timing of cardiac events, but in order to reconstruct a fuller image of the movement of the cardiac dipole in space, multiple leads are required. Three planes are used to describe the heart's electrical activity. The frontal plane views the body from the front using the horizontal X-axis (right-to-left) and the vertical Y-axis (from head to foot). The horizontal plane views the body from above with the horizontal X-axis (right to left) and an inward Z-axis (anterior to posterior). The sagittal plane views the body from the side with a vertical Y-axis (head to foot) and an inward Z-axis (anterior to posterior) (see Fig. 11.13). All of the three-dimensional information can be described by two planes. Standard electrocardiography has selected the frontal and horizontal planes. 6 leads reflect the projection of cardiac activity on the frontal plane, and 9 leads reflect the projection in the horizontal plane. In recent years, attempts have been made to simplify electrocardiography by reducing the number of leads to a total of three. The concept of an X, a Y, and a Z lead was originally described by Frank (1955). This is not in general use, and at the present time in a pediatric electrocardiogram, 12–15 leads are recorded (Fig. 11.14).

DERIVATION OF THE ELECTROCARDIOGRAM

Atrial depolarisation and repolarisation

The P wave and Ta wave

Atrial excitation propagates as if the atria were a two-dimensional sheet of cells (Spach et al, 1980; Weidman,

1965). Thus the impulse normally begins in the sinus node and travels radially, similar to oil spreading over a flat surface, throughout the right and left atria.

While the electrocardiogram records and summates mean vectors continually, it is often helpful to examine the vectors as if depolarisation were frozen at a particular instant. In this way, the direction of depolarisation can be seen closely in 'stop action'. In the atria of a child, approximately 60 ms are required for the impulse to conduct from the high right atrium in the region of the sinus node to the lateral left atrium. It is convenient to examine atrial depolarisation in three phases: early (the first 20 ms), middle (20–40 ms) and late (40–60 ms). In the early phase, depolarisation has spread approximately halfway through the right atrium and the mean vector of the dipoles points straight anteriorly, slightly to the left and inferiorly (Fig. 11.15A). As the rest of the right atrium is depolarised in the middle period of depolarisation, the mean vector points anteriorly, leftward and inferiorly. In the terminal portion, the left atrium is activated and since the left atrium is posterior to the right atrium, the terminal vector points posteriorly, left and inferiorly (Figs. 11.15B, C). If the direction and amplitude of all the instantaneous vectors throughout atrial depolarisation are averaged, the mean vector or 'axis' can be calculated. For the normal P wave, the mean vector points anteriorly, inferiorly and to the left.

Atrial repolarisation is manifested on the surface electrocardiogram by a slowly inscribed small deflection, the Ta wave, which is opposite in direction to the P wave (Burch & DePasquale, 1967). The mean electrical vector of the Ta wave is therefore directed posteriorly, superiorly and to the right. It can be seen that, in the relatively simple structure of the atria, the processes of depolarisation and repolarisation proceed sequentially and have opposite polarities. Depolarisation is a positive wave-front moving toward lead II, and results in a positive deflection (Fig. 11.15). Repolarisation is a negative wave-front moving towards lead II, and results in a negative deflection (Fig. 11.16A). Since the end of the Ta wave is inscribed within 0.20–0.30 s after the onset of the P wave, the Ta wave is usually superimposed upon the QRS complex and ST segment (Fig. 11.16B). The Ta wave is most easily seen when there is atrioventricular dissociation and P waves are found without following QRS complexes (Fig. 11.17). When the Ta wave is superimposed on the QRS complex (since the Ta wave is opposite in polarity to the P wave) the Ta wave is generally negative and may result in both PR and ST depression. ST depression due to ventricular disease without atrial disease is not associated with depression of the PR segment. For this reason, when measuring ST segment changes, the PR segment should be used as the baseline. This is despite the fact that the PR segment may not be truly isoelectric.

LIMB LEADS **AUGMENTED LIMB LEADS** **PRECORDIAL LEADS**

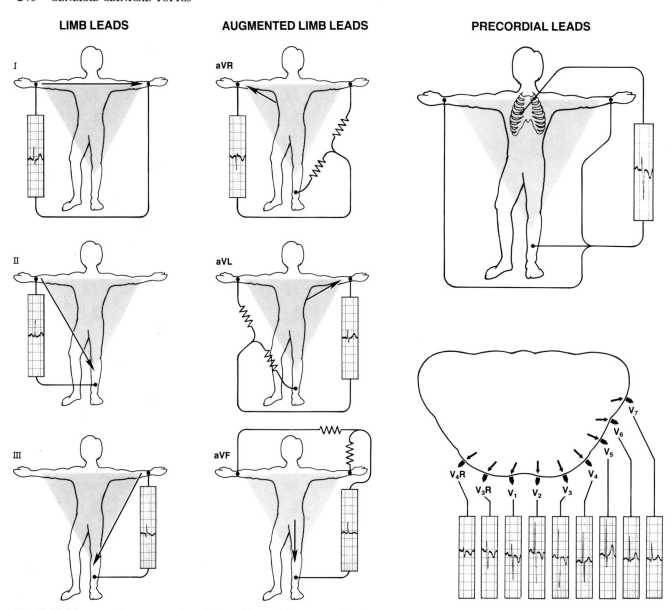

Fig. 11.14 Diagrammatic representation of the position and instrumentation for obtaining a 15 lead electrocardiogram in a child (see text). The tracings are taken from a normal 3-year-old.

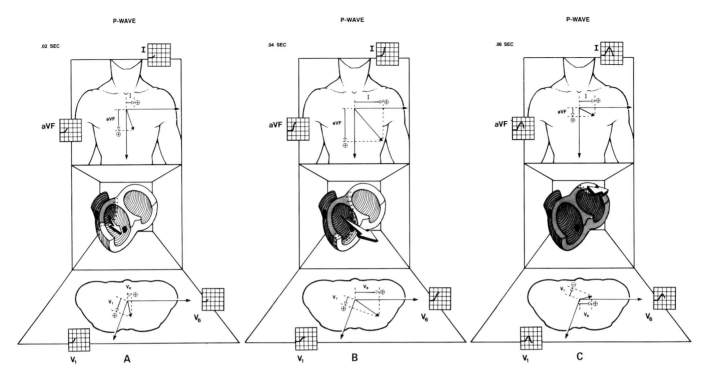

Fig. 11.15 Atrial depolarisation. (A) 0–20 ms vector. (B) 20–40 ms vector. (C) 40–60 ms vector. In each diagram, in the middle, a three-dimensional representation of the atria is shown with the position of the activation front at the end of each time period. The vector in three dimensions is shown as an arrow in the middle diagram. Above this, the projection of the three-dimensional vector on the frontal plane is shown on lead I and aV$_F$ axes. The horizontal component of the vector is designated by the length of the arrow in lead I and the vertical component of the vector is designated by the length of the arrow in lead aV$_F$. A diagrammatic P wave is shown on the graphs. The timing and standardisation are the same as those for a standard electrocardiogram. These graphs show the position of the P wave at each of the three successive time periods. Since the P wave duration may be longer than 60 ms, the terminal portion of the P wave is indicated by dotted lines in (C). At the bottom of the diagrams, a similar analysis is applied to the horizontal plane.

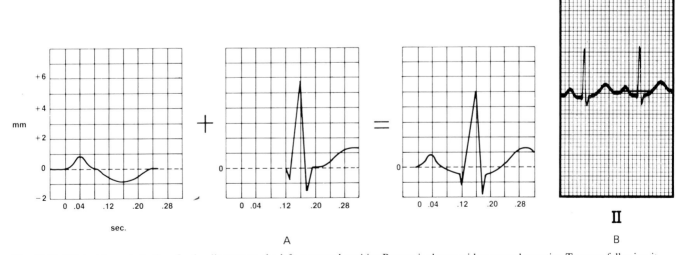

Fig. 11.16 (A) Atrial repolarisation. In the diagram on the left, a normal positive P wave is shown with a normal negative Ta wave following it. The diagram is similar to normal electrocardiographic paper. In the middle diagram, a normal QRS complex and T wave are shown without the preceding P or Ta wave. On the right side of the diagram, the combination of the preceding two drawings is shown. This demonstrates how the Ta wave can result in both PR and ST depression. (B) Lead II electrocardiogram from a 3-year-old child. The true isoelectric line has been extended through the PR and ST segments showing the depression produced by the Ta wave.

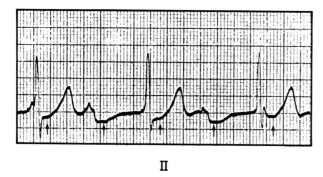

II

Fig. 11.17 Atrioventricular dissociation. The P waves (arrowed) are not followed by QRS complexes.

Ventricular depolarisation: the QRS complex

The QRS complex on the body surface is much more complicated than the P wave because ventricular depolarisation occurs in several different directions simultaneously. It has been estimated that only 5–10% of the electrical forces generated by ventricular depolarisation are reflected in the QRS complex; all others cancel each other (Scher, 1976). The QRS complex can best be divided into four time periods which correspond to the different major directions of activation (Fig. 11.18). The first is the 0.01 s initial vector (Fig. 11.18A). At the onset of the QRS, three areas on the left ventricular endocardium are activated simultaneously. The central part of the interventricular septum on the left side results from early branches of the main left bundle branch. The high anterior paraseptal wall at the base of the anterior papillary muscle is excited from the left anterior fascicle. The posterior-inferior ventricular septum one-third of the distance from the apex to the base is activated from the left posterior fascicle (Fig. 11.19; Durrer et al, 1970). Therefore, the initial vector is made up of three components of activation: septal depolarisation to the right, anterior left ventricular activation proceeding radially towards the anterior chest wall and left posterior endocardial spread moving away from the anterior chest wall. The anterior and posterior left ventricular forces tend to cancel in the normal heart, leaving the left-to-right septal vector. The base-apex axis of the ventricular septum is most often parallel to the diaphragm with the apex slightly more inferior and tilted such that the left side of the septum is caudad. Thus, left to right activation of the septum results in a vector which is anterior, to the right and superior. This usually produces a Q wave in leads I, aVF and V_6 and an R wave in lead V_1 (Fig. 11.18A). The second time period is the 0.02 s apicoanterior vector. Approximately 0.01 s after the endocardial surface of the left ventricle is activated, the endocardial surface of the right ventricle is activated in the region of the moderator band at the termination of the right bundle branch. Since the right bundle branch is longer than the left bundle

branch and is insulated to this point, activation occurs later. The spread of the wave orginating in the moderator band is primarily left-to-right as the anterior wall of the right ventricle is activated. Simultaneously, the lower two-thirds of the septum have depolarised via the left bundle branch with one activation front meeting the anterior right ventricular wall and the other spreading to the anteroapical left ventricle. In summary, the right ventricular free wall and left ventricular free wall are being activated in opposite directions. The left ventricle is thicker and so the resultant vector is to the left, anterior and inferior, along the long axis of the heart. Thus, the 0.02 s vector is approximately + 60° in the frontal plane, causing an R wave in leads I, aVF. In the horizontal plane, the vector contributes to the downstroke of the R wave in lead V_1 as the QRS returns toward the isoelectric line (Fig. 11.18B). The third period is the 0.04 s left ventricular endocardial-epicardial vector. All of the right ventricular endocardium and most of the left ventricular endocardium have been activated. Since activation spreads from the endocardium to the epicardiun, there is very little actual spread of impulses across the epicardium. Epicardial activation occurs approximately 25 ms later than the corresponding endocardium. There are three almost simultaneous areas of epicardial breakthrough: the anterior right ventricle, the left anterior basal left ventricle near the obtuse marginal coronary artery and the mid-posterior paraseptal left ventricle near the posterior descending coronary artery (Fig. 11.20). The majority of right ventricular free wall activation is completed before left ventricular activation because the left ventricle is thicker. This leaves the activation of certain parts of the left ventricular posterior and lateral unopposed and the resultant vector is to the left, posterior and slightly inferior (Fig. 11.18C). This is the peak of the R wave in leads I and V_6 and the bottom of the S wave in lead V_1. The final period is the 0.06 s terminal vector. The last parts of the heart to be activated are the posterobasal left ventricle and the pulmonary outflow tract. This is because of a paucity of ventricular conduction tissue cells in these areas. Terminal activation thus proceeds from apex to base. The resultant vector is directed superiorly and posteriorly causing an S wave in leads aVF and V_1. Depending upon the age of the child, and therefore the degree of right ventricular dominance, this vector may be directed slightly to the right or to the left. In younger children, it is directed to the right causing an S wave in leads I and V_6 (Fig. 11.18D). In older children, it is directed more to the left and there may be no S waves in leads I or V_6.

Ventricular muscle repolarisation: the T wave

Whereas ventricular depolarisation relies on multiple waves of cell-to-cell conduction, it appears that ventricular repolarisation is an individual process of each cell and probably does not proceed as a propagated wave. Thus, although

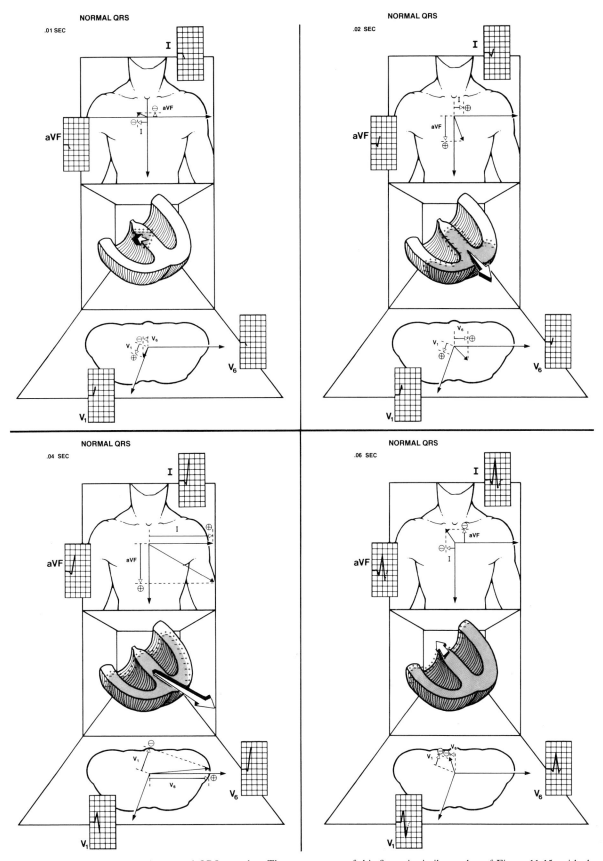

Fig. 11.18 Ventricular depolarisation: the normal QRS complex. The arrangement of this figure is similar to that of Figure 11.15, with the exception that the diagram in the middle shows the inner surfaces of the ventricles. (A) 0.01 s initial vector. (B) 0.02 s apicoanterior vector. (C) 0.04 s left ventricular endocardial-epicardial vector. (D) 0.06 s terminal vector.

ENDOCARDIAL ACTIVATION
0–5msec after QRS onset

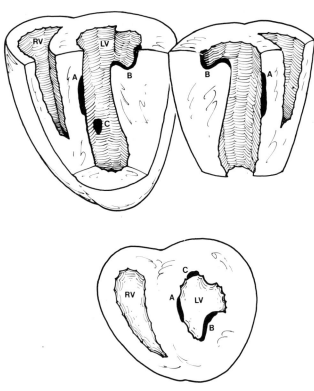

Fig. 11.19 Onset of ventricular endocardial activation. Top – coronal section through the ventricles with the inner surface exposed. Bottom – cross-section through the ventricles midway between the base and apex. The three simultaneous areas of activation of the left ventricle are shown: A – left side of the interventricular septum; B – anterior paraseptal wall; C – posterior-inferior ventricular septum.

repolarisation is represented by a single wave and vector on the surface electrocardiogram, it is much more complex than depolarisation. The ventricular recovery properties are systematically distributed such that areas activated first have the longest refractory periods and recover last. The endocardium has a longer refractory period than the epicardium, and the apex has a longer refractory period than the base. This tends to cause all portions of the ventricles to recover at approximately, but not exactly, the same time. Nevertheless, net repolarisation appears to proceed from epicardium to endocardium. This may be due to the shorter epicardial action potentials. Since the epicardium recovers slightly before the endocardium, the extracellular potential in the epicardium is positive with respect to the unrecovered endocardium. The vector of repolarisation (T wave) points toward the positive, or already recovered areas with short action potential duration (Fig. 11.21). This has been shown experimentally. It is known that warming a cell decreases its action potential duration and refractory period. If the epicardium is warmed, the action potentials shorten further and the T wave amplitude increases (Surawicz, 1972; Burgess, 1972).

Repolarisation is electrically the opposite process of depolarisation. In the atrium, since depolarisation and repolarisation follow the same sequence, the polarity of the P and Ta waves are opposite, reflecting the different electrical properties (Fig. 11.22A). In the ventricles, however, the sequence of depolarisation and repolarisation are reversed: depolarisation proceeds from endocardium to epicardium and repolarisation from epicardium to endocardium (Fig. 11.22B). Thus the opposing electrical properties of depolarisation and repolarisation occur in opposite

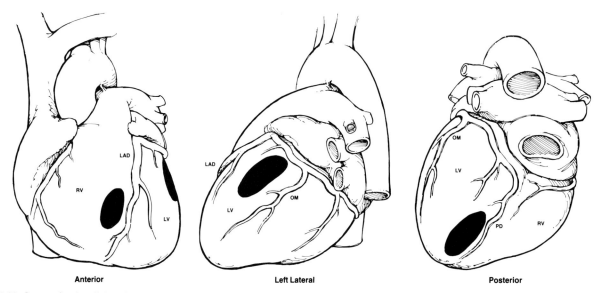

Anterior   Left Lateral   Posterior

Fig. 11.20 Onset of epicardial activation (which begins 25–35 ms after the onset of the QRS complex). Three areas are activated simultaneously: the anterior right ventricle, the left anterior basal left ventricle and the midposterior paraseptal left ventricle. Abbreviations: LAD – left anterior descending coronary artery; LV – left ventricle; OM – obtuse marginal coronary artery; PD – posterior descending coronary artery; RV – right ventricle.

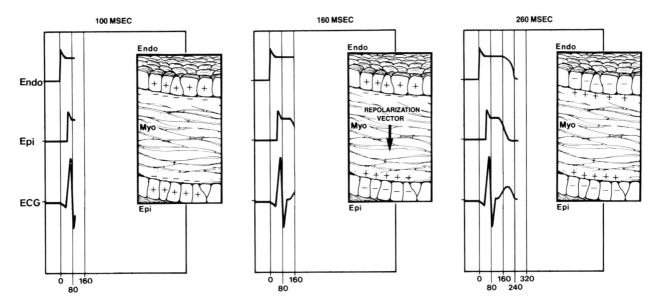

Fig. 11.21 Genesis of the normal T wave. Three phases of cardiac activity are shown. In each of the diagrams, an idealised action potential from the ventricular muscle is shown for the endocardium and the epicardium and, corresponding in time, the surface electrocardiogram. The timing in milliseconds is at the bottom of each diagram. On the right side of each diagram, the endocardium and epicardium are diagrammed, with the relative polarities of the cells in this region. In the left hand diagram, 100 ms after the onset of the QRS complex, both the endocardium and the epicardium are depolarised with the inside of the cell positive relative to the outside. This generates the ST segment. In the middle diagram, 160 ms after the onset of the QRS complex, the epicardium has begun to repolarise and the endocardium is still depolarised during the plateau phase. The epicardium is therefore relatively negative compared to the endocardium and the repolarisation vector extends from endocardium to epicardium. This generates the onset of the T wave. In the right hand diagram, repolarisation of both the endocardium and epicardium is complete and the T wave has ended.

directions in the ventricles and the net effect is QRS-T concordance: the mean QRS vector and T vector have a similar direction.

Ventricular Purkinje repolarisation: the U wave

The U wave is apparently due to normal repolarisation of ventricular Purkinje cells. Watanabe (1975) measured the action potential duration in ventricular muscle and Purkinje cells and found that the U wave corresponds to repolarisation in those parts of the ventricle with the longest action potential duration. In the normal heart, the Purkinje cells have the longest action potential duration; the end of the T wave corresponds to the end of ventricular muscle repolarisation and the end of the U wave corresponds to the end of Purkinje repolarisation. In the abnormal heart, an increased amplitude of the U wave implies that certain portions of the ventricular muscle or Purkinje cells are repolarising later than normally. Therefore, if the onset of the T wave occurs at the normal time, and there is a large U wave, this implies that parts of ventricular muscle are repolarising on time. Other parts are delayed and this increased 'dispersion of refractoriness' may lead to arrhythmias. Factors which prolong phase 3 of the action potential are associated with increased U waves: hypokalaemia, bradycardia, hypothermia, and quinidine. In the Jervell-Lange-Neilsen syndrome of

congenitally prolonged QT interval, the original description stated, 'It can be discussed as to whether the end deflections in these cases should be interpreted as T waves, U waves, or perhaps T-U waves. The electrocardiograms in our cases did not give any possibility to decide this question. The abnormal complexes were, in our opinion, caused by delayed repolarisation of the heart. The nomenclature, therefore, seems to be of less importance' (Jervell & Lange-Nielsen, 1957). We and others (Karhunen et al, 1970; James, 1967) agree that if the terminal vector of repolarisation has an increased magnitude, whether this is called a 'long T wave' or an 'enlarged U wave', the significance is the same: a vulnerability to ventricular arrhythmias.

The normal U wave has the same polarity as the preceding T wave. This may be accounted for by the observation that the action potential duration in Purkinje cells is longest at the left ventricular cavity and gets shorter toward the subendocardium. Thus, the cells closest to the cavity are repolarised last, giving a negative vector of repolarisation directed toward the cavity or a positive vector of the U wave directed away from the cavity toward the chest wall. An inverted U wave may have the same implications as an inverted T wave (see p. 290). In adults, inverted U waves are most often associated with conditions causing stretch in either ventricle: chronic volume overload, acute hypertension or acute pulmonary embolism (Lepeschkin, 1969; Lepeschkin & Surawicz, 1952).

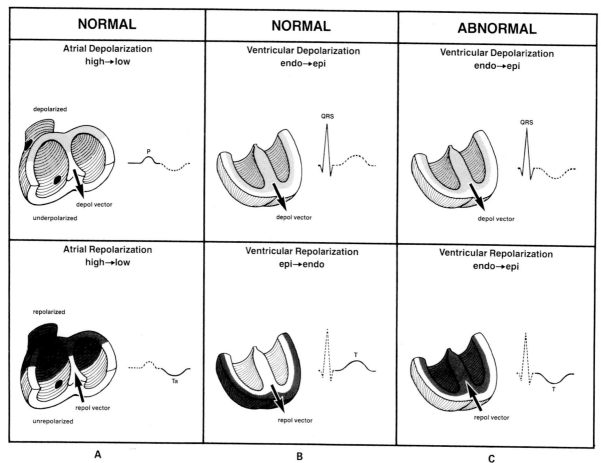

Fig. 11.22 Comparison of atrial and ventricular depolarisation and repolarisation. (A) Atrial depolarisation begins in the high right atrium and is directed inferiorly causing a positive P wave in lead II. Atrial repolarisation extends in the same direction but has an opposite polarity causing a negative Ta wave in lead II. (B) Normal ventricular depolarisation is shown to occur from endocardium to epicardium. This results in a positive depolarisation vector directed towards lead II. Since ventricular repolarisation occurs in the opposite direction and also has the opposite sign, the repolarisation vector has the same direction as the depolarisation vector and the QRS and T wave are both positive in lead II. (C) In an abnormal repolarisation sequence of the ventricles, the endocardium is depolarised before the epicardium, and the direction of depolarisation and repolarisation are the same. The situation in the abnormal ventricle is analogous to the normal atrium where the depolarisation vector and repolarisation vector have the same direction but opposite polarities. In the normal atrium, the P and Ta waves have different polarities; in the abnormal ventricle, the QRS and T waves have different polarities.

MEAN VECTOR ('AXIS')

The vector of cardiac forces changes in direction and magnitude from instant to instant as different regions of the heart activate and recover. For each of the four processes of atrial and ventricular depolarisation and repolarisation, a *mean* vector can be calculated which is the average direction and magnitude of all instantaneous vectors during that interval. We are concerned in standard electrocardiography with the direction of the mean vector as it projects on the frontal and horizontal planes. The three mean vectors most often considered are for the P wave, QRS complex and T wave.

QRS mean vector

Frontal plane

The most commonly calculated mean vector is for the QRS complex in the frontal plane. The term 'QRS axis' has become a popular substitute phrase for this term. The frontal plane QRS mean vector can be calculated in three ways.

The most accurate and most tedious method of determining the QRS mean vector is to determine the area subtended by each wave of the QRS deflection (Figs. 11.23, 11.24). Each component is measured as if it were a triangle. The formula used is for the area of a triangle (one-half of the base in seconds multiplied by the height in millimeters). The area of the deflections below the baseline are subtracted from the area of the deflections above the baseline yielding the algebraic sum of the areas. The algebraic sums in leads I and aVF can be plotted and the angle calculated (Dubin & Staib, 1977).

The second most accurate method for determining mean vector is to use the algebraic sum of the *amplitudes* of the components rather than the areas (Fig. 11.25).

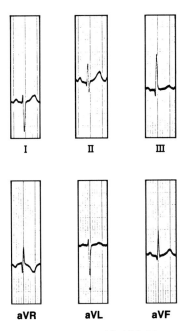

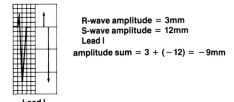

R-wave amplitude = 3mm
S-wave amplitude = 12mm
Lead I
amplitude sum = 3 + (−12) = −9mm

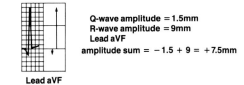

Q-wave amplitude = 1.5mm
R-wave amplitude = 9mm
Lead aVF
amplitude sum = −1.5 + 9 = +7.5mm

Fig. 11.23 Limb leads from a 4-year-old child. These tracings are used in the calculation of mean vector in Figures 11.24–11.26.

The most practical method for estimation of the mean vector is to determine the most isoelectric complex (Fig. 11.26). This is defined as the lead in which the sum of positive and negative deflections equals zero. The QRS mean vector is directed perpendicular to this lead. There are, however, two possible perpendiculars. For example, if lead aVR is isoelectric, this implies that the mean vector is directed 90° away from (perpendicular to) lead aVR.

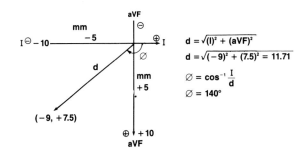

$d = \sqrt{(I)^2 + (aVF)^2}$

$d = \sqrt{(−9)^2 + (7.5)^2} = 11.71$

$\varnothing = \cos^{-1}\dfrac{I}{d}$

$\varnothing = 140°$

Fig. 11.25 Calculation of QRS frontal plane mean vector by the amplitude method (see text).

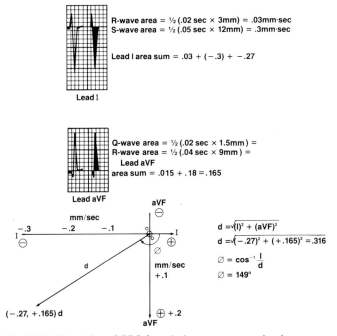

R-wave area = ½ (.02 sec × 3mm) = .03mm·sec
S-wave area = ½ (.05 sec × 12mm) = .3mm·sec

Lead I area sum = .03 + (−.3) + −.27

Q-wave area = ½ (.02 sec × 1.5mm) =
R-wave area = ½ (.04 sec × 9mm) =
Lead aVF
area sum = .015 + .18 = .165

$d = \sqrt{(I)^2 + (aVF)^2}$

$d = \sqrt{(−.27)^2 + (+.165)^2} = .316$

$\varnothing = \cos^{-1}\dfrac{I}{d}$

$\varnothing = 149°$

Fig. 11.24 Calculation of QRS frontal plane mean vector by the area method (see text).

1. **Inspection: Isoelectric to leads II and aVR**
   maximum positive : lead III

2. **Deduction:**
   a. isoelectric to II:
      either −30° or +150°
   b. maximum in III:
      +150°

   a. isoelectric to aVR:
      either −60° or 120°
   b. maximum in III:
      +120°

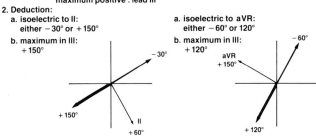

3. **Fine Tuning:**
   a. II slightly positive (Q (−2mm) + R (+8mm) + S (−4mm) = +2mm)
      ∴ slightly towards II from +150°
   b. aVR slightly positive (R (+1mm) + S (−4mm) + R' (+6mm) = +3mm)
      ∴ slightly towards aVR from +120°

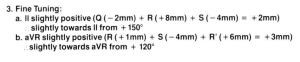

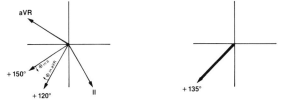

4. **Conclusion = Mean vector between +120° and +150° = +135°**

Fig. 11.26 Calculation of QRS frontal plane mean vector by the perpendicular method (see text).

Table 11.1 Frontal plane QRS mean vector (degrees)

Age	Min*	2%*	Mean	98%	Max	No. subjects
Less than 1 day	38	59	137	−167	−160	189
1–2 days	27	64	134	−161	−160	179
3–6 days	−8	77	132	−167	−162	180
1–3 weeks	−43	65	110	161	−176	117
1–2 months	−77	31	74	113	113	114
3–5 months	−7	1	60	104	112	108
6–11 months	−3	1	56	99	118	136
1–2 years	−2	1	55	101	115	191
3–4 years	−10	1	55	104	145	209
5–7 years	−48	1	65	143	200	224
8–11 years	−35	1	61	119	145	232
12–15 years	−13	1	59	130	198	245

*The limits of 'normal' include the 2nd and 98th percentile. 'Min' and 'max' are the minimum values in the sample of normal children. Statistically, these would be considered 'abnormal'.

Since lead aVR points toward −150°, the mean vector would be directed toward either −60° or +120°. To determine which of the two perpendiculars is the true mean vector, the lead with the maximum net positive deflection is examined. If lead III has the maximum net positive deflection, the frontal plane mean QRS vector is +120°. It is more accurate to base the calculation on the perpendicular to the isoelectric lead rather than simply on the direction of the largest deflection. This is because of the true difference in lengths of the lead axes. When all the QRS complexes in the frontal plane are equiphasic the mean vector is termed 'indeterminate'. No calculation can then be made.

The calculation of mean vector based upon each of these three methods may differ by up to 35°. This is because the three standard leads do not truly form an equilateral triangle and the adjacent axes are not separated by exactly 30°. The normal values for the QRS frontal plane mean vector given in Table 11.1 were based upon the area method.

'Axis deviation'

If the value for the QRS mean vector falls outside the range of normal values for age (see Table 11.1), 'axis deviation' is diagnosed. In the 1st month of life, 'right axis deviation' occurs when the mean vector is between the upper limit for age and −90° (see p. 255). In older children, right axis deviation occurs when the mean vector is between the upper limit for age and ±180°. For a 3-month-old, right axis deviation is between +105° and +180°. In a 10-year-old, right axis deviation is between +120° and +180° (Fig. 11.27). Using logic from the 'method of perpendiculars', right axis deviation is diagnosed if the QRS complex is isoelectric or positive in lead aVR (and isoelectric and positive in aVF) in a 10-year-old. The most common cause of right axis deviation in children is right ventricular hypertrophy.

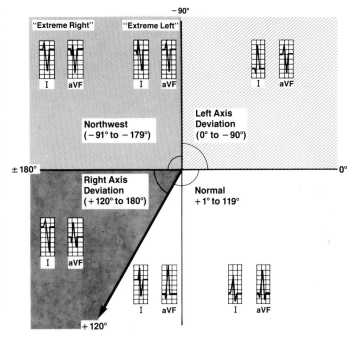

Fig. 11.27 'Axis deviation'. Limits for normal and abnormal frontal plane mean vector in a 10-year-old child. The electrocardiograms have been drawn to reflect the mean vector in each of the quadrants.

'Left axis deviation' occurs when the mean vector is between the lower limit for age and −90°. Above the age of 2 months, left axis deviation is between 0° and −90° (Fig. 11.27). Using logic from the method of perpendiculars, left axis deviation is diagnosed if the QRS complex is isoelectric or negative in lead aVF (and isoelectric or positive in lead I) in a child above 2 months of age. The most common causes of left axis deviation in childhood are those due to abnormal intraventricular conduction associated with congenital heart disease (atrioventricular septal defect and univentricular connexion to a dominant left ventricle due either to double inlet or absent connexion –

see p. 284). Concentric left ventricular hypertrophy generally does not cause left axis deviation.

If the frontal plane QRS mean vector is between $-90°$ and $\pm 180°$, a 'northwest axis' is diagnosed (Fig. 11.27). This may either be an extreme form of right axis deviation or left axis deviation. If, in northwest axis only, the initial QRS forces are directed at $+120°$ (Q wave in lead I or aVL), left anterior hemiblock coexists with the northwest axis and this is a form of extreme *left* axis deviation. On the other hand, if the initial forces are directed at $-60°$ (Q waves or QS pattern in leads II, III and aVF) this is extreme right axis deviation.

Horizontal plane

The QRS mean vector in the horizontal plane is not routinely calculated.

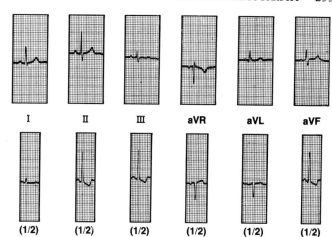

Fig. 11.28 T wave mean vector. Top tracings – normal 7-year-old; QRS frontal plane mean vector $+17°$, T wave mean vector $+34°$; the QRS-T angle is $17°$. Bottom tracings – seven-year-old with severe aortic stenosis; frontal plane QRS mean vector $+85°$, T wave mean vector $-90°$; the QRS-T angle is $175°$.

T Wave mean vector

Frontal plane

The T wave mean vector in the frontal plane can be calculated by the same methods as for the QRS complex. Generally, the T wave mean vector and QRS mean vector point in the same direction: positive QRS complexes have positive T waves. The amount of deviation between these mean vectors is called the QRS-T angle and the maximum allowable QRS-T angle varies with age (see Table 11.2). In early infancy, the QRS-T angle in the frontal plane is quite variable, but by 6 months, an angle greater than $75°$ is abnormal; after 6 months, the upper limit of normal is $60°$ (Liebman & Plonsey, 1978). If the QRS-T angle is abnormally large, this is called 'QRS-T discordance' and indicates either a primary or secondary T wave change (see p. 290). In practice, rather than calculating the QRS-T angle, it is helpful to remember that the T waves should be upright in normal children in leads I and II (above 48 hours of age), upright in lead aVF (above 5 days of age) and inverted in lead aVR (at all ages) (Fig. 11.28).

Horizontal plane

The QRS-T angle in the horizontal plane can be calculated. In practice, this is not done and the far right and far left chest leads are examined. Between approximately 5 days of age and adolescence, the T waves should be inverted in leads V_1 and V_3R (Hait & Gasul, 1963). If they are positive, this is usually a sign of right ventricular hypertrophy. In infants less than approximately 5 days of age or in adults, the T waves in lead V_1 or V_3R are variable The T waves in lead V_6 should be positive at all ages. T wave inversion in lead V_6 may be a primary or secondary T wave change (see p. 290).

P wave mean vector

Frontal plane

The P wave mean vector is directed away from the site of origin of atrial depolarisation. While it is possible to calculate the exact P wave mean vector, in practice only the quadrant of the vector in the frontal plane is determined. If the P wave is isoelectric or positive in lead I and isoelectric or positive in lead aVF (P wave mean vector between $0°$ and $+90°$), we infer that the atria begin depolarisation from the high right atrium, in other words from the sinus node (Fig. 11.29). If the P wave is negative in lead aV_F and isoelectric or positive in lead I (P wave mean vector between $-1°$ and $-90°$), the atria begin depolarisation from the low right atrium. If the P wave is negative in lead I (P wave mean vector between $+91°$ and $-91°$), the atria begin depolarisation from the left atrium (see p. 268).

Horizontal plane

The P wave mean vector in the horizontal plane is variable and is not helpful in determining the site of origin of atrial depolarisation.

THE NORMAL ELECTROCARDIOGRAM

Different patterns of normality occur in the electrocardiograms as the transition is made from the fetus to the neonate and through the stages of infancy and childhood to the adult. The variations are due to changes in physiology; changes in the size and position of the heart relative to the body, and changes in the overall body habitus. The major changes in amplitudes and direction of depolaris-

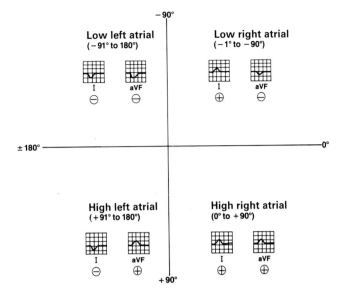

Fig. 11.29 Frontal plane P wave mean vector.

ation and repolarisation occur in the first year of life. Changes occur slowly thereafter in the timing of cardiac events as reflected in the electrocardiographic intervals. Since the majority of the measurements made on a neonatal electrocardiogram would be abnormal in an adult (Fig. 11.30), it is important to refer to the tables of normal values (Tables 11.1–11.17) which are given by age. In the following discussion, we will consider the normal electrocardiogram from the newborn at term through to that of the adolescent. Discussion of the normal premature (Sreenivasan, 1973), and adult (Cooksey et al, 1977) electrocardiograms can be found elsewhere.

Normal values

Normal values included in Tables 11.1–11.17 are those

collected and published by Davignon et al (1979). This population consisted of 2141 white children. Each had a normal physical examination. The total population was divided into 12 age-groups. 7 of these groups were in the 1st year of life, reflecting the greater changes in the electrocardiogram during this time. There are at least 100 children in each age-group. The data were analysed by computer. In addition, the electrocardiograms which fell in the upper or lower 10th percentile were displayed with an electrocardiograph and were verified visually by a physician. If the computer and physician disagreed, the visually determined value by the physician was substituted in the data file. These normal values are therefore applicable to all tracings recorded from an electrocardiograph which meets the standards of the American Heart Association. The limits of 'normal' include the 2nd and 98th percentile in each age range. A summary of normal values is presented in Table 11.17.

Heart rate

The heart rate in sinus rhythm is measured by determining the interval between successive P or R waves on the electrocardiogram. The onset of each deflection should be used for timing rather than the peak, since a change in the shape of a complex may result in a faulty measurement if the peak occurs at a different time relative to the beginning of the complex (Fig. 11.31). The exact heart rate can be calculated by dividing the RR intervals (in seconds) into 60. For example, assuming an RR of 0.46 s, the heart rate is 60/0.46 or 130/min. An approximation can be made by counting the number of 0.2 s blocks (large boxes on the electrocardiogram paper) which are contained in the RR interval. If the RR interval is approximately one box (0.2 s), the heart rate is 300/min; for two boxes, it is 150/min and so on: 300, 150, 100, 75, 60, 50, 43, 38. For a more exact heart rate, it is helpful to remember that the small boxes (0.04 s) between 100 and 150 represent 10 beats/min and those

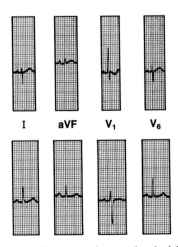

Fig. 11.30 Comparison of the normal neonatal and adolescent electrocardiogram. The neonate is shown in the top row and the adolescent is shown in the bottom row.

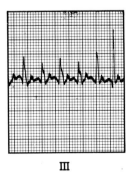

Fig. 11.31 Measurement of heart rate. In this patient with supraventricular tachycardia with varying intraventricular conduction, the QRS morphology changes sufficiently that the peak of each complex does not occur at the same time relative to the onset of each beat. Therefore, in measuring heart rate, rather than measuring from peak to peak, the onset of the QRS complex should be used at all times.

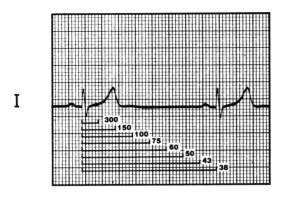

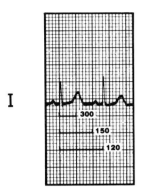

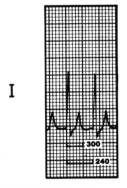

between 150 and 300 represent 30 beats/min (Fig. 11.32). This can be committed to memory.

The normal heart rate increases from the 1st day of life to a maximum between 1 and 2 months of age and then slowly declines (Table 11.2). The reason for this has not been demonstrated but probably is related to the relative immaturity of the sympathetic nervous system at birth.

P wave

The P wave is generally symmetrical in leads I and II. The normal shape is of a bullet, and not of a steeple (right atrial enlargement) or a bent staple (left atrial enlargement – see Fig. 11.33). Because of the improved frequency response of most electrocardiographic machines, over 25% of normal children will have a notch in the middle of the P wave. Notching by itself must therefore be considered a normal finding. The P wave may normally be biphasic in lead V_1, but the terminal negative portion should be less than 0.04 s

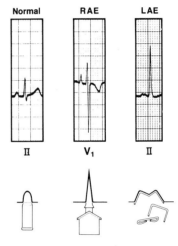

Fig. 11.33 P wave shape. On the left, the normal P wave shape is shown similar to that of a bullet. In the middle, the P wave of right atrial enlargement (RAE) is shown. This is similar to a church steeple. On the right, the P wave of left atrial enlargement (LAE) is shown. This is similar to a bent staple.

Fig. 11.32 Calculation of heart rate. Top tracing – a heart rate of 38/min. This is exactly nine large boxes on the electrocardiogram. The method of counting large boxes is illustrated. Middle tracing – sinus rhythm at a rate of 120/min. The QRS complexes are separated by two large boxes and three small boxes. Lower tracing – supraventricular tachycardia at 240/min. The QRS complexes are separated by one large and three small boxes.

Table 11.2 Heart rate (beats/min)

Age	Min	2%	Mean	98%	Max	No. subjects
Less than 1 day	88	93	123	154	168	189
1–2 days	57	91	123	159	170	179
3–6 days	87	91	129	166	166	181
1–3 weeks	96	107	148	182	188	119
1–2 months	114	121	149	179	204	112
3–5 months	101	106	141	186	188	109
6–11 months	100	109	134	169	176	138
1–2 years	68	89	119	151	165	191
3–4 years	68	73	108	137	145	210
5–7 years	60	65	100	133	139	226
8–11 years	51	62	91	130	145	233
12–15 years	51	60	85	119	133	247

in duration and less than 1 mm deep (less than one small box by one small box). The overall *duration* of the P wave in lead II should be between 0.03 and 0.09 s in children 3 years old and younger. The normal duration over the age of 3 years is between 0.05 and 0.10 sec. The normal P wave *amplitude* is less than 2.5 mm at all ages. The mean vector of the P wave is normally directed between 0° and +90° in sinus rhythm when there is usual atrial arrangement (situs solitus).

PR interval

The PR interval is measured from the beginning of the P wave to the beginning of the QRS complex. The true onset of atrial or ventricular depolarisation may not be recorded in a lead because the initial forces are directed perpendicular to the lead. The initial portion of the P wave or QRS complex may therefore be isoelectric in that lead. Thus the PR intervals measured in different leads may vary by as much as 0.04 s (Fig. 11.34). Usually they vary only by 0.02 s or less (Cooksey et al, 1977). It has been the practice to measure either the longest PR interval or the PR interval in lead II. Standards are available in children only for lead II (Table 11.3). If a 'delta wave' is present (see p. 288), the shortest 'PR interval' (actually a P-delta interval) should be sought in the diagnosis of the Wolff-Parkinson-White syndrome. With an isoelectric delta wave, the PR interval may be normal. Only in certain leads will the truly short PR interval be observed (Fig. 11.35) (see p. 288). A more common cause for a short PR interval in a normal heart is a low right atrial pacemaker. The P wave is then negative in lead aVF and positive or isoelectric in lead I. When the impulse originates low in the atrium, the normal high to low right atrial conduction time (which accounts for up to 0.04 s of the PR interval) is eliminated and therefore low right atrial pacemakers may have a PR interval up to 0.04 s less than normal. The PR interval normally increases with age and decreases with heart rate. The increase in PR interval with decreased heart rate can be accounted for by the fact that heart rate decreases normally with age. In Table 11.3,

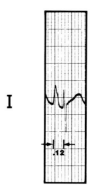

I

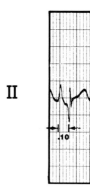

II

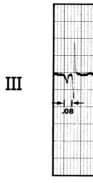

III

Fig. 11.34 PR interval. Simultaneous leads I, II and III. The PR interval in lead I is 0.12 s, in lead II, 0.10 s, and in lead III, 0.08 s. The reason for the seemingly short PR interval in lead III is that the early part of the P wave is isoelectric in that lead.

Table 11.3 PR interval (s) in lead II

Age	Min	2%	Mean	98%	Max	No. subjects
Less than 1 day	0.07	0.08	0.11	0.16	0.17	188
1–2 days	0.07	0.08	0.11	0.14	0.15	176
3–6 days	0.07	0.07	0.10	0.14	0.14	181
1–3 weeks	0.06	0.07	0.10	0.14	0.14	115
1–2 months	0.06	0.07	0.10	0.13	0.13	106
3–5 months	0.06	0.07	0.11	0.15	0.15	104
6–11 months	0.04	0.07	0.11	0.16	0.18	127
1–2 years	0.08	0.08	0.11	0.15	0.15	192
3–4 years	0.08	0.09	0.12	0.16	0.20	210
5–7 years	0.08	0.09	0.12	0.16	0.18	219
8–11 years	0.08	0.09	0.13	0.17	0.21	227
12–15 years	0.08	0.09	0.14	0.18	0.22	237

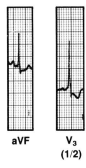

aVF   V₃
(1/2)

Fig. 11.35 PR interval in the Wolf–Parkinson–White syndrome. In lead aV_F, the PR interval is normal and there is no delta wave. The short PR interval and delta wave are only apparent in lead V₃, taken from the same patient.

therefore, the PR interval is correlated with age and not heart rate.

PR segment

The PR segment is measured from the end of the P wave to the beginning of the QRS complex. The length of this segment is variable and depends upon the duration of the P wave. Normal values for the duration of the PR segment in children are not available. A short PR segment is most often due to a long P wave with a normal PR interval, rather than due to the Wolff-Parkinson-White syndrome.

The importance of the PR segment in paediatrics is that it may provide the only estimation of the *isoelectric line* on the electrocardiogram. The true isoelectric line is the TP segment. But, in children at rapid heart rates, the T and P waves may merge without the electrocardiogram returning to the baseline between waves. In this case, the PR segment can be used as the isoelectric line. The PR segment, however, may be depressed from the true base-line by as much as 0.8 mm (or elevated in aVR by 0.5 mm) by a normal Ta wave of atrial repolarisation. When the Ta wave depresses the PR segment, the ST segment may be depressed to the same extent (see p. 266). It has been argued, therefore, that (although the PR segment is not the true isoelectric line) when diagnosing ST segment shifts,

the ST segment should be compared to the PR segment (Chou, 1979).

QRS complex

Duration

The QRS duration is measured from the beginning to the end of the ventricular depolarisation complex. It should be measured in a lead with a Q wave. The precordial leads may have a QRS duration which is 0.01–0.02 s longer than that measured in the limb leads (Cooksey et al, 1977). Lead V₅ was chosen to measure the duration for the normal values included in Table 11.4 because, in this lead, there usually is a Q wave and a defined termination to the QRS complex. As ventricular muscle mass increases, the QRS duration increases. Since the muscle mass increases with age, the QRS duration tends also to increase with age.

QRS mean vector

The measurement of the QRS mean vector in the frontal plane has been considered on page 253. The QRS frontal mean vector moves to the left with age as shown in Table 11.1.

QRS morphology

Depending upon the lead and orientation of the initial forces, a Q wave may or may not be present. The remainder of ventricular depolarisation is written as an R wave followed by an S wave. This is true in all normal precordial leads and limb leads other than lead aVR with one exception. An R wave without an S wave may be present normally in lead V₁ up to 5 months of age and in lead V₆ at any age. In approximately 7% of normal children, a second R wave or R′ may follow the S wave in the right chest leads giving an RSR′ pattern (Burch & DePasquale, 1967). The overall QRS duration in these normal children may be prolonged by 0.01 s above the normals given in Table 11.4, but the R′ wave has a rapid

Table 11.4 QRS duration (s) in V₅

Age	Min	2%	Mean	98%	Max	No. subjects
Less than 1 day	0.018	0.031	0.051	0.075	0.078	187
1–2 days	0.030	0.032	0.048	0.066	0.069	176
3–6 days	0.027	0.031	0.049	0.068	0.072	180
1–3 weeks	0.036	0.036	0.053	0.080	0.084	117
1–2 months	0.033	0.033	0.053	0.076	0.084	115
3–5 months	0.027	0.032	0.054	0.080	0.081	108
6–11 months	0.030	0.034	0.054	0.076	0.081	135
1–2 years	0.033	0.038	0.056	0.076	0.078	192
3–4 years	0.039	0.041	0.057	0.072	0.078	210
5–7 years	0.042	0.042	0.059	0.079	0.090	223
8–11 years	0.039	0.041	0.062	0.085	0.087	229
12–15 years	0.027	0.044	0.065	0.087	0.099	224

Table 11.5 Q amplitude in lead III (mm at normal standardisation)

Age	Min	2%	Mean	98%	Max	No. subjects
Less than 1 day	0.0	0.0	1.4	4.5	4.5	189
1–2 days	0.0	0.0	1.4	5.1	6.6	179
3–6 days	0.0	0.0	1.6	4.8	5.4	181
1–3 weeks	0.0	0.0	1.5	5.6	5.8	119
1–2 months	0.0	0.0	1.5	5.4	7.5	113
3–5 months	0.0	0.0	1.8	6.6	6.6	109
6–11 months	0.0	0.0	2.1	6.3	8.5	133
1–2 years	0.0	0.0	1.5	5.3	5.8	192
3–4 years	0.0	0.0	1.0	4.2	5.0	212
5–7 years	0.0	0.0	0.9	3.2	4.3	214
8–11 years	0.0	0.0	0.6	2.6	3.0	222
12–15 years	0.0	0.0	0.5	3.0	3.3	244

deflection and has the same duration as the preceding R and S waves. The S wave usually has a greater amplitude in normals (with an RSR′ pattern) than either the R or R′ wave. The RSR′ pattern can be found in complete right bundle branch block and right ventricular hypertrophy. In complete right bundle branch block, the total QRS duration is increased and there is a true terminal conduction delay with an increase in the duration of the slurred R′ compared to the normal duration of the initial R and S waves (see p. 281). In mild to moderate right ventricular hypertrophy, the R and especially the R′ waves have a greater amplitude than the S wave. With a normal duration QRS complex, right ventricular hypertrophy can be diagnosed by an R′ amplitude greater than 15 mm in an infant under 1 year of age, or 10 mm over 1 year of age. In children with a normal duration QRS complex and an RSR′ pattern with a small R′ wave (since the distinction between mild to moderate right ventricular hypertrophy, incomplete right bundle branch block and normal is difficult) we would prefer the designation 'RSR′ pattern in right chest leads' without a further attempt at diagnosis.

QRS amplitude

Q wave

A normal Q wave may be present in almost any lead. A QS pattern (or initial S wave) may be normal in lead aV_R at any age and in V_3R and V_4R in older children. A QR pattern (Q wave followed by an R wave) is not normal in lead aV_R or the right chest leads, and if present, this usually indicates right ventricular hypertrophy (see p. 274). If Q waves are present in the midprecordial leads, this generally implies counterclockwise rotation of the heart (see p. 271).

The distinguishing points between normal and abnormal Q waves are the duration and the amplitude of the Q wave. A normal duration Q wave is 0.01–0.015 s. Any Q wave greater than 0.03 s is definitely abnormal (Marriott, 1972; Burch & DePasquale, 1967). The normal amplitude of Q waves varies with the lead and with age (Davignon et al, 1979). Lead aVL normally is less than 2 mm; lead I less than 3 mm; lead II and aVF less than 4 mm. Leads III and V_6 are the most variable with all ages (Tables 11.5, 11.6) (Gerard et al, 1971). The implications of abnormal Q waves are further discussed on page 296.

R and S wave

Since the ventricles overlie each other in the frontal plane, to a great extent, the attempt at separation of right ventricular from left ventricular forces is best made in the horizontal plane. Therefore R wave and S wave amplitude will only be considered in the horizontal plane. In the normal

Table 11.6 Q amplitude in V_6 (mm at normal standardisation)

Age	Min	2%	Mean	98%	Max	No. subjects
Less than 1 day	0.0	0.0	0.3	2.0	2.6	189
1–2 days	0.0	0.0	0.4	2.4	3.4	179
3–6 days	0.0	0.0	0.6	3.1	4.0	181
1–3 weeks	0.0	0.0	0.8	3.1	3.1	119
1–2 months	0.0	0.0	0.7	2.9	4.0	115
3–5 months	0.0	0.0	0.8	2.9	4.0	109
6–11 months	0.0	0.0	0.8	3.2	3.6	138
1–2 years	0.0	0.0	1.0	3.1	4.6	192
3–4 years	0.0	0.0	1.2	3.5	4.6	210
5–7 years	0.0	0.0	1.2	4.7	6.0	222
8–11 years	0.0	0.0	1.0	3.0	3.2	221
12–15 years	0.0	0.0	0.8	3.1	5.0	243

heart with normally related ventricles the right ventricular forces are directed anteriorly and to the right. The anterior forces are reflected by the height of the R wave in lead V_1 and the rightward forces by the depth of the S wave in lead V_6. Conversely, the posterior forces generated by the left ventricle are reflected by the depth of the S wave in lead V_1 while the leftward forces are reflected by the height of the R wave in lead V_6. Left ventricular forces can also be represented by the sum of the posterior and leftward forces (or the sum of the depth of the S wave in lead V_1 plus the height of the R wave in lead V_6). The normal values by age for the amplitudes and ratios of R waves and S waves in

leads V_1 and V_6 are given in Tables 11.7–11.13.

The transition leads are the precordial leads in which the QRS complexes are approximately equiphasic (R and S wave equal amplitude). These leads record activity from both ventricles. If the total amplitude of the R wave plus S wave in the transition leads is increased, there is biventricular hypertrophy. The normal total amplitude of R plus S in lead V_4 is given in Table 11.4.

The mean amplitudes of the waves reflecting the right ventricle decrease while those reflecting the left ventricle increase with age. The variability of these amplitudes also decreases with age. With adolescence (in the 12–16-year-

Table 11.7 R amplitude in V_1 (mm at normal standardisation)

Age	Min	2%	Mean	98%	Max	No. subjects
Less than 1 day	3.6	5.2	13.8	26.1	29.2	189
1–2 days	0.9	5.3	14.4	26.9	38.0	177
3–6 days	1.0	2.8	12.9	24.2	27.2	181
1–3 weeks	2.5	3.2	10.6	20.8	23.0	119
1–2 months	2.8	3.3	9.5	18.4	20.6	115
3–5 months	0.7	2.7	9.8	19.8	25.2	109
6–11 months	1.4	1.4	9.4	20.3	24.0	138
1–2 years	2.0	2.6	8.9	17.7	34.4	192
3–4 years	0.4	1.0	8.1	18.2	20.6	211
5–7 years	0.0	0.5	6.7	13.9	14.8	219
8–11 years	0.0	0.0	5.4	12.1	15.4	230
12–15 years	0.0	0.0	4.1	9.9	12.6	244

Table 11.8 S amplitude in V_1 (mm at normal standardisation)

Age	Min	2%	Mean	98%	Max	No. subjects
Less than 1 day	0.0	0.0	8.5	22.7	28.4	189
1–2 days	0.0	0.0	9.1	20.7	30.0	178
3–6 days	0.0	0.0	6.6	16.8	21.4	181
1–3 weeks	0.0	0.0	4.2	10.8	14.2	119
1–2 months	0.0	0.0	5.0	12.4	13.4	115
3–5 months	0.0	0.0	5.7	17.1	26.6	109
6–11 months	0.0	0.4	6.4	18.1	24.4	138
1–2 years	0.0	0.7	8.4	21.0	33.0	191
3–4 years	0.6	1.8	10.2	21.4	26.2	212
5–7 years	0.8	2.9	12.0	23.8	29.4	219
8–11 years	1.8	2.7	11.9	25.4	28.8	226
12–15 years	1.4	2.8	10.8	21.2	23.0	235

Table 11.9 R amplitude in V_6 (mm at normal standardisation)

Age	Min	2%	Mean	98%	Max	No. subjects
Less than 1 day	0.0	0.0	4.2	11.1	22.8	189
1–2 days	0.0	0.0	4.5	12.2	17.0	179
3–6 days	0.0	0.3	5.2	12.1	14.5	181
1–3 weeks	1.2	2.6	7.6	16.4	24.0	119
1–2 months	3.1	5.2	11.6	21.4	24.2	115
3–5 months	5.0	6.4	13.1	22.4	25.0	109
6–11 months	5.8	5.8	12.6	22.7	24.6	138
1–2 years	3.7	5.9	13.3	22.6	24.6	192
3–4 years	7.6	8.1	14.8	24.4	36.0	209
5–7 years	6.4	8.4	16.3	26.5	28.4	223
8–11 years	7.0	9.2	16.3	25.4	33.0	233
12–15 years	5.5	6.5	14.3	23.0	32.2	246

Table 11.10 S amplitude in V_6 (mm at normal standardisation)

Age	Min	2%	Mean	98%	Max	No. subjects
Less than 1 day	0.0	0.0	3.2	9.6	16.3	189
1–2 days	0.0	0.0	3.0	9.4	12.4	179
3–6 days	0.0	0.0	3.5	9.8	10.4	181
1–3 weeks	0.0	0.0	3.4	9.8	13.0	119
1–2 months	0.0	0.0	2.7	6.4	6.4	115
3–5 months	0.0	0.0	2.9	9.9	12.8	109
6–11 months	0.0	0.0	2.1	7.2	14.2	138
1–2 years	0.0	0.0	1.9	6.6	10.4	192
3–4 years	0.0	0.0	1.5	5.2	5.4	210
5–7 years	0.0	0.0	1.2	4.0	4.3	217
8–11 years	0.0	0.0	1.0	3.9	4.6	232
12–15 years	0.0	0.0	0.8	3.7	4.4	241

Table 11.11 R/S ratio in V_1

Age	Min	2%	Mean	98%	Max	No. subjects
Less than 1 day	.04	.1	2.2	U	U	178
1–2 days	.03	.1	2.0	U	U	171
3–6 days	.06	.2	2.7	U	U	174
1–3 weeks	.9	1.0	2.9	U	U	103
1–2 months	.2	.3	2.3	U	U	104
3–5 months	.03	.1	2.3	U	U	97
6–11 months	.02	.1	1.6	3.9	5.2	130
1–2 years	.01	.05	1.4	4.3	5.2	185
3–4 years	.01	.03	.9	2.8	4.6	209
5–7 years	0.0	.02	.7	2.0	4.4	212
8–11 years	0.0	0	.5	1.8	2.2	225
12–15 years	0.0	0	.5	1.7	3.0	234

Note: U = undefined (S wave may equal zero)

Table 11.12 R/S ratio in V_6

Age	Min	2%	Mean	98%	Max	No. subjects
Less than 1 day	0.0	0.0	2.0	U	U	174
1–2 days	0.0	0.0	2.5	U	U	168
3–6 days	0.0	0.1	2.2	U	U	177
1–3 weeks	0.0	0.1	3.3	U	U	118
1–2 months	0.08	0.2	4.8	U	U	113
3–5 months	0.1	0.2	6.2	U	U	106
6–11 months	0.1	0.2	7.6	U	U	132
1–2 years	0.2	0.3	9.3	U	U	187
3–4 years	0.3	0.6	10.8	U	U	207
5–7 years	0.3	0.9	11.5	U	U	205
8–11 years	0.9	1.5	14.3	U	U	208
12–15 years	0.8	1.4	14.7	U	U	209

Note: U = undefined (S wave may equal zero)

old age-group) sex differences in the electrocardiogram become manifest (Table 11.15). R waves, especially in the left chest leads, are smaller in girls. This may represent either breast development or the smaller cardiac size in women. Changes in race and body habitus become more manifest with adolescence. Larger midprecordial voltages are found in blacks and those with thin chests (Chou, 1979).

Lower limit of QRS amplitude

We have been concerned heretofore with the upper limits for QRS amplitude. The lower limit is also important because low voltage QRS-complexes are usually a sign of myocardial oedema (for example, in myocarditis, myxoedema or generalised oedema), loss of functioning myocardium (in congestive heart failure, tumour or amyloid), or

Table 11.13 R amplitude in V_6 plus S amplitude in V_1 (mm at normal standardisation)

Age	Min	2%	Mean	98%	Max	No. subjects
Less than 1 day	1.4	1.4	12.6	28.0	40.8	189
1–2 days	1.6	1.6	13.7	28.7	32.8	179
3–6 days	2.8	2.8	11.7	24.7	27.2	181
1–3 weeks	2.7	3.0	11.7	21.0	24.0	119
1–2 months	6.8	6.8	16.5	29.1	30.2	115
3–5 months	6.6	7.2	18.6	34.9	42.2	109
6–11 months	6.1	7.3	19.0	32.2	34.4	138
1–2 years	5.8	7.7	21.7	39.0	51.8	192
3–4 years	10.4	13.0	25.1	41.8	45.4	210
5–7 years	12.4	13.6	28.2	47.1	52.4	217
8–11 years	14.1	15.3	28.1	45.5	57.4	225
12–15 years	6.9	11.4	25.1	41.1	43.6	235

Table 11.14 R plus S amplitude in V_4 (mm at normal standardisation)

Age	Min	2%	Mean	98%	Max	No. subjects
Less than 1 day	5.0	9.2	31.9	52.5	55.6	189
1–2 days	14.8	16.0	32.6	52.2	54.2	179
3–6 days	6.7	10.2	31.4	49.0	52.5	181
1–3 weeks	12.3	15.1	30.5	49.1	51.2	119
1–2 months	19.0	19.6	36.4	53.5	54.2	115
3–5 months	14.2	18.0	37.8	61.4	63.0	109
6–11 months	18.0	18.0	33.6	52.8	58.0	138
1–2 years	10.7	15.9	33.6	49.5	53.0	192
3–4 years	16.8	17.8	35.1	53.5	73.4	209
5–7 years	9.8	16.6	35.8	54.1	57.4	211
8–11 years	14.6	16.9	34.9	53.1	54.2	214
12–15 years	7.7	8.9	29.0	50.3	53.6	233

Table 11.15 Sex differences in R wave amplitudes in age-group 12–15 years

Lead	Sex	2%	R wave amplitude (mm at normal standardisation)	
			Mean	98%
V_1	Girls	0.1	3.5	9.6
	Boys	0.2	4.2	10.3
V_5	Girls	6.3	16.3	29.9
	Boys	10.9	24.1	34.7
V_6	Girls	5.9	12.2	19.1
	Boys	8.0	15.9	24.1

Notes
1. Based upon 105 boys and 142 girls.
2. Difference between boys and girls highly significant ($p < 0.0001$) for each lead.

else of an increased distance between the heart and chest wall (in obesity, pneumothorax, constrictive pericarditis, pericardial or pleural effusion) (see p. 295). The criterion for abnormally low voltage of QRS complexes is a total amplitude of R+S of 5 mm or less in each of the limb leads or 8 mm or less in each of the chest leads (Marriott, 1972).

ST segment

The ST segment is that portion of the electrocardiogram between the end of the S wave and the beginning of the T wave. The ST segment normally gently curves into the proximal limb of the T wave and is not perfectly horizontal. When determining ST segment deviation above or below the baseline, it is best to consider the PR segment as the baseline (see p. 266). The ST segments in children should not be elevated greater than 1 mm or depressed greater than 0.5 mm in any lead. The exception is the 'early repolarisation' syndrome of adolescence, in which the ST segment can be elevated to 4 mm in the mid-precordial leads (see p. 291).

The T wave

The T wave is normally asymmetrical with the upstroke having a more gradual slope than the downstroke (Fig. 11.36A). It usually has a smooth and curved form but may have a notch near its summit (Fig. 11.36B). Its amplitude is generally not measured in specific leads, since it is so variable in normal children. Low voltage or 'flattened' T waves in several leads, however, may indicate an abnormality (see p. 290). The T waves in leads I, II and V_6 should be greater than 2 mm in all children over 48 hours old. An abnormally tall T wave is generally defined at any age as greater than 7 mm in a limb lead or 10 mm in a precordial lead. The T wave mean vector generally parallels the QRS mean vector. Hence there are positive T waves in leads I, II and V_6 in children over 48 hours old (see p. 252).

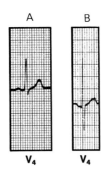

Fig. 11.36 T waves. (A) Normal smooth T wave. (B) Normal notched T wave.

The U wave

The normal U wave has the same polarity as the preceding T wave but the normal U wave has only 2–24% of the T wave amplitude. There is a wide variation of normal. Nonetheless, the normal U wave should not be more than 50% of the amplitude of the T wave (Fig. 11.37). The largest amplitude U waves are recorded in leads V_2–V_4. The shape of a normal U wave is different from the normal T wave. The upstroke is steeper than the downstroke in the U wave (Lepeschkin, 1969; Marriott, 1972).

Differentiating T, U and P Waves

It is important to differentiate between T waves and normal U waves so that the U wave can be discounted in

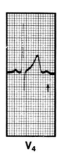

Fig. 11.37 U wave (arrow).

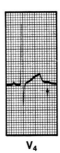

Fig. 11.38 Notched T wave followed by a U wave.

the measurement of the QT interval. A normal U wave is one with an amplitude no more than 50% of the preceding T wave. The T and U waves are usually separated at slow heart rates by a distinct isoelectric line. But, at rates over 90/min, there may be no intervening isoelectric line and it may be difficult to determine whether the terminal portion of the deflection is a U wave or the second half of a notched T wave. If, in the same or a different lead, another wave is seen later in timing than the questionable wave, then the questionable wave is a notched T wave (Fig. 11.38). It may be possible to bring out a U wave by recording the electrocardiogram in the sitting position. This tends to decrease the T wave and increase the U wave amplitude in the left precordial leads (Lepeschkin & Surawicz, 1952).

If there is a single wave in all leads, it is not possible to determine whether this represents a T wave or fusion of a T wave and U wave. If there is not a notch in any lead (but this wave is smooth throughout) this should be considered as a T wave (Fig. 11.39). If there is a notch in the terminal part of the wave and the amplitude is 50% or less of the peak, then the downstroke of the early portion of the wave should be extrapolated as the T wave (see Fig. 11.40). If the terminal portion of the wave in any lead (usually V_4 is the clearest) is more than 50% of the amplitude of the peak, the terminal portion of the wave should be included as part of the T wave (Fig. 11.41). Whether this terminal portion should be called a T wave is a question of semantics (Jervell & Lange-Nielsen, 1957). The important electrocardiographic question to be answered is whether there is a significant increase in the amount of late

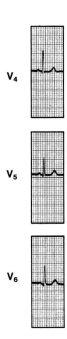

Fig. 11.39 There is no notch in any of the waves following the QRS complex and so these should all be considered as T waves. Simultaneous leads V₄, V₅ and V₆.

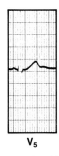

Fig. 11.40 T wave followed by a notch with an amplitude less than 50% of the peak of the T wave. In this case, the T wave is considered to have merged with the U wave and the T wave ends at the extrapolated downslope of the larger wave.

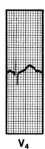

Fig. 11.41 T wave with a notch and the peak of the terminal segment is greater than 50% of the peak of the T wave. In this case, both of these waves should be considered as part of the T wave.

repolarisation. This can be indicated either by a separate U wave with an amplitude more than 50% of the T wave, or by a single fusion wave whose terminal portion is more than 50% of the amplitude of the peak. The causes and consequences of increased late repolarisation are the same. The same consideration should therefore be given to long T waves as to excessively large U waves.

The distinction of P waves from T or U waves in sinus rhythm is simplified by examining multiple leads. P waves are most obvious in lead II and least obvious in leads V₄–V₇. T and U waves are most obvious in leads V₄–V₇. A synthesis can therefore be made of the different waves by using the timing from different leads (Fig. 11.42). The P wave in sinus tachycardia may begin before the T wave has been completed. At rapid rates, P waves become much more pointed than T waves. Again, in leads V₆ or V₇ almost all of the wave is likely to be a T wave while in lead II, the maximum P wave is likely to be visible. In supraventricular tachycardia, the most pointed of the waves are P waves. P waves can also be identified as discrete deflections usually lasting 0.06 s or less which occur with an improper timing for a QRS complex or a T wave (Fig. 11.43). Using this type of analysis, we have found it possible to distinguish P waves in 55% of children during supraventricular tachycardia (Garson et al, 1981b).

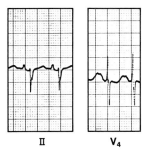

Fig. 11.42 Distinction of P waves from T waves. In lead V₄, it is not possible to tell whether these waves are merged P waves with T waves or T and U waves. It is apparent from examination of lead II in the same patient that the second notch in lead V₄ is caused by the P wave.

QT interval

The QT interval begins at the onset of the QRS complex and terminates at the end of the T wave. The longest interval in any lead should be used. As noted in the previous section, it may be difficult in certain conditions to choose the proper end of the T wave. We agree with James (1967) that 'In electrocardiography, there is no more nebulous measurement than the QT interval'. Some rules may nonetheless be helpful (Fig. 11.44). If a separate T and U wave are visible and the U wave amplitude is 50% or less than the T wave amplitude, the QT interval ends at the end of the T wave. If a single wave is visible and there is no notch in any lead, the entire wave is included

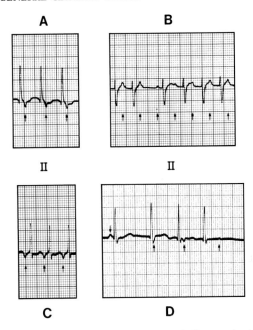

Fig. 11.43 Identification of P waves (arrows). (A) P waves in the early part of the ST segment. (B) P waves directly on top of T waves. The only way of distinguishing these waves was to observe an episode of spontaneous type I second degree atrioventricular block in which the P wave was not followed by a QRS complex. This allowed observation of the P wave preceding the next QRS complex with a lengthening PR interval in subsequent beats. (C) P waves on the downslope of the T wave. (D) P waves with differing relation to the QRS and T wave. In the second QRS complex, the widened S wave is caused by a superimposed P wave.

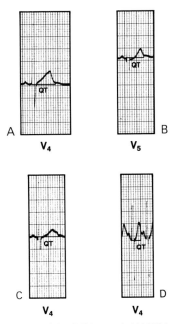

Fig. 11.44 Measurement of the QT interval. (A) With a notched T wave followed by a U wave, the downslope of the T wave is extrapolated to the baseline. (B) With a notch less than 50% of the peak of the T wave, the early segment is extrapolated to the baseline. (C) With a notch greater than 50% of the peak of the T wave, the second portion of the wave is extrapolated to the baseline. (D) With superimposed P waves, the downslope of the T wave is extrapolated to the baseline.

in the QT interval. If a single wave is visible but a notch is present in the wave and the terminal portion of the wave has an amplitude 50% or less than the peak, then the initial downslope should be extrapolated and the extrapolation used for the QT interval. If a single wave is visible with a notch and the terminal portion has an amplitude more than 50% of the peak, then the entire wave is included as the T wave. If a P wave is superimposed, the T wave is extrapolated back to the baseline from the initial downstroke (Fig. 11.44).

The QT interval varies with heart rate. It can be 'corrected' by Bazett's (1918) formula. The corrected QT interval is equal to the QT interval (in seconds) divided by the square root of the RR interval (in seconds). The corrected QT interval is abnormal if it is prolonged beyond 0.40 s under 12 years of age or is greater than 0.43 s in those 12 years of age or older. Alternatively, a patient's data can be compared with the normal QT interval derived from a plot of Bazett's data (Fig. 11.45). The actual measured QT interval in lead V_5 in children as it varies with heart rate is shown in Table 11.16.

Q-OT interval

The interval from the onset of the QRS complex to the onset of the T wave is the Q-OT interval. This interval may be corrected for heart rate in a similar way to the QT interval thus determining the Q-OTC interval. The entire T wave in hypocalcaemia is shifted later in the cardiac cycle (due to a prolonged ST segment). The Q-OTC interval provides a measure of this prolongation (Fig. 11.46). The normal corrected Q-OTC is 0.20 or less in premature infants, while in full-term infants it is 0.19 or less (Colletti, 1974).

TP interval

The TP interval is that segment between the end of the T wave (or U wave) and the beginning of the P wave. This is the true isoelectric segment of the electrocardiogram between the last ventricular repolarisation and the onset of atrial depolarisation (Fig. 11.47). It is best in cases with both PR and ST segment depression to use the PR segment as the isoelectric reference for the ST segment (see p. 263).

MALPOSITION OF THE HEART IN THE THORAX

Atrial arrangement (situs)

In the majority of cases, the atrial arrangement may be determined from the electrocardiogram. With usual arrangement of the atria and the bodily organs, the P wave mean vector in the frontal plane is approximately $+60°$. It points away from its site of origin in the high right atrium

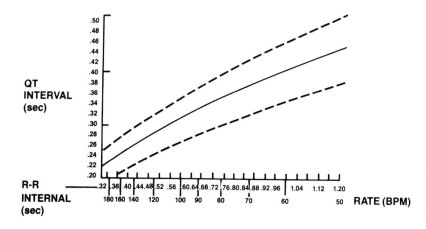

QT INTERVAL (sec)

R-R INTERNAL (sec)

RATE (BPM)

Fig. 11.45 Plot of Bazett's (1918) data for QT interval. The solid line shows the mean QT interval for each heart rate and cycle lenght. The dotted lines mark the upper and lower limits of normal calculated as ±2 standard deviations for the mean.

Table 11.16 QT duration (s) according to heart rate in lead V_5

Heart rate	Min	2%	Mean	98%	Max	No. subjects
80–90/min	0.222	0.293	0.343	0.380	0.396	168
90–95/min	0.273	0.280	0.329	0.372	0.378	101
95–100/min	0.270	0.290	0.325	0.361	0.432	111
100–105/min	0.267	0.274	0.318	0.364	0.423	143
105–110/min	0.255	0.264	0.307	0.355	0.417	139
110–115/min	0.228	0.247	0.300	0.367	0.372	168
115–120/min	0.207	0.245	0.293	0.344	0.360	159
120–125/min	0.222	0.233	0.289	0.351	0.363	137
125–130/min	0.198	0.228	0.280	0.334	0.345	175
130–135/min	0.204	0.212	0.273	0.331	0.336	121
135–140/min	0.210	0.228	0.272	0.325	0.330	139
140–150/min	0.195	0.218	0.263	0.308	0.318	164

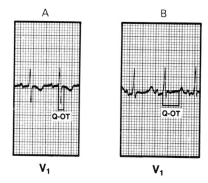

Fig. 11.46 Q-OT interval. (A) Q-OT interval in a normal newborn infant. The Q-OT interval is 0.10 s and the PR interval is 0.45 s. Therefore, the Q-OTC interval is 0.15. A normal Q-OT interval is 0.20 or less. (B) Q-OT interval in an infant with hypocalcaemia. The Q-OT interval is 0.27 s and the RR interval is 0.47 s. The Q-OTC interval of 0.39 is prolonged.

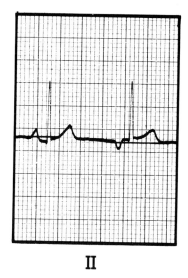

II

Fig. 11.47 Importance of using the TP segment as the baseline. In the beat at the left, in sinus rhythm, using the TP segment as the baseline, there is PR segment depression of approximately 1 mm due to an inverted Ta wave. In the beat at the right, with a low atrial rhythm, there is PR segment and ST segment elevation due to an upright Ta wave. In this tracing, the TP segment remains constant while the PR segment and ST segments change.

and away from the right shoulder. This results in a positive P wave in leads I and aVF (Fig. 11.48). In individuals with mirror-image atrial arrangement ('inversus'), a normal sinus impulse still originates high in the morphologically right atrium but since this chamber is on the patient's left, the origin of the P wave appears to be from the left shoulder. The P wave mean vector in the frontal plane,

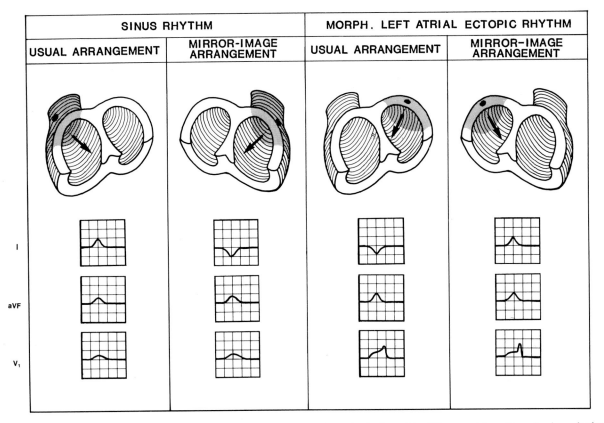

SINUS RHYTHM		MORPH. LEFT ATRIAL ECTOPIC RHYTHM	
USUAL ARRANGEMENT	MIRROR-IMAGE ARRANGEMENT	USUAL ARRANGEMENT	MIRROR-IMAGE ARRANGEMENT

Fig. 11.48 P wave morphology in sinus rhythm and morphologically left atrial ectopic rhythm with different atrial position. In sinus rhythm, the P wave is positive in lead I, with usual arrangement and negative in lead I with mirror-image arrangement. If the morphologically right atrium is depolarised before the left atrium, there is a normal P wave in lead V_1. If the morphologically left atrium is activated before the right atrium, a 'dome-and-dart' P wave is found in lead V_1. Therefore, in usual atrial arrangement (solitus) with morphologically left atrial ectopic rhythm, there is a negative P wave in lead I and a dome and dart P wave in lead V_1. With mirror-image atrial arrangement (inversus) and morphologically left atrial ectopic rhythm, there is a positive P wave in lead I and dome-and-dart P wave in lead V_1.

pointing away from the site of origin, is $+120°$. This results in a P wave which is negative in lead I and positive in aVF. The P wave mean vector in the horizontal plane is generally not helpful, because activation proceeds posteroanteriorly in this plane.

It may be impossible to determine atrial arrangement in the presence of an ectopic atrial rhythm (Hoffman, 1975a). In patients with normal arrangement and left atrial ectopic rhythm, however, despite the negative P wave in lead I, there may be a dome-and-dart P wave in lead V_1 (Fig. 11.48). This indicates that the morphologically left atrium is activated before the right atrium (Mirowski et al, 1963). In the rare case of a patient with mirror-image atrial arrangement and an ectopic rhythm originating from the right-sided morphologically left atrium, there would be a normal frontal plane P wave axis ($+60°$) but a dome-and-dart configuration in lead V_1 (Fig. 11.48).

In cases of atrial isomerism ('splenic syndromes'; visceral heterotoxy), the P waves may be characteristic. In right atrial isomerism there are two sinus nodes (Van Mierop & Wiglesworth, 1962; Momma & Linde, 1969). In such cases, competition between the sinus nodes may occur

with two P waves (one positive in lead I and one negative in lead I), each having a slightly different rate (Fig. 11.49). In left atrial isomerism there may be absence of any sinus node (Dickinson et al, 1979). The pacemaker is characteristically located in the low atrium giving a frontal plane P wave mean vector which is directly superior ($-90°$) (Fig. 11.50).

Ventricular position

Since ventricular position is independent of atrial arrangement, the P waves and QRS complexes should be interpreted independently (that is, a negative P wave in lead I suggests mirror-image atrial arrangement but not necessarily a right-sided heart). There are four major electrocardiographic patterns which describe ventricular position. These are the normal, the mirror-image arrangement, the rightward rotated arrangement and that associated with discordant atrioventricular connexion and usual arrangement (Fig. 11.51). Of great significance in the generation of these patterns is the ventricular topology (see Ch. 3). In the normally positioned heart, the maximal biphasic

R Atrial

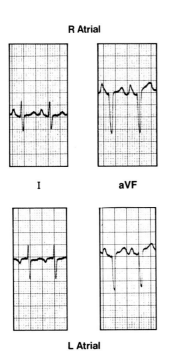

I   aVF

L Atrial

Fig. 11.49 P waves in right atrial isomerism (asplenia). In the top two tracings, the patient has positive P waves in leads I and aV$_F$ indicating the site of origin of the P waves high in the atrium on the right side. In the bottom two tracings, taken several minutes later, the P waves have changed such that they are negative in lead I and positive in aV$_F$ indicating the origin of the P wave high and on the left side. The QRS complexes are identical.

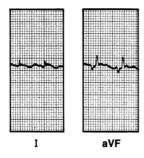

I   aVF

Fig. 11.50 P waves in left atrial isomerism (polysplenia). The P wave mean vector is $-90°$.

QRS voltage in the chest leads (transition) is at the left midclavicular line at lead V$_3$ or V$_4$. The initial forces in the frontal plane are directed superiorly and to the right (Q wave in leads I, aVF and V$_6$). The major forces are directed inferiorly and to the left (tall R wave in leads, I, aVF and V$_6$). The terminal forces are directed superiorly and to the left (small S wave in lead aVF, R wave in leads I and V$_6$) (Fig. 11.52).

Mirror-image arrangement with concordant atrioventricular connexion and left hand topology

When the ventricular mass is in the right chest with left

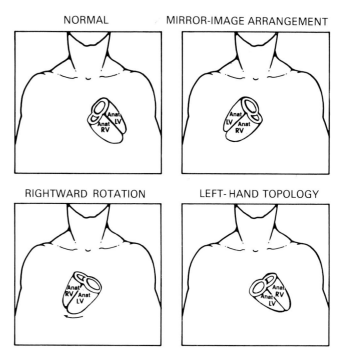

Fig. 11.51 Ventricular position. In the normal, the morphologically right ventricle is to the right and anterior relative to the morphologically left ventricle (right hand topology). The cardiac mass is in the left chest. In the mirror-image arrangement (left hand topology), the morphologically right ventricle is to the left and anterior relative to the morphologically left ventricle. The ventricular mass is in the right chest. With rightward rotation, the morphologically right ventricle is to the right and posterior relative to the morphologically left ventricle. The ventricular mass is in the right chest to a varying degree. With discordant atrioventricular connexion and left hand topology, the morphologically right ventricle is to the left and usually side-by-side relative to the morphologically left ventricle. The ventricular mass can be (indeed, usually is) in the left chest.

hand ventricular topology, there is usually a reversal of the anatomic left–right relationship but the anteroposterior relationships are maintained. Thus, the morphologically right ventricle is to the left and anterior. Whenever the ventricles are predominantly in the right chest, the maximal biphasic voltage is recorded in one of the *right* chest leads. *If the total voltage (top of the R wave to bottom of the S wave)* in leads V$_3$R or V$_4$R is larger than the total voltage in lead V$_3$ or V$_4$, the patient has a right-sided heart. When this is also associated with mirror-image atria, the QRS morphologies in all the right chest leads (V$_1$, V$_3$R–V$_7$R) should be the same as those found when recording the left chest leads in a normally situated heart. In a patient with mirror-image arrangement and right-sided heart, the initial forces in the frontal plane are directed superiorly and to the left (initial deep Q wave in leads I, aVF, and V$_6$). The major forces are directed inferiorly and to the right (small R, deep S in leads I and V$_6$, tall R in aVF). The terminal forces are directed superiorly and to the right (S wave in leads I, aVF and V$_6$) (Figs. 11.52, 11.53). A mirror-image arrangement with a right-sided heart

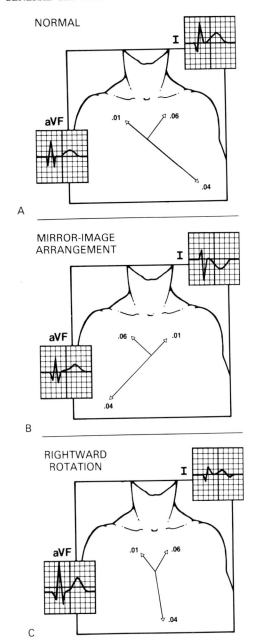

Fig. 11.52 Frontal plane QRS vectors in different ventricular positions. In the top tracing, the directions and amplitudes of the early (0.01 s), middle (0.04 s) and terminal (0.06 s) vectors are shown. In the normal (A), the early vector is to the right and superior, the middle vector is to the left and inferior and the terminal vector is to the left and superior. In mirror-image arrangement with left hand ventricular topology (B), the initial vector is to the left and superior, the middle vector is to the right and inferior, and the terminal vector is to the right and superior. With right hand rotation and right hand topology (C), the initial vector is to the right and superior, the middle vector is inferior, and the terminal vector is to the left and superior.

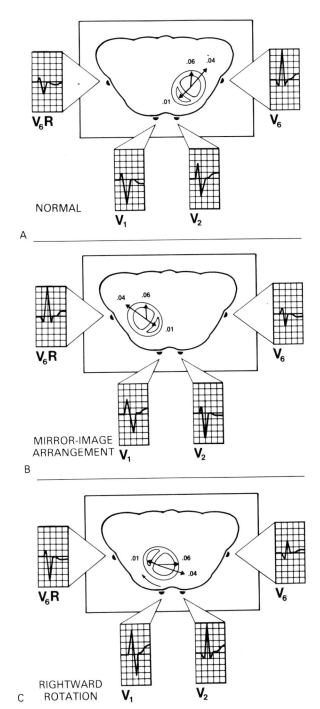

Fig. 11.53 Horizontal plane vectors in different cardiac positions. In the normal (A), the middle (0.04 s) vector points left and posterior. In mirror-image arrangement with left-hand topology (B), the middle (0.04 s) vector points to the right and posterior and in rightward rotation with right hand topology (C), the middle (0.04 s) vector points left and slightly anterior.

should be suspected if the magnitude of the total QRS deflection is greater in leads V_3R or V_4R than in lead V_3 or V_4, if lead I has a deep Q wave and a small R wave, or if, in leads V_3–V_7, the QRS complexes become progressively smaller with a small R, deep S, or QS, configuration (Burch & DePasquale, 1967).

The same criteria can be applied in assessing ventricular hypertrophy with this arrangement as with normally situated ventricles. The difference is that, instead of lead V_6, lead V_6R should be substituted. Similarly instead of lead V_1, lead V_2 should be substituted (Fig. 11.54). Even in the absence of a tracing with all the right chest leads, therefore,

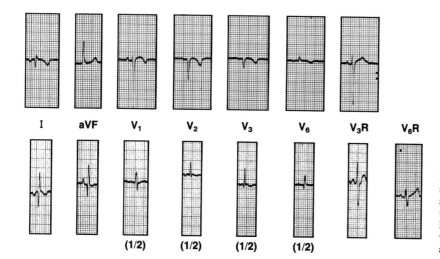

I	aVF	V₁	V₂	V₃	V₆	V₃R	V₆R

| | | (1/2) | (1/2) | (1/2) | (1/2) | | |

Fig. 11.54 Top tracings –7-year-old with mirror-image arrangement, concordant atrioventricular connexion with an otherwise normal heart in the right chest. Bottom tracings –6 month-old with mirror-image arrangement, left hand topology, a right-sided heart and anterior ventricular hypertrophy. There is a QR pattern in lead V_2 and a deep S wave in lead V_6R.

ventricular hypertrophy can be assessed by interpreting lead V_2 as if it were lead V_1 in a normaly situated heart.

Rotation of the heart to the right with right hand topology

In rotation, the anatomic relationships between the ventricles are preserved (that is, the right ventricle is on the right and the left ventricle is on the left-right-hand topology), but the heart is *shifted* to a varying degree into the right chest. This shift is usually accompanied by a counterclockwise rotation of the heart (viewed from the apex) such that the morphologically left ventricle is anterior to the right ventricle (Fig. 11.51). Since the amount of rightward shift is variable, the classic signs of a right-sided heart (greater voltage in the right chest leads than the left) may be missing. The direction of the initial, major and terminal deflections in the frontal plane may be similar to those found with normally situated ventricles. The mean frontal plane QRS vector is inferior and slightly to the left or right (Fig. 11.52). The major effect is on the precordial leads. The transition is found in leads more to the right than normal, i.e. in lead V_3R or V_4R (Fig. 11.53). The far right chest leads (lead V_6R) appear similar to the normal V_1, and the anterior leads (V_3) appear similar to the normal V_6. This can be suspected in a routine electrocardiogram when the anterior chest leads (V_2–V_4) have small Q waves and tall R waves (similar to the normal V_6) and the transition is just beginning in lead V_1 or V_3R (Fig. 11.55).

Ventricular hypertrophy is less accurately assessed when the heart is rotated to the right since the degree of rotation is unknown. Similar criteria to those used for mirror-image arrangement and a right-sided heart may be applied with caution.

Discordant atrioventricular connexion with usual atrial arrangement and left-hand ventricular topology

One other condition in which the ventricles are malposed is in discordant atrioventricular connexion ('ventricular in-

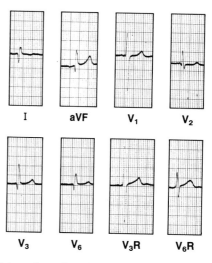

I	aVF	V₁	V₂

V₃	V₆	V₃R	V₆R

Fig. 11.55 Rightward rotation with right hand topology in a 12-year-old patient with mild pulmonary stenosis. The transition occurs in lead V_3R, and there are Q waves in leads V_2 through V_6. Lead V_6R in this patient appears similar to lead V_1 in a patient with normally positioned ventricles and mild pulmonary stenosis.

version'). When this occurs with otherwise normal cardiac position (usual atrial arrangement, left-hand ventricular topology and a left-sided heart), the ventricular septum is oriented straight anteroposteriorly. It is parallel to the diaphragm when the ventricles are side-by-side and the morphologically right ventricle is to the left of the morphologically left ventricle (Fig. 11.51). Since the left bundle branch is on the right, there is reversed septal depolarisation with a Q wave in lead V_1, and an absent Q wave in lead V_6 (Fig. 11.56). The other characteristics of a discordant atrioventricular connexion and an otherwise normal heart are left axis deviation in the frontal plane and atrioventricular block – (first, second or third degree). Usually, a discordant atrioventricular connexion is accompanied by additional cardiac malformations and the electrocardiogram may reflect these additional abnormalities.

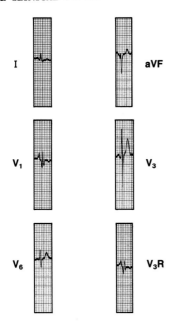

Fig. 11.56 Usual atrial arrangement with discordant atrioventricular connexion, left hand topology and a left sided heart. Note the deep Q waves in lead V_1 with a relatively small R wave. There are no Q waves in lead V_6.

Pectus excavatum and straight back syndrome

The mediastinum in both of these conditions is shortened in the anteroposterior dimension. This causes the heart to shift to the left and rotate clockwise as viewed from the apex. The morphologically right atrium is then more anterior relative to the left. The mean vector of atrial depolarisation is therefore oriented straight posteriorly. The P wave in lead V_1 may be entirely negative (Chou, 1979) (Figs. 11.57, 11.58). Clockwise rotation moves the left side of the heart posteriorly and superiorly, causing some patients to have left-axis deviation of the QRS in the frontal plane (De Leon et al, 1965). The right side of the heart is rotated anteriorly and inferiorly such that the vector of depolarisation in the pulmonary outflow tract is shifted from its normal superior and rightward position to a straight anterior position. This is responsible for the normal duration RSR' pattern in V_1 often found in these patients (De Oliveira et al, 1958). The transition is shifted to the left and there may be a persistent S wave in lead V_7. Abnormally deep QS waves followed by a normal duration R wave and inverted T wave in the anterior and midprecordial leads may occur rather than the RSR'. This can simulate anterior myocardial infarction. These changes can be explained by the clockwise rotation shifting the major QRS forces even more posteriorly and causing the deep QS and concordantly inverted T wave. The terminal R wave has the same genesis as the R' which may be found in this condition, namely normal terminal depolarisation of the right ventricular outflow tract.

Pneumonectomy

The chronic electrocardiographic changes following pneumonectomy result from shift and rotation of the heart. Following a right pneumonectomy, the findings are similar to those of rightward rotation with the transition moved to the right in the chest leads (Calleja, 1966). In over 90% of children after a left pneumonectomy, the heart was rotated clockwise with findings similar to those reported in pectus excavatum.

Pneumothorax and pneumomediastinum

Since air is a poor conductor of electrical activity, air between the heart and the recording electrode will decrease the voltage of the P, QRS and T waves. In pneumomediastinum the voltage may be decreased in all leads. In pneumothorax, the voltage may be decreased only in certain leads corresponding to the location of the air. Depending upon the amount of air, a pneumothorax may cause shift or rotation of the heart similar to that found following pneumonectomy on the opposite side. Depending upon the amount of hemodynamic compromise caused by the condition, non-specific ST and T wave changes as well as arrhythmias may occur. If the patient with pneumothorax is placed in a sitting position, the electrocardiogram may normalise as the air moves superiorly away from the heart.

Kyphoscoliosis

There may be virtually any positional abnormality with kyphoscoliosis (Chou, 1979). Both rotation and shift occur in severe cases, thus making it even more difficult to interpret the electrocardiogram. Since respiratory insufficiency and cor pulmonale may occur in these children (and cause right atrial enlargement, right axis deviation and right ventricular hypertrophy), an electrocardiographic diagnosis may be helpful in the management of the patient. As a general rule, a P wave amplitude of more than 2.5 mm in any lead constitutes right atrial enlargement. Right ventricular hypertrophy should be considered if a complex is found in any precordial lead to the right of the transitional leads with a tall R wave and a small S wave, and the height of the R wave is greater than the normal value for age given for lead V_1.

CHAMBER ENLARGEMENT AND HYPERTROPHY

The electrocardiogram can be helpful in the diagnosis of enlargement or hypertrophy of the cardiac chambers. While the electrocardiogram correlates with chamber size better in paediatric patients than adults, there is still only

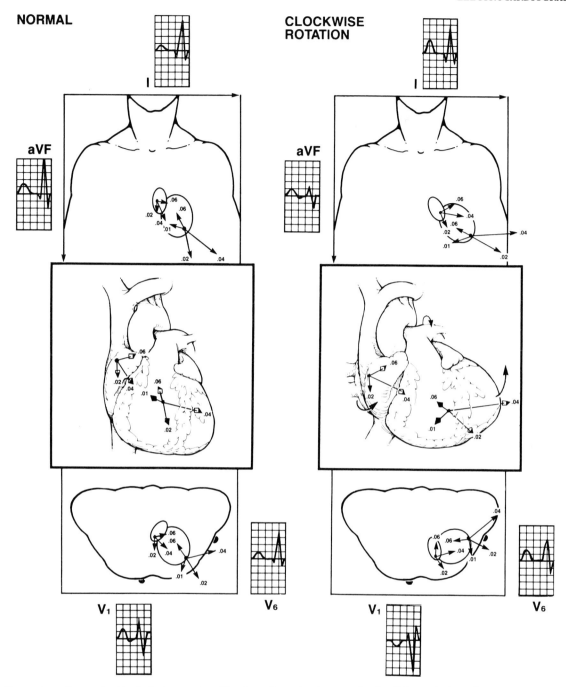

Fig. 11.57 Comparison of normal with clockwise rotation. The three-dimensional vectors for the different timings of the P wave are shown overlying the atrium and for the QRS complex are shown overlying the ventricles. In the top part of the diagrams, the projections of the vectors on the frontal plane are shown. The small circle denotes the atria and the larger circle denotes the ventricles. In the frontal plane with clockwise rotation, both the P wave and QRS vectors are shifted to the left and superiorly. In the bottom parts of the diagrams the horizontal plane vectors are shown. In the horizontal plane, the vectors are shifted to the left and posteriorly.

about a 60–70% predictive value of the electrocardiogram in children (Ellison et al, 1977; Wagner et al, 1977). If either the presence or absence of an abnormality on an electrocardiogram does not agree with the clinical or echocardiographic findings, the electrocardiogram should be viewed quite critically. In the following discussion,

criteria are listed for chamber enlargement or hypertrophy with the most reliable signs presented first.

Right ventricular hypertrophy

The electrocardiogram can provide important data on right

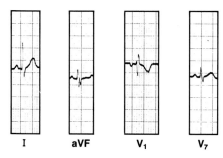

Fig. 11.58 Electrocardiogram from a 4-year-old patient with pectus excavatum. The frontal plane QRS mean vector is −45°. There is an RSR′ pattern in lead V_1 and a persistent S wave in lead V_7.

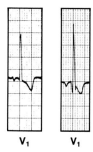

Fig. 11.59 Left – typical QR pattern in lead V_1 with a small Q wave. This is from a 9-month-old patient with unoperated complete transposition. Right – deep Q wave with a tall R wave and ST depression in a 4-year-old after Mustard operation for complete transposition.

ventricular hypertrophy or elevated right ventricular systolic pressure which are not currently available by non-invasive means. There are several criteria for right ventricular hypertrophy.

The first criterion is a QR pattern in the right chest leads (Fig. 11.59). The Q wave is due to a dominant early wave of excitation moving posteriorly. This may be due to the hypertrophied and dilated right side of the septum providing a larger surface area for a normally insignificant posterior vector. In this case, left-to-right septal activation occurs normally but is overshadowed by a stronger posterior vector. Alternatively, in right ventricular hypertrophy, the inferior wall of the right ventricle directly contiguous to the septum may bulge posteriorly and to the left of the septum. Therefore, instead of the earliest activation continuing left-to-right, the initial septal depolarisation may begin normally towards the right for a few milliseconds but then change orientation and move to the left as those parts of the inferior wall of the right ventricle which are situated to the left of the septum depolarise (Liebman & Plonsey, 1978).

The Q wave in the QR pattern of right ventricular hypertrophy is generally only 0.5–1 mm deep in infants but may become 3–5 mm deep in older children. The QR pattern is quite reliable and implies a right ventricular systolic pressure of 70 mmHg or more at any age (Cayler

et al, 1958). A QR pattern may also be seen in discordant atrioventricular connexion and usual atrial arrangement with reversed septal depolarisation. In general, in the QR pattern of right ventricular hypertrophy in lead V_2 or V_4R, the R wave is tall (15–20 mm). In discordant atrioventricular connexion, the Q wave may be slightly deeper than the usual Q wave seen in right ventricular hypertrophy and the R wave may not be as tall (Fig. 11.56). This distinction may not be possible in an individual patient. A final cause of a QR pattern in lead V_1 and V_3R is the rare case of an anterior myocardial infarction involving either the right ventricle or the anterior ventricular septum. Before making the diagnosis of a QR pattern, it is important to be certain that the QRS complex does not begin with a tiny R wave and thus the complex is an RSR′ pattern rather than QR pattern.

The second criterion concerns T wave changes. Between 1 week of age and the onset of adolescence, the T waves in the right chest leads should be negative. In mildly increased right ventricular systolic pressure, the electrocardiogram is normal with a small R wave and a symmetrically inverted T wave in lead V_1 (Fig. 11.60A). With increasing severity of pulmonary stenosis (usually before the R wave height is abnormal) the T wave becomes iso-electric or upright (Fig. 11.60B). The upright T wave is due to elevated right ventricular systolic pressure and not necessarily right ventricular hypertrophy. In a patient with increased right ventricular systolic pressure due to upper airway obstruction and hypoxia, the upright T waves may invert immediately with intubation and ventilation. In general, if the height of the R wave in lead V_1 is less than 10 mm, an inverted T wave is associated with less severe disease than an isoelectric or upright T wave (Fig. 11.60C). When the R wave height increases above 10 mm, the upright T wave may become asymmetrically inverted with a concave upward terminal portion (Fig. 11.60D). The progression and severity is therefore as follows: normal R

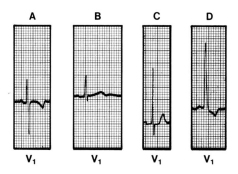

Fig. 11.60 Progression of T wave changes in lead V_1 in right ventricular hypertrophy. (A) Normal T wave in a 4-year-old child. (B) Upright T wave in a 7-year-old child with mild pulmonary stenosis. The R wave is 9 mm tall. (C) Tall R wave with upright T wave in a 2-year-old with severe pulmonary stenosis. (D) Tall R wave with asymmetrically inverted T wave ('right ventricular strain') in a 3-year-old patient with critical pulmonary stenosis.

with symmetrically inverted T; normal or slightly increased R with upright T; tall R with upright T; tall R with asymmetrically inverted T. The asymmetrically inverted T wave in lead V_1 is called the 'right ventricular strain' pattern. It may be associated with ST depression in the same lead. This is thought to be a primary T wave change due to the reversed direction of repolarisation which occurs from endocardium to epicardium in hypertrophy (Cooksey et al, 1977). The right ventricular strain pattern generally indicates a right ventricular systolic pressure equal to or greater than systemic pressure (Cayler et al, 1958; Burch & DePasquale, 1967). The deeply asymmetrically inverted T waves in the right ventricular strain pattern may extend as far to the left as lead V_4 and rarely V_5 but usually not to V_6 (Liebman & Plonsey, 1978). Conversely, the T wave inversion found in leads V_5 and V_6 which indicates 'left ventricular strain' may cause reciprocally *upright* T waves in the right chest leads (Fig. 11.61). Before the diagnosis of right ventricular hypertrophy is made on the basis of an upright T wave in lead V_1, leads V_5 and V_6 should be examined for left ventricular strain. One other T wave change of severe right ventricular hypertrophy is T wave inversion in lead aVF (Cayler et al, 1958). This is a non-specific sign since it may also be indicative of left ventricular strain or other condition (see p. 278). But in the presence of other signs of right ventricular hypertrophy, T wave inversion in lead aVF indicates severe right ventricular hypertrophy.

lar systolic pressure equals 5 times the R wave in V_1 (Cayler et al 1958; Liebman & Plonsey, 1978). If the R wave in V_1 is 20 mmHg or more at any age, the right ventricular systolic pressure is equal to or more than systemic pressure. One other reason for an abnormally tall R wave in lead V_1 in a patient without right ventricular hypertrophy is ventricular septal hypertrophy. This may cause deep Q waves in leads V_5 and V_6 with reciprocally tall R waves in lead V_1. Since septal depolarisation is completed relatively early in the QRS complex, the tall R wave in lead V_1 due to septal hypertrophy is 'narrow' and usually lasts 0.03 s or less. Conversely, in right ventricular hypertrophy ventricular activation is slightly prolonged and the R wave of right ventricular hypertrophy in lead V_1 generally lasts 0.04 s or longer (Chou, 1979). A similar pattern of a tall narrow R wave in V_1 may occur with Q waves in the left chest leads in patients with muscular dystrophy. This is thought to be due to posterobasal left ventricular fibrosis (Fig. 11.62).

The S wave amplitude in lead V_6 provides the fourth criterion. If the depth of the S wave in lead V_6 exceeds the 98th percentile for age (see Table 11.10), right ventricular hypertrophy is suspected. This is more sensitive and less specific. That is, a deep S wave in lead V_6 may be associated with conditions other than right ventricular hypertrophy. One of these is left ventricular hypertrophy localised to the superior septum. This part of the left

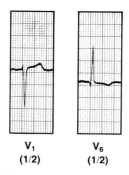

Fig. 11.61 Left ventricular strain with T wave inversion in lead V_6 causing upright T waves in lead V_1.

The third criterion is the R wave amplitude in lead V_1. If the amplitude of the R wave in lead V_1 exceeds the 98th percentile for age (Table 11.7) right ventricular hypertrophy is suspected. This sign is more specific but less sensitive, i.e. there may be children with right ventricular hypertrophy with a normal R wave in lead V_1 (Chou, 1979). The magnitude of the R wave in lead V_1 is directly proportional to the right ventricular systolic pressure. Two correlative formulas have been devised from children with pulmonary stenosis. Right ventricular systolic pressure equals 3 times the R wave in V_1 plus 47, or right ventricu-

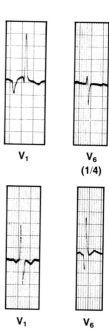

Fig. 11.62 Tall R wave in lead V_1. In the top tracings, the patient has right ventricular hypertrophy due to pulmonary atresia. In the bottom tracings, the tall R wave in lead V_1 is caused by the deep Q wave in lead V_6 in a patient with muscular dystrophy. The duration of the R wave in lead V_1 in the top tracing is 0.07 s in the patient with right ventricular hypertrophy, and in the bottom tracing is 0.04 s in the patient with muscular dystrophy.

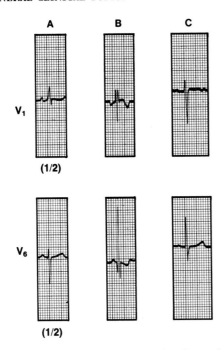

Fig. 11.63 Deep S wave in lead V_6. (A) The deep S wave is caused by right ventricular hypertrophy in a 2-year-old. (B) The deep S wave is caused by hypertrophy of the anterior part of the left ventricle in a 1-year-old patient with coarctation of the aorta. (C) The deep S wave is caused by left anterior hemiblock in an 8-year-old patient.

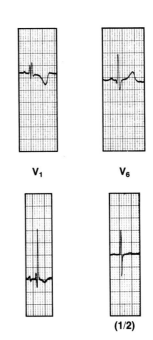

Fig. 11.64 The RSR′. Top tracings – normal duration QRS complex with RSR′ pattern in V_1 in a 6-year-old child. The R′ is not tall. No specific diagnosis can be applied. Bottom tracings – normal duration QRS complex with an RSR′ pattern in lead V_1. The R′ wave is tall. This is a 6-month-old child with right ventricular hypertrophy.

ventricle is the last to be activated. Since it is usually in the anterior part of the left ventricle, this may cause a delayed vector directed anteriorly causing an S wave in lead V_6 or even a normal duration RSR′ in lead V_1. This has been termed the 'incomplete right bundle branch block of aortic coarctation or stenosis' (Liebman & Plonsey, 1978). One other cause of a deep S wave in lead V_6 is left anterior hemiblock caused by delayed activation of the anterior left ventricle (Fig. 11.63) (see p. 284).

The fifth criterion relates to the RS ratio in lead V_1. This ratio suffers the inaccuracies of each of the single measurements. Nonetheless, an abnormally large RS ratio does correlate with right ventricular hypertrophy (see Table 11.11).

The sixth criterion is the RSR′ in V_1. In over 90% of children with a 'secundum' atrial septal defect, there is a normal duration RSR′ pattern in lead V_1. This correlates well with the mild right ventricular hypertrophy found in these children (Burch & DePasquale, 1967). Thus, the RSR′ pattern is quite sensitive for mild right ventricular hypertrophy but also quite non-specific since it may be found in normal children and those with incomplete right bundle branch block (see p. 259, p. 282). In right ventricular hypertrophy, the S wave tends to be smaller and the R′ wave larger than in normal children. With a normal duration QRS complex, right ventricular hypertrophy is usually the cause of an R′ wave greater than 15 mm in an infant under 1 year of age, or an R′ greater than 10 mm over 1 year of age (Fig. 11.64). The diagnosis

could be normal if the R′ is small with a normal duration RSR′ complex. Alternatively, there could be incomplete right bundle branch block pattern or right ventricular hypertrophy. We prefer the description 'RSR′ pattern in right chest leads' rather than attempting to make a specific diagnosis.

The final criterion is that of right axis deviation. Over the age of 3 months, right axis deviation correlates with right ventricular hypertrophy (Okuni, 1975). In adults, one of the common causes of right axis deviation is left posterior hemiblock (see p. 285). Left posterior hemiblock is very rare in children and so right ventricular hypertrophy is by far the leading cause of right axis deviation in children. Nonetheless, right axis deviation should be considered as supporting evidence. The electrocardiogram should then meet one of the other criteria for right ventricular hypertrophy. The diagnosis of right axis deviation may be stronger, supporting evidence for right ventricular hypertrophy in the patient with an RSR′ pattern in lead V_1 (Gerard et al, 1969).

Left ventricular hypertrophy

Recent echocardiographic and autopsy studies have shown that the electrocardiographic diagnosis of left ventricular hypertrophy is accurate only about half of the time. The greater the number of the following criteria met by an electrocardiogram, the more certain is the diagnosis of left ventricular hypertrophy (Cooksey et al, 1977).

Table 11.17 Summary of normal values

Age-group	Heart rate (BPM) *	Frontal plane QRS vector (degrees)	PR interval (sec)	Q III (mm)† **	Q V6 (mm) **	RV1 (mm)	SV1 (mm)	R/S V1	RV6 (mm)	SV6 (mm)	R/S V6	SV1 + RV6 (mm) **	R + S V4 (mm) **
Less than 1 day	93–154 (123)	+59 to −163 (137)	0.08–0.16 (0.11)	4.5	2	5–26 (14)	0–23 (8)	0.1–U (2.2)	0–11 (4)	0–9.5 (3)	0.1–U (2.0)	28	52.5
1–2 days	91–159 (123)	+64 to −161 (134)	0.08–0.14 (0.11)	6.5	2.5	5–27 (14)	0–21 (9)	0.1–U (2.0)	0–12 (4.5)	0–9.5 (3)	0.1–U (2.5)	29	52
3–6 days	91–166 (129)	+77 to −163 (132)	0.07–0.14 (0.10)	5.5	3	3–24 (13)	0–17 (7)	0.2–U (2.7)	0.5–12 (5)	0–10 (3.5)	0.1–U (2.2)	24.5	49
1–3 weeks	107–182 (148)	+65 to +161 (110)	0.07–0.14 (0.10)	6	3	3–21 (11)	0–11 (4)	1.0–U (2.9)	2.5–16.5 (7.5)	0–10 (3.5)	0.1–U (3.3)	21	49
1–2 months	121–179 (149)	+31 to +113 (74)	0.07–0.13 (0.10)	7.5	3	3–18 (10)	0–12 (5)	0.3–U (2.3)	5–21.5 (11.5)	0–6.5 (3)	0.2–U (6.2)	29	53.5
3–5 months	106–186 (141)	+7 to +104 (60)	0.07–0.15 (0.11)	6.5	3	3–20 (10)	0–17 (6)	0.1–U (2.3)	6.5–22.5 (13)	0–10 (3)	0.2–U (6.2)	35	61.5
6–11 months	109–169 (134)	+6 to +99 (56)	0.07–0.16 (0.11)	8.5	3	1.5–20 (9.5)	0.5–18 (4)	0.1–3.9 (1.6)	6–22.5 (12.5)	0–7 (2)	0.2–U (7.6)	32	53
1–2 years	89–151 (119)	+7 to +101 (55)	0.08–0.15 (0.11)	6	3	2.5–17 (9)	0.5–21 (8)	0.05–4.3 (1.4)	6–22.5 (13)	0–6.5 (2)	0.3–U (9.3)	39	49.5
3–4 years	73–137 (108)	+6 to +104 (55)	0.09–0.16 (0.12)	5	3.5	1–18 (8)	0.2–21 (10)	0.03–2.8 (0.9)	8–24.5 (15)	0–5 (1.5)	0.6–U (10.8)	42	53.5
5–7 years	65–133 (100)	+11 to +143 (65)	0.09–0.16 (0.12)	4	4.5	0.5–14 (7)	0.3–24 (12)	0.02–2.0 (0.7)	8.5–26.5 (16)	0–4 (1)	0.9–U (11.5)	47	54
8–11 years	62–130 (91)	+9 to +114 (61)	0.09–0.17 (0.13)	3	3	0–12 (5.5)	0.3–25 (12)	0–1.8 (0.5)	9–25.5 (16)	0–4 (1)	1.5–U (14.3)	45.5	53
12–15 years	60–119 (85)	+11 to +130 (59)	0.09–0.18 (0.14)	3	3	0–10 (4)	0.3–21 (11)	0–1.7 (0.5)	6.5–23 (14)	0–4 (1)	1.4–U (14.7)	41	50

* – 2%–98% (mean); ** – 98th percentile; † – mm at normal standardisation; U – undefined (S wave may equal zero).

We are concerned first with T wave changes. The T waves are normally upright in leads V_5 and V_6 after 48 hours of age. The most reliable sign of left ventricular hypertrophy is asymmetric T wave inversion with an upward convexity in the terminal portion of the T wave in leads V_5 or V_6. This is the so-called 'left ventricular strain' pattern (Figs. 11.28, 11.61, 11.65) which may coexist with ST depression in the same leads. These changes become more prominent in children with an increasing left ventricular to aortic gradient in aortic stenosis. In all children with a gradient less than 50 mmHg, the T waves in lead V_6 were upright, whereas half of those with gradients of 80 mmHg or more had inverted T waves in lead V_6. The T waves in lead aVF also became inverted with increasing gradient in aortic stenosis, but the findings in leads V_5 and V_6 were more reliable (Wagner et al, 1977). The ST-T wave changes of 'left ventricular strain' are the opposite of what would be expected in hypertrophy. In mild hypertrophy, the R wave in lead V_6 is increased in amplitude and the positive T waves are also increased in amplitude. In severe left ventricular hypertrophy, there is a variable amount of conduction delay and endocardial repolarisation begins before epicardial depolarisation has ended. This causes T wave inversion and ST depression (Fig. 11.65). Left ventricular strain is therefore a primary change unrelated to the height of the R wave. T wave inversion in the inferior and lateral leads is found in conditions other than severe left ventricular hypertrophy (see p. 290). But if no other cause is found for the T wave inversion (even in the absence of other criteria) the diagnosis of severe left ventricular hypertrophy should be suspected on the basis of the T waves.

The R wave amplitude in lead V_6 or S wave amplitude in lead V_1 provide the second criterion. An R wave in lead V_6 or an S wave in lead V_1 which is greater than the 98th percentile for age (Tables 11.8, 11.9) should be designated as 'left ventricular hypertrophy by voltage criteria' (Fig. 11.65A). Morganroth et al (1975) reported 11 teenagers with either an abnormally deep S wave in lead V_1 or an abnormally tall R wave in lead V_6. All had a normal echocardiogram and no other evidence of cardiac disease. All also had normal T waves. An individual adolescent, therefore, may have prominent voltage without an increased left ventricular mass. In the absence of T wave changes, the diagnosis of left ventricular hypertrophy based entirely on voltage criteria must be viewed critically.

The third criterion is the amplitude of the R wave in lead V_6 plus the amplitude of the S wave in lead V_1. This measurement suffers from the same problem as the individual measurements, but it does correlate with left ventricular hypertrophy. This should also be considered as 'left ventricular hypertrophy by voltage criteria' if greater than the 98th percentile for age (Table 11.13). The RS ratio in the precordial leads is less helpful in left ventricular hypertrophy than right ventricular hypertrophy.

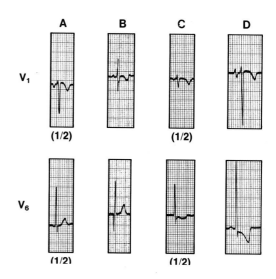

Fig. 11.65 Left ventricular hypertrophy. (A) Voltage criteria with deep S wave in V_1 and tall R wave in V_6. (B) Deep Q waves in lead V_6. (C) Absent Q wave in lead V_6. (D) T wave inversion in lead V_6 with ST depression ('left ventricular strain').

The final criterion relates to Q wave abnormalities. The 0.01 s vector consists of the net result of almost simultaneous activation of the anterior left ventricle, posterior left ventricle, and left side of the septum. If any of these areas is hypertrophied, the normal balance of forces may be upset and the initial portion of the QRS may change. The Q waves may vary independently from the R and S waves.

In left ventricular hypertrophy due either to a dilated left ventricle (aortic insufficiency or ventricular septal defect), septal hypertrophy (hypertrophic cardiomyopathy) or mild aortic stenosis, the initial forces may be increased in the right anterior-superior direction causing abnormally deep Q waves in the inferior and lateral leads (leads II, III, aVF, V_5, V_6) (Cabrera & Monroy, 1952) (Fig. 11.65B) (see p. 259). The other causes for abnormally deep Q waves are discussed on page 296. In advanced concentric left ventricular hypertrophy with increased thickness of the posterior wall and septum, the QRS vector shifts to the left and posteriorly causing the initial forces to be directed more to the left. This may cause the absence of a Q wave in lead V_6 (Fig. 11.65C). In children with aortic stenosis, an absent Q wave in lead V_6 was more than twice as common in those with a severe gradient than in those with a gradient less than 50 mmHg (Wagner, 1977). Nonetheless, more than half of those with a gradient of at least 80 mmHg had a 1 or 2 mm Q wave in lead V_6. The terms 'volume overload' and 'pressure overload' type of left ventricular hypertrophy have been associated with deep Q waves and absent Q waves respectively (Cabrera & Monroy, 1952). Since there is so much overlap, we would prefer not to use this terminology. Nonetheless, the absence of a Q wave or the presence of an abnormally deep

Q wave may be supportive evidence of left ventricular hypertrophy.

Biventricular hypertrophy

The first criterion is abnormal voltages in both the right and left chest leads. In the presence of isolated hypertrophy of one ventricle, the forces reflecting the other normal ventricle usually appear diminished on the electrocardiogram. For example, in isolated right ventricular hypertrophy with a tall R wave in lead V_1 and a deep S wave in lead V_6, the forces reflecting the left ventricle (S-wave in lead V_1, or R wave in lead V_6) are usually diminished because of the dominance of the other ventricle. Biventricular hypertrophy, therefore, can be diagnosed if (in the presence of voltage criteria for hypertrophy of one ventricle) the other ventricle generates at least normal forces. On this basis, it can be diagnosed in the presence of right ventricular hypertrophy (abnormally tall R wave in lead V_1 or deep S wave in V_6) together with either an S wave in lead V_1 or an R wave in lead V_6 exceeding the *mean* for age; or when signs of left ventricular hypertrophy (abnormally tall R wave in lead V_6 or deep S wave in lead V_1) coexist with either an S wave in lead V_6 or an R wave in lead V_1 exceeding the *mean* for age (Figs. 11.66A, 11.66B). Biventricular hypertrophy should not be diagnosed based upon Q wave or T wave morphology.

A second criterion is abnormal voltages in the midprecordial leads. Prominent midprecordial voltage is a sign of biventricular hypertrophy. Katz & Wachtel (1937) originally described large biphasic QRS complexes in the limb leads of patients with congenital heart disease. The 'Katz-Wachtel' criterion has become broadened to refer to increased midprecordial voltage in patients with biventricular hypertrophy (Fig. 11.66C). In lead V_4, the voltage from the top of the R wave to the bottom of the S wave varies with age (Table 11.14). Biventricular hypertrophy can be diagnosed if the total R plus S wave exceeds the 98th percentile. The 'Katz-Wachtel' criterion of increased midprecordial voltage may be inaccurate because of proximity effects enlarging the midprecordial QRS voltage or cancellation effects reducing the voltage.

Right atrial enlargement

Right atrial depolarisation is responsible for the early part of the P wave. When right atrial enlargement occurs this is manifest in the first 0.04–0.06 s of the P wave. The major sign is an increased amplitude of the P wave. The right atrium enlarges anteriorly and inferiorly causing an enlarged P wave of normal duration. The increased early vector causes the P wave to appear peaked. If the P wave in any lead is greater than 2.5 mm in amplitude at any age, right atrial enlargement is diagnosed (Fig. 11.67A) (Reynolds, 1971; Liebman & Plonsey, 1978). The

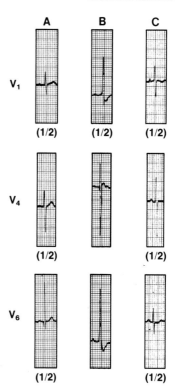

Fig. 11.66 Biventricular hypertrophy. (A) The R wave in lead V_6 is 42 mm high. This meets the criterion for left ventricular hypertrophy. The R wave in lead V_1 is 15 mm high. This exceeds the mean voltage for the R wave in lead V_1 for this 1½-year-old child, and therefore the diagnosis of biventricular hypertrophy is made. (B) The R wave in lead V_1 is 40 mm high. This meets the voltage criteria for right ventricular hypertrophy. The R wave in lead V_6 is 12 mm high. This exceeds the mean for the R wave in lead V_6 at 1 week of age and so the diagnosis of biventricular hypertrophy is made. (C) The voltage in V_1 and V_6 are not distinctly abnormal for a 1-week-old baby, however the voltage in lead V_4 constitutes abnormally prominent midprecordial voltage, and the diagnosis of biventricular hypertrophy is made on this basis. This is the 'Katz–Wachtel' criterion.

atrium may occasionally enlarge and wrap around the caval veins posteriorly as well as anteriorly. In this case, there is an early negative deflection in the first 0.04–0.06 s which is usually pointed (Fig. 11.67B). This negative deflection is not by itself a criterion for right atrial enlargement. It needs to be distinguished from the more rounded late

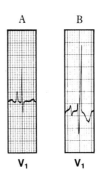

Fig. 11.67 Right atrial enlargement. Left – tall peaked P wave. Right – early (first 0.04 s) pointed, negative deflection in lead V_1.

terminal negative deflection which is a criterion of left atrial enlargement. If the mean vector of the P wave is such that atrial depolarisation is though to originate from an area other than the sinus node, the electrocardiogram should not be interpreted for atrial enlargement. The electrocardiographic criteria of right atrial enlargement are related both to high pressure and to high volume in the right atrium of children (Reeves et al, 1981). The presence of these changes immediately after an episode of supraventricular tachycardia or pulmonary embolism (and their absence after several hours have elapsed) implies that haemodynamics rather than hypertrophy are responsible for the changes.

Left atrial enlargement

Left atrial depolarisation is responsible for the terminal portion of the T wave. When left atrial enlargement occurs this is manifest in the latter part of the P wave. The signs are first an increase in the terminal posterior forces. The most reliable indicator of left atrial enlargement is a late negative deflection in lead V_1. This deflection begins later than 0.04 s after the onset of the P wave. If the terminal deflection in lead V_1 in children and adults is greater than 1 mm in depth and greater than 0.04 s in duration, left atrial enlargement is present (Fig. 11.68A) (Morris et al, 1964). As the left atrial enlargement gets more severe, the depth and duration of the terminal segment increase such that, in the most severe left atrial enlargement in children, the mean depth of the P terminal segment in lead V_1 was 2.8 mm and the duration 0.08 s (Sanyal et al, 1973). Increased terminal posterior forces are related more to left atrial volume than pressure. Similar to the changes in right atrial enlargement, the P waves may become abnormal with an abrupt increase in left atrial volume such as acute mitral insufficiency. They may then return to normal shortly after the stress is removed. This again implies that hypertrophy is not necessary for these changes. The increase in P terminal forces is generally a specific sign of left atrial enlargement but there may be false-negatives (Biancaniello

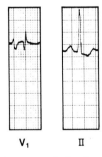

Fig. 11.68 Left atrial enlargement. Left – increased terminal negative deflection. The terminal portion of the P wave is 2.5 mm deep and 0.06 s wide. Right – increased P wave duration.

et al, 1980). As with right atrial enlargement, if the pacemaker does not originate in the sinus node, left atrial enlargement should not be diagnosed on the electrocardiogram.

The second criterion is an increased P wave duration. This is a more non-specific sign either of left atrial enlargement or of the interatrial conduction delay which may be found when the atrial myocardium is damaged by myocarditis, fibrosis or ischaemia (Sodi-Polares & Calder, 1956). An abnormal P wave duration is defined as being longer than 0.09 s in children younger than age 3 and longer than 0.10 s in children 3 years of age or older (Fig. 11.68B). This sign, similar to the increased terminal negative deflection, indicates abnormality when present. It is not sensitive enough to diagnose most cases of left atrial enlargement detected echocardiographically in children (Biancaniello et al, 1980).

Biatrial enlargement

Since the right and left atria depolarise sequentially causing different parts of the P wave, and since the signs of enlargement of one atrium do not distort the changes of enlargement in the other atrium, biatrial enlargement is diagnosed when the signs of right atrial enlargement coexist with the signs of left atrial enlargement. There is therefore both abnormal voltage and duration. If the first 0.04 s of the P wave are greater than 2.5 mm tall and the P wave is either prolonged for age or has a late terminal deflection in lead V_1 which is greater than 1 mm deep and 0.04 s in duration, the diagnosis is biatrial enlargement (Fig. 11.69).

INTERVENTRICULAR CONDUCTION DISTURBANCE

Conduction through the ventricles can be disturbed either by delay or by pre-excitation resulting in an abnormal sequence of ventricular activation.

Conduction delay

Right bundle branch block

Right bundle branch block results from delay in right ventricular activation. The right ventricle is activated sequentially after the left ventricle rather than simultaneously. The delay can occur in the distal conduction axis in fibres destined for the right bundle branch, or it may occur in the main portion of the right bundle branch (both are considered 'central' lesions). Alternatively, the delay may be localised to the peripheral ramifications of the right bundle branch (a 'distal' lesion). Regardless of the site of origin, the pattern is the same on the surface electrocardiogram. There is a delayed and slurred activation oriented

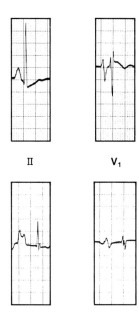

Fig. 11.69 Biatrial enlargement. Top tracings show P waves with increased positive amplitude in lead V_1 as well as a large terminal negative deflection in lead V_1. The P waves also have prolonged duration in addition to increased positive amplitude in lead II. Bottom tracings show P waves which are larger than the QRS complexes. The P wave is the first complex in each lead. The P wave in lead II begins with the sharp positive upstroke and is 6 mm tall. The P wave is 0.16 s in duration. In lead V_1, there is also a large terminal negative deflection.

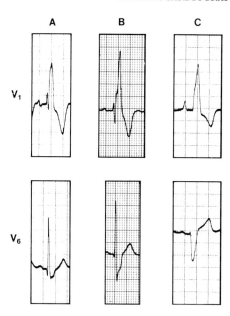

Fig. 11.70 Variations of complete right bundle branch block. (A) A large R wave and small S wave. (B) A small R wave and deeper S wave. (C) An R wave without an S wave. The latter part of all three complexes has a slurred component which is the R′ wave. All three tracings have broad terminal S waves in lead V_6.

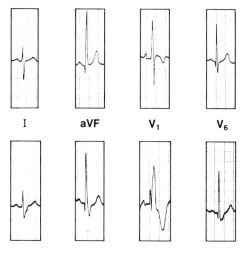

Fig. 11.71 Preoperative–postoperative comparison. In the top tracings, the preoperative electrocardiogram of a patient with tetralogy of Fallot is shown. There is right ventricular hypertrophy. In the bottom tracings, from the same patient, taken postoperatively, there is complete right bundle branch block. The first 0.04 s are the same comparing the preoperative with the postoperative tracing in each lead.

anteriorly and rightward (Gumbiner, 1981; Gelband et al, 1971).

Complete right bundle branch block. The pattern of the QRS is most important for the diagnosis of complete right bundle branch block. There is an initial rapid deflection, followed by a slurred, slower terminal deflection. In lead V_1, the rapid component consists of an R wave and an S wave of varying magnitudes followed by a slurred tall R wave. There may be no S wave, resulting in an RR′ complex (Fig. 11.70). In leads I and V_6, the late slurred terminal deflection causes a broad S wave. The rapid part of the complex results from normal left ventricular activation and is not changed by right ventricular surgery (Fig. 11.71).

The criteria for complete right bundle branch block are first a QRS duration prolonged for age (greater than 0.09 s up to the age of 4 years, and over 0.10 sec for 4–16 years), secondly the presence of normal initial forces (first 0.04 s), and finally terminal conduction delay directed anteriorly and to the right. The mean vector (or 'axis') in complete right bundle branch block considers the frontal plane QRS axis calculated based upon the 'fast' initial portion of the complex. Generally this is the first 0.04 ms; but, the initial rapid portion before the 'break' to the terminal slow portion should be used, regardless of the specific timing (Fig. 11.72). If the frontal plane axis of the initial 'unblocked' portion is between −30° and −90°, this is

considered to be left axis deviation in addition to complete right bundle branch block. This distinction is important in the diagnosis of bifascicular block and will be further discussed on page 286.

Attempts have been made to use the mean vector, as well as the absolute height and proportions of the R, S and R′ components to diagnose hypertrophy in the presence of complete right bundle branch block. The correlation of

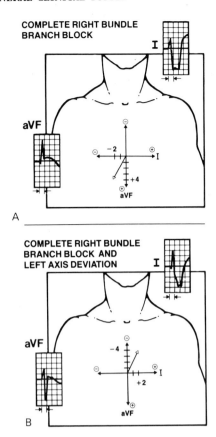

Fig. 11.72 Mean vector in right bundle branch block. The amplitude method has been applied to the first 0.04 s (see Fig. 11.25). (A) The frontal plane mean vector of the first 0.04 s is +120°. Depending upon the age, this is designated either 'complete right bundle branch block' or 'complete right bundle branch block with right axis deviation'. (B) The mean frontal plane QRS vector of the first 0.04 s is −60°. This is designated 'complete right bundle branch block with left axis deviation'.

these parameters with the ventricular pressure or free wall thickness is insufficient to permit the diagnosis of either right ventricular or left ventricular hypertrophy in the presence of complete right bundle branch block (Brohet et al, 1978; Wasserburger, et al 1962).

The T wave changes in complete right bundle branch block are secondary to the abnormal sequence of depolarisation. The T waves are opposite in direction to the QRS complexes. In right bundle branch block, ventricular repolarisation proceeds in the same direction as depolarisation. Opposite electrical processes occurring in the same direction result in discordant QRS and T waves. The major uncancelled voltage of the QRS consists of the terminal R' which is directed anteriorly and to the right. The T waves in complete right bundle branch block are therefore directed posteriorly and to the left. Since normal left ventricular repolarisation is occurring at the same time as depolarisation and repolarisation of the right ventricle, there is an ST segment shift caused by the T wave of the left ventricle. Therefore, in complete right bundle branch block in lead V_1, there is a positive R' with a negative T

wave and depressed ST segment. In lead V_6, there is a deep S wave with an elevated ST segment and a positive T wave.

The most common cause of complete right bundle branch block is surgery involving closure of a ventricular septal defect or right ventriculotomy (Gelband et al, 1971). In approximately half of the patients with right bundle branch block operated upon for repair of tetralogy of Fallot, the complete right bundle branch block is 'central' due to injury occurring during closure of the ventricular septal defect. In the other half it is 'peripheral', occurring during ventriculotomy (Garson et al, 1982). Congenital complete right bundle branch block is rare in children, but may occur with autosomal dominant inheritance. Isolated congenitally complete right bundle branch block does not appear to progress to further conduction disturbances (Husson et al, 1973; Esscher et al, 1975). Complete right bundle branch block may also be a manifestation of inflammation from myocarditis or endocarditis and may progress to complete block (Gumbiner, 1981). Functional right bundle branch block or left bundle branch block may occur in normal children, due to ventricular aberration of a supraventricular rhythm. Rate-dependent bundle branch block is extremely rare in children, however, and occurred in only 2% of children reported with supraventricular tachycardia (Garson, 1981).

'Incomplete right bundle branch block' pattern. The RSR' pattern in lead V_1, in which the duration of the R' is approximately equal to the duration of the RS wave (i.e. no terminal conduction delay) had been referred to as the 'incomplete right bundle branch block' pattern (Fig. 11.73). The duration of the QRS may be normal or slightly prolonged for age (up to 0.09 s under the age of 4 years or 0.10 s for 4–16 years). Approximately 7% of normal children over the age of 6 months have this pattern (Burch & DePasquale, 1967). The only major pathologic cause of an imcomplete right bundle branch block pattern in childhood is right ventricular diastolic volume overload. This is found in almost all children with a secundum atrial septal

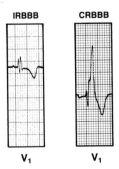

Fig. 11.73 Distinction of 'incomplete' from 'complete' right bundle branch block. Left – normal duration RSR' complex. There is no 'break'. The duration of the R wa e and R' wave are almost the same. This is the 'incomplete right bundle branch block pattern'. Right – In the 'complete right bundle branch block pattern', there is a definite break and the R' is three times the duration of the R wave.

defect. In children with atrial septal defect, it has been demonstrated that the central right bundle conduction time is normal, therefore implying that the pattern is due to more peripheral factors (Sung et al, 1975). This pattern of terminal activation directed anteriorly and rightward is currently explained either by selective hypertrophy of the right ventricular outflow tract or by stretching of the peripheral specialised conduction fibres due to distention of the right ventricular outflow tract (Boineau et al, 1964). Numerous attempts have been made first to distinguish normal children from those with atrial septal defect and secondly to predict the size of the shunt or right ventricular pressure among those with atrial septal defect. These attempts have been unsuccessful with a few exceptions. In atrial septal defects, the R′ tends to be slightly wider than normal. In those with a small shunt through an atrial septal defect there is a deep S wave compared to those with larger shunts or high pulmonary pressure where both the R and R′ waves become taller and the S wave disappears. Atrial septal defect was more common in those less than 1 year of age if the R′ was greater than 15 mm and in those older than 1 year if the R′ was greater than 10 mm (Wasserburger, 1963; Tapia & Proudfit, 1960). Despite these generalities, it may be impossible to distinguish normal from atrial septal defect by the electrocardiogram in an individual patient (Perloff, 1970).

Left bundle branch block

Complete left bundle branch block. Complete left bundle branch block results from delay in left ventricular activation. Since fibres of the left bundle branch initiate normal ventricular depolarisation, the entire QRS is aberrant if there is delay in left bundle branch conduction. This is different from the situation in right bundle branch block where only the terminal portion is aberrant. In left bundle branch block, the right ventricle is activated first, therefore, the normal initial vector, due to left-to-right septal spread, is absent. The slow activation of the left ventricle occurs from the right ventricle and the resultant slurred QRS is directed to the left, posteriorly and superiorly. The criteria for complete left bundle branch block are an abnormally wide QRS complex (greater than 0.09 s less than 4 years of age, or greater than 0.10 s from 4–16 years); a absence of normal initial forces (absent Q wave in leads I, aVL and V₆); and the presence of notched, slurred QRS complexes directed leftward and posterior (in lead V₁ a QS or small R–deep S, and in lead V₆ a tall, notched R wave – Fig. 11.74).

The frontal plane QRS mean vector in complete left bundle branch block is calculated based upon the major deflection of the QRS (Fig. 11.75). If the initial and terminal part have different vectors, the terminal part of the QRS should be used. Adults with left bundle branch

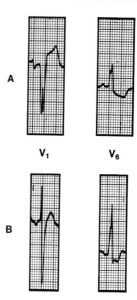

Fig. 11.74 Variations of complete left bundle branch block. (A) In the top tracings, there is a QS pattern in lead V₁ and in the bottom tracings (B) there is an RS pattern in lead V₁. In lead V₆, both tracings are similar and marked by the absence of a Q wave.

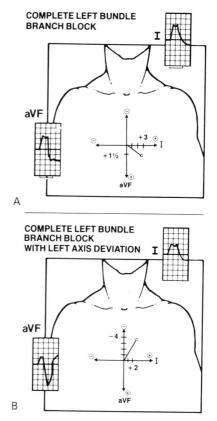

Fig. 11.75 Calculation of mean vector and left bundle branch block. The entire QRS complex is used for the calculation. The amplitude method (Fig. 11.25) was used. (A) Frontal plane mean QRS vector + 30°. This is designated 'complete left bundle branch block'. (B) Frontal plane QRS mean vector −60°. This is designated 'complete left bundle branch block with left axis deviation'.

block and left axis deviation are more likely to develop complete block than those without left axis deviation (Scher, 1976). These data are not available for children.

Left bundle branch block is rare in children. The most common cause is surgery on the aortic valve or subvalve area. It may occur as a result of myocarditis, endocarditis, hypertrophic cardiomyopathy or myocardial infarction (Gumbiner, 1981).

'Incomplete left bundle branch block' pattern. Left ventricular hypertrophy may cause delayed left ventricular activation or stretching of the fibres of the conduction tissues and produce a pattern of 'incomplete left bundle branch block'. The QRS duration may be normal or prolonged by 0.01 s for age. There are absent Q waves and tall slurred R waves in leads I and V_6 (Fig. 11.76). On the surface electrocardiogram, it is not possible to distinguish patients with incomplete left bundle branch block on the basis of left ventricular hypertrophy from those with mild conduction system disease.

Fascicular block

Although the anatomic correlation is not exact, there are patterns on the surface electrocardiogram which correspond to lesions in the anterior and posterior ramifications of the left bundle branch. These patterns are called 'left anterior hemiblock' and 'left posterior hemiblock' respectively.

Left anterior hemiblock. The pattern of left anterior hemiblock results from asynchronous left ventricular activation where the posterior-inferior wall is activated before the anterior-superior wall, and there are two sequential vectors. The 'earlier' activation of the posterior-inferior diaphragmatic surface of the left ventricle is directed inferiorly and slightly to the right at +120° in the frontal plane. The 'later' activation occurs in the opposite direction when the anterior-superior wall is activated at −60° in the frontal plane (Fig. 11.77A). The QRS duration is prolonged by less than 0.02 s in pure left anterior hemiblock because part of the left ventricle is activated normally and spread to the rest of the left ventricle occurs relatively rapidly

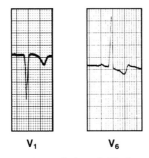

V_1 V_6

Fig. 11.76 'Incomplete left bundle branch block pattern'. There is an absent Q wave in lead V_6, a normal QRS duration for this 11-year-old child and no R wave in lead V_1.

through the endocardium. The criteria for left anterior hemiblock are:

1. Presence of initial forces directed inferiorly and slightly to the right at +120°.
2. Major QRS forces directed superiorly and leftward. Left axis deviation resulting from a horizontal heart position may give a QRS axis of −30°; therefore, for the diagnosis of left anterior hemiblock, the frontal plane QRS axis must be to the left of −30°, i.e. negative in lead II; in most children with left anterior hemiblock, the QRS axis is −60°.
3. Normal or minimally prolonged QRS duration (Fig. 11.78A).

The most common cause of the left anterior hemiblock pattern in children is that found in association with congenital heart disease. This may be due either to elongation of the left anterior fibres, or to shortening of the left posterior fibres, or to a different orientation of the conduction system such that the posterior left ventricular wall is activated before other parts of the heart (Rosenbaum et al, 1970). These mechanisms may explain the left axis deviation found in atrioventricular septal defects, double inlet left ventricle and double outlet right ventricle. Observations on tricuspid atresia suggest a different mechanism (Boineau et al, 1973). The activation times of the proximal left anterior and posterior ramifications were found to be normal and it has been postulated that in tricuspid atresia, selective hypertrophy of the basal anterolateral left ventricle is responsible for sufficient conduction delay to cause the pattern of left anterior hemiblock on the surface electrocardiogram (Kulangara et al, 1981). In anomalous left coronary artery, the left axis deviation frequently observed may also be due to selective hypertrophy of non-infarcted superior portions of the left ventricle. This mechanism may also account for the occasional left axis deviation found in aortic stenosis, aortic insufficiency or cardiomyopathy. Isolated injury to the left anterior radiation resulting in left anterior hemiblock from myocarditis has been postulated as the cause of the left axis deviation observed in up to 50% of infants with the rubella syndrome. Left anterior hemiblock may also result from myocardial infarction, ventricular septal myectomy, aortic valve surgery or subvalve aortic resection. In closure of a ventricular septal defect, the left anterior hemiblock is usually accompanied by right bundle branch block (see p. 282). Left anterior hemiblock may rarely be familial and occur in otherwise normal children (Husson et al, 1973).

Left posterior hemiblock. The activation sequence in left posterior hemiblock is exactly the opposite to that found in left anterior hemiblock (Fig. 11.77B). The anterior-superior wall is activated first with a frontal plane QRS axis of −60° and then the posterior-inferior wall is activated last with a frontal plane QRS axis of +120°. The

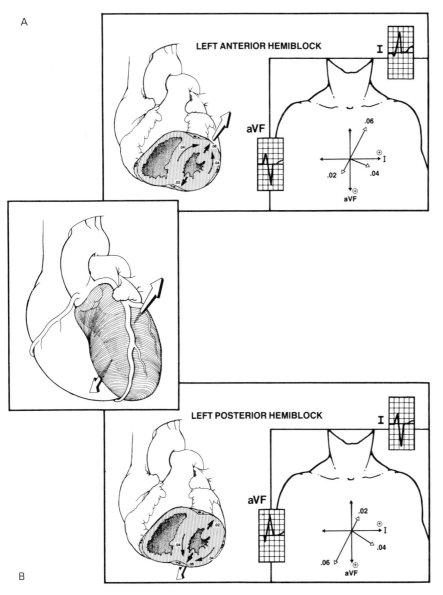

Fig. 11.77 Comparison of activation in left anterior hemiblock and left posterior hemiblock. (A) Left anterior hemiblock. The initial 0.02 s vector is directed at +120° and the terminal 0.06 s vector is directed at −60°. This causes an initial Q wave in lead I and a deep S wave in lead aV$_F$. A coronal section through the heart is shown with the posterior-inferior wall activated before the anterior-superior wall. The mean QRS vector is directed superiorly as shown by the large arrow in the top diagram. (B) Left posterior hemiblock. The initial 0.02 s vector is directed at −60° and the terminal 0.06 s vector is directed at +120°. This causes a Q wave in lead aV$_F$ and a deep S wave in lead I. The anterior-superior well is activated before the posterior-superior wall. The mean QRS vector in the frontal plane is directed at +120° as shown by the large arrow in the bottom diagram. The orientation of the posterior-inferior and antero-superior walls are shown in the middle diagram.

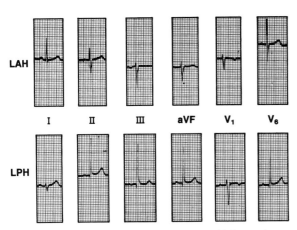

Fig. 11.78 Comparison of the electrocardiograms of left anterior hemiblock and left posterior hemiblock. Top tracings – left anterior hemiblock. Bottom tracings – left posterior hemiblock. Note the absence of right ventricular hypertrophy in this 15-year-old child with left posterior hemiblock.

criteria for left posterior hemiblock are: initial forces directed superiorly (Q waves in leads II, III, aVF); major frontal plane QRS forces directed inferiorly and rightward with an axis of +90° to +180°; normal or minimally prolonged QRS duration (Fig. 11.78B). This constitutes a normal electrocardiogram in most children and so left posterior hemiblock is difficult to diagnose. Left posterior hemiblock can be diagnosed if the frontal plane QRS axis is between +120° and +180° in a child over the age of 1 year who does not have right ventricular hypertrophy or right atrial enlargement (i.e. another reason for right axis deviation). Left posterior hemiblock is quite rare in children and has been diagnosed mainly in cases due to surgical trauma, myocarditis or endocarditis (Schatz et al, 1976).

Bifascicular block

The trifascicular conduction system is considered in terms of the left anterior fascicle, the left posterior fascicle and the right bundle branch. Bifascicular block can result from block in any two of the three fascicles. In the strict sense of the term, complete left bundle branch block is a form of bifascicular block. The combination of right bundle branch and left posterior hemiblock is practically never diagnosed in children because the right bundle branch block is most often due to an operation on a lesion with pre-existent right ventricular hypertrophy and right axis deviation. In children, therefore, the term 'bifascicular block' is almost synonymous with right bundle branch block plus left anterior hemiblock.

Right bundle branch block–left anterior hemiblock pattern. Left anterior hemiblock changes the first 'fast' part of the QRS complex and right bundle branch block changes the terminal 'slow' part. The criteria are: initial forces (first 0.02 s) directed inferiorly and rightward at +120° in the frontal plane giving a Q wave in lead aVL and possibly lead I; presence of the major axis of the 'unblocked' initial part of the QRS to the left of −30° giving a dominant S wave in the initial part of lead II and possibly leads V_5 and V_6; slurred terminal portion of right bundle branch block directed to the right (Fig. 11.79).

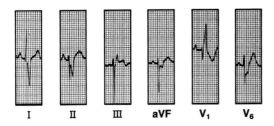

Fig. 11.79 Right bundle branch block with left axis deviation.

The most common cause of right bundle branch block and left anterior hemiblock in children is surgery for tetralogy of Fallot. It occurs in approximately 10% of such patients (Garson et al, 1981a). The pattern may also occur in any injury to the area of the distal conduction axis or proximal right bundle branch since the right bundle branch and left anterior fascicle lie in such close proximity. It may also be seen following other intracardiac operations involving surgery near the atrioventricular junction, or it may be found in myocarditis, cardiomyopathy and endocarditis. Familial bifascicular block occurs and may progress to complete block (Schaal et al, 1973).

Trifascicular block

Trifascicular block is defined as delay in all three fascicles. It can only be diagnosed by intracardiac electrograms as a prolonged H-V interval. It cannot be diagnosed on the surface electrocardiogram. The combination of right bundle branch block, left anterior hemiblock and first degree atrioventricular block has been erroneously termed 'trifascicular block.' This combination has many different possible causes. Most children with this pattern have atrioventricular nodal delay and bifascicular block with a normal H-V interval (Neches et al, 1979; Gillette et al 1977).

Diffuse interventricular conduction delay

The QRS complex is prolonged for age but without a specific pattern of right bundle branch block or left bundle branch block. This may be found in children with quinidine or procainamide toxicity, myocarditis, hypoglycaemia, myocardial ischaemia or hyperkalaemia (Fig. 11.80) (Garson et al, 1980).

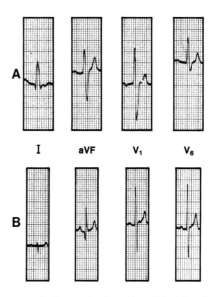

Fig. 11.80 Interventricular conduction delay. (A) Taken from a 1-month-old child with renal failure who was hyperkalaemic. (B) Taken from the same child after dialysis. The QRS complexes are similar in comparing the same leads but they have a prolonged duration in the top tracings.

Pre-excitation

'Pre-excitation' is defined as an abnormally rapid transit of the wave of depolarisation from atria to ventricles. In most cases of pre-excitation the ventricles are activated asymmetrically from a point other than the atrioventricular conduction axis in addition to being activated via the normal conduction system. Since conduction can then occur by two possible pathways, usually with different properties, one of the possible consequences of pre-excitation is reciprocating supraventricular tachycardia.

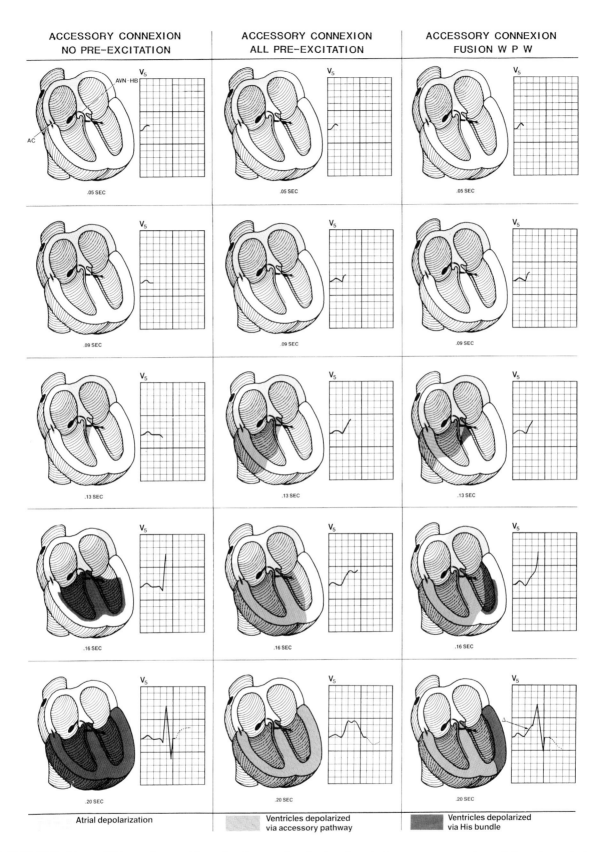

Fig. 11.81 Wolff–Parkinson–White syndrome with varying degrees of conduction through the accessory connexion and the atrioventricular node. The numbers refer to timing after the onset of the P wave. The left column of diagrams indicates the activation sequence in the patient with an accessory connection who is not conducting through the accessory connexion but entirely through the atrioventricular node. Note the normal PR interval, the Q wave and the lack of the delta wave. In the middle column, the activation sequence of a patient who is conducting entirely through the accessory connexion are shown. Note the short PR interval and the wide QRS complex. There is no real 'delta' wave because the entire QRS complex is wide. In the right column, the usual situation of Wolff–Parkinson–White syndrome is shown in which there is a 'fusion' complex resulting from conduction through both the accessory connexion and the atrioventricular node. The parts of the ventricles activated through the atrioventricular node are shaded differently in the diagrams from those activated by the accessory connexion. Note that there is a short PR interval and a delta wave (indicated by the 'delta' at 0.16 s in the column on the right). The delta wave occurs because there is fusion of the completely wide QRS with the completely narrow QRS causing an abrupt change in slope.

Wolff-Parkinson-White syndrome

Wolff, Parkinson and White first described the syndrome of short PR interval with a prolonged QRS duration in 1930. It has since been demonstrated that the cause of this pattern is a direct muscular connexion between the atria and the ventricles – an accessory atrioventricular connexion. The accessory connexion runs perpendicular to the atrioventricular ring and can be located anywhere around either valve orifice, but occurs only rarely across the fibrous continuity between the mitral and aortic valves. Most accessory connexions conduct much faster than the atrioventricular node. The atrial depolarisation is therefore transmitted to the ventricles prematurely resulting in a short PR interval. The ventricles then begin to depolarise from the point of insertion of the connexion. If there were no atrioventricular nodal conduction and the ventricles were completely excited by the accessory connexion, the QRS complex would appear similar to a premature ventricular contraction which originated at the site of insertion of the connexion. In the majority of cases, however, the node *also* conducts the impulse from atria to ventricles and the depolarisation waves resulting from the two pathways collide in the ventricles causing a 'fusion' QRS complex (Fig. 11.81). The characteristics of this complex are that the beginning is more slurred (resulting from eccentric slow ventricular activation by the accessory connexion) and the end of the complex is more normal (resulting from normal ventricular activation via the atrioventricular conduction axis). In any individual child, the amount of the ventricles activated via the different pathways can vary from day to day. This accounts for our observation that one-third of children with Wolff-Parkinson-White had at least one electrocardiogram without any pre-excitation (normal PR interval and normal QRS complex) which was later followed by the reappearance of the Wolff-Parkinson-White syndrome.

The criteria for Wolff-Parkinson-White syndrome are a short PR interval for age (see Table 11.4) and a QRS complex with initial slurring, the 'delta wave'. All electrocardiographic leads may not show the short PR interval and the delta wave if the vector of the delta wave is perpendicular to that lead (see Fig. 11.35). Rosenbaum classified the Wolff-Parkinson-White pattern on surface electrocardiogram into types A and B in an attempt to predict the localisation of the accessory connexion (Rosenbaum et al, 1945). In type A, the major QRS deflection is positive in lead V_1 predicting a left lateral accessory connexion (Fig. 11.82A). This simulates right bundle branch block. The two can be distinguished since the initial forces in Wolff-Parkinson-White syndrome are slow in comparison to the rapid initial forces in right bundle branch block. In type B, the major QRS deflection is negative in V_1, predicting a right-sided accessory connexion (Fig. 11.82B). This simulates left bundle branch block except that the

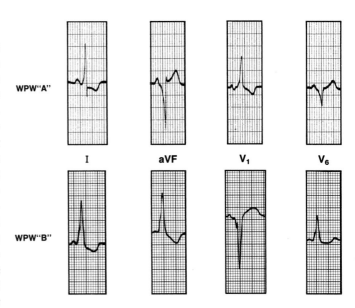

Fig. 11.82 Wolff–Parkinson–White syndrome. (A) Rosenbaum 'type A'. (B) Rosenbaum 'type B'.

Wolff-Parkinson-White syndrome usually has normal terminal forces. Despite the general helpfulness of this classification scheme, we have found that the exact site of the accessory connexion cannot be predicted from the 15 lead surface electrocardiogram. Since Wolff-Parkinson-White syndrome is more common in children than left bundle branch block, the PR interval should be measured carefully in any child with a pattern similar to left bundle branch block.

Lown-Ganong-Levine syndrome

Lown, Ganong and Levine described the syndrome of short PR interval without a delta wave in sinus rhythm in 1952. All their cases had associated supraventricular tachycardia. Although it does not cause interventricular conduction disturbance, we have included Lown-Ganong-Levine syndrome in this section because (by our definition) it results in ventricular pre-excitation. The anatomic substrate for the syndrome is thought to be an atriofascicular connexion between the atrium and the penetrating atrioventricular bundle (an atrio-His fibre – Brechenmacher, 1975). This results in bypass of the atrioventricular node and therefore a short PR interval is observed (Figs. 11.83, 11.84). Since there are two possible pathways from atria to ventricles, supraventricular tachycardia may occur. The criteria for a short PR interval are age-related (see Table 11.3). Lown-Ganong-Levine syndrome should probably not be diagnosed in the absence of supraventricular tachycardia, since a short PR interval may be found in normal children without a predisposition to supraventricular tachycardia (Thapar et al, 1979). It is

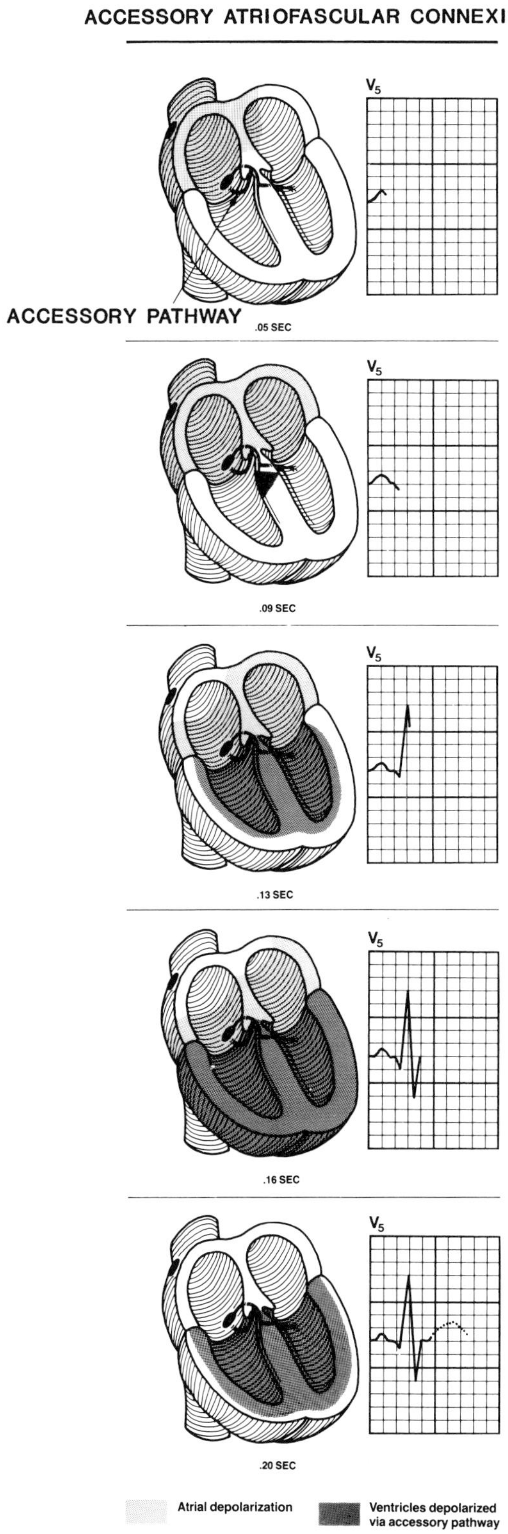

ACCESSORY ATRIOFASCULAR CONNEXION

ACCESSORY PATHWAY

.05 SEC

.09 SEC

.13 SEC

.16 SEC

.20 SEC

Atrial depolarization | Ventricles depolarized via accessory pathway

Fig. 11.83 Lown–Ganong–Levine syndrome. The ventricular activation sequence is shown in a manner similar to Figure 11.81. The PR interval is short but the ventricular activation sequence is entirely normal.

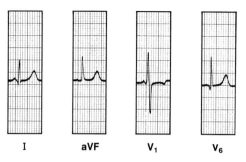

Fig. 11.84 Lown–Ganong–Levine syndrome. The PR interval is short and the QRS complex is normal in all leads.

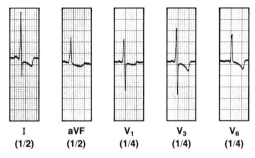

Fig. 11.85 Pompe's disease. Note the short PR interval and the extreme biventricular hypertrophy. There is 118 m of deflection (at normal standardisation) from the top of the R wave to the bottom of the S wave in lead V_3.

not currently possible to distinguish those with an anatomic bypass tract from those with rapid nodal conduction.

Short PR intervals are also observed in mannosidosis, Fabry's disease, and Pompe's disease (Fig. 11.85) (Mehta & Desnick, 1978; Roudebush et al, 1973; Gillette et al, 1974a; Rodriguez-Torres et al, 1971). All these diseases may have in common an increase in cell size in the atrioventricular node. This may be related to rapid nodal conduction (Gillette et al, 1974a). Since conduction is uniformly enhanced throughout the conduction axis and there is no bypass tract, patients with these diseases do not appear to be at risk for supraventricular tachycardia.

Nodo- and fasciculoventricular conduction

Mahaim first described muscular connexions between the conduction axis and the ventricular septum in 1938. The definition of a Mahaim fibre has been broadened to include a fibre which originates in the atrioventricular node, bundle or proximal bundle branches and inserts into the ventricular muscle. This is a 'bundle branch bypass' tract and results in pre-excitation. The bundle usually inserts into the right ventricle, giving a left bundle branch block morphology to the QRS complex (Gallagher et al, 1981). As conduction can also occur via the normal pathway and through the anomalous fibre, there may be a fusion QRS complex similar to that seen in the Wolff-Parkinson-White

MAHAIM FIBER FUSION

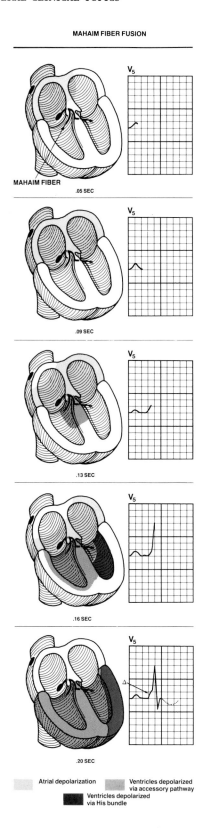

MAHAIM FIBER

.05 SEC

.09 SEC

.13 SEC

.16 SEC

.20 SEC

Atrial depolarization

Ventricles depolarized via accessory pathway

Ventricles depolarized via His bundle

Fig. 11.86 'Mahaim' conduction. Interventricular conduction is shown for a fasciculo-ventricular fibre. The PR interval is normal and there may be a delta wave resulting from fusion of the impulse passing through both the anomalous pathway and the atrioventricular node.

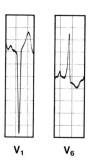

V₁   **V₆**

Fig. 11.87 'Mahaim' conduction. The PR interval is normal and there is a delta wave in lead V₆. The morphology of this complex is similar to left bundle branch block.

syndrome. With a Mahaim fibre, however, the PR interval is normal (Figs. 11.86, 11.87). Since two pathways exist with different properties, reciprocating supraventricular tachycardia can occur.

ISCHAEMIA, INJURY AND INFARCTION

The major changes that occur with ischaemia, injury and early infarction involve the T waves and ST segments.

Primary and secondary T wave changes

Primary T wave changes occur when repolarisation is affected, independent of changes in depolarisation. These may occur with uniform alteration in the shape or duration of all action potentials without a change in the sequence of depolarisation (e.g. hyperkalaemia). Alternatively, they may be found with non-uniform changes in the shape or duration of the action potentials in different parts of the ventricle resulting in an altered sequence of repolarisation (e.g. localised ischaemia). The majority of the primary T wave changes occur with ischaemia or other systemic alterations which have an effect on the heart.

Secondary T wave changes occur when altered repolarisation is caused by an abnormal sequence of depolarisation. These are much more common in children than primary changes. They occur in such conditions as bundle branch block, pre-excitation and hypertrophy. A secondary T wave change is frequently mistaken for a primary change because the minor QRS abnormality responsible for the secondary change is not recognised. Minor changes in the duration and shape of the QRS (especially in the terminal portion) may be responsible for significant secondary T wave changes. Before assigning a T wave change to the primary category, it is important to be sure the changes cannot be explained by an abnormal QRS complex (Cooksey et al, 1977).

Functional T wave changes

The majority of these changes appear to have a link to the sympathetic nervous system. Fear and anxiety are known to cause inverted T waves without a change in coronary blood flow (Awa et al, 1970). Sympathetic mechanisms are thought to be responsible for the T wave changes in hyperventilation. 10% of teenagers inverted the T wave in at least one chest lead after 10–15 s of hyperventilation. 70% inverted their T waves after 45 s (Thomsen & Wasserburger, 1967). The degree of alkalosis or hypocarbia could not be related to the T wave changes. Orthostatic T wave changes have been described in the inferior leads in 3% of normal adults who stand up after lying down for several minutes (Cooksey et al, 1977). It is not known whether the postural change is due to catecholamines or a physical shift of the heart. Approximately 4% of normal adults develop flat or inverted T waves in several leads within 30 min of eating a high carbohydrate meal or drinking a high concentration glucose solution. If a child has flat or inverted T waves without known cause, the electrocardiogram might be repeated in the postabsorptive state (Chou, 1979).

There are two other functional changes which are most common in adolescence. The 'early repolarisation syndrome' is recognized by J point elevation in several leads and may mimic true ST elevation. The T waves in early repolarisation are usually very large. This pattern is due to the early appearance of the T wave while the ventricles are still depolarising (Hoffman, 1975b). This eliminates the ST segment. Sympathetic stimulation either by exercise or proterenol infusion generally normalises the J point elevation (Fig. 11.88). Alternatively, in the asymptomatic patient, one can wait for several days and check another electrocardiogram. In early repolarisation, the J point elevation is persistent, whereas in pericarditis, the other common cause of elevated ST segments in children, the changes evolve.

The second functional T wave change found in adolescence is the isolated inverted T wave in a midprecordial lead with an upright T wave in the leads on either

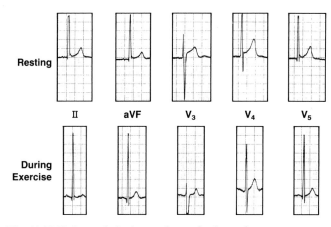

Fig. 11.88 Early repolarisation syndrome. In the resting electrocardiogram shown in the top, there is J point elevation in the inferior and lateral leads. In this patient, leads I and aV$_L$ were normal. There was 1 mm of J point depression aV$_R$. After 6 min of treadmill exercise, the bottom tracings were recorded. Note the normalisation of all the J point elevation. Without the exercise test, this would be difficult to distinguish from the ST elevation of pericarditis.

side. This occurs in 1% of adolescents and has no pathologic correlate (Awa et al, 1971). In general, benign T wave changes are labile (Sleeper & Orgain, 1963).

Ischaemia

Myocardial ischaemia is manifest electrocardiographically by distortion of the T wave amplitude, configuration and mean vector. In ischaemic tissue, the action potential duration is prolonged by a long plateau. Therefore, ischaemic tissue recovers more slowly than the surrounding normal tissue. The ischaemic tissue is negatively charged relative to the surrounding tissue which has already recovered. Thus, the T wave vector points away from the ischaemic tissue toward the positive potentials of the

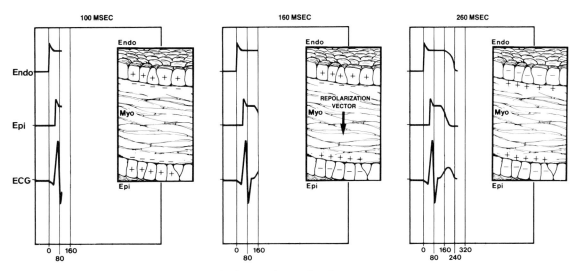

Fig. 11.89 Genesis of the normal T wave. See Figure 11.21 for complete explanation.

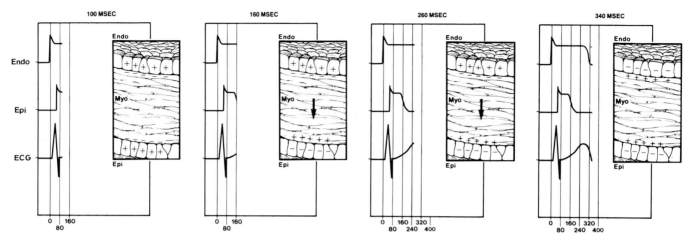

Fig. 11.90 Subendocardial ischaemia. The action potential duration is prolonged such that at 260 ms after the onset of the QRS complex, the endocardium is still depolarised and a vector remains from the endocardium to the epicardium causing a peaked T wave. The prolonged endocardial activation also results in a prolonged QT interval.

normal tissue. The first area to become ischaemic in the heart is generally the subendocardium. In cases of subendocardial ischaemia, the T wave points toward the normal epicardial tissue overlying the ischaemic area. In subendocardial ischaemia, the T waves are symmetrical and peaked with an increase in amplitude and duration in the leads overlying the ischaemic area (Figs. 11.89, 11.90). In subepicardial ischaemia, the T waves are inverted and overlie the ischaemic area. In transmural ischaemia, the sequence of repolarisation is abnormal and follows the depolarisation sequence from endocardium to epicardium. This is the reverse direction from normal and therefore the T waves are inverted overlying an area of transmural ischaemia (Fig. 11.91).

Myocardial ischaemia is rare in children. It can occur in the early stages of reduced coronary blood flow from neonatal stress, an anomalous left coronary artery arising from the pulmonary trunk or in the mucocutaneous lymph node syndrome (Kawasaki's disease) before infarction occurs. Subendocardial ischaemia may occur in children with aortic stenosis or pulmonary stenosis. The flattened or inverted T waves which accompany rapid sinus tachycardia or supraventricular tachycardia may be due to ischaemia. They may also be secondary T wave changes due to minor degrees of ventricular aberration obscured by the rapid rate. The persistence of these T wave changes up to days after the event may be related to potassium loss with slow replenishment of metabolic stores (Hoffman, 1975b). There is T wave inversion in the inferior and lateral leads in 10% of children with mitral valve prolapse. These changes may be explained either by the presence of small ischaemic areas due to traction interfering with the vascular supply or by uneven repolarisation (Chou, 1979). Other changes with mitral prolapse include a prolonged

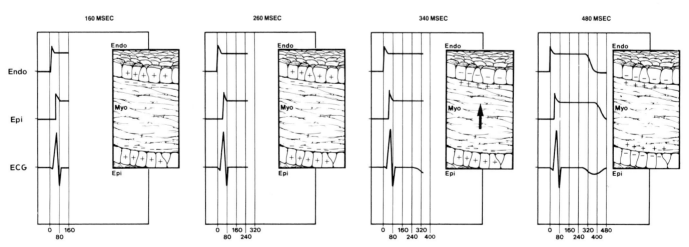

Fig. 11.91 Transmural ischaemia. The epicardial action potentials are prolonged longer than the endocardial action potentials resulting in a vector of repolarisation directed in the opposite direction to normal. This causes T wave inversion in leads overlying transmural ischaemia. There is also QT prolongation.

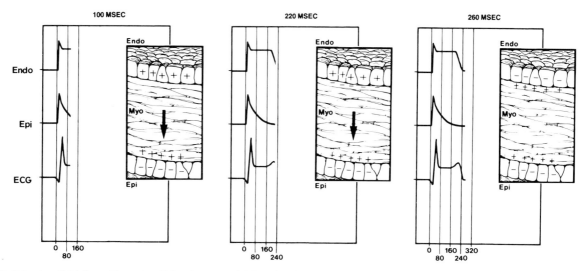

Fig. 11.92 Subepicardial injury. The epicardial action potential duration is shortened with a shortened plateau resulting in early repolarisation of the epicardium. This causes an ST segment shift toward the epicardial area of injury. The QT interval is normal because endocardial repolarisation proceeds on schedule.

QT interval and prominent U waves (Bissett et al, 1980).

The usual electrocardiographic pattern in pure left ventricular hypertrophy, is an increase in the T wave amplitude. There is ST depression with inverted T waves in advanced left ventricular hypertrophy, the 'strain' pattern (Mashima et al, 1969). Thus, 'strain' is different from subendocardial ischaemia where there is ST depression and upright or flat T waves. It has been suggested that 'strain' is a primary T wave abnormality, that it is due to a difference in endocardial and epicardial conduction times and that it has a different mechanism from ischaemia (Grant et al, 1951). Alternatively, the ST-T wave changes observed in hypertrophy and strain may be simply more severe changes in a spectrum from sub-endocardial to transmural ischaemia.

Injury

Myocardial injury is evidenced electrocardiographically both by deviations from the baseline and changes in the contour of the ST segment. In injured cells there is a release of potassium resulting in shortening of phase 2 of the action potential. This affects the ST segment. In subepicardial injury, the injured area is relatively positive compared to the underlying normal myocardium, and an electrode immediately over the area of subepicardial injury shows ST elevation (Fig. 11.92). In subendocardial injury, the positive injured area has overlying normal myocardium which is relatively negative and the electrode immediately over this area shows ST depression (Fig. 11.93). Thus, with injury, the ST segment is displaced toward the injured

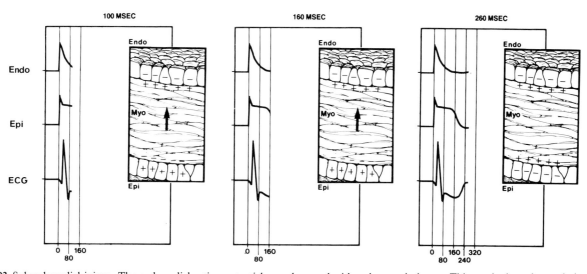

Fig. 11.93 Subendocardial injury. The endocardial action potentials are shortened with a shortened plateau. This results in early repolarisation and an ST segment shift towards the endocardium, or ST depression in leads overlying subendocardial injury.

surface. When the ST segment is elevated, the contour may be either upwardly convex or concave. The contour is usually concave or flat with ST depression. Injury patterns in children which are not due to systemic alterations are found most frequently in pericarditis and ischaemic episodes.

Injury due to ischaemia

It is rare to obtain an electrocardiogram from an infant or child who is undergoing an acute myocardial infarction. This diagnosis should be entertained when considering ST elevation (Fig. 11.94). A more common kind of ST segment shift seen in children is the ST depression found in some infants with patency of the arterial duct (Fig. 11.95). ST depression of 2.5–10 mm was found in leads. V_1 and V_2 in severely ill infants requiring ligation of the arterial duct. The depression disappeared after ligation. The explanation for these changes is a marked myocardial oxygen supply-demand imbalance primarily in the right ventricle. The supply is reduced due to the low aortic diastolic pressure with reduced coronary flow and the myocardial oxygen demand is increased due to the high pulmonary artery systolic pressure (Way et al, 1979).

Injury due to myocarditis

Cellular injury occurs with myocarditis. Approximately 70% of children with myocarditis have electrocardiographic

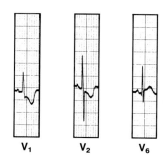

Fig. 11.95 ST segment shift with patent arterial duct. This tracing was taken from an 840 g infant with cardiomegaly because of the duct. Note the ST depression the V_1 and V_2 and ST elevation in lead V_6. The ST-T wave changes resolved after ductal ligation.

changes (Sachder & Puri, 1967). An abnormal electrocardiogram implies myocardial damage. A normal electrocardiogram does not preclude severe injury. The electrocardiogram may normalise within 2–3 weeks of the onset of the disease, but it may remain abnormal for up to 4 months with later reversion to normal. A normal electrocardiogram after myocarditis also does not preclude severe residual damage (Hoffman, 1975b). The most prominent electrocardiographic changes are flat or inverted T waves (primarily in the left chest leads) and 'low voltage' QRS complexes (see p. 262). The T wave changes are probably due to altered repolarisation of injured cells through the myocardium rather than to true ischaemia. The QT interval may be prolonged. The low voltage QRS results from myocardial oedema. Myocarditis also commonly results in ST depression due to extensive subendocardial injury. ST elevation is rare in myocarditis without pericarditis (Rodriguez-Torres et al, 1969). There have been several reports of the appearance of new Q waves in association with myocarditis. These have mostly been in children who have later died. The Q waves were accompanied by ST elevation in those patients. There was no characteristic electrocardiographic location for these changes. In different children, the Q waves were in the inferior, lateral or anterior leads (Fig. 11.96). Pathologic studies have documented extensive areas of necrosis and scarring which correlate with the electrocardiographic location of the Q waves in these patients (Gross, et al 1967; Dominguez et al 1959). Atrioventricular block and interventricular conduction delay may occur in any type of myocarditis, but right bundle branch block is particularly common to the myocarditis due to Chagas' disease. Premature ventricular contractions occasionally occur in myocarditis (Hoffman, 1975b).

Injury due to pericarditis

Pericarditis is by far the most common pathologic cause of ST elevation in children. Other causes of primary ST changes include myocardial infarction, cor pulmonale,

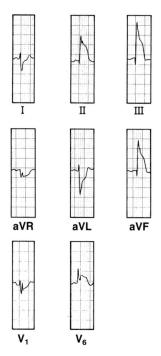

Fig. 11.94 Acute inferior myocardial infarction in a 3-month-old child with staphylococcal sepsis. At autopsy, there was extensive abscess in the left ventricle. There is considerable ST elevation in leads II, III and aV_F. There is reciprocal ST depression in leads I, aV_L, aV_R and V_1.

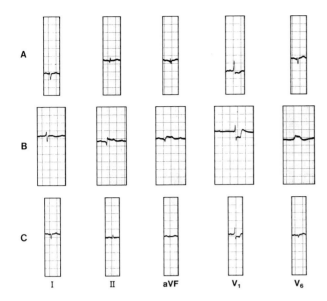

Fig. 11.96 Myocarditis in a 1-week-old infant. (A) Low voltage QRS complexes are shown in both the limb leads and precordial leads. The T waves are concordant but decreased in amplitude. (B) 12 hours later, there is development of complete atrioventricular block and deep, wide Q waves in leads III and aV_F accompanied by ST elevation in leads III, aV_F and V_6 with ST depression in lead V_1. This is compatible with an inferolateral myocardial infarction. (C) The bottom row shows the infant on the next day with even less voltage in the inferior and lateral leads. He died the following night and was shown at autopsy to have diffuse areas of myocarditis and areas of necrosis throughout both ventricles.

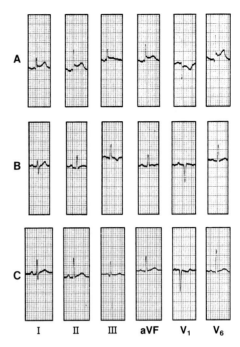

Fig. 11.97 Evolution of pericarditis in a 12-year-old. (A) In the top row, there is ST elevation with upright T waves in all leads except V_1. (B) In the middle row, the ST elevation is resolving and is replaced with T wave inversion in leads III and aV_F. This electrocardiogram was taken 4 days after the first electrocardiogram. (C) In the bottom row, 2 weeks later, the ST-T wave changes are resolved but there is a Q wave in lead III which is wider than on previous tracings. This could indicate a small area of old inferior myocardial infarction.

head injury, digitalis, hyperkalaemia, emetine intoxication, pneumothorax, pneumopericardium, early ventricular repolarisation, and normal atrial repolarisation. The electrocardiogram in pericarditis characteristically evolves through four stages (Fig. 11.97). The first stage is ST elevation. This is thought to be due to subepicardial myocarditis. The ST elevation occurs in leads facing the epicardium (leads II, aVF, V_3–V_6). Depending upon the position of the heart, lead I or III may also be involved. The leads without epicardial representation which are usually facing away from the left ventricle (leads aVR and V_1) may show reciprocal ST depression. The right ventricle in neonates constitutes more of the epicardial surface and the right chest leads may show ST elevation with the left chest leads showing ST depression (Hoffman, 1975b).

Pericarditis can usually be differentiated from acute myocardial infarction. In pericariditis, the ST elevation is found in numerous leads whereas in myocrdial infarction it is generally limited to a few leads; also, the ST elevation in pericarditis is associated usually with an upright T wave whereas in myocardial infarction, beyond the hyperacute phase, the T wave is usually inverted. In pericarditis during the time of ST elevation, it may also be possible to detect PR segment elevation (greater than 0.8 mm) due to atrial subepicardial injury in leads overlying the right atrium (aVR and V_1) and reciprocal PR depression (greater than 0.5 mm) in those leads normally showing ST elevation (Chou, 1979).

The second stage is characterised by normalisation of ST segments with T wave flattening. In the third stage there is T wave inversion in the same leads in which the ST elevation previously appeared. The fourth stage is resolution. In a prospective study of adults, 92% had electrocardiographic changes in pericarditis. In only half of these, typical ST elevation occurred followed by T wave inversion. In those without preceding ST elevation, T wave inversion did not occur. PR segment elevation occurred in 64% of these adults and in 10% this was the only change of pericarditis (Bruce & Spodick, 1980). The QRS complex is generally not affected by pericarditis. Even in the presence of a large pericardial effusion, the QRS have normal voltage in pericarditis (Chou, 1979).

Injury due to cardiac tumours

ST elevation and T wave inversion are the most common findings in metastatic tumors to the heart. This is because the pericardium is the most likely site for metastasis (see Ch. 48). If a primary cardiac tumour causes significant destruction of functioning myocardium, Q waves may appear. If the tumour is large enough, the QRS voltage may be decreased. Primary tumours of the heart can cause

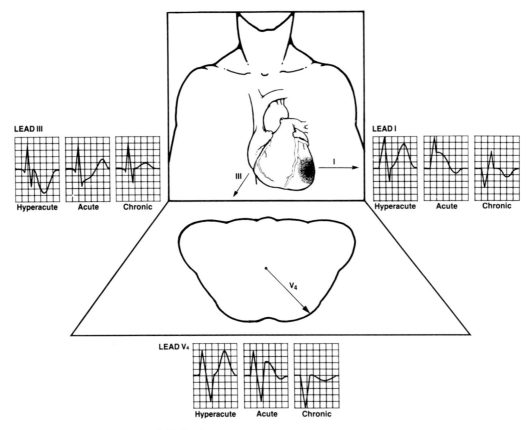

Fig. 11.98 Evolution of an anterolateral myocardial infarction.

any type of arrhythmias, most notably ventricular tachycardia and atrioventricular block (Chou, 1979).

Infarction

Infarcted muscle is electrically inert. The loss of electrical forces normally generated by the region of infarcted myocardium leaves unbalanced forces of unaltered magnitude in the opposite direction resulting in Q waves overlying the area of infarction (Fig. 11.98). The earliest electrocardiographic manifestations of myocardial infarction are 'hyperacute' very tall, peaked T waves. These occur because, in freshly infarcted tissue, the refractory periods have shortened considerably. The T wave points toward areas of shorter refractory period. Hyperacute T waves occur in the first minutes, and are therefore infrequently observed. Soon thereafter, ST elevation is observed in leads overlying the infarction and a current of injury to that area is displayed. There may be reciprocal ST segment depression in leads opposite the infarction. Within several hours to days the ST elevation is typically followed by the development of Q waves and inverted T waves in leads overlying the infarction. T wave inversion is due to eventual lengthening of the refractory periods of surviving cells in the region of the infarction. Q waves of myocardial infarction in children are wide (0.04 s or more)

and similar to those found in adults (Fig. 11.99). Q waves related to myocardial infarction in children may disappear. As growth occurs the infarcted area may become relatively smaller compared to the greater total mass of the heart.

Anomalous left coronary artery originating from the pulmonary trunk

Anomalous left coronary originating from the pulmonary trunk is the most common congenital anomaly causing myocardial infarction in childhood. Most of the infants and children with anomalous left coronary artery have already infarcted some areas of the left ventricle by the time of their first electrocardiogram. The electrocardiograms may variously reflect healed myocardial infarction, ventricular growth around the infarction, and varying degrees of acute and chronic ischaemia. Wide Q waves in infancy are more prominent than in later childhood (Puri et al, 1966). Q waves are almost invariably present in lead I and usually in lead aVL, and may extend from the mid to the lateral precordial leads (V_3–V_6). There may be an abrupt loss of R wave in the midprecordium with a normal R wave in V_1, V_6 and V_7. In the frontal plane, the QRS mean vector is usually +90° (Perloff, 1970). The T waves are usually inverted in leads I, aVL and the lateral precordial leads. In older children, the Q waves become less prominent

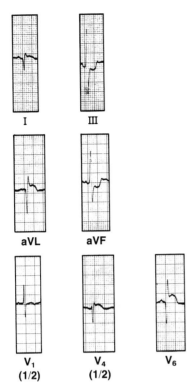

Fig. 11.99 Acute lateral myocardial infarction in a 4-month-old infant with anomalous left coronary artery originating from the pulmonary trunk. The 'acute' and 'chronic' stages diagrammed in Figure 11.98 occurred simultaneously in this patient. There is both ST elevation and the development of deep, wide Q waves in leads I, aV$_L$ and V$_6$.

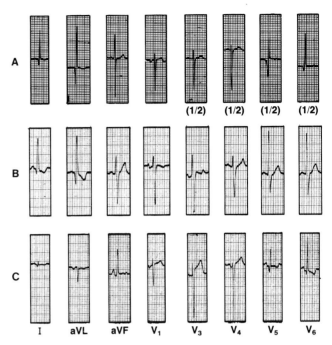

Fig. 11.100 Old myocardial infarction in three children with anomalous left coronary artery originating from the pulmonary trunk. (A) Tracings from a 7-month-old child. They demonstrate left axis deviation of the QRS mean vector in the frontal plane, a diminished R wave between lead V$_3$ and lead V$_6$, deep, wide Q waves in leads I, aV$_L$, V$_5$ and V$_6$. In the middle row, the tracings are from a 7-year-old girl. The findings are similar to those in the 7-month-old infant, with the exception that there are no Q waves in leads V$_5$ and V$_6$, but deep S waves in those leads. (B) Corresponds more to the 'adult' type of electrocardiogram in anomalous left coronary artery. (C) Taken from another 7-year-old. There is no left axis deviation, but there are deep Q waves in leads aV$_L$, V$_5$ and V$_6$. This is more consistent with the 'infantile' pattern. This demonstrates that the labels may not be helpful. In all these electrocardiograms there is a loss of R wave in lead V$_4$, and both Q waves and T wave inversion in leads I and aV$_L$.

resulting in compensatory hypertrophy of the posterobasal left ventricle. The major terminal QRS vector is superior, left and posterior frequently causing left axis deviation in the frontal plane. There may be loss of the normal right ventricular dominance and deep S wave in leads II, III, aVF and V$_1$ with tall R waves in leads aVL, V$_5$ and V$_6$. The T waves are discordant in leads I, V$_1$ and V$_6$. While this evolution is characteristic, an individual patient may present with any combination of these findings (Fig. 11.100).

Papillary muscle infarction

Newborn infants with severe neonatal stress or infants with severe pressure or volume overload may develop papillary muscle infarction. Characteristic electrocardiographic findings have been found in infants with aortic stenosis or total anomalous pulmonary venous connexion who were proven at autopsy to have had anterior papillary muscle infarction of either the right or left ventricle. In these infants, Q waves were present in lead V$_3$R. There was also a progressive diminution of the R wave in lead V$_3$R on serial electrocardiographic tracings (Kangos et al, 1969). This is to be distinguished from the other major causes of Q waves in the right chest leads in infancy, namely severe right ventricular hypertrophy or reversed septal depolarisation from left hand ventricular topology.

Kawasaki's disease

Kawasaki's disease (or mucocutaneous lymph node syndrome) is the most common acquired cause of myocardial infarction in infants and children (see Ch. 44). Approximately 15% of such patients develop coronary artery aneurysms associated with a pancarditis occurring in the first 2 weeks of the illness. In half of these the aneurysms regress. Sudden death occurs in 2% of these patients, presumably due to myocardial infarction and resultant arrhythmia (Fukushige et al, 1980). The Q waves which occur in Kawasaki's disease are abnormally deep and are usually abnormally wide (Fujiwara et al, 1980). Abnormally deep Q waves are defined on page 260. Q waves may develop in the first 2 weeks of the illness and may be due to severe myocarditis. These may subsequently resolve. If Q waves develop later than 2 weeks into the illness, this is usually associated with a coronary artery aneurysm and myocardial necrosis. In some patients, a serial deepening of the Q waves was the only sign of infarction (Fig. 11.101). The absence of Q waves does not imply

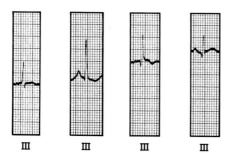

III   III   III   III

Fig. 11.101 Myocardial infarction in Kawasaki's disease. These tracings are from a 9-year-old boy who was hospitalised on the 7th day of the illness. The first tracing is from the day of admission. He was asymptomatic at the time. The second tracing was taken 3 days later. Note the development of small Q waves which were not present previously and the T wave inversion in lead III. 4 days later, the Q waves have deepend and are now slightly wider. There is also ST elevation with the terminal portion of the T wave inverted. The day following the third tracing, the Q wave remains and the T waves have normalised. By radionuclide imaging, the entire inferior wall of the left ventricle was shown to be infarcted. This points out the subtle changes which may occur in an extensive myocardial infarction in a child. While the depth of the Q wave in the last tracing is not distinctly abnormal, the new appearance of the Q wave is abnormal and the width of the Q wave is also abnormal.

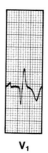

V_1

Fig. 11.102 Pseudoinfarction. This tracing was taken from a 20-year-old patient who had undergone intracardiac repair of tetralogy of Fallot. There is a deep, wide Q wave preceding the wide slurred terminal activation of the right bundle branch block. This Q wave was most likely due to the 3 cm by 8 cm patch which extended from the right ventricular anterior wall up to the pulmonary artery bifurcation. However, there was no clinical evidence for myocardial infarction, nor was there electrocardiographic evolution of an infarction.

an absence of aneurysms nor an absence of significant areas of myocardial necrosis at autopsy (Fujiwara et al, 1980).

Aneurysm

The most common electrocardiographic feature of a ventricular aneurysm is persistent ST elevation in leads overlying the aneurysm (Dubnow et al, 1965). This has been found in children with anomalous left coronary artery after myocardial infarction (Keith, 1959). In a congenital aneurysm of the posterior left ventricular base there was ST depression in the anterior chest leads (reciprocal from the posteriorly directed ST elevation) as well as diminished QRS voltage and T wave inversion in leads, I, II, aVL, V_5 and V_6 (Franco-Vasquez et al, 1970).

Pseudoinfarction

There are several other causes of abnormal Q waves, both with and without ST-T wave changes. They can be produced by left ventricular hypertrophy with strain and a QS pattern in lead I along with ST elevation, with reciprocal ST depression in V_6 or by right ventricular hypertrophy with a QR pattern in lead V_1. The ventricular topology of left hand pattern gives a left ventricular to right ventricular activation pattern occurring in a right-to-left direction and results in a narrow Q wave in lead V_1 and absent Q wave in V_6. Clockwise rotation of the heart from lung disease or pneumothorax may move the transition leads leftward to leads V_5 or V_6 and therefore lead V_1 may have a QS pattern. Hypertrophic cardiomyopathy with asymmetric septal hypertrophy can result in deep and usually not wide Q waves in the lateral leads. Replacement of myocardium by non-functioning living tissue can occur in myocarditis, progressive muscular dystrophy, Friedreich's ataxia, scleroderma and cardiac tumours. Replacement with prosthetic material can produce pseudoinfarction. For example, when a large prosthetic patch is used on the right ventricular outflow tract, deep and wide Q waves may occur in the anterior chest leads (Fig. 11.102). Left bundle branch block (causing a QS pattern in lead V_1), left anterior hemiblock (with Q waves in the lateral precordial leads), or the Wolff-Parkinson-White syndrome with wide Q waves in the inferior leads can all simulate infarction. Finally, intracranial haemorrhage may produce a QS pattern in leads V_1 or V_2.

EFFECT OF SYSTEMIC ALTERATIONS ON THE ELECTROCARDIOGRAM

Action potential changes reflected in the electrocardiogram

The majority of systemic alterations exert their effect on the electrocardiogram by changing all the action potentials in a similar manner. It is therefore important to understand how changes in action potentials cause changes in the electrocardiogram. The most important alterations are diagrammed in Figure 11.103 which was adapted from Surawicz (1966). A decrease in the upstroke velocity of the action potential (V_{max} of phase 0) causes a decrease in ventricular conduction velocity and uniform QRS widening (e.g. hyperkalaemia).

Since the end of the ventricular action potentials corresponds to the end of the T wave, prolonged action potential duration causes a long Q-T interval (e.g. quinidine). A short action potential duration causes a short Q-T interval (e.g. epinephrine). A long plateau (phase 2) causes a long ST segment (e.g. hypocalcaemia) while a short plateau causes a short ST segment (e.g. hypercalcaemia). Increased velocity of the initial phase of repolarisation abolishing the plateau causes disappearance of the isoelectric

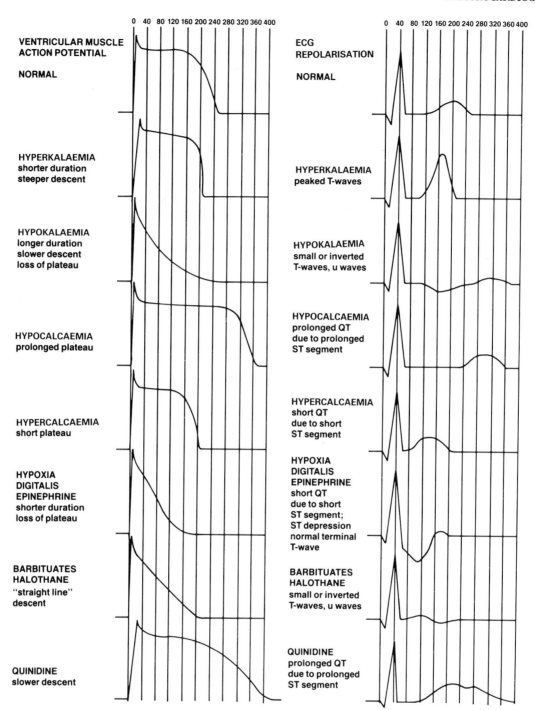

Fig. 11.103 Action potential and electrocardiographic changes in systemic alterations (see text).

portion of the ST segment and therefore deviation of the ST segment from the baseline (e.g. digitalis).

An abrupt transition from phase 2 to phase 3 combined with an increase in the slope of phase 3 results in an abrupt onset of the T wave with an increased amplitude and decreased duration. This causes the T wave to appear peaked (e.g. hyperkalaemia). Loss of plateau caused by uniform repolarisation approaching a straight line causes

a decrease in T wave amplitude (e.g. barbiturates). Prolonged terminal repolarisation of the ventricles causes U waves (e.g. hypokalaemia).

Body chemistry

Hyperkalaemia

Hyperkalaemia is most commonly due to renal failure, salt-losing adrenogenital syndrome, or iatrogenic overdose (Miller et al, 1970). The serum potassium level can be predicted from the electrocardiogram because of the different effects on the action potential. At a level of 5.5–6.5 mEq/l, the velocity of phase 3 of the action potential increases and the T waves on the electrocardiogram become tall and peaked. This is a poor sign because many normal children have 'peaked' T waves and many children with hyperkalaemia do not have peaked T waves. At a serum potassium over 6.6 mEq/l, the cellular resting membrane potential is decreased (more toward zero) and therefore the conduction velocity (and V_{max}) is decreased. This causes interventricular conduction delay. This may be manifested as diffuse QRS widening or it may have a specific bundle branch block or fascicular block pattern. These are generally very bizarre QRS complexes and may be combined with ST elevation leading to the mistaken diagnosis of ventricular tachycardia if preceding P waves are missed (Fig. 11.104). If P waves are seen, these complexes may also be mistaken for acute myocardial infarction or pericarditis. At a level over 7.0 mEq/l, intra-atrial conduction delay becomes manifest with prolongation of the P wave. At a level over 8.5 mEq/l, the P wave may disappear. Direct conduction from the sinus node through physiologically specialised atrial fibres to the atrioventricular node and the ventricles has been hypothesised. The sinus node and physiologically specialised atrial fibres are most resistant to hyperkalaemia. Since the ordinary atrial muscle fibres are depressed by the hyperkalaemia they neither conduct nor contract. Therefore, there may be no P wave despite conduction through the atrium. This has been termed 'sinuventricular conduction'. At approximately 9.0 mEq/l, arrhythmias begin, usually atrioventricular block, ventricular tachycardia and ventricular fibrillation.

Hypokalaemia

Hypokalaemia is seen most often in vomiting, diarrhoea, endocrine disease (Cushing's disease, hyperaldosteronism, cortisone treatment), acquired renal disease, iatrogenic lack of intake, and most importantly to cardiologists, diuretic treatment. Hypokalaemia causes a lengthening of phase 3 of the action potential with a loss of the plateau and a slower descent. At a level of 2.7–3.0 mEq/l, the electrocardiograms in 35% of adults have demonstrated abnormalities of hypokalaemia and at a level below 2.7 mEq/l, 78% are abnormal (Surawicz, 1967). The most prominent changes are the decrease in the T wave amplitude (occasionally with ST depression) and an increase in the U wave amplitude. Hypokalaemia therefore causes a broadened T wave and U wave with a normal onset to the T wave (Fig. 11.105). Other causes of prominent U waves are bradycardia, ischaemia, left ventricular hypertrophy, quinidine, procainamide, phenothiazines and cerebrovascular accidents. Hypokalaemia may cause a minimally prolonged QRS duration. Arrhythmias are rare with hypokalaemia unless the patient is receiving digitalis. In this case, hypokalaemia enhances the arrhythmogenic effects of digitalis.

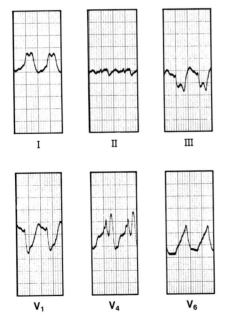

Fig. 11.104 Hyperkalaemia. These tracings are from a 2-day-old infant with renal failure and hyperkalaemia. The QRS complex is similar to left bundle branch block. The small P waves are marked with an arrow in lead I, indicating that this is sinus rhythm.

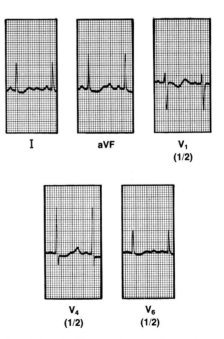

Fig. 11.105 Hypokalaemia. These tracings are from a 4-year-old with the nephrotic syndrome. Note the prominent U waves in all leads with ST depression and T wave inversion in leads I, aV$_F$, V$_4$ and V$_6$.

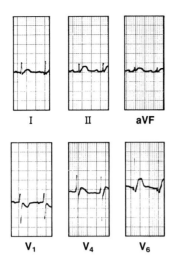

Fig. 11.106 Hypercalcaemia in a 1-year-old who had an iatrogenic overdose of calcium. The QT interval is short due to the absence of the ST segment.

Hypercalcaemia

Hypercalcaemia may be due to hyperparathyroidism, hypophosphatasia, hypervitaminosis D, idiopathic hypercalcaemia or iatrogenic overdose with rapid infusion of calcium. Hypercalcaemia shortens phase 2 of the action potential and therefore shortens the Q-T interval by shortening the ST segment. It may be difficult to diagnose hypercalcaemia on the electrocardiogram in sinus rhythm, because the Q-T interval may be normal and only the ST segment is shortened (Fig. 11.106). The most common effect of hypercalcaemia is on the sinus node, with slowing of the sinus rate, sinu-atrial block or sinus arrest. Atrioventricular block and ventricular arrhythmias are uncommon unless the patient is taking digitalis. In this case, hypercalcaemia potentiates digitalis effect and digitalis-induced arrhythmias.

Hypocalcaemia

Hypocalcaemia can be due to malabsorption, hypoparathyroidism, vitamin D deficiency, stress in the newborn period or iatrogenic lack of intake. This causes a prolongation of phase 2 of the action potential and prolongation of the ST segment on the electrocardiogram. Hypocalcaemia, therefore, has a different effect from hypokalaemia which prolongs phase 3. In hypokalaemia, the onset of the T wave occurs at the normal time, the T wave duration (including the U wave) is prolonged, and the Q-T (or QU) interval is prolonged. In hypocalcaemia, the T wave duration is normal and the Q-T interval is prolonged because there is a prolonged ST segment and a prolonged *onset* of the T wave (Fig. 11.107). The interval from the onset of the QRS to the onset of the T wave (Q-OT interval) correlates well with serum calcium in newborn babies (see Fig. 11.46). In

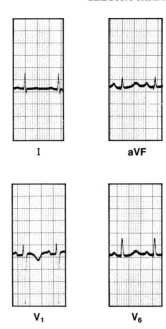

Fig. 11.107 Hypocalcaemia in a 13-year-old with the nephrotic syndrome. The ST segment is long. The Q-OTC interval is prolonged at 0.24 and the Q-TC interval is prolonged at 0.46.

prematures, the normal corrected Q-OT (Q-OT/square root of the RR) is 0.20 or less, and in full-term infants it is 0.19 or less (Colletti et al, 1974). Using these parameters, if the Q-OTC interval is normal, the serum calcium concentration is normal in 98% of babies; if the Q-OTC is prolonged, 70% are hypocalcaemic with a total serum calcium concentration less than 7.5 mg/dl. The remainder of the infants with a prolonged Q-OTC interval have undergone severe neonatal stress (Giacoia & Wagner, 1978). Although patients with hypocalcaemia have a prolonged Q-T interval, arrhythmias are rare, perhaps because repolarisation is uniformly prolonged throughout the ventricles. Atrioventricular block may occasionally occur.

Hypermagnesaemia

Hypermagnesaemia decreases the upstroke velocity of the action potential and shortens the duration of phase 2, simulating hypercalcaemia. Isolated hypermagnesaemia produces few changes on the electrocardiogram although individual cases of prolonged PR interval and interventricular conduction delay have been reported (Cooksey et al, 1977).

Hypomagnesaemia

The effects on the action potential and the electrocardiogram are similar to those of hypokalaemia. In newborns, hypomagnesaemia may coexist with hypocalcaemia. In these infants, the electrocardiographic pattern is similar to combined hypocalcaemia and hypokalaemia. There is a prolonged plateau and a slower descent. These produce a summation of effects to delay repolarisation and therefore large U waves are observed with flattened T waves.

Hypernatraemia and hyponatraemia

The effects of sodium on the action potential in the tissue bath are considerable. There is an increased sodium concentration causing an increase in the slope of phase 0 (increased V_{max}) and prolonged phase 3. A decrease in sodium concentration causes the opposite effect. In the range of serum sodium concentrations which are physiologically possible in the body, however, these effects are not usually seen on the electrocardiogram. The effects of sodium may be demonstrated in the patient with a prolonged QRS duration due to quinidine or hyperkalaemia. Sodium infusion improves interventricular conduction and shortens the QRS duration.

Hypoglycaemia

The electrocardiographic changes of hypoglycaemia are thought to be caused by the associated hyperkalaemia which is frequently present. In hypoglycaemia, insulin secretion is inhibited and hyperkalaemia may result.

Hypoxia and acidosis

The effects on the action potential of hypoxia and acidosis are similar to those of increased extracellular potassium and the changes may be due, in part, to leakage of potassium out of the cell (Hoffman, 1975b). The QRS duration prolongs, as does the Q-T interval. All types of atrial and ventricular arrhythmias may occur in addition to atrioventricular block.

Anti-arrhythmic drugs

Digitalis

Digitalis shortens phase 2 of the action potential and also shortens the action potential duration. The ST-T wave changes can be explained by the effect of digitalis to hasten repolarisation. Digitalis tends to cause all layers of the ventricle to repolarise simultaneously resulting in greater cancellation of the repolarisation vector and flat T waves. With moderate amounts of digitalis effect, the onset of repolarisation is primarily affected as represented in the ST segment. This segment is depressed most in the leads facing the left ventricle. Taller R waves are generally associated with more ST depression (Hoffman, 1975b). The late part of repolarisation is still unaffected. The terminal parts of the T waves are, therefore, normal and concordant with the QRS complex, although the overall QTC interval

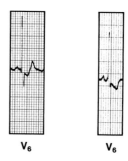

Fig. 11.108 Digitalis effect. Left–ST depression with normal terminal portion of the T wave. Right–coved initial portion, with complete inversion of the T wave.

may be shortened (Fig. 11.108A). With increasing amounts of digitalis effect the entire process of repolarisation is reversed (from endocardium to epicardium). The same leads with ST depression also show T wave inversion. The T waves are coved and the descending limb of the ST segment and T wave has an angle of 90° with the ascending limb (Fig. 11.108B) (Surawicz, 1967).

The effect of digitalis on impulse formation and conduction results from a combination of direct and vagotonic effects. The cellular basis of these effects has been reviewed by Reder & Rosen (1981). The overall effect of digitalis is to slow the sinus rate, speed intra-atrial conduction, decrease atrial automaticity and prolong atrioventricular conduction. This may be manifest on the electrocardiogram as sinus bradycardia and a prolonged PR interval.

Digitalis toxicity results in further slowing of the sinus rate, sinoatrial block or sinus arrest and second degree atrioventricular block (usually type 1 – Wenckebach) or third degree block. These manifestations are more common in children than those which result in increased atrial, junctional or ventricular automaticity, namely premature atrial contractions, supraventricular tachycardia, non-paroxysmal junctional tachycardia, premature ventricular contractions or ventricular tachycardia (Larese & Mirkin, 1974; Hayes et al, 1973). If atrioventricular block and premature ventricular contractions occur on the same electrocardiogram, digitalis toxicity should be suspected (Fig. 11.109).

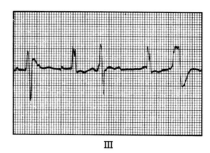

Fig. 11.109 Digitalis intoxication. There is complete atrioventricular block with an idioventricular escape rhythm (second and fourth QRS complexes).

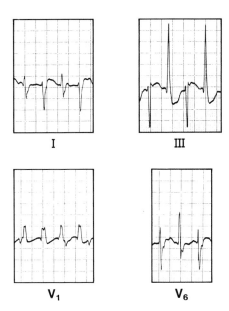

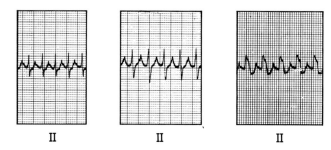

Fig. 11.111 Procainamide effect and toxicity. Left – before medication, this 5-month-old girl had supraventricular tachycardia due to an atrial ectopic focus at a rate of 270/min. The QRS duration was 0.05 s. Centre – after 70 mg of procainamide, the rate slowed to 225/min and the QRS duration increased to 0.08 s. Right – after 80 mg of procainamide, the rate did not change, but the QRS duration has increased to 0.10 s with a pattern of left bundle branch block.

Fig. 11.110 Bidirectional tachycardia. This was due to digitalis intoxication and hypokalaemia in a 5-year-old child. There is constant right bundle branch block in lead V_1 with alternating right axis and left axis deviation shown in the limb leads.

Digitalis toxicity (especially associated with hypokalaemia) has been associated with 'bidirectional tachycardia'. This has the morphology of constant complete right bundle branch block with alternating right axis deviation and left axis deviation (Fig. 11.110). Bidirectional tachycardia is probably ventricular tachycardia with alternating exit pathways, rather than junctional tachycardia with alternating bundle branch block (Morris & Zipes, 1973).

Quinidine, procainamide and disopyramide

These drugs are class I anti-arrhythmic agents and have similar actions. Quinidine's effects will be used as examples of the other type I agents. Quinidine decreases the upstroke velocity (reduced V_{max}) of all action potentials, prolongs phase 3 (resulting in a prolonged action potential duration) and reduces automaticity. The decreased upstroke velocity results in interventricular conduction delay and a prolonged QRS duration. This may result in a diffusely widened QRS, or a specific right or left bundle branch block pattern. The effects on the T waves are both 'secondary' (to the interventricular conduction delay) and 'primary' (due to prolongation of the action potential). Since the terminal part of repolarisation is most affected, the early part of the T wave may have decreased amplitude and the terminal part may be increased. This is difficult to distinguish from a U wave. The Q-T (or QU) interval is prolonged. Because of its vagolytic properties, quinidine may shorten the PR interval slightly.

Quinidine toxicity is manifest on the electrocardiogram as: a decreased atrial rate usually due to sinu-atrial exit block; prolongation of the P wave duration due to intra-atrial conduction delay; prolongation of the PR interval due to prolongation of His-Purkinje conduction; prolongation of the QRS complex to 125% or more of the original QRS duration (Fig. 11.111); further prolongation of the Q-T interval due to an increase in refractory period dispersion throughout the ventricles (DiSegni et al, 1980) and premature ventricular contractions and ventricular tachycardia (Castellanos & Salhanick, 1967). The ventricular tachycardia in quinidine toxicity may have a similar morphology to that sometimes found in other patients with prolonged Q-T intervals and is called 'torsades de pointes' (Fig. 11.112) (Horowitz et al, 1981).

Lidocaine and phenytoin

These drugs increase the slope of phase 0 (increase V_{max}) in diseased tissue (improving conduction) and shorten action potential duration but have very little effect on the surface electrocardiogram. Rarely with high doses of phenytoin the PR and Q-T intervals may shorten due to accelerated atrioventricular conduction and shortened ventricular refractoriness. If phenytoin is given to a patient with a prolonged Q-T interval for prevention of ventricular tachycardia, effective anti-arrhythmic treatment may occur without shortening the Q-T interval (Schwartz et al, 1975).

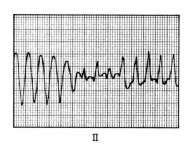

Fig. 11.112 Torsades de pointes due to quinidine toxicity. There are two different polarities to the tachycardia separated by a narrower transition QRS.

Propranolol

Propranolol decreases the upstroke velocity of phase 0 (reduces V_{max}), shortens the action potential duration, and decreases automaticity. The effects of propranolol in the patient are mainly anti-adrenergic. The sinus rate is slowed, the PR interval is prolonged and the Q-T interval may be shortened. As with phenytoin, propranolol may not shorten the Q-T interval in a patient with a prolonged Q-T interval but it may be effective in preventing ventricular tachycardia and sudden death (Schwartz et al, 1975).

Verapamil

Verapamil is a calcium antagonist with primary effects on the sinus node and atrioventricular node. It decreases the slope of phase 0 (reduced V_{max}), prolongs the action potential duration and reduces automaticity. The electrocardiographic findings are a slowed sinus rate and prolonged PR interval.

Anaesthetic agents

Halothane decreases the action potential duration slightly by increasing the slope of phase 2 and phase 3. These effects are rarely seen on the electrocardiogram but occasionally the Q-T interval is shortened and there may be a decrease in T wave amplitude. Halothane sensitises the heart both to vagal and sympathetic stimulation. Bradycardia and ventricular arrhythmias may therefore occur. Methoxyflurane, teflurane and enflurane have similar effects on the electrocardiogram to those of halothane.

Chloroform, ethyl chloride (given by inhalation), trichloroethylene and cyclopropane all may cause ventricular arrhythmias. Diethyl ether and other ethers have no effect on the electrocardiogram (Rollason, 1976).

Psychotropic drugs

Phenothiazines cause shift of potassium inside the cell thus decreasing the extracellular potassium and therefore prolong phase 3 of the action potential (Wolpert & Farr, 1975). These changes are similar to those found with quinidine. The T waves have reduced amplitude with prominent terminal depolarisations. It is difficult to distinguish a U wave from broad notched T waves with an increased terminal component. The Q-T (or QU) interval is prolonged (Burda, 1968). Arrhythmias are rarely observed with phenothiazines in therapeutic doses but ventricular arrhythmias may occur in overdosage.

The electrocardiographic changes with tricyclic antidepressants occur in 20% of adult patients taking the drugs. The most common manifestations are sinus tachycardia, prolonged PR interval and flat T waves. Less commonly observed are QRS prolongation, Q-T prolongation and ST-T wave changes. Overdosage with tricyclic antidepressants may cause any atrial or ventricular arrhythmias or atrioventricular block (Chou, 1979).

Imipramine (Tofranil) causes an imbalance of intracellular and extracellular potassium with an increase in serum potassium. Atrial flutter, atrioventricular block, interventricular conduction delay and ventricular tachycardia were all observed in one child suffering an overdose (Fouron & Chicoine, 1971).

Central nervous system effects

Congenital prolongation of the Q-T interval

Jervell & Lange-Nielsen (1957), Romano (1963) and Ward (1964) described syndromes which have in common congenital prolongation of the Q-T interval, syncope or sudden death and hereditary transmission. In the Jervell-Lange-Nielsen syndrome, the hearing is abnormal and the heredity is autosomal recessive. The hearing is normal in the Romano-Ward syndrome and the heredity is autosomal dominant. The electrocardiograms are similar. The T waves may be inverted, biphasic and vary in both shape and amplitude from minute to minute. The T waves frequently have bizarre shapes with greater amplitude at the terminal portion of the T wave (Fig. 11.113).

Although the exact mechanism of the prolonged Q-T

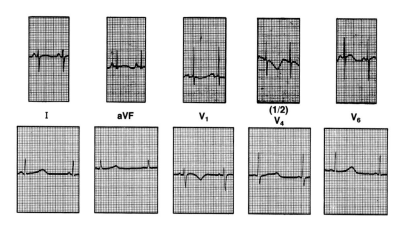

I   aVF   V₁   (1/2) V₄   V₆

Fig. 11.113 Congenital prolongation of the QT interval. Top tracings from a 9-day-old infant with a history of ventricular tachycardia and ventricular fibrillation at the age of 4 days. All the T waves are abnormal, however the T waves in lead V₄ (at half standard) are especially bizarre. Bottom tracings from a 12-year-old who had his first episode of syncope at the age of 10 years. He was being treated for a familial seizure disorder. Note that the terminal portion of the T wave in lead V₄ is greater in amplitude than the initial portion.

interval is uncertain, central and peripheral nervous system sympathetic imbalance is involved. Innervation to the heart is normally asymmetric. Fibres project from the right hypothalamus to the right stellate ganglion and supply the anterior surface of the cardiac ventricles. Fibres from the left hypothalamus project to the left stellate ganglion and supply the left lateral and posterior wall of the cardiac ventricles. Experimental stimulation of the left stellate ganglion prolongs the Q-T interval and causes ST depression (Hoffman, 1975b). In patients with a congenitally prolonged Q-T interval, left stellate ganglionectomy may shorten the Q-T interval. This may eliminate episodes of syncope, adding strength to the concept of neural imbalance as a cause of this syndrome.

Central nervous system injury

The electrocardiogram has been reported to be abnormal in 75% of children with moderate to severe head trauma or those who have undergone neurosurgical procedures (Rogers et al, 1980). The most common abnormalities are a prolonged Q-T interval with either notched, bizarre-shaped T waves or prominent U waves. The T waves are occasionally diffusely flattened in the lateral leads or even inverted with ST depression (Millar & Abildskov, 1968). ST elevation is rare in central nervous system lesions but has been reported (Anderson et al, 1973). 'J' or 'Osborne' waves are sometimes found (see below). These repolarisation changes are thought not to be due to increased intracranial pressure but rather to differential stimulation or suppression of the cortical representations of the sympathetic fibres. There is evidence at autopsy for cardiac abnormalities in some patients with central nervous system lesions, primarily subendocardial ischaemia. Identical lesions can be produced by catecholamine infusion (Bordiuk et al, 1969). Any arrhythmias can occur with central nervous system injury. Vagal tone is enhanced and there may be alternating sympathetic stimulation. The bradyarrhythmias (sinus bradycardia, wandering atrial pacemaker, junctional rhythm and type 1 second degree atrioventricular block) generally respond to atropine. This supports the theory of their central vagal origin. Sinus tachycardia may occur in addition to any of the pathologic tachyarrhythmias.

Hypothermia

A J wave (or Osborne wave) occurs on the electrocardiogram of patients with a body temperature below 25°C. This is a slowly inscribed extra deflection between the QRS and the early ST segment (Fig. 11.114) (Emslie-Smith et al, 1959). The PR and Q-T intervals prolong and there may be ST depression or ST elevation. The sinus node initially slows but at approximately 29°, 50–60% of adult patients with hypothermia have atrial fibrillation.

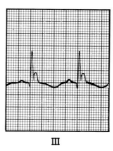

III

Fig. 11.114 Hypthermia. This tracing was taken from a 3-month-old with hypothermia and severe brain damage. The J wave is the rounded, second portion of the QRS complex. The heart rate is slow for an infant of this age. The PR interval, QRS duration and QT interval are also prolonged.

Neuromuscular disorders

The electrocardiogram in Duchenne's progressive muscular dystrophy is abnormal in about 75% of patients. The abnormalities are most specific to Duchenne's dystrophy and occur less frequently in the other forms of muscular dystrophy (Durnin et al, 1971). The usual findings are tall R waves in the right precordial leads (with or without interventricular conduction delay) and deep narrow Q waves in the left precordial leads (see Fig. 11.62). These changes are thought to be due to selective scarring of the postero-basal left ventricle rather than right ventricular hypertrophy, pulmonary hypertension or septal hypertrophy (Perloff et al, 1967). The scarring could be due to continued stress on the left atrioventricular ring due to poor support of the mitral valve from abnormal cardiac muscle. These electrocardiographic changes do not correlate with the degree of involvement in the skeletal muscles or the degree of cardiomyopathy. Late in the disease, when cardiomyopathy is present, any type of active arrhythmias may occur. Sinus tachycardia, premature atrial contractions, atrial flutter, premature ventricular contractions or ventricular tachycardia have all been described.

The electrocardiogram is abnormal in 90% of the patients with Friedreich's ataxia. Most commonly there is QRS-T discordance. 25% have asymmetric septal hypertrophy as the cause of deep Q waves in the lateral precordial leads (Chou, 1979). Either left ventricular hypertrophy or right ventricular hypertrophy may occur. The arrhythmias are similar to those in muscular dystrophy. The electrocardiogram in myotonic dystrophy is abnormal in about half of the patients, with low voltage P wages, prolonged PR interval, left axis deviation, left bundle branch block and ST-T wave changes. Atrial fibrillation is common.

Connective tissue disease

In patients with scleroderma or systemic lupus erythematosus, pulmonary hypertension may cause right ventricular hypertrophy and systemic hypertension may cause left

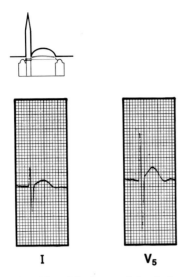

I   V₅

Fig. 11.115 Hypothyroidism. The 'mosque' sign is demonstrated with an absence of the ST segment and a symmetrically rounded T wave.

ventricular hypertrophy. In addition, ST elevation and T wave changes may occur from pericarditis. Chronic pericarditis with fibrin insulation or diffuse myocardial fibrosis may lead to low voltage QRS complexes. Supraventricular tachycardia, ventricular tachycardia, atrioventricular block and bundle branch block are all common in later stages of these diseases.

Metabolic diseases

Hypothyroidism

The classic sign of hypothyroidism is the 'mosque' sign (appropriately originally described in Turkey by Ertugrul in 1966). There is a dome-shaped symmetric T wave with an absent ST segment (Fig. 11.115). This was present in 37% of children with hypothyroidism. If present, therefore, the mosque sign is helpful in the diagnosis. If it is absent, the patient still may have hypothyroidism. Low voltage of the P waves, QRS complexes and T waves is also common, and most likely due to myocardial oedema rather than myxomatous pericarditis which is exceedingly rare (Malecka-Dymnicka & Bittel-Dobrzynska, 1966). Sinus bradycardia occurs in children with hypothyroidism, usually after 3 years of age.

Hyperthyroidism

The majority of children with hyperthyroidism have sinus tachycardia. Approximately 50% have left ventricular hypertrophy (Pilapil & Watson, 1970). Less commonly observed are prolonged PR interval, non-specific ST-T wave changes and right bundle branch block. These changes may take up to a year to reverse after the patient becomes euthyroid.

Adrenal insufficiency

Patients with adrenal insufficiency may have Q-T prolongation with inverted T waves. These changes can be reproduced in adrenalectomised animals. But, when the hearts are removed from the body, the cardiac action potentials are normal (Surawicz, 1967). These changes are therefore thought to be due to autonomic imbalance.

Pheaochromocytoma

Excess catecholamines are responsible for the prolonged Q-T interval and T wave inversion occasionally encountered in patients with pheaochromocytoma.

Miscellaneous diseases

Peritoneal inflammation

Peritonitis, appendicitis and ileitis may be associated with non-specific ST-T wave changes. These are thought to be due to vagally mediated reflexes (Surawicz, 1967).

Sarcoid

The granulomas of sarcoidosis have a predilection for the conduction system. The most common lesions are complete atrioventricular block and right bundle branch block. Premature atrial contractions and premature ventricular contractions also occur (Chou, 1979).

ARTEFACTS

Recognition of artefacts is both important and satisfying. It is exercise in mind over matter. Causes of artefacts can be classified into various major categories (Stanger et al, 1977).

Causes of artefacts

Incorrect positioning of the electrocardiogram leads

The most common cause is reversing the right arm with the left arm or the right leg with the left leg. Only the limb leads on the electrocardiographic tracing are affected. If the arm leads are reversed, the P wave, QRS complex and T wave are inverted in lead I. This can be checked by examining lead V₆, since V₆ has approximately the same vector as lead I. If the complexes in lead I and V₆ are completely different and the P waves are inverted in lead I, the limb leads are reversed (Fig. 11.116A, B). If the right leg and the left leg leads are switched, there is practically no change in the electrocardiogram (Fig. 11.116C). If the right leg and the right arm leads are switched, lead II is entirely isoelectric. Secondly, the complexes in aVR and

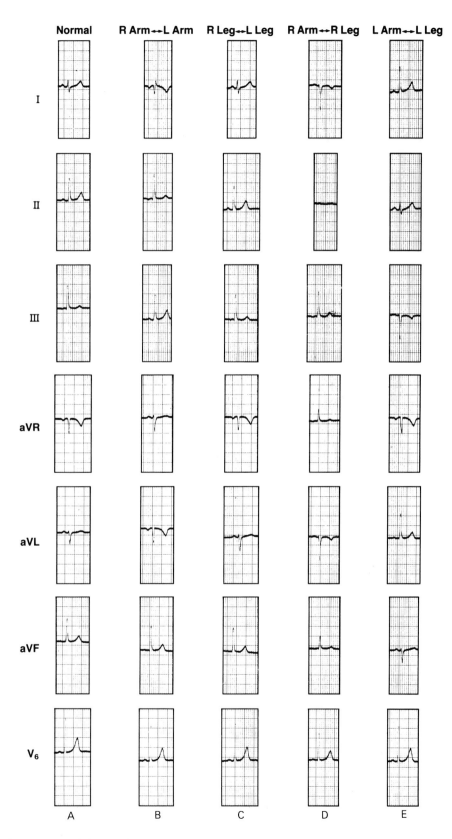

Fig. 11.116 Artefacts due to incorrect limb lead placement. (A) Limb leads in the normal positions. (B) Right arm and the left arm reversed. (C) Right leg and left leg reversed. (D) Right arm and right leg reversed, (E) Left arm and left leg reversed.

aVF are completely positive. It is not possible to calculate a mean vector which is entirely positive in aVR and aVF at the same time. Finally, lead I is entirely different from lead V₆. These leads should record similar complexes (Fig. 11.116D). If the left leg and left arm leads are switched, unlike the other errors, the resultant electrocardiogram is not obviously faulty. This error in position results in abnormal left axis deviation (Fig. 11.116E).

The chest leads may be positioned in an incorrect interspace (Fig. 11.117). If all the leads are placed one interspace too high (i.e. 3rd instead of 4th interspace) the R waves are diminished and the S waves are augmented in leads V₄–V₇. If the leads are placed one interspace too low, the R waves are augmented and the S waves are diminished. If electrode paste is not cleaned between chest lead placement, the entire anterior chest will become a conductor. The same 'average' QRS complex will then be recorded from each lead. This is a common problem in infants. It should be suspected if every chest lead appears similar (Fig. 11.118).

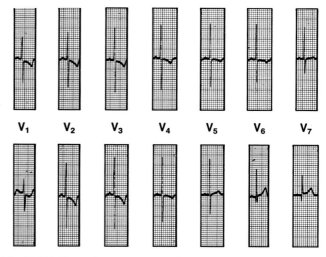

Fig. 11.118 Electrode paste not properly removed between applications of the chest electrodes. Top row with paste smeared on the anterior chest wall causing all complexes to appear the same. Bottom row with proper application of the paste showing a difference between complexes.

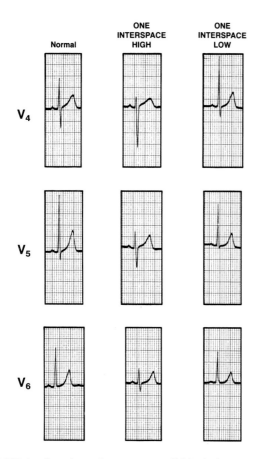

Fig. 11.117 Artefacts due to incorrect precordial lead placement. The first column is with the leads in the normal position. The second column is with the leads placed one interspace too high and the third column is with leads placed one interspace too low.

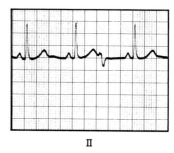

Fig. 11.119 Hiccough. The artefact can be best described as being midway in size between a P wave and a QRS complex. It is too large for a P wave. If it were a QRS complex, it should be followed by a T wave.

Patient-initiated movement

Hiccoughs produce monophasic or biphasic deflections which occur randomly throughout the cardiac cycle. They are usually midway in size between a P wave and QRS complex. There is no alteration in the basic rhythm (Fig. 11.119). Purposeful movement may be responsible for any random depolarisation on the electrocardiogram which does not affect the basic rhythm and should be suspected as an artefact. If the movement is repetitive (e.g. waving of the hand) it may simulate ventricular tachycardia. Non-purposeful movement (convulsions, 'jittery' newborns and somatic tremors) may simulate tachyarrhythmias (Fig. 11.120). The size of the QRS complex may also change with normal deep inspiration (Fig. 11.121).

Therapeutic manipulation of the patient

Chest percussion can occur at a rate of approximately 5/s

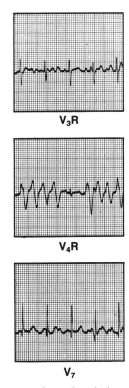

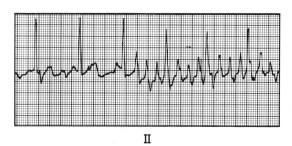

Fig. 11.122 Chest percussion. This is recorded from a 24-hour electrocardiogram and the artefact occurs at a rate of approximately 300/min. Note that the RR interval is unchanged before and during the artefact.

Fig. 11.120 Simultaneous tracings taken during a seizure. In lead V₄R, the tracing appears to be ventricular tachycardia but in the other two tracings, it is apparent that this is an artefact and that there is a regular supraventricular rhythm at a rate of 120/min. This demonstrates the value of having three simultaneous leads to aid in the identification of artefacts.

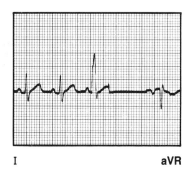

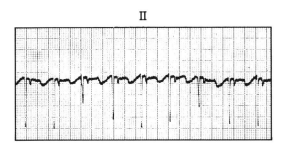

Fig. 11.121 Respiration. The QRS amplitude changes cyclically with approximately 2 s between the smallest QRS complexes. This corresponds to a respiratory rate of 30/min.

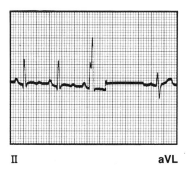

Fig. 11.123 Calibration fusion. These leads were recorded simultaneously. Most apparent in lead II is the onset of a normal QRS complex and then a further spike is introduced on top of the QRS complex. This is followed by an isoelectric segment when the electrocardiograph is not recording. This stimulates a premature ventricular contraction.

and result in an artefact at a rate of 300/min (Fig. 11.122). Open or closed chest massage adds artefactual complexes with each depression of the chest.

Properly functioning electrocardiographic system with 'built-in' artefact

In certain electrocardiographic recording machines, the calibration signal is provided automatically without stopping the paper. Thus, the calibration spike may be confused with parts of the true electrocardiogram and form an artefact (Fig. 11.123).

Malfunctioning electrocardiographic system

Loss of electrode contact is usually marked by an abrupt change in the baseline with an absence of cardiac depolarisations. In true asystole the baseline usually does not change (Fig. 11.124). Faulty cable shielding can result in movement artefact appearing on the electrocardiogram when the cable is moved. Faulty cable attachment may produce a repetitive artefact due to low-amplitude vibration in the environment (Fig. 11.125). Interference from 60 cycle leakage can give artefacts as can faulty paper drive. Uneven stylus marks may be present causing the paper to

II

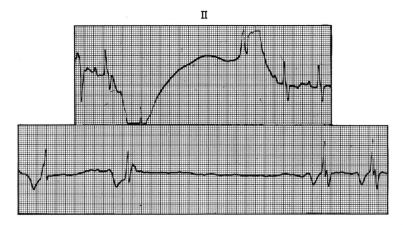

Fig. 11.124 Asystole versus loss of electrode contact. In the top tracing, there is asystole and in the bottom tracing, there is loss of electrode contact. Note the change in the baseline with the loss of electrode contact.

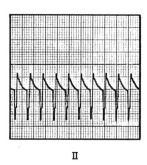

II

Fig. 11.125 Faulty cable attachment. This artefact was eliminated when the connector between the patient cable and the electrocardiograph was secured. This presumably resulted from repetitive vibrations in the pins which were placed loosely in the slots of the connector.

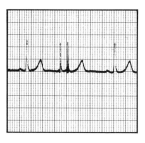

II

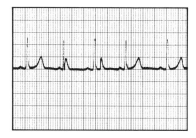

II

Fig. 11.126 Paper drag due to faulty paper drive. In the top tracing, the middle two QRS complexes are too narrow compared to the others and indicate that the paper is dragging. Also, there is an uneven stylus mark causing the paper to appear burned in the third complex. In the bottom tracing, in the middle three complexes, the PR, QRS and QT intervals are all shortened to a variable degree.

appear 'burned'. As the paper speed varies, all parts of the P wave, QRS complex and T wave shorten and prolong with the apparent increase or decrease in heart rate respectively (Fig. 11.126). At the slowest abnormal paper speeds, the heart rate may appear to be faster than physiologically possible, giving a hint that this may be an artefact (Fig. 11.127). A faulty stylus may draw an arc rather than a straight line for the R wave. Incorrect stylus position or improper gain may have the 'isoelectric' line unusually flat, indicating that the stylus is at the limit of its excursion or 'pegged' (Fig. 11.128A). This can be suspected by the lack of any deflection on one side of the isoelectric line, or a heavy mark at the peak of the QRS complex (Fig. 11.128B)

Current produced from external sources

Either an overhead warmer or respirator may cause cyclic production of 60 cycle current which may be printed on the electrocardiogram. The source of the current or electrical interference may not be identified. The 'infusion pump artefact' was originally described as a biphasic spike of 30 ms duration with a repetitive rate of 135/min (Sahn & Vaucher, 1976). This artefact is similar to, but wider than, a normal bipolar cardiac pacemaker artefact. The control plunger in a defective infusion pump was the source of current leak which was transmitted via the intra-

II

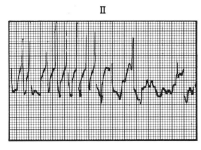

Fig. 11.127 Tape drag causing rapid and irregular rate. In this tracing from a 24-hour electrocardiogram, the rhythm is artifactually irregular, and the rate of 428/min is unphysiologic for a 14-year-old child.

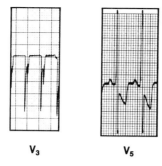

V₃   V₅

Fig. 11.128 Improper stylus position. Left – the isoelectric line is unusually flat and there are no complexes above this line. This indicates that the upper limit for the stylus was being reached at this point. The patient had ventricular tachycardia. Right – an improper gain setting has been applied such that the QRS complex is clipped at both the top and the bottom of the tracing. In cases such as these, it is impossible to tell how much larger the QRS complex would have been without changing the gain setting.

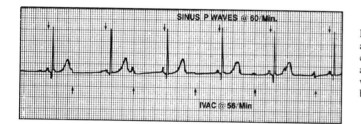

Fig. 11.129 The infusion pump artefact. The arrows on top of the tracing demonstrate the sinus P waves occuring at a rate of 60/min. The arrows on the bottom of the tracing indicate an artifact occurring at a constant rate of 56/min which is due to current leak from an improperly shielded infusion pump.

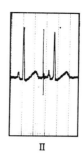

II

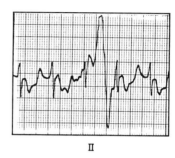

II

Fig. 11.130 Improper duration for QRS complex. Top tracing – the artefact between the two QRS complexes is too narrow to be a QRS complex and it is also not followed by a T wave. Bottom tracing – the artefact in the middle of the tracing is too wide to be a premature ventricular contraction in a 1-month-old child. It is also accompanied by a baseline shift.

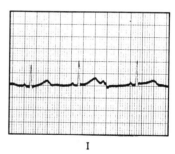

I

Fig. 11.131 Absence of a T wave following a 'QRS complex'. This artefact has the appearance of a QRS complex but is not followed by a T wave.

venous tubing and scalp vein to the patient and detected on the electrocardiogram. We have recently found an artefact which even more closely resembled P waves. This was again due to current leakage from an infusion pump down a nasogastric tube, through the patient and recorded on the electrocardiogram at a rate of 56/min (Fig. 11.129).

Systematic approach for the recognition of artefacts

A systematic approach is necessary for the recognition of artefacts. The following eight points are helpful in their identification.

1. The shape, amplitude or duration of the wave is atypical for a P wave or a QRS complex. The normal limits for P waves and QRS complexes are defined on pages 258–9. For example, many artefacts are 'narrower' than a normal QRS and some artefacts last longer than even the most prolonged bundle branch block pattern (Figs. 11.125, 11.130).

2. If a wave has the appearance of a 'QRS complex' but is not followed by a T wave, an artefact should be suspected (Fig. 11.131).

3. Artefacts may be accompanied by a shift in the baseline (Fig. 11.132).

4. An artefact which repeats itself must be differentiated from tachycardia. In a repetitive artefact the rate may be too rapid to be physiologically possible. The maximum regular atrial or ventricular rate is approximately 450/min in an infant (130 ms between waves) and 300/min in a child (200 ms between waves). Therefore, if there is less than 130 ms between successive regular waves in an infant, or less than 200 ms in a child, an artefact should be suspected (Fig. 11.133).

A single artefact must be distinguished from a premature beat. Some artefacts occur 'too early' to be physiologically possible. The normal atrial or ventricular effective

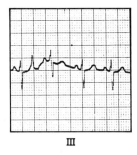

Fig. 11.132 Baseline shift. This hiccough is suspected as an artefact because it is too large for a P wave, is not followed by a T wave and results in a baseline shift.

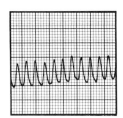

Fig. 11.133 Unphysiologically rapid rate. This tracing was recorded on a 24-hour electrocardiogram from a 6-year-old child. While these artefacts may appear similar to QRS complexes, the rate of 480/min is not physiologic.

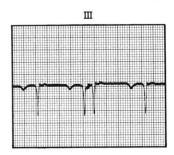

Fig. 11.134 Unphysiologically premature. This tracing was recorded from a normal 14-year-old. The third QRS complex occurs 180 ms after the last QRS. This is not physiologic. The cause of the artefact can be established by the shift in the baseline and the burned appearance to the paper. The electrocardiograph was stopped and started at this time.

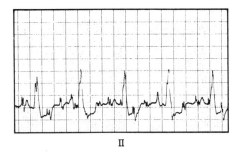

Fig. 11.135 Artefact parasystole. This tracing was recorded on a telemetry unit while a patient was brushing her teeth. The QRS complexes are regular and the artefact is somewhat irregular and occurs approximately 300 times per minute. The artefact, which simulates P waves, has a fairly regular interval between spikes, but is unrelated to the QRS complexes. Also, preceding the first, third and fifth QRS complexes, the true P wave can be seen in the tracing.

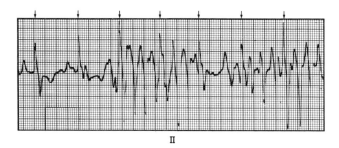

Fig. 11.136 QRS 'seen through' the artefact. The arrows mark the QRS complexes which continue undisturbed through the movement artefact.

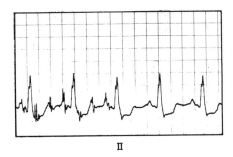

Fig. 11.137 QRS 'marches through' the artefact. In the patient who was brushing her teeth during the recording in Figure 11.134, the toothbrushing stopped in this recording and the basic rhythm continued unaffected.

refractory period is approximately 200 ms in an infant and 250 ms in a child. Thus, at least this amount of time is necessary before the atrium or ventricle can depolarise again. If there is, for example, a wave that follows a QRS complex by 180 ms in a 14-year-old child, this second wave is unlikely to be a QRS complex (Fig. 11.134).

5. Repetitive artefacts may simulate parasystole. The artefact will usually occur at a variable interval from the preceding P wave or QRS complex, but there may be a constant interval between the artefacts (Fig. 11.135).

6. The basic rhythm is unaffected by the artefact. An artefact may only affect part of the QRS, in which case the QRS may be 'seen through' the artefact (Fig. 11.136). Alternatively, the basic RR interval may be entirely unaf-

fected by the artefact and the QRS 'marches through' with the artefact present or absent (Fig. 11.137). In general, following an episode of supraventricular or ventricular tachycardia, the sinus node is suppressed and takes a few beats to regain its normal regular rate. Following a repetitive artefact, the sinus rate does not change, making preceding tachycardia less likely (Fig. 11.138). If a T wave is the first complex to follow a pause, the pause must have been artefactual since a T wave is unlikely without a preceding QRS complex (Fig. 11.139).

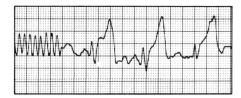

Fig. 11.138 Lack of 'sinus pause'. The absence of a pause in the rhythm following a rapid rate may be an indication that the rapid rate was an artefact. In this tracing, the rapid artefact stops and there is no pause in the QRS rate.

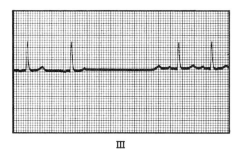

III

Fig. 11.139 Pause ends with a T wave. The pause in this tracing might have been real except for the undue evenness of the baseline, and the fact that the pause ends with a T wave, implying that there must have been a QRS complex preceding the T wave which was not recorded.

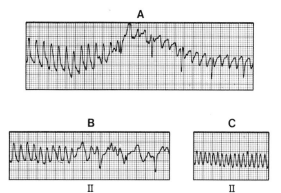

Fig. 11.140 Identification of an artefact at a different point in time. These tracings were both recorded from a 24-hour electrocardiogram. In the first tracing (A), it is not possible to identify the rhythm. It appears that there is a rapid, wide QRS rhythm which inexplicably changes to a rhythm simulating atrial flutter with block. In (B), 4 hours later, the artefact has a similar morphology but actually disappears before the last QRS complex in the tracing. Finally, in (C), the artefact has become even smaller in size and now has an unphysiologic rate, identifying the entire process as an artefact.

7. Artefacts may be phasic with external influences. Knowledge of the rate of the artefact may help to predict the external source. The infusion pump artefact shown in Figure 11.129 occurred at the same rate as the infusion: 56 times/min (interval 1.07 s between artefacts). Muscle movement related to respiration should occur between 15 and 60 times/min (interval every 1–4 s) (see Fig. 11.121); or toothbrushing occurs at approximately a rate of 300/min (interval of 200 ms) (Fig. 11.135).

8. Artefacts usually occur more than once. Even if a wave on the electrocardiogram cannot be positively identified as either due to depolarisation of the heart or due to an artefact, further observation of the remainder of the tracing or a subsequent tracing (perhaps under different circumstances with a more rapid or slower heart rate) will usually reveal the true identity (Fig. 11.140).

Despite all the guidelines, occasionally it is impossible to distinguish artefact from arrhythmia (Fig. 11.141). In these cases clinical correlation is mandatory. A faulty interpretation of an artefact may cause an 'electrocardiographic casualty'. Sometimes these casualties are fatal.

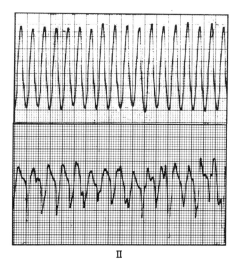

II

Fig. 11.141 Which is the artefact? The top tracing is ventricular tachycardia; the bottom tracing is the artefact.

ACKNOWLEDGEMENTS

The figures in this chapter are reproduced with permission from A. Garson Jr: The electrocardiogram in infants and children: A systematic approach. Lea & Febiger.

I would like to thank my assistant, Candy Killebrew, in general for her support throughout this endeavour, and in specific for typing and editing the manuscript several times. I would also like to thank Dr Andre Davignon and Pentii Rautaharju for supplying their tables of the normal values for the electrocardiograms. Finally, I would like to thank the staff of the Electrocardiographic Laboratory, Texas Children's Hospital: Pat McVey, Americo Simonelli, Donalee Cushman, Sandra Jordan, Alice Mast and Pauline Rousch. They recorded the high quality electrocardiograms displayed in the figures; they helped to find the examples which were included and refiled the majority which were not.

REFERENCES

Anderson G J, Woodburn R, Fisch C 1973 Cerebrovascular accident with unusual electrocardiographic changes. American Heart Journal 86: 395–398

Awa S, Linde L M, Oshima M, Okuni M 1970 The significance of late-phased dart T wave in the electrocardiogram of children. American Heart Journal 80: 619–628

Awa S, Linde L M, Oshima M, Momma K, Nakamura N, Yanagisawa M, Yoshiro K 1971 Isolated T wave inversion in the electrocardiogram of children. American Heart Journal 81: 158–165

Bachmann G 1916 The inter-auricular time inverval. American Journal of Physiology 41:309

Bazett H C 1918 An analysis of the time relations of electrocardiograms. Heart 7: 353–370

Biancaniello T M, Bisset G S, Gaum W E, Meyer R A, Kaplan S 1980 Left atrial size in childhood. Journal of Electrocardiology 13: 11–16

Bissett G S, Schwartz D C, Meyer R A, James F W, Kaplan S 1980 Clinical spectrum and long-term followup of isolated mitral valve prolapse in 119 children. Circulation 62: 423–428

Boineau J P, Spach M S, Ayers C R 1964 Genesis of the electrocardiogram in atrial septal defect. American Heart Journal 68: 637–642

Boineau J P, Moore E N, Patterson D F 1973 Relationship between the electrocardiogram, ventricular activity and the conduction system in ostium primum atrial septal defect. Circulation 48: 556–562

Boineau J P, Schuessler R B, Hackel D B, Wylds A C, Miller C B, Brockus C W 1980 Multicentric distribution and rate differentiation in the atrial pacemaker system. In: Little R C (ed) Physiology of Atrial Pacemakers and Conductive Tissues, Futura Publishing Inc., Mt. Kisco, New York, p 221–260

Bordiuk J M, Gelband H, Steeg C N, Tasker W 1969 Electrocardiographic changes in children undergoing pneumoencephalography. Neurology 19: 1217–1222

Brechenmacher C 1975 Atrio-His bundle tracts. British Heart Journal 37: 853–855

Brohet C R, Styns M, Arraud P, Brasseur L A 1978 Vectorcardiographic diagnosis of right ventricular hypertrophy in the presence of right bundle branch block in young subjects. American Journal of Cardiology 42: 602–612

Bruce M A, Spodick D H 1980 Atypical electrocardiogram in acute pericarditis: characteristics and prevalence. Journal of Electrocardiography 13: 61–66

Burch G E, DePasquale N P 1967 Electrocardiography in the diagnosis of congenital heart disease. Lea & Febiger, Philadelphia, p 30–105

Burda C D 1968 Electrocardiographic abnormalities induced by thioridazine (Mellaril). American Heart Journal 76: 153–156

Burgess M J 1972 Physiologic basis of the T wave. In: Schlant R C, Hurst J W (eds) Advances in electrocardiography. Grune & Stratton, New York, p 367–375

Cabrera C E, Monroy J R 1952 Systolic and diastolic loading of the heart. II. Electrocardiographic data. American Heart Journal 43: 669–680

Calleja H B 1966 Diagnostic value of electrocardiographic changes in pneumonectomies. Cardiologia 49: 228–238

Castellanos A, Salhanick P 1967 Electrocardiographic patterns of procainamide toxicity. American Journal of the Medical Sciences 253: 52–60

Cayler G C, Ongley P, Nadas A S 1958 Relation of systolic pressure in the right ventricle to the electrocardiogram. New England Journal of Medicine 258: 979–982

Chou T 1979 Electrocardiography in clinical practice. Grune & Stratton, New York, p 114–150

Colletti R B, Pan M W, Smith E W P, Genel M 1974 Detection of hypocalcemia in susceptible neonates: the QOTC interval. New England Journal of Medicine 290: 931–935

Cooksey J D, Dunn M, Massie E 1977 Clinical vectorcardiography and electrocardiography, 2nd Edn. Year Book, Chicago

Cranefield P 1975 The conduction of the cardiac impulse: The slow response and cardiac arrhythmias. Futura Publishing, New York, p 3–25

Davignon A, Rautaharju P, Boisselle E, Soumis F, Megelas M,

Choquette A 1979 Normal ECG standards for infants and children. Pediatric Cardiology 1: 123–131

De Leon A C, Perloff J K, Twigg H 1965 The straight back syndrome. Clinical cardiovascular manifestations. Circulation 32: 193–200

De Oliveira J M, Sambi M P, Zinnerman H A 1958 The electrocardiogram in pectus excavatum. British Heart Journal 20: 495–499

Di Segni E, Klein H O, David D, Libhaber C, Kaplinsky E 1980 Overdrive pacing in quinidine syncope and other long QT interval syndromes. Archives of Internal Medicine 140: 1036–1040

Dickinson D F, Wilkinson J L, Anderson K R, Smith A, Ho S Y, Anderson R H 1979 The cardiac conduction system in situs ambiguus. Circulation 59: 879–885

Dominguez P, Lendrum B L, Pick A 1959 False 'coronary patterns' in the infant electrocardiogram. Circulation 19: 400–419

Drory Y, Ouaknine E, Kosary I Z, Kellermann J J 1975 Electrocardiographic findings in brain death; description and presumed mechanism. Chest 67: 425–432

Dubin S, Staib J 1977 Numerical calculation of the mean electrical axis of electrocardiographic deflections. Journal of Electrocardiology 10: 77–78

Dubnow M H, Burchell H B, Titus J L 1965 Postinfarction ventricular aneurysm. American Heart Journal 70: 753–760

Durnin R E, Ziska J H, Zellweger T 1971 Observations on the electrocardiogram in Duchenne's muscular dystrophy. Helvetica Paediatrica Acta 26: 331–339

Durrer D, Van Dam R, Freud G, Janse M J, Meijler F L, Arzbaecher R C 1970 Total excitation of the isolated human heart. Circulation 41: 899–912

Ellison R C, Freedom R M, Keane J F, Nugent E W, Rowe R D, Miettinen O S 1977 Indirect assessment of severity in pulmonary stenosis. Circulation 56: 15–20

Emslie-Smith D, Sladden G E, Stirling G R 1959 The significance of changes in the electrocardiogram in hypothermia. British Heart Journal 21: 343–355

Ertugrul A 1966 A new electrocardiographic observation in infants and children with hyperthyroidism. Pediatrics 37: 669–672

Esscher E, Hardell L, Michaelson M 1975 Familial isolated complete right bundle branch block. British Heart Journal 37: 745–747

Fouron J, Chicoine R 1971 ECG changes in fatal imipramine (Tofranil) intoxication. Pediatrics 48: 777–781

Franco-Vasquez S, Sutherland R D, Fowler M, Edwards J E 1970 Congenital aneurysm of the left ventricular base. Chest 57: 411–415

Frank E 1955 Determination of the electrical center of ventricular depolarization in the human heart. American Heart Journal 49: 670–676

Fujiwara H, Chen C, Fujiwara T, Nishioka K, Kawai C, Hemashima Y 1980 Clinicopathologic of abnormal Q waves in Kawasaki disease. American Journal of Cardiology 45: 797–805

Fukushige J, Nihill M R, McNamara D G 1980 The spectrum of cardiovascular lesions in the mucocutaneous lymph node syndrome. American Journal of Cardiology 45: 98–107

Gallagher J J, Smith W M, Kasell J H, Benson D W, Sterba R, Grant A O 1981 Role of Mahaim fibers in cardiac arrhythmias in man. Circulation 64: 176–189

Garson A, 1981 Supraventricular tachycardia. In: Gillette P C, Garson A (eds) Pediatric cardiac dysrhythmias. Grune & Stratton, New York, Ch 7, p 177–254

Garson A, Gillette P C, McNamara D G (eds) 1980 A guide to cardiac dysrhythmias in children. Grune & Stratton, New York, p 10

Garson A, McNamara D G, Cooley D A 1981a Postoperative tetralogy of Fallot. In: Engle M A (ed) Pediatric cardiovascular disease. F.A. Davis, Philadelphia, p 407–430

Garson A, Gillette P C, McNamara D G 1981b Supraventricular tachycardia in children: clinical features, response to treatment, and long-term follow-up in 217 patients. Journal of Pediatrics 98: 875–882

Garson A, Porter C J, Gillette P C 1986 Ventricular tachycardia induction during electrophysiologic study after repair of tetralogy of Fallot. Pediatric Cardiology (in press)

Gelband H, Waldo A L, Kaiser G A, Bowman F O Jr, Malm J R,

Hoffman B F 1971 Etiology of right bundle branch block in patients undergoing total correction of tetralogy of Fallot. Circulation 44: 1022–1033

Gerard R, Lasry F, Seichter J, Malfroy P, Jouve A 1969 Les criteres electrocardiographiques de surcharge ventriculaire droite chez l'enfant. I. Les surcharges systoliques. Archives des Maladies de Coeur et des Vaisseaux 62: 1049–1071

Gerard R, Seichter J, Lasry F, Jouve A 1971 Les criteres de surcharge ventriculaire gauche distonique chez l'enfant dans le canal arteriel et la communication interventriculaire. Archives des Maladies de Coeur et des Vaisseaux 64: 1590–1612

Giacoia G P, Wagner H R 1978 Q-TC interval and blood calcium levels in newborn infants. Pediatrics 61: 877–882

Gillette P C, Nihill M R, Singer D B 1974a Electrophysiologic mechanism of the short PR interval in Pompe's disease. American Journal of Diseases in Children 128: 622–626

Gillette P C, El-Said G M, Sivarajan N 1974b Electrophysiologic abnormalities after Mustard's operation for transposition of the great arteries. British Heart Journal 36: 186–191

Gillette P C, Yeoman M A, Mullins C E 1977 Sudden death after repair of tetralogy of Fallot: electrocardiographic and electrophysiologic abnormalities. Circulation 57: 566–577

Grant R P, Estes E H, Doyle J T 1951 Spatial vector electrocardiography. The clinical characteristics of ST and T vectors. Circulation 3: 182–197

Gross H, Rubin I L, Dardick I 1967 Abnormal Q waves in a child with myocarditis. New York State Journal of Medicine 67: 283–287

Gumbiner C H 1981 Bundle branch and fascicular block. In: Gillette P C, Garson A (eds) Pediatric cardiac dysrhythmias. Grune & Stratton, New York, p 405–419

Haas G 1911 Ueber die gefassversorgung des reizleitungssystems des herzens. Anat Hefte 43: 629–635

Hait G, Gasul B M 1963 The evaluation and significance of T wave changes in the normal newborn during the first seven days of life. American Journal of Cardiology 28: 494–504

Hayes C J, Butler V P, Gersony W M 1973 Serum digoxin studies in infants and children. Pediatrics 52: 561–568

Ho S Y, Anderson R H 1985 Conduction tissue in congenital heart surgery. World Journal of Surgery 9: 550–567

Hoffman J I E 1975a The place of electrocardiography in pediatric cardiology. Praxis 64: 816–822

Hoffman J I E 1975b Primary T wave changes in children. Praxis 64: 803–811

Horowitz L N, Greenspan A M, Spielman S R, Josephson M E 1981 Torsades de Pointes: electrophysiologic studies in patients without transient pharmacologic or metabolic abnormalities. Circulation 63: 1120–1128

Husson G S, Blackman M S, Rogers M C 1973 Familial congenital bundle branch system disease. American Journal of Cardiology 32: 365–369

James T N 1963 The connecting pathways between the sinus node and AV node and between the right and left atrium in the human heart. American Heart Journal 66: 498–508

James T N 1967 Congenital deafness and cardiac arrhythmias. American Journal of Cardiology 19: 627–643

James T N 1977 The sinus node. American Journal of Cardiology 40: 965–986

Janse M J, Anderson R H 1974 Specialized internodal atrial pathways, fact or fiction. European Journal of Cardiology 2: 117–136

Jervell A, Lange-Nielsen F 1957 Congenital deafmutism, functional heart disease with prolongation of the Q-T interval and sudden death. American Heart Journal 54: 59–68

Kang P S, Gomes J A C, Kelen G, El-Sherif N 1981 Role of autonomic regulatory mechanisms in sinoatrial conduction and sinus node automaticity in sick sinus syndrome. Circulation 64: 832–838

Kangos J J, Ferrer I, Franciosi R A, Blanc W A, Blumenthal S 1969 Electrocardiographic changes associated with papillary muscle infarction in congenital heart disease. American Heart Journal 23: 801–809

Karhunen P, Ludmanmaki K, Heikkila J, Eisalo A 1970 Syncope and QT prolongation without deafness: the Romano-Ward syndrome. American Heart Journal 80: 820–823

Katz L N, Wachtel H 1937 The biphasic QRS type of electrocardiogram in congenital heart disease. American Heart Journal 13: 202–206

Keith J D 1959 Anomalous left coronary artery from the pulmonary artery. British Heart Journal 21: 149–156

Kugler J D 1981 Sinoatrial node dysfunction. In: Gillette P C, Garson A (eds) Pediatric cardiac dysrhythmias. Grune & Stratton, New York, ch. 9 p 265–293

Kulangara R J, Boineau J P, Moore H V, Rao P S 1981 Ventricular activation and genesis of QRS in tricuspid atresia. Circulation 64:225

Kulbertus H, Demoulin J 1975 The conduction system: anatomical and pathologic aspects. In: Krikler D, Goodwin S (eds) Cardiac arrhythmias. The modern electrophysiologic approach. Saunders, London, p 16–38

Kulbertus H E, Demoulin J 1976 Pathological findings in patients with left anterior hemiblock. In: Hoffman I, Hamby R I (eds) Vectorcardiography 3. North-Holland, Amsterdam

Larese R J, Mirkin B L 1974 Kinetics of digoxin absorption and relation of serum levels to cardiac arrhythmias in children. Clinical Pharmacology and Therapeutics 15: 387–396

Lepeschkin E 1951 Modern electrocardiography. Williams & Wilkins, Baltimore, p 1

Lepeschkin E 1969 The U wave of the electrocardiogram. Modern Concepts of Cardiovascular Disease 38: 39–45

Lepeschkin E, Surawicz B 1952 The measurement of the QT interval of the electrocardiogram. Circulation 6: 378–388

Lev M, Bharati S 1977 Anatomy of the conduction system in normal and congenitally abnormal hearts. In: Roberts N K, Gelband H (eds) Cardiac arrhythmias in the neonate, infant and child. Appleton Century Crofts, New York, p 29–50

Liebman J, Plonsey R 1978 Electrocardiography. In: Moss A J, Adams F H, Emmanovillides G C (eds) Heart disease in infants, children and adolescents, 2nd Edn. Williams & Wilkins, Baltimore, p 18–61

Lown B, Ganong W F, Levine S A 1952 The syndrome of short P-R interval, narrow QRS complex and paroxysmal rapid heart action. Circulation 5: 663–670

Mahaim I, Benatt A 1938 Nouvelles recherches sur les connexions superieures de la branche gauche du faisceau de His-Tawara avec cloison interventriculaire. Cardiologia 1: 61–71

Malecka-Dymnicka S, Bittel-Dobrzynska N 1966 Electrocardiographic changes in children with hyperthyroidism. Polish Medical Journal 5: 540–545

Marriott H J L 1972 Practical electrocardiography, 5th Edn. Williams & Wilkins, Baltimore, p 16–50

Mashima S, Fu L Fukushima K 1969 The ventricular gradient and the vectorcardiographic T loop in left ventricular hypertrophy. Journal of Electrocardiology 2: 55–62

Mehta J, Desnick R J 1978 Abbreviated PR interval in mannosidosis. Journal of Pediatrics 92: 599–600

Merideth J, Titus J L 1968 The anatomic atrial connections between sinus and AV node. Circulation 37: 566–571

Millar K, Abildskov J A 1968 Notched T waves in young persons with central nervous system lesions. Circulation 37: 597–603

Miller B L, Dumas P A, Victorica B E 1970 Office electrocardiography in general pediatrics VII: electrolyte effects. Clinical Pediatrics 9: 72–78

Mirowski M, Neill C A, Taussig H B 1963 Left atrial ectopic rhythm in mirror image dextrocardia and in normally placed malformed hearts. Report of 12 cases with 'dome and dart' P waves. Circulation 27: 864–877

Momma K, Linde L M 1969 Abnormal P wave axis in congenital heart disease associated with asplenia and polysplenia. Journal of Electrocardiology 2: 395–405

Morganroth J, Maron B J, Krovetz L J, Henry W L, Epstein S E 1975 Electrocardiographic evidence of left ventricular hypertrophy in otherwise normal children: clarification by echocardiography. American Journal of Cardiology 35: 278–281

Morris J J Jr, Estes E H Jr, Whalen R E 1964 P wave analysis in valvular heart disease. Circulation 29:242

Morris S N, Zipes D P 1973 His bundle electrocardiography during bidirectional ventricular tachycardia. Circulation 48: 32–38

Neches W H, Park S C, Mathews R A 1979 Management of surgical complete atrioventricular block in children. American Journal of Cardiology 43: 1175–1180

Okuni M 1975 A proposal of new pediatric electrocardiographic criteria for ventricular hypertrophy. Japanese Heart Journal 23: 189–195

Perloff J K, Roberts W C, DeLeon A C, O'Doherty D 1967 The distinctive electrocardiogram of Duchenne's progressive muscular dystrophy. American Journal of Medicine 42: 179–188

Perloff J K 1970 The clinical recognition of congenital heart disease. Saunders, Philadelphia, p 237

Pilapil V R, Watson D G 1970 The electrocardiogram in hyperthyroid children. American Journal of Diseases in Children 119: 245–248

Puri P S, Rowe R D, Neill C A 1966 Varying vector cardiographic patterns in anomalous left coronary artery arising from the pulmonary artery. American Heart Journal 71: 616–626

Reder R F, Rosen M R 1981 Basic electrophysiologic principles: application to treatment of dysrhythmias. In: Gillette P C, Garson A (eds) Pediatric cardiac dysrhythmias. Grune & Stratton, New York, Ch 4, p 121–143

Reeves W C, Hallahan W, Schwiter E J, Citiola T J, Buonocore E, Davidson C O 1981 Two dimensional echocardiographic assessment of electrocardiographic criteria for right atrial enlargement. Circulation 64: 387–391

Reynolds J L 1971 The electrocardiographic recognition of right atrial abnormality in children. American Heart Journal 81: 748–759

Rodriguez-Torres R, Lin J, Berkovitch S 1969 A sensitive ECG sign in myocarditis associated with viral infection. Pediatrics 43: 846–851

Rodriguez-Torres R, Schureck L, Klienberg W 1971 Electrocardiographic and biochemical abnormalities in Tay-Sachs disease. Bulletin of the New York Academy of Medicine 47:717

Rogers M C, Zakha K G, Nugent S K, Gioia F R, Epple L 1980 Electrocardiographic abnormalities in infants and children with neurological injury. Critical Care Medicine 8: 213–214

Rollason W N 1976 Electrocardiography for the anesthetist, 3rd Edn. Blackwell, London, p 63–80

Romano C, Gemme G, Pongiglione R 1963 Aritmie cardiache rare dell'eta' pediatrica. II. Accessi sincopali per fibrillazione ventricolare parossistica. Clinical Pediatrics 45: 656–683

Rosenbaum F F, Hecht H H, Wilson F N, Johnston F D 1945 The potential variations of the thorax and esophagus in anomalous atrioventricular excitation (WPW syndrome). American Heart Journal 29: 281–300

Rosenbaum M B, Elizari M V, Lazzari J O 1970 The hemiblocks, Tampa tracings. Oldsmar, Florida, p 30–60

Roudebush C P, Foerster J M, Bing O H L 1973 The abbreviated PR interval of Fabry's disease. New England Journal of Medicine 289:357

Sachder J C, Puri D 1967 Electrocardiographic alterations in diphtheria. Indian Journal of Pediatrics 34: 429–431

Sahn D J, Vaucher Y E 1976 Electrical current leakage transmitted to an infant via an IV controller: an unusual ECG artifact. Journal of Pediatrics 89: 301–302

Sanyal S K, Vijayalaxmi B, Sharma S, Vaishnava S, Madhavan S 1973 Evaluation of terminal P-V$_1$ index in assessment of left atrial enlargement in childhood. Indian Journal of Medical Research 61:1868

Schaal S F, Seidensticker J, Goodman R 1973 Familial right bundle branch block, left axis deviation, complete heart block, and early death. A heritable disorder of cardiac conduction. Annals of Internal Medicine 79: 63–66

Schatz J, Krongrad E, Malm J R 1976 Left anterior and left posterior hemiblock in tricuspid atresia and transposition of the great arteries. Circulation 54: 1010–1013

Scher A M 1976 Excitation of the heart. In: Nelson C V, Geselowitz D B (eds) The theoretical basis of electrocardiography. Clarendon, Oxford, p 44–95

Schwartz P J, Periti M, Malliani A 1975 The long Q-T syndrome. American Heart Journal 89: 378–390

Sleeper J C, Orgain E S 1963 Differentiation of benign from pathologic T waves in the electrocardiogram. American Journal of Cardiology 11: 338–348

Smith R E, Hyde C M 1969 Computer analysis of the electrocardiogram in clinical practice. In: Manning G W, Ahuja S P (eds) Electrical activity of the heart. Thomas, Springfield, p 305

Sodi-Polares D, Calder R M 1956 New bases of electrocardiography. Mosby, St Louis, p 23–28

Spach M S, Barr R C 1976 Cardiac anatomy from an electrophysiologic viewpoint. In: Nelson C V, Geselowitz D B (eds) The theoretical basis of electrocardiography. Clarendon Press, Oxford, p 1–23

Spach M S, Miller W T, Barr R C, Geselowitz D B 1980 Electrophysiology of the internodal pathways. In: Little R C (ed) Physiology of atrial pacemakers and conductive tissues. Futura, New York, p 367–380

Sreenivasan V, Fisher B J, Liebman J, Downs T D 1973 Longitudinal study of the standard electrocardiogram in the healthy premature infant during the first year of life. American Journal of Cardiology 31: 57–71

Stanger P, Lister G, Silverman N H, Hoffman J I E 1977 Electrocardiograph monitor artifacts in a neonatal intensive care unit. Pediatrics 60: 689–695

Sung R J, Tamer D M, Agha A S, Castellanos A, Myerburg R J, Gelband H 1975 Etiology of the electrocardiographic pattern of 'incomplete right bundle branch block' in atrial septal defect: an electrophysiologic study. Journal of Pediatrics 87: 1182–1186

Surawicz B 1966 Primary and secondary T wave changes. Heart Bulletin 15: 31–35

Surawicz B 1967 Relationship between the electrocardiogram and electrolytes. American Heart Journal 73: 814–825

Surawicz B 1972 The pathogenesis and clinical significance of primary T wave abnormalities. In: Schlant R C, Hurst J W (eds) Advances in electrocardiography. Grune & Stratton, New York, p 377–421

Tapia F A, Proudfit W L 1960 Secondary R waves in right precordial leads in normal persons and in patients with cardiac disease. Circulation 21: 28–35

Ten Eick R E, Singer D H 1979 Electrophysiological properties of diseased human atrium. I. Low diastolic potential and altered cellular response to potassium. Circulation Research 44: 545–557

Thapar M K, Gillette P C 1979 Dual atrioventricular nodal pathways: a common electrophysiologic response in children. Circulation 60: 1369–1374

Thomsen J H, Wasserburger R H 1967 Effect of hyperventilation on precordial T waves of children and adolescents. Circulation 36: 700–707

Thorel C 1910 Ueber den aufbau des sinusknotens und seine verbindung mit der cava superior und den Wenkebachschen bundeln. Munchener Medizinische Wochenschrift 57: 183–191

Van Mierop L H S, Wiglesworth F W 1962 Isomerism of the cardiac atria in the asplenia syndrome. Laboratory Investigation 11: 1303–315

Wagner H R, Weidman W H, Ellison R C, Miettinen O S 1977 Indirect assessment of severity in aortic stenosis. Circulation 56: 20–23

Waldo A L, Bush H L Jr, Gelband H, Zorn G L, Vitikainen K J, Hoffman B F 1971 Effects on the canine P wave in discrete lesions in the specialized atrial tracts. Circulation Research 29: 452–460

Ward O C 1964 A new familial cardiac syndrome in children. Journal of the Irish Medical Association 54: 103–106

Wasserburger R H 1963 The normal and abnormal unipolar electrocardiogram in infants and children. Williams & Wilkins, Baltimore, p 64–100

Wasserburger R H, Young W P, Siebecker K, Hawkins L K, Banforth B, King J T 1962 Further electrocardiographic observations on direct epicardial potentials in congenital heart lesions. Differential features of right ventricular preponderance and right bundle branch block. Circulation 26: 561–573

Watanabe Y 1975 Purkinje repolarization as a possible cause of the U wave in the electrocardiogram. Circulation 51: 1030–1037

Watanabe Y, Dreifus L S 1977 Cardiac arrhythmias. Grune & Stratton, New York, p 208–209

Way G L, Pierce J R, Wolfe R R, McGrath R, Wiggins J, Merenstein G B 1979 ST depression suggesting subendocardial injury in neonates with respiratory distress syndrome and patent ductus arteriosus. Journal of Pediatrics 95: 609–611

Weidmann S 1965 The functional significance of the intercalated discs. In: Taccardi B, Marchetti G (eds) Electrophysiology of the heart. Pergamon Press, London, p. 43–72

Wolff L, Parkinson J, White P D 1930 Bundle branch block with short PR interval in healthy young people prone to paroxysmal tachycardia. American Heart Journal 5: 686–692

Wolpert A, Farr D 1975 Psychotropics and their effect on the electrocardiogram in children. Diseases of the Nervous System 36: 435–436

Echocardiography

Of all the technical advances in paediatric cardiology during the last two decades, echocardiography has made the most impact on clinical practice. A basic understanding of the physics of ultrasound is an advantage for the paediatric cardiologist. For this, reference can be made to the reviews of Wells (1978) and Bom et al (1981). Two systems are in use for cardiac ultrasound, namely M-mode and cross-sectional echocardiography. M-mode echocardiography employs a single ultrasound beam directed to the heart. The beam is reflected from the cardiac structures and received back by the transducer. Reflected signals are displayed in 'motion mode' with time along the horizontal axis. This presentation permits the recording of amplitudes, pattern and rate of motion of moving objects with great accuracy, the sampling rate being essentially the pulse frequency of the transducer. Although occasionally described as 'one-dimensional', this is incorrect, as time is the second dimension on M-mode tracings. The M-mode beam may be moved to obtain different 'slices' through the heart or a continuous sweep can be recorded between different positions by moving the transducer through an arc.

While M-mode echocardiography has proved very valuable for recording the motion of cardiac structures parallel to the ultrasound beam, it has major limitations. It cannot provide information on motion at right angles to the beam and cannot provide a composite picture of the intracardiac anatomy. As a result it has never made a major impact on the management of patients with congenital heart disease, in whom knowledge of the anatomy is all important. Cross-sectional echocardiography, in contrast, has enormous advantages for the paediatric cardiologist. With this technique, the ultrasound beam is moved rapidly through an arc so that a series of lines is built up into a composite picture. This can be recorded in real-time, resulting in a recognisable moving picture of the cardiac structures. The ultrasound beam can be moved mechanically or be steered electronically using multiple ultrasound elements (phased array). The images are generally recorded on video-tape so that the temporal sampling frequency is significantly poorer than in M-mode recordings. The choice of ultrasound frequency is influenced by the size of the patient. When penetration is important, as in the older child or adult, a low frequency (e.g. 3 MH) transducer is required. Higher frequency transducers (5 or 7 MH and even higher) can be used in smaller patients with improved spatial resolution. Although M-mode echocardiography pre-dates the cross-sectional techniques, the principles of M-mode scanning are best described by reference to the cross-sectional images. We therefore think it will be more informative if the two techniques are described side-by-side. Both are valuable. The strength of the cross-sectional format is its display of anatomical relationships. M-mode comes into its own for the study of dynamics and the measurement of dimensions. This introductory chapter will be concluded with a brief review of the more recently developed Doppler techniques, which have much to offer for evaluation of function.

NORMAL CARDIAC ANATOMY

For the first time, with cross-sectional echocardiography, the clinician has at his disposal the technique to illustrate cardiac anatomy in the detail seen by the morphologist. To appreciate this detail, he must understand the morphology. This has not always been made easy for him. It has been rare to find cardiac anatomy presented as the heart is orientated within the body. For example, the mitral valve is usually illustrated by incising the atrioventricular junction and 'spreading' the valve leaflets and papillary muscles. This gives a totally false impression of the papillary muscle disposition. In life, they are adjacent. The echocardiographic sections display the anatomy in cross-section. It is helpful, therefore, if the morphologist displays the anatomy in similar fashion (Walmsley & Waston, 1978; Tajik et al, 1978; Edwards et al, 1981; Silverman et al, 1983). Understanding is helped further by illustrating the anatomical sections in the normal orientation of the heart in life (Silverman et al, 1983; Gutgesell,

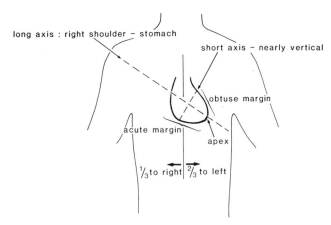

Fig. 12.1 The orientation and position of the cardiac silhouette relative to the thorax.

1985). Normally the long axis of the heart is oblique, extending more or less from the left subcostal region to the right shoulder (Fig. 12.1). This means that the heart does not stand on its apex in St. Valentine's fashion (Anderson & Becker, 1980; Edwards et al, 1981). In addition to the long axis being oblique, the cardiac chambers, particularly the ventricles, are arranged so that the morphologically right structures are anterior to their morphologically left counterparts. Thus, the left atrium is the most posterior of the cardiac chambers. Only its appendage projects to the border of the cardiac silhouette. The right ventricle lies anterior to the left ventricle. It swings across the front of the ventricular mass from the inferior and right-sided tricuspid valve to the anterosuperiorly positioned pulmonary valve (Fig. 12.2). The pulmonary valve is left-sided in relation to the aortic valve, which is embedded within the centre of the heart and related to all four cardiac chambers.

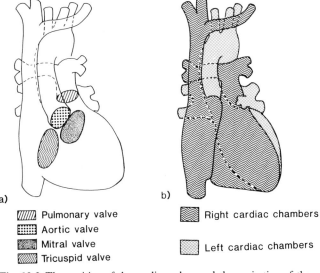

Pulmonary valve

Aortic valve

Mitral valve

Tricuspid valve

Right cardiac chambers

Left cardiac chambers

Fig. 12.2 The position of the cardiac valves and the projection of the cardiac chambers relative to the cardiac silhouette.

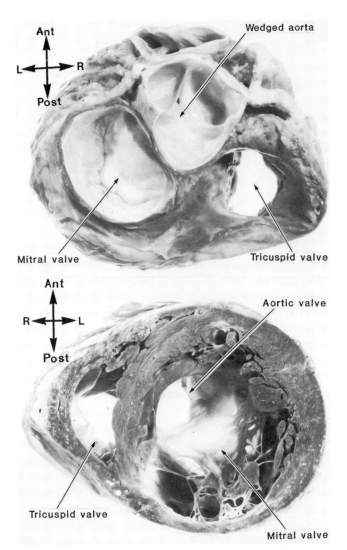

Fig. 12.3 The short axis sections of the atrioventricular junction. (a) The anatomic orientation, viewing the atrial surfaces of the atrioventricular valves and the aortic surface of the aortic valve. Note the deeply wedged position of the aorta. (b) The view as would be seen by the echocardiographer. Note how the wedged aorta lifts the mitral valve away from the septum.

This central position of the aortic valve, wedged between the tricuspid and mitral valves, is the key to the understanding of cardiac anatomy.

Careful study of the short-axis section of the heart as viewed from the atrial aspect (Fig. 12.3a), although not displayed in an orientation in keeping with our philosophy of correlating with echocardiographic images, does provide the necessary understanding to appreciate the echocardiographic short axis view (Fig. 12.3b). Because of the wedge position of the aortic valve, the posterior extension of the subaortic outflow tract lifts away the 'septal' leaflet of the mitral valve from the inlet septum. The orientation of the mitral orifice in the normal heart is consequently oblique, with papillary muscles in anterolateral and postero-medial position (Fig. 12.4a). There are no direct attach-

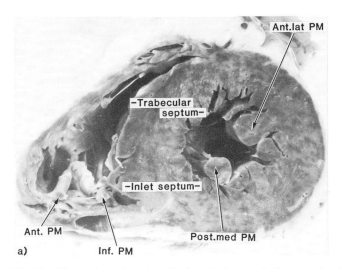
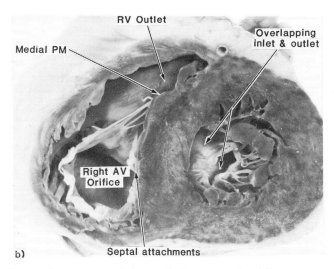

Fig. 12.4 Short axis sections (a & b) through the ventricular mass showing the curved arrangement of the ventricular septum, the oblique orientation of the left ventricular papillary muscles, and the close apposition of the septal leaflet of the tricuspid valve to the inlet septum.

ments of tension apparatus to the inlet septum in the left ventricle. In contrast, the septal leaflet of the tricuspid valve truly hugs the inlet septum and is attached to it by tension apparatus along its length (Fig. 12.4b). The short axis cuts emphasise other significant differences between the right and left sides of the normal heart. The arterial and atrioventricular valves in the right ventricle are separated by the posterior part of the subpulmonary infundibulum – the ventriculo-infundibular fold. This fold in the left ventricle, which represents the inner curvature of the heart wall, is attenuated so that the aortic and mitral valves are in fibrous continuity. One further vital (but poorly understood) area of the normal heart is intimately connected with the wedge position of the aorta. This is the area of the atrioventricular septum. This part of the septum has two components. One is made of fibrous tissue and is an integral part of the central fibrous body – the atrioventricular membranous septum. This interposes between the medial wall of the subaortic outflow tract and the right atrium (Fig. 12.5b). The other septum is a muscular structure (Fig. 12.5a). It exists because the attachment of the tricuspid valve leaflet to the septum is more towards the ventricular apex than that of the mitral valve. Consequently, in the area between these attachments (very much towards the crux of the heart), the atrial and ventricular septal structures overlap and form the

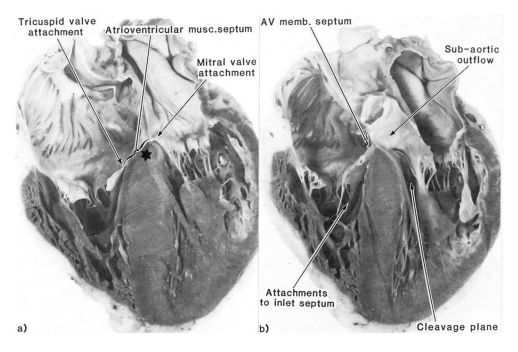

Fig. 12.5 Simulated four chamber sections through the heart showing (a) the atrioventricular muscular septum, and (b) the wedged position of the subaortic outflow tract and the membranous septum.

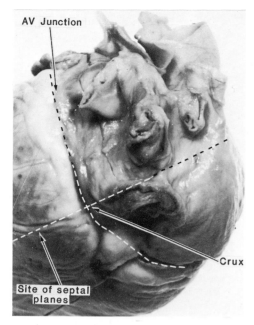

Fig. 12.6 A normal heart photographed from its posterior aspect to illustrate the anatomic crux. This is the crossing point of the atrioventricular junction with the planes of the atrial and ventricular septal structures.

muscular atrioventricular septum. In this respect, the anatomist refers to the crux as the area on the diaphragmatic surface of the heart where the plane of the normal septal structures crosses the atrioventricular groove (Fig. 12.6).

The echocardiographer cannot see this point on the heart surface, but he can identify the equally important echocardiographic crux (Magherini et al, 1983; Russo et al, 1986). This is the area of the atrioventricular muscular septum, where it is the attachment of the valves that produces the cruciate appearance.

THE ECHOCARDIOGRAPHIC EXAMINATION

All of the cardiac anatomy described above is potentially amenable to dissection with the ultrasonic beam. The beginner will, however, immediately become aware that the ultrasound beam is obstructed both by bony structures and the air-filled lungs. Because of this, pictorial access from the body surface is limited, although fortunately the heart can be viewed from many different aspects. Unobstructed views can be obtained from the cardiac apex, from alongside the sternum via the intercostal spaces (the parasternal windows), from beneath the rib-cage (the subcostal approach), from the suprasternal notch, and from the supraclavicular regions (Fig. 12.7). More recently the heart has been visualised using a transducer placed within the oesophagus (Hanrath et al, 1983). From these various approaches, the heart and great vessels, according to their position within the chest, can be cut in most planes. Although in the normal heart it is possible to define 'standard' approaches (and these will be described below), visualisation and understanding of the

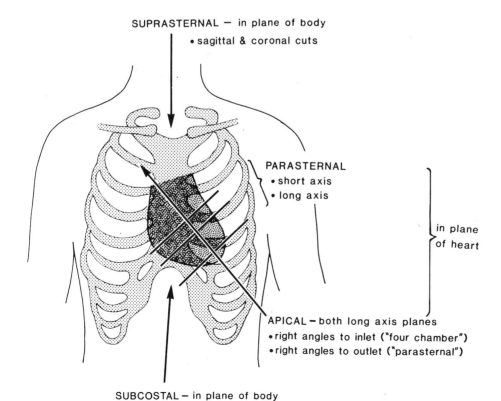

Fig. 12.7 The echocardiographic windows to the heart and the type of cuts that are obtainable through these windows.

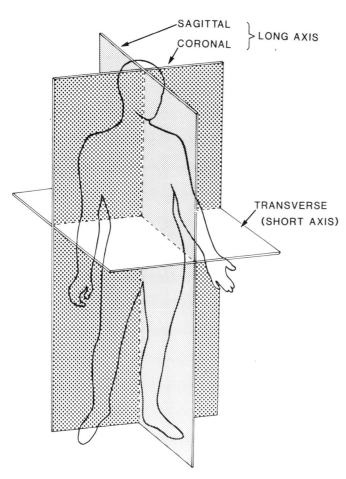

Fig. 12.8 The three orthogonal planes of the body which form the frames of reference for its description.

congenitally malformed heart is facilitated if the examiner develops a technique of orientation and identification based on points of reference which are internal to the heart and great vessels. For example, the sections obtained from the 'standard' approaches will be of little value when examining a heart in the right chest even though it may be structurally normal. The key to a universal system is to describe the heart, whatever its position, in terms of its three orthogonal planes. The three orthogonal planes of the body are the sagittal, coronal and short axis planes (Fig. 12.8). The axis of the heart rarely corresponds to the axis of the body. Nonetheless, it has its own orthogonal planes. There are again two long axis planes and a short axis plane, shown for the normally positioned heart in Figure 12.9. The index planes cannot all be obtained from a single echocardiographic window. Simple geometric principles dictate that from any given window it is possible to obtain only two basic planes, although intermediate cuts can be taken towards the third plane.

In the simplest terms, scanning from the apical window provides the two long axis planes of the heart itself (Fig. 12.10). The long axis plane at the right angles to the inlet septum is conventionally termed the 'four chamber plane' (Fig. 12.11). This is the plane which shows the anatomy of the atrioventricular septum. When taken through the membranous atrioventricular septum the section also incorporates part of the subaortic outflow tract (Fig. 12.5). Hence most of these cuts show more than the four basic cardiac chambers. Nonetheless, the 'four chamber' designation is a useful one. The long axis plane at right angles to the outlet part of the septum can, by analogy to the

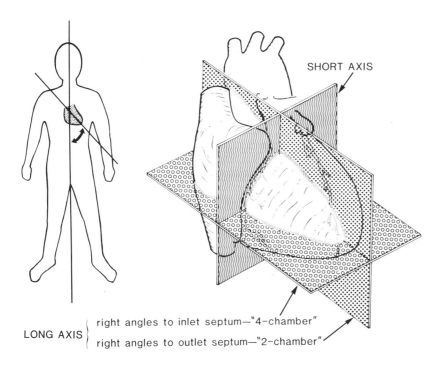

LONG AXIS { right angles to inlet septum—"4-chamber"
right angles to outlet septum—"2-chamber"

Fig. 12.9 The heart can also be described in terms of its orthogonal planes, but note the difference in orientation between the long axis cardiac planes and the long axis planes of the body.

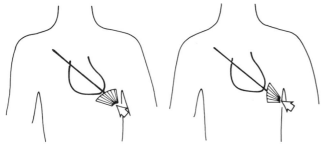

Sections along cardiac long axis

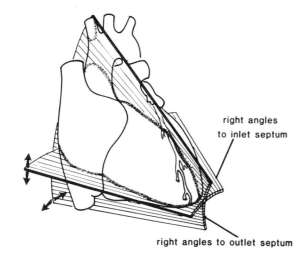

right angles
to inlet septum

right angles to outlet septum

Fig. 12.10 Sectioning from the apex permits both long axis planes to be obtained at right angles to the inlet septum (four chamber) and at right angles to the outlet septum (two chamber).

four chamber plane, be considered as a two-chamber plane (Fig. 12.12b). It also, in most cases, visualises part of the right ventricular outlet and illustrates more than the two basic chambers (Fig. 12.12a). The long axis two-chamber plane is one of the standard planes obtained from the parasternal window (Fig. 12.13), together with the series of short axis planes. When scanning from subcostal and suprasternal windows, it is no longer possible to cut a normally positioned heart in its own axes. This may be possible when the heart is malpositioned. The usually located heart, however, is cut in paracoronal and parasagittal planes (Fig. 12.14). From subcostal position this produces sections which are similar to, but differ subtly from, four chamber and short axis planes. For example, a paracoronal cut can on occasions replicate a heart with absent right atrioventricular connexion (Fig. 12.15), even when two normal atrioventricular valves are present. The parasagittal cuts show the ventricular outflow tracts to great advantage (Marino et al, 1984; Fig. 12.16). They also illustrate the long axis view of the aortic arch, although this is probably better seen from the suprasternal window (Smallhorn et al, 1982a). To obtain a complete impression of cardiac structures, many views must be used. Despite the need for presentation and description of echocardiographic findings in terms of 'cuts', the key to successful evaluation is to obtain continuous scans from one view to another. In practice, the echocardiographer builds up a three-dimensional whole from a series of two-dimensional parts. The experienced investigator will use any view, no matter how unorthodox, to attain this objective.

ECHOCARDIOGRAPHIC IDENTIFICATION OF CARDIAC STRUCTURES

Echocardiographic anatomy as discussed above has taken as its starting point the heart of the subject without any congenital cardiac malformations. Certain simple anomalies (such as persistence of the arterial duct) may be

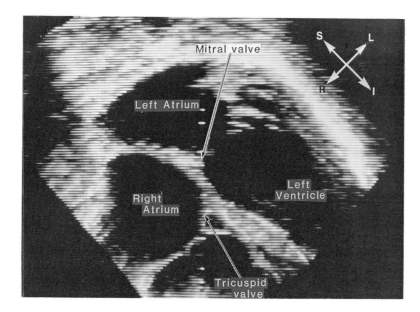

Fig. 12.11 The echocardiogram in the four chamber plane (right angles to the inlet septum). Note the offsetting of the attachments of the valves which produce the atrioventricular muscular septum (compare with Fig. 12.5).

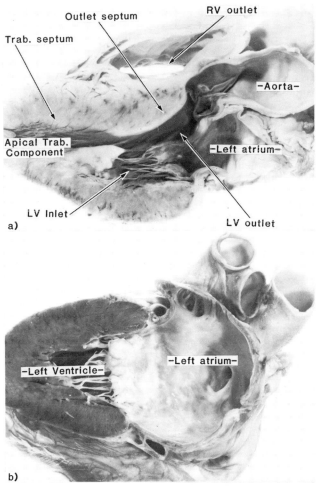

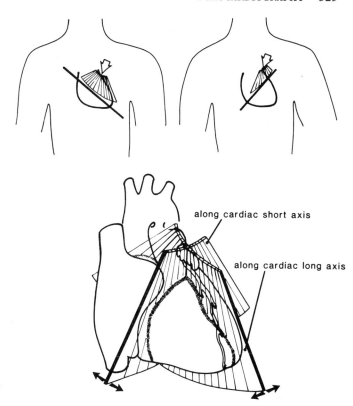

Fig. 12.13 Scanning from parasternal position permits the heart to be cut in the long axis plane at right angles to the outlet septum and in the cardiac short axis.

Fig. 12.12 Two simulated sections at right angles to the outlet septum. The upper panel (a) is the standard parasternal long axis section. The lower panel (b) is more towards the left cardiac border and shows a two chamber view of the left-sided structures.

Fig. 12.14 When scanning from subcostal position, the transducer beam moves more in the planes of the body than in the planes of the heart. Thus a series of paracoronal and parasagittal cuts are obtained.

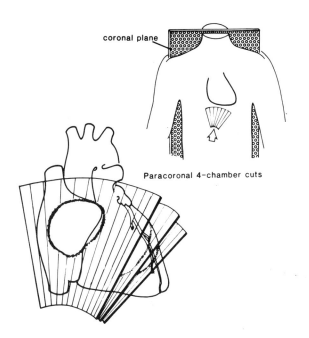

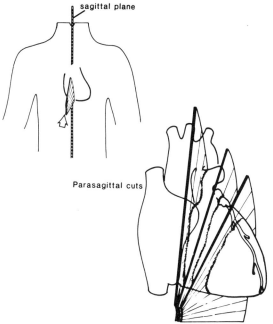

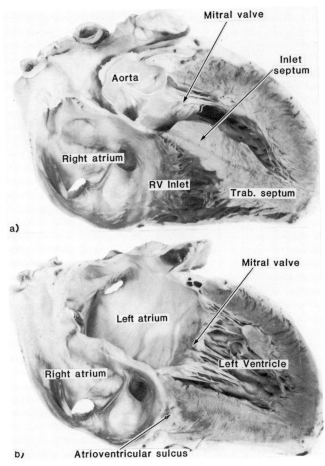

a)

b)

Fig. 12.15 Simulated paracoronal cuts of the heart as might be seen in subcostal position. Although they approximate to the four chamber cuts there are significant differences. The lower panel is particularly important, since it suggests absence of the right atrioventricular connexion.

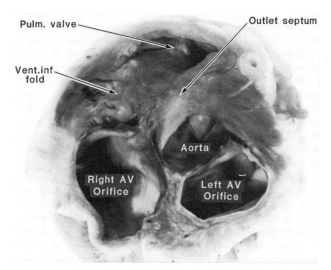

Fig. 12.16 A simulated parasagittal cut through the heart as might be seen from the subcostal window. It shows to advantage the outlet septum and the outflow tract of the right ventricle.

present without affecting the normal echocardiographic appearances of the heart. Other lesions (such as aortic or pulmonary stenosis or incompetence) may result in myocardial hypertrophy or chamber dilation. In other anomalies, such as an atrioventricular septal defect, the whole anatomy of the affected portion of the heart is altered. The alteration is then the essential morphology of the lesion. The more complex malformations can themselves coexist with other simple lesions such as pulmonary stenosis. The echocardiographer must therefore recognise both normal and abnormal morphology as well as any associated lesions. The best way of accomplishing this demanding task is to apply the sequential segmental approach (see Ch. 3). The anatomy of each cardiac segment is recognisable echocardiographically and we will now set out the basic criteria. Following this we will describe the echocardiographic aspects of sequential analysis.

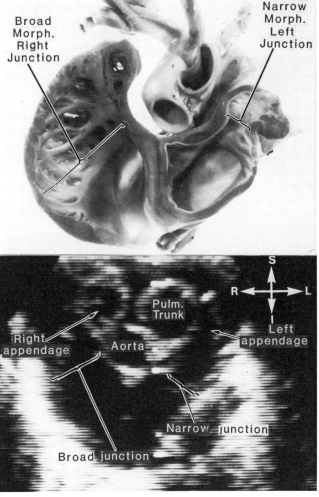

Fig. 12.17 A simulated short axis cut together with an echocardiogram which show the different morphology of the right and left atrial appendages.

Atrial arrangement and the atrial chambers

The first step in examination of any patient suspected of having congenital heart disease should be to establish atrial arrangement ('situs'). Ideally this should be done using the intrinsic features of the atrial chambers themselves. It is the characteristic morphology of the atrial appendages at their junction with the smooth venous atrial component which enables most reliable distinction of a morphologically right versus a morphologically left atrial chamber. The feature seen echocardiographically is a broad junction in a morphologically right atrial chamber versus a narrow junction in a morphologically left atrium. This is seen from either the suprasternal or precordial short axis approaches (Fig. 12.17). Although we know that the features can usually be seen in patients with lateralised atrial chambers, their reliability in predicting atrial arrangement needs to be established. A more firmly established (and probably easier) means is to infer the atrial arrangement from ultrasonic examination of the abdominal great vessels (Huhta et al, 1982). The basis of this technique is the presence in short axis abdominal cuts in the normal individual of the aorta to one side of the spine and the inferior caval vein to the other. When such a lateralised arrangement is found, then the morphologically right atrium is on the same side as the caval vein. When the inferior caval vein is lateralised and to the right, there is almost always usual atrial arrangement (atrial situs solitus) (Fig. 12.18). When it is lateralised and to the left, almost invariably there is mirror-image arrangement (situs inversus). Findings other than of a relatively symmetrical and lateralised relationship of the great vessels to either side of the spine are highly indicative of atrial isomerism. Presence of the inferior caval vein anterolateral to the aorta and on the same side of the spine nearly always indicates right atrial isomerism (Fig. 12.19; Elliott et al, 1966). This diagnosis is reinforced when, in addition, the hepatic veins can be shown to join the inferior caval vein. When the hepatic veins drain directly to the atria (Fig. 12.20), but the aorta and inferior caval vein are still on the same side of the spine, almost always there is left atrial isomerism. It is more usual, however, to fail to demonstrate the inferior caval vein in short axis cuts close to the diaphragm of patients with left isomerism. Another venous channel, the azygos

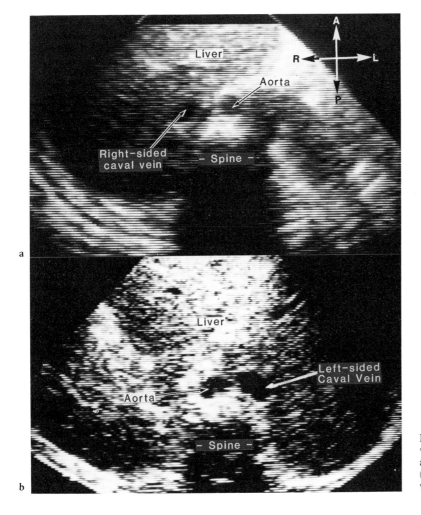

Fig. 12.18 The arrangements of the abdominal great vessels with lateralised bodily arrangement. (a) The usual arrangement with the caval vein to the right (solitus). (b) The mirror-image arrangement with a left-sided caval vein (inversus).

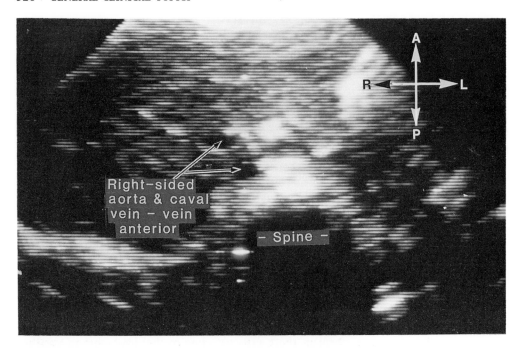

Fig. 12.19 The arrangement of the abdominal great vessels with right atrial isomerism. Both are on the same side of the spine, with the caval vein in anterior position.

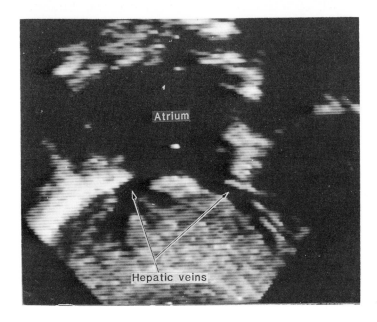

Fig. 12.20 The connexion of the hepatic veins directly to the atrium is indicative of left atrial isomerism.

or hemiazygos vein, is seen posterior to the aorta and on the same side (Fig. 12.21). Through this, the abdominal inferior caval venous return drains to a superior caval channel. A long axis abdominal cut will show the abdominal course of the inferior caval vein and its anomalous continuation. In addition, in most patients with left atrial isomerism there is direct connexion of the hepatic veins to the atria. This helps distinguish left atrial isomerism from those cases with lateralised atrial arrangement in whom a large portion of the abdominal venous return drains via an azygos continuation. In these latter cases, the hepatic veins continue to join a common venous

channel (the terminal portion of the inferior caval vein) which then joins the morphologically right atrium. Since atrial arrangement can reliably be diagnosed on the basis of orientation of the abdominal vessels and connexion of the hepatic veins, the first step in echocardiographic examination of the heart (at least conceptually) should be to place the transducer in the subxiphoid position.

Having identified atrial arrangement, venous connexions must be further clarified. In four chamber cuts from either the subcostal or apical approach (and in suprasternal cuts demonstrating the left or right atrium), the connexions of the superior and inferior caval veins (Fig. 12.22), the

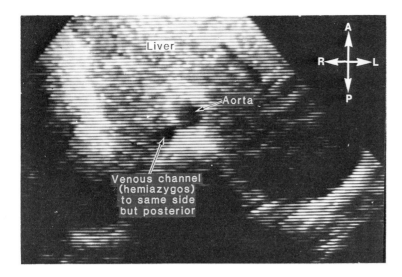

Fig. 12.21 The arrangement of the abdominal great vessels in left atrial isomerism. Both are to the same side of the spine. There is hemiazygos continuation of the inferior caval vein, which is posterior to the aorta.

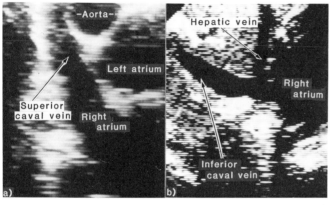

Fig. 12.22 The connexions of the superior (a) and inferior (b) caval veins to the right atrium. Note that the hepatic vein joins the inferior caval vein before it in turn joins the right atrium.

coronary sinus, and the pulmonary veins (Fig. 12.23) can all be seen. The subcostal parasagittal cuts are best for demonstrating the morphology of the atrial septum. Frequently these show the precise arrangement of the oval fossa, with the rim ('septum secundum') on the morphologically right atrial side and the flap valve extending into the morphologically left atrium (Fig. 12.24). The resolution of the ultrasound equipment is often inadequate, however, to demonstrate this fine detail. Subcostal views also show the arrangement of the valves of the inferior caval vein and coronary sinus (Eustachian and Thebesian valves). These are found only in the morphologically right atrium. When assessing the integrity of the atrial septum, it should be remembered that drop-out from the apical approach may give a false impression of an atrial septal

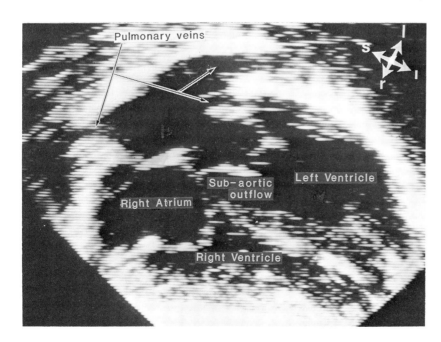

Fig. 12.23 The connexion of the pulmonary veins to the left atrium. The two left-sided and one right-sided pulmonary veins are visualised. Note also how the subaortic outflow tract lifts the mitral valve away from the septum.

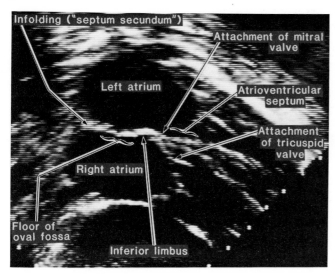

Fig. 12.24 A four chamber echocardiogram demonstrating the typical morphology of the atrial septum.

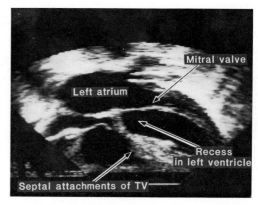

Fig. 12.25 The different morphology of the ventricular inlet portions as seen in a four chamber echocardiogram.

defect. M-mode echocardiographic examination gives no specific anatomical information about the atrial chambers. Systemic venous connexions can be shown to some extent by contrast echocardiography (see below).

The ventricular mass

It should always be possible using the various cross-sectional echocardiographic approaches to distinguish a morphologically right from a morphologically left ventricle. In hearts with biventricular atrioventricular connexions (each atrium connected to its own ventricle) the most reliable means of distinguishing the ventricles is from the morphology of the atrioventricular valves. We have never seen any heart with a biventricular atrioventricular connexion in which the mitral valve was not in the morphologically left ventricle and the tricuspid valve in the morphologically right ventricle. There are several anatomical features which permit the echographic distinction of these valves. The mitral valve leaflets are never attached by tendinous chords or papillary muscles to the inlet septum. There is always a discrete cleavage plane in the morphologically left ventricle between the inlet septum and the tension apparatus (Figs. 12.4, 12.25). In contrast, the tricuspid valve septal leaflet always has septal chordal attachments except when the entire septal leaflet is part of the septum in Ebstein's malformation. In the latter anomaly, however, the apical displacement of the leaflet attachment to the ventricular septum will in itself identify the valve as morphologically tricuspid. A second discriminating feature of the valves is the more apical attachment of the normal tricuspid valve to the inlet septum as compared with the mitral valve. When present, this feature is diagnostic. Unfortunately, in many hearts the valves will be attached to the septum at

the same level because of associated anomalies (Smallhorn et al, 1982b). Attention must then be directed to the tension apparatus. Details of both tension apparatus and leaflet septal attachments are best seen in the long axis four chamber sections. When the ventricular inlets are studied in the short axis plane, it is often possible to distinguish the pattern of opening of the valves. The mitral valve opens in typical fish-mouth fashion (Fig. 12.26). Scanning more apically will show the paired papillary muscles of similar size arising from the parietal wall of the morphologically left ventricle. In contrast, the tricuspid valve opens in trifoliate fashion and has an asymmetrical arrangement of papillary muscles of discernably different size (Fig. 12.27). The septal leaflet is tethered to the inlet septum.

Further valuable information for ventricular identification is obtained by studying the ventricular apical trabecular components. From the anatomical point of view, the ventricular trabecular pattern is the absolute determinant of ventricular identification. Thus, the morphologically right ventricle can be recognised by its coarse apical trabeculations. It is often possible to recognise also the moderator band, characteristically appearing as a blob in the centre of the right ventricular cavity, together with the septomarginal trabeculation running onto the septal surface (Fig. 12.27). The morphologically left ventricle has smooth apical trabeculations and a smooth septal surface. These features can be seen on long and short axis sections, but are probably best seen from the subcostal approach. This can also demonstrate well the differences between the triangular shape of the right ventricle and the ellipsoid or boot-like shape of the left ventricle. The distinctive apical ventricular trabecular pattern, however, is not so easily recognised with echocardiography as with selective ventricular angiocardiography.

The apical ventricular trabecular patterns are also the distinguishing feature for the morphologist to identify the ventricles when each is not connected to its own atrium (univentricular atrioventricular connexion). In contrast,

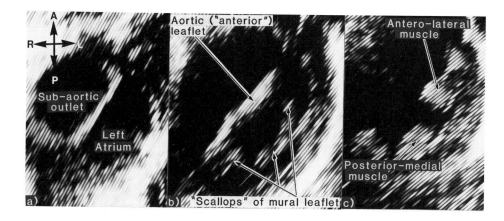

Fig. 12.26 A series of short axis echocardiograms illustrating the 'fish-mouth' appearance of the mitral valve and the oblique arrangement of its papillary muscles.

the echocardiographer may find it difficult to use this feature to identify the nature of a rudimentary ventricle. This is particularly true when it is small. Here the relationship of the septum and the atrioventricular valve or valves is the best guide. Finding a rudimentary ventricle anterior to the atrioventricular valve or valves is indicative of its right ventricular morphology. The dominant ventricle (the valve-receiving chamber) is then of left morphology (Fig. 12.28a). In contrast, when a rudimentary ventricle is behind the atrioventricular connexion or connexions it

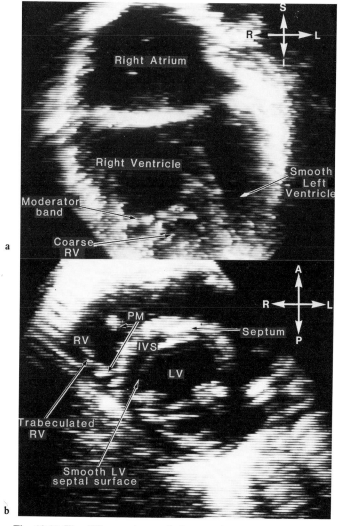

Fig. 12.27 The difference in ventricular morphology as seen (a) in four chamber section and (b) in short axis section. Note the papillary muscle arrangement in the right ventricle.

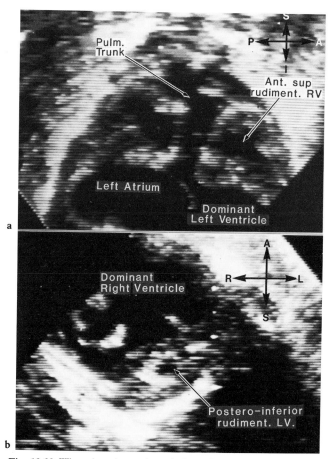

Fig. 12.28 When there is a univentricular atrioventricular connexion, the relationship of the rudimentary ventricle (if present) indicates ventricular morphology. (a) A dominant left ventricle with an anteroposterior rudimentary right ventricle, as seen in subcostal four chamber cut. (b) A dominant right ventricle with a postero-inferior rudimentary left ventricle, as seen in short axis cut.

will be of left ventricular type. The dominant ventricle connected to the atria will then be a morphologically right ventricle (Fig. 12.28b). No matter what the situation, one ventricle must be compared to the other when assessing ventricular trabeculation. Septal trabecular pattern is the most helpful. When only one ventricle is identified, therefore, it is often difficult to judge whether it is of indeterminate, right ventricular or left ventricular pattern. An apparently solitary left ventricle may be differentiated by its smoothness and general shape. The distinction between a ventricle of indeterminate type and an apparently solitary right ventricle may be impossible. When a ventricle gives rise to a great artery, the infundibular morphology also gives clues to the ventricular type. This is less reliable than the other features described above. In the majority of hearts, the great artery arising from the morphologically left ventricle will have echocardiographic continuity between its valve and the mitral valve. This is best seen in the parasternal long axis section (Fig. 12.29a). In contrast, the artery arising from the morphologically right ventricle usually has a complete muscular infundibulum.

This is best appreciated from the subcostal or high parasternal long axis approaches (Fig. 12.29b).

M-mode techniques have strictly limited value in distinguishing right from left ventricular morphology in terms of the anatomy of the atrioventricular valve or the trabecular pattern. When there is a univentricular atrioventricular connexion, however, M-mode scanning itself will distingish the morphology. Those hearts with the septum in front of the valve will have a dominant left ventricle (Mortera et al, 1977). Those with the septum posterior to the valves will have a dominant right ventricle (Fig. 12.30). Whatever the atrioventricular connexion, the M-mode examination will give information about the arterial-atrioventricular valve relationships along with the inferential information this provides for ventricular identification. The finding of atrioventricular-arterial valve continuity in the long axis parasternal sweep (by its exclusion of a complete infundibulum) suggests the presence of a morphologically left ventricle. Failure to demonstrate such continuity suggests that one is looking at a morphologically right ventricle. When everything else in the M-

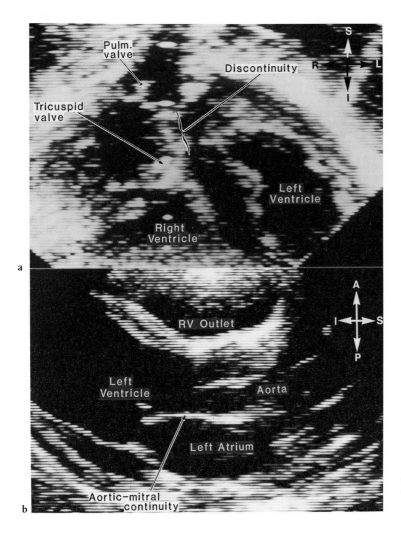

Fig. 12.29 The different arrangements of the normal ventricular outflow tracts as seen (a) in subcostal four chamber, and (b) parasternal long axis views.

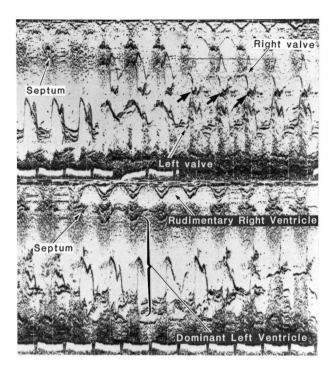

Fig. 12.30 M-mode echocardiogram illustrating how both atrioventricular valves are positioned behind the septum. This is indicative of univentricular connexion to a left ventricle. If the valves were both in front of the septum it would be diagnostic of double inlet right ventricular with postero-inferior rudimentary left ventricle.

mode study is normal, this is useful supportive evidence of ventricular morphology. The variability of the ventricular location of the infundibulum, however, renders this of limited value in complex malformations. Furthermore, the wedge position of the posterior great artery between the two atrioventricular valves means that, on occasions, when the ventricular septum is not normally aligned to the parasternal beam, continuity may be seen between the posterior great artery and the valve in the ventricle from which it does not take origin. This is exemplified by the arrangement in congenitally corrected transposition. The echoes from the pulmonary valve can be demonstrated in continuity with an atrioventricular valve. This might be presumed to be the right-sided morphologically mitral valve. It is the left-sided morphologically tricuspid valve (Keutel & Hagenmueller, 1978).

The ventricular septum

Before making judgements about abnormal septal orientations, it is necessary to understand that the echocardiographic examination of the normal interventricular septum is a complicated procedure. The normal interventricular septum can be divided into four segments, each with a characteristic normal orientation. The 'inlet septum' lies close to the sagittal plane and is best seen in the four chamber cuts (Fig. 12.31a). In the normal heart

it is an inlet-outlet septum, since it interposes between the inlet of the right ventricle and the subaortic outflow tract. It is not seen in the parasternal long axis cut. In this cut the outlet portion of the septum is seen because it lies close to the coronal plane (Fig. 12.31b). In this section, since the outlet septum is insignificant when the rest of the septum is intact, a portion of the trabecular septum is also seen. A different portion of this septum appears in the four chamber cut. This is because the trabecular portion curves between inlet and outlet segments and cannot be visualised in its entirety in one single cut. The septum also extends to the cardiac apex. Multiple short axis cuts together with a subcostal sweep (Fig. 12.32) may be required to examine it completely.

These inlet, outlet and trabecular portions together make up the muscular ventricular septum. The fourth component, the membranous septum, is small but is a vital echocardiographic landmark. It is seen in short axis and four chamber aortic root cuts but not in the parasternal long axis cut. The membranous septum usually has the septal leaflet of the tricuspid valve attached to its right ventricular aspect. This divides it into interventricular and atrioventricular portions. Nothing is attached to the left ventricular aspect. Here the membranous septum forms part of the fibrous aortic root. Thus, the entirety of the aortic root, including this important contribution from the membranous septum, can only be examined fully by sweeping from the subcostal four chamber view through the aortic valve. The structures seen will be, posteriorly, the atrioventricular muscular septum (Figs. 12.5a, 12.33a), the components of the membranous septum (Figs. 12.5b, 12.33b) and finally the muscular outlet septal and free wall origins of the aorta (Fig. 12.32). When considering ventricular septal defects (see Ch. 25) a combination of all these septal views allows complete anatomical characterisation of any defect large enough to be visualised. The importance of echocardiographic demonstration of the components of the atrioventricular septum lies in the clues it provides to the relationship of the atrioventricular conduction axis to the margins of the defects.

The atrioventricular junction

Echocardiography is a technique without peer for investigation of the atrioventricular junction. At this level, study should be made of the type of connexion, the mode of connexion, and the morphology of the atrioventricular septum. From the stance of the type of connexion, the important feature is whether each of the atrial chambers connects to its own ventricle (biventricular atrioventricular connexion) or whether only one ventricle is connected to the atrial chambers (univentricular atrioventricular connexion). With a biventricular connexion and lateralised atrial chambers (usual or mirror-image arrangement), the connexion can be concordant or discordant. It will be

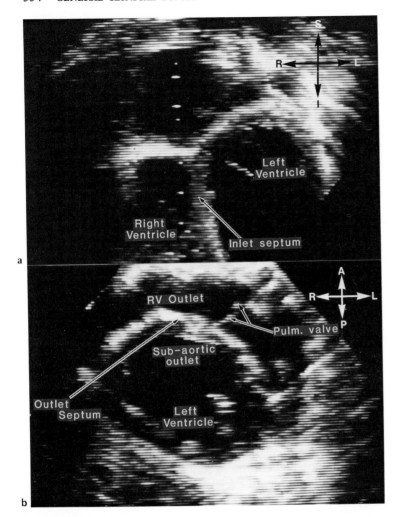

Fig. 12.31 The inlet and outlet parts of the septum are normally at right angles to each other. The inlet septum (a) is therefore cut in the four chamber sections, whilst the outlet septum (b) is cut in paracoronal subcostal sections.

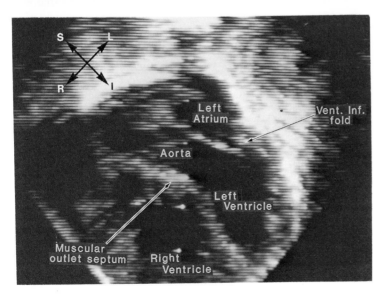

Fig. 12.32 A subcostal intermediate section reveals the muscular outlet septum together with the parietal origin of the aorta from the ventriculo-infundibular fold. The apical trabecular septum is also seen.

demonstrated by identifying the morphology of the atrial and ventricular chambers as described above. With isomeric atrial chambers, each connected to its own ventricle, the connexion of necessity is ambiguous. Then it is important to characterise also the ventricular topology, which may be of right-hand or left-hand pattern. Identification of topological pattern may be difficult echocardiographically. In practice, a right-hand pattern may be

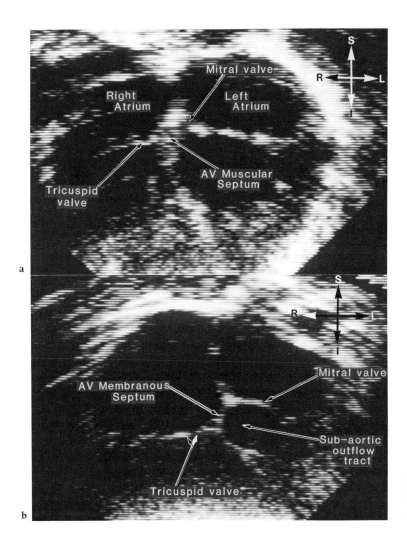

Fig. 12.33 Four chamber sections showing the muscular (a) and membranous (b) parts of the atrioventricular septum. The muscular septum is only seen in the most posterior cuts of the heart.

presumed when the right-sided atrial chamber is connected to a morphologically right ventricle. Similarly, a left-hand pattern will almost invariably be present when the right-sided atrium is connected to a morphologically left ventricle (see Ch. 3). Distinguishing these patterns is important, since it gives a guide to the conduction tissue disposition (Dickinson et al, 1979).

When only one ventricle is directly connected to the atria, the possibilities are either double inlet ventricle or absence of the right or left atrioventricular connexion. Either connexion can exist with lateralised or isomeric atrial chambers. Echocardiographic demonstration of double inlet ventricle is simple, be the connexion through a common valve or two separate valves. It can be achieved using cross-sectional or M-mode techniques (Fig. 12.34). Demonstration of the double inlet connexion amounts to demonstration that the interventricular septum is missing or abnormally positioned. The cross-sectional method is more accurate, since the M-mode appearances of a double inlet connexion may mimic those of a large perimembranous inlet ventricular septal defect. As indicated above,

the relationship of the double inlet connexion to the septum enables the ventricular morphology to be determined. Recognition of an absent atrioventricular connexion is limited to the cross-sectional technique, since failure to demonstrate a structure by M-mode examination cannot be taken as proof that it is not there. The essence of an absent connexion is the separation by atrioventricular sulcus tissue of the muscular floor of the blind-ending atrium from the underlying ventricular mass (Fig. 12.35a). Echocardiographically, it gives the impression of an open-sandwich of dense echoes from the sulcus tissue on the layer of the ventricular myocardium (Fig. 12.35b). Absence of an atrioventricular connexion should be distinguished from an imperforate atrioventricular valve (see below). Since an absent connexion is always associated with a solitary atrioventricular valve draining the other atrium, it must also be distinguished from double inlet via a common atrioventricular valve. A common valve by definition is connected to both atrial chambers. When an absent connexion is identified, the relation between the ventricular septum and the persisting atrioventricular

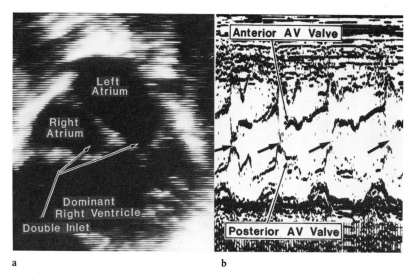

Fig. 12.34 A double inlet atrioventricular connexion as seen (a) in cross-sectional format (to a right ventricle) and (b) with the M-mode technique (to a left ventricle). Note that the valves meet during diastole in the M-mode tracing, as shown by the arrows.

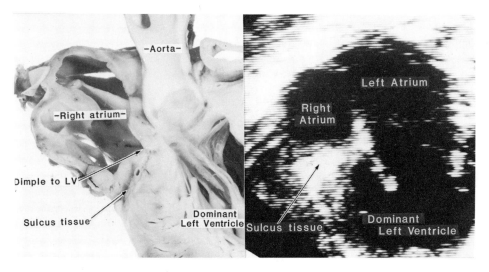

Fig. 12.35 The anatomy of absent right atrioventricular connexion as seen in a specimen and an echocardiogram.

connexion indicates once more the morphology of the ventricle connected to the atria. This is a particularly valuable point when only M-mode examination is available.

Mode of connexion

When studying the mode of connexion, the first step (having determined that both atria connect to the ventricular mass) is to establish whether they do so through a common atrioventricular valve or two atrioventricular valves. As with the identification of an absent connexion, this judgement is made using four chamber sections. When there are two valves, then each valve will guard one atrioventricular junction. The only time when it will be difficult to determine if one or two valves are present is when the valve guarding a common atrioventricular junction in an atrioventricular septal defect is divided into two orifices (see below). Aside from this, it will be easy matter to distinguish two valves from a common valve. This is the case when the atrioventricular junctions are committed to

separate ventricles or the same ventricular chamber. (Fig. 12.36). When two valves have been identified, it is important to show that each valve is patent. Imperforate valves form one type of atrioventricular valve atresia. This type of atresia must be distinguished from an absent atrioventricular connexion. In the case of an imperforate valve, the atrioventricular junction will be normally structured with parietal and septal components, but the orifice will be blocked by fused leaflet tissue. Usually the entire junction will be hypoplastic (Fig. 12.37a), but occasionally large imperforate membranes may be encountered, particularly in association with Ebstein's malformation. Either the right or left atrioventricular valve can be imperforate, and imperforate valves can exist with concordant (Fig. 12.37a), discordant, ambiguous, or double inlet (Fig. 12.37b) connexions. The imperforate valve will be visualised as echo-dense structure which usually has considerable mobility. Although sometimes the membrane is supported by tension apparatus, this is not always the case, particularly when the valve is hypoplastic. Although

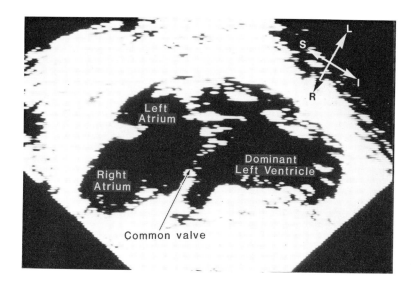

Fig. 12.36 A cross-sectional echocardiogram illustrating a common valve connecting both atria to a dominant left ventricle.

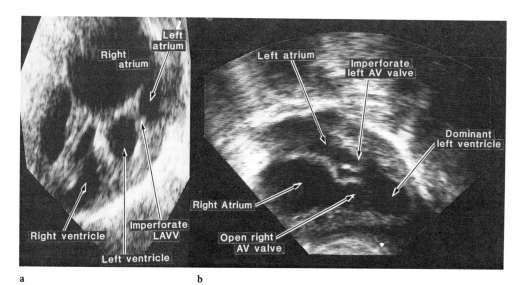

Fig. 12.37 Cross-sectional echocardiograms showing an imperforate left atrioventricular valve (a) in the setting of a concordant atrioventricular connexion and (b) in the setting of double inlet ventricle. (Reproduced by kind permission of Dr George Sutherland, Southampton General Hospital, UK.)

rare, it is also possible for the right or left components of a common valve to be imperforate.

Having ascertained whether the valves are patent or imperforate, and having examined their function, the commitment of the valve to the ventricular mass must be studied. This will already have been done during the diagnosis of the type of connexion. In some hearts this will have shown commitments of the valves which are intermediate between biventricular and univentricular atrioventricular connexions. This occurs when the valve orifice overrides a septum or its tension apparatus straddles. Cross-sectional echocardiographic study in the long axis or four chamber cuts is the best technique for detecting straddling (Fig. 12.38b) or overriding (Fig. 12.38a) of an atrioventricular valve. Adjudication of the precise degree of straddle or override may be difficult when the valve is more-or-less equally connected to two ventricular chambers. A judgement can usually be made by combining long axis and short axis sweeps. Either the right or the left valve can straddle or override (and occasionally both) with any possible chamber combination. This gives a formidable permutation of types of straddling or overriding valves (see Ch. 28). Problems may arise because the two valves may be malorientated with respect to each other when one is straddling or overriding. It may be difficult to obtain views of both valves in a single cut. Alternatively, one valve is seen in its short axis and the other in its long axis in the same cut. A common valve usually straddles and overrides, but not always. Thus, in double inlet ventricle (see Ch. 26) a common valve can be exclusively committed to one ventricle. When a common valve straddles, it is not always equally committed to the ventricular chambers. Echocardiography is an invaluable tool for diagnosing ventricular dominance of an atrioventricular septal defect and for distinguishing double inlet from biventricular atrioventricular connexions in the presence of a common valve (Small-

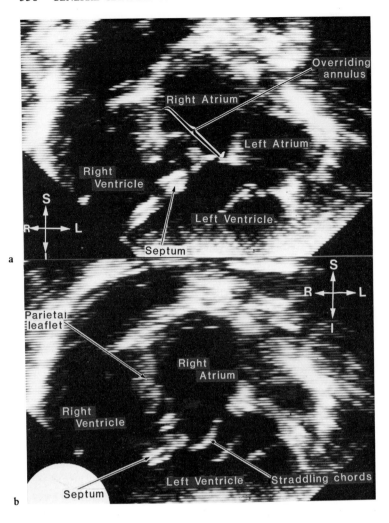

Fig. 12.38 Echocardiograms from the same heart showing (a) the overriding annulus and (b) the straddling tension apparatus of a straddling and overriding right atrioventricular valve.

horn et al, 1981). Straddling and overriding of a solitary valve can also occur when one atrioventricular connexion is absent. Echocardiography will readily distinguish this rare mode of connexion. Although of limited value in the diagnosis of the type of atrioventricular connexion, M-mode echocardiography is well suited to the diagnosis of the mode of connexion. From both parasternal and subcostal approaches a common valve can be distinguished from two separate valves (Fig. 12.39). An imperforate valve can be detected (Fig. 12.40), as can the leaflet motion of a straddling valve (Fig. 12.41). The M-mode technique, though superseded in almost all respects by cross-sectional echocardiography, remains without peer for quantitative study of valve function (see Ch. 7).

The septal atrioventricular junction

When determining the type and mode of atrioventricular connexion, the echocardiographer will perforce have studied the septal atrioventricular junction. Obvious abnormalities in this junction will direct attention to major anomalies. Double inlet ventricle will be recognised when

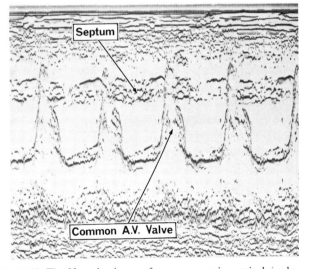

Fig. 12.39 The M-mode picture of a common atrioventricular valve. The valve gives the impression of passing through the septum.

the atrial septum supports both atrioventricular valve 'septal' leaflets but there is no underlying ventricular septum. More subtle abnormalities should direct attention

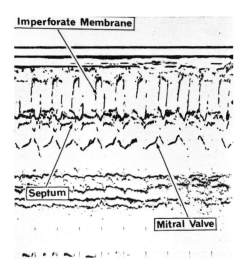

Fig. 12.40 An M-mode tracing showing an imperforate right atrioventricular valve of good dimensions. The valve does not open. The tracing has been retouched.

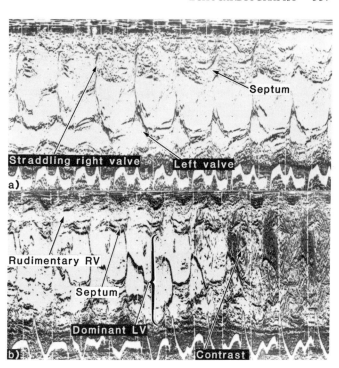

Fig. 12.41 An M-mode tracing showing the pattern of movement of a straddling right atrioventricular valve. (a) The valve seems to pass through the septum and illustrates the two valves meeting in diastole as in double inlet (see Fig. 12.34). (b) A tracing following a peripheral systemic venous injection of contrast. The dominant and rudimentary ventricles are opacified simultaneously.

to other equally important anomalies. As described above, the key to a normal atrioventricular junction is the deeply wedged position of the aortic valve. Thus, in the normal heart it is only over a very short distance of the septum that the mitral valve and the tricuspid valve can be echoed with opposing septal attachments (Fig. 12.33a). When the transducer beam is angled anteriorly from this section, almost immediately it transects the posterior extension of the subaortic outflow tract which 'lifts' the mitral valve from its septal attachment (Fig. 12.33b). This section can then be traced into the four chamber aortic plane. Here the full width of the left ventricular outflow tract separates the mitral valve from the septum. In this plane in the normal heart the right border of the outflow tract will be seen to be formed by the membranous septum. This is crossed on its right ventricular aspect by the septal leaflet of the tricuspid valve, dividing it into atrioventricular and interventricular components (Fig. 12.33b). If the echocardiographer finds that this septal morphology is abnormal, but that there is no defect of the inlet septum (Fig. 12.42), he should suspect the presence of one of the malformations in which the posterior great artery loses its normal wedged position. These include double outlet right ventricle or, to a lesser extent, complete transposition. In contrast, finding the entire atrioventricular septal structures to be lacking

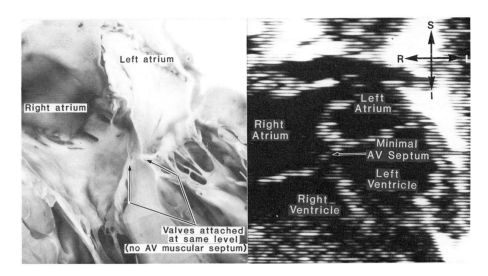

Fig. 12.42 When there is no wedging of the posterior great artery such as in complete transposition or double outlet right ventricle, the valves are attached to the septum at very much the same level, so that there is no atrioventricular muscular septum. This is illustrated by an anatomic cut and an echocardiogram from a patient with complete transposition.

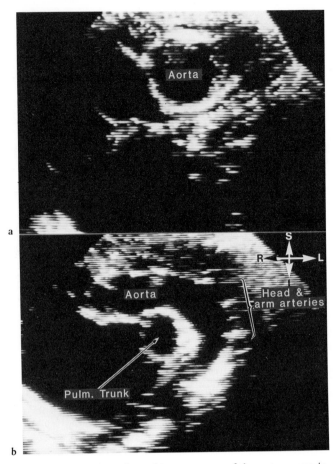

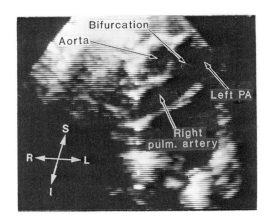

Fig. 12.44 The typical branching pattern of the pulmonary trunk as seen in a short axis section.

Fig. 12.43 The echocardiographic appearances of the aorta as seen in short axis (a) and long axis (b) sections.

The great arteries

Unlike the atria and ventricles, the great arteries have no intrinsic features to permit their recognition. The trunks which arise from the ventricular mass must be identified by following them to their branches. In this way the aorta will be recognised because it gives rise to the coronary arteries and the head, neck and arm arteries (Fig. 12.43). The pulmonary trunk hardly ever gives rise to coronary arteries and can be easily traced to its characteristic bifurcation (Fig. 12.44). A common arterial trunk is identified because it has a common valve and gives rise directly to coronary, systemic and pulmonary arteries (Fig. 12.45). The process of tracing the arteries from their ventricular origins can be done in either the subcostal or apical long axis cuts. Invaluable information about the arteries themselves is obtained by using the suprasternal approach. In this way the arterial duct is readily recognised and its course and character mapped (Fig. 12.46). Obstructive

is pathognomonic for an atrioventricular septal defect. In this anomaly, there is a characteristic common atrioventricular junction which is readily recognised by cross-sectional echocardiography (see Ch. 24).

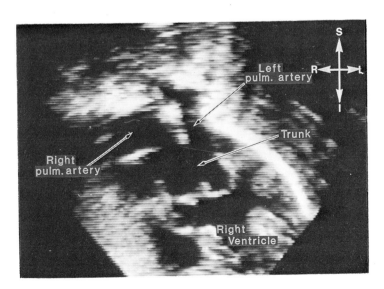

Fig. 12.45 The branching pattern of a common arterial trunk as seen in paracoronal subcostal section.

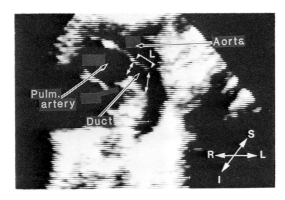

Fig. 12.46 The echocardiographic appearance of a duct which has considerable length (L) and is widely patent (white arrows).

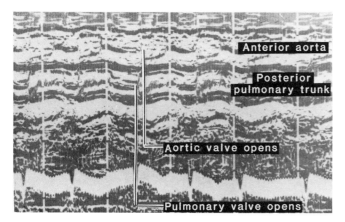

Fig. 12.47 M-mode tracings illustrating the different valve motions of the aortic and pulmonary valves.

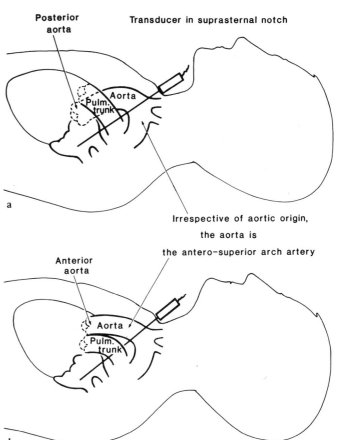

Fig. 12.48 The arrangement of the great arteries (a) is such that when viewed from the suprasternal window the aorta is always the artery closest to the transducer, irrespective of the ventriculo-arterial connexion. This fact is useful since contrast injected into a peripheral vein fills the pulmonary trunk (the posterior artery) in cases of normal connexions (a), but predominantly opacifies the aorta (anterior artery) when there is ventriculo-arterial discordance (b).

lesions of the aortic arch are easily seen (Smallhorn et al, 1982a, 1983).

M-mode echocardiographic identification of the great arteries depends on inferential evidence. At their origins from the heart, they can only be differentiated by the differing patterns of valve motion (Fig. 12.47) and by the differing systolic time intervals which exist because the pulmonary vascular resistance is normally lower than that in the systemic circuit. From the suprasternal notch the aorta can be identified as that artery closest to the transducer (Fig. 12.48). When there is a single arterial trunk its nature cannot reliably be deduced using the M-mode technique.

The ventriculo-arterial junction

During identification of the great arteries they will have been traced from their ventricular origin. This will have enabled the ventriculo-arterial connexions to be determined. At the same time, the mode of connexion will be identified as the echo beam crosses the arterial valves which guard the junction. In this way sophisticated cross-

sectional examination permits the diagnosis of concordant, discordant and double outlet connexions and the distinction between the various types of single outlet ventriculo-arterial connexion. Again, although often difficult, identification of the commitment of overriding arterial valves makes it possible for the echocardiographer to assign them to one or other ventricle. By combining the information obtained from long axis sweeps with that seen in short axis cuts, the echocardiographer is also able to assess the relationships of the ascending arterial trunks. During these various manoeuvres, information will undoubtedly have emerged concerning the nature of the infundibular morphology. This is of very limited therapeutic significance once the connexions have been clearly defined.

As with the atrioventricular junction, the M-mode examination of the ventriculo-arterial junction is limited by the lack of morphological information imparted by this technique. Overriding valves (Fig. 12.49) can, however, reliably be identified. A high index of suspicion can be

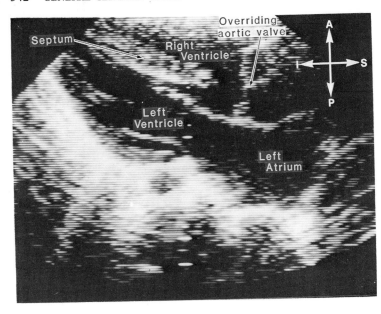

Fig. 12.49 A parasternal long axis echocardiogram illustrating overriding of the aortic valve.

engendered concerning discordant, double outlet and single outlet connexions.

CONTRAST ECHOCARDIOGRAPHY

This technique involves rendering 'opaque' to ultrasound those spaces which are normally echo-free. This is achieved, in the case of vascular cavities, by the injection of dextrose, saline or indocyanine green, which all contain microbubbles due to microcavitation following injection. The microbubbles cause multiple reflections, thus filling the vascular cavity with echoes. The opacification produced can be visualised by either M-mode or cross-sectional techniques. Injections may be made into peripheral veins, thus providing more information in an almost non-invasive fashion. Alternatively, selective injections into cardiac chambers, arteries or veins may be made during cardiac catheterisation. Contrast echocardiography was initially used with the M-mode technique to validate the origin of the cardiac echoes recorded (Gramiak & Shah, 1968). Now it is used in the demonstration of segmental cardiac connexions (Tajik & Seward, 1978; Silverman & Snider, 1982) and in the demonstration of shunts and valvar insufficiency (Seward et al, 1975; Valdes-Cruz et al, 1976; Serwer et al, 1978).

In practice the transducer is positioned to visualise the desired structures. A rapid injection of 0.5–2 ml of 5% dextrose is made and the passage of the 'opacifying' bolus observed. In the normal heart a four chamber subcostal view shows opacification of the right heart chambers (Fig. 12.50). An M-mode echocardiogram in the parasternal view will show right ventricular opacification. From the suprasternal view, the pulmonary trunk is shown

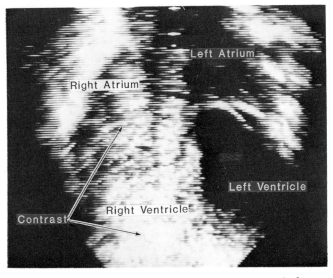

Fig. 12.50 Opacification of the right-sided chambers as seen in four chamber section following injection of contrast into a systemic vein.

to opacify. There will be no opacification whatsoever of the left heart chambers and the aorta. This is because the microbubbles are removed during passage through the lungs. When the septal structures are intact and the investigator limited to M-mode studies, contrast echocardiography is invaluable for the diagnosis of discordant ventriculo-arterial connexions. This is because, when studied from the suprasternal window, the aorta is almost invariably the superior arterial trunk irrespective of its ventricular origin. Thus, complete transposition can be confidently diagnosed if this superior trunk is shown to opacify following a peripheral venous injection (Fig. 12.51). When the cardiac septa are intact, no contrast material is demonstrated in the

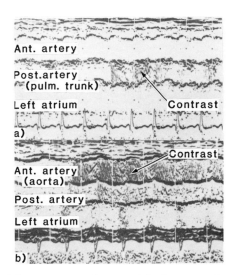

Fig. 12.51 The appearances of contrast injection as seen by the M-mode technique, illustrating the appearances with (a) a concordant ventriculo-arterial connexion, when the posterior vessel opacifies, and (b) with a discordant connexion when it is the anterior artery which is filled by the contrast. See Figure 12.48.

left heart chambers. The finding of left-sided echoes therefore indicates the presence of a right-to-left shunt. Furthermore, the site where the contrast material appears indicates the site of the shunt. This can be judged using either cross-sectional (Fig. 12.52) or M-mode techniques. The existence of intracardiac shunts in association with abnormal ventriculo-arterial connexions makes the use of the suprasternal approach less reliable. With practice it is still possible to derive much information from contrast studies (Mortera et al, 1979).

The interpretation of contrast studies with peripheral injection may be difficult. Such difficulties can be overcome if contrast echocardiography is combined with cardiac catheterisation. Selective injections in known cardiac chambers are then of particular value in the demonstration or exclusion of shunts in small infants.

Multiple injections of angiographic contrast may otherwise approach or exceed a toxic dose. Selective contrast injections are also useful in the demonstration of valvar regurgitation (Fig. 12.53) as well as in many other situations (such as determining whether a valve membrane is imperforate). The combination of contrast echocardiography with catheterisation is now well tried and tested (Seward et al, 1975). A further use of cross-sectional echocardiography in combination with catheterisation is to identify the position of the catheter. Established in this role during balloon septostomy (Allan et al, 1982), it is also useful in a technique such as myocardial biopsy (Fig. 12.54).

DOPPLER ULTRASOUND

Both M-mode and cross-sectional echocardiography provide anatomical information about vascular and cardiac structures and their movement. The application of the Doppler shift principle to study the pattern of blood flow within the cardiovascular system has greatly increased the physiological information that can be obtained using diagnostic ultrasound. Thus, rather than representing alternative techniques, cross-sectional echocardiography and Doppler ultrasound are complementary. When used together, the need for invasive investigation in the assessment of congenital heart lesions may be further reduced. Christian Johann Doppler (1803–1853) was the first to describe the shift in frequency of a wave-form when the source and receiver are moving relative to one other. The frequency is increased when the source moves towards the receiver and decreased when it moves away. In medical practice, Doppler echocardiography, like conventional imaging ultrasound, uses a piezo-electric crystal to emit an ultrasound beam of known frequency which is reflected back from moving objects within the body. In the case of Doppler echocardiography these are the red blood cells.

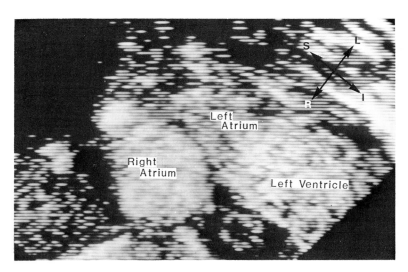

Fig. 12.52 Contrast material injected into the right atrium in four chamber projection shows the presence of an interatrial communication and subsequent opacification of the left ventricle.

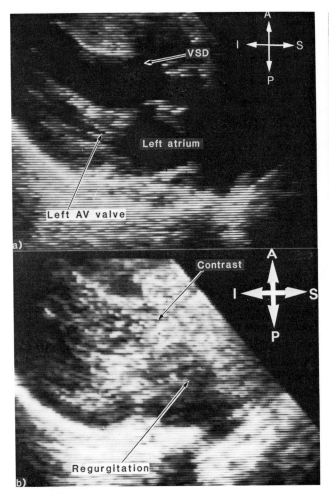

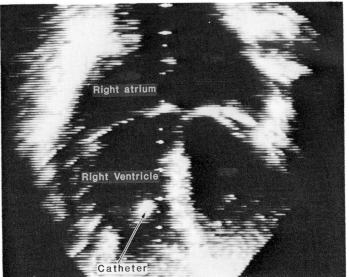

Fig. 12.53 (a) The appearance before injection of contrast material. (b) The post-injection frame illustrating regurgitation through the left atrioventricular valve.

Fig. 12.54 This four chamber cross-sectional echocardiogram shows how it is possible to visualise catheter position within the heart.

The difference in frequency between the transmitted and reflected beams (the Doppler shift) is proportional to the component of velocity in the line of the beam.
This is expressed as

$$\text{Velocity} = \frac{\text{velocity of sound in blood} \times \text{Doppler shift}}{2 \times \text{carrier frequency} \times \cos \theta}$$

(θ is the angle between the ultrasound beam and the velocity vector). This Doppler shift can be used to study several clinically useful features of blood flow. Qualitative information can be obtained regarding flow direction and type (laminar or turbulent). In addition, velocity of flow can be quantified.

Practical considerations

There are two basic Doppler techniques. One uses a continuous wave and the other uses pulsed beams. The emitting crystal is continuously excited in continuous wave systems and a second crystal within the same transducer is used to detect the reflected ultrasound (Hatle & Angelsen, 1982). This is simple and relatively cheap and has the advantage of being able to measure a very high flow velocity. There are two major disadvantages. Firstly, it is not possible to determine where a given velocity was generated along the beam (that is, there is 'range ambiguity'). Secondly, simultaneous imaging with the same transducer is not possible. In pulsed Doppler systems a single transducer acts both as emitter and receiver. The emitter produces rapid repetitive pulses and, during the interval between the pulses, it receives reflected ultrasound. Since ultrasound travels at a known speed in soft tissues, the location of the sample can be detected with great accuracy from the time delay between emission and reception. This ability to define the exact location of a sample is called 'range-gating' and enables flow at a particular location in the cardiac chamber or vessel lumen to be studied. This can be controlled by a cross-sectional echocardiographic display (Fig. 12.55). The main disadvantage of pulsed Doppler ultrasound is that the rate of pulsing and the frequency of the transducer limit the maximum velocity that can be detected. The maximal Doppler shift that can be displayed without ambiguity is equal to half the pulse repetition frequency (the Nyquist frequency: Hatle & Angelsen, 1982). Ambiguity is introduced when Doppler shift exceeds the Nyquist frequency. This artefact is termed 'frequency aliasing'. When displayed, the spectrum initially has directional character but disappears off the edge of the display. It then 'wraps around', reappearing at the other edge of the frequency as if coming from the opposite direction (Fig. 12.56). This problem can be improved by choosing a lower Doppler carrier frequency or by shifting the zero calibration line

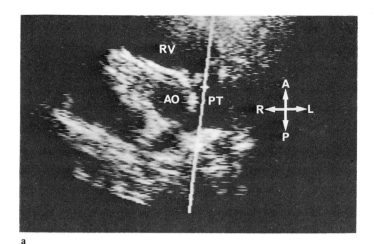

a

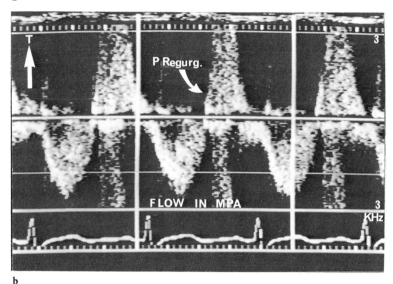

b

Fig. 12.55 The value of 'range-gating' in Doppler echocardiography is illustrated in this study in a patient suspected of having pulmonary valve incompletence. (a) The sample volume is placed within the pulmonary trunk. (b) Demonstrates regurgitant flow.

from the centre to the edge of the display. The upper velocity information that can be obtained without ambiguity has been further extended recently by increasing the pulse repetition frequency. If the transducer is pulsed rapidly, more than one pulse will be in the heart at any given time and more than one range-gate will therefore be present. Higher velocities can then be measured without aliasing by summating velocity information from several range-gates. This introduces some 'range ambiguity' towards that of continuous wave system and thus represents a compromise. Essentially there is a trade-off between the range-gating of pulsed Doppler ultrasound and the disadvantage of aliasing at high velocities. For simple lesions with predictable cardiac anatomy, range-gating may not be necessary. It is clearly advantageous when dealing with complex congenital heart disease. Ideally, instrumentation should have both continuous waves and pulsed Doppler facilities.

Doppler signals can be monitored both visually (by spectral analysis) and audibly. Analysis of the spectrum has been greatly improved by fast Fourier analysis which allows instantaneous observations on the whole spectrum (Greene et al, 1980; Goldberg et al, 1982). Concurrent display of the electrocardiogram and phonocardiogram may be required to aid interpretation of the spectral signal.

Clinical applications

Qualitative information regarding the direction and pattern of blood flow is often of great value in paediatric cardiac diagnosis. Demonstration or exclusion of turbulent flow may be useful in the differential diagnosis of systolic murmurs (Kawabori et al, 1980). The Doppler ultrasound is an extremely sensitive means of detecting the presence of regurgitation and stenosis of arterial and/or atrioventricular valves (Figs. 12.55, 12.57). Abnormal extracardiac structures, such as a left superior caval vein or an anomalous pulmonary venous connexion, which may be confused on the echocardiogram, may be differentiated by the directions and patterns of flow (Stevenson et al, 1979a). A further advantage of Doppler ultrasound is its ability to document the presence of multiple areas of flow disturbance

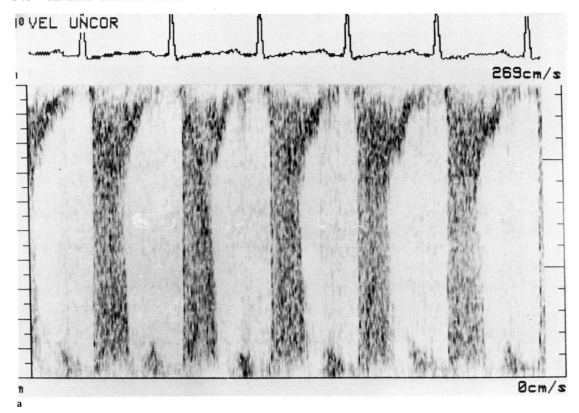

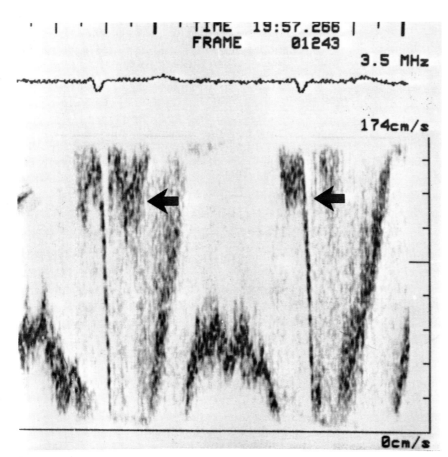

Fig. 12.56 (a) A case of aortic stenosis studied from the suprasternal notch. It shows the high velocity turbulent blood flow seen in systole which has exceeded the velocity measurement capability of the instrument. It is, thus 'off the scale'. (b) A case of pulmonary stenosis studied from the parasternal approach. Again the high velocity blood flow has exceeded the velocity scale, but in this instance, it has 'wrapped around', reappearing at the top of the frame (arrowed). (Reproduced by kind permission of Dr Neil Wilson, Killingbeck Hospital, Leeds, UK).

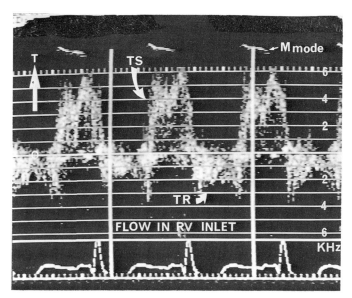

Fig. 12.57 This trace shows both rapid forward (TS) and regurgitant (TR) flow in a patient with tricuspid valve disease. The sample volume was placed in the inlet of the right ventricle (RV).

when auscultation is dominated by the murmur from only one of the lesions. Surgical applications are numerous and include the detection of obstruction after intra-atrial repair of complete transposition (Stevenson et al, 1979b; Wyse et al, 1979), differential diagnosis of residual flow disturbances and murmurs in the postoperative period (Stevenson et al, 1977), and demonstration of surgical shunt patency (Stevenson et al, 1983). The qualitative information obtained from Doppler has been extended by recent technical developments of colour flow mapping. This codes flow towards and away from the transducer into different colours which are then superimposed on the cross-sectional echocardiogram (Miyatake et al, 1984). The resulting visually appealing picture may have some advantages, for example in the detection of minor lesions such as small ventricular septal defects (Ortiz et al, 1985), for mapping of valve regurgitation and demonstration of anomalous pulmonary venous return.

Reliable accurate non-invasive quantitation of intracardiac pressure or flow is a highly desirable goal since this is often the major indication for cardiac catheterisation. Quantitative Doppler ultrasound is being used increasingly with varying degrees of success to predict gradients across obstructive lesions, valve regurgitation, flow (including cardiac output) and pulmonary pressures and resistance. The most widely accepted current use is for predicting gradients across obstructive lesions. This relies on the increase in maximal velocity of flow which occurs across the obstruction. The relation between this increase in velocity and the pressure drop across the obstruction can be described by the simplified Bernoulli equation.

$$P_1 - P_2 = 4 (V_2^2 - V_1^2) \text{ (in mmHg)}$$

Where P_1 = pressure prior to the obstruction; P_2 = pressure after the obstruction; V_1 = velocity prior to the obstruction; V_2 = maximal velocity after the obstruction. Friction and flow acceleration are ignored, but this is valid in most clinical situations. In practice, the equation can be still further simplified to:

$$P_1 - P_2 = 4 V_2^2$$

since the velocity prior to the obstruction (V_1) is relatively low (Hatle & Angelsen, 1982). The biggest potential error is that ideally the highest velocity jet should be aligned with the ultrasound beam. When this is not possible, the angle between the two must be estimated and corrected for in the equation. This is not really possible with continuous wave techniques. It may be difficult even with pulsed systems, largely because the jet of flow cannot be imaged in three dimensions. Other factors influencing assessment of velocity include the shape or length of the obstruction and the presence of a small orifice. Nevertheless, excellent correlations have been reported between predicted gradients using continuous wave Doppler and those measured at cardiac catheterisation in relatively discrete lesions such as aortic and pulmonary stenosis and aortic coarctation (Fig. 12.58). The technique has found widespread acceptance (Hatle et al, 1980; Wyse et al, 1984). Results, however, have been less reliable in more complex lesions where cardiac connexions are abnormal or when obstructive lesions occur in series. This is particularly the case in neonates, where the technique should be interpreted with caution. The same principle has been applied in mitral stenosis (Holen et al, 1976; Hatle et al, 1978) and used to predict the right ventricular pressure in ventricular septal defect. In the latter situation, the velocity of the jet through the ventricular septal defect and the blood pressure are measured. Assuming there is no left ventricular outflow tract obstruction, the left ventricular pressure is equal to the systolic blood pressure. An estimate of the right ventricular pressure may be obtained by subtracting the pressure drop predicted by the peak flow velocity across the ventricular septal defect from this left ventricular pressure. Obvious potential errors are introduced by this technique (particularly that from angle correction for the jet across the ventricular septal defect). As underestimation of the jet will lead to overestimation of the right ventricular pressure, any errors will be in a 'clinically safe' direction.

Quantitative estimation of valvar regurgitation has proved more difficult. Several approaches have been tried, including pulsed Doppler ultrasound to map the spatial distribution of the regurgitant flow (Veyrat et al, 1984) and the derivation of a variety of regurgitation indices. Most of these have proved semiquantitative at best and have been disappointing in clinical practice.

Doppler ultrasound can be used to obtain a quantitative estimate of flow both in normal hearts and in patients with

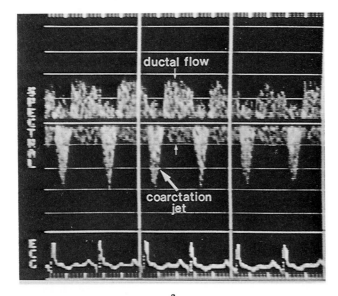

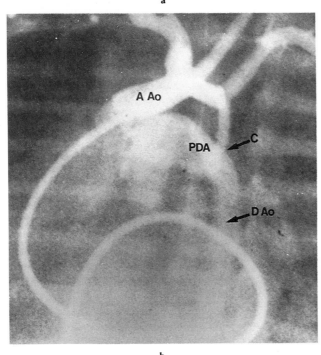

Fig. 12.58 (a) Shows the flow of blood through the duct (PDA) along with a jet through the narrowed aortic isthmus (C) in the patient whose angiogram is shown in (b). AAo – ascending aorta; DAo – descending aorta.

intracardiac shunting. Methods are based on the measurements first of blood velocity, as already described, and second of the area through which that velocity has occurred. Volume flow is then derived from the equation:

$$Q(cc/min) = \frac{\text{mean velocity (cm/sec)} \times \text{area (cm)}^2 \times \text{heart rate}}{\text{Cos } \theta}$$

The greatest source of error (in addition to those already discussed with regard to estimation of blood velocity) is inherent in the measurement of the area through which flow is occurring. This has been attempted at several sites, including the ascending aorta, pulmonary trunk and the mitral and tricuspid valve orifices. Additional assumptions implicit in the calculation include a flat velocity profile and an orifice of constant diameter through the cardiac cycle. In artificial experimental situations, despite numerous assumptions, good correlations have been obtained with electromagnetic flow measurements (Valdes-Cruz et al, 1983; Fisher et al, 1983). A more pragmatic approach using the method to predict pulmonary-to-systemic flow ratios in patients has also yielded encouraging data (Stevenson & Kawabori, 1984). This application of the Doppler technique will no doubt receive further attention. There is now considerable experience using continuous wave Doppler ultrasound to measure cardiac output in the aortic arch and ascending aorta in a variety of physiological and pathological situations, including intensive care. The technique could prove invaluable for documenting serial changes in cardiac output, particularly in unstable clinical situations (Alverson et al, 1982; Haites et al, 1984).

The use of transcutaneous Doppler ultrasound in paediatric cardiology has proliferated dramatically in the last few years. This has been associated with significant improvement in technology, expertise and imaginative applications. The examinations are usually quick, atraumatic and inexpensive. In some situations they may obviate the need for invasive investigations. As the technique can be repeated, it should provide valuable serial physiological assessment of cardiovascular function to complement the anatomic information derived from cross-sectional echocardiography.

REFERENCES

Allan L D, Leanage R, Wainwright R, Joseph M C, Tynan M 1982 Balloon atrial septostomy under two dimensional echocardiographic control. British Heart Journal 47: 41–43

Alverson D C, Eldridge M, Dillon T, Yabek S M, Berman W Jr 1982 Noninvasive pulsed Doppler determination of cardiac output in neonates and children. Journal of Pediatrics 101: 46–50

Anderson R H, Becker A E 1980 Cardiac anatomy – An integrated text and colour atlas, Gower-Churchill Livingstone, London, p 1.14–1.18

Bom N, Gussenhoven W J, Roelandt J 1981 Ultrasonic diagnostic

methods and their limitations. In: Becker A E, Losekoot T G, Marcelletti C, Anderson R H (eds) Paediatric cardiology, Vol 3. Churchill Livingstone, Edinburgh, p 355–370

Dickinson D F, Wilkinson J L, Anderson K R, Smith A, Ho S Y, Anderson R H 1979 The cardiac conduction system in situs ambiguus. Circulation 59: 879–885

Edwards W D, Tajik A J, Seward J B 1981 Standardized nomenclature and anatomic basis for regional tomographic analysis of the heart. Mayo Clinic Proceedings 56: 479–497

Elliott L P, Cramer G C, Amplatz K 1966 The anomalous relationship of inferior vena cava and abdominal aorta as a specific angiographic sign of asplenia. Radiology 87: 859–863

Fisher D C, Sahn D J, Friedman M J, et al 1983 The mitral valve orifice method of noninvasive two-dimensional echo Doppler determination of cardiac output. Circulation 67: 872–877

Goldberg S J, Sahn D J, Allen H W, Valdes-Cruz L M, Hoenecke H, Carnahan Y 1982 Evaluation of pulmonary and systemic blood flow by two-dimensional Doppler echocardiography using fast Fourier transform spectral analysis. The American Journal of Cardiology 50: 1394–1400

Gramiak R, Shah P M 1968 Echocardiography of the aortic root. Investigative Radiology 3: 356–366

Greene E R, Hoekenga D E, Richards K L, Davis J G 1980 Pulsed Doppler echocardiographic audio spectrum analysis: time interval histogram versus multifilter spectrogram and fast Fourier transform. Biomedical Sciences Instruments 16: 139–147

Gutgesell H P 1985 Cardiac imaging with ultrasound: rightside up or or upside down? The American Journal of Cardiology 56: 479–480

Haites N E, Mowat D H R, McLennan F M, Rawles J M 1984 How far is the cardiac output? Lancet 1: 1025–1027

Hanrath P, Schluter M, Langenstein B A, et al 1983 Detection of ostium secundum atrial septal defects by transoesophageal cross-sectional echocardiography. British Heart Journal 49: 350–358

Hatle L, Angelsen B A 1982 Doppler ultrasound in cardiology. Lea & Febiger, Philadelphia

Hatle L, Brubakk A, Tromsdal A, Angelsen B 1978 Noninvasive assessment of pressure drop in mitral stenosis by Doppler ultrasound. British Heart Journal 40: 131–140

Hatle L, Angelsen B, Tromsdal A 1980 Non invasive assessment of aortic stenosis by Doppler ultrasound. British Heart Journal 43: 284–293

Holen J, Aaslid R, Landmark K, Simonsen S 1976 Determination of pressure gradient in mitral stenosis with a noninvasive ultrasound Doppler technique. Acta Medica Scandinavica 199: 455–460

Huhta J C, Smallhorn J F, Macartney F J 1982 Two dimensional echocardiographic diagnosis of situs. British Heart Journal 48: 97–108

Kawabori I, Stevenson J G, Dooley T K, Guntheroth W G 1980 Evaluation of ejection murmur by pulsed Doppler echocardiography. British Heart Journal 43: 623–628

Keutel J, Hagenmueller H 1978 Echocardiography in diagnosis of corrected transposition. In: Anderson R H, Shinebourne E A (eds) Paediatric cardiology 1977. Churchill Livingstone, Edinburgh, p 515–523

Magherini A, Azzolina G, Careri J 1984 Anatomy of the echocardiographic crux-cordis in the evaluation of the spectrum of atrioventricular valve atresia. International Journal of Cardiology 5: 163–172

Marino B, Ballerini L, Marcelletti C, et al 1984 Right oblique subxiphoid view for two-dimensional echocardiographic visualization of the right ventricle in congenital heart disease. The American Journal of Cardiology 54: 1064–68

Miyatake K, Okamoto M, Kinoshita N, et al 1984 Clinical applications of a new type of real-time two-dimensional Doppler flow imaging system. American Journal of Cardiology 54: 857–868

Mortera C, Hunter S, Tynan M 1979 Contrast echocardiography and the suprasternal approach in infants and children. European Heart Journal 9: 437–454

Mortera C, Hunter S, Terry G, Tynan M 1977 Echocardiography of primitive ventricle. British Heart Journal 39: 847–855

Ortiz E, Robinson P J, Deanfield J E, Franklin R, Macartney F J, Wyse R K H 1985 Localisation of ventricular septal defects by simultaneous display of superimposed colour Doppler and cross sectional echocardiographic images. British Heart Journal 54: 53–60

Russo P A, Rigby M L, Anderson R H, Magherini A, Ho S Y 1986 The significance of the echocardiographic crux in the diagnosis of congenital heart disease. Journal of Cardiovascular Ultrasonography (in press)

Serwer G A, Armstrong B E, Anderson P A W, Sherman D, Benson D W Jr, Edwards S B 1978 Use of contrast echocardiography for evaluation of right ventricular hemodynamics in the presence of ventricular septal defects. Circulation 58: 327–336

Seward J B, Tajik A J, Spangler J G, Ritter D G 1975 Echocardiographic contrast studies: initial experience. Mayo Clinic Proceedings 50: 163–192

Silverman N H, Snider A R 1982 Two-dimensional echocardiography in congenital heart disease. Appleton-Century-Crofts, Norwalk, Connecticut, p 47–66

Silverman N H, Hunter S, Anderson R H, Ho S Y, Sutherland G R, Davies M J 1983 Anatomical basis of cross sectional echocardiography. British Heart Journal 50: 421–430

Smallhorn J F, Tommasini G, Macartney F J 1981 Two-dimensional echocardiographic assessment of common atrioventricular valves in univentricular hearts. British Heart Journal 46: 30–34

Smallhorn J F, Huhta J C, Anderson R H, Macartney F J 1982a Suprasternal cross-sectional echocardiography in assessment of patent ductus arteriosus. British Heart Journal 48: 321–330

Smallhorn J F, Sutherland G R, Anderson R H, Macartney F J 1982b Cross-sectional echocardiographic assessment of conditions with atrioventricular valve leaflets attached to the atrial septum at the same level. British Heart Journal 48: 331–341

Smallhorn J F, Huhta J C, Adams P A, Anderson R H, Wilkinson J L, Macartney F J 1983 Cross-sectional echocardiographic assessment of coarctation in the sick neonate and infant. British Heart Journal 50: 349–361

Stevenson J G, Kawabori I 1984 Noninvasive determination of pressure gradients in children: two methods employing pulsed Doppler echocardiography. Journal of The American College of Cardiology 3: 179–192

Stevenson J G, Kawabori I, Guntheroth W G 1977 Differentiation of ventricular septal defects from mitral regurgitation by pulsed Doppler echocardiography. Circulation 56: 14–18

Stevenson J G, Kawabori I, Guntheroth W G 1979a Pulsed Doppler echocardiographic detection of total anomalous pulmonary venous return: resolution of the left atrial line. The American Journal of Cardiology 44: 1155–1158

Stevenson J G, Kawabori I, Dooley T K, Dillard D H, Guntheroth W G 1979b Pulsed Doppler echocardiographic detection of obstruction of systemic venous return following repair of transposition of the great arteries. Circulation 60: 1091–1095

Stevenson J G, Kawabori I, Bailey W W 1983 Noninvasive evaluation of Blalock-Taussig shunts: Determination of patency and differentiation from patent ductus arteriosus by Doppler echocardiography. The American Journal of Cardiology 106: 1121–1132

Tajik A J, Seward J B 1978 Contrast echocardiography. Cardiovascular Clinics 9: 317–341

Tajik A J, Seward J B, Hagler D J, Mair D D, Lie J T 1978 Two dimensional real time ultrasonic imaging of the heart and great vessels. Mayo Clinic Proceedings 53: 271–303

Valdes-Cruz L M, Pieroni D R, Roland J-M A, Varghese P J 1976 Echocardiographic detection of intracardiac right-to-left shunts following peripheral vein injections. Circulation 54: 558–561

Valdes-Cruz L M, Horowitz S, Mesel E, et al 1983 A pulsed Doppler echocardiographic method for calculation of pulmonary and systemic flow: accuracy in a canine model with ventricular septal defect. Circulation 68: 597–602

Veyrat C, Ameur A, Bas S, Lessana A, Abitbol G, Kalmanson D 1984 Pulsed Doppler echocardiographic indices for assessing mitral regurgitation. British Heart Journal 51: 130–138

Walmsley R, Watson H 1978 Clinical anatomy of the heart. Churchill Livingstone, Edinburgh

Wells P N T 1978 Unit 1. Physics. In: Leech, Sutton G C (eds) An introduction to echocardiography. Medi-Cine, London

Wyse R K H, Haworth S G, Taylor J F N, Macartney F J 1979 Obstruction of superior vena caval pathway after Mustard's repair. Reliable diagnosis by transcutaneous Doppler ultrasound. British Heart Journal 42: 162–167

Wyse R K H, Robinson P J, Deanfield J E, Tunstall Pedoe D S, Macartney F J 1984 Use of continuous wave Doppler ultrasound velocimetry to assess the severity of coarctation of the aorta by measurement of aortic flow velocities. British Heart Journal 52: 278–283

13

Prenatal detection of congenital heart disease

In the last fifteen years techniques for the prenatal diagnosis of congenital diseases have been extensively explored and developed. Ultrasonography is particularly attractive for this field as it carries no fetal risk or maternal discomfort. The early static B scanners developed in the 1960s only allowed determination of the number of fetuses, fetal position, placental localisation and estimation of fetal age and growth. But improved resolution, producing better image quality in the more recent scanners and the addition of real-time cross-sectional display, has allowed fetal anatomy to be seen in previously unimaginable detail. As early as 1970 the prenatal diagnosis of renal abnormality was made (Garrett et al, 1970). Since then abnormality in nearly every system in the fetus has been described, neural tube defects (Campbell et al, 1972), gastrointestinal tract atresia (Houlton et al, 1974), limb deformities (O'Brien et al, 1980), to name but a few. During this period of rapid development of ultrasound as a reliable technique for prenatal diagnosis, those involved in this field avoided the cardiovascular system, partly because of the apparent anatomical complexity of the heart, and partly because of the infinite variety of structural abnormalities. It was not until paediatric cardiologists became aware of the quality of prenatal imaging that several workers in different centres made a systematic study of the fetal heart. (Kleinman et al, 1980; Sahn et al, 1980; Allan et al, 1980). The fetal heart was found to be easier to visualise than the heart in postnatal life and prediction of structural abnormality was also found possible (Kleinman et al, 1980; Allan et al, 1981a, b).

FETAL CARDIAC ANATOMY

The fetal heart is much more accessible to study by ultrasound than is the heart in postnatal life. This is because visualisation is unobstructed by the sternum, rib cage or by the unaerated lung fields. This means that the heart is seen in unusual projections which are initially difficult to interpret. There are also some intrinsic anatomical differences between the heart in prenatal and postnatal life. For these reasons and in order to validate our early echocardiographic interpretation we used anatomical sections of preserved fetal specimens to imitate echocardiographic planes of section. The anatomical studies also allowed the transducer orientation to be discovered for each described section relative to the whole fetus. Figure 13.1 shows the transducer orientation necessary to visualise five planes of section which will illustrate all the features of cardiac anatomy that must be identified in the normal heart. This is, of course, an artificial method of dividing up the heart, but essential for description. When scanning the maternal abdomen, the ease of swivelling the transducer from plane to plane means that the cardiac connexions can be followed in a continuous fashion.

In the fetus, the large fetal liver displaces the apex of the heart cranially so that the inlet portion of the right ventricle lies directly anterior to the inlet portion of the left ventricle. In postnatal life by contrast the inlet portion of the right ventricle lies below the inlet of the left ventricle. This means that a four chamber view of the fetal heart is achieved in a completely transverse section of the fetal thorax. This is seen in Figure 13.2, the corresponding anatomical section being displayed alongside the echocardiogram. Figure 13.2 also demonstrates some of the other intrinsic anatomical differences between pre- and postnatal echocardiography. The right ventricle can be seen to be approximately equal to the left ventricle in size and the foramen ovale flap is widely patent. These anatomical differences reflect the haemodynamic differences in the circulation in prenatal life. Firstly the oxygenated blood in the inferior caval vein is preferentially streamed across the right atrium, through the oval foramen, to the left heart and head and neck vessels. Secondly the right and left ventricles eject a similar volume of blood against a similar arterial pressure (Dawes et al, 1955; Dawes & Mott, 1964) and therefore are of approximately equivalent size. The other features to be noted in this section are the mitral and tricuspid valves, and the normal feature of differential insertion of their septal attachment; the integrity of the inlet and trabecular septum; the differential trabeculation

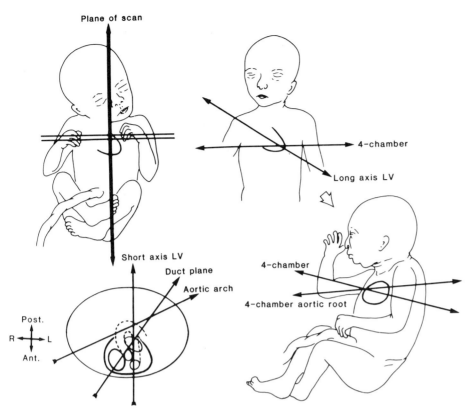

Fig. 13.1 Diagram illustrating the basic planes used for determination of normal fetal cardiac anatomy. The top right-hand panel shows the transverse scans which produce, first the four chamber plane, and then, with angulation towards the right shoulder, the long axis of the left ventricle. The lower right-hand panel shows the cranial angulation required to produce the four chamber plus aortic root plane (see Fig. 13.3). The other planes are taken in the long axis of the fetus, as shown in the left-hand panel. These are, respectively, the aortic arch plane (see Fig. 13.4); the short axis of the left ventricle (see Fig. 13.5) and the ductal plane (see Fig. 13.6).

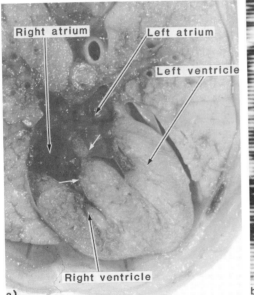

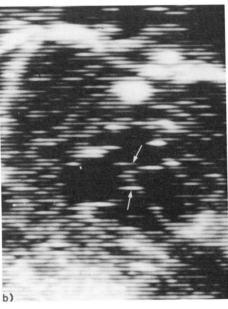

Fig. 13.2 The heart is seen within the fetal thorax in the four chamber projection with the spine anterior. The right ventricle lies closer to the anterior chest wall than does the left. Differential septal insertion of the tricuspid and mitral valve and differential trabeculation between the ventricular chambers can be seen.

between the two ventricular chambers; the integrity of the primary and secondary atrial septal structures and the entrance of two pulmonary veins into the left atrium. The orientation of the heart relative to the spine and the relative size of the heart to the thorax should also be observed. The descending aorta can be seen between the left atrium and the spine.

Angling the transducer from this plane of section so that the beam passes between the right fetal shoulder and left hip will allow the origin of the aorta from the left ventricle to be visualised. Figure 13.3 shows the right atrium connecting to the right ventricle, with the left ventricle giving rise to the aorta posteriorly. The aortic valve can be well seen as can the area of the central fibrous body.

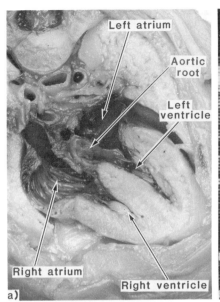

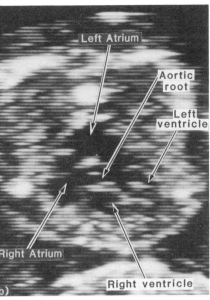

Fig. 13.3 Angulation of the transducer from the four chamber projection towards the fetal head allows the aortic root to be seen arising from the posterior left ventricle. The anatomical specimen has been dissected so as to correspond with the echocardiogram. (This, and the other normal fetal specimens, were dissected and photographed by kind permission of Dr J.L. Wilkinson and Mrs Audrey Smith, University of Liverpool.)

The left atrium lies behind the aortic root. Aortic-mitral and aortic-septal continuity can be noted. Unless this great artery has been followed to the arch of the aorta, however, it has not been positively identified as the aorta. Head and neck vessels must be identified arising from the aortic arch as seen in Figure 13.4. The connexion of left ventricle to ascending aorta and thence to the arch of the aorta can be readily illustrated by continuous transducer angulation.

The connexions of the right heart can be demonstrated by the plane of section, illustrated in Figure 13.1, that cuts the fetus in a sagittal plane to the left of the midline. This shows the left ventricle in short axis, the right ventricle, the muscular infundibulum supporting the pulmonary valve and the pulmonary trunk arching around the left ventricle (Fig. 13.5). Angling the transducer from this plane so that the beam lies between the left fetal shoulder and right hip will demonstrate the connexion of the pulmonary trunk to the arterial duct as seen in Figure 13.6. Several normal features can be observed in this plane of section. The inferior caval vein enters the right atrium and the Eustachian valve can be seen directing flow across the oval foramen. The left atrium lies behind the aortic root. The tricuspid valve, pulmonary outflow tract, and pulmonary valve can be seen together with the pulmonary trunk 'wrapping around' the centrally positioned aorta. The pulmonary valve is seen to be anterior and cranial to the aortic valve. The ductal connexion can be identified to be just below, and in a slightly different plane of section from, the arch of the aorta.

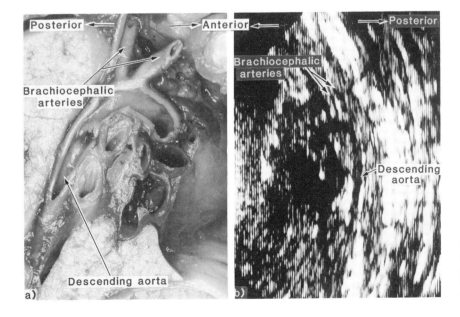

Fig. 13.4 The artery arising from the left ventricle can be followed to the arch of the aorta, which gives rise to the head and neck vessels, confirming that it is the aorta. The anatomic specimen has been dissected in reciprocal orientation.

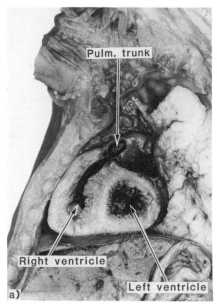

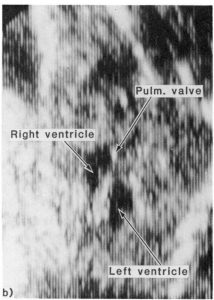

Fig. 13.5 The muscular infundibulum of the right ventricle supporting the pulmonary valve is seen arching over the left ventricle when is a circular structure in this projection. The anatomical specimen is dissected in directly comparable fashion.

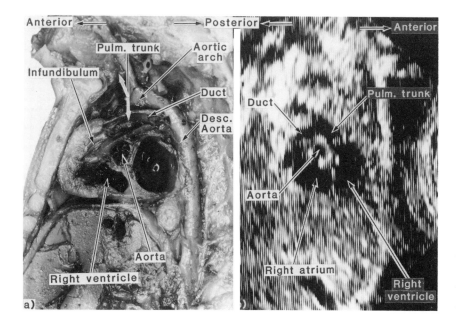

Fig. 13.6 The pulmonary outflow tract is seen wrapping around the central aorta seen in cross-section. The tricuspid valve, pulmonary valve and pulmonary trunk connecting to the duct can be seen. The comparable anatomic specimen is dissected in reciprocal fashion.

M-MODE ECHOCARDIOGRAPHY IN THE FETUS

The M-mode echocardiogram has been used to acquire measurement data for intracardiac structures in preference to a frozen frame cross-sectional image preferred by other workers (Sahn et al, 1980). This is because, using single beam echocardiography, there is better definition of endocardial surfaces and more accurate timing within the cardiac cycle. Measurement and functional data can also be compared with already documented postnatal data.

Standard projections of the fetal heart must be used to acquire the measurements so as to achieve reproducible results. A short axis view of the left ventricle as seen in Figure 13.5 is used to measure the right ventricle, septum, left ventricle and posterior left ventricular wall. Measurements can be made in systole or diastole as illustrated in Figure 13.7. Measurement of the aortic root and left atrium can be made in the short axis projection of the aorta such as were shown in Figure 13.6. Growth charts have been constructed for these parameters between 16 weeks gestation and term (Figs. 13.8–13.13). These charts have proved of particular use when a measurement anomaly is suspected on the cross-sectional study. A structural defect can be more precisely defined if accurate measurements can be made.

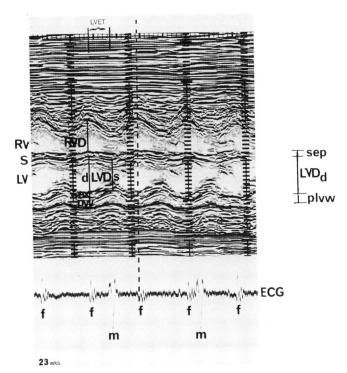

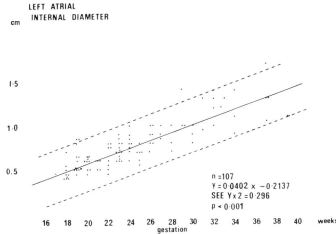

Fig. 13.9 The growth of the left atrium between 16 weeks gestation and term.

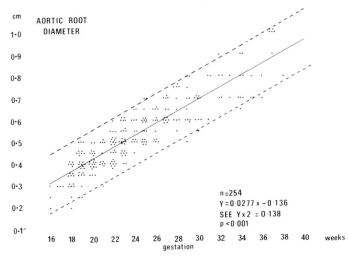

Fig. 13.7 The M-mode echocardiogram of a 23-week-old fetus taken across the two ventricular chambers with the beam perpendicular to the septum.

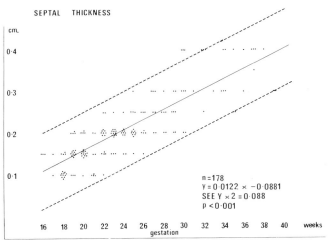

Fig. 13.10 The increase in septal thickness between 16 weeks gestation and term.

Fig. 13.8 The growth of the aortic root between 16 weeks and term. The mean and two standard deviations for the mean are plotted on the graph.

Pregnancies at increased risk of congenital heart disease

Ideally all pregnancies should be screened for congenital anomalies using cross-sectional ultrasound at around 18 weeks gestation. At this stage many major abnormalities can be detected or excluded. As the cost of good image quality scanning equipment becomes progressively less, this is not an unreasonable future prospect. At the present time, however, resources in services and equipment dictate that fetal echocardiography be confined to high risk pregnancies. Table 13.1 lists the high risk groups which should be selected for study. When a previous baby has been affected by congenital heart disease the risk of recurrence in a subsequent pregnancy is 1 in 50 (Nora, 1968). The risk in those pregnancies where a parent is affected is 14% (Whittemore et al, 1982). Diabetic mothers are reported to have double the risk of the normal population of congenital heart disease, although this may not be true of a well-controlled diabetic population such as we have studied.

Fetal ascites can be due to intra-uterine cardiac failure (Allan et al, 1981). Kleinman et al (1982) found structural cardiac abnormality in over one-half of their referred cases of fetal ascites. If an abnormality is detected in any system in the fetus, then the fetal heart should be studied as there

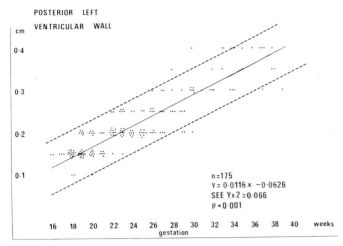

Fig. 13.11 Posterior left ventricular wall thickness parallels septal growth with increasing gestational age.

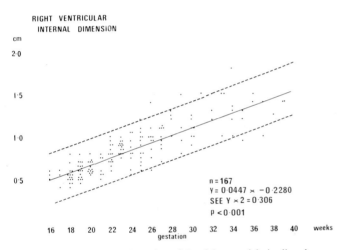

Fig. 13.12 The internal dimension of the right ventricle in diastole between 16 weeks gestation and term.

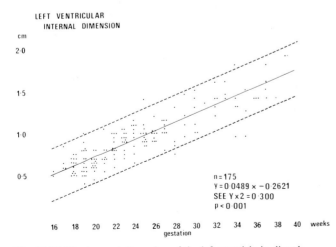

Fig. 13.13 The internal dimension of the left ventricle in diastole between 16 weeks gestation and term.

Table 13.1 High risk groups of pregnancies

Family history of congenital heart disease
Maternal diabetes
Fetal arrhythmia
Fetal ascites
Fetal anomaly
Miscellaneous groups e.g. – drugs such as lithium, steriods, etc.
– infections, e.g. rubella

is an increased incidence of congenital heart disease in association with other anomalies. Some drugs such as cortisone or oral contraceptives have been reported to increase the incidence of congenital heart disease if taken in early pregnancy. Lithium, a drug not uncommonly used in healthy young women for depression, has been associated with an increased incidence of Ebstein's anomaly (Nora et al, 1974). Rubella infection of the fetus can cause com-

Table 13.2 Structural cardiac abnormalities predicted

Echocardiographic diagnosis	Gestational age first seen (weeks)	Outcome of pregnancy
Primum atrioventricular septal defect	16	TOP for trisomy 21
Hypoplastic aortic arch	18	TOP for XO
Primum atrioventricular septal defect, interrupted aortic arch, complete heart block	20	TOP for congenital heart defect
Rhabdomyoma	22	TOP for congenital heart defect
Mitral atresia	22	Catheter confirmation. NND
Ebstein's anomaly	24	NND. Anatomical confirmation
Hypertrophic cardiomyopathy (3 cases)	22, 24, 26	TOP for renal anomalies × 3
Cardiac tumour	27	Intra-uterine death
Common arterial trunk	27	Catheter confirmation postnatally
Tetralogy of Fallot (3 cases)	32, 33, 37	NND anatomical confirmation
Aortic stenosis	32	NND anatomical confirmation
Aortic atresia	32	NND anatomical confirmation
Right ventricular hypertrophy	35	NND anatomical confirmation
Complete atrioventricular septal defect, DORV, complete heart block	38	Catheter confirmation

TOP – termination of pregnancy; NND – neonatal death

plex congenital heart disease but much more commonly it damages the arterial duct so that it does not close postnatally (Hardy, 1968). This, of course, would not be predictable prenatally.

Detection of abnormalities

During our study we have, to date (March 1984), examined over 1000 pregnancies. The first 200 studies were of unselected normal pregnancies. No abnormality was seen in this group. All the predicted abnormalities have been seen in high risk groups. Altogether, thirty-four abnormalities were observed (Allan et al, 1984; Table 13.2). (*Editors' note*: In the period up to September 1986, a further 100 cases were successfully diagnosed during intrauterine life.)

Four of the abnormalities detected are illustrated in Figures 13.14–13.17. Figure 13.14 shows a rhabdomyoma filling the right ventricle. The anatomical specimen displayed alongside is cut in the same projection. Figure 13.15 shows the displacement of the tricuspid valve that occurs in Ebstein's anomaly. The four chamber projection of the heart is seen in both the anatomical and echocardiographic section.

Figure 13.16 shows a common arterial trunk sectioned in the long axis. The aorta overrides the ventricular septum and a large ventricular septal defect is present. Angling the transducer from this section showed that the pulmonary trunk arose directly from the common trunk. Figure 13.17 shows another heart sectioned in its long axis. The aortic root was small, being below the 5th percentile for the gestational age. The left ventricle and left atrium are grossly dilated. The left ventricle was contracting poorly and the mitral valve excursion was diminished. This was considered to be aortic atresia or critical aortic stenosis with

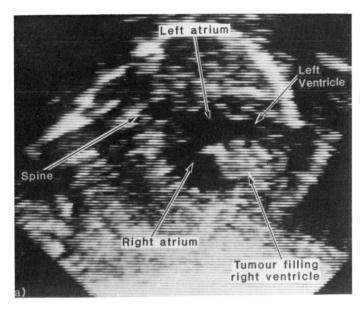

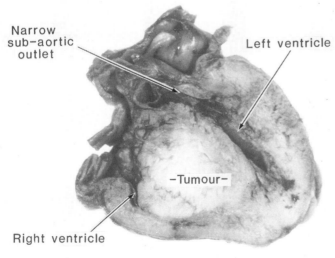

Fig. 13.14 A large tumour is seen filling the right ventricular cavity in the four chamber projection. The same heart is dissected to show the appearance as seen at autopsy.

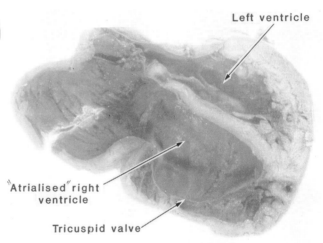

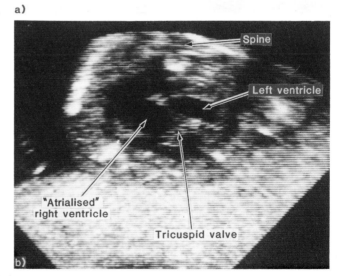

Fig. 13.15 The heart is seen in the four chamber projection at 24 weeks gestation (upper). The septal leaflet of the tricuspid valve is displaced. The right atrium is dilated. The heart therefore shows Ebstein's anomaly, as confirmed by dissection of the autopsy specimen.

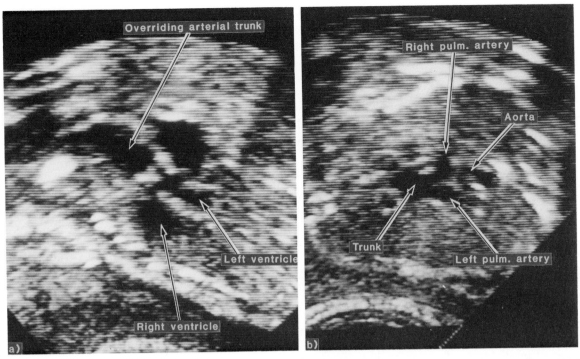

Fig. 13.16 The aorta was found to arise astride the ventricular septum and appeared dilated (a). (b) Angulation of the transducer from this view revealed the pulmonary trunk arising from the back of this artery, which was a common arterial trunk.

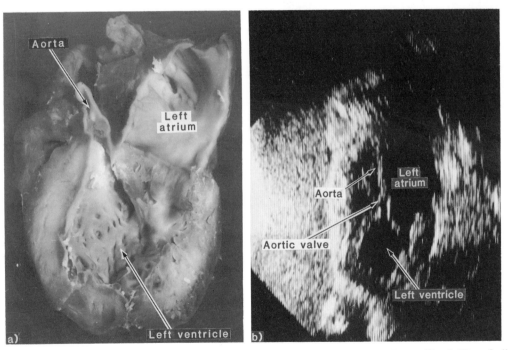

Fig. 13.17 The aortic root is small for the gestational age (0.4 cm at 32 weeks). The left atrium and ventricular are dilated. These findings were confirmed by dissection of the autopsy specimen.

associated dilatation and hypertrophy of a left ventricle probably affected by endocardial fibrosis. These findings were confirmed at autopsy. The aortic valve was disorganised but patent and endocardial fibrosis was present affecting the left ventricle and left atrium.

In addition to the abnormalities shown in Table 13.1, ten further cases were seen at around 24 weeks gestation when a ventricular septal defect was apparently present in the perimembranous region. Nine of the cases were reviewed at 36 weeks gestation when the septum was seen

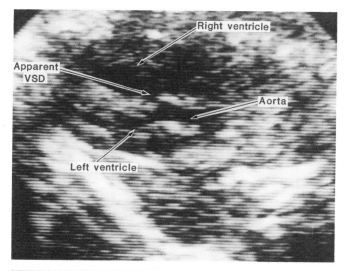

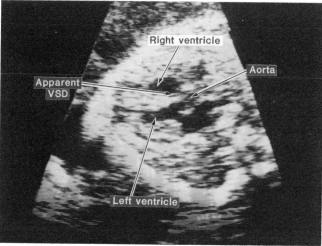

Fig. 13.18 Both echocardiograms display the heart in long axis, both pregnancies around 24 weeks gestation. The top picture shows the apparent perimembranous ventricular septal defect which was confirmed at autopsy. The bottom picture shows a similar septal discontinuity. This however had disappeared before term.

to be intact. The tenth case was not reviewed because the patient lived at a distance. This fetus died in neonatal life of associated renal anomalies. A small perimembranous ventricular septal defect was found at autopsy. The echocardiogram from this case is seen as the top panel of Figure 13.18. The lower panel shows one of the other cases of ventricular septal defect which closed in intra-uterine life.

Right ventricular dilation was seen in six cases. This was a consequence of cardiac failure due to extracardiac anomalies, for example rhesus iso-immunisation. It was also seen if cardiac failure was caused by a fetal arrhythmia. Global cardiac dilation and diminished left ventricular function was seen in two cases just prior to death in utero.

In over 1000 pregnancies a normal fetal heart was predicted echocardiographically and this was confirmed postnatally. False negative diagnoses were made in three cases. All died of a chromosomal trisomy and the cardiac

specimens were examined at autopsy. In the first case, a small ostium primum atrioventricular septal defect, between 2 and 3 mm in size, was found which had not been detected echocardiographically. But good pictures were obtained and, since this heart showed all the stigmata of an atrioventricular septal defect, it should not have been overlooked. In the second case, studied echocardiographically at 22 weeks gestation, poor quality images were interpreted as showing a normal heart. At autopsy tetralogy of Fallot was found. Although the ventricular septal defect was small and the aortic override and pulmonary outflow tract obstruction not yet marked, the defect should again have been detected. In the third case, studied at 38 weeks gestation, image quality was poor because of the late gestational age. Again the heart was considered to be normal, but at autopsy complete transposition with interrupted aortic arch was found. Retrospectively it proved very difficult to trace either great artery away from the heart because of rib shadowing, but their relative orientation appeared to be normal. These three cases demonstrate the difficulties in detecting even major anomalies. It is to be hoped that rigid adherence to the rules of establishing connexions completely, together with restudy of any case in which image quality is inadequate, will eradicate false negative results. In none of the three cases was a repeat examination possible, despite unacceptable image quality in two cases, as each pregnancy was subsequently interrupted.

Two false positive diagnoses have been made, namely aortic stenosis at 34 weeks and a ventricular septal defect at 18 weeks gestation. In the first case the right ventricle was dilated and the left ventricle and aortic root were small for the gestational age. A persistent sinus bradycardia was recorded and the aortic valve did not appear to open normally. Postnatally the underdeveloped, poorly functioning left ventricle was confirmed, as was the small aortic root. A valve abnormality was not demonstrable. Since then two similar cases of right ventricular dilation in association with left ventricular underdevelopment and bradycardia have been detected. In both cases the mitral valve excursion again appeared limited but these findings have been interpreted as perhaps secondary to functional limitation of left heart flow. This may be due to alteration for some reason, as yet unknown, of the volume of right to left atrial shunting. In the second false positive case, an inlet perimembranous ventricular septal defect was thought to be present in a Down's fetus examined at 18 weeks gestation. Autopsy revealed no abnormality.

Fetal arrhythmias

Twenty nine cases were referred for evaluation of suspected fetal arrhythmias (Allan et al, 1983). Seven were thought to show only normal variation in fetal heart rate and rhythm (i.e. they either showed runs of sinus bradycardia

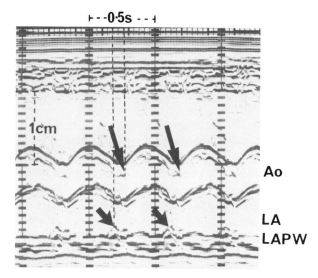

Fig. 13.19 The M-mode echocardiogram crosses the aortic root and left atrium. Ventricular contraction can be inferred from aortic valve opening; left atrial wall contraction can be seen posteriorly.

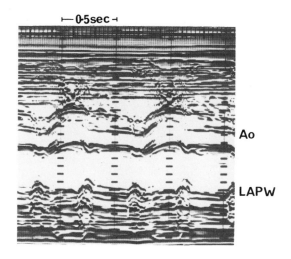

Fig. 13.21 The aortic root and left atrial wall are seen. The aortic valve opens about 80 times per min. It is unrelated to atrial contraction at around 140 beats per min.

or sinus tachycardia, neither rhythm being sustained for more than a few minutes). There were ten cases which showed irregularity of rhythm with frequent premature atrial or ventricular contractions. 'Frequent' was arbitrarily defined as there being more than one premature contraction in ten sinus beats. The origin of the premature beats could be assessed by the M-mode echocardiogram. Atrial and ventricular contraction and their relationship to each other could be compared. Figure 13.19 shows the M-mode beam crossing the atrial and ventricular walls. Normally atrial contraction precedes ventricular contraction by approximately 100 ms at the normal fetal heart rate of around 140 beats per min. Figure 13.20 demonstrates a

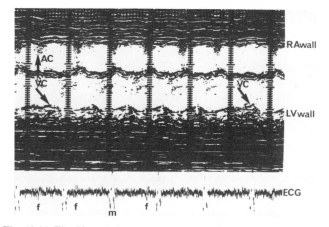

Fig. 13.20 The M-mode beam crosses atrial and ventricular wall simultaneously allowing the relationship between atrial and ventricular contraction to be observed. The first premature ventricular contraction (VC) is preceded by a premature atrial contraction (AC). The second premature ventricular contraction is unassociated with atrial contraction. The first premature beat therefore originates in the atria, the second in the ventricles.

premature atrial contraction with a normal time relationship to a ventricular beat, but later in the tracing a premature ventricular contraction occurs unassociated with atrial contraction. Premature contractions were not found to give rise to tachycardias and were not associated with fetal morbidity or mortality. This is consistent with larger series from other centres (Komaromy et al, 1977; Southall et al, 1980). The comparison of atrial and ventricular contraction is also used for the evaluation of a bradycardia or tachycardia. Figure 13.21 shows complete heart block. The atrial contraction at 140 beats per min is unrelated to ventricular contraction occurring at 80 beats per min. Five cases of isolated complete heart block were detected and two associated with structural cardiac malformation. In three of the five cases of isolated block there was serological evidence of maternal connective tissue disease. Isolated heart block was associated with a good prognosis. Five cases were referred because of the detection of a fetal heart rate of over 200 beats per min. Three were found to be in atrial flutter while the other two had supraventricular tachycardias. Figure 13.22 shows atrial flutter waves of 480 beats per min with a ventricular rate of 240 beats per min. One case had gross intra-uterine cardiac failure as evidenced by right ventricular dilatation, fetal ascites and subcutaneous oedema. One early case was delivered prematurely. The other cases were all treated with maternal anti-arrhythmic drugs. All converted to sinus rhythm before delivery. Three responded satisfactorily to digoxin, the case with cardiac failure also required verapamil and frusemide. There was a good outcome in all fetuses. It is important that antenatal therapy is tried aggressively in these cases in order to avoid the premature delivery of a hydropic infant. There is a high mortality in fetal hydrops which is increased if prematurity is also present.

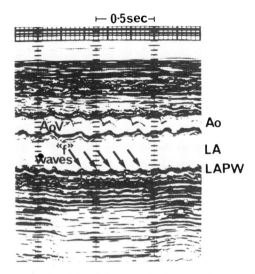

Fig. 13.22 The left atrial wall is seen behind the aortic root and contracts 480 times per min. The aortic valve opens at half this rate, 240 times per min.

PLACE OF FETAL ECHOCARDIOGRAPHY

Our results (Allan et al, 1981b) and those of other workers in the field (Kleinman et al, 1980; Silverman et al, 1982) suggest that fetal echocardiography can predict structural cardiac anomaly with accuracy. Initial routine screening, with referral of suspected abnormal pregnancies to a specialist centre, is already starting in the UK. It is hoped that this will increase in the future. It is relatively easy to predict cardiac normality, but often very difficult to 'sort out' accurately all the components of a complex lesion. This requires specialist knowledge of paediatric echocardiography. Concentration of the experience of anomalies in a referral centre will hopefully increase accuracy. It is also preferable that selected centres gather experience with any therapy which might be given during pregnancy. This can become necessary in cases of intra-uterine arrhythmia. Termination of a pregnancy where an inoperable lesion is detected is one application of the technique. We have now seen three cases in which a major abnormality was detected early enough for termination of pregnancy to be considered. Termination has taken place in two cases. This application raises many technical and ethical problems. For example, how accurate is the echocardiogram alone at defining operability? Which defects should be considered inoperable or associated with a very high operative risk? Only a team approach involving paediatric cardiologists, surgeons and the parents, the team together considering the case on its individual merits, will solve these problems. Where abnormality is detected late in pregnancy or where pregnancy is electively continued, the chances of infant survival will be optimised if the pregnancy is delivered in centres where paediatric cardiac investigative and surgical facilities are available.

REFERENCES

Allan L D, Tynan M J, Campbell S, Wilkinson J L, Anderson R H 1980 Echocardiographic and anatomical correlates in the fetus. British Heart Journal 44: 444–451

Allan L, Little D, Whitehead M I 1981a Fetal ascites associated with congenital heart disease. British Journal of Obstetrics and Gynaecology 88: 453–455

Allan L D, Tynan M J, Campbell S, Anderson R H 1981b Identification of congenital cardiac malformations by echocardiography in mid-trimester fetus. British Heart Journal 46: 358–362

Allan L D, Anderson R H, Sullivan I D, Campbell S, Holt D W, Tynan M 1983 Evaluation of fetal arrhythmias by echocardiography. British Heart Journal 50: 240–245

Allan L D, Crawford D C, Anderson R H, Tynan M 1984 Echocardiographic and anatomical correlates in fetal congenital heart disease. British Heart Journal 52: 542–548

Campbell S, Holt E M, Johnstone F D, May P 1972 Anencephaly: Early ultrasonic diagnosis and active management. Lancet 2: 1226–1227

Dawes G S, Mott J C 1964 Changes in O₂ distribution and consumption in foetal lambs with variations in umbilical blood flow. Journal of Physiology 170: 524–540

Dawes G S, Mott J C, Widdicombe J G 1955 The fetal circulation in the lamb. Journal of Physiology 128: 384–395

Garrett W J, Grimwald G, Robinson D E 1970 Prenatal diagnosis of fetal polycystic kidney by ultrasound. Australian and New Zealand Journal of Obstetrics and Gynaecology 10: 7–9

Hardy J B 1968 Viruses and the fetus. Postgraduate Medicine 43: 156

Houlton M C C, Sutton M, Aitken J 1974 Antenatal diagnosis of duodenal atresia. Journal of Obstetrics and Gynaecology of the British Commonwealth 81: 821

Kleinman C S, Hobbins J C, Jaffe C C, Lynch D C, Talner N S 1980 Echocardiographic studies of the human fetus: Prenatal diagnosis of congenital heart disease and cardiac dysrhythmias. Paediatrics 65: 1059–1067

Kleinman C S, Donnerstein R L, De Vore G R, et al 1982 Fetal echocardiography for evaluation of in utero congestive heart failure. New England Journal of Medicine 306: 568–575

Komaromy B, Gaal J, Lampe L 1977 Fetal arrhythmias during pregnancy and labour. British Journal of Obstetrics and Gynaecology 43: 719–721

Nora J J 1968 Multifactorial inheritance hypothesis for the etiology of congenital heart diseases. Circulation 38: 604

Nora J J, Nora A H, Toews W H 1974 Lithium, Ebstein's anomaly and other congenital heart defects. Lancet 2: 594–595

O'Brien G D, Rodeck C, Queenam J T 1980 Early prenatal diagnosis of diastrophic dwarfism by ultrasound. British Medical Journal 280: 1300

Sahn D J, Lange L W, Allen H D, et al 1980 Quantitative real-time cross-sectional echocardiography in the developing normal human fetus and newborn. Circulation 62: 588–597

Silverman N H, Snider A R, Golbus N S, Stanger P 1982 Perspectives on fetal echocardiography. In: 1ᵉʳ symposium international d'echocardiologie foetale. Strasbourg 23 & 24 Avril, 1982. Milupa diététique, p 95–110

Southall D P, Richards J, Hardwick R A, et al 1980 Prospective study of fetal heart rate and rhythm patterns. Archives of Disease in Childhood 55: 506–511

Whittemore R, Hobbins J C, Engle M A 1982 Pregnancy and its outcome in women with and without surgical treatment of congenital heart disease. American Journal of Cardiology 50: 641–651

14

Cardiac catheterisation and angiocardiography

Facilities for cardiac catheterisation and angiocardiography are essential for any centre which undertakes surgical management of patients with congenital heart disease. The cost of a cardiac catheterisation laboratory or laboratories will be the single greatest capital outlay required for such a unit, and therefore bears close examination. In this chapter we will consider the basic requirements for a cardiac catheterisation laboratory, and the general approach to the investigation of children with heart disease. Special techniques related to specific diseases will be dealt with under those diseases.

BASIC EQUIPMENT

It is important when planning a cardiac catheterisation laboratory to ensure that it is of adequate size. As new techniques develop, it is almost certain that these will require extra pieces of equipment, and provision for space for these should be 'planned into' the original specification. It should also be recognised that some equipment will come into and out of the cardiac catheterisation laboratory, for example the trolley on which the patient is transported. While there are strong arguments for having a dedicated cross-sectional ultrasound scanner in the cardiac catheterisation laboratory, if this is not possible, it is essential that the layout of the laboratory permits the scanner easily to be brought into the laboratory and alongside the patient. The same can be said for isotope scanning equipment.

The room should be built with as much attention to sterility as is any operating theatre. This means that, in general, technicians and radiographers should be separated by glass panels from the catheterisation laboratory, so far as is possible, which dictates that there be an efficient intercom system between the catheterisation table and the technicians and radiographers.

A defibrillator and anaesthetic trolley will be required. Some catheterisation laboratories have the facilities of projecting moving pictures onto the roof of the catheterisation laboratory, so as to soothe the patient. Soft background music is often helpful for inducing calm both in the child and in the operators.

Equipment for screening and angiocardiography

Standard equipment for the mid 1980s would consist of facilities for biplane screening and biplane angiocardiography. If biplane screening is used intelligently, it can greatly reduce the risk of cardiac perforation, since it prevents, for example, manipulation of the catheter within the right atrial appendage under the false impression that it is pointing towards the left atrium. Techniques such as trans-septal and supra-sternal puncture are also made much safer if performed with biplane screening, since there can be no doubt as to where the tip of the needle is in relation to the cardiac chambers if orthogonal planes of screening are used.

From the angiocardiographic point of view, there is considerable advantage in having the two planes not locked at right angles to one another. Having to move the patient for an angiocardiogram carries the risk that they will wake up from sleep and become distressed. So, if it is at all possible to have the X-ray equipment moved rather than the table or the patient, this is beneficial. As a minimum requirement, it should be possible to rotate one or other plane round the long axis of the patient, which is in turn parallel to the long axis of the table. If axial views are to be obtained, it is also valuable to be able to have caudocranial angulation applied to one or both planes. However, the benefits of built-in capacity for caudocranial tilt can be overemphasised. This is because while the patient lies flat on the table, his chin gets in the way of applying caudocranial tilt to the degree of steepness required for the best possible pictures. The angle can be steepened somewhat if the head is rotated to one side or the other, but in practice, the optimal orientation can only be achieved if the patient's shoulders are lifted off the table with a wedge so that his head can fall back. If this kind of manoeuvre is needed, one might as well not have built in caudocranial tilt in the first place.

Another problem with X-ray equipment is that the more versatile it is in terms of possible projections, the bulkier it tends to be, and the more difficult it is to gain access to the child. Ideally, the operator wants to be able to perform catheterisation from either leg, either arm, or the neck, without breaking his own neck while looking at the monitors during cardiac catheterisation. Very few installations are designed so that the operator can sit anywhere he likes round the catheterisation table. If he cannot do this, it is essential that he should be able to reach the necessary position relative to the child by turning the child round on the table. Movement of the child should not prejudice making any of the measurements or looking at the monitors. Furthermore, the safety of the child during cardiac catheterisation demands that there should be easy access to the airway by an anaesthetist in case of a cardiac arrest. In practice, having the way to the patient's head clear means that, normally, a nurse familiar to the child can sit by his head during the catheterisation and soothe him if necessary. Babies can be given a dummy coated with brandy and honey to suck.

The advent of digital vascular imaging will probably result in a major change in the planning of cardiac catheterisation laboratories, because it is cheaper to install digital vascular imaging for a single plane device than to add a second plane. From the angiocardiographic point of view, this will probably not matter, because digital vascular imaging will permit multiple selective injections in the same site with small doses of contrast medium in different projections. Provided that one does not wish to measure, say, ventricular volumes by biplane techniques, the second plane will become dispensible, and this will take away most of the problems of access to the child that have been already mentioned. However, the aspects of safety already mentioned will be compromised by complete removal of the second plane, although this will be mitigated to some extent by use of cross-sectional echocardiography rather than X-rays for screening.

It should be clear from the description above that equipment for studying congenital heart disease differs very significantly from that needed for coronary arteriograms. Though it is inevitable that adult and paediatric cardiologists will have to share facilities in smaller centres, this is far from ideal.

To inject contrast medium, some kind of pressure injector is essential. The most important requirement of any machine is that it should be able to deliver contrast medium so fast that it almost, but not quite, bursts the cardiac catheter. All other considerations are secondary, such as the capability of performing multiple and/or electrocardiogram-triggered injections.

Pressure measurements

It should be possible to measure at least two pressures simultaneously, and preferably four. Transducers for fluid-filled catheters are standard, but ideally, it should also be possible to measure pressures with catheter-tip micromanometers. A pressurised flush system containing no air helps to keep catheters free of clot, and a system of slow heparin infusion into arterial pressure lines is also valuable.

Blood gas analysis

Correct interpretation of haemodynamic data depends upon knowing the acid-base state of the child at the time the measurement was made. Furthermore, if the child is (or becomes) sick during catheterisation, it is essential to be able to measure blood gases repeatedly and swiftly. Automated blood gas analysers have proved very valuable in this respect.

Oximetry

Cuvette oximetry used to be very popular in cardiac catheterisation laboratories, because once the oxygen saturation in the cuvette had been measured, the blood could be returned to the patient, thereby sparing blood loss. Such oximetry was never particularly accurate, and nowadays it is best to use an accurate machine even if it does not permit blood replacement, since these can provide measurements on as little as 0.1 ml of blood, and therefore do not present a significant risk of blood loss. Though oxygen content can be determined indirectly from oxygen saturation and haemoglobin concentration, this involves multiplication of errors. For measurement of blood flow by the Fick method, it is preferable to buy a machine which measures oxygen content directly.

Oxygen uptake

Use of the flow-through method has meant that it is extremely easy to measure oxygen uptake in babies and children of any age breathing room air (Kappagoda & Linden, 1972; Kappagoda et al, 1973). Measurement of oxygen consumption during anaesthesia or during breathing of mixtures other than room air is more complicated, but methods have been described (Jones et al, 1972). As will be argued below, the Fick method is so central to the measurement and comprehension of the haemodynamics of congenital heart disease that some means of measuring oxygen uptake is essential in any cardiac catheterisation laboratory.

Optional extras

Electrophysiological studies are probably best carried out in a laboratory dedicated to that purpose. Nonetheless, they can be incorporated in a general purpose catheterisation laboratory. Six to eight channels are required for recording intracardiac electrograms, and a unit for programmed electrical stimulation is essential.

Many cardiac catheterisation laboratories now have the facility for on-line computer recording of data. This is a mixed blessing. If this does what the manufacturers say it will do, cardiologists in training will no longer have to measure pressures for themselves, or perform the calculations necessary to determine, for example, pulmonary blood flow. They will therefore miss out an important educational exercise as far as understanding cardiac function is concerned. More importantly, many pressure recordings from fluid-filled catheters in babies with very rapid heart rates contain too much artefact for the computer programme to deal with. As a result, measurements of pressure frequently have to be made by old-fashioned methods. If this has to be done, the on-line computer is not paying its way. In our view, the off-line archiving of cardiac catheterisation data is far more important, if less exciting, than on-line acquisition. Probably the most valuable use of the computational capabilities of the computer in the vicinity of the cardiac catheterisation laboratory is in calculating ventricular volumes and mass. This kind of analysis, however, can almost always be done perfectly satisfactorily directly from video tape rather than on-line.

Facilities for thermodilution and dye-dilution

These are useful, but certainly not essential when Fick measurements of cardiac output are available together with facilities for cross-sectional contrast echocardiography. On the other hand, if exercise-studies are to be carried out in, for example, postoperative patients, measurement of cardiac output by thermodilution or dyedilution is preferable, since these methods compare most favourably with the Fick method at high cardiac outputs. The simplest way of applying a fixed workload within the catheterisation laboratory is to exercise patients in the supine position using a bicycle ergometer.

PRELUDE TO CARDIAC CATHETERISATION

In-patient or out-patient investigation?

Traditionally, children requiring elective cardiac catheterisation are admitted for two nights – one before and the other following cardiac catheterisation. This practice is justified on the grounds that it ensures that the child is relaxed and fasting on the day of catheterisation, and also provides in-hospital monitoring of problems following cardiac catheterisation. This approach has been effectively challenged by at least two groups of workers (Cumming, 1982; Waldman et al, 1982). Older children who feel well after catheterisation are sent home 30–120 minutes after the procedure if limb circulation is normal and there is no

indication of bleeding at the catheterisation site. Infants and young children are often more heavily sedated, and need to be kept in hospital for somewhat longer, until they are awake or easily aroused, and have been fed at least once. Selection of patients for out-patient cardiac catheterisation would appear to be the key to this policy, but Cumming (1982) stated that for the past several years, neither disease severity nor type of procedure had influenced the decision to perform catheterisation on an out-patient basis. Patients sent home after cardiac catheterisation included some with primary pulmonary hypertension, complete transposition with severe cyanosis, and patients with tetralogy of Fallot and cyanotic spells. The last group were discharged home on propranolol, however. No-one would advocate out-patient catheterisations for desperately ill neonates, but both of the above-mentioned teams have increased the proportion of patients catheterised as out-patients to 80%. The incidence of complication was extremely low in both series, and where problems did occur, they were easily treated by return of the child to the hospital. The advantages of this policy are that both patient and parents are much happier, and that it saves money. Such a programme demands very great efficiency on the part of the medical staff concerned, and may not be so appropriate in centres where a large proportion of cardiac catheterisations are carried out by doctors in training, where the complication rate can be higher.

We believe that it cannot be stressed too much that cardiac catheterisation and angiocardiography are but parts of the entire investigation of the child. This means that, before beginning the procedure, the operator should have examined the child himself, and have reviewed the electrocardiogram and chest X-ray, together with all previous cross-sectional echocardiograms, cardiac catheterisations and angiocardiograms. Cardiac catheterisation can kill the patient. It is tragic if death should occur during a manoeuvre designed to gain information which has already been obtained in a previous investigation. The operator, having considered all the information that has already been obtained, must decide precisely what information is lacking, and develop a strategy for obtaining those data in the safest and quickest possible way. One of the most important parts of the training of a paediatric cardiologist is time spent in thinking these matters over and discussing them with a senior colleague before he embarks on the catheterisation itself. One additional advantage of out-patient cardiac catheterisation may be that it encourages this planning to be carried out at leisure a day or two before the cardiac catheterisation, rather than immediately before the study.

Premedication

There is much to be said for performing cardiac catheterisation under a general anaesthetic. It causes much less distress to the child, and permits the procedure to be carried out much more quickly and therefore safely. The only disadvantage is that the conditions under general anaesthesia are far removed from those pertaining in normal life. This disadvantage can be largely mitigated if standard gas mixtures are employed, e.g. 30% oxygen and the remainder nitrous oxide, with as much fluothane as is necessary to induce light general anaesthesia. Sick infants very often require intubation, paralysis and ventilation for shock and heart failure; these conditions are ideal for cardiac catheterisation. An alternative to general anaesthetic which produces similar ideal conditions for cardiac catheterisation is ketamine; with this agent the child is entirely quiet and still, yet breathing room air. The systemic hypertension that occurs shortly after administration of the drug resolves after 20 minutes or so (Faithfull & Haider, 1971). The depth of anaesthesia is such that an anaesthetist should be in the catheterisation laboratory throughout the procedure.

When anaesthetists cannot spare the time to assist with cardiac catheterisation, or the cooperation of the patient is necessary, or it is felt important that conditions should be as 'physiological' as possible, all children (except babies in the first three months of life) require premedication.

The most widely used is 0.1 ml/kg of 'Toronto mix', which consists of pethidine (25 mg/ml), phenergan (6.25 mg/ml) and chlorpromazine (6.25 mg/ml) (Smith et al, 1958). In dogs, this causes pulmonary vascular resistance to rise and systemic vascular resistance to fall (Goldberg et al, 1969). It by no means always produces adequate sedation during catheterisation; supplementary intravenous diazepam is often required.

An alternative is droperidol (62.5 μg/kg) and fentanyl (1.25 μ/kg). This sedates better than Toronto mix, but occasionally causes nightmares and athetoid movements which make cardiac catheterisation impossible despite the use of diphenhydramine. Indices of left ventricular function are not different from those obtained with light general anaesthesia (Graham et al, 1974b).

APPROACH TO THE HEART

Up until 1963, cardiac catheterisation in infants and children was almost entirely carried out by the cut-down approach. Then Lurie and colleagues (1963) demonstrated the possibility of percutaneous catheterisation in children. Their methods were refined (Kirkpatrick et al, 1970; Takahashi et al, 1970) and also adopted by others (Boijsen & Lundstrom, 1968; Simovitch et al, 1970). Further technological improvement resulted from the use of percutaneous sheaths (originally introduced by Desilets & Hoffman in 1965), as described by Neches and colleagues (1972). The advantage of using a sheath during percutaneous cardiac catheterisation is that it facilitates changing catheters, and means that catheters without end-holes, which are safer for angiocardiography, can be used. Furthermore, long sheaths reaching the heart or great vessels can be used to direct unwieldy catheters such as those used for closing ducts to the appropriate spot. The result of all these improvements is that, now, percutaneous catheterisation is easily the most popular method of approach to cardiac catheterisation both in infants and children. It will therefore be described first.

Percutaneous catheterisation

Use of the percutaneous technique in children is almost entirely restricted to femoral vein and artery catheterisation. This is because entry to them is simple, and they provide the easiest access to the heart, certainly for the transvenous approach. The pulses are felt prior to the beginning of the catheterisation, and if the femoral pulses are feeble or impossible to palpate, they may be located using a Doppler probe (Sunderland et al, 1976). Once the position of the femoral artery is found, a scratch on the skin with the needle can be used to mark it. The groins are then scrubbed and prepared, and the skin and vessels anaesthetised with 1% lignocaine. It is important to place the local anaesthetic in strategic sites, otherwise the whole area becomes so bulky with injectate that the vessels become difficult to feel. Accordingly, the needle of the local anaesthetic is introduced in the same direction as will be the needle for percutaneous catheterisation. The solution is infiltrated round the anticipated site of entry to the femoral artery and vein and around the site of the skin puncture (Fig. 14.1).

Percutaneous femoral venous catheterisation

In infants, we have found it extremely helpful for a nurse to exert manual pressure on the abdomen (J. Endrys, personal communication, 1977). This distends the femoral vein, increasing the size of the target. Pressure is maintained while the dilator and/or sheath are being advanced into the vein, but then relaxed, so as not to produce back bleeding. The femoral artery is palpated, and the point at which it begins to dip posteriorly is identified. The femoral vein will then lie medially to the femoral artery, at a distance varying from 1 cm in a patient over 40 lb to 2 mm in a newborn baby. In difficult cases, the femoral vein may actually lie behind the femoral artery. Since there is no clear-cut relationship between the distance of vein from artery and the size of the patient, exploration of a sizeable region medial to the femoral artery may be needed. The needle is advanced at a shallow angle along the anticipated line of the vein until dark venous blood flows back freely through it without spurting. Abdominal compression in infants greatly assists identification of penetration of the vein, because it increases the amount of bleeding back

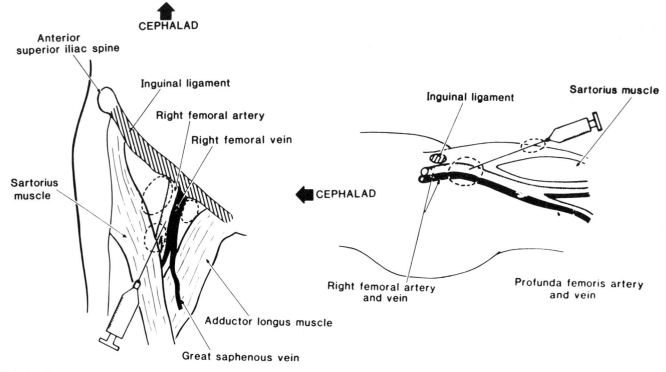

Fig. 14.1 Percutaneous femoral arterial and venous catheterisation. The diagram shows the relevant landmarks. The dotted lines enclose regions where infiltration of local anaesthetic is necessary. (Redrawn after Takahashi et al, 1970.)

through the needle. The soft end of the guide-wire is then introduced through the needle, with as little force applied to the needle as possible. With luck, it will pass without difficulty into the vein. If any difficulty is experienced in advancing the wire beyond the tip of the needle, it is essential to use no force. The needle should be angled to and fro, and possibly rotated, with gentle movements in and out of the guide-wire until the vein is satisfactorily entered. If force is used, the result will almost certainly be a false passage of the guide-wire outside the vein. If the guide-wire cannot be passed beyond the end of the needle, then both needle and wire should be withdrawn and digital pressure kept on the site of puncture for a minute or two before starting again. Sometimes, the guide-wire enters the vein satisfactorily from the needle, but becomes stuck a little way further on. In this case, the best thing to do is to pass a dilator over the guide-wire into the vein, remove the guide-wire, and then inject a little dilute contrast medium while screening the end of the dilator. This usually demonstrates the problem, which can be overcome by choice of a suitable guide-wire.

With the guide-wire satisfactorily positioned in the vein, it is held in place by digital pressure upstream of the puncture site, and the needle is pulled back and off the end of the guide-wire. A sharp scalpel blade is used to enlarge the puncture site in the skin to 2 or 3 mm across, so that entry to the skin does not impede insertion of dilators. A dilator is now passed over the guide-wire, and advanced into the

vein. It is often helpful to twist the dilator as it penetrates the vein wall. As it enters the vein, a slight 'give' is usually felt. A succession of dilators can now be used if a large catheter is required. The last dilator used has a sheath over it. Dilator and sheath are passed into the vein, the catheter is then prepared and flushed, the dilator is withdrawn and the catheter is introduced into the sheath. Blood loss after withdrawing the dilator can easily be controlled by digital pressure on the sheath. It is most important not to use any force in advancing the catheter through the sheath; otherwise, the very fine sheath may be avulsed from its Luer lock. If the catheter size is matched to the sheath size, then blood loss is usually minimal. It sometimes happens that one wants to change from a larger to a smaller catheter, or else that one wants to use a catheter which is not of uniform diameter, such as a balloon catheter. In this case, it is wise to connect a grommet to the percutaneous sheath. The grommet can then be tightened round the shank of the catheter to prevent blood loss. It should not be over-tightened, since this would impede catheter manipulations.

The great advantage of percutaneous sheath catheterisation is that it makes changes of catheters extremely easy. If a larger catheter is desired, then the original dilator has to be introduced into the sheath, and the guide-wire advanced into the vein. Sheath and dilator are then withdrawn and replaced with a larger dilator and sheath. The catheter is then exchanged for the dilator as before.

Percutaneous femoral arterial catheterisation

This is preferably carried out after femoral vein catheterisation, particularly if systemic heparinisation is employed (Girod et al, 1982). It seems logical to give the heparin prior to attempted entry to the femoral artery so that the heparin will assuredly reach the limb distal to the point of arterial puncture. The artery is carefully palpated as it emerges from under the inguinal ligament, and then as it bends posteriorly during its descent into the inguinal fossa. This 'bend' is the target. For obvious reasons, no abdominal pressure is applied. The needle is advanced until arterial blood spurts back through it, signifying entry to the appropriate vessel. Occasionally, it is helpful to 'spear' the artery by rapidly advancing the needle, and then watch for blood returning during withdrawal of the needle, signifying entry. While blood spurts back through the needle, the guide-wire is advanced carefully through it. All the precautions already listed for venous catheterisation are observed. In the first instance, it is probably best to introduce a fine plastic dilator into the artery and nothing else. This manoeuvre in itself results in a very low rate of arterial complication (Neches et al, 1972) while providing an invaluable means of monitoring the state of the patient throughout the cardiac catheterisation, as well as having a systemic arterial pressure as a reference point for comparison with other pressures. Then, if it is clear that retrograde catheterisation is going to be required, the appropriate sized catheter can be introduced by dilation of the artery and the percutaneous sheath method as already described.

Consideration of the size and description of needles and guide-wires to be used has deliberately been left until last, since it is so much a matter of personal preference. The needle should be disposable (i.e. sharp), preferably with a short bevel, since it is then less likely to lie half in the wall of the vessel and half in the lumen. It should be big enough to hold easily, and for this reason some prefer butterfly needles. Most operators use a 20 gauge needle and a 0.018 or 0.21 inch guide-wire in young infants, a 19 gauge needle with a 0.021 or 0.025 inch guide-wire in older infants and an 18 gauge needle with a 0.025 or 0.035 guide-wire in children. The guide-wire must have a flexible tip and the only mandatory requirement is that the operator checks that the guide-wire will go through the needle and dilator, and the dilator and catheter through the sheath, **before** he punctures the skin.

As fine guide-wires are easily kinked if too large a dilator is passed over them, it is helpful in small infants to use a stepwise progression of fine guide-wire, tight-fitting dilator, loose-fitting dilator that will accept the next size up of guide-wire, that guide-wire, tight fitting larger dilator and so on.

Complications of percutaneous catheterisation

Percutaneous transvenous catheterisation has a very low complication rate indeed, whatever the age of the patient. It is safer than cutdown approaches to the veins, because there is much less risk of bleeding, and no risk of avulsion of the vein. Most importantly, the incidence of venous thrombosis after venous catheterisation is much lower than after a cutdown approach. Thus the femoral vein can be used over and over again in patients who for any reason require repeated catheterisations. Fortunately, the patient with no veins left for cardiac catheterisation has become a historical curiosity.

Regrettably, there is much higher rate of complications from percutaneous arterial catheterisation, particularly in neonates and small infants. Table 14.1, taken from the work of Girod and colleagues (1982), shows the incidence of decreased pulses at various intervals after catheterisation as noted by different workers. The study by Freed and colleagues (1977) is noteworthy in that a double blind controlled study of the use of heparin was carried out, which demonstrated a 7% incidence of decreased pulses at 4 hours after catheterisation in the group treated with heparin, as opposed to a 40% incidence in the group treated without. This proportion was statistically highly significantly different. This may explain the remarkably good results achieved by Girod and colleagues, with a 3% incidence of decreased pulses at 6 hours in patients below 10 kg and a 0.4% incidence in patients above 10 kg. On the basis of this and their previous experience (Hurwitz et al, 1977), these authors believe that absent pedal pulses 6 hours after cardiac catheterisation denote femoral arterial thrombosis. Though this is usually compensated for by the development of collateral circulation, it can very rarely

Table 14.1 Incidence of decreased femoral pulses after percutaneous catheterisation. (After Girod et al, 1982).

Authors	Hours after catheterisation	Patients heparinised	<10 kg	%	>10 kg	%	All patients	%
Girod et al, 1982	6	Yes	7/258	3	4/958	0.4	11/1316	0.8
Kirkpatrick et al, 1970	12	No					19/122	1.5
Simovitch et al, 1970	24	No	7/21	33	59/835	7	66/856	8
Neches et al, 1978	4	No	6/24	25	4/236	2	10/260	4
Freed et al, 1974	4	No	0		15/37	40	15/37	40
Freed et al, 1974	4	Yes	0		3/40	7	3/40	7

lead to the necessity for amputation of the lower extremity (Mansfield et al, 1970; White et al, 1968). Claudication can also occur as a result of femoral artery thrombosis (Mansfield et al, 1970). The excellence of the results by Girod and his colleagues are probably in part due to the fact that all percutaneous arterial catheterisations were carried out by experienced paediatric cardiologists and not by doctors in training.

Cut-down catheterisation

If a cut-down approach to cardiac catheterisation is going to be used, consideration should first be given to the prime purpose of the cardiac catheterisation. This is because the best site of cut-down depends upon whether one wants primarily to carry out antegrade transvenous or retrograde arterial catheterisation. Antegrade venous catheterisation is almost always preferable from the leg in children, because of the high incidence of patency of the oval foramen, which permits access to the left side of the heart. The only exception to this is when there is no easy access to the heart via the inferior caval vein. This can occur for two reasons. One is absence of the suprarenal inferior caval vein with azygos continuation to the superior caval vein, which should have been recognised before catheterisation by cross-sectional echocardiography (Huhta et al. 1982). The other is thrombosis of both iliac veins or the inferior caval vein itself, usually the result of previous catheterisation.

By contrast, if the principal objective is a retrograde arterial catheterisation, there is much to be said for cut-down to the axillary artery. Damage to the axillary artery has much less serious consequences than damage to the femoral artery, since there is a plentiful collateral arterial blood supply round the shoulder joint. We have never seen problems in a child even after complete occlusion of the axillary artery at cardiac catheterisation. Furthermore, the short and direct route from the axillary artery to the aortic valve means that crossing the aortic valve, and consequent manipulation of the catheter within the heart is somewhat easier than it is from a femoral artery approach. A disadvantage of the axillary approach is that the venous approach to the heart is less satisfactory, both because it is more difficult to cross the oval foramen, and because in small babies, unless the incision is made high in the axilla, a vein of adequate size may not be found. Before contemplating the axillary approach, the side of the aortic arch should be established either from chest radiography, or from cross-sectional echocardiography, because one usually does not want to pass down the axillary and subclavian artery into the descending aorta. It is extremely difficult to reach the ascending aorta having traversed the more distal of the two subclavian arteries, whereas if the innominate artery has been traversed, entry to either ascending or descending aorta is straightforward. Cross-sectional echocardiography using a scanner with a good near field and high resolution permits identification of the bifurcating innominate artery, and indicates that the cut-down should be carried out on the same side.

Femoral cut-down

The femoral artery is located in the groin, as described above. If it is impalpable, and no Doppler equipment is available, its position should be anticipated as a third of the way from the pubic tubercle to the anterior superior iliac spine. After infiltration with local anaesthetic, a skin crease incision should be made with its centre over the anticipated site of the femoral artery. In small babies, this incision will be at or immediately below the inguinal crease, whereas in older children, it needs to be a little further down the leg. Using blunt dissection, the saphenous vein is identified by its appropriate size for the patient, and its direction, which is more or less parallel with the leg, but running slightly medially as it ascends. If any other smaller vein running in a different direction is encountered, it should be followed, because one end of it will terminate in the saphenous vein (Fig. 14.2 – top panel).

In children beyond 6 months of age, the saphenous vein is usually adequate to take a catheter big enough for optimal angiocardiography. However, in neonates, even of normal birth weight, it is unusual to be able to introduce a catheter of greater than 5 French calibre into the vein, and therefore impossible to carry out a balloon atrial septostomy, or, sometimes, to obtain adequate results with angiocardiography. Under such circumstances, the saphenous vein should be followed to its junction with the femoral vein.

Sometimes, of course, the femoral vein is encountered before the saphenous vein, lying in the femoral sheath along with the femoral artery. It is vital to dissect out both of these vessels and clearly identify them, because, if this is not done, it is very easy in a cyanotic baby whose femoral pulses are weak for any reason, to confuse the femoral artery for the femoral vein, and therefore make an unnecessary femoral arteriotomy (Fig. 14.2 – lower panel).

It is usually possible to introduce an adequate sized catheter into the saphenous vein of a neonate just before it enters the femoral vein. This should never be done until complete haemostatic control of the femoral vein has been achived. Otherwise, avulsion of the saphenous vein from the femoral vein, which sometimes occurs when there is a spasm of the saphenous vein round the catheter, will result in considerable bleeding, which may be difficult to control. Thus it is necessary to dissect behind the femoral vein both above and below the entrance of the saphenous vein. This must be done with great care, because the profunda vein enters the common femoral vein from behind, and it is easy to lacerate this vein even during blunt dissection. Only when untied ligatures have been

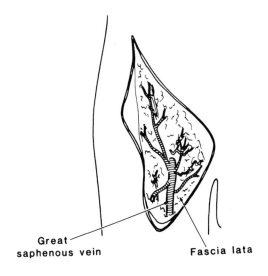

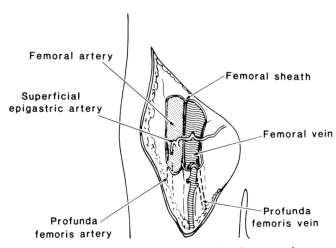

Fig. 14.2 Anatomy of the femoral triangle, as it relates to cutdown catheterization of the femoral vein or artery, and the great saphenous vein. The upper panel demonstrates more superficial anatomy than the lower panel, and the incision is clearly far more generous than is necessary for a cut-down.

placed around the profunda vein, and the common femoral vein above and below the entry of the saphenous vein, is it safe to ligate the saphenous vein, and introduce the catheter just downstream to the ligature.

Sometimes, the saphenous vein is at no point large enough to accept the required catheter. In such a case, the venotomy should be made in the femoral vein, and the catheter introduced directly into it. It is frequently possible to repair the femoral vein after femoral venotomy using a continuous suture (interrupted sutures usually do not provide adequate haemostasis), but if this proves impossible, the femoral vein can simply be ligated. The leg will swell up and look very blue for a day, but after that, provided that the arterial supply to that leg has in no way been compromised, it will return to normal because of the development of collateral venous channels.

We have found it quite useful to introduce a dilator and sheath into the vein, having carried out a venotomy, rather than a catheter, because once the dilator has been removed, changing of catheters is much easier. Whether a catheter or a dilator is introduced, it is useful to have a 'shoe horn' to dilate the vein while the catheter is being introduced into it.

If femoral arteriotomy is to be used, the technique is the same as for axillary arteriotomy (see below).

Axillary cut-down

This approach appears more alarming to the uninitiated than does the groin approach, because of anxiety about dissecting among the nerves of the brachial plexus. It is in fact in many ways simpler, because the axillary vein and artery are so easy to find.

The patient's arm is fully extended to lie beside his head, and the axillary artery is palpated over the head and neck of the humerus. The distal boundary of the axilla is marked by a U-shaped skin fold or depression, the apex of the U being distal. In any child over 6 months of age, the incision will be made over the line of the axillary artery immediately distal to this U-shaped boundary (strictly speaking, beyond the axilla) (Fig. 14.3 – top panel). In small babies, one needs to go higher up into the axilla. This has the disadvantage that the vein and artery will be much deeper, but if the incision is made more distal, frequently a plexus of veins is found, none of which is big enough to accept a catheter. This plexus of veins tends to fuse into a single adequate sized vein deeper in the axilla.

After infiltration with local anaesthetic in the appropriate spot, the incision is made. Access to the vein and artery is made easier if the incision is in line with them, but a better scar will result if a skin crease incision is made at right angles to the axillary artery. No attempt is made to infiltrate the brachial plexus at this point. The object is simply to anaesthetise the skin and subcutaneous tissues. Blunt dissection is then used to pass through the subcutaneous tissue and superficial fascia, and before long the deep fascia comes into view. Because it is transparent, the nerves of the brachial plexus can easily be seen through this structure. Provided this deep fascia is still intact, it is then a simple matter to anaesthetise the entire region by infiltration underneath it under direct vision, injecting into the space between the nerves and vessels, rather than into them.

Once the brachial plexus and vessels have been adequately anaesthetised, blunt dissection is continued by parting the deep fascia in the line of the arm. All that then needs to be done is to separate the structures within the brachial plexus. The nerves, recognised by their white, glistening appearance and lack of pulsation, are identified one by one and kept to one side with a retractor until the axillary artery is found. This is of a much creamier colour,

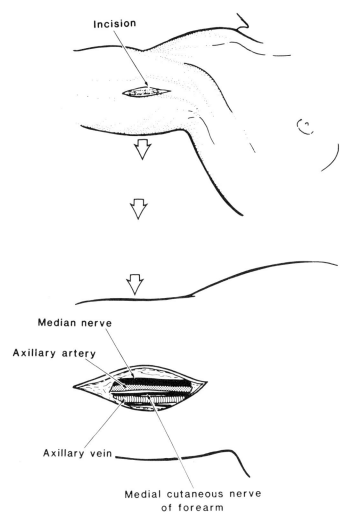

Fig. 14.3 Site of incision for axillary cut-down in an older child. The initial incision does not go through the deep fascia. When the deep fascia is divided, the brachial plexus comes into view as demonstrated in the lower panel.

has tiny blood vessels in its wall, and pulsates unless the patient is desperately ill. The axillary vein usually lies alongside and beneath it, but as mentioned earlier, veins of all shapes and sizes may be found intermingled with the nerves of the brachial plexus (Fig. 14.3 – lower panel). Provided they are of adequate size, any will do for cardiac catheterisation. Mobilisation of a length of axillary artery is usually a straightforward matter. In older children, the axillary vein frequently assumes quite awesome proportions. If this is so, the first thing to do is to look around for something smaller. Otherwise, it is not difficult to mobilise and control even a very large vein with safety, provided that one is always aware of the possibility of other veins entering it from behind, just as the profunda femoris vein enters the common femoral vein (see above).

A catheter is introduced into the vein, and 0.1 mg/kg of heparin is given if an axillary arteriotomy is contemplated. Then elastic bands or umbilical tapes are placed

around the axillary artery, making quite sure that any side branches are also adequately controlled. Using a very sharp pair of scissors, a tiny transverse incision is made in the artery. If too large an incision is made, back bleeding will be a problem throughout the catheterisation, and attempts to control it by tightening the rubber band round the proximal end of the artery will probably result in trauma to the intima, thereby lessening the chance of successful arterial repair.

Both arterial and venous catheters should be chosen with a sharp bend at the tip in order to assist turning the right-angled bend necessary to enter the innominate artery and superior caval vein respectively.

Upon termination of the catheterisation, the vein can be tied off. The artery should be controlled with good atraumatic clamps, preferably arranged so that they lift the artery out of the wound without putting tension on the arteriotomy (Fig. 14.4 – lower panel). A purse-string suture has an innate tendency to constrict the artery and should be

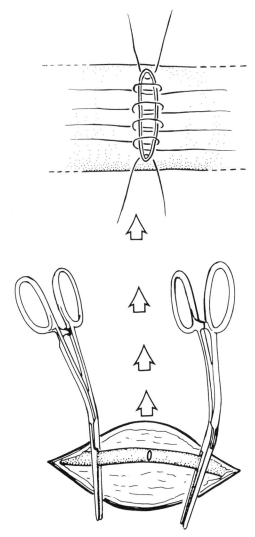

Fig. 14.4 Repair of arteriotomy. For further details see text.

avoided. The artery should be repaired with a transverse suture line. A compromise has to be made between using interrupted sutures, which are naturally less haemostatic, and a single continuous suture, which provides excellent haemostasis, but also tends to narrow the artery. Our compromise is to place a stay suture at either end of the incision, and then use interrupted continuous sutures, each interrupted suture consisting of two passages through the wall of the artery (Fig. 14.4 – top panel). Each suture should be placed 1 mm from the edge of the arteriotomy and they should be spaced 1 mm apart. The needle should pass through all three layers of the artery with each bite. It is obviously most important to avoid inadvertent inclusion of the posterior wall of the artery in a suture. This is best achieved by using each suture to lift the anterior wall of the artery forwards during insertion of the next suture. The sutures are not tied until all have been inserted. If they are, undue tension may be placed upon a single suture which cuts out as a result. The arterial clamps are then pushed together by an assistant while they still grasp the artery, so as to minimise tension on the suture line. Each suture is tied, but not cut. When the clamps are removed, a trickle of blood or a slight spurt can usually be controlled by digital pressure for 5 minutes. Any more serious leak will require placement of more sutures. The fact that the ones already used have not been cut means that they can be used to lift forward the wall of the artery, thus ensuring that further sutures inserted do not catch the back wall of the artery and occlude it when they are tied.

At the end of all this, there should be a good arterial pulse distal to the suture line. If not, surgical assistance should be called for. In the exceptionally rare circumstance that a distal pulse cannot be produced, though the arm may be cold for a few hours, the collateral circulation around the shoulder joint is in our experience always sufficient to restore satisfactory circulation to the limb.

Other approaches

During the first few days of life, **umbilical vein catheterisation** is well worthy of consideration, particularly when the diagnosis of complete transposition has been established by cross-sectional echocardiography and all that is required is balloon atrial septostomy (Newfeld et al, 1974). The umbilical stump is freshened up if necessary, and the umbilical vein identified as the single structure, in contrast to the usually paired umbilical arteries. Control on the umbilical vein is usually best achieved with umbilical tape round the entire umbilicus, and the catheter is introduced into the vein. The course into the inferior caval vein involves passing the catheter first posteriorly and then superiorly. Is a little more tricky than other approaches to the heart, but once the catheter is there, it crosses from right to left atrium with considerable ease, since it is following the course of fetal umbilical venous return. This is why balloon septostomy is particularly appropriate from this approach. On the other hand, it is sometimes rather more difficult to enter the right side of the heart and catheterise the pulmonary artery. However, this approach saves a vein, which is no bad thing. **Umbilical arterial catheterisation** is of some value if all that is required is an aortogram, particularly in the descending aorta. The tortuous course of the catheter from umbilical artery into common iliac artery and descending aorta requires the use of a very flexible catheter, which in turn makes further manipulation within the heart much more difficult. Thus this approach is not really of any particular value under most circumstances. The umbilical artery is useful as a route for monitoring arterial pressure, but thrombosis of the aorta and its main branches is a hazard (Tyson et al, 1976).

The usual approach to adults via **brachial cut-down** has, in our view, no advantages over axillary cut-down except for being slightly quicker. It has the considerable disadvantage in most children that the only catheters that can be introduced are small ones, inadequate for high quality angiocardiography. There is also a high incidence both of venous and arterial spasm if an attempt to use larger catheters is made.

If there are no other veins, it is possible to cut down on the **jugular vein** and the **carotid artery** (Azzolina et al, 1973). Good results have been reported with this technique, but to us it is used as a last resort because of the risk of interference with cerebral blood supply.

Entry to an otherwise complete inaccessible left atrium, pulmonary trunk or ascending aorta is possible by **suprasternal puncture** (Radner, 1955). If single plane fluoroscopy only is available, first a direct lateral angiocardiogram must be obtained to demonstrate the position of the structure of interest relative to the chest and the supra-sternal notch. The patient is given a general anaesthetic and his shoulders are propped up on a wedge to permit his head to fall back and rotate away from the operator. A long, flushed 21 gauge needle attached via flexible tubing to a transducer is then inserted through the skin and advanced under fluoroscopic control into aorta, pulmonary trunk or left atrium, whichever is required. This is straightforward with biplane fluoroscopy; otherwise the lateral angiocardiogram is used with frontal fluoroscopy. Most beginners direct the needle too far anteriorly; the correct angle is about 45° to the long axis of the trunk. Arrival at the correct site is detected by the pressure trace and checked by injection of small amounts of contrast medium.

It is frequently necessary to traverse the aortic arch with a needle, since the course has to be through mediastinum, not lung, but this does not seem to matter. After this procedure chest X-rays should be taken at regular intervals. Some mediastinal widening often occurs, but otherwise the procedure is remarkably safe. It is simpler than transbronchial puncture of the left atrium, which is virtually obselete.

The innaccessible left ventricle is best approached by **direct ventricular puncture**, which requires no general anaesthetic in a quiet patient. The apex beat is localised by palpation and marked with a cross. This region is infiltrated with local anaesthetic and a fine flexible intra-cardiac needle is flushed and attached to a transducer. It is advanced from the point marked with a cross towards the back of the left shoulder. Fluoroscopic control is of value in difficult cases, but is not usually necessary. As soon as the needle contacts the left ventricle, it begins to move vigorously with the heart, which may become lacer-ated, so the trick is to advance the needle confidently and rapidly and then let go of it. If entry to the left ventricle (signalled by pressure monitoring) has not been achieved, it is probably safer to withdraw the needle and start again than to advance it further. The main risk of this procedure is tamponade due to coronary artery laceration, so the patient should be monitored by repeated cross-sectional echocardiograms after the procedure.

Neither supra-sternal nor direct ventricular puncture should be used unless the information is vital for the management of the patient.

It is possible to obtain aortograms by countercurrent injection into the radial artery (Ueda et al, 1982), but this procedure is unlikely to give information that cannot be obtained by cross-sectional echocardiography and/or digital subtraction angiography with venous injection.

MANIPULATION AND CHOICE OF CARDIAC CATHETERS

The wise director of a cardiac catheterisation laboratory stocks a very broad range of products indeed, because individual preferences vary greatly between different oper-ators. Furthermore, a particularly difficult manoeuvre may be accomplished by one particular shape of catheter and no other. Most manufacturer's catalogues are full of cath-eters which are of no use at all to the paediatric cardi-ologist because they are designed to manoeuvre round adult sized hearts. For example, the standard adult cardiac cath-eter, with a 30° bend about 5 cm from its end, is virtually useless in a newborn baby, whose heart measures only 5 cm from one side to the other. For a catheter to be of any use it must have a bend at a distance of about half the maximum diameter of the cardiac chamber through which it is being manipulated. Besides being of the wrong shape, most standard catheters are far too long for paediatric use. In order to achieve adequate flow rates of contrast medium during angiocardiography, the catheter ideally should be such that at most 10–15 cm of the catheter is outside the patient when the angiocardiogram is being shot.

In past days, one of the rituals of cardiac catheterisation involved sampling of blood from all over the heart in order to localise left-to-right and right-to-left shunts. In order to do this more accurately, catheters were used which had only an end-hole, or at most an end-hole and two side holes very close to the tip. Nowadays, with proper preoperative evaluation by cross-sectional echocardio-graphy, it is hardly necessary to be accurate in this fashion. All that is important is to obtain representative samples of blood from the great arteries and veins, so that calculations of flows can be made. Given that this is the case, catheters suitable for angiocardiography (i.e. those with multiple side holes towards the tip, and usually a closed end) are almost always perfectly adequate for sampling blood.

For the reasons stated above, our main armamentarium consists of a series of preformed polyethylene catheters specifically designed for paediatric use (Fig. 14.5). General

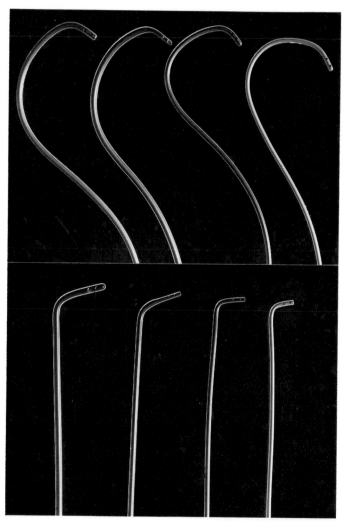

Fig. 14.5 Purpose-built catheters for paediatric cardiac catheterisation (Cook, Bloomington, Indiana). Each row contains 8,7,6 and 5 French catheters in order. Open or blind-ended versions can be obtained for each catheter.

purpose catheters have an almost right-angled bend varying from 0.8 to 3 cm from the tip, depending upon the size of the patient. There is in addition a series of cobra-shaped catheters, again with the bend beginning at various distances from the tip, but all with a fairly sharp bend at about 0.5 cm from the tip. Largely for sentimental reasons, we maintain a stock of woven Dacron catheters which are steam sterilised around a U-shaped former for the particular purpose of entering the pulmonary trunk in transposition of the great arteries. These could just as well be made of polythene. All of the catheters come with a choice of either closed or open ends. A manoeuvre is first tried with the closed ended catheter, but if it seems as though a guide-wire would be advantageous, the catheter is changed to one with an open end.

Special preformed catheters are particularly useful for retrograde catheterisation, e.g. pigtail catheters for traversing the aortic arch and aortic valve from the femoral arterial approach, and specially designed coronary artery catheters for children from the same approach (Takahashi et al, 1983). Another catheter which is useful from the axillary artery approach is a Shirey transvalvar catheter (Shirey & Sones, 1966), which is made of woven Dacron, but with a taper quite a long way from the tip so that it is very flexible. This is useful for retrograde catheterisation of the left atrium (Morrison et al, 1977). From the femoral arterial approach, entry to the left atrium in retrograde fashion can usually be achieved without such a specialised catheter since the catheter tends naturally to pass posteriorly having traversed the aortic valve. Catheters with firm shanks and flexible tips are also useful for retrograde catheterisation of the pulmonary trunk in complete transposition with ventricular septal defect (Mullins et al, 1972). Here, the catheter is passed across a ventricular septal defect first, and then looped in the left ventricle to pass up to the pulmonary trunk. Sometimes it is easier to loop the catheter in the right ventricle first and then advance it across the ventricular septal defect.

The catheter with a simple curve near the tip is quite adequate for catheterising the right side of the heart and entering the pulmonary trunk, and also for crossing the oval foramen into the left atrium and entering the pulmonary veins. With gentle pressure on the junction between the right pulmonary vein and left atrium, a tighter loop can usually be produced which enables the catheter to be turned down into left ventricle. In general, it is better to enter the left ventricle with the cobra-shaped catheter, since it sits better in the centre of the left ventricular cavity, thereby reducing the risk of intra-myocardial injection of contrast medium. Furthermore, this catheter can with ease be passed on up into the pulmonary trunk in almost all cases of complete transposition (Macartney et al, 1975) and into the aorta in most cases where that artery arises from the left ventricle. The cobra-shaped catheter is also useful in crossing ventricular septal defects. These

should have been recognised preoperatively by cross-sectional echocardiography. The shape of the catheter is such that, in the case of typical perimembranous ventricular septal defect, it is a simple matter, having crossed the ventricular septal defects, either to turn the tip of the catheter down towards the apex of the left ventricle for a left ventriculogram, or to turn it up towards the great artery which originates from the left ventricle.

In our experience, this collection of catheters is adequate to achieve whatever the operator desires. Many would be equally enthusiastic about flow-directed balloon catheters (Swan et al, 1970; Jones & Miller, 1973). These double lumen catheters have a lumen for pressure measurement, which either terminates in an end-hole, or in side-holes for angiocardiography proximal to the balloon. The second lumen is used to introduce carbon dioxide into the balloon. In paediatric use, the balloon is usually not inflated until it is in a strategic position within the heart. For example, to enter the normally positioned pulmonary trunk, the balloon is best inflated in the right atrium. As soon as it is advanced, it often floats straight into the pulmonary trunk. On the other hand, if the left ventricle is to be entered the balloon should be inflated in the left atrium. It then normally shoots to the apex of the left ventricle in a very good position for an angiocardiogram, but stays there. If the objective is to enter the great artery coming from the left ventricle, it is usually beter to form a loop with the catheter in the left atrium, advance the catheter on the loop into the left ventricle, and then inflate the balloon, whereupon it will usually sail out of the left ventricle with the greatest of ease. Balloon flotation catheters are particularly useful in tricuspid atresia, when they may be the only catheters which can be persuaded to pass from left ventricle to right ventricle across the ventricular septal defect and out of the artery originating from there.

When a catheter can be persuaded to go almost, but not quite all of the way required, guide-wires come into their own. These should be available in a variety of shapes, particularly straight and J-shaped. It is also of some value to have a guide-wire whose curve can be altered by movement of the central core relative to the outside winding. The disadvantage of using guide-wires is that one can no longer monitor the pressure. This is a pity, in that an important clue is lost as to the catheter position, increasing the risk of unwitting perforation of the cardiac wall.

For the most difficult intracardiac manoeuvres, a steerable catheter system, such as the Müller handle, is of occasional value. The heart of this system is a guide-wire whose shape can be varied from straight to completely bent back on itself. Over this guide-wire fits a rather flexible catheter with side-holes near its tip. There is a complicated valve system at the proximal end of the catheter which permits one to obtain a rather damped pressure trace through the catheter while the guide-wire is inside it. The other key feature of this system is that, once the curve of the guide-wire has been fixed, it is very rigid. The catheter can be advanced over the curve. To illustrate how this system is used, consider entering the pulmonary trunk in a case of simple complete transposition. The catheter alone is passed up into the right atrium from the transvenous groin approach, and can frequently be persuaded to enter the left atrium without using the guide-wire. If this is impossible, the guide-wire is simply inserted into the catheter, a gentle bend put on it, and the catheter and guide-wire then advanced into the left atrium in normal fashion. To enter the left ventricle, the bend is increased, and the catheter is then advanced over the guide-wire, so that its flexible and atraumatic tip enters the left ventricle. The bend on the guide-wire is then relaxed, and the guide-wire passed on, while still inside the catheter, into the left ventricle. Once the tip of the catheter is sitting in the middle of the left ventricular cavity, the guide-wire is advanced to a point just short of the tip. A sharp bend is then made in the guide-wire, such that the tip of the catheter then points towards the pulmonary trunk. The catheter is then advanced over the guide-wire and, with luck, goes straight out into the pulmonary trunk. The guide-wire is then relaxed and carefully withdrawn completely from the catheter. The disadvantage of the Müller handle is that it is difficult to clean, and that the wires controlling curvature of the guide-wire frequently break at the crucial moment. Most seriously, the catheter sometimes loses position as the guide-wire is withdrawn, making measurement of an undamped pressure impossible. The catheter is too floppy to use for angiocardiography without the risk of recoil of the catheter from its chosen position. On the other hand, the ability of the Müller guide-wire to bend right back on itself and form a closed loop makes it extremely useful for removing foreign bodies from the circulation (see below).

Recognition of catheter position

The two immediate guides to catheter position are the pressure measured and the shape of the catheter (Fig. 14.6). In cases of doubt, oxygen saturation may be measured and recordings of the injection of small amounts of contrast medium made.

Trans-septal puncture

This old and largely forgotten technique (Ross, 1966) has recently been resuscitated by the remarkable report of 520 trans-septal punctures in adults and children using a special trans-septal introducer set (Mullins, 1983). This consists of a long straight dilator and a tight fitting sheath 4 cm shorter than the dilator, with a U-bend at the end. When one is inside the other, both become gently curved at the tip, and can be advanced over a guide-wire previously positioned after femoral vein puncture in the superior caval vein.

At the proximal end of the introducer set are two plastic hubs, one belonging to the sheath and the other to the dilator. The guide-wire is removed and the dilator aspirated. Separating the two hubs by 1 cm permits the dilator to be bent so as to admit the curved end of the needle, which is advanced until it is just short of the tip of the dilator, its proximal end being attached to a flexible tube and transducer. Under biplane fluoroscopic control the entire assembly is pointed backwards and to the left and withdrawn into the right atrium. It is usually possible then to engage the tip of the dilator in the superior rim of the oval fossa, but if this is not possible the dilator tip is placed against the atrial septum at about its mid-point, again pointing backwards and to the left. Trans-septal puncture is achieved by advancing the needle through the dilator.

If, and only if, an acceptable left atrial pressure trace is obtained immediately after feeling the needle 'pop' through the septum, the dilator, needle and sheath can be advanced as a single unit until the dilator enters the left atrium with a slight give. Otherwise, a small volume of contrast medium is injected through the needle while observing the fluoroscope. If the left atrium opacifies, well and good. If the tip is within the atrial septum, a 'tag' of contrast medium spreads through a small area of the septum. This 'tag' can then be used as a target for a further attempt at trans-septal puncture.

Once the dilator is in the left atrium, the needle is withdrawn to a point just inside the dilator. The sheath is then advanced approximately 4 cm so as to lie well within the left atrium. The distance from sheath hub to skin is measured and recorded, because as the needle and dilator are withdrawn one by one, it becomes difficult to see the sheath. As catheters are exchanged, it is important that they are never withdrawn unless the sheath is in the left atrium, and this measurement is the best guide to the position of the sheath tip. The sheath is then gently aspirated, and the required catheter introduced. Despite the fact that 149 of the 520 patients in Mullins' series (1983) were under 10 kg in weight, there were only 4 unsuccessful punctures.

Two patients developed haemopericardium with tamponade, but survived emergency surgery. The needle alone entered the pericardium in one patient and the aortic root in another. The erroneous position was recognised, the needle withdrawn and trans-septal puncture accomplished without incident. Trans-septal puncture is not a technique for the occasional operator, but if used regularly, it is a valuable means of entry to the otherwise inaccessible left atrium.

Endomyocardial biopsy

This is still a research technique in children, and will

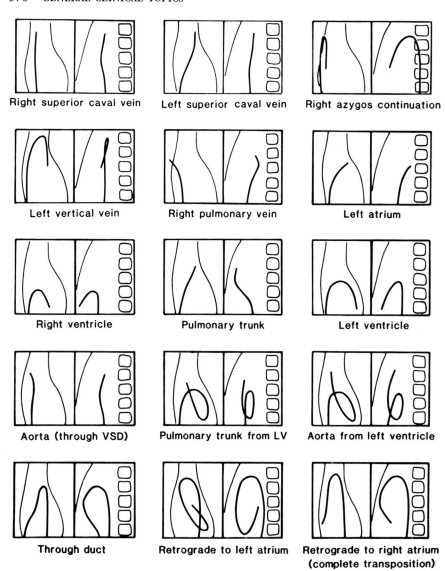

Right superior caval vein

Left superior caval vein

Right azygos continuation

Left vertical vein

Right pulmonary vein

Left atrium

Right ventricle

Pulmonary trunk

Left ventricle

Aorta (through VSD)

Pulmonary trunk from LV

Aorta from left ventricle

Through duct

Retrograde to left atrium

Retrograde to right atrium (complete transposition)

Fig. 14.6 Assorted catheter positions as seen in frontal (left) and lateral (right) projections for each panel.

therefore be described only briefly. A special technique suitable for use in infants and children has been developed by Lurie and colleagues (1978), designed to permit biopsy from either side of the ventricular septum. Stylets which act as templates for construction of the guide catheters are hand-moulded to the desired shape based on the frontal and lateral plain chest X-rays. Over the stylet goes a teflon catheter and over the catheter an ultra-thin teflon sheath. Immersion in boiling water shapes catheter and sheath. The stylet is removed and the catheter and sheath advanced to the desired position for biopsy. The catheter is then removed and replaced with 4F or 5F biopsy forceps which are guided via the sheath to their destination. The sheath is then withdrawn 1 cm to free the jaws of the bioptome, which are then opened. The bioptome is advanced to the septum and the jaws are closed, thus obtaining a biopsy. The bioptome is withdrawn and cleaned with heparinised saline in an ultrasonic cleaner once the biopsy

sample has been removed. The bioptome is then ready to obtain another sample.

The indications for this technique have not yet been defined.

ANGIOCARDIOGRAPHY

The choice of sites for angiocardiography is of key importance, and should be based, wherever possible, on previous cross-sectional echocardiography. In general, the more selective the angiocardiogram, the more information it will give, because the fewer structures are opacified, the less likely is overlap between structures. Such overlap makes interpretation far harder.

Another means of reducing overlap is to choose the angle of projection with care. Since the heart and pulmonary arteries lie with their long axis in a plane running from back to front as it passes downward, caudocranial tilt will always reduce overlap of cardiac chambers and pulmonary arteries. Because the long axis of the heart also normally runs from right to left as it passes downwards, left superior or right inferior oblique projections also reduce foreshortening. Since the interventricular and interatrial septa normally lie in an oblique plane, passing from front to back as it moves left to right, some degree of left anterior or right posterior obliquity will improve demonstration of these structures and any defects in them. The right ventricle usually wraps around the left ventricle, so the interventricular septum is normally curved. This means that, if it is desired to profile a particular region of ventricular septum, the more anterior it is, the steeper must be the degree of obliquity. While it is possible to investigate the majority of patients using standard 'long axial', 'four-chamber' and 'head-up tilt' projections (Bargeron, 1981), readers are encouraged to modify the degree of obliquity to frontal, horizontal and sagittal planes according to the individual patient: if this is done routinely, it becomes much easier to decide the appropriate planes in patients with cardiac malposition, particularly if good cross-sectional echocardiograms have been obtained.

The faster contrast medium can be injected into the patient, the better will be the angiocardiograms, so the first necesssity is to use a catheter as large as possible, and the second is to inject with as high a pressure as feasible. The latter consideration is secondary, since high pressure of injection has two adverse effects – namely, a higher risk of recoil of the catheter from its chosen position, and a greater likelihood of intramyocardial injection. Both these complications are less likely if the catheter position is carefully chosen. This is particularly true in ventricles. In general the catheter tip should be as near the apex as possible without risking intra-myocardial injection (see below). The dose of contrast medium required depends on the volume of the chamber injected into and the flow of blood through that chamber. The greater these are, the more dilute will become the contrast medium, and the less satisfactory will be the pictures. Thus 1 ml is sufficient to opacify densely a major aortopulmonary collateral artery in a newborn baby, 0.75 ml/kg produces enough opacification for a normal aorta, 1 ml/kg is required for a normal left or right ventricle, 1.5 ml/kg will be necessary for volume overloaded left or right ventricles or ventricles from which contrast medium will escape to the other side of the heart, and up to 2 ml/kg may be needed to opacify a double inlet ventricle in the presence of increased pulmonary blood flow.

However carefully these simple rules are adhered to, the results of cineangiocardiography in particular will be suboptimal unless meticulous attention is given to the correct selection of X-ray factors and processing of the films. Bargeron (1981) has written an excellent practical guide to this subject, which is highly recommended.

Cardiac radiologists can be enormously helpful in these matters, but if they are slapdash, or obsessed with reducing radiation dose at the expense of all considerations of film quality, they will compromise the accuracy of anatomical diagnosis.

INTERVENTIONAL CARDIAC CATHETERISATION

Over the past few years, there has been a dramatic increase in the possibilities for interventional cardiac catheterisation. It is now possible not only to create defects, as with balloon atrial septostomy, but to dilate stenosed vessels and valves and occlude vessels. The specific techniques to be used are related to specific conditions, and will therefore be described in the chapters devoted to those topics, but the range of possibilities will be briefly surveyed here.

Balloon angioplasty

This technique and balloon valvoplasty both depend upon the use of sausage-shaped balloons which are made of polythene such that, when inflated, they reach a predictable diameter. As they are inflated with dilute contrast medium, there is initially very little resistance to filling. Once the required balloon diameter has been acquired, resistance to filling increases sharply. Thereafter, increasing the pressure in the balloon produces very little change in diameter, but simply permits the balloon to exert a greater force on the wall of the vessel in which it has been placed. At about $4\frac{1}{2}$ atmospheres, these balloons rupture, though stronger balloons have recently been developed. In order to prevent rupture occurring, the pressure in the balloon may be monitored through a side-arm in the catheter.

Because larger balloons have a larger surface area, they also occupy a greater volume when collapsed. Thus, in practice it is difficult to obtain a balloon which will inflate to above 15 mm in diameter and yet pass through a No. 10 sheath. If greater diameters are required, the solution is to use two balloon catheters, introduced into different veins, side by side in the vessel to be dilated (D'Souza et al, 1984). The contrast medium used to dilate the balloon should be so diluted that it can only just be seen on the screen. In this way, a more rapid deflation rate of the balloon can be achieved, which is important if it compromises cardiac output.

The technique has been effectively applied in coarctation of the aorta (and particularly recoarctation) (Sperling et al, 1983; Kan et al, 1983, 1984; Lock et al, 1983a; Finley et al, 1983; Lababidi et al, 1984b), and in obstruction of the pulmonary venous, inferior caval venous and superior caval venous pathways after baffle operations for complete transposition of the great arteries (Lock et al, 1984). A particularly important application is relief of stenosis

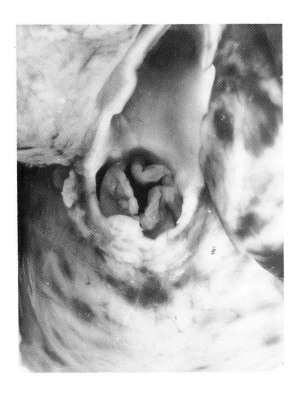

Fig. 14.7 The appearance of a previously stenotic valve relieved by balloon angioplasty. The stenotic leaflets have been split cleanly along the commissures and the valve does not appear to be regurgitant. The patient died from a cause unrelated to the valvoplasty (multiple hepatic arteriovenous fistulas).

of the intrapulmonary arteries, which are inaccessible to surgery (Lock et al, 1983b; Rocchini et al, 1984a). The one condition where balloon angioplasty has been demonstrated to be useless is in pulmonary vein stenosis (Driscoll et al, 1982; Lock et al, 1984). It is important to realise that angioplasty succeeds in children because it usually tears the intima and part or all of the media (Lock et al, 1982; Kan et al, 1983; Edwards et al, 1985). Thus it is the adventitia which prevents vascular rupture. The intima and media heal over the course of 2–6 weeks with reconstitution of normal-appearing intima and replacement of the media with vasculalr scar tissue (Lock et al, 1981, 1982; Edwards et al, 1985). Dilation of a functionally closed duct in 8 piglets produced patency in 6 up to six months later (Lund et al, 1983, 1984).

Balloon valvoplasty (Fig. 14.7)

Here the basic techniques are exactly as for angioplasty, except that the balloon will almost certainly completely occlude either pulmonary or systemic output or both. Thus, it is even more important to ensure rapid deflation of the balloon. The technique has been most profitably employed in pulmonary valve stenosis (Kan et al, 1982, 1984; Lababidi & Wu, 1983; Rocchini et al, 1984b; Tynan et al, 1984, 1985). It is important to recognise that there may be very little immediate reduction in gradient across the pulmonary valve. Presumably, this is because of infundibular stenosis, which disappears over the next few months

in exactly the same way as it does after surgical pulmonary valvotomy. Furthermore, a second balloon valvoplasty at 6 months where the initial result is suboptimal often produces a further reduction in gradient (Sullivan et al, 1985). More controversial is the use of balloon valvoplasty in congenital aortic stenosis (Lababidi, 1983; Lababidi et al, 1984a). We find it difficult to believe that balloon valvoplasty can be better than aortic valvotomy under direct vision, and we already have ample evidence of the deficiencies of that surgical procedure. Certainly, to create pulmonary incompetence matters little (though this is extremely rare after valvoplasty), whereas to create aortic incompetence is serious. Furthermore a transverse aortic wall tear has been reported after an appropriate size balloon burst during attempted valvoplasty in a 2-day-old infant (Waller et al, 1984).

One use of balloon valvoplasty of great potential value is mitral valvoplasty in patients with rheumatic mitral stenosis who have a pliable valve. The balloon is filled with carbon dioxide and is cleverly designed so as to inflate first on the ventricular side of the valve and then on both (Inoue et al, 1984). The technique is obviously of great potential, particularly in developing countries where cardiac surgery cannot be afforded.

Embolisation of vessels

Transcatheter closure of vessels can be achieved with a number of materials, each of which has its own advocates and advantages. The simplest method is probably the steel coil, which consists of a tightly bound steel spring to which are attached tassles of wool (Gianturco, et al, 1975). This steel coil is purchased inside a straight pod. In order to introduce the coil into the patient, the pod is apposed to the end of the catheter, and the stiff end of a guide-wire is used to push it out of the pod into the catheter. The coil is then pushed through the catheter with the floppy end of the guide-wire, and on emerging from its tip, wraps into a tight ball which embolises the vessel. Occlusion is never immediate, because it depends upon the formation of clot on the tassels. If, after about 10 minutes, occlusion has not occurred, then small pieces of gelfoam can be passed through the catheter in order to seal the remaining lumina. Alternatively, further coils can be inserted, preferably placed in such a way that they interlink (Fuhrman et al, 1984).

The advantage of steel coils is their ease of use. The disadvantage is that the positioning of the catheter and the choice of size of balloon is absolutely critical to success. If the tip of the catheter is not positioned correctly, the wrong vessel may be embolised, or the correct vessel embolised in the wrong place. If the size of the coil chosen is too small, it will pass further down the vessel than was planned. If on the other hand, it is too large, as it is pushed out, it may fail to coil in the vessel. Continued pushing on the guide-wire will then result in retrograde movement of the catheter tip, possibly into a main blood vessels such as the descending aorta, where embolisation would be disastrous. Once this happens, it is very difficult to retrieve the situation, because even if the catheter can be withdrawn with the spring still inside it, as soon as it enters a larger vessel such as the aorta, the distal end will coil into a ball and it may be very difficult to extract the coil from the patient.

An alternative approach to embolisation is the use of detachable balloons (White et al, 1979; Barth et al, 1982; Grinnell et al, 1982; Reidy et al, 1983; Florentine et al, 1984). These have the great advantage over coils that trial inflation of the balloon can be carried out. If the position is unsatisfactory, the balloon can then be deflated and repositioned. The situation only becomes irreversible when the balloon has been detached by a sharp tug. There are broadly two varieties of balloons – standard and mini balloons. The mini balloons are made of silicone, and are inflated with isotonic contrast medium such as metrizamide. The silicone will permit air to leak out of the balloon, which makes removal of all air from the balloon a simple matter. Because diffusion of solute can also occur through the silicone, it is important to use isotonic solution to fill the balloon, otherwise the balloon will either expand or shrink, which is not desirable. Latex balloons are larger than mini balloons, and are filled initially with contrast medium until the position achieved is satisfactory. The contrast medium is then exchanged for a mixture of the two silicone modified reactive monomers, which solidify in about 20 minutes when polymerisation and vulcanisation has occurred.

Whichever type of balloon is used, the mode of insertion is the same. A large catheter is placed with its end-hole in the appropriate position, and the balloon is then advanced through this catheter. In the case of mini balloons, with their very flexible fine polythene catheters, some kind of injection device is useful to direct the mini balloon down the catheter (White et al, 1979). When the balloon reaches the tip of the catheter it is inflated and floated to the appropriate occlusion site. Contrast medium is then injected until the vessel is completely occluded. This is easily checked for in the case of the mini balloons since, with gentle traction on the balloon, it should be possible to establish that the balloon is firmly stuck. Only when satisfactory occlusion has been proved by this method is the sharp tug given which then detaches the balloon from the catheter. The only disadvantage of the latex ballon system is that it is not easy to check for wedging of the balloon, since only very light traction is required to detach the balloon. The mini balloons carry a small valve which prevents their deflation when the catheter is detached. Mini balloons up to 8–9 mm in external diameter are obtainable. If the vessel is larger, then latex balloons should be used.

Warnecke and colleagues (1984) created beagle 'ducts' by inserting a length of subclavian artery between pulmonary trunk and descending aorta. They then closed them with a detachable double balloon from the venous side.

With the catheter through the duct, the distal 'position' balloon was inflated with contrast medium and then pulled back against the aortic end of the duct. The proximal 'occlusion' balloon was then inflated with radio-opaque silicone rubber until this was cured, when the position balloon was deflated. The results, while promising, have not yet been reported as extending to humans.

Umbrellas

One major limitation of balloons and coils is that the vessel needs to be of an appropriate shape to hold the balloon or coil firmly. For this reason, closure of a patent arterial duct requires a rather more subtle approach than simple balloons or coils, for example the double balloon technique just described. Porstmann and colleagues (1967, 1971) first described transcatheter closure of patent arterial duct using a wedge-shaped plug of Ivalon. The plug is sized from angiographic demonstration of the duct. Percutaneously (or sometimes using a cut-down) a long guide-wire and catheter are advanced into the femoral artery and through the duct into the pulmonary trunk and right heart. This catheter is then snared (see below) with a catheter introduced percutaneously into the femoral vein. Its tip is pulled through the femoral vein out of the patient. The guide-wire and catheter now form a long loop through the duct, with both ends outside the patient. Using a special introducer, the plug is then introduced into the femoral artery over the guide-wire and pushed on until it occludes the duct with first a long needle and then a second catheter. The original catheter and guide-wire are then withdrawn through the femoral vein. Successful treatment has been carried out in more than 200 patients (Rashkind, 1985). This method has the great disadvantage of requiring cut-down on the artery with the complications thereby involved. Accordingly, Rashkind (1983, 1985) developed a special catheter which has a pod at the end containing a double disc prosthesis. Each of the two discs has three stainless steel struts supporting a disc of polyurethane foam. The catheter is introduced transvenously and passed through the pulmonary trunk across the duct. The device is then pushed out at the end of the pod so that the aortic disc sits in the aortic end of the duct. Then the catheter is withdrawn, thus permitting the second disc to occlude the pulmonary end of the duct. The catheter is then detached.

The duct has to be of the right size for this technique, and Rashkind was obliged to reject a quarter of patients on this criterion. In those in whom the device was placed, complete occlusion of the duct occurred in 23 out of 30 patients. This is obviously an experimental technique, and not advised for general use at present, given the very low surgical risk of closure of a duct. Nonetheless, Mullins had, by mid 1986, successfully closed over 100 ducts in this fashion (personal communication, July 1986). Two patients have been successfully treated at Guy's Hospital, London.

A similar device has been used for attempted closure of atrial septal defect, first by King and colleagues (1976), and subsequently by Rashkind (1985). The device currently favoured by Rashkind consists of six radiating stainless steel arms projecting from a central hub. At the end of alternate ribs are small barbed hooks. The whole steel frame carries a foam rubber matrix. Again, the device is enclosed in a pod. The atrial septal defect is sized by seeing when it will just accept an inflated balloon, and then the catheter is advanced into the left atrium. The pod is then extruded and the device pulled against the atrial septum. The hooks then engage in the atrial septum, hopefully holding the prosthesis fast at this point.

Using the six rib, three hook prosthesis, Rashkind was obliged to turn down 10 patients either because the defect was too small or too large. Of the remaining 23 patients, the defect was adequately closed in 14 patients and the result was unsatisfactory in 9. Again, this is obviously a highly experimental procedure, not recommended for general use because of the very low risk of surgical closure of the atrial septal defect.

Balloon atrial septostomy

This was first described in 1966 by Rashkind & Miller. It has now become standard treatment for complete transposition and for other circumstances where the patient's life may depend upon the presence of an atrial septal defect. With the passing of years, balloon design has improved considerably so that balloons are now easy to introduce into the saphenous vein in most instances, or else percutaneously into the femoral vein. They are precurved to permit easy crossing of the patent oval foramen. Under either cross-sectional echocardiographic or biplane fluoroscopic control, the catheter is advanced into the left atrium and then inflated with up to 3.5–4 ml of contrast medium. With a sharp tug on the catheter, the balloon is then pulled down towards the inferior caval vein. If the septostomy is satisfactory, this tears the interatrial septum. It is a good idea to start with about 2.5 ml of contrast medium in the balloon. If smaller amounts are used, they may simply dilate the oval foramen rather than tear the interatrial septum. Usually, the balloon is withdrawn across the atrial septum five to ten times, and the size of the defect is then checked with cross-sectional echocardiography.

Blade atrial septectomy

This adjunct to balloon atrial septostomy was first described by Park and colleagues in 1978. In patients above 3 months of age, the interatrial septum is too tough to be torn with a balloon. The object of blade atrial septectomy is to make a cut in the inferior margin of the flap valve in order to start a tear in the interatrial septum which can be completed with balloon atrial septostomy. The end of the catheter contains a small knife hinged at its distal end to the catheter and at its proximal end to a firm wire passing down the catheter. This is a stiff and awkward catheter to use, and it is frequently necessary to use a long sheath to position the catheter in the left atrium. The left atrium is first entered with a conventional catheter. A guide-wire is then passed through the catheter and left with its tip in the left atrium. The long sheath is passed over the guide-wire, the guide-wire removed, and the blade septectomy catheter passed through the long sheath. With the catheter in the left atrium, its curve is pointed towards the left shoulder, and the blade is slowly pushed out of the catheter by advancing the wire. It should only be pushed out if it opens easily. The safest blade position in infants with complete transposition is with it open end towards the left diaphragm on the frontal view and the blade slightly anterior as seen on lateral fluoroscopy. To cut the atrial septum, the blade is placed in its fully open position and withdrawn slowly through the atrial septum with gentle, but firm pressure. The operator's hands should be steadied on the table as the catheter is pulled down to prevent a sudden cut too far inferiorly.

The main disadvantage of blade atrial septectomy is that it is of least use when it is most needed, such as in patients with absent left connexion. Here it is potentially particularly useful because thepatient may have survived infancy without too much in the way of symptoms, but then developed severe pulmonary venous hypertension in early or mid childhood. The problem is that most of these patients have a very small left atrium and therefore a small interatrial septum. It is difficult to introduce the catheter into the left atrium, and very difficult to make an adequate cut in the interatrial septum. This procedure carries quite a high risk even in expert hands (Park et al, 1982).

Removal of foreign bodies from the circulation

As this subject will not be dealt with elsewhere in this book, it will be covered in somewhat more detail than the other forms of interventional catheterisation. An excellent review has been provided by Bloomfield (1978). The commonest foreign bodies in the circulation are fragments of polyethylene central venous pressure catheters which have been cut in two by the sharp edge of the inserting needle. Other possibilities are fragments of standard catheters, guide-wires, ventriculo-atrial shunts, bits of permanent pacing catheters, and a miscellaneous category including bullets and catheter shapers.

The catheter fragment is usually introduced on to the venous side, and passes such that its proximal end most commonly is in the right atrium or superior caval vein. Its distal end is usually in the right ventricle or pulmonary trunk. It is important that such foreign bodies be removed from the circulation as soon as possible. Once both ends migrate to the pulmonary trunk, retrieval becomes more difficult.

The variety of methods used is a tribute to the ingenuity of operators. Broadly, these may be divided into four categories: snares, ureteric stone catchers, endoscopic forceps, and adjunctive techniques.

Snares

These are usually 'home-made' from an open-ended catheter and a long stainless steel suture or guide-wire. Either the suture or the guide-wire has to be pushed through the catheter doubled, so it is important that the doubled guide-wire or stainless steel suture should be able to be advanced down the catheter without kinking. It is often helpful to remove the stiffening wire from the guide-wire, leaving just the flexible coil part, because this is less likely to kink. A 3.0 stainless steel suture will pass satisfactorily down a 6 French catheter.

The snare is advanced to the proximal end of the fragment, provided that this is lying free in the blood stream. If it is stuck into the wall of the heart, then the snare should be positioned near the distal end of the fragment. By moving the tip of the catheter around in the region of the fragment, one hopes to encircle the fragment in the snare. In order to check that this has been achieved, the snare is advanced a little way down the fragment from the end which has been snared, and then advanced in order to demonstrate that the fragment moves with the snare. Once encirclement has been achieved, the snare is then tightened and the fragment withdrawn. As with all other techniques, the fact that what is withdrawn from the body is usually a rather irregular shaped object means that it is better to use a cut-down than a percutaneous technique for introducing the snare.

Ureteric stone catcher

This is a somewhat sophisticated snare and has the advantage that the added planes of sweep provided by the wires of the basket give better coverage and an increased possibility of being able to snare the foreign body quickly.

Endoscopic forceps

The most useful aspect of these devices is that they can catch the fragment at any point along its length, making it unnecessary to pass the instrument over the end of the fragment. The great disadvantage is the lack of manoeuvrability, which limits the scope of the endoscopy forceps to the removal of foreign bodies in the caval veins or the right atrium. Furthermore, there is a risk of perforation with these instruments.

Adjunctive techniques

Sometimes, the primary instrument for catching the fragment does not work on its own, and one has to use another device to reposition the fragment so that it can be caught by the primary instrument. Balloon catheters, hooked catheters and catheters with multiple loops have all been used for this purpose. If the object is to dislodge the fragment with the adjunctive device, it is important that the primary retriever is immediately adjacent to the dislodger in order to prevent migration of the fragment to the pulmonary trunk before it is caught.

Despite the wide variety of techniques used, and the limited experience of any one operator, these techniques have proved to be highly successful and complication-free.

Miscellaneous

Reimenschneider and colleagues (1983) have investigated laser atrial septectomy (Bommer et al, 1983). At present, there seems to be no advantage of this technique over balloon atrial septostomy or blade atrial septectomy. As it has been demonstrated that arrhythmogenic foci and the penetrating atrioventricular bundle can be obliterated using electric shock or cryotherapy and a catheter, it may be anticipated that this technique will be used in children for the occasional treatment of arrhythmias.

COMPLICATIONS OF CARDIAC CATHETERISATION

Problems with the approach to the heart have already been covered. Manipulation of the catheter can produce cardiac perforation, arrhythmias, blockage of normal channels, and knotted or broken catheters. Balloon catheters can tear atrioventricular valves.

Perforation of the heart

This is a serious complication, often causing death (Ho et al, 1972). The usual site of the perforation is in the atria, particularly the atrial appendages, though perforation of the right ventricular outflow tract has been reported. Perforation should be suspected whenever there is sudden hypotension, enlargement of the cardiac silhouette or entry of the catheter to a site from which blood cannot be withdrawn. The diagnosis may be confirmed by cross-sectional echocardiography, which demonstrates the catheter outside the heart and fluid in the pericardial cavity if this is the site of perforation. Treatment consists of leaving the catheter where it is to plug the perforation if possible, and performing emergency thoracotomy. A better policy is to avoid perforation by using atraumatic catheters when possible and always staying away from the atrial appendages. This necessitates the use of biplane screening. Catheters should only be flexed in the atria by gentle pressure on the right wall of the right atrium and a pulmonary vein/left atrial junction.

Tachyarrhythmias

These are often precipitated by catheter manipulation, and are a particular problem in patients with corrected transposition and Ebstein's anomaly.

Supraventricular tachycardias

These can usually be terminated by manipulation of the catheter within the atria, since production of an appropriately timed atrial extrasystole will 'break' a re-entrant tachycardia. In patients with frequent bouts of tachycardia, an electrode catheter with a central lumen may be used instead of a standard catheter so that overdrive pacing may be employed to terminate the tachycardia. If these simple measures fail, the usual methods of increasing vagal tone,

such as carotid sinus massage, may be tried. Very rarely, synchronised countershock is necessary.

Ventricular tachycardia

This is usually self-terminating after three or four beats, but if it persists, should be treated like ventricular fibrillation with immediate defibrillation.

Bradycardias

These are badly tolerated in small babies. They are usually due to manipulation in the region of the atrioventricular node and conduction axis, producing all degrees of heart block. Sinus bradycardia is usually the result of partial or complete penetration of the ventricular myocardium. Whatever the cause of the bradycardia, the catheter should at once be withdrawn from the site at which manipulation produced the bradycardia. Atropine 0.01 mg/kg should be given down the catheter for sinus bradycardia. The catheter should not be manipulated again until the heart rate has returned to normal for a minute or two and, if possible, the spot where the bradycardia was induced should be avoided. If the bradycardia persists for more than two minutes, the patient should be dealt with as if a cardiac arrest had occurred.

Blockage of a normal channel

Advancing the catheter across a critically stenotic pulmonary or aortic valve, into a coronary artery not much bigger than the catheter, or into a duct upon which pulmonary or systemic circulation depends, may virtually occlude it and produce sudden bradycardia and hypotension. Sometimes manipulation of the catheter in the subpulmonary outflow tract provokes a cyanotic spell. The treatment is immediate withdrawal of the catheter and desisting from further attempts at traversing the obstruction. Cyanotic spells are best treated by propranol 2 mg in 10 cc saline given as a slow infusion, titrating the dose against the systemic arterial saturation and pressure. It appears that the incidence of spells during catheterisation can be reduced by premedication with 0.15 mg/kg morphine sulphate in at risk patients (Stanger et al, 1974). These have tetralogy of Fallot or tricuspid atresia with normally connected great arteries and no functioning shunts.

Knotted catheters

These are a serious problem if they cannot be unravelled, because surgery may be required to remove the catheter. The best treatment is preventive. Complex loops should be avoided if at all possible, and if a knot looks as though it is beginning to form, a guide-wire should be passed to straighten out the catheter.

Broken catheters

These are fortunately extremely rare and are managed as for removal of any foreign body from the circulation.

Balloon catheters may produce torn atrioventricular valves if they are withdrawn across them while inflated. This is particularly likely during balloon atrial septostomy if the right ventricle is mistaken for the left atrium. The method of avoiding this has already been detailed.

Angiocardiography

This carries the particular hazards of air embolism, intra-myocardial injection of contrast medium, and contrast medium toxicity.

Air embolism

Air embolism will not occur if meticulous attention is paid to flushing catheters and removing all air from syringes before injection.

Intramyocardial injection

Intramyocardial injection of contrast medium is serious because it may either cause immediate death or depression of ventricular function sufficient to prejudice the result of emergency surgery. Any angiocardiogram must be **immediately** preceded by a test injection of a small volume of contrast medium to ensure that it clears rapidly from the injection site. As already mentioned, the use of balloon catheters probably reduces the risk of intramyocardial injection by keeping the catheter away from the wall of the cardiac chamber where injection is made.

With the advent of isotonic contrast media such as metrizimide, the risk of overdose of contrast medium is now greatly reduced, but it is unwise to exceed the dose of 2 ml/kg of contrast medium in a single injection or 4 ml/kg in all. By using angiocardiography intelligently (in other words, as an adjunct to cross-sectional echocardiography) the total dose injected can be reduced considerably. Allergic reactions are rare.

General hazards of cardiac catheterisation

These include blood loss, hypothermia, metabolic acidosis and hypoglycaemia.

Blood loss

Blood loss can be reduced by meticulous attention to detail and micro-methods for blood gas and oxygen saturation determination. It is treated by transfusion.

Hypothermia

Hypothermia is only a problem in young babies and can be largely prevented by wrapping the baby in warm cotton-wool and placing it on a thermostatically controlled warm water circulating pad.

Metabolic acidosis

Metabolic acidosis can be reduced by speed of operation and is corrected with sodium bicarbonate or THAM administration.

Hypoglycaemia

Hypoglycaemia should be tested for in newborns with dextrostix and treated with glucose infusion.

Risk of death from cardiac catheterisation

Beyond 1 month of age, the risk is extremely small, being variously quoted as 0/96 (Taylor, 1978), 2/942 (0.2%) (Stanger et al, 1974) and 2/1605 (0.1%) (Ho et al, 1972). One group of older patients at risk from angiocardiography comprises patients with pulmonary vascular obstructive disease (Keane et al, 1978). For neonates the risk of catheterisation is extremely difficult to assess accurately, since many of them have an appreciable chance of dying within 24 hours of any procedure, including auscultation. Defining death from cardiac catheterisation as any death within 24 hours of the procedure, the mortality of cardiac catheterisation is variously reported as 33/215 (15.1%) (Stanger et al, 1974) and 10/104 (9.6%) (Taylor, 1978). Including deaths where deterioration began during catheterisation, Ho et al (1972) reported a mortality of 2/66 (3%). If, on the other hand, the first week of life is considered, but death due to catheterisation is imprecisely defined as 'death at or shortly after the study' (presumably before any operation) the mortality has been reported to be as low as 2/118 (1.7%) (Miller, 1974). In the New England Infant Cardiac Program report, death rate within the first 24 hours of cardiac catheterisation in infants varied from 0% for atrial septal defect to 22% for hypoplastic left heart syndrome (Fyler et al, 1980). The most important determinants of mortality related to catheterisation in neonates are therefore the definition of mortality, the nature of cases studied and the policy and results of surgery. It is quite impossible to determine what is the mortality **due** to catheterisation, except to say that it must be lower than any figure based upon the first 24 hours after catheterisation.

CALCULATIONS MADE FROM CATHETERISATION DATA

The power of modern computing makes calculation of a bewildering number of variables possible with the greatest ease. This makes it more important, not less, that the underlying calculations should be understood, and particularly that the assumptions behind them should be recognised. There is no uglier sight than the reverence with which some clinicians view the list of derived variables on a computer output, deluding themselves that because a variable is called 'wall stress', it is by some magic scientific, or worse, that it actually measures rather than estimates wall stress. We are not suggesting that no measurement should be made unless a precision of $\pm 1\%$ is possible; all we ask is that any measurement should be valued in proportion to its accuracy either in measuring what it purports to measure, or in predicting some future event which will permit rational decision making. There is an inescapable paradox here, which is that some of the most accurate measurements are the least useful in decision making and vice versa. The greater the number of original measurements involved in the calculation of some variable, the less precise it is likely to be (because of propagation of errors), but the end result may be a more accurate predictor than any of its components.

Mean atrial and arterial pressures are usually obtained directly by heavy electronic damping of the pressure trace. Should this have been omitted, diastolic pressure plus one-third of the pulse pressure (the difference between systolic and diastolic pressure), gives a good approximation of arterial mean pressure.

Pulmonary venous and arterial and systemic arterial mean oxygen saturations are normally taken as a mean of the values obtained in, say right and left pulmonary veins or arteries, or ascending and descending aorta. Should these readings be significantly different in different sites, it should be appreciated that in making the calculations which follow, assumptions are being made that are not necessarily valid. For example, suppose that the right pulmonary artery oxygen saturation is 80% and the left is 60%, while pulmonary veins are fully saturated. It is only strictly legitimate to calculate total pulmonary blood flow using 70% as the mean pulmonary artery saturation if oxygen uptake in the two lungs is equal.

In the case of mixed systemic venous oxygen saturation a problem arises, because normally the oxygen saturation is higher in the inferior than the superior caval vein. Since blood mixes well in the right ventricle, the appropriate point at which to measure mixed systemic venous oxygen saturation is the last cardiac chamber before any left-to-right shunt. If there is an atrial septal defect (as seen on cross-sectional echocardiography) then mixed venous oxygen saturation may be calculated as $(3 \times SCV + ICV)/4$ where SCV is superior caval venous and ICV is inferior

caval venous oxygen saturation (Flamm et al, 1969; Miller et al, 1974).

One gram of haemoglobin can carry 1.34 ml of oxygen, so oxygen capacity (ml/100 ml) is haemoglobin concentration (g/dl) multiplied by 1.34. The oxygen content of haemoglobin (ml/100 ml) may then be calculated as oxygen capacity times oxygen saturation (%) divided by 100. Blood also contains oxygen dissolved in the plasma. If the patient is breathing room air this may be simply approximated by adding 0.1 ml/100 ml to the oxygen content for oxygen saturations between 75 and 85%, 0.2 ml/100 ml for saturations of 85–95% and 0.3 ml/100 ml for saturations above 95% (Kelman & Nunn, 1966). If, on the other hand, the patient is breathing oxygen in higher concentration than room air, it is essential to be more accurate in calculating blood oxygen content by including the oxygen content of the plasma. This is achieved accurately enough by multiplying the P_{O_2} (mmHg) by 0.003. Plasma oxygen content is then added to haemoglobin oxygen content to give blood oxygen content. The calculations thus far may be bypassed entirely with a resultant improvement in accuracy if oxygen content is measured directly.

The Fick equation then states that:

$$\text{Qp} = \frac{\text{VO}_2/10}{\text{Cpv} - \text{Cpa}} \quad \text{and} \quad \text{Qs} = \frac{\text{VO}_2/10}{\text{Csa} - \text{Csv}}$$

where Qp and Qs are pulmonary and systemic blood flow (1/min), VO_2 is oxygen consumption (ml/min), Csa is systemic arterial oxygen content, Csv systemic venous content, Cpv pulmonary venous content and Cpa pulmonary arterial content. The mysterious division by ten is necessary because the answer of 1/min is based upon oxygen content measured in g/100 ml rather than g/l.

If there is no shunt, Cpa = Csv and Cpv = Csa, so that Qp = Qs.

In the presence of shunts, the concepts of effective and recirculated pulmonary and systemic blood flow have proved of great value. Consider Figure 14.8a which represents diagrammatically a bidirectional shunt. Both pulmonary and systemic circulations are shown as consisting of two theoretical components, effective and recirculated. Effective pulmonary and systemic flow (Qpe and Qse) must on average be equal, despite temporary differences, or else the pulmonary or systemic circulation would run dry. They are termed 'effective' as they are responsible for the entire uptake and release of oxygen in the circulation. Since Qpe is raised from systemic to pulmonary venous oxygen content in the lungs, and Qse is lowered from pulmonary venous to systemic venous saturation in the body,

$$\text{Qse} = \text{Qpe} = \frac{\text{VO}_2/10}{\text{Cpv} - \text{Csv}}$$

Knowing total and effective pulmonary and systemic blood flows, it is possible to calculate recirculated pulmonary and systemic flows by subtracting effective from total. Left-to-right shunt is then given by recirculated pulmonary blood flow expressed as a percentage of total pulmonary blood flow. Similarly right-to-left shunt is recirculated systemic flow as a percentage of total systemic flow.

This general derivation is applicable to all conditions involving recirculation of either systolic or pulmonary blood flow or both. It is important to realise that, for example, the right-to-left shunt so calculated does not necessarily quantify flow from right-sided to left-sided cardiac chambers. This is because congenital heart disease may produce cyanosis by one of two basic mechanisms: first, a right-to-left shunt in the presence of 'normal connection haemodynamics', and secondly, 'complete transposition haemodynamics'.

In 'normal connection haemodynamics' systemic venous blood still tends to be directed appropriately to the pulmonary trunk, and pulmonary venous blood to the aorta. Thus systemic arterial oxygen content is higher than that in the pulmonary arteries. By contrast, in 'complete-transposition haemodynamics', since pulmonary venous blood tends to be directed to the pulmonary trunk and systemic venous blood to the aorta, pulmonary arterial oxygen content is higher than aortic.

As Figure 14.8 demonstrates, the general considerations of bidirectional shunts apply as much to 'normal connection haemodynamics' (Fig. 14.8b) as to 'complete transposition haemodynamics' (Fig. 14.8c), except that with 'complete transposition haemodynamics', **the shunted blood is the effective flow**, whereas in 'normal connection haemodynamics' **the shunted blood is in the recirculated flow**. Complete transposition haemodynamics may also be termed 'unfavourable streaming', whereas normal connection haemodynamics may be termed 'favourable streaming'. In between these two lies 'complete mixing'.

Assuming that the pulmonary and systemic circuits behave like a simple direct current electrical circuit (this is quite an assumption!) resistances may be calculated as follows:

$$\text{Total pulmonary resistance} = \frac{PA}{Qp} \text{ units}$$

$$\text{Pulmonary vascular resistance} = \frac{PA - LA}{Qp} \text{ units}$$

$$\text{Total systemic resistance} = \frac{SA}{Qs} \text{ units}$$

$$\text{Systemic vascular resistance} = \frac{SA - RA}{Qs} \text{ units}$$

where PA = mean pulmonary artery pressure (mmHg),

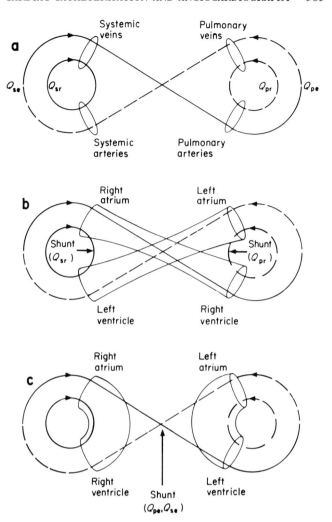

Fig. 14.8 Diagrammatic representation of bidirectional shunting. In each panel the body is to the left, the lungs to the right, and the heart central. (a) Any bidirectional shunt can be represented in terms of effective systemic flow (Q_{se}), effective pulmonary blood flow (Q_{pe}), recirculated systemic flow (Q_{sr}) and recirculation pulmonary flow (Q_{pr}). The portals of entry to and exit from the heart are also shown. This picture is the basis of the other two. (b) Where the cardiac connections are normal, the left and right sides of the heart transmit effective flow. Recirculated flow is shunted from one side of the heart to the other. (c) In complete transposition each side of the heart transmits recirculated flow. Effective flow is shunted from one side of the heart to the other. (Reproduced by kind permission from Godfrey S, Baum J D (eds) (1979) Clinical paediatric physiology. Blackwell Scientific, Oxford.)

LA = mean left atrial pressure (mmHg), SA = mean systemic arterial pressure (mmHg) and RA = mean right atrial pressure (mmHg).

Calculating ratios between the pulmonary and systemic resistances is attractive because one does not need to know the oxygen consumption (it cancels out) nor even the haemoglobin concentration (it cancels out if one ignores oxygen dissolved in plasma). It should not be imagined that this ratio in any comprehensive way 'normalises' total pulmonary or pulmonary vascular resistance, since systemic vascular resistance is inversely proportional to systemic arterial oxygen saturation (Morrison & Macartney, 1981). In other words, in two patients with the same pulmonary vascular resistance, one cyanotic and the other acyanotic, the pulmonary/systemic resistance ratio will be higher in the cyanotic patient.

When oxygen consumption has not been measured, it is often predicted from the size and age of the patient (Kappagoda et al, 1973) or from these measurements and heart rate (LaFarge & Miettinen, 1970). The advantage of the latter is that it gives the result in ml/min/m², so that one does not need to know the body surface area of the patient. The disadvantage is that the equation does not apply to children under 2 years of age. The weakness of predicting oxygen consumption is that it generates a large random error in any calculation derived from it. The estimated standard deviation of the differences between measured values and the values implied by the model of LaFarge & Miettinen was a massive 28.0 ml/min/m², and the predictive accuracy of Kappagoda's model was no better.

Providing that there is no shunt, or a shunt at only one level in the heart it is then possible to estimate the areas of the heart valves. For any valve, it is necessary to know the time from opening to closing of the valve and the mean pressure gradient across the valve during that time. The time the valve is open is known as the 'systolic ejection period' (SEP) for semilunar valves, and 'diastolic filling period' (DFP) for atrioventricular valves. These are measured in seconds. The mean pressure gradient is calculated by planimetering the area between the pressure traces during the DFP or SEP. This area of course depends upon the scale of the recording both with regard to horizontal and vertical displacement. The area is then divided by the length of the DFP or SEP **as it appears on the recording paper**. This gives the mean gradient **as it appears on the recording paper** which must then be converted to mmHg in the same way as any other pressure is measured, i.e. by taking account of the scale used to make the recording.

The estimated valve area (cm²) is then calculated as

$$\frac{\text{Flow through valve (l/min)} \times 1000}{\text{SEP (or DFP)} \times \text{constant} \times 44.5 \times \text{mean gradient}}$$

This constant is 0.85 for the mitral valve and 1 for the rest.

Clearly, estimation of valve areas requires high fidelity, simultaneous, pressure records on either side of the valve.

Dilution curves

If a substance is introduced rapidly into the circulation at one point and its concentration is measured at another, the result is a dilution curve. The method for introduction may be by injection (as with thermodilution, ascorbate radionuclide or indocyanine green) or by inhalation (as with hydrogen). To quantitate blood flow, it is necessary to assume that the indicator is injected instantly and mixes completely in blood before it is sampled. Furthermore, its concentration is measured instantaneously. In practice the requirement most obviously violated is usually that of complete mixing; it only occurs when the indicator is introduced upstream to a ventricle and sampled downstream. Injection into the apex of a ventricle and sampling downstream gives very good mixing, but any other injection (e.g. ascending aorta with sampling in femoral artery) gives highly inaccurate results.

In the absence of intracardiac shunts the theory is extremely simple. Let us suppose that I mg of injectate are administered and that a fraction f of this is sampled. Let us further suppose that no recirculation of injectate occurs, and that 1 cm on the recording of the dilution curve corresponds to S_c mg/l of injectate and S_t seconds. Then if A is the actual area under the dilution curve and t is the time from beginning to end of the dilution curve, the mean concentration of injectate will be $S_c S_t A/t$ (mg/l). But this corresponds to fI mg of dye dissolved in v ml of blood.

$$\text{Hence} \quad \frac{fI}{v} = S_c S_t A/t$$

$$\text{so} \quad \frac{v}{t} = \frac{fI}{S_c S_t A}$$

Since blood is fully mixed with injectate, $v/t = fQ$ where Q is the cardiac output in l/min.

$$\text{Hence} \quad Q = \frac{I}{S_c S_t A}$$

For a given dose of injectate, cardiac output is inversely proportional to the area of the dye curve. In a very large circulatory system one can therefore imagine a series of widely separated dye curves, each corresponding to successive transits through the circulation and lower but wider than the previous one. Injectate disappears completely between each curve. The cardiac output could be measured off any of the curves.

In practice, these successive dilution curves overlap, so some approximation has to be made to establish what would have been the area under the dye curve had recirculation not occurred. The classical way of doing this for indocyanine green curves is to assume that the decay of concentration on the downslope of the curve is exponential. Thus the concentrations at equal successive intervals (say seconds) on the dye curve are measured. Those on the downslope of the curve are plotted on semi-logarithmic paper. This should produce a plot that is linear in its central section, corresponding to the period of exponential decay. The central straight section is extrapolated downwards and concentration at successive intervals read off until the concentration is less than 1% of peak concentration. These concentrations correspond to those that would have been obtained had no recirculation occurred. The concentrations at one-second intervals are summed to give the area.

In the past, dilution curves were widely used to localise shunts, but have now been replaced by cross-sectional echocardiography with injection of contrast microbubbles into the cardiac chambers. This method has the great merit of demonstrating unequivocally in most instances the precise site of the shunt. Problems only occur when the echocardiographic section does not pass through the communication. For this reason, the appearance of dilution curves in the presence of shunts will not be discussed except for one particular application.

In patients with some degree of pulmonary vascular obstructive disease, accurate measurement of pulmonary venous oxygen content is essential for precise measurement of pulmonary blood flow and resistance. If the left atrium cannot be entered, and systemic arterial blood is desaturated, pulmonary venous saturation cannot be assumed, because the desaturation of systemic arterial blood may either be due to pulmonary venous desaturation or to a right-to-left shunt or to both. A right-to-left shunt may be excluded by contrast echocardiography, injecting in both caval veins and imaging the aorta. If it is present, then its magnitude must be calculated. The dye curves obtained by injection into both caval veins and sampling in a systemic artery will usually have a small early appearing peak of injectate corresponding to the right-to-left shunt, followed by the main first circulation peak. The ratio between the areas under both peaks corresponds to the right-to-left shunt. By substituting into the equation previously given for right-to-left shunt, one can solve for pulmonary venous oxygen saturation or content. To avoid problems with recirculation, instead of comparing the entire areas under the curves, the area of the two forward triangles are compared, these being constructed by dropping a perpendicular from each peak concentration and drawing a straight line from that peak to the point of onset of the relevant portion of the dye curve (in other words, either the right-to-left shunt or the normally circulating dye).

Quantitative angiography

This is now a well-established technique in children. Though it is possible to use single-plane right anterior oblique projections for measurement of ventricular volumes, no satisfactory single-plane technique for the right ventricle has been described. The method relies upon using timed cineangiograms exposed in the frontal and lateral planes. It is helpful if the timing can be related to the electrocardiogram. The faster the frame rate the better, though the calculations become more laborious. Because most cineangiograms are pulsed (that is, the frontal and lateral tubes fire alternately), the pairs of frames that are used to calculate the volume are not quite synchronous, which introduces a slight error.

All X-ray pictures are magnified because of divergence of rays from the source. This magnification factor is usually calculated by filming a wire grid or metal sphere of standard size immediately before or after the angiocardiogram with the grid or sphere being placed where the child's heart was while the film was running.

During injection of contrast medium, it is important that as few extrasystoles as possible are provoked. This necessitates careful placement of the catheter tip in midcavity, and possibly injection at a lower rate than usual. These considerations, together with the need to film in two orthogonal planes (and as yet volumes have been validated in children only for frontal and lateral planes), mean that there is an inescapable conflict between the requirements of quantitative angiography and the need for optimal demonstration of cardiac anatomy.

The most widely used methods of estimating ventricular volume are the area-length method for the left atrium and left ventricle, and Simpson's rule for the right atrium and ventricle (Graham et al, 1971, 1973, 1974a). These will therefore be described although other workers have obtained equally accurate results by different methods (Arcilla et al, 1971, 1973; Thilenius & Arcilla, 1974; Lange et al, 1978a, b, c, 1982).

Whichever method is used, the first step is to trace the outlines of the chambers in paired frontal and lateral images, including trabeculations and papillary muscles within the ventricular outlines, and drawing straight lines across the cavoatrial junctions or the base of the semilunar valves as appropriate.

Simpson's rule

Simpson's rule is nothing more than a standard method for integrating otherwise non-integrable functions, in this case summing the volumes of horizontal slices of the right ventricle. As described by Graham and colleagues (1973), ten slices are created by eleven horizontal lines. Each slice is then assumed to be an ellipsoid with axes the same length as the horizontal lines and the volumes are summed. Clearly horizontal slices through the right ventricle are **not** ellipsoids, since the right ventricle wraps around the left. This method is bound to overestimate volume. Fortunately by comparing the known volume of right ventricular casts with volume estimated by Simpson's rule, Graham and colleagues (1973) were able to show that a good estimate of right ventricular volume could be obtained by multiplying the result of the Simpson's rule calculation by

0.649. For the right atrium the model corresponds more to real life and the correction factor is 0.991.

The area-length method

This method is used for the left heart chambers partly for historical reasons. Simpson's rule is as accurate, but much more time-consuming. In the days when these calculations had to be done by hand, this was very important. Nowadays, with so many automated systems around, this is unimportant.

In each projection the longest possible straight line is drawn within the left ventricle, running from apex to base of aortic valve. Having allowed for magnification factors, the shorter of the two lengths (1 cm) is chosen. The model assumes that the longer of the lengths is the major axis of the prolate ellipsoid (the rugby-ball-shaped left ventricle or more spherical left atrium). The volume V (ml) is then given by the following formula

$$V' = \frac{0.847 \times Af \times Al}{1}$$

where Af and Al are the areas (in cm²) of the frontal and lateral images of the left atrium or ventricle.

This volume has now to be corrected as was that of the right ventricle to give the true volume V (cm³). For the left atrium and ventricle two equations are necessary:

$$V = 0.974V' - 3.1 \quad (V' > 15 \text{ cm}^3)$$
$$V = 0.733V' \quad\quad\quad (V' \leq 15 \text{ cm}^3)$$

Left ventricular mass is calculated by measuring left ventricular wall thickness (t) from the lateral wall of the left ventricle on the frontal projection at end-diastole. The volume of cavity and wall is then calculated as that of a prolate ellipsoid having major and minor axes longer by 2t cm than those of the left ventricular cavity at end-diastole. Subtraction of cavity volume from the volume of cavity and wall gives wall volume. Multiplying this by the specific gravity of heart muscle (1.05) gives left ventricular mass.

For calculation of end-systolic and end-diastolic volumes, it is now necessary to plot the volumes against time for as many cycles as possible. Post-extrasystolic beats should certainly be ignored and it is best not to analyse any records containing extrasystoles during opacification of the heart. The volume/time curves are then smoothed either by hand or by a computer curve fitting routine. The end-diastolic volume is normally taken to be the average maximum volume and the end-systolic volume the average minimum volume over the cycles studied. Subtracting the two gives the stroke volume and dividing this by the end-diastolic volume gives the ejection fraction.

Multiplying stroke volume by heart rate gives total right and left ventricular output. If there is no valvar regurgi-tation and no intracardiac shunt these correspond to cardiac output. If there are no shunts and there is regurgitation of one valve on either side of the heart this provides a method of quantitating regurgitation, for the difference between forward stroke output calculated from an indicator dilution curve or the Fick method and total stroke output calculated from the ventricular volume represents the volume regurgitating with each heart beat. If this is divided by end-diastolic volume, one obtains regurgitant fraction.

Contrariwise, if there is no valvar regurgitation but there is a shunt, this can, with certain qualifications, be calculated. For example, the difference between total right and left ventricular outputs in atrial septal defect corresponds to the net left-to-right shunted flow. In an isolated ventricular septal defect, with or without a duct, total left ventricular output equals pulmonary blood flow. As soon as shunting occurs both upstream and at or beyond ventricular level (as in atrial and ventricular septal defect) calculation of shunt flows becomes impossible because of the assumptions necessary.

There are many other more complex measures of function that can be made once ventricular volume and wall thickness have been measured, such as wall stress and the study of pressure-volume loops, but these are beyond the scope of this chapter.

ESTABLISHMENT OF NORMAL VALUES, ALLOWING FOR THE SIZE OF THE PATIENT

This is a central problem for all paediatricians, and one about which there is a great deal of muddled thinking. How can one compare the same measurement made in two children of different sizes, and how can we know whether a given value is outside the normal range for a person of that size?

The ideal method is exemplified by height and weight charts, familiar to every paediatrician. These are obtained by examining heights and weights in very large numbers of normal children. More important still, large numbers of children are measured at each specific age for a given sex. Because of this, the percentiles are directly derived from the data. These percentiles are then plotted for each sex and each age as points, and the points are then joined up to permit interpolation. Because such large numbers are used, no assumptions are made either as to the distribution at any particular age or as to the general shape of the relationship between weight and height and age. Within the cardiological field, a good example of this kind of approach is that of derivation of normal standards for electrocardiographic measurements (Davignon et al, 1979, 1980a,b).

Where the necessary data can be collected from normal children without harming them, there is really no excuse for establishing normal standards in any other way. It is laborious, but worth all the toil involved if one really wants to know the probability of obtaining a particular value from a normal individual.

Data from cardiac catheterisation are in quite another category because of the ethical problems involved in obtaining the information in normal children. Because of the paucity of data it is necessary to make far-reaching assumptions both as to the distribution of a variable among children of a particular size or age, and as to the overall relationship between that variable and size or age. Furthermore, what is meant by size, and how is this best measured?

The first assumption made is that at any particular size the variable under consideration has an approximately normal distribution. Only if that is the case is it possible to state that, if the value obtained is more than two standard deviations from the mean, the two-tailed probability of obtaining such an extreme measurement from a normal individual is less than 1 in 20. **Without knowledge of the underlying distribution it is not possible to know the probability of lying at a particular point in the distribution.** The fact that this key point is hardly ever spelt out by laboratories when tests are reported does not in any way authenticate the practice. There is a further fundamental problem which is far too little appreciated. Even if the underlying distribution has been shown to be normal, the only information obtained from the use of standard deviations is the probability of obtaining such an extreme measurement given that the individual is normal. What you, the clinician would really like to know is the probability that the patient is normal, given the measurement obtained. These probabilities are **not the same**. The latter probability can only be obtained from the former if the prevalence of disease and the probability of obtaining such an extreme measurement (given that the disease is present), are known. Space does not permit further discussion of this key point, but interested readers are commended to study Galen & Gambino (1975).

The second assumption (or strictly, set of assumptions) comes when a mathematical model is fitted to the data to express the relationship between the variable under consideration and size. This is where the question of choice of measure of size becomes important. Ideally, the size variable should be chosen in such a way that the relationship is a straight line passing through or very close to the origin, and this model should have the least variance not explained by the regression. If, and only if, this model fits, it then becomes possible to express the variable as a ratio equally applicable to patients of any size. One example of this kind of fit is the relationship between cardiac output and body surface area (Cayler et al, 1963). Because the relation is to a straight line passing through origin, it is meaningful to express cardiac output as an index $(l/min/m^2)$ which should be the same whatever the body surface area. Another example is left ventricular mass related to body surface area (Graham et al, 1971).

If the relationship of the variable to body size is linear, but does not pass through the origin, then indexing is fraught with peril, as pointed out long ago by Tanner (1949). To illustrate this point, let us consider the relationship between normal left ventricular end-diastolic volume and body surface area given by Graham and colleagues (1971)

$$LVEDV = 88.7 \times BSA - 13.3$$

If we substitute values into the equation, this tells us that the mean LVEDV for a $0.2\ m^2$ baby is 4.44 ml whereas that of a $1.8\ m^2$ adult is 146.36 ml. The corresponding indexed figures are $22.2\ ml/m^2$ and $81.3\ ml/m^2$. For no other reason than that the straight line misses the origin by 13.3 ml, the expected 'indexed' value for the adult is nearly four times as great as that of the baby. With this in mind, it is instructive to look at the comparison between normal values in patients under and over two years published by Graham and colleagues (1971), for in every case where there is a significant difference between the groups and a plot of the data is provided, the straight line fails to pass through or near the origin, whereas in the only case where there is no significant difference between the two groups and a plot is provided, the straight line goes virtually through the origin. In providing indexed values, these authors were merely following a long established precedent, so we do not single them out for criticism. Indeed they are to be congratulated on two counts. First they provided multiple regression estimates of normal values (see below) and second, they largely avoided ascribing these differences at different ages to **biological** causes. As should now be clear, most if not all of the difference can be explained as a mathematical artefact.

Indexed values are useful because they can be retained in the memory, and because it is possible to define more accurately the normal range by lumping all subjects together into one category. For this reason, we find it hard to follow the logic of the repeated attacks launched by Krovetz on the use of body surface area (Krovetz, 1965; Krovetz et al, 1967). It is true that the Dubois formula (Du Bois & Du Bois, 1916) is less accurate in measuring body surface area than the method of Sendroy & Cecchini (1954), but this is strictly irrelevant to the task of establishing normal values from catheterisation. If the relationship between body surface area and the variable concerned is a straight line through the origin with low residual variance whereas the relation with height and weight is not, then it seems to us that there is every reason to index by body surface area and no reason not to use the Dubois formula (body surface area = 0.007184 × weight (kg) 0.425 × height (cm) since this is computationally easier. All we have to understand is that we must not imagine that we have actually measured the body surface area. Perhaps if *body surface area* was enclosed in quotes, it would emphasise this point.

If, on the other hand, the same straight line through the origin can be obtained using weight, height or even age, and the residual variance is as small, then we can see no reason to use 'body surface area'. Finally, if a curvilinear model has to be fitted, or the straight line does not go through the origin, then we would agree with Krovetz and colleagues (1967) that multiple regression is the method of choice. A brief description of this is given in Chapter 59. The main criterion of a useful multiple regression model is that it uses as few predictors as possible consistent with a low residual variance. A further factor must be considered which in practice rules out the use of reciprocals to predict pulmonary and systemic vascular resistance as advocated by Krovetz and colleagues (1967). This is that when the residuals (the differences between actual and predicted values) are plotted against the predictors, the variance of the residuals should be, if possible, constant (Draper & Smith, 1966). This is highly unlikely to happen when reciprocals are used, because the variance in small subjects is inevitably far greater than that in large ones (Morrison & Macartney, 1981).

Let us suppose that we have obtained a particular measurement of, say, systemic vascular resistance, together with values for the variables which have been shown to predict it in normal individuals. Only if the variance of the residuals is approximately constant (and approximately normally distributed) is it possible to determine the probability of obtaining such an extreme value of systemic vascular resistance, given that the patient is normal and that the predictors are as measured. This is mathematically quite a complex task, because one needs to take account not only of the variance about the regression line, but also of the variance of the regression line itself. The confidence limits for patients at the extremes of the distribution of predictors will be wider than for those of average size.

It should now be clear that the establishment of normal ranges for catheterisation data is a much more difficult matter than most cardiologists imagine. Table 14.2 presents what information we do have on the matter. Fortunately, deciding whether a patient is normal or not quite normal is relatively unimportant compared with obtaining information which is of value in predicting the outcome of particular interventions, notably cardiac surgery. One example is pulmonary/systemic resistance ratio in ventricular septal defect (Cartmill et al, 1966), but this book is full of others.

INTERPRETATION OF DATA OBTAINED FROM CARDIAC CATHETERISATION

This is the most important stage of all. The details depend on what exactly is wrong with the patient, and are covered in chapters devoted to specific defects of diseases. It is often extremely helpful to have made measurements before and during interventions. At this point we will simply enumerate some broad principles.

First, in congenital heart disease in particular, the

Table 14.2 Comparison of selected haemodynamic data (Krovetz & Goldbloom, 1972).

| | Units | Present report | | | | Literature | | | |
		No.	Mean	S.D.	Range	No.	Mean	S.D.	Range
Age	Years	30	8.7	5.8	0.003–19.9	123	9.0	5.8	0.001–19
Arterio-venous difference	ml/l	23	44.3	15.0	20–78	90	39.1	8.2	24–26
Cardiac index	l/min/m^2	21	4.32	0.7	3.5–5.7	72	4.5	1.3	2.5–9.2
Stroke volume index	ml/m^2	21	44.3	15.0	22.7–82.6	52	48.1	13.3	26.2–81.8
Oxygen cons/m^2	ml/m^2	8	141.8	20.1	114.0–165.4	68	167.7	32.3	87.1–268.2
PA/SA mean	–	28	0.15	0.03	0.11–0.23	35	0.21	0.12	0.04–0.93
Systemic artery									
systolic	mmHg	29	111.1	13.0	77–138	36	110.3	26.2	48–152
diastolic	mmHg	29	64.2	9.8	48–88	36	63.2	14.2	28–84
mean	mmHg	29	80.5	11.6	57–109	42	79.0	18.0	38–112
Pulmonary artery									
systolic	mmHg	28	21.8	6.2	12–42	86	22.4	9.5	6–60
diastolic	mmHg	28	8.7	2.8	4–18	86	9.6	6.0	2–42
mean	mmHg	28	12.4	3.1	6–22	92	14.2	7.1	3–49
Right ventricle									
systolic	mmHg	27	28.0	5.9	9–42	48	32.9	14.7	16–80
end-diastolic	mmHg	26	5.0	1.9	1–8	48	3.3	3.1	−1–13
left atrial mean or pulmonary artery wedge mean	mmHg	18	7.0	2.3	3–12	39	6.8	3.9	−2–14
right atrial mean	mmHg	8	3.8	2.0	1–8	47	2.6	2.8	−3–9
Left ventricle									
end-diastolic	mmHg	13	7.5	2.2	4–11	No data			

PA = pulmonary artery; SA = systemic artery; S.D. = standard deviation.

physiological disturbance must be interpreted in terms of the underlying pathological anatomy. It is many years since it was necessary to deduce pathological anatomy from the haemodynamic disturbance present.

Secondly, because of the difficulty of establishing normal values for data measured at catheterisation, it is generally more fruitful to compare one measurement with another in the same patient (e.g. peak left ventricular and aortic systolic pressure) than to compare one measurement in a patient with 'normal'.

Thirdly, as a general rule, individual measurements should be interpreted in the light of other measurements rather than in isolation (e.g. pressure gradients in the light of flow).

In conclusion, cardiac catheterisation, done well, is of enormous value in decision-making, therapy and research. Done badly, it is a menace.

REFERENCES

Arcilla R A, Tsai P, Thilenius O, Ranniger K 1971 Angiographic method for volume estimation of right and left ventricles. Chest 60: 446–454

Arcilla R A, Thilenius O G, Chiemmongkoltip P, Ranniger K 1973 Left atrial volume calculation by angiocardiography in children. Chest 63: 189–197

Azzolina G, Eufrate S A, Allela A 1973 New approach to catheterization of the heart in infants and children. British Heart Journal 35: 643–646

Bargeron L M Jr 1981 Angiographic recognition of specific anatomic structures. In: Becker A E, Losekoot G, Marcelletti C, Anderson R H (eds) Paediatric cardiology, Vol 3. Churchill Livingstone, Edinburgh, p 33–47

Barth K H, White R I Jr, Kaufman S L, Terry P B, Roland J-M 1982 Embolotherapy of pulmonary arteriovenous malformations with detachable balloons. Radiology 142: 599–606

Bloomfield D A 1978 The nonsurgical retrieval of intracardiac foreign bodies – an international survey. Catheterization and Cardiovascular Diagnosis 4: 1–14

Boijsen E, Lundstrom N R 1968 Percutaneous catheterization and angiocardiography in infants and children. American Journal of Cardiology 22: 572–575

Bommer W J, Lee G, Riemenschneider T A, et al 1983 Laser atrial septostomy. American Heart Journal 106: 1152–1156

Cartmill T B, DuShane J W, McGoon D C, Kirklin J W 1966 Results of repair of ventricular septal defect. Journal of Thoracic and Cardiovascular Surgery 52: 486–499

Cayler G C, Rudolph A M, Nadas A S 1963 Systemic blood flow in infants and children with and without heart disease. Pediatrics 32: 186–201

Cumming G R 1982 Cardiac catheterization in infants and children can be an outpatient procedure. American Journal of Cardiology 49: 1248–1253

Davignon A, Rautaharju P, Boisselle E, Soumis F, Megelas M, Choquette A 1979/80a Percentile charts. ECG standards for children. Pediatric Cardiology 1: 133–152

Davignon A, Rautaharju P, Boisselle E, Soumis F, Megelas M, Choquette A 1979/80b Normal ECG standards for infants and children. Pediatric Cardiology 1: 123–131

Desilets D T, Hoffman R 1965 A new method of percutaneous catheterization. Radiology 85: 147–148

D'Souza V J, Velasquez G, Weesner K M, Prabhu S 1984 Transluminal angioplasty of aortic coarctation with a two-balloon technique. American Journal of Cardiology 54: 457–458

Draper N R, Smith H 1966 Applied regression analysis. Wiley, New York

Driscoll D J, Hesslein P S, Mullins C E 1982 Congenital stenosis of individual pulmonary veins: clinical spectrum and unsuccessful treatment by transvenous balloon dilatation. American Journal of Cardiology 49: 1767–1772

Du Bois D, Du Bois E F 1916 A formula to estimate the approximate surface area if height and weight be known. Archives of Internal Medicine 17: 863–871

Edwards B S, Lucas R V Jr, Lock J E, Edwards J E 1985 Morphologic changes in the pulmonary arteries after percutaneous balloon angioplasty for pulmonary arterial stenosis. Circulation 71: 195–201

Faithfull N S, Haider R 1971 Ketamine for cardiac catheterisation. Anaesthesia 26: 318–323

Finley J P, Beaulieu R G, Nanton M A, Roy D L 1983 Balloon catheter dilatation of coarctation of the aorta in young infants. British Heart Journal 50: 411–415

Flamm M D, Cohn K E, Hancock E W 1969 Measurement of systemic cardiac output at rest and exercise in patients with atrial septal defect. American Journal of Cardiology 23: 258–265

Florentine M, Wolfe R R, White R I Jr 1984 Balloon embolization to occlude a Blalock-Taussig shunt. Journal of the American College of Cardiology 3: 200–202

Freed M D, Keane J F, Rosenthal A 1977 The use of heparinizationn to prevent arterial thrombosis after percutaneous cardiac catheterization in infants and small children. Circulation 56: 102–105

Fuhrman B P, Bass J L, Castaneda-Zuniga W, Amplatz K, Lock J E 1984 Coil embolization of congenital thoracic vascular anomalies in infants and children. Circulation 70: 285–289

Fyler D C, Buckley L P, Hellenbrand W E, Cohn H E 1980 Report of the New England Regional Infant Cardiac Program. Pediatrics 65 (Suppl): 376–461

Galen R S, Gambino S R 1975 Beyond normality: the predictive value and efficiency of medical diagnoses. Wiley, New York

Gianturco C, Anderson J H, Wallace S 1975 Mechanical devices for arterial occlusion. American Journal of Roentgenology 124: 428–435

Girod D A, Hurwitz R A, Caldwell R L 1982 Heparinization for prevention of thrombosis following pediatric percutaneous arterial catheterization. Pediatric Cardiology 3: 175–180

Goldberg S J, Linde L M, Wolfe R R, Griswold W, Momma K 1969 The effects of meperidine, promethazine and chlorpromazine on pulmonary and systemic circulation. American Heart Journal 77: 214–221

Graham T P Jr, Jarmakani J M, Canent R V Jr, Morrow M N 1971 Left heart volume estimation in infancy and childhood. Reevaluation of methodology and normal values. Circulation 43: 895–904

Graham T P Jr, Jarmakani J M, Atwood G F, Canent R V Jr 1973 Right ventricular volume determinations in children. Normal values and observations with volume or pressure overload. Circulation 47: 144–153

Graham T P Jr, Atwood G F, Faulkner S L, Nelson J H 1974a Right atrial volume measurements from biplane cineangiocardiography. Methodology, normal values, and alterations with pressure or volume overload. Circulation 49: 709–716

Graham T P Jr, Atwood G F, Werner B 1974b Use of droperidol-fentanyl sedation for cardiac catheterization in children. American Heart Journal 87: 287–293

Grinnell V S, Mehringer C M, Hieshima G B, Stanley P, Lurie P R 1982 Transaortic occlusion of collateral arteries to the lung by detachable valved balloons in a patient with tetralogy of Fallot. Circulation 65: 1276–1278

Ho C S, Krovetz L J, Rowe R D 1972 Major complications of cardiac catheterization and angiocardiography in infants and children. Hopkins Medical Journal 131: 247–258

Huhta J C, Smallhorn J F, Macartney F J 1982 Two dimensional echocardiographic diagnosis of situs. British Heart Journal 48: 97–108

Hurwitz R A, Franken E A Jr, Girod D A, Smith J A, Smith W L 1977 Angiographic determination of arterial patency after percutaneous catheterization in infants and small children. Circulation 56: 102–105

Inoue K, Owaki T, Nakamura T, Kitamura F, Miyamoto N 1984 Clinical application of transvenous mitral commissurotomy by a new balloon catheter. Journal of Thoracic and Cardiovascular Surgery 87: 394–402

Jones R S, Meade F, Owen-Thomas J B 1972 Oxygen and nitrous oxide uptake during general anaesthesia for cardiac catheterization in infants with congenital heart disease. British Heart Journal 34: 53–57

Jones S M, Miller G A H 1973 Catheterization of the pulmonary artery in transposition of the great arteries using a Swan-Ganz flow-directed catheter. British Heart Journal 35: 298–300

Kan J S, White R I Jr, Mitchell S E, Gardner T J 1982 Percutaneous balloon valvuloplasty: a new method for treating congenital pulmonary-valve stenosis. New England Journal of Medicine 307: 540–542

Kan J S, White R I Jr, Mitchell S E, Farmlett E J, Donahoo J S, Gardner T J 1983 Treatment of restenosis of coarctation by percutaneous transluminal angioplasty. Circulation 68: 1087–1094

Kan J S, White R I Jr, Mitchell S E, Farmlett E J, Donahoo J S, Gardner T J 1984 Treatment of restenosis of coarctation by percutaneous transluminal angioplasty. Circulation 68: 1087–1094

Kappagoda C T, Linden R J 1972 A critical assessment of an open circuit technique for measuring oxygen consumption. Cardiovascular Research 6: 589–598

Kappagoda C T, Greenwood P, Macartney F J, Linden R J 1973 Oxygen consumption of children with congenital diseases of the heart. Clinical Science and Molecular Medicine 45: 107–113

Keane J F, Fyler D C, Nadas A S 1978 Hazards of cardiac catheterization in children with primary pulmonary vascular obstruction. American Heart Journal 96: 556–558

Kelman G R, Nunn J F 1966 Nomograms for correction of blood P_{O_2}, P_{CO_2}, pH, and base excess for time and temperature. Journal of Applied Physiology 21: 1484–1490

King T D, Thompson S L, Steiner C, Mills N L 1976 Secundum atrial septal defect: nonoperative closure during cardiac catheterization. Journal of American Medical Association 235: 2506–2509

Kirkpatrick S E, Takahashi M, Petry E L, Stanton R E, Lurie P R 1970 Percutaneous heart catheterization in infants and children. Circulation 42: 1049–1056

Krovetz, L J, 1965 The physiologic significance of body surface area. Journal of Pediatrics 67: 841–862

Krovetz L J, Goldbloom S 1972 Normal standards for cardiovascular data. II. Pressure and vascular resistances. Johns Hopkins Medical Journal 130: 187–195

Krovetz L J, McLoughlin T G, Mitchell M B, Schiebler G L 1967 Hemodynamic findings in normal children. Pediatric Research 1: 122–130

Lababidi Z 1983 Aortic balloon valvuloplasty. American Heart Journal 106: 751–752

Lababidi Z, Wu J-R 1983 Percutaneous balloon pulmonary valvuloplasty. American Journal of Cardiology 52: 560–562

Lababidi Z, Wu J-R, Walls J T 1984a Percutaneous balloon aortic valvuloplasty: Results in 23 patients. American Journal of Cardiology 53: 194–197

Lababidi Z A, Daskalopoulos D A, Stoeckle H Jr 1984b Transluminal balloon coarctation angioplasty: experience with 27 patients. American Journal of Cardiology 54: 1288–1291

LaFarge C G, Miettinen O S 1970 The estimation of oxygen consumption. Cardiovascular Research 4: 23–30

Lange P E, Onnasch D, Farr F L, Heintzen P H 1978a Angiocardiographic right ventricular volume determination.

Accuracy, as determined from human casts, and clinical application. European Journal of Cardiology 8: 477–501

Lange P E, Onnasch D, Farr F L, Heintzen P H 1978b Angiocardiographic left ventricular volume determination. Accuracy, as determined from human casts, and clinical application. European Journal of Cardiology 8: 449–476

Lange P E, Onnasch D, Farr F L, Malerczyk V, Heintzen P H 1978c Analysis of left and right ventricular size and shape, as determined from human casts. Description of the method and its validation. European Journal of Cardiology 8: 431–448

Lange P E, Onnasch D G W, Schaupp G H, Zill C, Heintzen P H 1982 Size and function of the human left and right ventricles during growth. Normative angiographic data. Pediatric Cardiology 3: 205–211

Lock J E, Niemi T, Einzig S, Amplatz K, Burke B, Bass J L 1981 Transvenous angioplasty of experimental branch pulmonary artery stenosis in newborn lambs. Circulation 64: 886–893

Lock J E, Niemi T, Burke B A, Einzig S, Castaneda-Zuniga W R 1982 Transcutaneous angioplasty of experimental aortic coarctation. Circulation 66: 1280–1286

Lock J E, Bass J L, Amplatz K, Fuhrman B P, Castaneda-Zuniga W 1983a Balloon dilation angioplasty of aortic coarctations in infants and children. Circulation 68: 109–116

Lock J E, Castaneda-Zuniga W R, Fuhrman B P, Bass J L 1983b Balloon dilation angioplasty of hypoplastic and stenotic pulmonary arteries. Circulation 67: 962–967

Lock J E, Bass J L, Castaneda-Zuniga W, Fuhrman B P, Rashkind W J, Lucas R V Jr 1984 Dilation angioplasty of congenital or operative narrowings of venous channels. Circulation 70: 457–464

Lund G, Cragg A, et al 1983 Patency of the ductus arteriosus after balloon dilatation: an experimental study. Circulation 68: 621–627

Lund G, Cragg A, Rysavy J, et al 1984 Long-term patency of the ductus arteriosus after balloon dilatation: an experimental study. Circulation 69: 772–774

Lurie P R, Armer R M, Klatte E C 1963 Percutaneous guide wire catheterization: diagnosis and therapy. American Journal of Diseases in Children 106: 189–196

Lurie P R, Fujito M, Neustein H B 1978 Transvascular endomyocardial biopsy in infants and small children: description of a new technique. American Journal of Cardiology 42: 452–453

Macartney F J, Scott O, Deverall P B, Hepburn F 1975 New preformed catheter for entry into pulmonary artery in complete transposition of great arteries. British Heart Journal 37: 525–529

Mansfield P B, Gazzaniga A B, Litwin S B 1970 Management of arterial injuries related to cardiac catheterization in children and young adults. Circulation 42: 501–507

Miller G A H 1974 Congenital heart disease in the first week of life. British Heart Journal 36: 1160–1166

Miller H C, Brown D J, Miller G A H 1974 Comparison of formulae used to estimate oxygen saturation of mixed venous blood from caval samples. British Heart Journal 36: 446–451

Morrison G W, Macartney F J 1981 Determinants of systemic vascular resistance in children with congenital heart disease. Cardiovascular Research 15: 245–253

Morrison G W, Scott O, Macartney F J 1977 Retrograde left atrial catheterization in children with congenital heart disease. American Heart Journal 94: 333–335

Mullins C E 1983 Transseptal left heart catheterization: experience with a new technique in 520 pediatric and adult patients. Pediatric Cardiology 4: 239–245

Mullins C E, Neches W H, Reitman M J, El-Said G, Riopel D A 1972 Retrograde technique for catheterization of the pulmonary artery in transposition of the great arteries with ventricular septal defect. American Journal of Cardiology 30: 385–387

Neches W H, Mullins C E, Williams R L, Vargo T A, McNamara D G 1972 Percutaneous sheath cardiac catheterization. American Journal of Cardiology 30: 378–384

Newfeld E A, Purcell C, Paul M H, Cole R B, Muster A J 1974 Transumbilical balloon atrial septostomy with transposition of the great arteries. Pediatrics 54: 495–497

Park S C, Neches W H, Zuberbuhler J R, et al 1978 Clinical use of blade atrial septostomy. Circulation 58: 600–606 ·

Park S C, Neches W H, Mullins C E, et al 1982 Blade atrial septostomy: collaborative study. Circulation 66: 258–266

Porstmann W, Wierny L, Warnke H 1967 Closure of persistent ductus arteriosus without thoracotomy. Thoraxchirurgie 15: 199–201

Porstmann W, Wierny L, Warnke H, Gerstberger G, Romaniuk P A 1971 Catheter closure of patent ductus arteriosus. Radiologic Clinics of North America 9: 203–218

Radner S 1955 Extended suprasternal puncture technique. Acta Medica Scandinavica 151: 223

Rashkind W J 1983 Transcatheter treatment of congenital heart disease. Circulation 67: 711–716

Rashkind W J 1985 Interventional cardiac catheterization in congenital heart disease. International Journal of Cardiology 7: 1–11

Rashkind W J, Miller W W 1966 Creation of an atrial septal defect without thoracotomy. Journal of the American Medical Association 196: 991–992

Reidy J F, Baker E, Tynan M 1983 Transcatheter occlusion of a Blalock-Taussig shunt with a detachable balloon in a child. British Heart Journal 50: 101–103

Riemenschneider T A, Lee G, Ikeda R M, et al 1983 Laser irradiation of congenital heart disease: potential for palliation and correction of intracardiac and intravascular defects. American Heart Journal 106: 1389–1393

Rocchini A P, Kveselis D, Dick M, Crowley D, Snider A R, Rosenthal A 1984a Use of balloon angioplasty to treat peripheral pulmonary stenosis. American Journal of Cardiology 54: 1069–1073

Rocchini A P, Kveselis D A, Crowley D, Dick M, Rosenthal A 1984b Percutaneous balloon valvuloplasty for treatment of congenital pulmonary valvular stenosis in children. Journal of the American College of Cardiology 3: 1005–1012

Ross J Jr 1966 Considerations regarding the technique for transseptal left heart catheterization. Circulation 34: 391–399

Sendroy J Jr, Cecchini L P 1954 Determination of human body surface area from height and weight. Journal of Applied Physiology 7: 1–12

Shirey E K, Sones F M Jr 1966 Retrograde transaortic and mitral valve catheterization. Physiologic and morphologic evaluation of aortic and mitral valve lesions. American Journal of Cardiol 18: 745–753

Simovitch H, Hohn A R, Wagner H R, Vlad P, Subramanian S, Lambert E C 1970 Percutaneous right and left catheterization in children. Circulation 41: 513–517

Smith C, Rowe R D, Vlad P 1958 Sedation of children for cardiac catheterization with an ataractic mixture. Canadian Anaesthetists Society Journal 5: 35–40

Sperling D R, Dorsey T J, Rowen M, Gazzaniga A B 1983 Percutaneous transluminal angioplasty of congenital coarctation of the aorta. American Journal of Cardiology 51: 562–564

Stanger P, Heymann M A, Tarnoff H, Hoffman J I E, Rudolph A M 1974 Complications of cardiac catheterization of neonates, infants, and children. A three-year study. Circulation 50: 595–608

Sullivan I D, Robinson P J, Macartney F J, et al 1985 Percutaneous balloon valvuloplasty for pulmonary valve stenosis in infants and children. British Heart Journal 54: 435–441

Sunderland C O, Nichols G M, Henken D P, Linstone F, Menashe V D, Lees M H 1976 Percutaneous cardiac catheterization and atrial balloon septostomy in pediatrics. Journal of Pediatrics 89: 584–587

Swan H J C, Ganz W, Forrester J, Marcus H, Diamond G, Chonette D 1970 Catheterization of the heart in man with use of a flow-directed balloon-tipped catheter. New England Journal of Medicine 283: 447–451

Takahashi M, Petry E L, Lurie P R, Kirkpatrick S E, Stanton R E 1970 Percutaneous heart catheterization in infants and children. I. Catheter placement and manipulation with guide wires. Circulation 42: 1037–1048

Takahashi M, Schieber R A, Wishner S H, Ritchie G W, Francis P S 1983 Selective coronary arteriography in infants and children. Circulation 68: 1021–1028

Tanner J M 1949 Fallacy of per-weight and per-surface area standards and their relations to spurious correlation. Journal of Applied Physiology 2: 1–15

Taylor J F N 1978 The investigation of congenital heart defects in small infants. Herz 3: 87–97

Thilenius O G, Arcilla R A 1974 Angiographic right and left ventricular volume determination in normal infants and children. Pediatric Research 8: 67–74

Tynan M, Jones O, Joseph M C, Deverall P B, Yates A K 1984 Relief of pulmonary stenosis in first week of life by percutaneous balloon valvuloplasty (letter). Lancet 1:273

Tynan M, Baker E J, Rohmer J, et al 1985 Percutaneous balloon pulmonary valvuloplasty. British Heart Journal 53: 520–524

Tyson J E, Desa D J, Moore S 1976 Thromboatheromatous complications of umbilical arterial catheterisation in the newborn period. Clinico-pathological study. Archives of Disease in Childhood 51: 744–754

Ueda K, Saito A, Nakano H 1982 Aortography by countercurrent injection via the radial artery in infants with congenital heart disease. Pediatric Cardiology 2: 231–236

Waldman J D, Young T S, Pappelbaum S J, Turner S W, Kirkpatrick S E, George L M 1982 Pediatric cardiac catheterization with same-day discharge. American Journal of Cardiology 50: 800–803

Waller B F, Girod D A, Dillon J C 1984 Transverse aortic wall tears in infants after balloon angioplasty for aortic valve stenosis: relation of aortic wall damage to diameter of inflated angioplasty balloon and aortic lumen in seven necropsy cases. Journal of the American College of Cardiology 4: 1235–1241

Warnecke I, Frank J, Hohle R, Lemm W, Bücherl E S 1984 Transvenous double-balloon occlusion of the persistent ductus arteriosus: an experimental study. Pediatric Cardiology 5: 79–84

White J J, Talbert J L, Haller J A 1968 Peripheral arterial injuries in infants and children. Annals of Surgery 167: 757–765

White R I Jr, Kaufman S L, Barth K H, DeCaprio V, Strandbert J D 1979 Embolotherapy with detachable silicone balloons. Technique and clinical results. Radiology 131: 619–627

Exercise and pulmonary function

Exercise is part of the normal life of children, even more than adults where habit often substantially curtails the desire and subsequently the ability to undertake strenuous physical exertion. The reserve capacity for exercise of normal children and young adults is quite considerable since at maximal levels of exercise the oxygen uptake may exceed 24 times the resting level (Saltin & Astrand, 1967) while cardiac output may reach 7 times the resting level. This means that oxygen transport (cardiac output multiplied by oxygen consumption) may be almost 170 times the resting level. This adaptation to exercise is dependent upon the synchronous adaptation of the cardiovascular, respiratory and neuromuscular systems.

The pulmonary reserve is substantial in normal children since at maximum levels of exercise they utilise only some 70% of their maximum breathing capacity (Godfrey, 1974). Gas transport between the lungs and the blood is also believed to be adequate to meet all requirements since oxygen and carbon dioxide diffusion never reach limiting values under normal atmospheric conditions (Johnson, 1967). We cannot be certain about the limiting role of the cardiovascular system in normal exercise since there is no comparable method to the voluntary determination of maximum breathing capacity. We do know, however, that heart rate does reach a plateau (Astrand, 1952) and so apparently does stroke volume (Godfrey et al, 1972) so that it is probable that cardiac output does reach a limiting value on strenous exercise. If this is true then the only possibility of a continuing increase in aerobic work is by widening the arterio-venous oxygen content difference and extracting more oxygen from the blood. This occurs pari passu with the normal increase in cardiac output but also seems to reach a limiting value in health (Eriksson, 1972). This means that ultimately exercise is limited by the inability to increase heart rate and to extract oxygen from blood above certain limits.

During growth from infancy to adulthood there is an integrated change in the dimensions of the body which includes the cardiovascular and respiratory systems. Not only are there increases in the physical dimensions of the

heart and lungs, but also changes in the rate of breathing and the heart rate. The adaptations to growth, as will be seen later, are such that certain basic parameters, notably arterial blood gases and the arterio-venous content difference, are held virtually constant throughout life. This not only applies to rest but also to the response to physical exercise. In order to determine the effects of disease of the heart or lungs on the response of children to physical exertion, it is necessary to take these normal adaptive processes into account.

Exercise testing and pulmonary function testing form an essential part of the investigation of children with heart or lung disease, and perhaps particularly for documenting normality in patients with symptoms but no objective evidence of disease at rest. The conduct of such tests of exercise or pulmonary performance presents certain problems in children because of their willingness or ability to cooperate during the tests. Attention must be paid to designing tests which are not painful or frightening, which are non-invasive and which above all give worthwhile information which will be of use in the management of the individual child. Probably the first non-invasive measurement of cardiac output in children during exercise was undertaken some fifty-five years ago by Galle (1926) using the nitrous oxide method which was then very tedious to perform. Fortunately, with the rapid advance in technology in recent years, it is possible to obtain quite sophisticated data during exercise in children in a manner which they can accept and even enjoy. In many cases the problem of cooperation does not arise since most children, if physically able to exercise, will do so provided they are suitably encouraged.

Ethical considerations are very important with regard to exercise testing, particularly in children who cannot give informed consent to the procedures. As far as studies in healthy children are concerned, provided the tests are safe and painless, one may equate the exertion to that undertaken during sports activities. In sick children there is less of an ethical problem as the tests are carried out to define the nature or severity of a particular problem. Indeed it could well be argued that failure to undertake exercise tesing in order to define the problem under controlled (safe) conditions is negligent since the child may be unnecessarily restricted in his activities, or may undertake potentially dangerous activities spontaneously.

From what has already been said it should be apparent that there is a need for the technology of exercise testing and pulmonary function testing in children. Children habitually take exercise and any limitation in this natural activity either for real or imaginary reasons imposes a serious physical and psychological handicap on the child (Bergman & Stamm, 1967; Caylor et al, 1973). The ability to compete with peers is so important that objective evaluation is well worthwhile in sick children so that clear guidelines may be given to the child, his parents and teachers. The extent to which conventional grading of effort intolerance by the questioning of the mother can be in error is shown in Figure 15.1. This shows the results of a study of children with Fallot's tetralogy carried out by Taylor (1972) in my laboratory at the Brompton Hospital. There was no correlation between the mothers' opinion of effort tolerance elicited by a standardised questionnaire and the fraction of predicted normal maximum working capacity (W_{max}) measured on a cycle ergometer. The error was in both directions, namely overoptimistic and overpessimistic.

Given that it is worthwhile to undertake exercise testing and lung function testing in children, we need to consider which children need such tests. Broadly speaking, there are two categories of patients needing such tests:

The 'Do they have it?' group
The 'How bad is it?' group.

In the first group we have patients with or without signs of organic heart or lung disease at rest who complain of shortness of breath on exercise or effort intolerance. In the present context, the problem of children without significant resting cardiovascular findings is particularly important. It must be remembered that the absence of such signs at rest is no guarantee of normal performance under stress, and so when in doubt an exercise test may resolve the problem. The child with the 'innocent' systolic murmur is a classic example of a patient for whom exercise testing may be helpful. It must also be remembered that lung disease may present to the paediatric cardiologist as effort intolerance. Simple lung function tests as well as, of course, the chest X-ray, may point in the right direction. Of particular interest is the child with exercise-induced asthma (Godfrey, 1978). Such patients may be totally well between attacks with no signs in the chest, but develop severe bronchospasm following strenuous exercise as shown in Figure 15.2. This can be confused with cardiac disease – even 'cardiac asthma' – but the changes shown in Figure 15.2 are only seen in patients with bronchial asthma (Godfrey, 1974) and can be abolished by premedication with sympathomimetic bronchodilator drugs and to a lesser extent with other agents, especially sodium cromoglycate (Anderson et al, 1975).

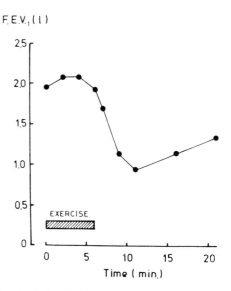

Fig. 15.2 Exercise-induced asthma resulting from 6 min of running. The major fall in lung function occurs 3–5 min after stopping exercise.

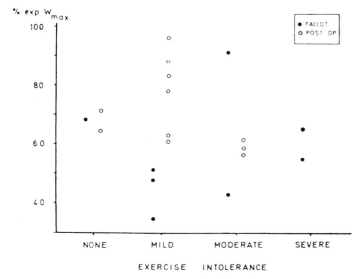

Fig 15.1 Maximum working capacity (W max) as percent of predicted compared with maternal grading of effort tolerance in two groups of children with Fallot's tetralogy, one before and the other after surgery. (From Taylor, 1972.)

The second group of patients comprises those with objective evidence of heart or lung disease at rest in whom it is desired to determine the nature or severity of any limitation of exercise. This may be a question of observing, under carefully controlled laboratory conditions, whether or not adverse and potentially harmful effects result from exercise, or exercise may be used to shed light on the nature of physiological disturbances which occur. The latter type of exercise testing requires a more sophisticated analysis than the former in that it is usually necessary to determine cardiac output, arterial blood gases and shunt in order to obtain the information. Children with aortic or pulmonary stenosis could be considered to be in the first category and exercise testing would be used to define the safety of their participation in sports, etc., given the potential risk of sudden unexpected death (Glew et al, 1969), although in children it seems that sudden death has not clearly been linked to exercise (Doyle et al, 1974; Lambert et al, 1974). Exercise could also be used as an additional guide to the timing of surgical intervention although this has not yet been widely used. Children who develop cyanosis on exertion but who are not cyanosed at rest, whether due to lung disease or cardiac disease, would fall into the category of those for whom exercise testing provided an explanation of their problem. This information would then be of use for determining prognoses or planning treatment.

In the following sections we shall consider the methods of measuring pulmonary function and exercise response in children, the growth and development of lung function and exercise physiology in health, and some of the disturbances which occur in disease.

LUNG FUNCTION TESTING IN CHILDREN

A large number of different tests of lung function are available but only a few of them are of practical importance in children with suspected heart or lung disease. Essentially, we require information about the size of the lungs, the resistance to flow in the airways and the adequacy of gas exchange. It is now possible to measure these parameters in children of all ages and even premature infants (Stocks & Godfrey, 1977) except for the small group aged 1 year to about 5 years who cannot cooperate with tests. Even in these children we can now obtain considerable information on lung function by the use of insoluble radio-isotopic lung scans (Ronchetti et al, 1975a).

The volume of the lungs is divided up into a number of components (Fig. 15.3) of which for practical purposes only three are of any importance: vital capacity (VC) which is the maximum volume of air which can be moved in and out of the lungs in one breath; total lung capacity (TLC) which is the absolute volume of gas in the lungs at full inspiration; and resting lung volume (thoracic gas volume, TGV, or functional residual capacity, FRC) which is the absolute volume of gas in the lungs at the end of a normal expiration. Whenever the lungs are significantly diseased in childhood the vital capacity is reduced. As this is the simplest parameter to measure in children (as distinct from infants), it is obviously a most useful index. Total lung capacity may or may not be affected depending upon the

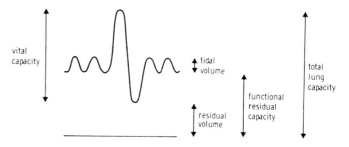

Fig. 15.3 Definition of lung volumes.

nature of the problem. Vital capacity is measured by having the children take a maximum inspiration and then exhale fully into a spirometer which may be of the conventional water-filled variety or a modern electronic device.

Absolute resting lung volume and other parameters derived from it such as total lung capacity and residual volume (the absolute volume of gas in the chest at the end of a full expiration, RV) can only be determined by either a gas dilution technique or whole body plethysmography. The simple helium dilution method requires the child to rebreathe a helium-oxygen mixture for 5–10 minutes to that resting lung volume can be determined from the known initial volume of the spirometer used and the reduction in helium concentration. It requires the cooperation of the child and is only really applicable over 5 or 6 years of age by which time they can already perform simple spirometry. Since for practical purposes an abnormal resting volume will usually be accompanied by changes in parameters measured by simple spirometry this helium dilution test is of no great value in paediatric cardiology.

Infants cannot cooperate by performing the maximum inspiration and expiration needed to measure vital capacity by spirometry and for these patients measurement of resting lung volume is important. Although inert gas dilution can be used (Ronchetti et al, 1975b) it is tedious and the whole body infant plethysmograph (Stocks et al, 1977) is much to be preferred as it enables airway resistance to be measured simultaneously. The plethysmograph consists of an airtight chamber in which the infant sleeps quietly and breathes through a respiratory circuit provided with a three-way tap system. By occluding the tap at the end of a normal expiration and measuring the pressure developed at the mouth and in the chamber as the infant makes a respiratory effort against the obstruction, resting lung volume can be calculated by applying Boyle's Law (Dubois et al, 1956a). This measurement is very accurate with a coefficient of variation of 3.7% (Stocks, 1977). It gives an excellent estimate of lung volume in infants up to about one year of age using minimal sedation. Above this age the infant is usually too alert and inquisitive to lie quietly in the plethysmograph and deep sedation is rarely justified in order to obtain results.

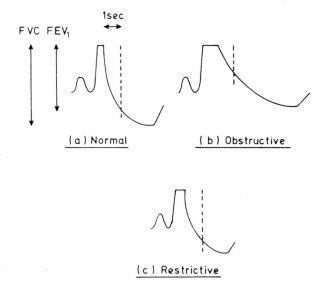

Fig. 15.4 Diagrammatic representation of a conventional forced expired vital capacity manouever in health, in obstructive lung disease and in restrictive lung disease.

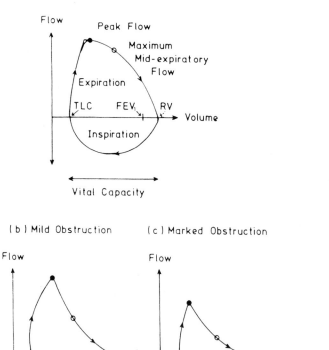

Fig. 15.5 Diagrammatic representation of the maximal inspiratory and expiratory flow–volume loop in health, airways obstruction chiefly affecting small airways, and generalised airways obstruction.

The other major parameter of lung function which can help distinguish pulmonary from cardiac disease is the airway resistance. While this can be measured plethysmographically (see below), a very good index can be obtained in older children by parameters derived from a forced vital capacity manoeuvre. All that is required is for the child to take a maximum inspiration and then blow the air out as hard and fast as he can. The simplest index measured is the forced expired volume in the first second of expiration (FEV$_1$). In the presence of airway disease, the velocity of expiration is reduced and hence the FEV$_1$ is reduced (Fig. 15.4). Generally there is much less reduction in the forced vital capacity (FVC) and hence in airways obstructive disease the FEV$_1$/FVC ratio is reduced below the normal 70–80% found in children. In diseases where the lungs are just small – restrictive lung disease – this ratio is normal because both the FEV$_1$ and the FVC are reduced proportionately (Fig. 15.4). A more modern and indeed more informative test of airway function which nevertheless uses the same simple forced expired vital capacity manoeuvre, is the expired flow-volume loop. During this test, both the expiratory flow rate and the expired volume are monitored simultaneously by suitable equipment and then displayed as a graph of expired flow rate on the Y-axis against expired volume on the X-axis (Fig. 15.5). From this graph it is possible to read off the peak expiratory flow rate (PEFR) – a simple index of airway function which is rather effort-dependent – and a much more useful parameter of maximum flow at low lung volumes – conventionally recorded most often as the maximum mid-expiratory flow rate (MMEF). It can be shown that the MMEF (and indeed the shape of the latter part of the flow-volume curve) is a relatively effort-independent test of airway function which re-

flects particularly the resistance in the smaller airways (Cotes, 1981). The FEV$_1$ is more effort-dependent than the MMEF and reflects both large and small airway functions.

The measurement of absolute airway resistance requires the use of a whole body plethysmograph and employs the technique first described by Dubois (1956b). In essence, during free breathing within the closed chamber, changes in chamber pressure reflect changes in alveolar pressure and can be related to the instantaneous air flow rate measured at the mouth to calculated airway resistance. The relationship between alveolar pressure change and chamber pressure change is obtained from the previously described measurement of resting lung volume during airway occlusion. Whole body plethysmographs suitable for children are readily available but the measurement is somewhat tedious and rarely, if ever, contributes more than the simple forced expiratory manoeuvre described above to the diagnosis of lung disease in children. Where the plethysmograph does become very valuable is in the detection of airway disease in the infant who cannot cooperate with forced expiratory manoeuvres. The whole body infant plethysmograph is a little more complex than the adult version in that the infant has to rebreathe heated humidified gas during the measurement to avoid artefacts due to temperature and humidity changes of respired air (Stocks et al, 1977). Even so this instrument has proved to be extremely valuable in detecting airway disease in infants and in helping to distinguish cardiac from pulmonary disease. As noted earlier, infant plethysmography is not generally practical over one year of age and other techniques must be used.

Another approach to measuring lung mechanics is to measure intrathoracic pressure changes recorded from a balloon placed in the midthoracic oesophagus. When related to airflow at the mouth, oesophageal pressure can be used (after an appropriate correction for changing lung volume) to derive pulmonary resistance which is airway resistance plus a small amount of pulmonary tissue frictional resistance. Although inherently much simpler than plethysmography, this measurement is far less accurate and in any case entails swallowing an oesophageal balloon which few infants and no children appreciate very much.

The oesophageal balloon can also be used to measure the elastic properties of the lung tissue – compliance and static recoil pressure. Compliance is the volume change produced by a given pressure change measured under static conditions, i.e. after airflow has ceased, while static recoil is the absolute pressure across the lungs (from oesophagus to mouth) at a nominal lung volume (usually resting lung volume) under static conditions. Although these parameters may well be abnormal in infants with cardiac disease, the difficulties of using oesophageal balloons after the first few months of life make such tests of little practical value – at least until adolescence.

Many other measurements of lung function such as the pulmonary diffusing capacity for carbon monoxide flow–volume loops expressed at absolute lung volumes, and inert gas washout time have little or no practical value in children and will not be considered further.

The absolute test of pulmonary function is the quality of arterial blood, since the function of the lungs is to convert systemic venous blood into arterial blood of normal composition. Measurement of arterial blood gas tensions is essential in solving all but the most elementary problems and requires that a good representative blood sample be obtained. This is a painful procedure unless local anaesthetic is used (which I strongly recommend) and may be quite frightening. Blood samples in children are usually best drawn from the radial artery (on the right side unless there is complete transposition). Arterialised capillary blood can give reasonable results if taken with great care except when high oxygen concentrations are being breathed (Godfrey et al, 1971b). Samples taken during crying or breath-holding may be highly misleading and there is no doubt that arterial blood sampling in children requires considerable skill. It is often best to insert a small cannula in the artery and return later, preferably when the child is asleep, to collect the sample.

Provided the arterial blood sample is properly obtained it may be very helpful in distinguishing cardiac from pulmonary problems (Jones et al, 1976). In lung disease there may be some alveolar hypoventilation with elevation of the arterial P_{CO_2} while this does not occur in heart disease. Of greater importance is the presence of hypoxia and its response to breathing a high concentration of inspired oxygen. In lung disease the hypoxia is due to alveoli which are poorly ventilated and by giving added oxygen the P_{O_2} rises in these alveoli so that the hypoxia is wholly or large corrected. In most cardiac conditions associated with hypoxia, the low P_{O_2} is due to the shunting of blood in the heart or great vessels. Since the shunted blood bypasses the lungs, no amount of added inspired oxygen makes any appreciable difference (Jones et al, 1976). Arterial blood should be sampled while the child breathes room air and after breathing as near as possible 100% oxygen for 10 minutes. It is essential to measure the concentration of inspired oxygen at the mouth in order to calculate the shunt. This calculation can be performed for practical purposes in simple stages. First the alveolar oxygen tension is calculated from a simplified alveolar air equation

$$P_{A}O_2 = P_{I}O_2 - Pa_{CO_2}/R \tag{1}$$

where $P_{A}O_2$ is alveolar oxygen, $P_{I}O_2$ is inspired oxygen tension = fractional concentration of O_2 inspired X (barometric pressure in mmHg – 47), Pa_{CO_2} is arterial CO_2 tension (which is assumed to equal alveolar CO_2 tension) and R is the respiratory exchange ratio (normally 0.8) which allows for the fact that more oxygen molecules are absorbed by the blood than carbon dioxide molecules are discharged into the alveoli. The ideal pulmonary capillary oxygen tension is assumed to be equal to the alveolar oxygen tension. Once alveolar (pulmonary capillary) oxygen tension is calculated and arterial oxygen tension is measured, they are converted into their equivalent oxygen contents using an appropriate dissociation curve. The shunt may then be calculated using the standard shunt equation on the (reasonable) assumption that the resting arterio-venous oxygen content difference in childhood is 40 ml/l, as follows, (all values in ml/l blood)

Shunt (%) =
$$\frac{\text{(Alveolar capillary } O_2 \text{ content } - \text{ Arterial } O_2 \text{ content)}}{\text{(Alveolar capillary } O_2 \text{ content } - \text{ Arterial } O_2 \text{ content)} - 40} \tag{2}$$

The shunt during air breathing can than be compared with the shunt during breathing of a high concentration of inspired oxygen in order to determine that part due to 'anatomical' shunt and that part due to ventilation-perfusion inbalance as follows:

Shunt breathing air = Anatomical shunt
+ Ventilation-perfusion imbalance shunt

Shunt breathing 100% O_2 = Anatomical shunt

(3)

Thus:

Shunt breathing air − Shunt breathing 100% O_2
= Ventilation-perfusion imbalance shunt

(4)

In lung disease the ventilation-perfusion imbalance predominates while in cardiac anomalies the anatomical shunt predominates.

In children between about 1 and 5 years it is quite difficult to undertake any meaningful lung function tests. Moreover, children with either heart or lung disease often have regional variations in the severity of the disease. For these reasons simple techniques of radio-isotopic lung scanning using inert isotopes of xenon or nitrogen have been developed. In my own studies the gas is given as bolus either by inhalation or intravenously after dissolving in saline and the lungs are scanned using a gamma camera-computer system (Ronchetti et al, 1975a). In the presence of lung disease the arrival and washout of isotope is disturbed by either route of administration. For practical purposes the intravenous route produces more striking results as well as being much easier to perform since it does not depend on synchronisation with the breathing of the child.

GROWTH AND DEVELOPMENT OF NORMAL LUNG FUNCTION

The chief parameters of lung function already discussed grow with the child in an orderly and predictable fashion from infancy to adult life. Thanks to a series of investigations in infancy using the whole body plethysmograph (Stocks & Godfrey, 1977) and a number of studies during childhood (Polgar & Promadhat, 1971) we now have an almost complete picture of the normal increase in parameters of lung function throughout childhood. As can be seen from Figure 15.6, all the measured indices of increase of lung volume vary in a curvilinear fashion with respect to height (which is probably the best index for comparison). The growth of total lung capacity, resting lung volume and residual volume is such that the proportionate relationships between them remain constant. Only the resting lung volume has been measured in infancy with accuracy and speculations on other parameters based on the 'crying' vital capacity are not really of much value.

Along with the growth of lung volume there is an increase in airway diameter and length. Since resistance is inversely related to the fourth power of diameter and only linearly to length, the net effect is a very substantial reduction in airway resistance from 20–30 sec^{-1} in the newborn infant to 2–3 $cmH_2O/l.sec^{-1}$ in the young adult. In practice it is often easier to relate the reciprocal of resistance (conductance, Gaw) to resting lung volume, measured plethysmographically (thoracic gas volume since they are almost linearly related throughout growth as shown in Fig-

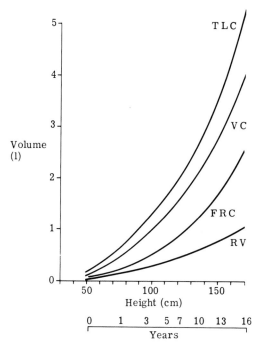

Fig. 15.6 The increase in the various subdivisions of lung volume with growth. (From Godfrey S 1981 Growth and development of the respiratory system. In: Davis J A, Dobbing J (eds) Scientific foundations of pediatrics. Heinemann, London, p 432–450.)

ure 15.7). In fact the ratio of conductance to thoracic gas volume (specific conductance, SGaw) is approximately 0.2–0.3 $sec^{-1}.cmH_2O^{-1}$ throughout infancy and childhood. Only in the premature infant is SGaw increased (Stocks & Godfrey, 1977) and this may be related to the earlier maturation of the airways compared to the alveoli. It should be noted that the infant up to some 3–6 months of age is an obligatory nose breather and nasal resistance accounts for some 49% of the total airway resistance in white infants and 30% in black infants (Stocks & Godfrey, 1978). Feeding a small sick infant through a nasogastric tube which causes occlusion of one nostril may place a very considerable burden on the respiratory system.

Indirect indices of airway resistance such as the FEV_1 and MMEF increase proportionately with lung volume as the airways grow. As mentioned earlier, FEV_1 remains at about 80% of the FVC. MMEF when divided by resting lung volume gives the functional residual capacity which, when expressed as FRCs per sec (instead of l per sec), remains at approximately 1.8–2.0 throughout childhood. Recent work in my laboratory suggests that this latter number might also hold true in infancy.

Consequent upon the orderly growth of the lungs, the proportionate increase in alveolar and dead space ventilation (discussed later) and the increase in pulmonary blood flow, the increasing metabolic demands of the growing body are met without any major changes in arterial blood gases. Apart from the first few minutes of life when

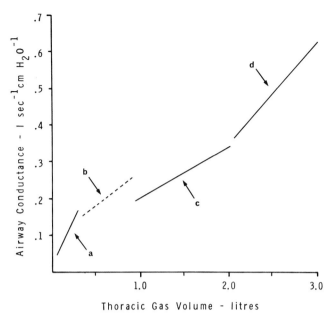

Fig. 15.7 Relationship between airway conductance (reciprocal of resistance) and lung volume throughout growth from infancy to adulthood. The four lines represent studies of different age groups. (From Stocks J 1977 Early Human Development 1: 285–309.)

cardiopulmonary adaptations are occurring very rapidly (Koch & Wendel, 1968), the arterial oxygen tension and carbon dioxide tension of children are in the low normal range for adults, i.e. P_{O_2} of 80–90 mmHg and P_{CO_2} of 33–36 mmHg. When given high oxygen concentrations to breathe, the normal child – just like the normal adult – should increase his arterial P_{O_2} to 550–600 mmHg, although in practice it may not exceed 300 mmHg unless great care is taken to ensure that 100% O_2 is breathed for 10 minutes at least. Neither the ventilation-perfusion shunt nor the anatomical shunt of the healthy child should exceed 3–4% of systemic blood flow.

Radio-isotopic lung scans have been used in children with suspected local lung disease and this has enabled some estimates to be made on the ability of the healthy lung areas to clear inhaled or injected isotope (McKenzie et al, 1977). It appears that, as predicted from their rather high alveolar ventilation per unit lung volume, infants clear isotope rather faster than older children. The fractional ventilation after inhalation of isotopic nitrogen expressed in $l/sec.l^{-1}$ lung volume decreases from 6 in newborn infants to 2 in adults. Fractional washout after intravenous injection is less affected by age – the normal range being from about 4 in infants to 2 in adults. In the presence of disease these washout results are usually very much slower and differ from zone to zone if the abnormality is localised.

EXERCISE TESTING IN CHILDREN

There are many different protocols for exercise testing in children which vary in terms of equipment, complexity and objective. Basically there are two types of test
1. Tests of maximum effort performance
2. Tests of adaptation to exercise at submaximal levels.

For the child suspected of having asthma, the objective is to determine if there is any change in lung function as a result of exercise (exercise induced asthma) and this is best done using treadmill running which has been fully reviewed elsewhere (Anderson et al, 1975).

Tests of maximum effort performance

In classical exercise physiology terms it is customary to attempt to measure the maximum oxygen uptake ($\dot{V}O_2$ max), sometimes called the maximum aerobic power, by having the subject exercise at higher and higher levels until there is no further increase in $\dot{V}O_2$ with increasing work (Fig. 15.8). This type of test can be performed on a treadmill or cycle ergometer and in most protocols the subject exercises in steady state conditions for four to six minutes at each of several increasingly severe work levels either in a progressive fashion or with rest between work loads (Cumming & Friesen, 1967). In order to satisfy the definition of $\dot{V}O_2$ max it is necessary to measure $\dot{V}O_2$ at each work level and demonstrate failure of any rise – or minimal rise (say less than 2%) between two loads which differ significantly. The implication is that the subject is working chiefly through anaerobic metabolism to achieve the increment in load and some workers would suggest that blood lactate should rise to about 8 mmol/l in younger children and 10 mmol/l or more in older children in order for the $\dot{V}O_2$ maximum to be acceptable. The technical details of measurement of $\dot{V}O_2$ will be considered later.

It should be obvious that the type of test described requires considerable will-power on behalf of the child and

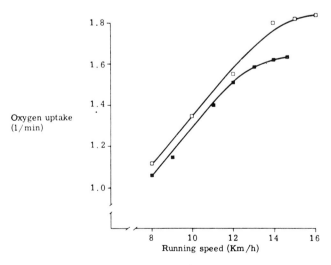

Fig. 15.8 Demonstration of attainment of a maximum oxygen uptake plateau in two subjects studied by Astrand (1972). (From Godfrey, 1981.)

may be tedious for both subject and investigator. For this reason various simpler techniques have been tried which give reasonable estimates of maximum performance. The one which I favour is termed the 'simple progressive exercise test' and consists of progressive increments of work load every minute using a cycle ergometer until the patient is unable to continue. The actual increment is so chosen that every subject should complete about five to eight work loads. Thus, for small but healthy children we should use an increment of 10 watts, for large healthy children 20 watts, and for medium-sized children, 15 watts. A reduced increment is used for patients who are expected to have a reduced working capacity so as to enable them to complete at least four or five levels of work.

At maximum levels of work there is a plateau of oxygen uptake and, since the subject is now exercising anaerobically, carbon dioxide production rises very rapidly and ventilation is stimulated. This means that there is a disproportionate increase in breathing towards the end of progressive test of maximum performance. Heart rate, like oxygen consumption, also tends to plateau at maximum levels of work. There are thus a number of parameters which may be used to judge the validity of maximum work and the various test protocols use all or some of these indices. In truth, this type of study is more appropriate for studies by exercise physiologists than clinical cardiologists and the determination of exact indices of maximum oxygen uptake is of little practical value. Moreover, there is very considerable doubt as to the best way in which to standardise the index for the growing child. As will be discussed later, simple correction based on body weight or surface area often implies differences between the sexes or between children of different races or sizes which a priori are unlikely to exist.

Tests of submaximum performance

The objective of submaximal exercise tests are generally to make detailed observations on cardiopulmonary performance under conditions of stress and to compare them with the situation at rest or at other levels of work. Submaximal testing is used to enable the child to attain and hold a steady physiological state for long enough so that meaningful measurements can be made. This is rarely, if ever, possible at maximal levels of work. It is generally helpful to choose the submaximal level as a given fraction of the maximum working capacity of the child rather than to use an arbitrary work load and thus to achieve some degree of intersubject standardisation. We have generally used one-third and two-thirds of maximum (Godfrey et al, 1971a) but others have used one-quarter and one-half or just one level. Experience suggests that good steady-state results are most difficult to achieve above about 70% of maximum.

What is measured during the submaximal test will depend upon the particular problem and on the facilities available. The range extends from the simple recording of heart rate of electrocardiogram through non-invasive measurements of cardiac output to the measurement of ventricular function by invasive techniques during cardiac catheterisation. This chapter will concentrate mainly on non-invasive technology as catheterisation is fully considered elsewhere. Moreover the normal growth and development of the response to exercise has largely been determined by non-invasive techniques and these serve as reference values for invasive studies in patients. Mention will also be made of the new and very exciting non-invasive techniques which are being developed for use during exercise in order to visualise cardiac chamber size, namely echocardiography and radio-isotopic cardiac scans (Alpert et al, 1980a, b).

In every submaximal exercise test it is essential to have a reference standard for the stress to which the child is being subjected. The most reliable measure is the oxygen consumption ($\dot{V}O_2$) and this is a direct reflection of the metabolic cost of all the work being performed by the subject in undertaking the task in hand. It does not matter what type of exercise is being performed – treadmill running, erect cycling, supine cycling, swimming, and so on – the VO_2 provides an absolute reference. Other measures such as the speed and slope of a treadmill, height and rate of stepping, nominal setting on a cycle ergometer, etc., give only very approximate measures of the rate of working and most will be very dependent on the size of the subject. Even the cycle ergometer setting will not accurately reflect the total cost of work since a fat person will use more energy moving his legs around then a thin person. The simple friction types of ergometer are very dependent on the rate of pedalling but even the very expensive electronically braked ergometers which are much less rate-dependent will not give a totally accurate measure of the energy expenditure because of differing body physique. However, the relationship between $\dot{V}O_2$ and work rate in upright cycling using a properly calibrated electronically braked cycle ergometer is remarkably constant and that for normal children is shown in Figure 15.9. The 95% confidence limits are approximately ±200 ml which means a variation of about ±20% at a low level of work corresponding to 50 watts (300 Kpm/min) and only 13% at a moderate work rate of 100 watts (600 Kpm/min). The reason for this constant relationship is that the mechanical efficiency of work in man is itself constant. The mechanical efficiency is the fraction of the metabolic energy cost (calculated from the oxygen consumption) which appears as external mechanical work (moving the ergometer, raising the body weight up a slope, etc.). In our studies we obtained a value for mechanical efficiency of 24.4% in normal children (Godfrey, 1974) which compares very well with the values of 23–24% in normal males and 22–23% in normal females obtained by Astrand (1952) and is almost identical to the value in adults obtained by Wahlund (1948). This relationship is so

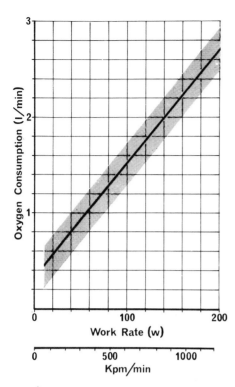

Fig. 15.9 Relationship between oxygen consumption and work rate. (From Godfrey, 1974.)

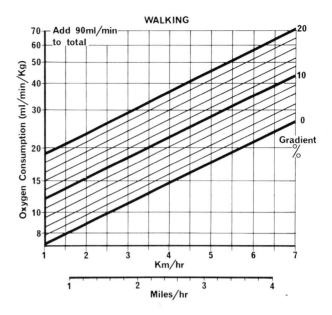

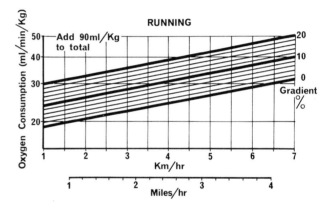

Fig. 15.10 Relationship between treadmill settings and oxygen consumption for both walking and running. Redrawn from the data of Silverman & Anderson (1972). (From Godfrey, 1974.)

constant that the VO_2 and the setting on the cycle ergometer serve as checks on each other. If they are outside the limits shown in Figure 15.9 it suggests that one or other parameter is in error. Of particular importance is the fact that mechanical efficiency of exercise also appears to be about 24% in sick children with lung, heart or other conditions (personal observations). This means that the prediction of $\dot{V}O_2$ from ergometer setting and vice versa applies in both health and disease and that the two parameters serve as checks on the techniques used in all subjects.

Prediction of work performed during treadmill exercise is far less certain because the work depends upon body weight, whether the subject runs, trots or walks and on his personal efficiency of walking (Silverman & Anderson, 1972). The relationship found in our laboratory for children by Silverman & Anderson (1972) is shown in Figure 15.10 as an approximate guide while standards for adults have been prepared by Givoni & Goldman (1971). There is really no alternative to measuring $\dot{V}O_2$ directly for accurate studies in forms of exercise other than those involving a properly calibrated electronically braked cycle ergometer.

We now have to consider a most important topic – namely the standardisation of parameters of body size measured during exercise. It is an almost universal custom amongst cardiologists to standardise their measurements by expressing results per square metre of body surface area.

The observation of a parameter such as oxygen consumption at rest ($\dot{V}O_1$) has some merit since the larger the subject, the higher the oxygen consumption. When we move on to exercise, as discussed above, mechanical efficiency is independent of size and since the resting $\dot{V}O_2$ forms a small part of the total $\dot{V}O_2$ once significant external work is being performed, absolute $\dot{V}O_2$ at a given level of external work varies little in relation to size. Thus dividing by surface area (or anything else) will not improve standardisation and indeed will be frankly misleading. It is better to report the absolute $\dot{V}O_2$ and perhaps to give this as a fraction of the subjects measured maximal oxygen uptake ($\dot{V}O_2$ max) in addition.

When we now consider standardisation of other parameters such as cardiac output in relation to size we need to be very clear about our objectives. It is essential to realise for a start that cardiac output ($\dot{Q}$) is merely the ratio of oxygen consumption ($\dot{V}O_2$) to the arterio-venous oxygen content difference ($C(a-\bar{v})O_2$)

Thus

$$Q = \frac{\dot{V}O_2}{C(a-\bar{v})O_2} \qquad (5)$$

Since at a given rate of exercising the $\dot{V}O_2$ is virtually independent of size and is the same in health or disease, there is no point in expressing Q per square metre of surface area. It is even more absurd when both $\dot{V}O_2$ and $\dot{Q}$ are expressed per square meter surface area since we are then dividing both sides of Equation 5 by the same number. The use of the cardiac index ($\dot{Q}/m^2$) at rest can be justified to the extent that $\dot{V}O_2/m^2$ is valid, as discussed above. In my view, provided VO_2 is measured directly, the most useful method for comparison between subjects at rest or on exercise is to relate absolute Q to absolute VO_2 or in other words to calculate the arterio-venous oxygen content difference.

Measurement of ventilation and gas exchange

For adequate standardisation and investigation of the response to exercise it is necessary to measure minute ventilation ($\dot{V}E$), tidal volume ($\dot{V}T$), frequency of breathing (f), oxygen consumption ($\dot{V}O_2$) and carbon dioxide production ($\dot{V}CO_2$). The classical method consists of collecting expired air in Douglas bags and measuring the volume of gas and the concentration of mixed expired oxygen ($Fe O_2$) and carbon dioxide ($Fe CO_2$) in the bag using a chemical analyser. This is the most accurate method but also the most tedious. Fortunately the rapid technological advances in recent years have substantially simplified and automated these measurements. All methods have one feature in common, the separation of inspired from expired air using some form of mechanical valve system. The volume of gas between the inspiratory and expiratory valve together with the volume of gas in the mouth piece from which the patient breathes constitutes instrumental dead space (i.e. this will be filled with expired gas during expiration and will have to be inspired before fresh air enters the mouth). It is important to keep this dead space volume as small as possible without making the tubing so narrow as to present a significant resistance. The physiological dead space of a newborn infant is about 7 ml, that of a 5-year-old child about 50 ml and that of an adolescent about 100 ml. The apparatus dead space should not be any more than the dead space of the patient and preferably less to avoid affecting the response.

There are two basic semi-automatic methods of measuring ventilation and gas exchange. A simple and relatively cheap method continuously measures expired ventilation using an electronic flow meter (pneumotachygraph) placed in the expiratory air line. This signal is integrated electronically to give tidal volume and minute ventilation. Expired air is passed into a mixing chamber to ensure thorough mixing of gases and the $Fe O_2$ and $Fe CO_2$ are measured from a port at the outlet of the mixing chamber. Infrared carbon dioxide analysers and paramagnetic oxygen analysers properly calibrated with accurate calibration gas mixtures are perfectly adequate for this purpose.

Since inspired air contains no carbon dioxide, its production is calculated simply by the formula:

$$\dot{V}CO_2 = \dot{V}E \times Fe CO_2 \qquad (6)$$

Oxygen consumption is calculated by the difference between total inspired and total expired oxygen. The equation is complicated by the fact that the total volume of gases expired is normally a little less than the volume inspired since a little less carbon dioxide is produced than oxygen is consumed (the respiratory quotient is less than 1.0). The complete equation is:

$$\dot{V}O_2 = \dot{V}E \times [0.2648 \times (1.0 - Fe CO_2 - Fe O_2)] - Fe O_2 \qquad (7)$$

and its derivation can be found elsewhere (Cotes, 1981).

Volumes of gases breathed, i.e. minute ventilation and tidal volume, are expressed at body temperature and pressure, saturated with water vapour (BTPS), while $\dot{V}O_2$ and $\dot{V}CO_2$ are expressed at standard temperature (0°C) and pressure (760 mmHg), dry (STPD). The correction equations can be found (Cotes, 1981) or derived by simple manipulation of the gas laws.

Fortunately for the average practising physician, all of these calculations can be performed simply by a microprocessor and systems are now available which give 'semi-online' print outs of $\dot{V}E$, $\dot{V}T$, f, $\dot{V}O_2$, $\dot{V}CO_2$ every 30 or 60 seconds. This has the very considerable advantage that the values can be scanned until they become constant and we then know that the patient has reached a steady state for the particular work load.

A more elegant but much more costly automatic method of undertaking this analysis uses a mass spectrometer to measure continuously the fluctuations of oxygen and carbon dioxide at the mouth. These concentrations are instantly multiplied by the flow signal using a more sophisticated computer program with appropriate correction equations and gives individual breath by breath results for ventilation and gas exchange. There are a number of centres using such systems with great success but, except for certain research purposes related to sudden changes of the work rate or the control of breathing, they have no significant advantages over the simpler and far cheaper systems.

One other method for measuring $\dot{V}O_2$ which has been used during cardiac catheterisation (Lees et al, 1967) is based on the principle of drawing air at a known (high) flow rate through a hood placed over the head of the subject and analysing the concentrations of carbon dioxide and oxygen. The great advantage is that no mouth piece, valve box or respiratory circuit is needed but the method does not measure $\dot{V}E$ or $\dot{V}T$ and is less accurate than other methods because of the very great accuracy demanded of the analysers and the requirement that all expired air is sucked away from the patient so that none escapes around the hood.

Measurement of cardiac output during exercise

Basic to almost every exercise study of significant cardiac (or pulmonary) disease in children is the measurement of cardiac output ($\dot{Q}$). During cardiac catheterisation $\dot{Q}$ is normally measured either by the direct ($\dot{O}_2$) Fick method or by dye or thermal dilution techniques. With careful attention to detail and proper calibration of equipment these are accurate methods, especially on exercise, and can be used with certain reservations even in the presence of left-to-right or right-to-left shunts. It is not intended to consider these techniques further as they are invasive but instead to concentrate on non-invasive techniques which do not require cardiac catheterisation and hence have been used to determine the response of normal children to exercise.

The indirect (CO_2) Fick method

The first method ever applied to man for the measurement of cardiac output was the Fick method using carbon dioxide

$$\dot{Q} = \frac{\dot{V}CO_2}{Cv_{CO_2} - Ca_{CO_2}} \qquad (8)$$

where Cv_{CO_2} and Ca_{CO_2} are the carbon dioxide contents (in ml/l of blood) of mixed venous (pulmonary arterial) and systemic arterial blood respectively. As we have seen $\dot{V}CO_2$ can be easily measured and the very considerable advantage of this technique is that mixed venous PCO_2 (Pv_{CO_2}) and hence Cv_{CO_2} can also be measured non-invasively by rebreathing (Collier, 1956).

The rebreathing technique relies on the principle that if the subject rebreathes a mixture of oxygen and carbon dioxide from a small bag and the concentration of carbon dioxide is correctly chosen, an identical concentration can occur in the bag, lungs and in mixed venous (pulmonary arterial) blood. Under these circumstances carbon dioxide will neither leave nor enter the blood and the concentration of gas measured at the mouth will remain unchanged as the subject breathes back and forth. This process is illustrated in Figure 15.11. There is an initial mixing phase followed by a plateau representing equality of carbon dioxide in bag, lungs and blood, i.e. the Pv_{CO_2}, and then after recirculation has occured the plateau breaks and carbon dioxide begins to rise. This technique has been described in great detail elsewhere (Ashton & McHardy, 1963; Jones et al, 1967; Godfrey & Wolf, 1972), together with a simply practical method of correcting for a less than perfect plateau (Denison, 1968). At rest the plateau should appear after

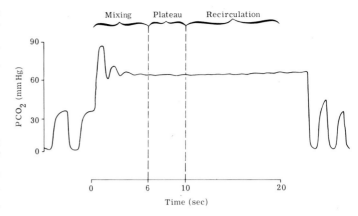

Fig. 15.11 P_{CO_2} recorded at the mouth during rebreathing while exercising. The three phases of mixing, mixed venous P_{CO_2} plateau and recirculation are indicated. (From Godfrey, 1981.)

6–8 seconds and break due to recirculation after 20–25 seconds, while on exercise these times would be 6 and 10 seconds respectively.

Another technique for measuring Pv_{CO_2} utilises the principle that if a subject rebreathes oxygen, the carbon dioxide in the bag will tend to rise exponentially towards Pv_{CO_2} (Defares, 1958). By measuring end-tidal Po_2 breath by breath before recirculation occurs it is possible to extrapolate to the Pv_{CO_2}. We have shown this method to be far less reproducible than the plateau technique (Godfrey & Wolf, 1972) and the values obtained for cardiac output are far less reliable.

Once Pv_{CO_2} is known, all we need is arterial Pco_2 (Pa_{CO_2}) in order to solve the CO_2 Fick equation. In children without lung disease we have found that the end-tidal (end-expired) CO_2 tension (Pet_{CO_2}) is very close to Pa_{CO_2}, especially on exercise (Godfrey & Davies, 1970), because the alveolar-arterial carbon dioxide tension difference is normally very small. The end-tidal carbon dioxide can be recorded at the mouth with an infra-red carbon dioxide analyser before rebreathing when the child has reached a steady state of VO_2 and $\dot{V}CO_2$. If lung disease is present it is necessary to measure arterial Pco_2. This can be done in some children by placing a radial artery catheter but this would be unacceptable to many children and certainly for studies in normal subjects. For this reason, various techniques have been developed to obtain arterialised capillary blood of which the most successful has been the sampling of capillary blood from the vasodilated lobe of the ear (Godfrey et al, 1971b). This method is illustrated in Figure 15.12 and is very easy to perform, almost painless, well accepted by children and accurate for measurement of carbon dioxide, oxygen and pH. A most important detail is the use of a flexible collection tube made from a cut off connexion cannula with the Luer cup being used to catch the drops of blood which are then allowed to run in to the heparinised tubing in a controlled fashion without bubbles.

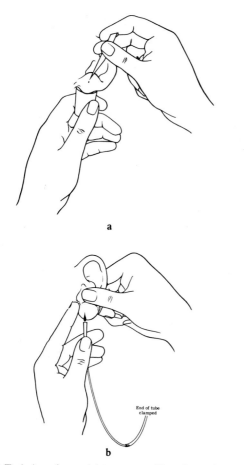

Fig. 15.12 Technique for ear lobe puncture (A) and sample collection (B) used to take arterialised ear lobe blood. (From Godfrey et al, 1971.)

Once Pv_{CO_2} and Pa_{CO_2} are known, they can be converted in carbon dioxide contents using an appropriate dissociation curve (McHardy, 1967) and cardiac output can then be calculated by Equation 8. A computer program has been developed (Godfrey, 1970) for solving the CO_2 Fick equation and exploring possible values for cardiac output and physiological dead space.

The great advantage of the carbon dioxide method is that it can be used in children with lung disease because poorly ventilated lung regions will already contain gas with a tension close to Pv_{CO_2} while the well ventilated regions will mix with the rebreathing bag gas. The chief disadvantage is that it cannot be used in children with left-to-right shunts because the rapid recirculation does not allow adequate time for rebreathing.

Soluble gas methods for measuring cardiac output

If the solubility of a gas in blood is known and we determine the rate of absorption of this gas from a bag during rebreathing, we can calculate the volume of blood which has absorbed the gas and hence the cardiac output. This is the basis of the soluble inert gas methods for measuring $\dot{Q}$ using such gases as nitrous oxide or acetylene. In practice a rebreathing bag of known volume is prepared containing a low concentration of nitrous oxide and an insoluble marker gas such as argon. The subject rebreathes this mixture and a record such as that shown in Figure 15.13 is obtained. The details have been fully described elsewhere (Godfrey, 1974). The concentration of nitrous

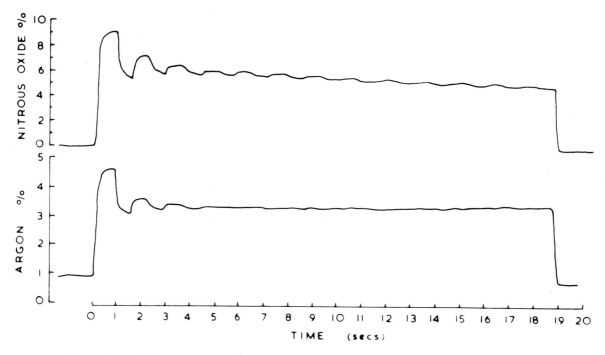

Fig. 15.13 Rebreathing a mixture of nitrous oxide and argon during exercise. The absorption of N_2O is reflected in the falling concentration while the shrinking of the lung/bag volume is shown by the rising concentration of argon. (From Zeidifard et al, 1976.)

oxide falls as the gas is absorbed and that of argon falls initially due to mixing of lung and bag gas and then rises steadily as the total lung-bag volume decreases. Gas concentrations are read off before recirculation could have occured (10 seconds on exercise) and plotted to enable extrapolation back to zero time. Knowing these zero time values and the values at 10 seconds, the cardiac output ($\dot{Q}$) can be calculated from the formula

$$\dot{Q} = \frac{\left(VB \times \dfrac{Fi_A}{Fe_A}\right) \times \dfrac{760}{PB - 47} + (\alpha_t \times V_t)}{\alpha b \times T}$$

$$\times \log_n\left(\frac{N_2O_T}{N_2O_O}\right) \times 60 \qquad (9)$$

where: VB = total initial volume of rebreathing bag and tubing (ml), FiA and FeA = initial and final argon fractional concentrations, PB = barometric pressure (mmHg), α_t = solubility of N_2O in lung tissue = 0.420 ml per ml per atmosphere (STPD), V_t = volume of lung tissue in ml = 5.8 × body weight in Kg, α_b = solubility of N_2O in blood = 0.474 ml per ml per atmosphere (STPD), T = rebreathing time (normally about 10 sec), $\log_n$ = natural logarithm, N_2O_T and N_2O_0 concentrations of N_2O extrapolated to time T and time zero respectively, 60 = factor to convert seconds to minutes.

The derivation of this equation is fully discussed by Cander & Forster (1959) and Zeidifard et al (1976). The chief advantage of the nitrous oxide method is that it is rapid and not critically dependent on a steady state. Its disadvantages are that it cannot be used in patients with lung disease because of poor mixing of lung and bag gas, and it requires a mass spectrometer for really accurate gas analysis. This method was the first ever used to determine $\dot{Q}$ in children (Galle, 1926) and the results agree closely with those obtained by the carbon dioxide Fick and dye dilution methods (Zeidifard et al, 1976).

Other non-invasive methods of measuring cardiac output

A most interesting non-invasive technique for measuring cardiac output is based on the measurement of the electrical impedance of the chest (Kubicek et al, 1970). A low alternating current is passed between electrodes which can be conveniently placed around the forehead or neck above and around the chest at the level of the xiphisternum below. Another pair of band electrodes placed around the chest between the outer pair measure the change in impedance which fluctuates with the cardiac cycle. There has been a great deal of discussion as to the exact cause of the impedance change but it seems likely that it is related to the ejection of blood into the pulmonary vessels with consequent lowering of electrical resistance. If the chest is considered as a cylinder, an equation can be derived which

relates the stroke volume to the changes in impedance as follows

$$sv = \rho . \left(\frac{L}{Zo}\right)^2 . \frac{dz}{dt} . T \; ml \qquad (10)$$

where ρ = resistivity of blood at 37°C in ohm/cm, L = mean distance between inner recording electrodes, Zo is mean (baseline) impedance in Ohms, $\frac{dz}{dt}$ = maximum negative rate of change of impedance with time during cardiac cycle in Ohm/sec, and T = ventricular ejection time.

The derivation of this equation can be found elsewhere (Kubicek et al, 1970). In our own studies on infants (Costeloe et al, 1977) and children (Edmunds et al, 1981) we found that, while the impedance cardiac output correlated well with either the nitrous oxide or carbon dioxide Fick cardiac output measurements, the results did not fall on the line of identity and a constant multiplication factor had to be used. We also found that it was important to use a value for blood resistivity derived from fresh human blood (Mohoptra et al, 1977) and not that of banked blood or animal blood which had previously been employed. Despite reservations as to the exact origin of the signal, we found that the impedance method could be used reliably in children during exercise. As the method involves no more invasion or cooperation than recording an electrocardiogram it is obviously very interesting for studies in children. Moreover, in our studies of infants (personal observations) it appeared that the impedance measurement in the presence of left-to-right shunting through a patent arterial duct more closely reflected pulmonary flow than systemic flow. This could mean that the impedance method might be applicable when other non-invasive (rebreathing) methods cannot be used but this has not yet been explored.

More recently attention has been focused on the use of radionuclide imaging of the heart as a non-invasive method of measuring cardiac output. By using a suitable position of the collimator, a view of the heart can be obtained which shows the two ventricles separated by the interventricular septum. After the injection of a suitable isotope, the changing gamma counts over each ventricle reflect the changing volumes (stroke volumes). By using a computer to gate the counting in relation to the electrocardiogram, a number of beats can be summed to give a very reliable index of stroke volume. If there is an independent measure of stroke volume (e.g. by the O_2 Fick method or dye dilution during cardiac catheterisation), the change in counts can be calibrated in terms of stroke volume. There is also the possibility of calculating cardiac output directly from the isotopic study during the first pass of the isotope after its injection just as in the classical dye dilution technique. This totally non-invasive method is currently being explored in relation to other studies of exercise during cardiac catheterisation in young patients and the results look promising.

Ventilation-perfusion relationships (shunt and dead space)

Besides measurement of cardiac output during exercise it is important to have an index of ventilation-perfusion matching. As a simple example it is well known that some 'acyanotic' Fallot's tetralogy patients become cyanotic on exercise due to an increase in right-to-left shunt. On the other hand, patients with lung disease may be very limited in their exercise performance by their large dead space. Shunt and dead space reflect different aspects of ventilation-perfusion mismatching (Figure 15.14) and provide useful practical indices. Their calculation requires a measurement of arterial blood Pa_{O_2}, Pa_{CO_2} and pH, of mixed expired Pe_{CO_2} (for dead space) and of arterio-venous oxygen content difference (for shunt). The equation for dead space (V_D) is given by

$$V_D = \frac{Pa_{CO_2} - Pe_{CO_2}}{Pa_{CO_2}} \qquad (11)$$

and includes the instrumental dead space which must be subtracted to calculate the dead space of the patient.

Shunt is calculated from the alveolar-arterial oxygen tension difference in the manner described above. This shunt will include both anatomical types of shunt and shunt due to ventilation-perfusion imbalance. As with resting studies, these can be differentiated to some extent by breathing high concentrations of oxygen during the test, though this is often very difficult to achieve during exercise. It is important when calculating shunt during exercise that the arterio-venous oxygen content difference be measured (or derived from the cardiac output and oxygen consumption). This difference changes with the work level and with disease, so that a constant value cannot be used for the equation as in the case of studies at rest.

THE GROWTH AND DEVELOPMENT OF THE RESPONSE TO EXERCISE IN NORMAL CHILDREN

Maximum exercise performance

As a child grows, so does his ability to work, and various methods can be used to assess this work capacity. We have found the simple progressive type of exercise test to be very practical and have undertaken studies in a large group of children aged 5–18 years of both sexes (Davies et al, 1972; Godfrey et al, 1971a). The maximum power output (W_{max}) was closely correlated to height and the relationship is shown in Figure 15.15. It can be seen that, at all levels, boys achieved higher W_{max} than girls but as discussed below this may partly be an artefact. The scatter amongst normal children makes prediction a little uncertain at the lower size range. Care is needed with the term 'working' capacity since this term has been applied to a number of other methods of expressing fitness. Of particular importance is the PWC_{170} – physical working capacity at a standardised heart rate of 170/min – first described by Wahlund (1948) but still very popular in the adult litera-

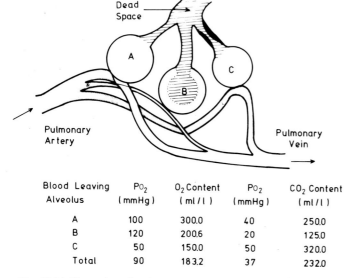

Blood Leaving Alveolus	P_{O_2} (mmHg)	O_2 Content (ml/l)	P_{O_2} (mmHg)	CO_2 Content (ml/l)
A	100	300.0	40	250.0
B	120	200.6	20	125.0
C	50	150.0	50	320.0
Total	90	183.2	37	232.0

Fig. 15.14 Illustration of various ventilation–perfusion relationships within the lungs ranging from the normal (A) to the high (B) and low (C), together with the effects of these relationships on the composition of pulmonary venous blood leaving the individual alveoli and the lung as a whole.

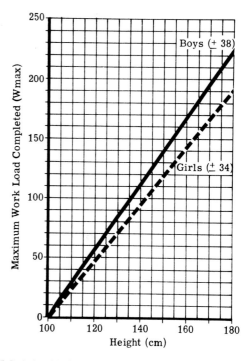

Fig. 15.15 Relationship between maximum work load completed in a progressive exercise test and height in normal children. The number in brackets gives the 95% range. (From Godfrey, 1974.)

ture. As will be seen, heart rate is very size-dependent and so the PWC_{170} is meaningless in children.

During the simple progressive exercise test we also recorded heart rate and minute ventilation. The maximum heart rate in normal children was 196 ± 13 (SD) for boys and 195 ± 13 (SD) for girls but this is a little lower than found under 'steady state' maximum exercise tests. In the latter case maximum heart rate is somewhat size-related as shown in Figure 15.16, reaching its peak of some 212/min in 12-year-old children (Astrand, 1952). There is no doubt that healthy children should be able to achieve peak heart rates of the order of 200/min which is substantially greater than one would expect from adults. Whereas in children maximum heart rate is only marginally size-dependent, maximum ventilation increases with maximum power output. It is instructive to relate maximum exercise ventilation to maximum voluntary ventilation from which it appears that healthy children utilise only some 60–70% of their pulmonary ventilatory reserve even at maximum levels of exercise (Godfrey, 1974).

The classical descriptor of maximum performance is the maximum oxygen uptake ($\dot{V}O_{2max}$). This has been measured in children in numerous studies dating from the extensive investigations of Robinson (1938) and Astrand (1952). The results from our own studies of $\dot{V}O_{2max}$ related to age are shown in Figure 15.17 (Davies et al, 1972) which agree generally with other published data. In common with other studies we found a difference between the $\dot{V}O_{2max}$ of boys and girls and considerable intersubject scatter. Attempts have been made to standardise $\dot{V}O_{2max}$ by various techniques of which the most common is to express it per kg of body weight. In children $\dot{V}O_{2max}$ remains reasonably constant at about 50 ml/min.kg^{-1} while above the age of 20 years there is a steady decline of about 0.5 ml/kg.year^{-1}. Females achieve rather lower levels than males and our own values for girls were around

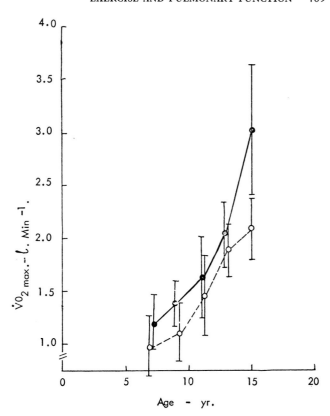

Fig. 15.17 Maximum oxygen uptake ($\dot{V}O_2$ max) in relation to age for boys (O) and girls (O). Redrawn from Davies et al, 1972. (From Godfrey, 1974.)

40 ml/min.kg^{-1}. Since there is no inherent reason, at least before puberty, to expect girls to be less fit than boys, Davies et al (1972) explored the possibility that leg muscle volume was a better indicator. Indeed, when $\dot{V}O_{2max}$ is expressed per litre of measured leg muscle volume there is no sex difference. However, the method of deriving leg muscle volume is tedious (Jones & Pearson, 1970) and only really suitable for research studies.

Before leaving the topic of maximum exercise performance we should just consider what eventually causes the child to stop. At high levels of work when, by definition, the $\dot{V}O_2$ has reached a plateau a large proportion of the total work is being performed anaerobically. Any further increment in work will be entirely anaerobic. This results in the formation of lactic acid which reaches levels of 8–12 mmol/l in children (and higher in adults). This lactate releases carbon dioxide and drives breathing so that the increment in ventilation is disproportionate to the increment in work. It may be that this imbalance is the cause of severe dyspnoea, which together with muscle discomfort causes the subject to stop. As seen above, the maximum ventilation does not reach the maximum ventilatory capacity in normal children. On the other hand we believe (see below) that stroke volume reaches an upper limit and since heart rate is also limited, maximum cardiac output

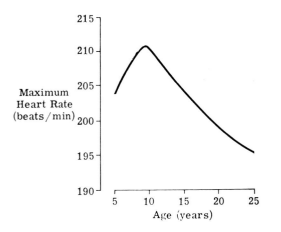

Fig. 15.16 Maximum heart rate on exercise in relation to age. (After Astrand, 1952. From Godfrey, 1974.)

must reach a limiting value. The only reliable study in children was undertaken in Sweden (Eriksson, 1972) using the dye dilution technique. He obtained a maximum cardiac output of 12.5 l/min at a maximum oxygen uptake of 1.7 l/min, giving a maximum arterio-venous oxygen content difference of 142 ml/l. This maximum arterio-venous difference in children is similar to the maximum in adults and may reflect the inability of exercising muscle to extract more than a certain quantity of oxygen from the blood. Once this point is reached exercise becomes predominantly anaerobic and the breaking point is soon reached.

Submaximal exercise performance

Ventilation

As children are subjected to higher and higher work loads, so their demand for oxygen and need to excrete carbon dioxide increases and minute ventilation ($\dot{V}E$) increases in proportion to the increasing oxygen consumption ($\dot{V}O_2$). Age and sex has a small effect on this relationship as shown in Figure 15.18 but the overall pattern is such that the $\dot{V}E$ at a given level of $\dot{V}O_2$ differs little between children. However, the manner in which this $\dot{V}E$ is achieved is markedly size-dependent. Small children have small lungs and breathe faster with a smaller tidal volume in comparison with larger children for a given $\dot{V}E$ (Godfrey, 1974). Thus a 6-year-old boy who is 120 cm tall working at a $\dot{V}O_2$ of 1 l/min will have a $\dot{V}E$ of 33 l/min, $\dot{V}T$ of 610 ml and frequency of 54/min while a 16-year-old boy who is 170 cm tall working at the same rate will have a $\dot{V}E$ of 27 l/min, $\dot{V}T$ of 950 ml and frequency of 28/min.

In the simple progressive exercise test described earlier $\dot{V}E$ increases linearly with increasing rate of working (W) but since steady-state levels are not achieved by 1 minute increments at submaximal levels, the absolute ventilation is 5–10% lower than would be predicted from Figure 15.18 at low levels of work but surprisingly similar at levels over 100 W.

Heart rate

Just as frequency of breathing is markedly size-dependent and to some extent sex-dependent, so is cardiac frequency. In fact the relationship between heart rate and $\dot{V}O_2$ (or W) is fan-like, with smaller children having higher rates than larger children at a given work level. In order to derive a simple graphical expression of this relationship we found that a semilogarithmic plot was useful and the full results for boys and girls in relationship to $\dot{V}O_2$ are given in Figure 15.19. As with ventilation, the heart rate tends to be about 5–10% lower in the relatively unsteady simple progressive exercise test compared with values predicted from these steady-state results.

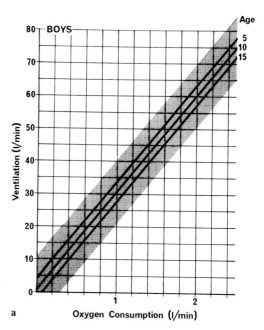

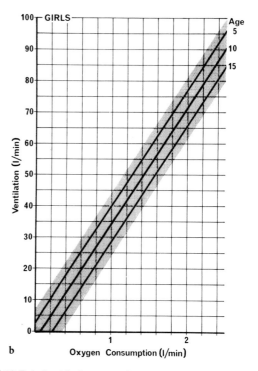

Fig. 15.18 Relationship between minute ventilation and oxygen consumption with the effect of age for boys (A) and girls (B). The shaded area represents the 95% confidence range for the 10 year old line. (From Godfrey, 1974.)

Cardiac output and stroke volume

By analogy with what has already been seen with ventilation and tidal volume, we might predict that cardiac output ($\dot{Q}$) on exercise would be relatively independent of size while stroke volume (SV) would be size-related. This is

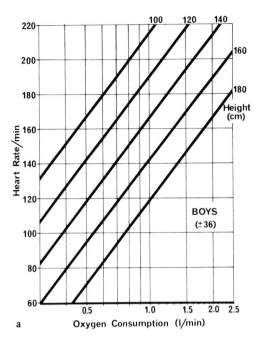

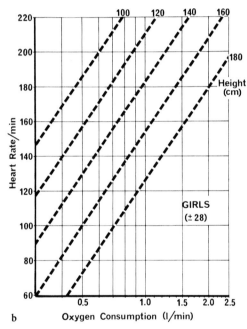

Fig. 15.19 Relationship between heart rate and oxygen consumption with the effect of age for boys (A) and girls (B). (From Godfrey, 1974.)

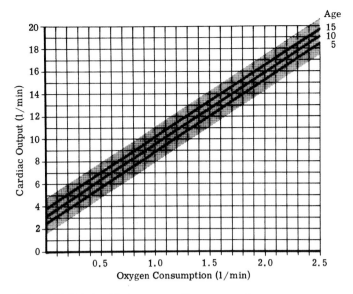

Fig. 15.20 Relationship between cardiac output and oxygen consumption in absolute terms with the effect of age. (From Godfrey, 1974.)

exactly what has been found by studies using non-invasive methods such as carbon dioxide or nitrous oxide rebreathing (Gadhoke & Jones, 1969; Godfrey et al, 1971a; Anderson & Godfrey, 1971; Bar-Or et al, 1971; Zeidifard et al, 1976) and by dye dilution (Eriksson et al, 1971; Eriksson & Koch, 1973). Our own observations, which are very similar to those in the literature, are summarised in Figure 15.20. As with ventilation, size has a small effect

on $\dot{Q}$ but in contrast we found no significant sex differences. Larger children and adults have a $\dot{Q}$ about 1 l/min greater than smaller children at levels of $\dot{V}O_2$ which both can achieve, which means that the arterio–venous oxygen content difference in small children is correspondingly a little greater. Thus over the range of $\dot{V}O_2$ from 500–1500 ml/min the anterio-venous oxygen content difference of smaller children will increase from about 90 to 125 ml/l compared with 70 to 110 ml/l in larger children – a difference of some 15–20%. The non-invasive techniques in older children also agree closely with invasive results (dye or direct O_2 Fick) methods in adults (Zeidifard et al, 1976) and curiously the results in smaller children agree with published data on exercising adult dogs using the direct O_2 Fick method (Barger et al, 1956). This may mean that the small size-related difference in $\dot{Q}$ at a given $\dot{V}O_2$ seen in children is a function of absolute physical size rather than maturity.

Stroke volume (SV) reflects the size of the heart and increases with the size of the child as does tidal volume. It has long been known that stroke volume increases in any one subject as he changes from rest to modest exercise and then remains relatively constant as work rate increases with the increase in cardiac output being due chiefly to the rising heart rate. In our studies of children we also noted this effect but resting studies are relatively unreliable so that the magnitude is not certain but was of the order of an increase of 40% when passing from rest to exercise. In adults, summarising a number of measurements, Rowell (1969) also reported an increase of about 40%. When looking at the exercise stroke volume at mild and hard levels of work there is a significant size-related and sex-related effect as

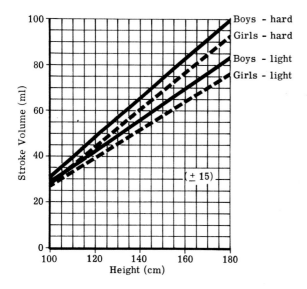

Fig. 15.21 Relationship between stroke volume in absolute terms and height during light (one-third W max) and heavy (two-thirds Wmax) work in boys and girls. (From Godfrey, 1974.)

shown in Figure 15.21. If we accept that stroke volume does not increase above the levels seen during hard work and that the maximum heart rate of all children is close to 200/min, we can calculate the maximum $\dot{Q}$ of a 170 cm boy as 18.4 l/min and that of a 110 cm boy as 8.0 l/min. A 12-year-old boy of 145 cm would have a maximum $\dot{Q}$ of 14.0 l/min at a predicted $\dot{V}O_2$max of 1.93 l/min giving a theoretical maximum arterio-venous oxygen content difference of 138 ml/l which is very close to the value of 142 ml/l measured during maximum exercise in the study of Eriksson (1972). These simple mathematical gymnastics nevertheless suggest that the results expressed in the graphs given in this chapter are internally consistent and reliably represent the cardiopulmonary responses of children to exercise.

Gas exchange

Exercise has relatively little effect on the arterial blood gases of healthy children. At higher levels of work there is a small fall in P_{CO_2} and pH as lactate rises but P_{O_2} shows no change either in children or adults. These relatively constant blood gases mean that the cardiopulmonary adaptation to exercise in healthy children must be exceedingly good and that the balance between ventilation and perfusion is preserved. This may be explored by considering dead space and shunt. Alveolar P_{CO_2} (which for all practical purposes is the same as arterial P_{CO_2}) is proportional to the ratio of CO_2 production ($\dot{V}CO_2$) to alveolar ventilation ($\dot{V}A$)

$$Pa_{CO_2} = k \times \frac{\dot{V}CO_2}{\dot{V}A} \qquad (12)$$

and for the rising VCO_2 during exercise P_{CO_2} remains more or less constant. Thus, the VA rises proportionately to the rising VCO_2. Now VA is the difference between total ventilation (VE) and dead space ventilation (VD)

$$\dot{V}A = \dot{V}E - \dot{V}D \qquad (13)$$

or

$$\dot{V}A = f(\dot{V}T - \dot{V}D) \qquad (14)$$

where f is the frequency of breathing and $\dot{V}T$ and $\dot{V}D$ are the tidal volume and dead space respectively. For a given level of work (and hence carbon dioxide production) children of different sizes have different tidal volumes and it therefore follows that dead space must also be closely related to size. This has been confirmed in measurements by Radford (1945) as well as by ourselves more recently (Godfrey & Davies, 1970). For any given subject, dead space also increases somewhat with increasing levels of exercise. In adults the increase is of the order of 8 ml/100 ml of tidal volume (Asmussen & Nielsen, 1956; Jones et al, 1966), while our figure for children was about 5 ml/100 ml tidal volume (Godfrey et al, 1971a). Exercise dead space varies greatly with the smallest children not having dead space volume values above about 50 ml because they also have very small tidal volumes, and a child of say 17 or 18 exercising with a tidal volume of 2000 ml having a dead space of 200 ml. However both these extremes are so finely adjusted that arterial P_{CO_2} will be about 35 mg in both cases.

Since arterial P_{O_2} remains at normal levels even during strenuous exercise it follows that any right-to-left shunt must be very small. The total shunt is about 4–5% of systemic blood flow at rest in healthy children or adults (Taylor, 1972; Eriksson, 1972) and actually falls a little to 2–3% on exercise. Thus normal children, even on strenuous exercise do not develop hypoxia. Any fall in P_{O_2} or saturation is pathological and represents abnormal cardiac shunting or ventilation–perfusion mismatching.

The electrocardiogram, blood pressure and ventricular function

So far we have considered what might be termed 'whole system' or 'whole body' responses to exercise in children. Recently there has been increasing interest in the evaluation of ventricular function during exercise in children. This may be measured by such simple, non-invasive techniques as electrocardiography and blood pressure recording, by more complex non-invasive techniques such as echocardiography and radionuclide cardiac scanning, and by invasive methods for recording directly from the left ventricle.

The form of the electrocardiogram changes during exercise and has been extensively investigated in adults but relatively little in children. A common problem has been the best way to evaluate changes in the waveform of the tracing to avoid artefacts. A coherent and apparently worthwhile method has been proposed by Thapar et al (1978) in which a (usually sloping) P–R isoelectric line was projected on to evaluate any J point depression while a (usually horizontal) PQ-PQ isoelectric line was used to evaluate the slope of the ST segment (beginning at the J point). They studied 170 healthy black children aged 7–14 years at rest and on graded exercise up to maximum levels with heart rates reaching 191/min on average. Recording from left chest leads, there was a small decrease in the R wave (27 to 22 mm) and increase in the S wave (6.9 to 7.8 mm) at maximum exercise indicating a small right shift of the QRS vector. Using their definition, J point depression of more than 1 mmHg was rarely seen (2.3% of children). ST segment slope increased on average from 1.5 to 4.3 mV/sec at maximum exercise and there were minor changes in T wave size and duration. Studies in white children (Riopel et al, 1979; James et al, 1980) gave very similar results but if J point and ST segment changes were measured from a conventional PQ-PQ isoelectric line, they found a very high incidence of ST depression of 1–2 mm in perfectly healthy children. Using the normal data, Alpert et al (1981a) were able to define definite characteristics of ischaemia based on J point depression and/or downsloping ST segment from the P–R isoelectric line and to apply them to a study of children with sickle cell anaemia.

Blood pressure changes with exercise with the systolic pressure rising and the diastolic remaining constant or even falling a little. The changes in blood pressure in a large group of children studied by Riopel et al (1979) during progressive treadmill exercise up to maximum levels are summarised in Figure 15.22. The smallest children showed a rise from a resting blood pressure of about 112/75 to about 145/75 on maximal exercise while the largest children showed a rise from about 130/85 to 200/80. Studies by

James et al (1980) using a cycle ergometer gave very similar results. The resting blood pressure and the rise on exercise is size-dependent with larger children having higher pressures and larger rises. Alpert et al (1981b) found that black children, especially the boys, tend to have resting and exercise blood pressure 10–15% greater than white children of the same size using upright cycling but Riopel et al (1979) found smaller differences using treadmill exercise.

Echocardiography can be used to define the size and motion of the cardiac chambers and this has now been used during exercise with a view to obtaining information on contractility. One index of contractility, E_{max}, is allegedly independent of preload or postload and a good index of ventricular function. It is normally calculated during cardiac catheterisation by the ratio of intraventricular pressure to volume but Alpert et al (1981a) have shown an excellent correlation between this index and the ratio of peak systolic pressure to smallest systolic volume, the volume being obtained by M-mode echocardiography. This index (corrected for body surface area) rose from about 1.2 mmHg/ml.m^{-2} at rest to 1.8 mmHg/ml.m^{-2} at 50% or maximal exercise intensity. They were able to use this index to separate groups of children with various cardiac problems. Recently the same group has been using radionuclide cardiac imaging in an effort to improve the reliability of non-invasive measurements of ventricular function, but the results are not yet available. Using a combination of direct intraventricular pressure recording and echocardiography they have been able to derive a number of other indices of contractility at rest and on exercise but of course no normal values are available for healthy children (Alpert et al, 1980b).

Thus we now have non-invasive techniques for a complete analysis of haemodynamic performance at rest and during exercise in children from about 5 years of age and upwards. We also have a substantial body of data on the responses of normal children to graded exercise. In general the use of direct invasive techniques during exercise is unacceptable to smaller children but in any case the results agree closely with those obtained non-invasively.

EXERCISE IN CHILDREN WITH CARDIAC DISEASE

General remarks

Breathlessness on exertion and effort intolerance are the hallmarks of a number of serious congenital and acquired types of heart disease and this is very much in the mind of physicians, parents and teachers alike. Bergman & Stamm (1967) undertook an extremely interesting study in which they evaluated the amount of disturbance to everyday life and activity caused by real or imaginary heart disease in children. They found a very large number of children with insignificant or non-existent heart disease

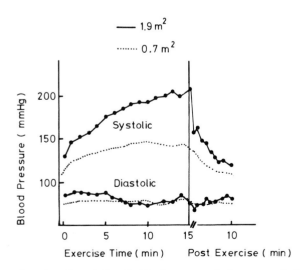

Fig. 15.22 Systolic and diastolic blood pressures during progressively increasing work and subsequent recovery in groups of large and small children. (After Riopel et al, 1979.)

were being prevented from undertaking normal physical activities on medical or parental advice. Nobody had ever considered undertaking an exercise test and they themselves found that the cycle ergometer proved to be an excellent tool for reassuring parents. Since that time, despite considerable technical advances, especially in the field of non-invasive exercise testing, there has remained a great paucity of exercise studies in children with heart disease. Unfortunately physicians seem prepared to base decisions concerning surgery for limitation of activity on measurements made at rest. It is worth noting that few children really restrict their activities even when ordered to do so and hence there may be a moral obligation to investigate exercise under controlled conditions.

Subjective estimates of effort intolerance are notoriously unreliable, even when dignified by the use of a scoring system. Taylor (1972), working in my laboratory, related the opinion of the mother concerning effort intolerance to maximum work achieved in a simple progressive exercise test on the cycle ergometer in children with Fallot's tetralogy. The results were shown in Figure 15.1 and emphasise the total lack of correlation between subjective and objective criteria. He obtained similar results in another group of children with aortic stenosis. It is particularly difficult to use subjective criteria to evaluate the effects of cardiac surgery since parents expect their children to be better and in any case would be rather reluctant to admit that improvement had not occurred. Goldberg et al (1967) thought there was some agreement between objective and subjective criteria of effort tolerance pre- and postoperatively in children with a variety of lesions. Careful inspection of their data suggests that any correlation is exceedingly poor.

A number of objective studies of maximum exercise performance have been undertaken in children with congenital heart disease but since a variety of different lesions were included they are of little value for individual problems. As expected these studies showed poor performance compared to normal children, the difference being more marked in those with more severe lesions (Duffie & Adams, 1963; Goldberg et al, 1966). Children with cyanotic lesions or who become cyanosed on exercise are generally more intolerant of exercise than children with acyanotic lesions. This may be due to the nature of the lesions or to the changes which occur with exercise. We measured arterialised ear lobe oxygen tension in a group of children with such lesions at rest and on exercise, breathing both air and 100% oxygen. As can be seen in Figure 15.23, there was a fall of P_{O_2} with exercise in every case totally unaffected by breathing a high concentration of oxygen. In contrast, children with acyanotic lesions remained with normal blood gas tensions on exercise. This hypoxia in the cyanotic patients causes stimulation of breathing and these patients consequently overbreathe on exercise. Taylor (1973) found this overbreathing to be

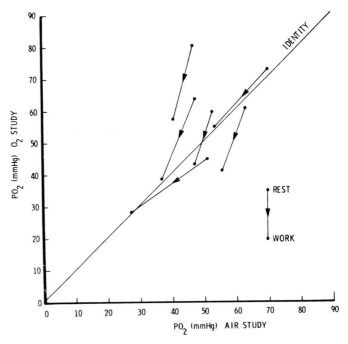

Fig. 15.23 Pattern of change in arterialised ear-lobe blood P_{CO_2} when passing from rest to exercise in children with cyanotic congenital heart disease. A comparison is made between air breathing and oxygen breathing showing that breathing a high concentration of O_2 had no appreciable effect on the result. (From Godfrey, 1974.)

directly proportional to the desaturation which occurred. It has been found that patients with cyanotic congenital heart disease have a blunted response to hypoxia at rest (Sorensen & Severinghaus, 1968) but it seems that their response to hypoxia on exercise is very brisk and may well contribute to their inability to achieve normal maximum levels of work.

Specific conditions

Detailed analysis of the cardiopulmonary response to exercise has been undertaken in a few conditions in children, namely Fallot's tetralogy, congenital heart block and left-sided lesions and these will be considered briefly.

Fallot's tetralogy

Taylor (1972) found effort intolerance in a preoperative group of children with Fallot's tetralogy with low pulmonary blood flow and large right-to-left shunt which increased on exercise. Other postoperative patients had on average greater effort tolerance, low normal and equal pulmonary and systemic blood flows and much less shunt. In a more recent study, Cumming (1979) investigated 29 children one to five years postoperatively by exercise testing during cardiac catheterisation. He found a low normal effort tolerance in 80% of subjects and occasionally even more severe intolerance. In the majority of patients peak right ventricular pressure was over 50 mmHg, right ventricular end diastolic pressure was over 15 mmHg in one-third of patients and pulmonary arterial pressure was abnormal in one-sixth of patients. In other words both these studies reveal significantly abnormal responses to exercise in postoperative Fallot's tetralogy patients. This work must surely be continued to judge the importance of these findings for ultimate prognosis.

Congenital heart block

Congenital heart block is an interesting condition haemodynamically, especially in children whose general well-being has allowed them to avoid the insertion of an artificial pacemaker. Early studies of adults suggested effort intolerance but Thoren et al (1974) studying children with a mean age of 11 years found normal maximum oxygen uptakes in the large majority of cases. Since ventricular rate increases only about twofold from rest to maximum exercise in this condition, normal levels of exercise must demand either a very large stroke volume or extraction of more than the normal quantity of oxygen from arterial blood – or both. We studied four subjects with congenital heart block, two of whom (aged 9 and 15 years) had normal effort tolerance and were active in sports (Taylor & Godfrey, 1972). In these subjects cardiac output was rather low on exercise but stroke volume was enormous, reaching 170 ml (twice normal) in one subject. Arterio-venous oxygen content difference was also much increased in the children with normal effort tolerance, reflecting greater oxygen extraction, and the calculated mixed venous oxygen saturations of 16–22% were well below those reported for top-class athletes. Thus, children with congenital heart block can achieve normal effort tolerance by having a very large stroke volume and extracting more than the usual amount of oxygen from the blood. All this can be measured by the non-invasive techniques described in this chapter.

Aortic stenosis

The basically straightforward nature of aortic stenosis has made it a subject of interest, as far as exercise response is concerned, for a number of years. At one time it was thought that exercise was contraindicated in aortic stenosis because of the risk of sudden death but this does not appear to be true for children (Glew et al, 1969; Doyle et al, 1974) and many exercise studies have been performed without ill-effects. Taylor (1972) found mild to moderate reduction in maximum working capacity (W_{max}) in aortic stenosis but no relation between W_{max} and resting outflow tract gradients. At one-third and two-thirds of W_{max} during steady-state exercise, cardiac output was in the low normal range (Fig. 15.24) exactly as found more recently by Alpert et al (1980a) using direct dye dilution measurements. Taylor (1972) found a correlation between reduc-

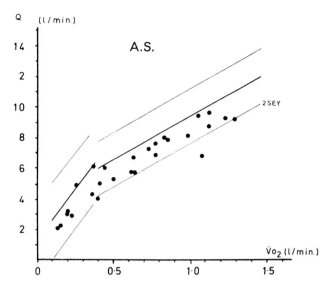

Fig. 15.24 Cardiac output at rest and on exercise in absolute terms in children with aortic stenosis superimposed on the mean relationship with 95% limits for normal children. (From Taylor, 1972.)

tion in stroke volume (the cause of the low cardiac output) and the gradient across the value at rest.

Other tests which are useful predictors in aortic stenosis include blood pressure and ventricular contractility. Alpert et al (1981b) showed a diminution in the normal rise of blood pressure on exercise in more severely affected patients such that if the rise was ⩾35 mmHg there was a 10% or less chance of the value gradient being greater than 50 mmHg. Whitmar et al (1981) investigated 23 children before and after surgical correction of aortic stenosis and found increased effort tolerance, less ST depression and increased peak systolic blood pressure. Indices of ventricular contractility such as the rate of change of ventricular pressure with time measured from direct intravascular recording show greater rises on exercise in children with aortic stenosis than other left-sided conditions (Alpert et al, 1980a), but even more interesting is the fact that the non-invasive index, E_{max}, determined from blood pressure and echocardiographic measurements, was also different (Alpert et al, 1981a). In this latter study, E_{max} in children with left ventricular pressure overload was elevated at rest and increased further with exercise, but with volume overload or combined lesions the resting levels were normal or elevated and failed to increase with exercise.

Thus aortic stenosis can be investigated very thoroughly from the cardiopulmonary and haemodynamic aspects by acceptable non-invasive techniques and these can be used to evaluate the severity of the lesion, the progression or otherwise during conservative management, and the response to surgery.

Other non-cyanotic lesions

Too few exercise studies have been reported to date for

other types of problem in children for any clear pattern to emerge. Taylor (1972) also studied pulmonary stenosis and found good effort tolerance with some reduction in stroke volume while Stone et al (1974) in a pre- and postoperative study also found rather low stroke volumes on exercise which improved after surgery together with a reduction in right ventricular end diastolic pressure and peak right ventricular pressure.

In a series of publications, Alpert and his colleagues described various invasive and non-invasive measurements at rest and during exercise in children with left-sided lesions (Alpert et al, 1980a, b, 1981a, b). From these it appears that effort tolerance was normal with pressure and/or volume overload but reduced with cardiomyopathy, that simple parameters such as cardiac output did not well distinguish between the groups, but more promising differences were found on exercise using invasive and non-invasive indices of ventricular contractility. This work clearly needs to be pursued in order to define the patterns of abnormality, preferably by non-invasive measurement

techniques, so that they may be used as an aid to the evaluation of these types of patient.

CONCLUSION

Lung function and exercise testing in children are safe and practical propositions both for those who are well and those who have heart or lung disease. Normal values have now been established for lung function from infancy to adult life and can be used to evaluate the nature of the problem in children with dyspnoea and to help distinguish lung from heart disease. Normal values for the cardiopulmonary and haemodynamic response to exercise in children have also been established and may be used to evaluate the severity and nature of cardiac disease. In particular such tests may be used serially during the conservative management of patients and for the evaluation of the effects of treatment, especially surgical treatment.

REFERENCES

Alpert B S, Bloom K R, Olley P M 1980a Assessment of left ventricular contractility during supine exercise in children with left-sided cardiac disease. British Heart Journal 44: 703–710

Alpert B S, Bloom K R, Newth C J, Olley P M, Williams C M, Kartodiharjo W 1980b Hemodynamic responses to supine exercise in children with left-sided cardiac disease. American Journal of Cardiology 45: 1025–1032

Alpert B S, Benson L, Olley P M 1981a Peak left ventricular pressure/volume (E max) during exercise in control subjects and children with left-sided cardiac disease. Catheterisation and Diagnosis 7: 145–153

Alpert B S, Kartodihardjo W, Harp R, Izukawa T, Strong W B 1981b Exercise blood pressure response – a predictor of severity of aortic stenosis in children. Journal of Pediatrics 98: 763–765

Anderson S D, Godfrey S 1971 Cardio-respiratory response to treadmill exercise in normal children. Clinical Science 40: 433–442

Anderson S D, Silverman M, Konig P, Godfrey S 1975 Exercise-induced asthma. British Journal of Diseases of the Chest 69: 1–39

Ashton C H, McHardy G J R 1963 A rebreathing method for determining mixed venous P_{CO_2} during exercise. Journal of Applied Physiology 18: 668–671

Asmussen E, Nielsen M 1956 Physiological dead space and alveolar gas pressures at rest and during muscular exercise. Acta Physiologica Scandinavica 38: 1–21

Astrand P O 1952 Experimental studies of physical working capacity in relation to sex and age. Munksgaard, Copenhagen

Barger A C, Richards V, Metcalf J, Gunther B 1956 Regulation of the circulation during exercise, cardiac output (direct Fick) and metabolic adjustments in the normal dog. American Journal of Physiology 184: 613–623

Bar-Or, Shephard R J, Allen C L 1971 Cardiac output of 10 to 13-year old boys and girls during submaximal exercise. Journal of Applied Physiology 30: 219–223

Bergman A B, Stamm S J 1967 The morbidity of cardiac non-disease in school children. New England Journal of Medicine 276: 1008–1013

Cander L, Forster R 1959 Determination of pulmonary parenchymal tissue volume and pulmonary capillary blood flow in man. Journal of Applied Physiology 14: 541–551

Caylor G G, Lynn D B, Stein E M 1973 Effect of cardiac 'nondisease' on intellectual and perceptual motor development. British Heart Journal 35: 543–547

Collier C R 1956 Determination of mixed venous CO_2 tensions by rebreathing. Journal of Applied Physiology 9: 25–29

Costeloe K, Stocks J, Mohapatra S N, Hill D W, Godfrey S 1977 Cardiac output in the neonatal period using impedance cardiography. Pediatric Research 11: 1171–1177

Cotes J E 1981 Lung function. Blackwell, Oxford

Cumming G R 1979 Maximal supine exercise haemodynamics after open heart surgery for Fallot's tetralogy. British Heart Journal 41: 683–691

Cumming G R, Friesen W 1967 Bicycle ergometer measurement of maximal oxygen uptake in children. Canadian Journal of Physiology and Pharmacology 45: 937–946

Davies C T M, Barnes C, Godfrey S 1972 Body composition and maximal exercise performance in children. Human Biology 44: 195–214

Defares J G 1958 Determination of P_vCO_2 from the exponential CO_2 rise during rebreathing. Journal of Applied Physiology 13: 159–164

Denison D 1968 Mixed venous blood gas tensions and respiratory stress in man. PhD Thesis, University of London

Doyle E F, Aromogham P, Lara E, Rutkowski M R, Kiely B 1974 Sudden death in young patients with congenital aortic stenosis. Pediatrics 53: 481–489

Dubois A B, Botelho S Y, Bedell G N, Marshall R, Comroe J H Jr 1956a A rapid plethysmographic method for measuring thoracic gas volume: A comparison with a nitrogen washout method for measuring functional residual capacity in normal subjects. Journal of Clinical Investigation 35: 322–326

Dubois A B, Botelho S Y, Comroe J H 1956b A new method for measuring airway resistance in man using a body plethysmograph: values in normal subjects and in patients with respiratory disease. Journal of Clinical Investigation 35: 327–335

Duffie E R, Adams F H 1963 The use of the working capacity test in the evaluation of children with congenital heart disease. Pediatrics 32: 757–768

Edmunds A T, Godfrey S, Tooley M 1981 Cardiac output measured by transthoracic impedance cardiography at rest, during exercise and at varying lung volumes. Clinical Science (in press)

Eriksson B O 1972 Physical training oxygen supply and muscle metabolism in 11–13 year old boys. Acta Physiologica Scandinavica (Supplement) 384: 1–48

Eriksson B O, Koch G 1973 Effect of physical training on

haemodynamic response during submaximal and maximal exercise in 11–13 year old boys. Acta Physiologica Scandinavica 87: 27–39

Eriksson B O, Grimby G, Saltin B 1971 Cardiac output and arterial blood gases during exercise in pubertal boys. Journal of Applied Physiology 31: 348–352

Gadhoke S, Jones N L 1969 The responses to exercise in boys aged 9 to 15. Clinical Science 37: 789–801

Galle P 1926 The oxygen consumption per litre of blood in children. Skandinavisches Archiv fur Physiologie 47: 174–187

Givoni B, Goldman R F 1971 Predicting metabolic energy cost. Journal of Applied Physiology 30: 429–433

Glew R H, Varghese P J, Krovetz L J, Dorst J P, Rowe R D 1969 Sudden death in congenital aortic stenosis. A review of eight cases with an evaluation of premonitory clinical features. American Heart Journal 78: 615–625

Godfrey S 1970 Manipulation of the indirect Fick principle by a digital computer programme for the calculation of exercise physiology results. Respiration 27: 513–532

Godfrey S 1974 Exercise testing in children. In: Applications in health and disease. Saunders, London

Godfrey S 1978 Exercise-induced asthma. Allergy 33: 229–237

Godfrey S 1981 Growth and development of cardio-pulmonary responses to exercise. In: Davies J A, Dobbing J (eds) Scientific foundations of paediatrics. Heinemann, London, p 271–280

Godfrey S, Davies C T M 1970 Estimates of arterial P_{CO_2} and their effect on the calculated values of cardiac output and dead space on exercise. Clinical Science 39: 529–537

Godfrey S, Wolf E 1972 An evaluation of rebreathing methods for measuring mixed venous P_{CO_2} during exercise. Clinical Science 42: 345–353

Godfrey S, Davies C T M, Wozniak E, Barnes C A 1971a Cardiorespiratory response to exercise in normal children. Clinical Science 40: 419–431

Godfrey S, Wozniak E R, Courtney-Evans R J, Samuels C S 1971b Ear lobe blood samples for blood gas analysis at rest and during exercise. British Journal of Diseases of the Chest 65: 58–64

Godfrey S, Katznelson R, Wolf E 1972 Gas to blood PCO_2 differences during rebreathing in children and adults. Respiration Physiology 13: 274–282

Goldberg S J, Weiss R, Adams F H 1966 A comparison of the maximal endurance of normal children and patients with congenital cardiac disease. Journal of Pediatrics 69: 46–55

Goldberg S J, Adams F H, Hurwitz R A 1967 Effect of cardiac surgery on exercise performance. Journal of Pediatrics 71: 192–197

James F W, Kaplan S, Glueck C J, Tsay J Y, Knight M J S, Sarwar C J 1980 Responses of normal children and young adults to controlled bicycle exercise. Circulation 61: 902–912

Johnson R L 1967 In: Chapman C B (ed) Physiology of muscular exercise. American Heart Association, New York, p 154–160

Jones N L, Campbell E J M, McHardy G J R, Higgs B E, Clode M 1967 The estimation of carbon dioxide pressure of mixed venous blood during exercise. Clinical Science 32: 311–327

Jones P R M, Pearson J 1969 Anthropometric determination of leg fat and muscle plus bone volumes in young male and female adults. Journal of Physiology 204: 63–66P

Jones R W A, Baumer J H, Joseph M C, Shinebourne E A 1976 Arterial oxygen tension and response to oxygen breathing in differential diagnosis of congenital heart disease in infancy. Archives of Disease in Childhood 51: 667–673

Koch G, Wendel H 1968 Adjustment of arterial blood gases and acid base balance in the normal newborn infant during the first week of life. Biology of the Neonate 12: 136–161

Kubicek W G, Patterson R P, Witsoe D A 1970 Impedance cardiography as a non-invasive method of monitoring cardiac function and other parameters of the cardiovascular system. Annals of the New York Academy of Sciences 170: 724–732

Lambert E C, Menon V A, Wagner H R, Vlad P 1974 Sudden unexpected death from cardiovascular disease in children. American Journal of Cardiology 34: 89–96

Lees M H, Bristow J D, Way C, Brown M 1967 Cardiac output by Fick principle in infants and young children. American Journal of Diseases of Children 114: 144–149

McHardy G J R 1967 The relationship between the differences in pressure and content of carbon dioxide in arterial and venous blood. Clinical Science 32: 299–309

McKenzie S A, MacArthur C G C, Godfrey S, Hallidie-Smith K A 1977 Hypertensive pulmonary vascular disease in children: detection by radioactive nitrogen (13N) inhalation and injection. British Heart Journal 39: 866–871

Mohoptra S N, Costeloe K L, Hill D W 1977 Blood resistivity and its implications for the calculation of cardiac output by the thoracic electrical impedance technique. Intensive Care Medicine 3: 63–67

Polgar G, Promadhat V 1971 Pulmonary function testing in children. Saunders, Philadelphia

Radford E P 1945 Ventilation standards for use in artificial respiration. Journal of Applied Physiology 7: 451–460

Riopel D A, Taylor A B, Hohn A R 1979 Blood pressure, heart rate, pressure-rate product and electrocardiographic changes in healthy children during treadmill exercise. American Journal of Cardiology 44: 697–704

Robinson S 1938 Experimental studies of physical fitness in relation to age. Arbeitsphysiologie 10: 251–323

Ronchetti R, Stocks J, Freedman N, Glass H, Godfrey S 1975a The clinical application of regional lung function studies in infants and small children using 13N. Archives of Disease in Childhood 50: 595–603

Ronchetti R, Stocks J, Keith I, Godfrey S 1975b An analysis of a rebreathing method for measuring lung volume in the premature infant. Pediatric Research 9: 797–802

Rowell L B 1969 Circulation. Medicine and Science in Sports 1: 15–22

Saltin B, Astrand P O 1967 Maximum oxygen uptake in athletes. Journal of Applied Physiology 23: 353–358

Silverman M, Anderson S D 1972 Metabolic cost of treadmill exercise in children. Journal of Applied Physiology 33: 696–698

Sorensen S C, Severinghaus J W 1968 Respiratory insensitivity to acute hypoxia persisting after correction of tetralogy of Fallot. Journal of Applied Physiology 25: 221–223

Stocks J 1977 The applications of whole body plethysmography to the study of cardiopulmonary function in infants. PhD Thesis, University of London

Stocks J, Godfrey S 1977 Specific airway conductance in relation to postconceptional age during infancy. Journal of Applied Physiology 43: 144–154

Stocks J, Godfrey S 1978 Nasal resistance in infancy. Respiration Physiology 34: 233–246

Stocks J, Levy N M, Godfrey S 1977 A new apparatus for the accurate measurement of airway resistance in infancy. Journal of Applied Physiology 43: 155–159

Stone F M, Bessinger F B, Lucas R B, Moller J H 1974 Pre- and post-operative rest and exercise hemodynamics in children with pulmonary stenosis. Circulation 49: 1102–1106

Taylor M R H 1972 The response to exercise of children with congenital heart disease. PhD Thesis, University of London

Taylor M R H 1973 The ventilatory response to hypoxia during exercise in cyanotic congenital heart disease. Clinical Science 45: 99–105

Taylor M R H, Godfrey S 1972 Exercise studies in congenital heart block. British Heart Journal 34: 930–935

Thapar M K, Strong W B, Miller M D, Leatherby L, Salebhai M 1978 Exercise electrocardiography of healthy black children. American Journal of Diseases of Children 132: 592–595

Thoren C, Herin P, Vavra J 1974 Studies of submaximal and maximal exercise in congenital complete heart block. Acta Paediatrica Belgium 28 (Supplement): 132–143

Wahlund H 1948 Determination of the physical working capacity. Acta Medica Scandinavica 215 (Supplement): 5–78

Whitmer J T, James F W, Kaplan S, Schwartz D C, Knight M J S 1981 Exercise testing in children before and after surgical treatment of aortic stenosis. Circulation 63: 254–263

Zeidifard E, Godfrey S, Davies E E 1976 Estimation of cardiac output by an N_2O breathing method in adults and children. Journal of Applied Physiology 41: 433–438

Management

Medical management

In this chapter we shall consider medical management at two levels: first, the general framework of medical decision-making which underlies management, and then specific details of drug treatments which are of general use in childhood heart disease.

GENERAL PRINCIPLES

There is really only one principle of medical treatment, and that is that it should either do good and no harm or else more good than harm. If the treatment is available, of proven benefit in the patient's disease, and does no harm, then it must be used. One such example would be the use of vitamin C to treat scurvy.

It is quite difficult to find examples of treatment which do no harm at all. Even the use of penicillin to treat acute lobar pneumonia involves some risk to the patient, who may be allergic to the drug. But in this, as in many other examples, the benefit of the treatment so far outweighs its risk that again, there is really no option but to use it.

The real challenge to a physician is to make the correct decision when the trade-off between risks and benefits is by no means so obvious. Here clinical intuition is at a premium. Some clinicians are better endowed with intuition than others, and their intuition is more closely related to reality. They therefore treat their patients better. The great disadvantage of intuition, however, is that it cannot be transferred from one doctor to another. What can be taught and learnt is the logical framework which underlies the decision-making process. The purpose of this chapter is to define one such framework, which is a branch of mathematics known as 'decision theory'. This relatively new subject has been widely applied to making business decisions. It is particularly appropriate for this purpose because sums of money are easy to handle mathematically. It has appeared briefly on the fringes of many medical and surgical specialties but, with rare exceptions, it is almost unknown in paediatric cardiology. No attempt will be made to provide a comprehensive account of this very large

subject. Those who wish to pursue the matter further are urged to read a book on the subject such as that by Weinstein and colleagues (1980). They should also examine articles in the new journal *Medical Decision Making*. We shall simply provide three examples of its use, in ascending order of complexity, trusting that they will serve at least to whet the appetite of the reader.

Don't do something, stand there

Intravenous prostaglandin therapy has become one of the most important forms of medical treatment in paediatric cardiology, and is widely accepted as such. The infusion is usually used simply to tide a very sick baby over at most a day or two, in the hope that the improved general condition of the patient will reduce the risk of operation. More controversial is the use of oral prostaglandin. Although this can be used in hospital treatment as a substitute for intravenous prostaglandin, its benefits when so used are marginal. They consist mainly of the avoidance of continuous intravenous therapy. The real potential benefit of oral prostaglandin is that it may permit patients to be sent home on oral therapy to grow. If this can be achieved, the hope is that subsequent surgical intervention, such as a shunt operation, can be carried out at a lower risk than would have been possible in the newborn period. The problem is that, even in hospital, patients receiving oral prostaglandin have been seen to die suddenly. The risk of death at home, therefore, is presumably substantial. Thus, the problem in essence is whether the benefits gained by the purchase of time before surgical intervention are greater than the risks of death while waiting for surgery. The first stage in analysing this problem is to construct a decision tree (Fig. 16.1).

Decision trees are conventionally drawn from left to right. They consist of lines which proliferate by branching at what are known as 'nodes'. Two kinds of nodes appear on a decision tree. Circles represent probability nodes, while squares represent decision nodes. A number of mutually exclusive and exhaustive decisions spring from

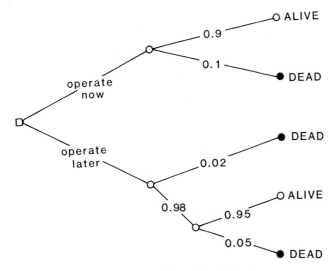

Fig. 16.1 Decision tree corresponding to the decision 'operate now or later?'. For further explanation, see text.

any decision node, while a set of probability branches arises at each probability node. The probabilities are those of exclusive and exhaustive events for the given node. Because of this requirement, the sum of the probabilities springing from any particular node must be one. Thus, in Figure 16.1 the first node is a decision node, having two branches – one corresponding to the decision 'operate now', and the other to the decision 'give 2 months medical treatment and then operate'. The lower branch then reaches a probability node. One branch of this node corresponds to the probability that the patient will die while on medical treatment and the other to the probability that he will survive. There is an outcome at each tip of the branch. That outcome is associated with a value which must behave like a probability if it is to be used in decision analysis. In this particular example, the outcome could be the probability of surviving surgery. This is mathematically equivalent to making the outcome dead or alive (as in Fig. 16.1) and setting the value of being alive to 1 and the value of being dead to 0, for reasons which will shortly become clear. It is important in any decision tree that the order of nodes reading from left to right should correspond to the temporal sequence of events. In other words, if two decisions are made, the first must lie to the left of the second. Similarly, the position of the probability nodes must be related temporally to the decision nodes. As an illustration, in the simple example given, it is no use starting off the decision tree with a probability node. This is because the effect of the probability of dying from medical treatment only takes place after the decision to use medical treatment has been made. Another way of expressing the same idea is to state that each probability or decision on the tree is conditional on the events to the left of it. For example, the probability of surviving surgery

at 2 months of age is conditional upon the fact that the patient has survived that long.

In the example given, we have assumed that the probability of surviving operation as a newborn is 0.9, and that the probability of surviving operation at 2 months is 0.95. In other words, the mortality of operation has been halved. But there is a 2% risk that the patient will die while on medical treatment. The probability of surviving medical treatment is consequently 0.98.

Taking as our criterion for the best decision that which gives the best probability of survival, the merits of the alternative decisions can now be assessed, by calculating the expected probability of survival for each decision. In the case of the decision to operate now, this is simply $0.9 \times 1 = 0.9$. In the case of the decision to apply medical treatment, we can ignore the branches ending in death, since these correspond to a 0% chance of survival. We simply multiply backwards down the branch from right to left to the origin. In this case, this means multiplying $1 \times 0.95 \times 0.98$, which gives 0.931. Since the expected survival of patients initially given two months medical treatment is 93.1%, as against 90% for those operated on immediately, the correct decision is clearly to treat with oral prostaglandin for two months, and then operate.

Note that, although this chapter purports to concern principles of medical treatment, this first and most simple example involves also the timing of surgical treatment. We make no apology for this. The place of medical treatment in isolation in paediatric cardiology is small indeed. Decisions about medical treatment almost always involve decisions about the timing of surgery. And, as we shall see, decision analysis provides a powerful means of analysing such problems.

The next question one might reasonably ask is at what point the mortality for medical treatment would be too high to justify deferral of surgery. In other words, what is the acceptable maximum mortality for surgical treatment? Many clinicians would intuitively argue that, since the surgical mortality in the neonatal period is 10% (as opposed to 5% at two months of age), the acceptable medical mortality would be up to 5%. This subtraction of risks is not strictly correct, though it is a good approximation when the risks are small. It is incorrect because it ignores the fact that, if you die during medical treatment, you are no longer available to undergo surgical treatment. The correct answer is obtained by calling the minimal acceptable medical survival probability m and solving the equation $0.95 \times m = 0.9$. This gives the answer 0.947, which corresponds to a 5.3% mortality from medical treatment. This critical probability is known as a 'threshold probability'. It corresponds to the point at which the optimal decision changes from one branch to another.

Two further points immediately arise. The first may be termed the 'problem of particularity'. This is that the reader may feel that the probabilities used in the example do not correspond to those pertaining in his own institution. Instead, he may feel that the correct decision for his own patients would be to institute immediate surgical treatment. The simple answer to this problem is for the reader to insert the probabilities which apply to his own institution and then see which decision gives rise to the highest expected survival proportion. An alternative approach is to provide what is known as a 'sensitivity analysis'. This leads to the second point, which is that the use of oral prostaglandin is but one example of a whole family of medical decisions whose structure corresponds precisely to this one. Should we operate now or defer operation until later? Thus, the idea of providing a generalised solution to this problem is attractive. This can be achieved by seeing what happens to the threshold probability when the three different probabilities in the decision tree vary with respect to one another. The result of this process is demonstrated in Figure 16.2. If one knows the probability of dying after immediate surgery, the probability of dying after delayed surgery, and the probability of dying during intermediate medical treatment, one may read off the appropriate decision from the graph. Sensitivity analysis of this kind is also important, as we shall see, because in more complex decision trees, some probabilities are known with greater certainty than others. If the effect on the decision is unchanged for a wide range of plausible probabilities of a particular event, we need not worry too much about the precision of that probability. If, on the other hand, a small change in the probability of a particular event produces a change in the optimal strategy, this may or may not be important. If the change in strategy is accompanied by little change in utility, then it matters little which of the two alternative strategies is

adopted. If, by contrast, the change in strategy is accompanied by a large change in utility, it does matter which strategy is adopted. It is important that the relevant probability be determined as accurately as possible.

Finally, we note that the optimal decision can be altered if we can find a way of changing one or more probabilities in the decision tree. This approach underlies what is generally accepted policy with infants with ventricular septal defect in heart failure, namely to give a trial of medical treatment. The patient is given maximal medical treatment for a variable length of time, usually two weeks. If improvement occurs, medical treatment is continued. If it does not, the ventricular septal defect is closed surgically. This decision requires no sophisticated analysis, provided that medical treatment carries no risk. If a trial of medical treatment results in a lower overall surgical mortality, either because the risk of operating is lower at a later age or because there is the possibility that the patient may turn out never to require surgery at all, then a trial of medical treatment is clearly justifiable. The decision falls into one of the obvious strategies of treatment discussed at the beginning of the chapter. It is certainly extremely unlikely that a child undergoing a trial of medical treatment will die in hospital. On the other hand, if the trial of medical treatment is carried out at home, then the decision becomes much more comparable to the use of oral prostaglandin. The problem then needs to be analysed as outlined above.

More complex decision trees

A patient is admitted to hospital with prosthetic valve endocarditis. Should we operate now, should we take blood cultures and treat with antibiotics blind for three weeks and then decide about operation, or should we wait up to three weeks for a positive blood culture and then decide about operation? The problem is much more complex than the previous one, not only because two decisions are involved, but also because the outcome involves use of a clinical test (namely blood culture). Operation may be more appropriate for certain kinds of infection than for others. If the difference between outcomes for different infective organisms is sufficiently striking, then we want to maximise the possibility of obtaining a positive blood culture. In this circumstance we will not commence administration of antibiotics immediately. The problem is further complicated by the fact that the patient may live but suffer permanent damage as, for example, from a cerebral embolus. There are still further possible long-term complications of endocarditis, such as renal infarction. There is no difficulty mathematically in incorporating all these problems into the model. For the sake of simplicity, however, we will concentrate on one outcome other than life or death, which is cerebral embolism. The alert reader will immediately observe that

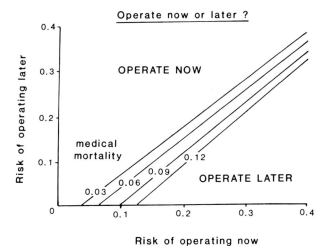

Fig. 16.2 Three-way sensitivity analysis for Figure 16.1. The diagonal lines correspond to borderlines between 'operate now' and 'operate later' for different medical mortalities. With a risk of 0.2 of operating now, 0.1 operating later and 0.06 of dying meanwhile (i.e. medical mortality), the correct strategy is to operate later, since (0.2, 0.1) lies to the right of the 0.06 line.

we can no longer use the straightforward probability of survival as a measure of the outcome of our decision. What is needed is to express the desirability of the outcome in terms which will obey the rules of probability. This is known as a 'utility'. How is it obtained?

Everyone would agree that a year of life without a cerebral embolus is worth more than a year of life with one. Most people would also agree that they would prefer living with a cerebral embolus to being dead. For the first example cited above, the value of 1 is given to the utility of the best possible outcome (alive without embolus), and the value of 0 to that of the worst possible outcome (dead). The utility of surviving a cerebral embolus must therefore be given an intermediate value somewhere between 0 and 1. If it is felt to be better to be dead than to live with an embolus, the state of being alive with an embolus is given a utility of zero and death becomes an outcome of intermediate utility. Let us return, however, to the original position, where death is the worst possible outcome.

The utility of the intermediate outcome (U_I) is obtained by a thought experiment involving a wager. Suppose that we are to assess your (the reader's) utility of living with a cerebral embolus. We offer you the alternatives of a *probability* of the best possible outcome (P_B) and the *certainty* of the intermediate outcome ($P_I = 1$). You have to make the choice. Most readers would prefer a probability of 0.99 of living without a cerebral embolus to the certainty of living with one. On the other hand, they would prefer the certainty of being alive with an embolus to a probability of 0.05 of living without one. Somewhere between 0.05 and 0.99 lies a point at which you find each alternative equally attractive (or repulsive). This point can be found by offering you repeated wagers at probabilities increasing progressively from 0.01 and decreasing progressively from 0.99. The intermediate probability at which you cannot make up your mind between one alternative and the other is the utility of the intermediate outcome (U_I). This is because at the point of indifference, the expected utilities are equal, i.e. $P_B U_B = P_I U_I$. But $U_B = P_I = 1$, so $U_I = P_B$. For the purpose of this example we have started with a utility of living with a cerebral embolus of 0.8.

Now we can begin to construct the decision tree (Fig. 16.3). The initial decision to the left of the figure is whether to operate immediately or to adopt one of two conservative strategies. The first is to wait up to 3 weeks for a positive culture. The second is to give initially blind antibiotic treatment for three weeks. If a positive culture is obtained, appropriate antibiotic therapy is instituted for two weeks prior to the decision about surgery. Either of the two decisions that postpone a decision about surgery incur a risk of embolus or death while waiting. The probability nodes for these two divisions split, therefore, into three branches. Those branches corresponding to death are end-points. By contrast, the decision tree continues in other figures in those corresponding to living with or without an embolus.

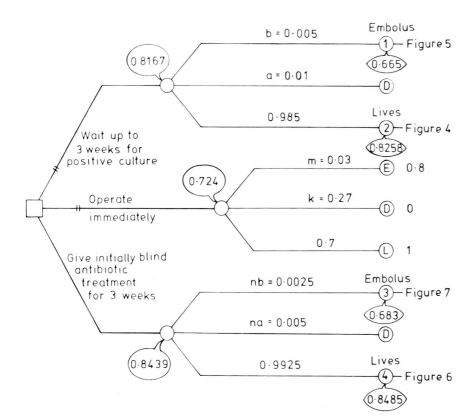

Fig. 16.3 Decision tree for management of prosthetic valve endocarditis. This is the left-hand end of the tree, extended to the right in Figures 16.4–16.7. For further explanation, see text. D – dead; E – embolus; L – lives. For other abbreviations, see Table 16.1.

The decision to operate immediately is entirely contained in Figure 16.3. There are three simple endpoints: death, survival without embolus, and survival with embolus. Expected utility for this decision is calculated by 'averaging out' (multiplying probabilities or utilities along each branch and then summing them). The utility of this decision is $0.03 \times 0.8 + 0.27 \times 0 + 0.7 \times 1 = 0.724$. The value is inserted on that branch, enclosed in a balloon, as are all other expected utilities. Similar values are inserted on the other branches in the figure. We cannot calculate them at this point, however, since calculations must always start at terminal nodes working from the right. The process of averaging out, nonetheless, is exactly the same.

Throughout this analysis, wherever possible, probabilities have been obtained from the literature. It is important, however, to think ahead to the crucial sensitivity analysis in which the effect is studied of varying different probabilities within the model. This is achieved by defining probabilities as variables rather than as constants. For example, a, b, m and k are defined as in Table 16.1. It is not necessary so to define the probabilities of surviving without embolus in the model, since this is one less than the probabilities of death and embolus. For example, the probability of surviving immediate operation $1 - k - m$.

Wherever possible, variables should be defined in a way that reflects risk ratios inherent in the model. For example, the risks of death and embolus in Figure 16.3 are defined for the strategy of waiting for a positive culture. The corresponding probabilities for blind antibiotic treatment are defined as na and nb. This reflects the idea that if blind antibiotic treatment reduces the risk of death while waiting for a decision about surgery, it reduces also the risk of embolisation proportionately. For the initial model n is set at 0.5. But, as n can take values above one, the possibility can be examined that the risk of death while waiting is greater for the strategy of blind antibiotic treatment than waiting for a positive culture. This use of risk ratios (Macartney et al, 1984) is also attractive because it reflects

Table 16.1 Definitions of probabilities and risk ratios.

Definitions of probabilities and risk ratios	Initial value
a = probability of dying while awaiting decision about surgery for strategy of waiting for positive culture.	0.01
b = probability of surviving a cerebral embolus while awaiting decision about surgery for strategy of waiting for positive culture.	0.005
c = probability of negative blood culture for strategy of waiting up to three weeks for positive culture.	0.1
d = probability of fungal blood culture for strategy of waiting up to three weeks for positive culture.	0.05
e = probability of death given choice not to operate after waiting three weeks for positive culture and culturing bacteria.	0.15
f = probability of embolus given choice not to operate after waiting three weeks for positive culture and culturing bacteria.	0.02
g = probability of death given choice not to operate after waiting three weeks for positive culture and culturing fungi.	0.9
h = probability of embolus given choice not to operate after waiting three weeks for positive culture and culturing fungi.	0.08
k = probability of death during or after immediate operation.	0.27
m = probability of embolus during or after immediate operation.	0.03
n = probability of death (or embolus) while awaiting decision about surgery for strategy of blind antibiotic treatments/same for waiting for positive culture.	0.5
p = probability of negative culture with blind antibiotic treatment/same probability with waiting for positive result.	2
q = probability of fungal culture with blind antibiotic treatment/same probability with waiting for positive result	1
r = probability of embolus after operation/probability of embolus with medical treatment for all types of culture and both conservative strategies.	1.5
s = probability of death after operation/probability of death with medical treatment for bacterial culture and both conservative strategies.	4/3
t = probability of death after operation/probability of death with medical treatment for fungal culture.	0.5
v = probability of death after operation/probability of death with medical treatment for negative culture.	5/6
w = probability of death (or embolus) with blind antibiotic therapy/same probability with waiting for positive culture, given that bacterial culture is obtained.	0.8
x = probability of death (or embolus) with blind antibiotic therapy/same probability with waiting for positive culture, given that fungal culture is obtained.	1
y = probability of death (or embolus) with blind antibiotic therapy/probability of death (or embolus) with waiting for positive culture for medical and surgical treatment with negative culture.	0.9
z = probability of death (or embolus) with negative culture/probability of death (or embolus) for bacterial culture for medical or surgical treatment.	1.5

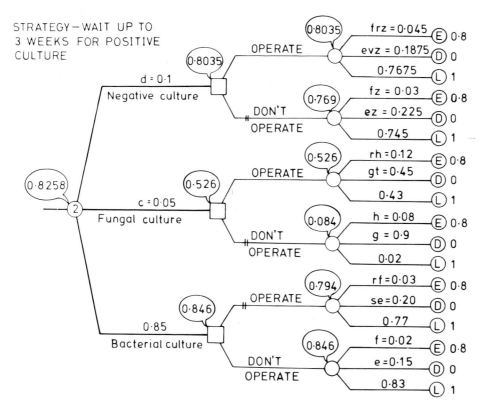

STRATEGY—WAIT UP TO
3 WEEKS FOR POSITIVE
CULTURE

Fig. 16.4 Decision tree for management of infective endocarditis. This section, related to Figure 16.3, refers to patients treated according to the strategy of waiting for a positive culture for up to 3 weeks, and who have not died or had a cerebral embolus. For abbreviations see Figure 16.3 and Table 16.1. For further explanation, see text.

the idea of proportional hazards inherent in the Cox model for risk factor survival analysis (see Ch. 59).

The analysis continues in Figure 16.4 for the strategy of waiting for a positive culture, given that the patient has survived so far without an embolus. To simplify matters, we assume that there are three exhaustive, and mutually exclusive possibilities, namely bacterial, fungal and negative culture. We have then to decide whether to operate or not, so there are three decision nodes in the centre of the figure. For each decision there are the familiar three outcomes of death, embolus or life. The probabilities have been assigned starting at the bottom right hand corner (which gives a kind of baseline), starting with the decision not to operate in the face of a positive bacterial culture. This particular probability has been chosen because it corresponds to the most likely event, bacterial infection. It can therefore be determined with more precision than other probabilities in the model. The probabilities of death and embolism after operation are presumed to be related to those without operation, so risk ratios r and s are used to modify probabilities e and f (for definitions, see Table 16.1). r and s are initially set to make the risk of surgical treatment somewhat higher than that of medical treatment.

The probabilities both of death and embolus with medical treatment after a negative culture are assumed to be related to those pertaining to bacterial culture by using risk ratio z. By contrast, these probabilities in the case of fungal infection are independently assigned as g and h. Just as in the case of bacterial culture, the risks of death and

embolism in fungal culture treated by operation are assumed to be related to those with medical treatment by the risk ratios r and t. r is assumed to be the same whatever the nature of the culture (since it applies to embolisation, which is rare, any departure from this ratio will have little effect on the model). The risk of death following operation is catered for separately in each culture group by using different ratios s, t and v.

Averaging out of each terminal triplet of branches is now carried out to give the expected utility of each decision. Taking these two at a time, it is seen that the decision not to operate has a lower utility for negative and fungal culture, while the decision to operate has a lower utility for bacterial culture. These branches are therefore each pruned by a double slash, and the expected utility of the unpruned branch is transferred to the decision node. This process is known as 'folding back'. If we have decided to wait up to three weeks for a positive culture, the correct decision is to operate if the culture is negative or fungal. The expected utility of the entire decision is now obtained by averaging out the expected utilities of the three decision nodes $(0.1 \times 0.8035 + 0.05 \times 0.526 + 0.846 \times 0.85 = 0.8258)$. This expected utility is then transferred to Figure 16.3.

If the patient has had an embolus while waiting for a positive culture, we assume that this does not affect any of the probabilities in Figure 16.4. Since there is no possibility of living without an embolus, however, the corresponding branches are removed. The probability of surviving with an embolus is calculated as 1 minus the probability of death. Figure 16.5 demonstrates the resultant tree. The recommended strategy is not affected and the overall expected utility of 0.665 is transferred to Figure 16.3.

The decision tree for the strategy of treating blind with antibiotics is displayed in Figure 16.6 and is very similar to Figure 16.4. It results in the same recommended strategy. Risk ratios w, x and y are introduced to relate the probabilities with this strategy to those with the other

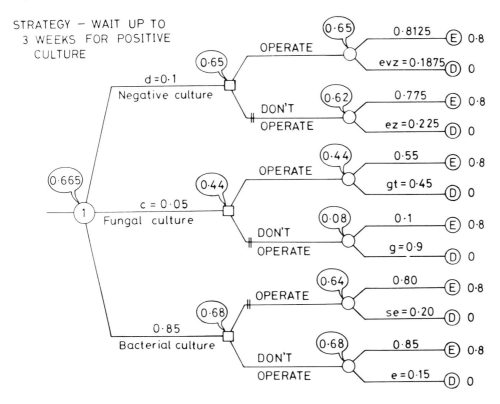

Fig. 16.5 Decision tree for management of infective endocarditis. This section, related to Figure 16.1, has exactly the same structure as Figure 16.4, except that, since it involves only patients who have already had a cerebral embolus, there is no possibility of living without an embolus.

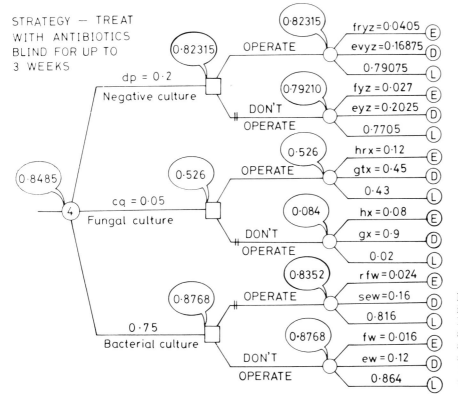

Fig. 16.6 Decision tree for management of infective endocarditis. This section, related to Figure 16.3, refers to patients given blind antibiotic treatment, who have not died or had a cerebral embolus while awaiting a decision about surgery. For abbreviations see Figure 16.3 and Table 16.1. For further explanation, see text.

conservative strategy (see Table 16.1) for each type of infection. Their initial values indicate no change in the risk with fungal infection. There is a reduction of risk with blind antibiotic therapy, this being greater in the case of bacterial infection. p and q are chosen so as to reflect the fact that blind antibiotic therapy doubles the chance of a negative blood culture, decreases the chance of a positive bacterial culture, and does not affect the chance of a fungal culture. The overall expected utility of 0.8485 is transferred to Figure 16.3.

Figure 16.7 is derived from Figure 16.6 just as Figure 16.5 was derived from Figure 16.4, so as to produce an expected utility of 0.683 if the patient has an embolus while waiting for a decision on surgery and on blind antibiotic therapy. This expected utility is transferred to Figure 16.3.

Returning to Figure 16.3 and averaging out the branches for the two conservative strategies, we obtain a maximum expected utility of 0.8439 for the strategy of blind antibiotic therapy followed by surgery if either a fungal or negative culture is obtained. This is therefore the recommended treatment. Its utility is higher by 0.0272 than that of waiting for a positive culture. It is particularly important, because this gap is quite small, to carry out a sensitivity analysis so as to identify which factors are particularly crucial to the decision. The easy way to do this is to write a simple computer programme which will change one or more parameters in the model continuously over a wide range of possible values and compute the necessary expected utilities. Such a programme will easily run on a very small microcomputer.

Effect on first decision varying one parameter at a time

The mortality of medical treatment of a patient who has a positive bacterial culture after waiting for this has to be over 30% before the appropriate strategy is to operate immediately. In contrast, k (the operative mortality for immediate operation) has to be below 15% before immediate operation is the preferred strategy. This critical probability is easily calculated from Figure 16.3 by setting equal the expected utilities of the optimal strategy and immediate operation, and solving for k.

$$0.03 \times 0.8 + (1 - 0.03 - k) \times 1 = 0.8439$$
$$\Rightarrow \quad k = 0.1503$$

The probability of obtaining a negative culture with blind antibiotic treatment has to be at least 7.1 times the same probability with waiting for a positive culture before the optimal strategy changes to the latter (ratio = p). Similarly, the probability of obtaining a fungal culture must be at least $2\frac{1}{2}$ times higher (ratio = q). The probability of death (or embolus) with blind antibiotic therapy (given that a bacterial infection is found) has to be at least 1.03 times the same probability with waiting for a positive culture before a change of strategy in that direction is

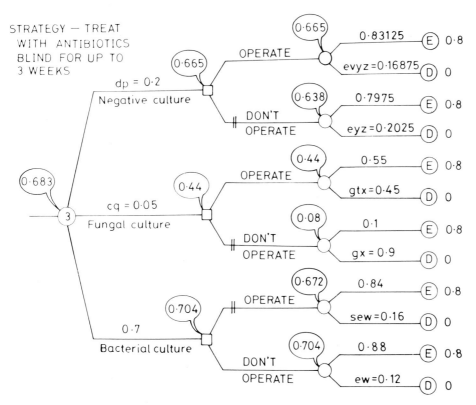

Fig. 16.7 Decision tree for management of infective endocarditis. This section, related to Figure 16.3, refers to patients given blind antibiotic treatment who have a cerebral embolus while awaiting a decision about surgery. For abbreviations see Figure 16.3 and Table 16.1. For further explanation, see text.

justified (ratio = w). Similar ratios for fungal and culture negative infection are (x) 2.2 and (y) 1.6. Finally, the probability of death (or embolus) with a negative culture has to be at least 4.5 times (ratio = z) the same probability for a bacterial culture before the correct decision is to wait for a positive culture.

None of the other parameters listed in Table 16.1 materially affect this decision.

Effect on second decision

If the operative mortality is less than 0.9867 of the medical mortality, *in presence of a bacterial culture*, then the correct decision is to operate rather than treat medically. This ratio s, is simple to calculate from Figures 16.6 or 16.4 by setting expected utilities of medical and surgical treatment equal and solving

$$0.8rfw + 1 - rfw - sew = 0.8fw + 1 - ew - fw$$
$$- 0.2rfw - sew = -0.2fw - ew$$
$$se = 0.2f(1 - r) + e$$
$$s = \frac{0.2f(1 - r) + 1}{e}$$
$$= 0.9867$$

Similarly, if the operative mortality is greater than 0.9867 of the medical mortality, *in presence of a negative culture*, then the correct decision is to treat medically. None of the other parameters listed in Table 16.1 materially affect this decision.

We conclude that the primary decision recommendation, to treat blind with antibiotics, is likely to be of general applicability, in particular because it seems improbable that blind antibiotic treatment can increase the risk of medical treatment in presence of bacterial infection. Fears about the effect of a lower likelihood of obtaining a positive culture after blind antibiotic treatment are shown to be groundless, in that gross deviations from what is likely to be found are required before the strategy is changed.

The second decision, on the other hand, is critically dependent on the relative mortalities of surgical and medical treatment. Thus, if we are to make recommendations for a particular centre, these are the pieces of information which are most needed.

Notice that the changes in the risk of embolism do not change the recommended decision. Varying the utility of embolisation all the way from 0 to 1 similarly has no effect on the decision. This is because a cerebral embolus is a rather rare complication. We conclude that it is not important to be precise in establishing probabilities or utilities of cerebral embolus.

Consideration of how critically a decision depends on particular probabilities is also helpful in deciding how to obtain these probabilities. Decision theory does not demand that all probabilities are established for long run

experiments, for example from retrospective studies. Informed clinical hunches are equally permissible. Long run probabilities are likely to be of more general validity, but carry the disadvantage of being based upon past experience. Today's decision demands today's probability, which may be different. Furthermore, there are probabilities in many decision trees which simply cannot be established by long run experiments. These must therefore be replaced by subjective judgements (Macartney et al, 1984).

Short-term versus long-term gains

The first two examples given have both required a more or less arbitrary decision on a time, namely the time for which medical treatment will be continued before surgical treatment is considered. This is often an extremely valuable approach, but it can also be an over-simplification. In many situations, the most important decision a paediatric cardiologist has to make about therapy is not what therapy to employ but when to institute it, and in particular, when to operate upon the patient. Of all subjects discussed at medical or surgical meetings, this is the one most likely to provoke furious discussion. The very heat of the argument demonstrates how tenuous are its logical foundations. Most operations have a higher risk in younger children. This phenomenon has some interesting consequences. Some referral centres for cardiac surgery stress the importance of waiting until the patient grows older and bigger before sending him to the centre for operation. The benefit of advocating such a policy is that it improves the surgical results of the institution, because death of patients before they arrive do not appear in the statistics. Even in centres where this paradox is fully understood, the possibility exists for unintentional manipulation of surgical results simply by refusing to operate on extremely sick patients. In any condition which has a poor natural history, there is always a trade-off between surgical and medical mortality. Our knowledge of the population of children with congenital heart disease would be greatly benefited if centres would report what happened to all the children who arrive on their doorstep with a particular condition rather than simply considering the results of those who reach the operating table.

Let us take as an example the optimal timing of operation for complete transposition with intact ventricular septum (see Ch. 34), since this carries a very poor natural history even after balloon atrial septostomy. Though some recent reports have shown that there is no change in immediate mortality irrespective of the age at which intra-atrial repair is carried out, for the purposes of this example, let us assume that young age is an incremental risk factor. Specifically, let us suppose that the mortality of baffle repair is 1% at three and six months, 2% at one month, and 4% at one week. When is the best time to

Table 16.2 Determination of optimal timing of baffle operation.

Probability of survival Time at end of interval	1 week	1 month	3 months	6 months	1 year
Natural history after septostomy	0.975	0.955	0.915	0.90	0.86
Baffle at 6 months	0.975	0.955	0.915	0.90	0.882
Baffle at 3 months	0.975	0.955	0.915	0.901	0.892
Baffle at 1 month	0.975	0.955	0.933	0.928	0.919
Baffle at 1 week	0.975	0.935	0.932	0.927	0.918
Banding at 6 months, then switch	0.975	0.955	0.915	0.90	0.731

operate? We shall assume that the late complication rate is independent of the age at operation.

Table 16.2 shows the probability of survival for the first year of life in patients who have been treated with balloon atrial septostomy alone. These figures have been obtained from the data collected from Great Ormond Street for a study published by Leanage and colleagues (1981). We can then calculate the overall probability of survival, taking into account the natural history of the condition, the risk of operation, and the risk of late death following operation (which for the purposes of this example is taken as 2% of the survivors per year). This figure corresponds to a probability of 0.817 of surviving to 10 years after operation, given that you have lived long enough to have an operation, which corresponds closely to that reported by Macartney and colleagues (1980).

Let us take, for example, operation at six months. We know from the natural history the probability of survival to the beginning of that interval. For the time interval 6–12 months, we have to take into account the operative mortality and the late mortality for that time interval. To do this we make the (not unreasonable) assumption that these risks are statistically independent. We then multiply together each of the conditional probabilities of survival and the probability of surviving up to the beginning of the interval. Thus, the probability of surviving to one year is $0.90 \times (1 - 0.01) \times 0.985^{5/12}$. The 5/12 is there because we count operative mortality as that occurring within one month of operation. We have, therefore, a postoperative hazard function lasting for five months (5/12 of a year). The probability of survival to six months after a baffle operation at three months is $0.915 \times 0.99 \times (0.98)^{1/6} = 0.901$, and of survival to one year is $0.901 \times (0.98)^{1/2}$, and so on.

This process has been repeated in the Table 16.2 for baffle operations at one month and at one week. As you see from Table 16.2, the probability of survival to one year for operation at six months is 0.882. The corresponding figure for operation at three months is 89.2%, at one month is 91.9% and at one week is 91.8%. Thus, by a short head, operation at one month is the preferred

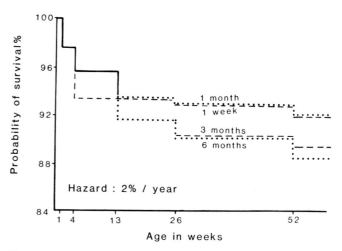

Fig. 16.8 Estimated survival curves for different ages of baffle operation for simple complete transposition. A solid line indicates overlap of two or more survival curves. For further explanation, see text.

strategy (Fig. 16.8). As we are assuming the same late death rate regardless of the time of surgery, the ranking of the options at one year will be the same as it would be at 10, 20 or 70 years.

The optimal timing of surgery will clearly depend critically upon the mortality of surgery at different ages. It should be clear from the example given, nonetheless, that the arguments for very early operation on patients with complete transposition and intact ventricular septum are very persuasive, providing that one is prepared to consider the complete results of management of the patient rather than simply the results of surgical management. For comparison, using the same strategy, we have calculated the results of a two-stage operation for complete transposition, consisting of pulmonary arterial banding as a first stage and arterial switch operation as a second, using the data from Yacoub et al (1980). We have simplified this slightly by taking banding at six months and arterial switch at a year, rather than banding at 8 months on average and a switch operation at 14 months on average as originally reported. The one year survival rate with this policy is

73.1%, which is decidedly unattractive (Table 16.2). This, therefore, raises the question of the value of an arterial switch operation for this condition in the neonatal period. This has been advocated by some authors, and has been the subject of hot controversy, both as regards medical common sense and medical ethics. At the heart of this debate is the question of relative merits of short-term and long-term gain. Given that the switch operation, being more physiological, is likely to have a lower late death rate than baffle repair, what is an acceptable mortality for the switch operation carried out in the neonatal period?

This question has been addressed using almost the same analytic methods as were used to determine the optimal age for atrial baffle repair. Before we carry out the analysis, the reader might care to think for a moment about what he would estimate as the immediate surgical mortality of a switch operation in the neonatal period that would give the same life expectancy as intra-atrial baffle repair at one month as described above, if the hazard rate after a switch operation were 15% of that after intra-atrial baffle repair.

In order to calculate life expectancy, we need to take into account the survival curve of the normal population (Fig. 16.9). For the purpose of this analysis, we have assumed that our patients with complete transposition are selected in that all they have wrong with them is complete transposition, and that the remainder of mortality in the first year of life is therefore irrelevant. For each time interval after one year, however, we assume that the patient is subject to two independent risks, that of dying because they are normal human beings, and that of dying because they have had a switch operation.

Table 16.3 shows part of the calculations required to calculate life expectancy. Each 5-year period beyond 35 years is treated in exactly the same way as the periods from 5 to 35 years, so the later period has been omitted for clarity.

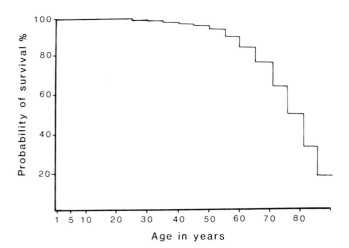

Fig. 16.9 Survival curve for normal population, weighted according to sex ratio in complete transposition, with deaths in the first year of live excluded.

In row 1 are probabilities of survival of a normal population, weighted towards males as is complete transposition. Strict accuracy would demand a separate analysis for each sex. This has been done, and does not materially affect the conclusions, so for simplicity's sake, a single weighted analysis is present. Row 2 is obtained by subtracting each probability of survival from the one before it to obtain an unconditional death density. The hazard rate (row 3) is obtained by dividing each unconditional death density by the probability of survival up to the start of the period for children surviving at least a year. Subtracting row 3 from 1 gives row 4, the probability of surviving that time interval, given that the subject has survived to the beginning of it. Row 5 contains the probability of surviving 30 days after operation (0.6 in this example), and row 6 contains the probability of surviving the time interval, given survival to the beginning of it and the assumed constant postoperative hazard (in this case 0.003/year). The conditional probability of survival is $1 - 0.003 = 0.997$. Each figure in row 6 is 0.997^t where t is the length of the interval in years. The overall conditional probability of survival is then obtained in row 7 as the product of row 4 and row 6 for all years after one. The first year of life is dealt with by transferring row 5 to row 7 for the probability of surviving 30 days after operation. Row 6 is transferred to row 7 for the next four cells, which is equivalent to our assumption that there is no risk of dying during this time simply because you are a human being but only because you have had a switch operation. Subtracting row 7 from 1 gives us finally our overall hazard rate in row 8 which reflects the immediate and late risk of the operation together with the risk of being alive, and dying from unrelated causes. If computing facilities are not available and the hazard rates are low, we may take advantage of the fact that $(1 - x)(1 - y) = (1 - x - y + xy) = (1 - (x + y))$ for x, y small in comparison to 1. The natural hazard (row 3) is added to the postoperative hazard $(1 - \text{row } 6)$ and subtracted from 1 to give overall hazard (row 8). We now work from this to obtain our anticipated life table.

The simplest way of thinking of the calculation of row 9 is to imagine starting with 10 000 patients. At the end of the first interval, with 40% dead there would be 6000 left. This is obtained by multiplying 10 000 by the 0.6 obtained from the first cell of row 7. All 6000 patients survive one month, but the probability of surviving the next two months is 0.9995 (from row 7). Thus there are $6000 \times 0.9995 = 5996$ survivors. The probability of these surviving the next interval is 0.9992 (row 7), i.e. there will be $59.96 \times 0.9992 = 5991$ survivors. This process is continued all the way to the end of the table. Row 9 then consists of the number of survivors divided by 10 000 to give the probability of survival (Fig. 16.10).

To calculate life expectancy we need to calculate the unconditional death density from the probability of

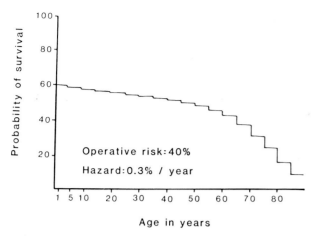

Fig. 16.10 Estimated survival curve for switch operation at birth with 40% mortality and late postoperative hazard of 0.3%/year. Unweighted life expectancy is 39.1 years.

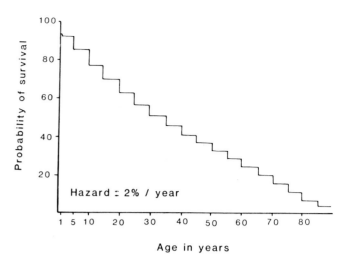

Fig. 16.11 Estimated survival curve for baffle operation at one month with 2% mortality and late postoperative hazard of 2%/year. Unweighted life expectancy is 35.3 years.

survival, just as we generated row 2. Row 10 is obtained by subtracting each probability of survival from the previous one, remembering that the probability at birth is 1. Row 11 is obtained by multiplying row 9 by the midpoint of the interval in years. Life expectancy is now obtained by summing all the values in row 11 out to 85 years of age and multiplying the unconditional death density in that cell by 90, which is 85 plus the life expectancy for that cell. The estimated life expectancy turns out to be 39.1 years.

To calculate life expectancy after our optimal baffle strategy (operate at one month) we go through precisely the same stages as for the switch (Table 16.3), except that we have to allow for deaths prior to operation. This is

simply done by calculating hazard rates for the first two cells of row 8 from the balloon septostomy data of Table 16.2, and including the risk of operation in the third cell of row 8. The estimated survival curve for a 2% operative mortality and a hazard rate of 2%/year is shown in Figure 16.11. Life expectancy is 35.3 years, which is 3.8 years less than for a neonatal switch operation with a 40% early mortality , but a 0.3%/year late hazard rate.

This result demonstrates very graphically that the main determinant of life expectancy is late rather than early mortality. To make a point of general validity, however, it is necessary to generalise this solution. This was achieved by writing a comparatively simple programme,

Table 16.3 Estimation of life expectancy after switch operation.

	Time at end of interval								
	1 week	1 month	3 months	6 months	1 year	5 years	10 years	15 years	20 years
Normals									
1. Probability of survival				0.9834	0.9806	0.9791	0.9777	0.9743	
2. Unconditional death density					0.0028	0.0015	0.0014	0.0034	
3. Hazard function					0.0028	0.0015	0.0014	0.0035	
4. 1-hazard function					0.9972	0.9985	0.9986	0.9965	
5. 1-operative hazard	0.6								
6. 1-postoperative hazard		1	0.9995	0.9992	0.9985	0.9880	0.9851	0.9851	0.9851
7. 1-overall hazard	0.6	1	0.9995	0.9992	0.9985	0.9852	0.9836	0.9817	0.9817
8. Overall hazard	0.4	0	0.0005	0.0008	0.0015	0.0148	0.0164	0.0183	
9. Overall probability of survival	0.6	0.6	0.5996	0.5991	0.5982	0.5894	0.5797	0.5703	0.5596
10. Overall unconditional death density	0.4	0	0.0004	0.0006	0.0009	0.0088	0.0097	0.0094	0.0105
11. Figures to be summed for life expectancy	0.0038	0	0	0.0002	0.0007	0.0264	0.0728	0.1175	0.1838
12. Switch operation in newborn (operative mortality = 40%: late postoperative hazard 0.5%/year)									

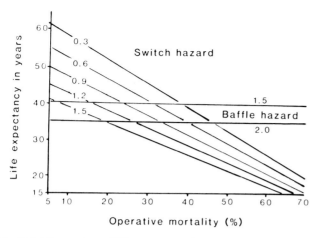

Fig. 16.12 Comparison of life expectancy after switch and baffle operations given a 2% mortality for a baffle operation at one month, and a variety of different operative mortalities for the switch operation (abscissa) and late postoperative hazards. For further explanation, see text.

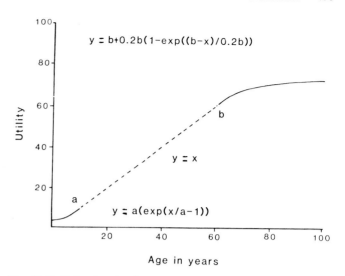

Fig. 16.13 Utility function for weighting life expectancy. For further explanation, see text.

again running on a very modest desk-top microcomputer, to calculate life expectancy in the manner already described. The computer programme was necessary because thousands of life expectancies needed to be calculated. The result is shown in Figure 16.12.

If the late hazard rate of the arterial switch procedure is greater than that of the baffle, then the problem does not merit discussion. The baffle operation is the one of choice. Thus we have only considered hazard rates for the arterial switch below or equal to 1.5%/year. The point at which the horizontal lines intersect with the sloping ones are those at which the corresponding operative mortality for the switch operation (read off the abscissa) will give the same life expectancy. This could be termed the 'maximum acceptable mortality' for the switch operation. If the baffle hazard is 2%/year (as has been assumed thus far) the maximum acceptable operative mortalities for a switch operation are 19%, 27%, 32%, 40% and 47% for hazards of 1.5%, 1.2%, 0.9%, 0.6% and 0.3% per year. If the hazard rate for the switch operation is only 1.5/year, these acceptable mortalities are all lower, but still remarkably high.

At this point it is worth considering what assumptions have been made. The only important one is that the postoperative hazard rate is constant. This can be justified for the baffle operation both on the grounds of what has been observed and an underlying model of death due to arrhythmia which is the result of a particular combination of adverse conditions coinciding. It is easy to introduce more complex late hazard functions into the model and recalculate the results.

It may be argued that life expectancy is not the best measure of outcome since, for example, it assumes that every year of added life is of the same value as any other. Most people would agree that a year of added life for a 30-

year-old parent of three children is more valuable than a year of added life to a newborn baby or a 95-year-old. This concept can be expressed mathematically as a utility function (Fig. 16.13). Between points a and b on the graph, each year of added life is as valuable as any other, so the slope of the line is 1. Below a and above b, curved lines are drawn according to the functions shown in the figure. These reflect the diminished values of years of added life in the very young and the very old. These functions are chosen so that they are monotonically increasing and fit smoothly onto the central straight line. a and b are selected by a thought experiment (at what ages do years of added life become less valuable?) or else by writing a computer programme to plot the curve interactively and permitting the subject to alter a and b until a curve corresponding to his/her utility function is obtained. The fact that a baby cannot do the thought experiment or choose a computer plot merely reflects real life, where others have to take decisions about the baby.

Weighted life expectancy is then calculated by taking the overall unconditional death densities (row 10 of Table 16.3). Instead of multiplying these by the mid-point of each interval, the utility of that age is read off the graph which forms Figure 16.13 (or better calculated), and this adjusted age is multiplied by the overall unconditional death density for that cell. The sum of these products is then the weighted life expectancy. The plot of Figure 16.12 has been redrawn in Figure 16.14 with weighted life expectancy on the ordinate, a and b having been set at 3 and 60 years. The maximum acceptable mortalities for a switch operation and a baffle hazard of 2%/year are now 18%, 26%, 31%, 39% and 44% for hazards of 1.5%, 1.2%, 0.9% and 0.6%. These figures are all slightly lower than with unweighted life expectancy, i.e. the balance is tilted slightly in favour of the baffle operation. Why is this?

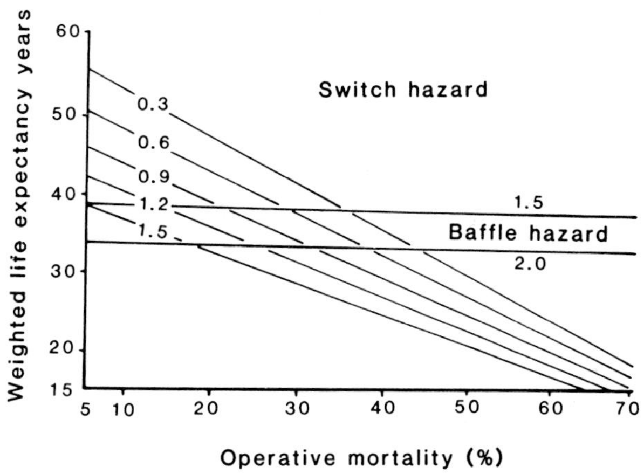

Fig. 16.14 Figure 12 redrawn with weighted life expectancy on the ordinate. a = 3 years; b = 60 years (see Fig. 16.13).

There are two opposing effects of weighting life expectancy as suggested. The flatter slope at young age means that one is more ready to take risks with a baby, which favours the switch operation. On the other hand, the flatter slope at old age favours the baffle operation since survivors of this procedure are less likely to reach old age (compare Figs. 16.10, 16.11). Clearly, with the parameters a and b chosen, the effect at old age outweighs that at young age. Wide alterations in a and b have relatively little effect on the result.

Much of the debate on the ethics of the arterial switch procedure has centred on the immediate mortality of that procedure. What really matters is late hazard rate and not the immediate mortality.

There is no subject more likely to raise the temperature of a medical audience than decision theory. Part of the angst is due to the perceived threat of a machine taking over one of the most treasured functions of the clinician, which is to make decisions. We do not regard the prospect of computers making decisions as likely or even desirable. The principle benefit of decision theory is that it forces the clinician to make explicit the assumptions underlying the decision. This is of enormous educational value, because it may well produce a profound change in the 'mind-set' of the clinician, thereby affecting all his/her future decisions in the same area. In practice, considerable resistance is often encountered to making assumptions explicit. Presumably this is because of fear that the process of decision-making by the clinician will be shown to be far more based on hunch than logic. Once it is understood that there is nothing wrong with hunch (provided that it is made explicit), decision analysis becomes immediately more acceptable. Undoubtedly, paediatric cardiologists will be hearing more of it.

PRINCIPLES OF DRUG TREATMENT

For infants and children with heart disease, the major circumstances requiring drug treatment are circulatory failure, hypoxia and cardiac arrhythmias. Arrhythmias themselves often give rise to circulatory failure, but in these circumstances the management of the rhythm disturbance is often the most important aspect. This problem has been dealt with extensively in Chapter 54.

Circulation provides a mechanism for transport of oxygen and metabolic substrates to the various tissues of the body so that specialised functions, cellular integrity and growth can be maintained. Because the demands of various organs vary considerably during exercise or disease, cardiac output must be able to change rapidly and adjustments of regional distribution of blood flow must be possible. This regional distribution can change within seconds through intrinsic and extrinsic control. Intrinsic control of cardiac output is predominantly by the Frank-Starling mechanism (Little & Little, 1982) together with the autoregulation of peripheral vascular tone. Extrinsic control is predominantly through neural regulation of heart rate, atrioventricular conduction, peripheral vascular resistance (afterload) and peripheral venous capacitance (preload). The function of the heart, therefore, is to pump sufficient blood to satisfy the metabolic requirements of the body tissues. Cardiac output is the product of stroke volume and heart rate. The latter is under adrenergic and cholinergic vagal control. The fundamental determinants of stroke volume are preload, afterload and intrinsic myocardial contractility (Mason, 1978). Preload may be somewhat imprecisely defined as myocardial end-diastolic fibre length or ventricular end-diastolic volume. Its relationship to cardiac output is governed by Starling's law. This is principally influenced by venous return to the heart which in turn depends on the circulating blood volume, venous capacitance and ventricular compliance. The end-diastolic ventricular pressures or the right and left atrial pressures most closely reflect preload (Little & Little, 1982). The term 'afterload' refers to the total force opposing ventricular ejection. It is difficult to define precisely, but is related to the tension of the ventricular wall developed during systole. It depends upon systemic vascular resistance, which is under neural and humoral control, and arterial wall compliance. These are two of the major components of aortic impedance. Thus, increasing the afterload reduces the stroke volume and cardiac output. Conversely, reducing afterload may increase stroke volume. Studies on isolated heart muscle have shown that afterloading conditions during ejection relate to instantaneous wall stress during contraction (Milnor, 1975; Ross, 1976). Wall stress develops during cardiac contraction and relates to intraventricular pressure, ventricular volume and wall thickness. It changes continuously throughout systole

(Mason, 1978; Milnor, 1975; Ross, 1976). In clinical practice, the measurement of afterload is extremely difficult. The value of aortic pressure is usually used, although this is a product of peripheral vascular resistance and cardiac output and comparable but opposite changes in resistance and cardiac output will not change blood pressure. But for practical purposes, clinical assessment of afterload depends on the measurement of arterial blood pressure and observations of heart rate and peripheral perfusion. Whilst most physicians would understand in general terms what is meant by the term 'myocardial contractility', there is no precise definition. There is, however, a full account of ventricular function in Chapter 7. In clinical practice, techniques used for the assessment of ventricular performance include M-mode and cross-sectional echocardiography, ventriculography and radionuclide studies.

Specific problems of the small infant

The myocardium of the newborn and small infant is unique in its inability to adapt to stress because of its small functional reserve capacity (Friedman, 1972; Romero & Friedman, 1979). There are numerous reasons for this frequently observed phenomenon. The myocardium has fewer myofilaments (Sheldon et al, 1976), ventricular compliance is reduced (McPherson et al, 1976) and consequently preload reserve or diastolic reserve is limited (Kirkpatrick et al, 1976). In addition, oxygen consumption and cardiac output in the newborn are relatively high. Thus, the systolic reserve for adaptation to the stress of hypoxia, acidosis, hypocalcaemia, hypoglycaemia, anaemia, sepsis or heart disease is extremely limited (Weber & Janicki, 1979). As well as the relatively low diastolic and systolic reserve, resting heart rate is high. Cardiac output is more dependent on heart rate in neonates and infants than in older children. Because of this, bradycardia may be poorly tolerated, but there is also a limited ability to increase cardiac output by increasing heart rate. This is because, at heart rates over 180, diastolic filling time and coronary blood flow are reduced and myocardial oxygen consumption and energy expenditure are increased (Kirkpatrick et al, 1975). Finally, the heart of the neonate and small infant is less able to tolerate pressure or volume overload (Berman & Christensen, 1983), is less responsive to inotropic agents (Hougan et al, 1982), and has an immature adrenergic nervous system. Thus, in view of the relative inability of the infant myocardium to adapt to stress, it is likely that pharmacological manipulation of preload and afterload may be beneficial in this group of patients.

The causes of circulatory failure (Table 16.4)

Circulatory failure is more common in neonates and infants

Table 16.4 Causes of circulatory failure.

Cardiogenic
Pump failure
  Cardiomyopathy
  Myocardial ischaemia
  Anomalous origin of left coronary artery
High pulmonary blood flow
  Total anomalous pulmonary venous connexion
  Atrioventricular septal defect
  Ventricular septal defect
  Heart with univentricular atrioventricular connexion
  Aortopulmonary window
  Arterial duct
  Common arterial trunk
Left heart obstruction
  Mitral stenosis
  Divided left atrium
  Hypertrophic cardiomyopathy (in infants)
  Critical aortic stenosis
  Infant coarctation
  Interrupted aortic arch
  Hypoplastic left heart syndrome
Severe valve insufficiency
Arrhythmias

Hypovolaemia
Blood loss
Plasma loss
Water loss

Loss of peripheral resistance
Sepsis
Anaphylaxis
Drugs

Negative inotropic factors
Hypoxia
Acidosis
Hypocalcaemia
Hypomagnesaemia
Hypoglycaemia

not only because major structural abnormalities are present at birth (so that decompensation occurs early in life) but also for the reasons already outlined. The major causes relate to pump failure, high pulmonary blood flow, left heart obstruction, severe valve insufficiency, arrhythmias, hypovolaemia, loss of peripheral resistance and negative inotropic factors. It is important to be aware that negative inotropic factors (such as acidosis, hypoxia, hypoglycaemia and hypocalcaemia or anaemia) may all aggravate existing circulatory failure or precipitate failure when there is coexisting heart disease.

Clinical features of circulatory failure

The regional distribution of blood flow is under neural and autoregulatory local control. Thus, when cardiac output falls, blood flow to the organs with the greatest metabolic demands (heart and brain) is maintained at the expense of the less essential tissues. When cardiac output is inadequate, increased adrenergic neurohumoral tone reduces blood flow to the skin, liver, kidneys and gastrointestinal tract. In addition to this, there is an increase in heart rate. The adrenergic effects account for the usual clinical signs of circulatory failure. The early signs are anxiety, restlessness and tachycardia with cool and pale extremities. Cardiogenic shock begins to develop with more severe failure so that tachycardia, pallor and cold extremities become more manifest and there is frequently pyrexia and oliguria. The common signs in the infant are feeding difficulties, failure to thrive, tachypnoea, tachycardia, rales, liver enlargement and cardiomegaly. Peripheral oedema, ascites, pulses alternans, gallop rhythm and sweating of the face and forehead are less frequent. These are more likely to occur when coexisting heart disease is aggravated by anaemia or negative inotropic features.

Treatment of circulatory failure

The general principles of treatment of circulatory failure are to increase tissue oxygen supply, to reduce tissue consumption and to correct anaemia and any metabolic abnormalities. The agents available include inotropic drugs, diuretics and vasodilators. It is important to correct for hypovolaemia by volume infusion and to control any cardiac arrhythmias.

The initial management of cardiogenic shock is to intubate and ventilate the patient using at least 50% oxygen. A central venous line is inserted percutaneously. Arterial blood gases, haematocrit, serum electrolytes, glucose and calcium are all determined so that acidosis, hypoxia and metabolic abnormalities can be corrected. If coexisting heart disease is likely, it may be possible to establish the diagnosis rapidly and to assess ventricular function by cross-sectional echocardiography. If the systemic blood flow is likely to be duct-dependent, prostaglandin E_1 or E_2 should be administered intravenously. Heart rate and the electrocardiogram should be monitored continuously and blood pressure measured either every 15 minutes (or preferably continuously by the use of an indwelling cannula placed in the radial artery). A routine infection screen should be performed and, if sepsis seems likely, broad spectrum antibiotics commenced.

Two major types of cardiogenic shock are encountered in practice. In the first, usually in the neonate or infant, major congenital heart disease is associated with hypovolaemia, often because of an excessive diuresis caused by the administration of diuretics. The same situation may occur when there has been excessive blood loss. Central venous pressure will be low. The initial treatment should be to give intravenous plasma (or dextrose-saline) 10 ml/kg over a period of 10 minutes. This can be repeated if the central venous pressure remains low. Replacement of blood volume should increase the systemic blood pressure, causing peripheral skin temperature to rise and core temperature to fall. An inotropic agent such as dopamine may also be helpful. The second clinical picture encoun-

tered is that of cardiogenic shock associated with a high central venous pressure. Initial treatment should be by intravenous frusemide or an inotropic agent such as dopamine and nitroprusside. When there is severe systemic obstruction or high pulmonary blood flow, medical management may produce only marginal improvement. Emergency surgery will almost certainly then be required. When cardiogenic shock complicates supraventricular or ventricular tachycardia, cardioversion is the preferred immediate treatment, since many anti-arrhythmic agents have a marked negative inotropic effect.

Drug treatment of circulatory failure

Digitalis

The modern history of digoxin began in 1775 when William Withering demonstrated the therapeutic effects of foxglove in dropsy. Much later, Gold & Cattell (1944) recognised that cardiac glycosides produced a direct positive inotropic action on heart muscle. There is convincing evidence that acute digoxin therapy enhances the contractility of the myocardium, resulting in a decreased end-diastolic volume and increased ejection fraction of the left ventricle (Weissler et al, 1964; Braunwald et al, 1965). It appears that digoxin increases cardiac output when there is heart failure but not in the normal heart. The greatest clinical improvement occurs when there is generalised depression of myocardial contractility (Mason et al, 1969). The benefits of chronic digoxin therapy have been questioned (Dall, 1970) but there is convincing evidence of its efficacy (Carliner et al, 1974; Kleiman et al, 1978). There are, however, theoretical objections to the use of digoxin in infants with high pulmonary blood flow and severe left ventricular volume overload. These patients already have an extremely high cardiac output and consequently the use of an inotropic agent is unlikely to be of any significant benefit.

There are numerous drug interactions with digoxin that are of note. Quinidine may significantly increase the serum digoxin concentration (Doering, 1979). Spironolactone actively inhibits the secretion of digoxin by renal tubules (Steiness, 1974). Recent information supports the use of lower doses of digoxin for premature and term infants than has often been recommended in the past (Hofstetter et al, 1979; Nyberg & Wettrell, 1978; Sandor et al, 1980). The recommendations listed in Table 16.5 are based upon these studies and should maintain a serum digoxin level within the therapeutic range of 1–3 ng/ml.

Diuretics (Table 16.6)

Diuretics are the mainstay of treatment for circulatory failure. Their effect is to remove excessive extracellular fluid. A variety of drugs are available, but the most

Table 16.5 Digoxin – dose regime.

Age/weight	Digitalising dose (μg/kg over 24 hours)		Maintenance dose (μg/kg twice daily)	
	i.v.	Oral	i.v.	Oral
Preterm under 1.5 kg	20	30	2	3
Preterm 1.5–2.5 kg	30	40	3	4
Term neonate to 2 years	35	50	3	5
Over 2 years	40	40	4	4

Note: Maximum dose 1.5 mg twice daily

Table 16.6 Diuretic agents – dose regime.

Drug	i.v.	Oral
Frusemide	0.5–1 mg/kg/dose 2 or 3 times daily	0.5–3 mg/kg/dose 2 or 3 times daily
Ethacrynic acid	0.5–1 mg/kg/dose 2 times daily	25 mg/m² BSA daily (Daily dose may be increased as required)
Bumetamide	10–20 μg/kg/dose 2 or 3 times daily	10–60 μg/kg/dose 2 or 3 times daily
Chlorothiazide		10–30 mg/kg/dose 12-hourly
Hydrochlorothiazide		1–3 mg/kg/dose 12-hourly
Spironolactone		1–3 mg/kg/dose 12-hourly
Mannitol	0.5–2.0 g/kg/dose	

Note: Information on the use of ethacrynic acid and bumetamide in infants and children is limited. They should probably not be used routinely. When they are indicated, relatively low starting doses are preferred.

commonly used in infants and children are frusemide, thiazides, spironolactone and mannitol. The newborn infant presents special problems because of the well-recognised inability to excrete a sodium load, thus increasing extracellular fluid and giving rise to oedema (Spitzer, 1978). The reasons for this frequently observed phenomenon are uncertain. It may be related to an extremely low glomerular filtration rate, to preferential blood flow to juxtamedullary nephrons or to the relatively high concentration of renin-angiotensin and aldosterone in the newborn compared with the adult.

The action of a diuretic is to promote the excretion of sodium and water in urine and thus decrease the extracellular fluid volume. The most important osmotic diuretic is mannitol (Mudge, 1970). Saliuretic diuretics directly promote the excretion of sodium and/or chloride with accompanying water. These drugs act along various segments of the renal tubule. Frusemide and thiazide preparations are those most commonly used in children. Richardson (1971) found that infants ranging in age from three days to six months with heart failure responded to 1.0–1.25 mg/kg of frusemide administered intramuscularly within 20–40 minutes of treatment. The mean urine volume was increased almost 4-fold and was accompanied by a 10-fold increase in sodium excretion, a 13-fold increase in chloride excretion and an almost 7-fold increase in free water clearance. Potassium excretion was not altered. The duration of response in infants is somewhat lengthened when compared to adults and may be up to 5–6 hours (Ross et al, 1978). Frusemide is highly bound to human albumin but this does not present a threat to the infant with hyperbilirubinaemia (Aranda et al, 1978). In contrast to frusemide, the thiazide diuretics cause only a modest diuresis. Walker & Cumming (1964) found that a standard dosage caused a 1.5-fold increase in urine volume, a 5-fold increase in sodium excretion, a 1.5-fold increase in potassium excretion and a 2.5-fold increase in chloride excretion in an 8-hour period of observation. Spironolactone has relatively little clinical efficacy when used alone and is best used in combination with thiazides

or frusemide in order to prevent potassium loss and hypokalaemia. It may be of particular use in the patient with liver failure when the metabolic breakdown of alderosterone is reduced. Mannitol is used primarily to reduce intracranial pressure in cases of cerebral oedema. Recommended dosages for the commonly used diuretics are shown in Table 16.6.

Diuretics have important complications. In neonates and infants they may induce an excessive diuresis leading to hypovolaemia which will exacerbate the existing low cardiac output. Hypokalaemia may occur following the use of proximal tube diuretics such as mannitol, loop diuretics or distal tube diuretics such as thiazides. Compensatory changes, however, will tend to minimise the continued loss of potassium in patients on long-term treatment. The use of excessive sodium or water will exacerbate potassium loss. It should be emphasised that the use of potassium-sparing diuretics (such as spironolactone) may be associated with hyperkalaemia, particularly in patients with reduced renal function. For this reason potassium supplementation in the form of fruit, orange juice or potassium preparations may be a much safer approach. Alkalosis is often seen in conjunction with total potassium depletion following the use of loop diuretics and thiazides. Hyponatraemia is a common complication, but it is important to avoid the temptation to administer excessive amounts of sodium supplements. Other complications of thiazides and frusemide include hyperuricaemia, hypercalcaemia, intestinal nephritis and hyperglycaemia. Ethnacrynic acid and frusemide have been associated with deafness. Most of these latter complications tend to be infrequent and should not preclude the use of the drugs.

Table 16.7 Vasodilators – dose regime.

Nitroglycerine	$0.5–20\ \mu g/kg/min$ i.v.
Nitroprusside	$0.5–8\ \mu g/kg/min$ i.v.
Salbutamol	$0.1–1\ \mu g/kg/min$ i.v.
Hydrallazine	$1–2\ \mu g/kg/min$ i.v. $0.1–1$ mg/kg/dose i.v. 6-hourly $0.5–1$ mg/kg/dose orally 8-hourly
Chlorpromazine	0.2 mg/kg i.v. bolus up to 3 times hourly
Captopril Under 1 month 1 month–1 year Over 1 years	$0.1–0.5$ mg/kg/dose orally up to 6-hourly $0.5–2$ mg/kg/dose orally up to 6-hourly $0.5–1$ mg/kg/dose orally 12-hourly
Prazosin	$5–25\ \mu g/kg/dose$ 6-hourly
Prostaglandin E_1	$0.05–1\ \mu g/kg/min$ i.v.
Prostaglandin E_2	$0.01–0.05\ \mu g/kg/min$ i.v.
Oral prostaglandin E_2	$20\ \mu g/kg/h$ may be given every 3–4 hours
Prostacyclin	$5–20$ ng/kg/min i.v.
Tolazoline	$0.5–1$ mg/kg dose i.v. $0.2–1$ mg/kg/h i.v.

Vasodilators (Table 16.7)

Vasodilators offer an alternative treatment in the management of congestive heart failure for patients who have not shown a satisfactory response to conventional treatment (Chatterjee & Parmley, 1977, 1980, 1983). A variety of drugs have been used successfully in patients with mitral or aortic regurgitation, myocardial ischaemia and following cardiopulmonary bypass (Benson et al, 1979). Myocardial failure is accompanied by ventricular dilation which increases ventricular end-diastolic volume resulting initially in an increased cardiac output. Systemic or pulmonary venous pressures rise with increased dilation, thus promoting peripheral or pulmonary oedema. As ventricular wall stress increases, myocardial oxygen requirements rise. The response to circulatory failure includes a rise in sympathetic tone (Burch, 1956) and an increase in circulating catecholamines (Pool & Braunwald, 1968). Changes in the renin-angiotensin system also occur which elevate the systemic vascular resistance in order to maintain systemic arterial pressure (Cohn, 1981). This in turn impairs left ventricular ejection.

Vasodilator drugs may be classified according to their site of action. Thus venodilators act predominantly by dilating systemic veins. Arteriolar vasodilators exert a more balanced effect on both veins and arteries.

Venodilators

Nitroglycerine and organic nitrates act directly to relax the smooth muscle in large veins and produce a significant reduction in systemic and pulmonary venous pressure. This reduces venous return to the heart and improves cardiac output (Mason, 1978). They are helpful in patients with pulmonary oedema occurring secondary to aortic or mitral regurgitation (Sniderman et al, 1974). Their principal use, however, is following cardiac surgery when low cardiac output is accompanied by elevated filling pressures (Benson et al, 1979). It is self-evident that they should not be administered to patients with a low preload, low capillary wedge or low ventricular end-diastolic pressures, because they will further reduce cardiac output.

Arteriolar and mixed dilators

Hydrallazine acts predominantly upon the precapillary arterioles, but also on venous capacitance vessels (Loggie et al, 1979). Bio-availability is greater following parenteral administration. It is useful in the treatment of hypertension and congestive heart failure. The most serious side-effect is a lupus-like syndrome which occurs in so-called 'slow hepatic acetylators' (Perry et al, 1970). This syndrome usually disappears spontaneously when administration of the drug is stopped.

Captopril exerts its action as a competitive inhibitor of angiotensin-converting enzyme (Ondetti et al, 1977). It is administered prior to meals or feeding and the dose must be reduced in patients with impaired renal function (Ferguson & Vlassis, 1981). Its action is to reduce systemic resistance. Occasionally proteinuria and neutropenia have been observed (Erslev et al, 1982; Gavras et al, 1978).

Sodium nitroprusside acts directly and equally on arterial and venous smooth muscle (Palmer & Lasseter, 1975). Thus, it reduces pulmonary and systemic vascular resistance and hence may be particularly useful in patients with an elevated pulmonary vascular resistance (Rubis et al, 1981). It is frequently used in infants and children who have undergone cardiac surgery, often in combination with dopamine. It is important to be aware of the complication of thiocyanate intoxication which may result in fatigue, nausea, anorexia and disorientation and even cyanide toxicity (Dillon et al, 1980). Of practical importance is the tendency to rapid photochemical degradation within 6 hours.

Prazosin is a post-synaptic alpha-adrenergic blocking agent which is administered orally and relaxes both arterial and venous smooth muscle (Chatterjee & Parmley, 1980). It is particularly useful for the treatment of chronic congestive heart failure (Mehta et al, 1978).

Tolazoline is an alpha-adrenergic blocking agent which may be particularly useful in lowering pulmonary vascular resistance, but may reduce systemic resistance as well (Ward, 1984). It is a histamine agonist and a direct vasodilator with sympathetic and cholinergic activity (Drummond & Lock, 1984). It has been used effectively for the management of pulmonary hypertensive crises following cardiac surgery in patients with an elevated pulmonary vascular resistance. Significant side-effects include increased gastrointestinal secretions, gastrointestinal, renal and pulmonary haemorrhage, seizures, hyponatraemia and thrombocytopaenia (Jones et al, 1981; Ward, 1984).

Prostacyclin is an arachidonic acid metabolite which is continuously secreted by vascular endothelial cells (Moncada et al, 1976). Almost alone among the prostagladins, it is not metabolised by the lungs. It has many putative local effects on blood vessels, platelets and their interactions (Data et al, 1981). Prostacyclin was thought to be a highly selective pulmonary vasodilator on the basis of animal experiments. Studies in infants with pulmonary hypertension confirm that it is a more selective pulmonary vasodilator than other prostaglandins (Kadowitz et al, 1978). Dose-response curves for the effects of prostacyclin on the pulmonary and systemic circulation in children with pulmonary hypertension complicating congenital heart disease have been obtained by Bush and his co-workers (1985). Results were obtained with children breathing both air and 100% oxygen. Prostacyclin caused a dose-dependent fall in pulmonary vascular resistance. When infused whilst the subjects were breathing 100% oxygen, prostacyclin caused additional dose-dependent pulmonary vasodilatation. Unlike 100% oxygen, prostacyclin was not selective and caused tachycardia and systemic hypotension at the higher dose.

The beneficial effects of the use of intravenous prostaglandin E_1 or E_2 in the treatment of neonates with duct dependent systemic flood flow is now well established (Heymann & Rudolph, 1977). These drugs are life saving in the treatment of infants with aortic coarctation, interruption of the aortic arch, critical aortic stenosis and the hypoplastic left heart syndrome. The major complications include hypotension, pyrexia, jitteriness, seizures, apnoea and diarrhoea. Most are, to some extent, dose-related. Certainly the advantages produced in this group of patients with duct-dependent systemic circulation far outweigh the risks of complications. The role of prostaglandins is to treat and prevent the development of a metabolic acidosis so that investigation and surgical treatment can be carried out with the infant in the best possible condition.

Table 16.8 Sympathomimetic agents – dose regime.

Isoprenaline (isoproterenol)	0.05–0.5 μg/kg/min i.v.
Adrenaline (epinephrine)	0.05–0.2 μg/kg/min i.v.
Noradrenaline (norepinephrine)	0.02–0.2 μg/kg/min i.v.
Dopamine	2–10 μg/kg/min i.v.
Dobutamine	2–10 μg/kg/min i.v.

Inotropic agents (Table 16.8)

The receptor sites in the cardiovascular system for catecholamines were described by Alquist in 1948. Adrenergically-induced arterial vasoconstriction of cutaneous, coronary, splanchnic and renal vessels is mediated by alpha receptors. Vasodilation is mediated by beta-2 receptors located predominantly in skeletal muscle. Beta-1 receptors

Table 16.9 Receptor response to adrenergic stimuli.

Tissue	Receptor	Response
Heart		
Sinus node	beta-1	Increased rate
Atrioventricular node	beta-1	Increased rate
Atria	beta-1	Increased contractility
Ventricles	beta-1	Increased contractility
Coronary circulation	alpha	Vasoconstriction
Cardiac metabolism	beta-1	Increased glycogenolysis and oxygen consumption
Peripheral vasculature		
Skin and mucosa	alpha	Vasoconstriction
Skeletal muscle	beta-2	Vasodilation
Renal, splanchnic	alpha	Vasoconstriction
	delta	Vasodilation

are located in the atria, the ventricles and the conduction system. They mediate increased heart rate, increased myocardial contractility and cardiac metabolism. Delta receptors mediate splanchnic and renal dilation and respond specifically to dopamine (Goldberg et al, 1972). The receptor responses to adrenergic stimuli are listed in Table 16.9.

Pure alpha agonists include phenylephrine and methoxamine and pure antagonists include tolazoline and phentolamine. Isoprenaline is a pure beta agonist whereas beta blockers such as propranolol are beta antagonists. Droperidol is a delta antagonist.

Sympathomimetic amines

The most common use of these drugs is in the intensive care unit following cardiac surgery. They are occasionally of use in patients with severe circulatory failure requiring intensive therapy. Noradrenaline is primarily an alpha agonist with mild beta-1 or cardiac effects (Goldberg et al, 1972). Its effect is to increase systemic resistance, but it is also a mild inotrope and may cause renal ischaemia. Adrenaline is primarily a beta agonist when given at low doses (up to 0.1 μg/kg/min). With increasing doses, it behaves as an alpha antagonist with only moderate beta-1 effects (Goldberg et al, 1972). Isoprenaline is a pure beta-adrenergic agonist that produces cardiac intropic and chronotropic effects with dilatation of skeletal muscle beds. It causes a fall in systemic vascular resistance (Gifford et al, 1968). The effect of vasodilatation is often to reduce venous return to the heart. It also increases myocardial oxygen consumption and may occasionally induce cardiac arrhythmias.

Dopamine activates delta, beta and alpha receptors in a dose-dependent fashion. At 2–4 μg/kg/min, its main effect is on renal and splanchnic vessels. It thus decreases systemic vascular resistance. In the dose range of 4–8 μg/kg/min, dopamine has a positive inotropic action (beta-1) together with systemic vascular (beta-2) effects. Significant alpha vasconstriction is produced with doses greater than 10 μ/kg/min.

Dobutamine, a synthetic catecholamine derived from chemical manipulation of isoprenaline, increases myocardial contractility with minimal peripheral vasconstriction (Akhtar et al, 1975). Its effect is to increase myocardial contractility by direct action on myocardial beta-1-adrenergic receptors. Beta-adrenergic blocking agents may make the drug ineffective. Dobutamine only occasionally causes tachycardia and produces little vasoconstriction at the usual therapeutic doses. It does not dilate renal and mesenteric vessels as dopamine does, although renal and splanchnic blood flow may increases as a consequence of improved cardiac output.

Table 16.10 Other useful inotropic agents.

Aminophylline	1 mg/kg i.v. bolus
Calcium chloride	0.025–0.1 mmol/kg/h i.v.

Other inotropic agents (Table 16.10)

Aminophylline has a mild positive inotropic and chronotropic effect. It relaxes smooth muscle and is a mild diuretic. It may produce a marked diuresis when used in combination with frusemide. Calcium chloride exerts a positive inotropic effect and produces a modest increase in systemic vascular resistance (Hardman, 1962). Hypocalcaemia occurs frequently in infants and children with circulatory failure. It is important to note that the total serum calcium does not reflect the ionised fraction in this unstable situation. Low cardiac output may respond dramatically to intravenous calcium given by bolus or continuous infusion.

Selection of the appropriate inotropic agent

The selection of the appropriate inotropic agent can be extremely difficult, particularly for infants and children following cardiac surgery. Noradrenaline is rarely used, since it produces such marked peripheral vasoconstriction. Adrenaline has a significantly greater beta-2 action and the vasoconstriction caused by its alpha-adrenergic stimulation is less. It is used primarily to treat low cardiac output after cardiac surgery. Isoprenaline causes an increase in myocardial oxygen consumption out of proportion to the increase in cardiac output. It is most useful when there is significant bradycardia or when other inotropic agents have failed. Dopamine has less chronotropic effects than isoprenaline and results in far less peripheral vasoconstriction than either adrenaline or noradrenaline. It is particularly useful in the treatment of circulatory failure following cardiac surgery. It is also valuable in treating transient myocardial ischaemia and other types of cardiogenic shock. Dobutamine improves myocardial contractility, but has

less chronotropic and vascular side-effects than isoprenaline. It does not exert any dopaminergic renal effects, but may be usefully be combined with a low dose of dopamine.

The drug treatment of hypoxia

The newborn infant with severe subpulmonary stenosis or pulmonary atresia depends upon patency of the arterial duct to provide adequate pulmonary blood flow and oxygen uptake. Infants with pulmonary atresia with ventricular septal defect, pulmonary atresia with intact ventricular septum, tetralogy of Fallot with severe infundibular stenosis and other types of congenital heart disease associated with severe subpulmonary stenosis or pulmonary atresia often present in the first week of life with severe hypoxia leading to acidosis. The intravenous administration of prostaglandin E_1 or E_2 dilates the arterial duct, thus increasing pulmonary blood flow and reducing the degree of hypoxia and preventing or reversing acidosis (Heymann & Rudolph, 1977). An intravenous infusion of prostaglandin should be commenced immediately whenever there is clinical suspicion of duct-dependent pulmonary blood flow. The arterial oxygen tension rises within 30 minutes of treatment. The complications of prostaglandins have already been listed and these should not be considered a contraindication to its administration. Oral prostaglandins may be used as long-term treatment (Silove et al, 1981), but in practice are rarely indicated, as a systemic to pulmonary artery shunt procedure is preferable.

Apart from infants with duct-dependent pulmonary blood flow, prostaglandins may also be of limited use in the neonate with hypoxia due to complete transposition. Dilation of the arterial duct in this setting increases pulmonary blood flow and improves mixing at atrial level and may also allow shunting from the pulmonary artery to the aorta. In some instances the increase in left atrial pressure gives rise to marked tachypnoea. Prostaglandin infusion should therefore be considered as a short-term palliative treatment.

When severe hypoxia is not associated with duct-dependent pulmonary blood flow, usually outside the neonatal period, drug treatment is rarely indicated and palliative or corrective surgery is required. The major exception is the occurrence of hypercyanotic spells in patients with tetralogy of Fallot (see Ch. 32). Although this complication is an absolute indication for surgery, acute or short-term treatment with propranolol is often effective. If severe hypoxia complicates pulmonary vascular disease as occurs in other patients with severe restriction in pulmonary blood in whom palliative or corrective surgery cannot be undertaken, heart and lung transplantation may be the only effective method of treatment.

REFERENCES

Akhtar N, Mikulic E, Cohn J N, Chaudhry M H 1975 Hemodynamic effect of dobutamine in patients with severe heart failure. American Journal of Cardiology 36: 202–205

Alquist R P 1948 Study of the adrenotropic receptor. American Journal of Physiology 153: 586–597

Aranda J V, Perez J, Sitar D S, et al 1978 Pharmacokinetic disposition and protein binding of furosemide in newborn infants. Journal of Pediatrics 93: 507–511

Benson L N, Bohn D, Edmonds J F 1979 Nitroglycerin therapy in children with low cardiac index after heart surgery. Cardiovascular Medicine 4: 207–215

Berman W Jr, Christensen D 1983 Effects of acute preload and afterload stress on myocardial function in newborn and adult sheep. Biology of the Neonate 43: 61–66

Braunwald E, Mason D T, Ross J Jr 1965 Studies on cardiocirculatory actions of digitalis. Medicine (Baltimore) 44: 233–248

Burch G E 1956 Evidence for increased venous tone in chronic congestive heart failure. Archives of Internal Medicine 98: 750–766

Bush A, Busst C M, Shinebourne E A 1985 The use of oxygen and prostacyclin as pulmonary vasodilators in congenital heart disease. International Journal of Cardiology 9: 267–270

Carliner N H, Gilbert C A, Pruitt A W, Goldberg L I 1974 Effects of maintenance digoxin therapy on systolic time intervals and serum digoxin concentrations. Circulation 50: 94–98

Chatterjee K, Parmley W W 1977 The role of vasodilator therapy in heart failure. Progress in Cardiovascular Diseases 19: 301–325

Chatterjee K, Parmley W W 1980 Vasodilator therapy in chronic heart failure. Annual Review of Pharmacology and Toxicology 20: 475–512

Chatterjee K, Parmley W W 1983 Vasodilator therapy for acute myocardial infarction and chronic congestive heart failure. Journal of the American College of Cardiology 1: 133–153

Cohn J 1981 Physiologic basis of vasodilator therapy for heart failure. American Journal of Medicine 71: 135–139

Dall J L C 1970 Maintenance digoxin in elderly patients. British Medical Journal 2: 705–706

Data J L, Moloney B A, Meinzinger M M, Gorman R R 1981 Intravenous infusion of prostacyclin sodium in man: clinical effects and influence on platelet adenosine diphosphate sensitivity and adenosine 3′:5′-cyclic monophosphate levels. Circulation 64: 4–8

Dillon T R, Janos G G, Meyer R A, Benzing G, III, Kaplan S 1980 Vasodilator therapy for congestive heart failure. Journal of Pediatrics 96: 623–629

Doering W 1979 Quinidine-digoxin interaction: pharmacokinetics, underlying mechanism and clinical implications. New England Journal of Medicine 301: 400–404

Drummond W H, Lock J E 1984 Neonatal pulmonary vasodilation drugs, current status. Developmental Pharmacological Therapeutics 7: 1–20

Erslev A V, Alexander J C, Caro J 1982 Hematologic side effects of captopril and associated risk factors. Cardiovascular Review Reports 3: 660–671

Ferguson R K, Vlassis P H 1981 Clinical pharmacology and therapeutic applications of the new oral angiotensin-converting enzyme inhibitor, captopril. American Heart Journal 101: 650–656

Friedman W F 1972 The intrinsic physiologic properties of the developing heart. Progress in Cardiovascular Diseases 1: 87–111

Gavras H, Faxon D P, Berkoben J, Brunner H R, Ryan T J 1978 Angiotensin-converting enzyme inhibition in patients with congestive heart failure. Circulation 58: 770–776

Gifford R M, MacCannell K L, McNay J L 1968 Changes in regional blood flows induced by dopamine and by isoproterenol during experimental hemorrhagic shock. Canadian Journal of Physiology and Pharmacology 46: 847–851

Gold H, Cattell M 1944 Clinical studies on digitoxin (Digitaline Nativelle): further observations as its use in the single average full dose method of digitalization. Journal of Pharmacology and Experimental Therapy 82: 187–196

Goldberg L I, Bloodwell R D, Braunwald E, Morrow A G 1972 The direct effects of norepinephrine, epinephrine and methoxamine on myocardial contractile force in man. Circulation 22: 1125–1132

Hardman H F 1962 Molecular form of theophylline responsible for positive inotropic activity. Circulation Research 10: 598–607

Heymann M A, Rudolph A M 1977 Ductus arteriosus dilatation by prostaglandin E1 in infants with pulmonary atresia. Pediatrics 59: 325–329

Heymann M A, Rudolph A M, Silverman N H 1976 Closure of the ductus arteriosus in premature infants by inhibition of prostaglandin synthesis. New England Journal of Medicine 295: 530–533

Hofstetter R, Land E, Von Bernuth G 1979 Effect of digoxin on left ventricular contractility in newborns and infants estimated by echocardiography. European Journal of Cardiology 9: 1–11

Hougan T J, Schuessler R, Friedman W F 1982 Age-related effects of digoxin on myocardial contractility and Na-K pump in sheep. American Journal of Physiology 243: H517–522

Jones O D H, Shore D F, Ribgy M L, et al 1981 The use of tolazoline hydrochloride as a pulmonary vasodilator in potentially fatal episodes of pulmonary vasoconstriction after cardiac surgery in children. Circulation 64 (Suppl II): 134–139

Kadowitz P J, Chapnick B M, Feigen L P, Hyman A L, Nelson P K, Spannhake E W 1978 Pulmonary and systemic vascular effects of the newly discovered prostaglandin PGI2. Journal of Applied Physiology 45: 408–411

Kirkpatrick S E, Nabiloff J, Pitlick P T, Friedman W F 1975 The influence of post-stimulation potentiation and heart rate on the fetal lamb heart. American Journal of Physiology 229: 318–323

Kirkpatrick S E, Pitlick P T, Nabiloff J, Friedman W F 1976 Frank-Starling relationship as an important determinant of fetal cardiac output. American Journal of Physiology 231: 495–500

Kleiman J H, Ingels W B, Daughters G, II, Stinson E B, Alderman E L, Goldman R H 1978 Left ventricular dynamics during long-term digoxin treatment in patients with stable coronary artery disease. American Journal of Cardiology 41: 937–942

Leanage R, Agnetti A, Graham G, Taylor J, Macartney F J 1981 Factors influencing survival after balloon atrial septostomy for complete transposition of the great arteries. British Heart Journal 45: 559–572

Little R C, Little W C 1982 Cardiac preload, afterload and heart failure. Archives of Internal Medicine 142: 819–822

Loggie J M H, New M I, Robson A M 1979 Hypertension in the pediatric patient: a reappraisal. Journal of Pediatrics 94: 685–699

Macartney F J, Taylor J F N, Graham G R, De Level M, Stark J 1980 The fate of survivors of cardiac surgery in infancy. Circulation 62: 80–91

Macartney F J, Douglas J, Spiegelhalter D 1984 To catheterise or not to catheterise? An approach based on decision theory. British Heart Journal 51: 330–338

Mason D T 1978 Afterload reduction and cardiac performance. Physiologic basis of systemic vasodilators as a new approach in treatment of congestive heart failure. American Journal of Medicine 65: 106–125

Mason D T, Spann J F Jr, Zelis R 1969 New developments in the understanding of the actions of the digitalis glycosides. Progress in Cardiovascular Diseases 6: 443–478

McPherson R A, Kramer M F, Covell J W, Friedman W F 1976 A comparison of the active stiffness of fetal and adult cardiac muscle. Pediatric Research 10: 660–664

Mehta J, Iacona M, Feldman R L, Pepine C J, Conti C R 1978 Comparative hemodynamic effects of intravenous nitroprusside and oral prazosin in refractory heart failure. American Journal of Cardiology 41: 925–930

Milnor W R 1975 Arterial impedance as ventricular afterload. Circulation Research 36: 565–570

Moncada S, Gryglewski R, Bunting S, Vane J R 1976 An enzyme isolated from arteries transforms prostaglandin endoperoxides to an unstable substance that inhibits platelet aggregation. Nature 263: 663–665

Mudge G R 1970 Diuretics and other agents employed in mobilization of edema fluid. In: Goodman L S, Gilman L (eds) The Pharmacological bases of therapeutics. Macmillan, New York, p 839

Nyberg L, Wettrell G 1978 Digoxin dosage schedules for neonates and infants based on pharmacokinetic considerations. Clinical Pharmacokinetics 3: 453–461

Ondetti M A, Rubin B, Cushman D W 1977 Design of specific inhibition of angiotensin converting enzyme: new class of orally active antihypertensive agents. Science 196: 441–444

Palmer R F, Lasseter K C 1975 Sodium nitroprusside. New England Journal of Medicine 292: 294–297

Perry H M Jr, Tan E M, Carmody S 1970 Relationship of acetyl transferase activity to antinuclear antibodies and toxic symptoms in hypertensive patients treated with hydralazine. Journal of Laboratory and Clinical Medicine 76: 114–125

Pool P E, Braunwald E 1968 Fundamental mechanisms in congestive heart failure. American Journal of Cardiology 22: 7–15

Richardson H 1971 Furosemide in heart failure of infancy. Archives of Disease in Childhood 46: 520–524

Romero T E, Friedman W F 1979 Limited left ventricular response to volume overload in the neonatal period. A comparative study with the adult animal. Pediatric Research 13: 910–915

Ross B S, Pollak A, Oh W 1978 The pharmacologic effects of furosemide therapy in the low-birth-weight infant. Journal of Pediatrics 92: 149–52

Ross J Jr 1976 Afterload mismatch and preload reserve: a conceptual framework for the analysis of ventricular function. Progress in Cardiovascular Diseases 4: 255–264

Rubis L J, Stephenson L W, Johnston M R, Nagaraj S, Edmunds L H Jr 1981 Comparison of effects of prostaglandin E1 and nitroprusside on pulmonary vascular resistance in children after open-heart surgery. Annals of Thoracic Surgery 32: 563–570

Sandor G G, Bloom K R, Izukawa T, Patterson M W, Rowe R D 1980 Noninvasive assessment of left ventricular function related to serum digoxin levels in neonates. Pediatrics 65: 541–546

Sheldon C A, Friedman W F, Sybers H D 1976 Scanning electron microscopy of fetal and neonatal lamb cardiac cells. Journal of Molecular and Cellular Cardiology 8: 853–862

Silove E D, Coe J Y, Shiu M F, et al 1981 Oral prostaglandin E_2 in ductus-dependent pulmonary circulation. Circulation 63: 682–688

Sniderman A D, Marpole D G G, Palmer W H, Fallen E L 1974 Response of the left ventricle to nitroglycerin in patients with and without mitral regurgitation. British Heart Journal 36: 357–361

Spitzer A 1978 Renal physiology and functional development. In: Edelmann C M Jr (ed) Pediatric kidney disease. Little, Brown & Co, Boston, p 25

Steiness E 1974 Renal tubular secretion of digoxin. Circulation 50: 103–7

Walker R D, Cumming G R 1964 Response of the infant kidney to diuretic drugs. Canadian Medical Association Journal 91: 1149–1153

Ward R M 1984 Pharmacology of tolazoline. Clinical Perinatology 17: 703–713

Weber K T, Janicki J S 1979 The heart as a muscle-pump system and the concept of heart failure. American Heart Journal 98: 371–394

Weinstein M C, Fineberg H V, Elstein A S, et al 1980 Clinical Decision Analysis. Saunders, Philadelphia

Weissler A M, Gamel W G, Grode H E, Cohen H, Schoenfeld C D 1964 The effect of digitalis on ventricular ejection in normal human subjects. Circulation 29: 721–729

Yacoub M, Bernhard A, Lange P, et al 1980 Clinical and hemodynamic results of the two-stage anatomic correction of simple transposition of the great arteries. Circulation 62 (Suppl I): 190–196

17

Principles of surgical treatment

The trends in cardiac surgery for congenital heart defects over the last two decades have been characterised by repair increasingly earlier in life along with the development of new procedures for most complex anomalies. After an overwhelming enthusiasm for primary intracardiac repair of congenital heart defect in early infancy, however, a more subtle attitude has been adopted by most surgical units in more recent years. There is no doubt that open heart surgery under 3 months of age carries a higher risk than later in life. Unless surgical treatment is mandatory and satisfactory palliation not available, cardiopulmonary bypass in that age-group is best avoided. With the exception of superb results obtained in a few isolated centres for repair of tetralogy of Fallot in infancy, for example, many surgeons are more confident of achieving consistently good results when the operation is performed in childhood. This example illustrates the paradoxical tendency to carry out more palliative operations now than perhaps were performed 10 years ago.

The development of ingenious intracardiac repairs for complex transpositions, double outlet ventricles, double inlet ventricles, the use of extracardiac valved conduits and the description of the Fontan operation made most complex congenital cardiac anomalies amenable to surgical treatment. Late complications following these formidable procedures are, unfortunately, not uncommon. Subarterial obstructions have been reported after insertion of complex intraventricular prosthetic baffles. The incidence of conduit stenosis due to heterograft valve degeneration is such that some surgeons are now advocating the use of valveless conduits. Alternatively, we would rather accept a moderate ventricular outflow tract gradient than incorporate an extracardiac valved conduit. The long-term results using fresh antibiotic preserved homografts are significantly better than those achieved with heterografts. Unfortunately they are not readily available. The Fontan operation became a valuable part of the surgical armamentarium for the treatment of several complex anomalies. The limitations of this circulation must, however, remain present in our minds. The necessity for the right atrial pressure to be significantly higher than the left atrial pressure so that blood flows through the pulmonary circulation provides the Fontan circulation with very little flexibility. An increase in the pulmonary vascular resistance, the development of left atrioventricular valve regurgitation and, more importantly, any increase in ventricular end-diastolic pressure are unlikely to be tolerated by these patients. Our future efforts should therefore be concentrated on a careful and meticulous analysis of the long-term results.

In this chapter, it is my aim to discuss briefly the current techniques and results of the most common operations. A number of these operations are open-heart procedures which are performed on cardiopulmonary bypass or under deep hypothermia and total circulatory arrest. Deep hypothermia and total circulatory arrest techniques provide the surgeon with a bloodless field and ideal working conditions. The limitations of this method relate to the potential side-effects of prolonged ischaemia. Studies in man have focused on the neurological changes after total circulatory arrest and on late psychomotor development. From the data currently available it appears to be safe to arrest the circulation for 45 minutes at a temperature of 18°C nasopharynx. We currently use the technique of deep hypothermia and total circulatory arrest in neonates and small infants with conditions such as total anomalous pulmonary venous connexion or other lesions which can be repaired within 45 mintues of circulatory arrest. Occasionally we use the same technique in larger patients with complex anomalies of systemic venous return.

Most intracardiac repairs, however, are now performed using hypothermic cardiopulmonary bypass. Hypothermia permits reduction of perfusion flow, thus improving visability and at the same time providing the surgeon with a margin of safety. The pump oxygenator consists of a venous reservoir, an oxygenator, a heat exchanger and an arterial pump. We currently use membrane oxygenators in infants and small children. They are supposed to produce less blood damage and require a smaller priming volume.

Direct caval cannulation for the venous return offers the same quality of total exposure as total circulatory arrest, which currently is less utilised. The superiority of cold cardioplegia as a means of myocardial protection has not been clearly demonstrated in infants. It appears, however, that cold cardioplegia increases the safe interval of aortic occlusion. For this reason, we use it more-or-less routinely in the majority of our patients.

PALLIATIVE PROCEDURES

Systemic to pulmonary and cavopulmonary shunts

The concept of improving systemic oxygen saturation in patients with cyanotic congenital heart disease and diminished pulmonary blood flow was introduced by Blalock & Taussig (1945) when they created a shunt between a systemic and a pulmonary artery. This was followed one year later by the description of an aortopulmonary anastomosis by Potts and colleagues (1946). In 1962, Waterston described an anastomosis between the ascending aorta and the right pulmonary artery as an alternative shunt procedure in infants. The use of prosthetic material for the construction of systemic to pulmonary artery shunts was reported by Redo & Ecker in 1963. With the development of microvascular surgical methods, the Blalock-Taussig operation continues to provide excellent palliation. This is even the case in infancy, when it can be performed on the side opposite to the aortic arch. The subclavian artery is then used as it takes origin from the brachiocephalic artery, thus minimising the risks of kinking its origin. The operation is performed through a lateral thoracotomy incision. An adequate length of pulmonary artery is dissected. The subclavian artery is mobilised and divided to be turned down and anastomosed to the pulmonary artery. With good mobilisation of the brachiocephalic and the carotid arteries, together with dissection of the deep groove between the superior caval vein and the trachea, it is possible in most instances to divide the subclavian artery at the level of its first branches (Fig. 17.1).

The Waterston anastomosis provided satisfactory palliation in small infants. It is not used frequently today, however, because of the relatively high incidence of distortion of the right pulmonary artery and the risk of creating too big a shunt. The latter results in the development of congestive heart failure and, later, pulmonary vascular disease. The Potts anastomosis has been almost completely abandoned because of the same risks and also because of the difficulties of closure at the time of the intracardiac repair. When the classical Blalock-Taussig anastomosis is not suitable, we now prefer the modified Blalock-Taussig shunt (de Leval et al, 1981). A prosthetic graft having a diameter greater than that of the origin of the subclavian artery is anastomosed end-to-side to the undivided subclavian artery and end-to-side to the pulmonary artery (Fig. 17.2). Blood flow through the shunt is limited by the diameter of the subclavian artery, thus preventing flooding of the lungs. The flow should increase with growth of the child.

Whereas these anastomoses are arterial in nature, Glenn & Patino (1954) described an experimental veno-arterial shunt for certain cyanotic heart defects. The operation involves connecting the distal end of the right pulmonary artery to the side of the superior caval vein, the venous channel then being ligated below the anastomosis. The main advantage of the cavopulmonary anastomosis is that approximately one-third of the systemic venous blood is

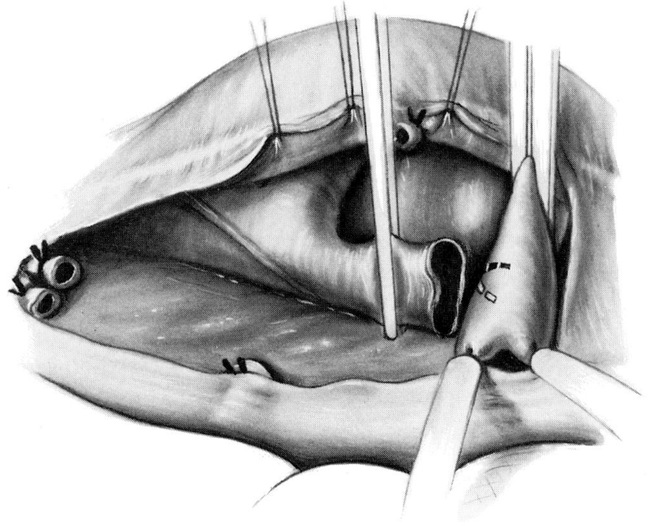

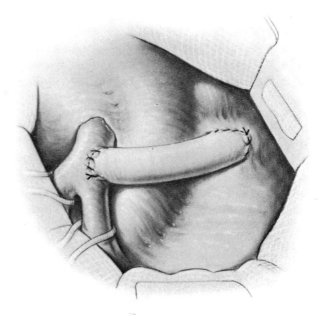

Fig. 17.1 Classical Blalock-Taussig shunt. The right subclavian artery is bowed down to the pulmonary artery.

Fig. 17.2 Modified Blalock-Taussig shunt interposing a prosthesis between the subclavian artery and the pulmonary artery.

directed to the right lung, bypassing the heart so that any overloading of the left ventricle is minimised. This has made it the procedure of choice for tricuspid atresia and other patients with hypoplastic right ventricles. The main current indication for the Glenn anastomosis is persistent systemic venous hypertension with a low cardiac output following an atriopulmonary anastomosis (Fontan procedure) for tricuspid atresia or double inlet ventricle.

Banding of the pulmonary trunk

Banding of the pulmonary trunk, suggested by Muller & Dammann in 1952, is currently indicated for patients with uncorrectable lesions who have a large left-to-right shunt at ventricular level, or in those in whom a palliative procedure is preferred to complete repair. This includes infants with multiple ventricular septal defects (swiss cheese septum) and others with coarctation of the aorta and large ventricular septal defects in whom the coarctation is relieved and the pulmonary trunk banded as a first stage procedure. Some surgeons continue to advocate banding of the pulmonary trunk for patients with complete transposition and ventricular septal defects who are under 3 months of age or those with atrioventricular septal defects who are in intractable congestive heart failure. The operation is done through a short left lateral or left anterior thoracotomy incision. The arterial duct (or ligament) is routinely dissected and ligated. Then a ligature of heavy plaited silk is passed around the pulmonary trunk and tied to produce an optimal degree of constriction. This is achieved when the systemic pressure reaches a plateau and the distal pulmonary pressure is 30–50% of the systemic pressure. This depends on the systemic arterial oxygen saturation and, therefore, on the underlying lesion.

Surgical atrial septectomy (Blalock-Hanlon procedure)

Surgical creation of an atrial septal defect was one of the milestones in the treatment of complete transposition (Blalock & Hanlon, 1950). Balloon atrial septostomy (Rashkind & Miller, 1966) has now, however, almost completely replaced surgical septectomy. Nonetheless, some surgeons perform surgical septectomies a few months after balloon atrial septostomy so as to delay the intra-atrial redirection of venous return (Mustard or Senning). This is not our practice, as we would rather proceed if necessary with an early intracardiac repair. We continue to do Blalock-Hanlon operations in patients with complete transposition and left ventricular outflow tract obstruction with or without a ventricular septal defect when it is advantageous to defer the repair for a few months (or even years). There are also some conditions not amenable to complete repair in which left atrial decompression may result in considerable improvement. This is the case for patients with severely hypoplastic or atretic left atrioven-

tricular connexions and intact atrial septum (or restrictive atrial septal defect). This applies also to occasional patients with right atrioventricular valve atresia, hypoplastic tricuspid valves and restrictive atrial septal defects.

Various techniques for the creation of an atrial septal defect have been suggested. We prefer the Blalock-Hanlon technique as modified by Aberdeen (1968). The pericardium is opened behind the right phrenic nerve through the fifth right intercostal space. Heavy ligatures are passed around the upper and lower pulmonary veins and around the right pulmonary artery. A partial occlusion clamp is placed with one jaw behind the pulmonary veins and the left atrium and the other anterior to the right atrium. When closed, portions of both the left and right atria are included in the clamp. An incision is made on the right and the left side of the septum which is grasped and excised. The atrial incision is then closed (Fig. 17.3). Surgical septectomy can also be performed under inflow occlusion or on cardiopulmonary bypass.

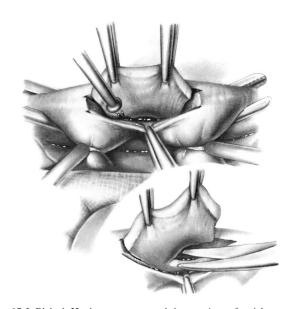

Fig. 17.3 Blalock-Hanlon septectomy. A larger piece of atrial septum is excised through an incision in the interatrial groove.

CORRECTIVE PROCEDURES

Persistent patency of the arterial duct (ductus arteriosus)

Intractable congestive heart failure is an indication for closure of a persistent arterial duct in infancy. Closure is indicated in childhood even in the absence of heart failure in order to prevent subacute bacterial endocarditis and pulmonary vascular obstructive disease. In the presence of increased pulmonary vascular resistance, we prefer not to operate on patients with a pulmonary arteriolar resistance greater than 8 units/m². We routinely close the arterial

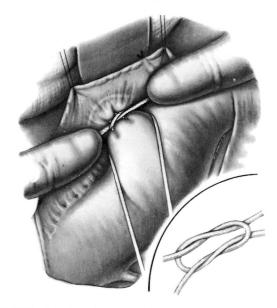

Fig. 17.4 Ligation of persistent arterial duct.

duct by ligation through a left lateral thoracotomy incision in the fourth intercostal space (Fig. 17.4). When the duct is particularly large, (and in the presence of severe pulmonary hypertension in older patients) it is preferable to use the technique of division between vascular clamps followed by suture. When the duct is associated with intracardiac lesions which are repaired at the same time, the dissection can be performed from a midline sternotomy incision. The duct is then ligated prior to or soon after initiation of cardiopulmonary bypass. The risk of closure as a single lesion is less than 0.5% (Panagopoulos et al, 1971). The risk increases if additional cardiac anomalies are present. The same applies when the pulmonary vascular resistance is increased. The operative mortality in premature infants has also remained higher than in older patients.

Coarctation of the aorta and interruption of aortic arch

Coarctation of the aorta

For practical purposes the surgeon has to deal with two groups of patients with aortic coarctation: the symptomatic infant and the asymptomatic older child.

If a clinical diagnosis of coarctation of the aorta is made in a neonate in severe heart failure (and if the cross-sectional echocardiogram shows continuity between ascending and descending aorta), the diagnosis is accepted without cardiac catheterisation unless associated intracardiac anomalies warrant further investigations. If at all possible, the surgical treatment is undertaken only if the patient is clinically stable, with a good cardiac output and in the absence of metabolic acidosis and/or renal failure.

When these are present (or if cardiac output is low) an intensive medical treatment is instituted. This consists of an infusion of prostaglandin E_1 (0.1 μg/K/min) and administration of digitalis and diuretics (Leanage et al, 1981). Mechanical ventilation and inotropic support may be necessary in the sickest infants prior to cardiac catheterisation (if indicated) and/or surgery. Patients in established renal failure are placed on peritoneal dialysis, often prior to surgery. Surgical treatment is indicated in all symptomatic infants as soon as they are clinically stable and in patients who continue to deteriorate in spite of maximum medical treatment. With increasing expertise in cross-sectional echocardiography, we have now reduced further the indications for cardiac catheterisation. This is so even in the presence of, for example, a large ventricular septal defect or a univentricular atrioventricular connexion. The size of a ventricular septal defect, if present, is assessed preoperatively and the probability of survival without banding is determined (Leanage et al, 1981).

If the probability of survival without banding is greater than 90%, repair is performed without banding the pulmonary trunk. Otherwise, banding is also carried out.

The surgical repair is performed through a left lateral thoracotomy in the fourth intercostal space. The arterial duct is routinely dissected and ligated. The aorta is dissected and mobilised proximally and distally. Resection of the stricture with restoration of continuity by end-to-end anastomosis is still occasionally used in infants. Most often we prefer the subclavian arterioplasty, as described by Waldhausen & Nahrwold, (1966). Hamilton and his colleagues (1978) have demonstrated the superiority of this method. The incision in the mediastinal pleura is extended superiorly along the left subclavian artery which is ligated and divided proximal to its first branch. The aorta is then incised well below the coarctation. The incision is continued across the narrow segment through the isthmus and along the lateral border of the subclavian artery. There is frequently a shelf of intimal tissue at the site of the coarctation. This should be carefully excised. The flap of subclavian artery is then turned down and sutured on the aortotomy incision across the site of the coarctation (Fig. 17.5). Compared to resection and end-to-end anastomosis, the subclavian flap angioplasty has reduced, but not abolished, the incidence of recoarctations. It also seems to provide a better relief of the obstruction. The mortality for repair of aortic coarctation in infancy is closely related to the presence or the absence of associated cardiac anomalies. In our institution, we performed 148 subclavian patch angioplasties for infants with aortic coarctation between 1974 and 1980. There were 3 deaths among the 48 isolated coarctations (6%) and 20 deaths among 100 complex coarctations (20%).

When coarctation is seen during childhood, most children are asymptomatic and surgical repair can be planned electively. The thoracotomy incision is extended posteriorly

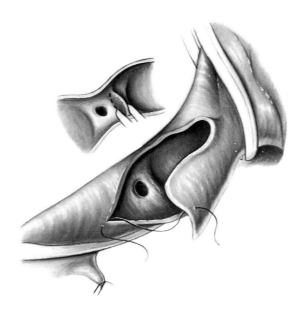

Fig. 17.5 Subclavian flap angioplasty to relieve coarctation of the aorta.

between the scapula and the vertebral column. Dissection and mobilisation of the aorta must be carried out, paying particular attention to the well developed collateral circulation. Special care must be taken in the posterior aspect of the aorta, where small arterial branches to posterior mediastinal structures (bronchial and oesophageal arteries) may be injured. These can cause distressing haemorrhages. Great attention must be paid inferiorly to the intercostal vessels. These are usually dilated and thin walled. They can bleed briskly if injured. Some of these may require division, but they should be preserved whenever possible. Excision and direct end-to-end anastomosis as originally described by Crafoord & Nylin (1945) remains our preferred operative technique. An alternative approach is the patch graft aortoplasty described initially by Vosschulte in 1957 and repopularised by Reul and colleagues in 1974. This technique has the advantage of limiting dissection, thus reducing the risks of haemorrhagic complications. A hospital mortality of less than 2–3% has been reported in several large series when the patients have been older than 1 year at operation. Spinal cord injury is the most non-lethal complication in this group of patients. It seems to occur in about 0.5% of the cases despite careful attention to surgical technique (Brewer et al, 1972). Paradoxical hypertension is a further common early complication and occurs in about 30% of patients (Pennington et al, 1979). Abdominal pain with ileus has been reported with an incidence which varies from 0–10%. This might be related to mesenteric vasculitides which, in very rare cases, may become necrotising and require surgical intervention. A better control of postoperative hypertension has reduced this complication. Residual permanent hypertension after repair of coarcta-

tion appears to become a significant problem only in patients operated upon after the age of 5 years (Liberthson et al, 1979). Our current policy is to operate on the asymptomatic child between the ages of 3 and 5 years. This is late enough to avoid recoarctation but early enough to correct the lesion before irreversible vascular changes leading to sustained hypertension occur.

Interruption of the aortic arch

The site of the interruption (and the associated intracardiac anomalies) dictate the surgical approach. The classification into three types of Celoria & Patton (1959) continues to be useful. Ventricular septal defect is the most frequent intracardiac anomaly. Left ventricular outflow tract obstruction, due to leftward displacement of the outlet septum (Van Praagh et al, 1971) or to an anterolateral muscle bundle of the left ventricle (Moulaert et al, 1976a) is often seen.

When the interruption is at the isthmus (so-called 'type A'), the distance between the proximal and distal segments is short. The situation is very similar to pre-ductal coarctation of the aorta. The aortic isthmus and descending aorta are widely mobilised. The arterial duct is ligated and divided and a direct end-to-end anastomosis is performed between the transverse aortic arch and the descending aorta. The pulmonary trunk is banded according to the criteria used in the treatment of coarctation with ventricular septal defect. If the distance between the two segments of the interrupted arch does not permit a direct anastomosis in spite of mobilisation, continuity can be established by turning down the left subclavian artery to the descending aorta, or by using a prosthetic graft.

When the interruption is proximal to the isthmus (types B and C), we believe that the chances of survival are greater if primary complete repair is carried out. From an anterior approach, the proximal descending aorta is widely dissected and mobilised. The arterial duct is divided and the ascending aorta is anastomosed to the back of the descending aorta. The ventricular septal defect is closed through the right atrium, right ventricle, or through the pulmonary trunk (Trusler & Izukawa, 1975; Bailey et al, 1978).

Palliative treatment may be considered in patients with left ventricular outflow tract obstruction (Litwin et al, 1972). Through a left thoracotomy in the fourth intercostal space, a vascular prosthesis is anastomosed end-to-side to the proximal pulmonary trunk and brought over the left hilum to be anastomosed on the upper descending aorta. The arterial duct is ligated and the pulmonary trunk is banded between the graft and the bifurcation. The mortality rate for correction of interrupted aortic arch has remained high in most institutions. Small series of more encouraging results have been published more recently (Monro et al, 1977).

Anomalies of the pulmonary venous connexion

Total anomalous pulmonary venous connexion

Most patients with total anomalous pulmonary venous connexion present very early in a critical condition and require surgical treatment in infancy. We believe that palliation using balloon atrial septostomy is not useful in the symptomatic neonate and infant presenting with extra-cardiac pulmonary venous obstruction. The repair is accordingly done using the technique of profound hypothermia and total circulatory arrest. The aim of the repair is to create a large opening between the pulmonary venous confluence and the left atrium and to close the arterial duct (if patent) and the atrial septal defect. The surgical technique depends on the anatomical type.

Supracardiac type. We prefer to repair this anomaly from the right side by making an incision in the posterior aspect of the right atrial wall. This is then carried posteriorly across the interatrial septum into the left atrium towards the orifice of the left atrial appendage. The ascending vertical vein is ligated and the pulmonary venous confluence is opened behind the heart. The anastomosis between the confluence and the posterior wall of the left atrium is started near the left atrial appendage and the pulmonary veins are connected to the left atrium (Fig. 17.6). The atrial septal defect is closed either directly or with a small patch of pericardium.

Infracardiac type. We prefer the posterior approach for this variety. The heart is lifted outside the pericardial sac so as to expose the posterior left atrium and the pulmonary venous confluence. An oblique incision is made in the left atrium starting at the base of the left atrial appendage. As the anomalous pulmonary venous channel is often oriented vertically, an oblique incision from the left upper

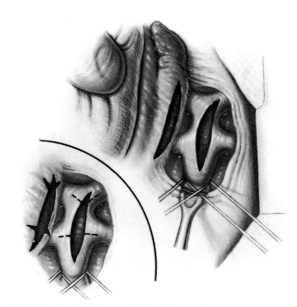

Fig. 17.7 Repair of an intracardial total anomalous pulmonary venous connexion. The heart is lifted up and the anastomosis between the left atrium and the pulmonary veins is performed from behind the heart.

pulmonary vein down to the descending common vein allows for a large anastomosis (Fig. 17.7).

Intracardiac type. Depending on the age of the patient, this type can be corrected on cardiopulmonary bypass or total circulatory arrest. The pulmonary veins drain either directly into the right atrium or, more commonly, into the coronary sinus. The principle of the correction is the same. One must ensure that the atrial septal defect is large enough to accept the full pulmonary venous return. If the pulmonary veins drain into the coronary sinus, a cut back is made from the sinus into the oval fossa or atrial septal defect. Care must be taken to avoid the area of the atrioventricular node, the patch being sutured within the mouth of the coronary sinus.

Partial anomalous pulmonary venous connexion

The most common form is that associated with a sinus venosus type of atrial septal defect. The atrial septal defect patch must be inserted so as to redirect the pulmonary venous blood to the left atrium. This must be accomplished while avoiding an obstruction of either pulmonary or systemic venous return and, at the same time, avoiding damage to the sinus node and its blood supply.

Anomalous connexion of all the veins of the right lung to the inferior caval vein is a rare anomaly. The preferred technique of repair is to tunnel the pulmonary venous blood to the left atrium through an enlarged atrial septal defect with a pericardial patch. Disconnexion of the anomalous venous channel and direct anastomosis to the left atrium has also been performed. Anomalous drainage of all the left pulmonary veins is a very rare anomaly. This

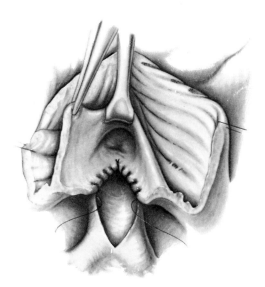

Fig. 17.6 Total anomalous pulmonary venous connexion. Anastomosis of the posterior wall of the left atrium with the common pulmonary venous channel.

can be corrected by anastomosing the left pulmonary venous trunk to the base of the amputated left atrial appendage. Isolated connexion of the left upper pulmonary vein to the left innominate vein may be left uncorrected.

Between 1971 and 1980, 77 infants with total anomalous pulmonary venous connexion underwent surgical repair in our Institution, with an overall mortality of 32%. Long-term results were excellent, as there was only 1 late death amongst 52 survivors of the operation.

Atrial septal defect

Surgical closure of atrial septal defect is indicated in all patients with a shunt of 1.5–2.0, or greater. The optimal age for the operation is probably between 3 and 5 years. Occasionally an atrial septal defect causes congestive heart failure and must be closed earlier.

Various methods have been utilised for repair. It is now widely accepted, however, that they are best closed using cardiopulmonary bypass with or without hypothermia. Air embolism is the most threatening complication of closure. The only absolute protection against it is the prevention of left ventricular ejection while the left side of the heart is open. This can be achieved either by cross-clamping the aorta or by induced ventricular fibrillation. The left atrium should not be emptied of blood. The defect is then closed before the left ventricle is allowed to eject blood into the aorta. Small and medium-sized defects are routinely closed by direct suture. Patch closure is preferred for large defects (and for the sinus venosus type of defect) so as to avoid obstruction to the systemic and/or pulmonary venous return. Care must be taken when the atrial septal defect is situated in the inferior aspect of the septum to prevent tunnelling the inferior caval venous blood into the left atrium. The hospital mortality rate is low, and the functional results are excellent in uncomplicated cases.

Ventricular septal defect

Operations for ventricular septal defects are performed through a midline sternotomy incision. Conventional hypothermic cardiopulmonary bypass with cold cardioplegia are used in the majority of patients above the age of 3 months. The technique of deep hypothermia and total circulatory arrest is often preferred in younger infants. Depending on their location in the interventricular septum (and the presence or absence of associated cardiac anomalies), the defects may be closed through the right atrium, the right ventricle, the left ventricle or one of the great arteries.

Closure through the right atrium

The right atrial approach is chosen to close most isolated defects of perimembranous or inlet muscular type. Apical trabecular and outlet muscular defects are not always accessible through the right atrium. Be that as it may, the anatomy of the defect is first assessed through the tricuspid valve. If the central fibrous body (area of continuity of the membranous septum and the annulus of the tricuspid, mitral and aortic valves) forms part of the rim of the defect, a perimembranous defect is present which is therefore closely related to the atrioventricular conduction tissue. From the atrioventricular node (apex of the triangle of Koch), the penetrating bundle passes through the central fibrous body and then continues as the branching bundle on the inlet side (right-hand side) of the defect (Fig. 17.8). Though small defects may be repaired by direct sutures, most of them are closed with a prosthetic patch. The patch is trimmed in an appropriate shape and size. The size must be greater than the actual defect, as part of the suture line is away from its margin. Deep stitches can be placed on the septomarginal trabeculation and on the cephalad margin of the defect (left-hand side) until the area of the central fibrous body is reached. Sutures are then placed through the base of the insertion of the septal leaflet of the tricuspid valve. If a deficiency is present in the septal leaflet, care must be taken to avoid the bottom of the 'cleft', which may reach back to the penetrating bundle. On the caudad (right-hand side) margin of the defect, the sutures cannot pass through the full thickness of the septum, but grasp only its right surface. They should be placed 3–5 mm away from the edge to avoid the branching bundle. The patch can be inserted with interrupted (Fig. 17.9) or continuous (Fig. 17.10) sutures..

Most apical trabecular muscular septal defects are positioned to either side of the body of the septomarginal trabeculation and can also be closed through the right atrium. The main problem in repairing these defects is the

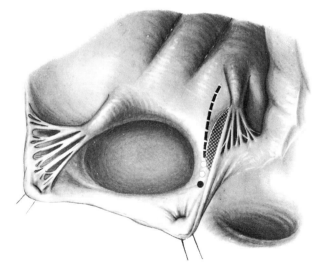

Fig. 17.8 Surgical anatomy of a perimembranous ventricular septal defect as seen through the tricuspid valve, showing the position of the conduction system.

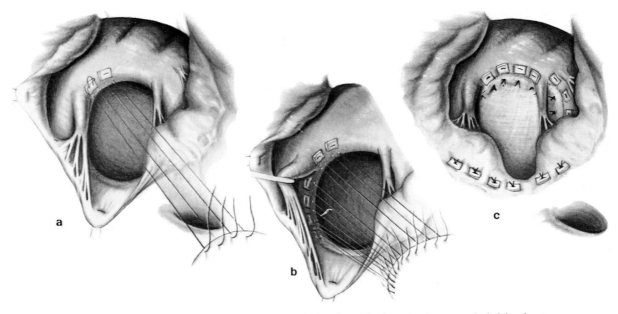

Fig. 17.9 Closure of a perimembranous ventricular septal defect through the tricuspid valve using interrupted pledgleted sutures.

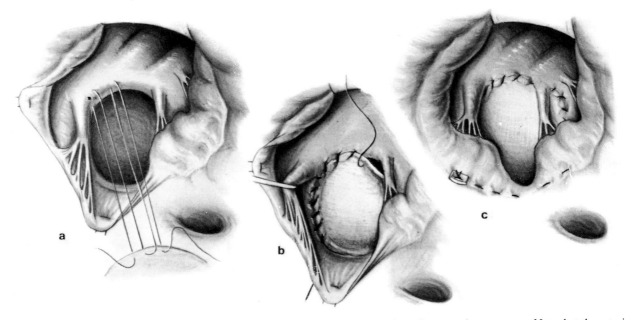

Fig. 17.10 Closure of a perimembranous ventricular septal defect through the tricuspid valve using a continuous suture. Note that the suturing is done so as to leave the area of the conduction behind the patch.

difficulty of identifying the true margin amongst the trabecular pattern of the right ventricular aspect of the septum. The defects have no direct relationship to the penetrating or branching segments of the conduction tissue, but may be related to terminal bundle branches. The stitches are placed along the margin of the defect on the right side of the septum.

Compared to perimembranous defects, the inlet muscular ventricular septal defects have a rim of muscular tissue on their atrial side. The atrioventricular conduction

axis penetrates into the ventricles on the outlet aspect of the defect (to the left-hand of the surgeon). In that area, the stitches are placed superficially on the right ventricular side of the rim of the defect.

Closure through the right ventricle

The right ventricular approach can be used for the perimembranous, outlet and some apical trabecular defects. This is the approach commonly used, for example, to close the ventricular septal defect in tetralogy of Fallot. If the defect reaches back to the tricuspid valve, one is again dealing with a perimembranous defect. The inferior margin is then in the vicinity of the conduction tissues. In these cases, the patch is first attached in that part of the tricuspid valve which forms the limit of the defect. The sutures are placed on the right side of the septum, 3–5 mm from the edge of the defect between the tricuspid ring and the medial papillary muscle, since this area may contain the penetrating bundle. Suturing then continues along the ventriculo-infundibular fold and the parietal extension of the outlet septum, taking deep bites in the muscle adjacent to the non-coronary leaflet of the aortic valve. Deep sutures are then placed through the full thickness of the outlet septum and its septal extension (Fig. 17.11). When bounded by entirely muscular rims, outlet muscular defects are closed with a prosthetic patch sewn on the free margin of the defect. This is separated inferiorly from the conduction tissue by the fusion of the posterior limb of the septomarginal trabeculation with the ventriculo-infundibular fold. The subarterial and doubly committed defect exists when the upper margin of an outlet defect is formed by the contiguous facing leaflets of the aortic and pulmonary valves. The chief challenge in repairing this type of defect is the accurate attachment of the patch between the arterial valves. Sutures are placed in this area first. They must avoid the adjacent semilunar leaflets but, at the same time, be anchored securely (although somewhat superficially) in the fibrous ridge separating the two valves. The rim of the tissue is sometimes non-existent, in which case, interrupted sutures are placed from inside the leaflets of the pulmonary valve.

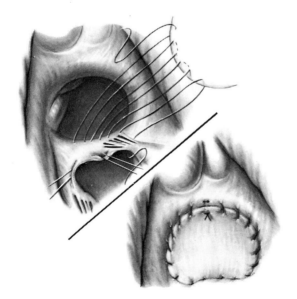

Fig. 17.11 Closure of a perimembranous outlet ventricular septal defect through the right ventricle.

Closure through a great artery

Doubly committed subarterial outlet defects can be closed through the pulmonary trunk when there is no right ventricular outflow tract obstruction. The trunk is incised longitudinally or transversely and the anterior leaflet of the pulmonary valve is retracted to expose the defect (typically situated beneath the facing pulmonary valve leaflets).

Closure through the left ventricle

A left ventriculotomy is performed to close trabecular muscular defects located in the lower part of the septum. They are often multiple and can be associated with higher defects that might need to be closed through the right atrium and/or through the right ventricle. A short 'fish mouth' type of incision is made at the apex of the left ventricle away from and parallel to the anterior descending coronary artery. Care must be taken to avoid damaging the anterolateral papillary muscle of the mitral valve. The margins of the defect are easily defined on the smooth left side of the ventricular septum. The defect is usually closed with a patch. If defects are multiple and near to each other, a large patch can be inserted with a continuous suture to cover them all. The high left ventricular pressure then keeps the patch against the septum.

The mortality for primary repair of isolated ventricular septal defects in infancy has been shown (McNicholas et al, 1979) to be significantly lower than the two-stage approach (consisting of banding the pulmonary trunk in infancy and closing the defect with debanding in childhood). In a series of 41 consecutive primary closures performed in infancy in our institution, we produced only 1 hospital death (2.4%). The safety of repair of isolated defects in childhood is primarily related to the pulmonary vascular resistance. Patients above 2 years of age with normal or only mildly elevated pulmonary vascular resistance can undergo repair with a risk of less than 1% (Blackstone et al, 1976).

Atrioventricular septal defects

Operation for atrioventricular septal defect with only interatrial shunting ('ostium primum') is advised electively for most patients at pre-school age unless symptoms of heart failure or growth failure occur earlier. Operation is then advisable at the onset of problems. This is the case for a small percentage of infants who may present with severe heart failure and regurgitation through the left atrioventricular valve. In view of the high mortality during the first year of life (and the risk of pulmonary vascular disease) it is now recognised that cases with common orifice should be repaired during the first year of life.

Atrioventricular septal defect with separate valve orifices ('ostium primum')

The repair is carried out on hypothermic cardiopulmonary bypass and cold cardioplegia unless the patient is an infant under 3 months of age. The technique of profound hypothermia and temporary circulatory arrest is preferred in the latter case. The repair of the left atrioventricular valve is best performed if it is considered as a trifoliate structure (Carpentier, 1978). The three leaflets are designated as mural, superior and inferior with an anterior, posterior and septal commissure. The septal commissure, if competent, is left untouched. If incompetent, it is usually best treated by placing a fine suture to approximate the superior and inferior leaflets nearest the septal attachment. In addition to an incompetent septal commissure (the so-called 'cleft'), regurgitation can be due to incompetence of the other commissures, to enlongation of tendinous chords or to annular dilation. These anomalies must be dealt with separately. The atrial septal defect is closed with a patch of pericardium, sewn anteriorly on the base of the attachment of the left atrioventricular valve and posteriorly on the base of attachment of the right valve. The coronary sinus and the area of the conduction tissue are left on the left side (Fig. 17.12). In a series of 164 patients with separate valve orifices operated at the University of Alabama Medical Center, there was a hospital mortality of 3.6% for patients without and 14% for those with major associated anomalies (Studer et al, 1982).

Atrioventricular septal defect with common valve orifice ('complete defect')

In this malformation, the atrioventricular valve is common to the right and left ventricles. It has five leaflets (left and right mural, superior and inferior bridging and a right anterosuperior leaflet). There is always a bare area beneath the bridging leaflets of varied extent (the ventricular septal defect), and there is also in 'ostium primum' type of interatrial communication. The surgical repair consists of closure of interventricular and interatrial communications with attachment of the bridging leaflets to the patch. This can be performed with a single or two separate patches. The architecture of the common valve must be studied carefully in each patient so as to divide it into left and right portions that are competent and not stenotic. We often prefer the two patch technique because this allows the surgeon more flexibility to avoid any significant alteration of the morphology and also to avoid completely suturing near the conduction tissues. A pericardial patch is preferred to close the interatrial communication. This avoids the postoperative haemolysis that can result from a jet of residual incompetence striking the patch. Figure 17.13 shows the line of insertion of the ventricular patch away from the area of the conduction tissue. If properly placed and trimmed, the patch should not interfere with the architecture of the left atrioventricular valve which is tested by injecting cold saline into the ventricles. The mortality for repair is about 10%.

Right ventricular outflow tract obstruction with intact ventricular septum

This can be divided into two surgical groups. The first includes patients with hypoplastic right ventricle and critical pulmonary valve stenosis or atresia. The second constitutes those with normal-sized or enlarged right ventricular cavities. The first group usually present to the surgeon in the neonatal period or early infancy, whereas the second group is more often encountered in childhood.

Critical pulmonary stenosis or atresia with intact ventricular septum and hypoplastic right ventricle

Our present management of these infants is based on a revised classification of the condition (Bull et al, 1982; de Leval et al, 1982). Once the diagnosis is suspected, the patient is immediately started on a prostaglandin infusion so as to improve arterial oxygen saturation and correct the acidosis. The degree and type of right ventricular hypoplasia must be defined preoperatively. A pulmonary valvotomy alone can be envisaged for a case having a tripartite right ventricle of good size. We currently prefer transpulmonary valvotomy performed under inflow occlusion. In theory, some of these patients could be candidates for a complete repair including a relief of the right ventricular outflow tract obstruction and closure of the atrial septal defect on cardiopulmonary bypass. It is because of a high mortality following these procedures that we have now

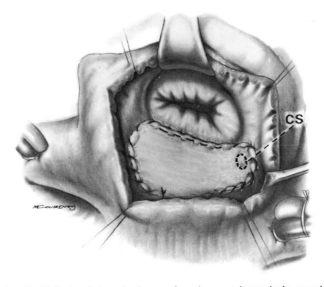

Fig. 17.12 Pericardial patch closure of a primum atrioventricular septal defect leaving the coronary sinus connecting into the pulmonary venous atrium.

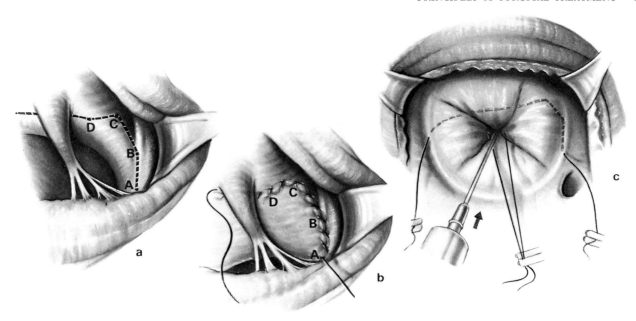

Fig. 17.13 Repair of the ventricular component of an atrioventricular septal defect staying away from the area of the conduction system (a, b). The common atrioventricular valve is then tested (c).

opted for valvotomy alone. For hypoplastic right ventricles lacking their apical trabecular component, we combine the transpulmonary valvotomy with a modified left Blalock-Taussig shunt. This is performed through a left thoracotomy. If the outlet component of the right ventricle is also absent, a systemic-to-pulmonary artery shunt is performed on the side opposite the arterial duct. It is for this last group that a balloon atrial septostomy could be performed if there is a significant preoperative interatrial gradient. A complete repair is rarely achieved in infancy. If the right ventricular cavity grows, a further relief of the right ventricular outflow tract obstruction with closure of the atrial septal defect may be considered. If the right ventricular cavity remains too small to cope with the whole cardiac output, a Fontan or modified Fontan procedure may constitute the best treatment (de Leval et al, 1985).

Pulmonary stenosis without right ventricular hypoplasia in the asymptomatic patient

We would advocate surgery or balloon valvoplasty (see Ch. 39) for right ventricular outflow tract gradients greater than 40 mmHg. This is best carried out before school age. Earlier relief of the stenosis is indicated whenever the patient becomes symptomatic (low exercise tolerance, right ventricular failure or cyanosis from shunting at atrial level) or whenever the right ventricular pressure is suprasystemic. This is to prevent endocardial fibroelastosis. Surgical treatment is routinely performed on hypothermic cardiopulmonary bypass with cold cardioplegia. If the semilunar attachments of the pulmonary valve are of normal size, the valvotomy is performed through a

pulmonary arteriotomy. Secondary right ventricular hypertrophy is common in patients with valvar pulmonary stenosis. Relief of the subvalvar obstruction might then be required. The infundibular area is examined through the pulmonary valve. If the outflow tract appears clear of any significant anatomic obstruction, the pulmonary trunk is closed and the cardiopulmonary bypass discontinued. If the right ventricular pressure remains elevated (greater than 80% of left ventricular pressures) 0.01 mg/kg propranolol is injected intravenously (Moulaert et al, 1976b). If the pressure ratio remains greater than 0.8 after the injection, cardiopulmonary bypass is reinstituted and a right ventricular outflow tract resection with patch enlargement is undertaken. The number of surgical valvotomies for isolated pulmonary valve stenosis has sharply decreased since the introduction of balloon dilation. The presence of a very dysplastic valve, the association of anatomic infundibular obstruction or of an atrial septal defect are unequivocal indications for surgical repair.

Right ventricular outflow tract obstruction and ventricular septal defect

In this section, I will consider the surgical management of patients with tetralogy of Fallot and pulmonary atresia with ventricular septal defect.

Tetralogy of Fallot (see Ch. 32)

Patients with mild cyanosis, mild polycythaemia and mild disability can be safely operated around the age of 3–5 years. The surgical approach for infants and small children who present with either severe cyanosis and polycythaemia or recurrent severe hypoxic spells varies from one institution to the other. Whereas some surgeons prefer a primary repair for all infants needing operation and have produced superb results (Castaneda et al, 1977), we continue to adopt a more conservative approach. Symptomatic infants with tetralogy of Fallot who need surgery before the age of 6 months of age undergo a preliminary shunt procedure. After the age of 6 months, an intracardiac repair is performed unless the pulmonary arteries are too small. In the latter case, a shunt operation is performed or the right ventricular outflow tract is enlarged without closure of the ventricular septal defect.

The intracardiac repair is routinely done using hypothermic cardiopulmonary bypass and cold cardioplegia. If the pulmonary valve is stenotic but the valve annulus is of adequate size, the pulmonary trunk is opened and the fused commissures are incised. A short vertical incision is made in the right ventricular outflow tract. If the pulmonary valve ring (measured with Hegar dilators) is smaller than normal, the incision is extended across the pulmonary valve annulus into the pulmonary trunk. For this purpose we use the table developed by Rowlatt and colleagues (1963) relating the size of the pulmonary valve ring to the mean normal values. The markedly hypertrophied parietal and septal extensions of the outlet septum are deeply incised and partially excised. After excision of these heavy muscular bands, the outlet septum (freed from its attachments to the free wall of the right ventricle), moves posteriorly and thus widens the right ventricular outflow tract. There is virtually no hypertrophy of these muscle bundles in infancy and little or no resection of the outflow tract is required. The ventricular septal defect is then repaired with a patch of Dacron velour. One can usually distinguish two anatomic variants of ventricular septal defects. The most common type is perimembranous, extending to the area of aortic-mitral-tricuspid valvar continuity. With this defect, the sutures must be kept on the right ventricular side and well away from the edge of the defect posteriorly and inferiorly. Several sutures are inserted along the base of attachment of the septal leaflet of the tricuspid valve. The defect is closed either by direct or continuous suture. Less frequently, the defect has a completely muscular rim as seen from the right ventricle which is formed by the fusion of the posterior limb of the septomarginal trabeculation with the ventriculo-infundibular fold. These defects can be closed by suturing the patch with stitches that are along the very edge of the defect on its right ventricular aspect. When present, a patent oval foramen or atrial septal defect is closed through a right atriotomy incision. In most cases we close the right ventriculotomy incision with a small patch of preclotted woven Dacron or pericardium. This patch is extended across the pulmonary valve ring when necessary as discussed above. Hospital mortality for repair of tetralogy of Fallot is around 5% in most large series. The incremental risk factors for hospital death include young age and transannular patching (Kirklin et al, 1983). A number of studies have documented the excellent late results that follow repair of tetralogy of Fallot, as shown for example from the Mayo Clinic experience (Poirier et al, 1977).

Pulmonary atresia and ventricular septal defect (see Ch. 33)

The outstanding feature in pulmonary atresia and ventricular septal defect is the anatomy of the pulmonary circulation and the source of blood supply. Preoperative investigations must include a detailed angiographic study of the central pulmonary arteries, their connexion with the right ventricle, their systemic sources of blood supply and their destination in the lungs. Similarly, the origin, course and destination of all major aortopulmonary collateral arteries must be demonstrated. The aims of the surgical repair are first to connect the right ventricle with as many bronchopulmonary segments as possible, and secondly, to avoid excessive residual right ventricular hypertension which has been shown to be an important determinant of hospital mortality. Thirdly, it is necessary to close the major aortopulmonary collateral arteries not connected to the right ventricle so as to prevent postoperative pulmonary overcirculation. The majority of these patients need surgical intervention in infancy or in early childhood. This is a systemic-to-pulmonary artery shunt in the great majority of the cases. Procedures needed to connect non-confluent pulmonary arteries or pulmonary arteries with major aortopulmonary collateral arteries are sometimes undertaken. The aim is to produce a unifocal blood supply.

The corrective procedures consist of control of the source of pulmonary blood flow. These include closure of major aortopulmonary collateral arteries in some cases, closure of the ventricular septal defect and connexion of the right ventricle to the pulmonary trunk or confluence. A patent arterial duct, surgically created shunts and/or large aortopulmonary collateral arteries are occluded as soon as the cardiopulmonary bypass is initiated. The ventricular septal defect is closed as for patients with tetralogy of Fallot. The establishment of continuity between the right ventricle and the pulmonary arteries may be achieved in several ways. These include infundibular resection with patch enlargement of the right ventricular outflow tract, placement of an extracardiac valved conduit, or extensive reconstruction of the pulmonary arterial pathways.

Results of palliative surgery for pulmonary atresia and ventricular septal defect have been rather disappointing. This is because surgical treatment is often needed during the neonatal period and carries a considerable mortality. The survivors may not reach the age of definitive repair. Even if they do, their anatomy may not be suitable for repair. This applies particularly to those patients with multifocal pulmonary blood supply. Between November 1963 and September 1981, 125 palliative operations for pulmonary atresia and ventricular septal defect were performed in 98 patients in our unit. There were 17 early and 10 late deaths (28%). In a series of 103 patients who underwent definitive repair at the Mayo Clinic between 1967 and 1975 (Olin et al, 1976), there were 10 hospital deaths (9.7%). Alfieri et al (1978) reported a 16% mortality rate in a group of 80 patients operated upon at the University of Alabama Medical Centre between 1967 and 1978.

Complete transposition (see Ch. 34)

Complete transposition without significant associated defects

A balloon atrial septostomy is performed in the neonatal period and an intra-atrial rearrangement of the venous return is carried out between 6 and 12 months of age. If the patient fails to improve after the balloon septostomy, or deteriorates, the atrial repair is carried out irrespective of age and weight. For several years we have performed the Mustard operation with satisfactory results (Stark et al, 1974). Our preference now, however, goes to the Senning procedure which in our hands is less likely to produce late systemic and/or venous obstructions. The Senning procedure also has the theoretical advantage of preserving the contractile function of the atria. We do not believe that the Senning procedure reduces the risks of postoperative arrhythmias.

The operation is performed under hypothermic cardiopulmonary bypass with direct cannulation of both caval veins. The technique of profound hypothermia and total circulatory arrest is preferred in the small infant. The operation consists of developing a flap of atrial septum which remains attached to the intra-atrial groove. Sometimes a small patch is sutured to the septal flap to make up for the deficiency created by an atrial septal defect. The flap is sutured between the left pulmonary veins and the left atrial appendage so as to separate the pulmonary venous return from the mitral valve. The posterior margin of the right atriotomy incision is then brought about the caval venous orifices and sutured to the remnant of the interatrial septum. This completes the caval pathways which are now directed to the mitral valve (Fig. 17.14). The anterior margin of the atriotomy incision is then brought down to the right pulmonary veins that have been widely opened in the interatrial groove (Fig. 17.15). The recent enthusiasm for reviving Senning's technique of interatrial transposition of venous return as initiated by Brom (1982) has been supported by excellent early results. In a composite surgical experience reported by Brom (1982), Stark (1982) and Locatelli and colleagues (1979), there was only 1 hospital death for 110 procedures for

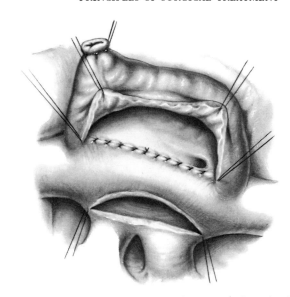

Fig. 17.14 Senning procedure. The systemic venous pathway has been completed. The right pulmonary veins are widely opened in the Waterston groove.

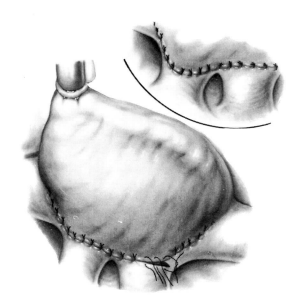

Fig. 17.15 Senning procedure completed, having brought the atrial wall posteriorly to the right pulmonary veins and on the lateral aspects of both caval veins.

'simple' complete transposition. Late cardiac catheterisation studies performed on patients operated following the early description of the Senning procedure have confirmed the appropriate course of each venous pathway (Senning, 1975).

A number of surgeons are now performing the arterial switch operation in neonates with simple complete transposition prior to the fall in pulmonary vascular resistance with encouraging early results (Castaneda et al, 1984; Yacoub et al, 1985; Quaegebeur, 1986; Quaegebeur et al, 1986).

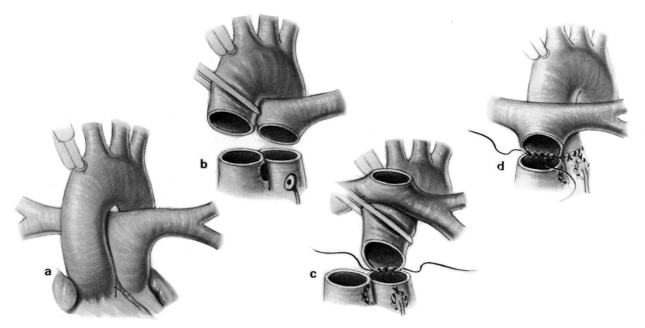

Fig. 17.16 Arterial switch operation for complete transposition. The great arteries are transected (b). The coronary arteries are transferred from the aorta to the pulmonary. The pulmonary trunk is brought in front of the aorta (Lecompte manoeuvre) (c). The distal pulmonary artery is anastomosed to the proximal aorta (d).

Complete transposition and large ventricular septal defect

It is now well recognised that severe pulmonary vascular disease can develop in these infants even within the first 6 months of life. Surgery is therefore recommended before that age. If heart failure and/or failure to thrive are unmanageable, the operation is performed regardless of the age or weight of the patient.

Atrial redirection with closure of the ventricular septal defect has been the treatment of choice for many years. The techniques are similar to those previously described in isolation. It is now largely accepted, however, that the procedure of choice is an arterial correction with closure of the ventricular septal defect. The great arteries are transected, the coronary arteries are excised from the aorta and transferred to the proximal pulmonary trunk. The distal aorta is then also anastomosed to the proximal pulmonary trunk. Finally, the distal pulmonary trunk is connected to the proximal aortic stump (Fig. 17.16). The ventricular septal defect is closed through one of the great arteries, the right atrium or the right ventricle. Encouraging early and medium-term results of this procedure are now available (Pacifico et al, 1983; Bical et al, 1984; Quaegebeur, 1986).

Complete transposition with left ventricular outflow tract obstruction and ventricular septal defect

When seen initially, these patients may need to be treated with a systemic-to-pulmonary artery shunt. The intracardiac repair described by Rastelli (1969) is usually performed between the ages of 4 and 6 years. The oper-ation consists of creating an intraventricular tunnel to connect the left ventricle to the aorta, closing the proximal pulmonary trunk and connecting the right ventricle with the distal pulmonary trunk using an extracardiac valved conduit (Fig. 17.17). In a series of 41 patients operated at Great Ormond Street between 1971 and 1978, we reported

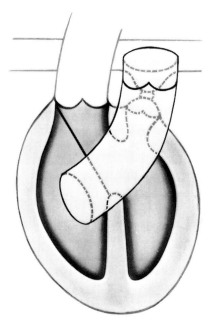

Fig. 17.17 The Rastelli procedure consists in closing the ventricular septal defect so as to connect the ventricle with the aorta, closing the proximal pulmonary artery and connecting the right ventricle with the distal pulmonary artery using an extracardiac valved conduit.

4 early deaths (10%) and we encountered a late mortality of 19%.

Complete transposition with left ventricular outflow tract obstruction and intact ventricular septum

A pressure gradient between the left ventricle and the pulmonary trunk does not necessarily mean that an anatomical obstruction is present. This gradient can be due to an increased blood flow across the left ventricular outflow tract. If anatomic obstruction is present, the left ventricular outflow tract is usually approached through the pulmonary trunk to resect fibrous shelves or to do a myotomy. If the obstruction cannot be directly relieved, it can be bypassed with an extracardiac valved conduit between the apex of the left ventricle and the pulmonary trunk.

Double outlet ventricles (see Ch. 36)

The type of repair depends on the position of the great arteries, the location of the ventricular septal defect and its relationship to the great arteries, the presence or absence of pulmonary stenosis and the presence or absence of additional intracardiac anomalies such as straddling of one or both atrioventricular valves.

Double outlet right ventricle

With subaortic ventricular septal defect. These can exist with or without pulmonary stenosis. They are amenable to an intraventricular repair in most cases. If the diameter of the ventricular septal defect is smaller than the aortic valve ring, the defect is enlarged by excision of the septum in its superior and lateral margin. A large patch of prosthetic material is then sewn around the margin of the ventricular septal defect and the aortic valve ring so as to connect the left ventricle to the aorta. The techniques to relieve the pulmonary stenosis are similar to the ones utilised in the repair of tetralogy of Fallot.

With subpulmonary ventricular septal defect (Taussig-Bing anomaly). In these patients, the great arteries may have either a side-by-side or an anterior-posterior relationship. When the great arteries are more or less side-by-side, pulmonary outflow tract stenosis is virtually non-existent but subaortic narrowing, pre-ductal hypoplasia and aortic coarctation are frequent. When the great arteries are antero-posterior, pulmonary outflow tract stenosis can occur but obstruction to the aortic outflow is very infrequent. These defects were in the past commonly repaired by closure of the ventricular septal defect so as to connect the left ventricle to the pulmonary trunk. This was combined with a redirection of the venous return following the Mustard or the Senning procedure. It is now generally accepted that one should correct the ventriculo-arterial connexion so that the morphologically left ventricle and the mitral valve serve the systemic circulation. In patients with side-by-side great arteries it is usually possible to perform an interventricular repair. This consists of a wide excision of the outlet septum to relieve any pre-existing subaortic obstruction and construction of an interventricular tunnel so as to connect the left ventricle to the aorta. In patients with anteroposterior relationship of the great arteries, anatomic correction can be achieved by diverting the blood from the left ventricle to the ventricular septum to the adjoining pulmonary trunk and switching the great arteries with coronary transfer as for patients with complete transposition (Yacoub & Radley-Smith, 1984).

With non-committed ventricular septal defect. The technical difficult in repairing these defects relate first to the necessity of constructing a long intraventricular tunnel which can easily become restrictive, and secondly to the presence of papillary muscles and chordal apparatus of the triscuspid valve between the ventricular septal defect and the great artery with which it should be connected. Cutting a patch from a woven Dacron tube as suggested by Stewart et al (1979) has the advantage of using a rather stiff material with corrugations that keep the required curve, thus preventing the obstruction of the intraventricular tunnel (Fig. 17.18). The ventricular septal defect must be

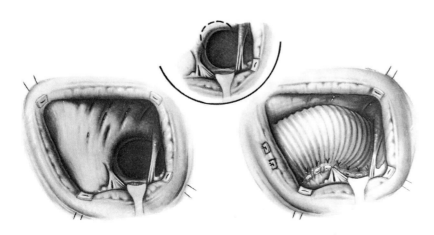

Fig. 17.18 Enlargement of a ventricular septal defect in a double outlet right ventricle and closure using a patch cut from a woven Dacron tube.

enlarged if smaller than the great artery to which it is connected. The suture line has to be placed around the papillary muscle of the antero-septal commissure of the tricuspid valve. In some hearts an intraventricular connexion of the ventricular of septal defect with one of the great arteries is not feasible. In these cases, it is preferable to close the ventricular septal defect, proceed with an interatrial redirection of the venous return and connect the left ventricle with the distal pulmonary trunk by means of extracardiac conduit.

Double outlet left ventricle

This is a much less common condition. The pulmonary trunk may be connected to the right ventricle, either with an intraventricular tunnel or an extracardiac conduit.

Common arterial trunk (see Ch. 37)

The results of palliative surgery for this condition have been so poor that it is now widely agreed that a primary repair performed in infancy (before pulmonary vascular changes occur) offers the best chances to these patients. The repair consists of detaching the pulmonary artery or arteries from the common trunk, closing the ventricular septal defect and establishing continuity between the right ventricle and the pulmonary artery or arteries (Fig. 17.18). Aortic homografts, when available, are the best extracardiac conduits to use in infants and children. It is a mistake to try to fit in very large conduits which can cause cardiac compression after the closure of the sternum. It is therefore recognised that the patients who survive this first surgical procedure will require replacement of the extracardiac conduit. Rather than using extracardiac conduits bearing a heterograft valve (which are known to calcify rapidly in the young age-group), it has been suggested that implantation of valveless tubes is better. After initial successful case reports of primary repair in infancy, larger series have now been reported. Among them, Ebert has undoubtedly produced the most remarkable results, with

an overall mortality of about 10%, (Ebert et al, 1984). In our own experience, very young age (under 3 months), truncal valve regurgitation and poor preoperative condition are all incremental risk factors. The mortality for conduit replacement has been low in most centres.

Left ventricular outflow tract obstruction

Cardiomegaly, congestive heart failure and left ventricular hypertrophy with left ventricular strain pattern are the main indications for surgical treatment in infancy. A systolic gradient of more than 50 mmHg or a strain pattern on electrocardiogram with demonstration of a discrete subvalvar, valvar or supravalvar stenosis are the main indications for surgery in childhood.

Subvalvar aortic stenosis

The obstruction can be made of a shelf or a fibromuscular obstruction. The shelf usually consists of fibrous tissue that forms a crescent-shaped wedge across the anterior two-thirds of the ventricular outflow tract. Characteristically the shelf inserts at each end along the base of the aortic leaflet of the mitral valve and beneath the right and non-coronary aortic cusps. The shelf is grasped with forceps and easily excised with a knife or pair of scissors (Fig. 17.19). To relieve a discrete fibromuscular obstruction, a myotomy with or without myectomy must be performed in addition to the excision of the fibrotic tissue. In order to avoid damaging the conduction system and the mitral valve, the muscular incisions must be confined to that area of the muscular septum situated beneath the commissure between the left and the right coronary leaflets of the aortic valve.

Severe diffuse subaortic obstructions remain a surgical challenge for which direct relief, aortoventriculoplasty, apical aortic bypass and aortic root replacement have all been advocated. As most of these patients also have a small aortic valve annulus, a direct relief of the obstruction is

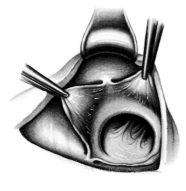
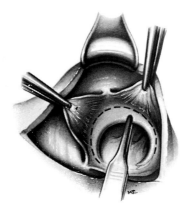

Fig. 17.19 Excision of subaortic shelf.

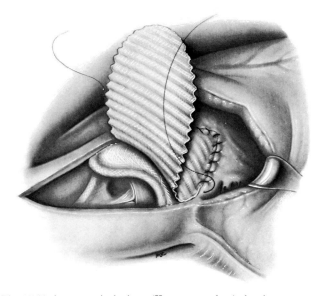

Fig. 17.20 Aortoventriculoplasty (Konno procedure) showing a prosthetic aortic valve and a patch enlargement of the interventricular septum and of the aortic root.

often inadequate. The aortoventriculoplasty was first suggested by Konno and colleagues (1975). It consists of incising the aortic valve leaflet attachments between the right and the left coronary cusps. The incision is extended onto the anterior wall of the right ventricle and the upper portion of the ventricular septum so as to open widely the left ventricular outflow tract. The aortic valve is then excised and replaced with a prosthesis, and the defects in the ventricular septum, the aorta and the right ventricular outflow tract are closed with patches (Fig. 17.20). Rather than employing such radical manipulations within the heart, an extracardiac procedure, such as the insertion of a conduit between the apex of the left ventricle and the aorta has been advocated by other authors. This type of procedure has tended to be abandoned in view of the high incidence of degeneration of these extracardiac valved conduits. In older children, aortic root replacement with a fresh aortic homograft and reimplantation of the coronary arteries is an excellent alternative (Somerville & Ross, 1982).

Valvar aortic stenosis

For the cases of critical aortic stenosis presenting in infancy, we now perform aortic valvotomy under inflow occlusion using a transaortic approach. In older children the operation is performed on cardiopulmonary bypass. The procedure consists in incising the fused commissure or commissures, taking care not to produce overwhelming aortic regurgitation. It must be noted that a short incision may result in an appreciable opening of the outflow orifice. It is sometimes difficult to differentiate a fused commissure from a raphe that represents a rudimentary commissure

without lateral support to the aortic valve. These ridges should not be incised as this will produce aortic insufficiency. If there is doubt as to whether a stenotic valve is trifoliate or bifoliate, it should always be treated as bifoliate.

Supravalvar aortic stenosis

Supravalvar aortic stenosis has been classified as localised and diffused. In the localised type the aortic narrowing is closed by an annular ridge protruding into the lumen of the aorta immediately above the commissural attachment of the aortic cusp. The outer diameter may be normal or reduced. In the diffuse type, narrowing of the lumen and abnormal thickness of the wall usually involves the ascending aorta and extends to the origin of the innominate artery.The surgical relief of the localised stenosis is done by partial resection of the stricture and a patch enlargement of the aortic root. This is best achieved using the aortoplasty recommended by Doty and colleagues (1977). This is illustrated in Figure 17.21, showing the opening of the aorta along a 'Y' incision and the shape of the Dacron prosthesis sewn to enlarge the left ventricular outflow tract.

Although it is a relatively simple procedure, the mortality for aortic valvotomy in infancy remains fairly high. In many instances, aortic valvotomy remains a palliative operation. About one-third of the patients will require a second operation within 10 years (Dobell et al, 1981). Early results of relief of subvalvar stenosis are generally satisfactory, with a low operative mortality. Encouraging results following aortoventriculoplasty (Rastan & Koncz, 1976) and aortic root replacement (Somerville & Ross, 1982) have been reported for the relief of diffuse subaortic obstructions.

Tricuspid atresia (see Ch. 27)

The great majority of patients with tricuspid atresia require surgical treatment during the first year of life. Cyanosis with decreased pulmonary blood flow is the most common indication for surgery. Our shunt of choice for these infants is the Blalock-Taussig anastomosis or its modification using a Gore-Tex prosthesis. Management of the infant with increased pulmonary blood flow remains difficult. If the great arteries are normally related, it is often possible to improve them with medical treatment, as they have a tendency to develop pulmonary stenosis with progressive cyanosis. In contrast, patients with discordant ventriculo-arterial connexion are often in severe congestive heart failure early in infancy and require banding of the pulmonary trunk. Recurrence of cyanosis, rising haemoglobin level and decreased exercise tolerance due to further reduction in the pulmonary blood flow are indications for a second surgical procedure. If the criteria for a successful

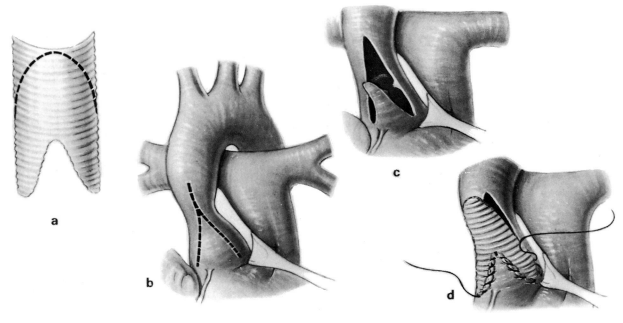

Fig. 17.21 Repair of a supravalvar aortic stenosis using the Doty technique.

Fontan procedure are fulfilled, this is currently our operation of choice. If not, a second palliation is carried out. From their early and extensive experience, Fontan's group suggested a set of rules (the ten commandments) within which the operation can be expected to be successful (Choussat et al, 1978). These are: a minimum age of 4 years; sinus rhythm; normal caval drainage; right atrium of normal volume; mean pulmonary artery pressure < 15 mmHg; pulmonary arteriolar resistance < 4 units/m²; pulmonary artery to aorta diameter ratio > 0.75; normal ventricular functions (ejection fraction 0.6); competent left atrioventricular valve; no impairing effects of previous shunt. The Fontan procedure itself consists of an atrioventricular or atriopulmonary connexion.

Atrioventricular connexion

This is the operation of choice for cases of tricuspid atresia with concordant ventriculo-arterial connexion having a rudimentary right ventricle sufficiently well developed to use as a pumping chamber and thus contribtue to pulmonary blood flow. The atrial septal defect must be closed meticulously to avoid a right to left shunt at atrial level. An incision is made on the anterior aspect of the rudimentary right ventricle and the septal defect is either closed directly or with a patch. We prefer to use fresh antibiotic preserved aortic homografts to connect the right atrium and the rudimentary right ventricle (Fig. 17.22), although valveless connections using Dacron tubes or an atrial flap augmented by a pericardial patch have been successfully utilised. We believe that a valve between the right atrium and the right ventricle is useful when the

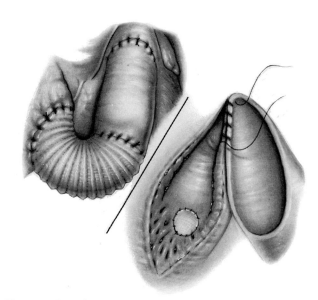

Fig. 17.22 An atrioventricular connexion for tricuspid atresia using a homograft conduit.

latter acts as a pumping chamber. When incorporating a rudimentary right ventricle in the Fontan circulation, it is mandatory to establish a gradientless connexion. If the right ventricle and/or the pulmonary valve are so small that an obstructionless connexion cannot be established, it is preferable to ignore the rudimentary ventricle and procede with an atriopulmonary connexion (Bull et al, 1983).

Atriopulmonary connexion

This operation is indicated for patients with tricuspid

atresia and discordant ventriculo-arterial connexion, or those with a concordant connexion and a rudimentary right ventricle so small that it would not contribute to the pulmonary circulation, but rather be an obstruction between the right atrium and the pulmonary trunk. We now prefer the direct atriopulmonary anastomosis behind the aorta as described by Doty and colleagues (1981).

Fontan and his colleagues (1983) reported 100 cases of tricuspid atresia operated between April 1968 and September 1981, with 12 deaths (12%). In our institution, among 28 Fontan procedures performed up to August 1981, there were 16 for tricuspid atresia, with 3 deaths (18.7%).

Corrected transposition (see Ch. 35)

The principles of repairing anomalies associated with a discordant atrioventricular connexion are influenced by the distribution of the coronary arteries and by the anatomy of the conduction system. Ventricular septal defect is the commonest intracardiac anomaly. Its closure is known to carry a risk of producing surgical heart block. As the penetrating and the branching bundle are always located on the morphologically left side of the septum, we have proposed (de Leval et al, 1979) a technique of closure of these defects which consists in placing the sutures on the morphologically right side of the septum without opening the systemic ventricle (Fig. 17.23). This illustration shows the ventricular septal defect closed with a patch, and the conduction system running in front of the pulmonary valve and descending on the interventricular septum along the anterior/superior aspect of the ventricular septal defect.

Relief of pulmonary stenosis presents a special problem, as the posterior location of the pulmonary trunk places it adjacent to the left coronary artery and to the conduction system. With the exception of valvar stenosis and subvalvar obstructions due to fibrous tags or aneurysms of the membranous septum, relief of significant pulmonary stenosis is best achieved with an extracardiac conduit placed between the morphologically left ventricle and the pulmonary trunk.

Tricuspid valve regurgitation is the third commonest anomaly associated with a discordant atrioventricular connexion. If the degree of regurgitation is more than moderate, the tricuspid valve must be repaired or replaced with a prosthetic valve.

A discordant ventriculo-arterial connexion is most commonly associated with the discordant atrioventricular connexion. Double outlet right ventricle comes next. As an intraventricular repair would necessitate a ventriculotomy incision on the systemic ventricle, we prefer using an extracardiac conduit to connect the left ventricle with the pulmonary trunk. A discordant atrioventricular connexion exceptionally exists with ventriculo-arterial concordance (Arciprete et al, 1985). This condition is best treated by a rearrangement of the venous return following the Senning or the Mustard procedure.

The early results of surgical repairs of anomalies associated with a discordant atrioventricular connexion have improved significantly over the last few years. The current early mortality varies between 15 and 20%. The incidence of surgically induced heart block has decreased. It must be remembered, however, that these patients continue to have a tendency to develop spontaneous heart block.

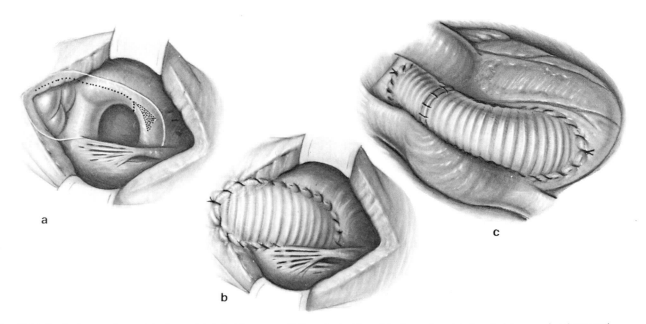

Fig. 17.23 Patch closure of a ventricular septal defect in a case of discordant atrioventricular and ventriculo-arterial connexion (corrected transposition). The position of the conduction system is indicated in panel (a). When associated with pulmonary stenosis, it may be necessary to use an extracardiac conduit between the left ventricle and the pulmonary trunk as shown in (b) and (c).

Double inlet ventricle (see Ch. 26)

Only palliative procedures can be offered to infants with double inlet ventricle and related lesions. They are the shunt procedures for patients with reduced pulmonary blood flow, banding of the pulmonary trunk for patients with excessive pulmonary blood flow and atrial septectomy for patients with absent left atrioventricular valve connexion and restrictive atrial septal defect. Two types of definitive repair, resulting in a complete separation of the pulmonary and the systemic circulations are available.

Septation

Patients with two atrioventricular valves and a left-sided rudimentary right ventricle giving rise to the aorta seem to be the only candidates for this procedure. Better results have been achieved when the septation is performed on a large heart with large pulmonary blood flow (Stefanelli et al, 1984).

Fontan procedure

A modification of the Fontan procedure can be performed for those patients with univentricular atrioventricular connexion whose pulmonary arterial and haemodynamics fulfil the criteria of the Fontan circulation. The right atrial exclusion may necessitate the closure of the right atrioventricular valve for patients with two atrioventricular valves or the septation of the atrial chamber for those patients with a common atrioventricular valve or an absent left atrioventricular connexion. In a group of 74 patients who underwent a Fontan procedure for a univentricular atrioventricular connexion at the Mayo Clinic (excluding tricuspid atresia), there was a 26% mortality (Danielson, 1983).

REFERENCES

Aberdeen E 1968 Blalock Hanlon operation and Rashkind procedure. In: Rob C, Smith R (eds) Operative surgery – cardiothoracic surgery, 2nd Edn. Butterworths, London, p 193

Alfieri O, Blackstone E H, Kirklin J W, Pacifico A D, Bargeron L M Jr 1978 Surgical treatment in tetralogy of Fallot with pulmonary atresia. Journal of Thoracic and Cardiovascular Surgery 76: 321–335

Arciprete P, Macartney F J, De Leval M, Stark J 1985 Mustard's operation for patients with ventriculoarterial concordance. Report of two cases and a cautionary tale. British Heart Journal 53: 443–450

Bailey L L, Jacobson J G, Vyhmeister E, Petry E 1978 Interrupted aortic arch complex: Successful total correction in the neonate. Annals of Thoracic Surgery 25: 66–70

Bical O, Hazan E, Lecompte Y, et al 1984 Anatomic correction of transposition of the great arteries associated with ventricular septal defect: midterm results in 50 patients. Circulation 70: 891–897

Blackstone E H, Kirklin J W, Bradley E L, DuShane J W, Appelbaum A 1976 Optimal age and results in repair of large ventricular septal defects. Journal of Thoracic Cardiovascular Surgery 72: 661–679

Blalock A, Hanlon C R 1950 The surgical treatment of complete transposition of the aorta and the pulmonary artery. Surgery Gynecology and Obstetrics 90: 1–15

Blalock A, Taussig H B 1945 The surgical treatment of malformations of the heart in which there is pulmonary stenosis or pulmonary atresia. Journal of the American Medical Association 128:189

Brewer L M 1903 Sur la lesion dite stenose congenitale de l'aorte dans la region de l'isthme. Review of Medicine Paris 23:108

Brom G 1982 The Senning procedure. In: Moulton A (ed) Current controversies and techniques in congenital heart disease. Appleton Davies, California

Bull C, De Leval M R, Mercanti C, Macartney F J, Anderson R H 1982 Pulmonary atresia and intact ventricular septum: a revised classification. Circulation 66: 266–272

Bull C, De Leval M R, Stark J, Taylor J F N, Macartney F J 1983 Use of a subpulmonary ventricular chamber in the Fontan circulation. Journal of Thoracic and Cardiovascular Surgery 85: 21–31

Carpentier A 1978 Surgical anatomy and management of the mitral component of atrioventricular canal defects. In: Anderson R H, Shinebourne E A (eds) Paediatric Cardiology 1977. Churchill Livingstone, Edinburgh, p 477–486

Castaneda A R, Freed M D, Williams R G, Norwood W I 1977 Repair of tetralogy of Fallot in infancy. Early and late results. Journal of Thoracic and Cardiovascular Surgery 74: 372–381

Castaneda A R, Norwood W I, Jonas R A, Colon S D, Sanders S P, Lang P 1984 Transposition of the great arteries and intact ventricular septum: anatomical repair in the neonate. Annals of Thoracic Surgery 38: 438–443

Celoria G C, Patton R B 1959 Congenital absence of the aortic arch. American Heart Journal 56: 407–426

Choussat A, Fontan F, Besse P, Vallot F, Chauve A, Bricaud H 1978 Selection criteria for Fontan's procedure. In: Anderson R H, Shinebourne E A (eds) Paediatric cardiology 1977. Churchill Livingstone, Edinburgh, p 559–566

Crafoord C, Nylin G 1945 Congenital coarctation of the aorta and its surgical treatment. Journal of Thoracic Cardiovascular Surgery 14:347

Danielson G 1983 Univentricular Heart. In: Stark J, de Leval M (eds) Surgery for congenital heart defects. Grune & Stratton, London, p 427–437

de Leval M R, Bastos P, Stark J, Taylor J F N, Macartney F J, Anderson R H 1979 Surgical technique to reduce risks of heart block following closure of ventricular septal defect in atrioventricular discordance. Journal of Thoracic and Cardiovascular Surgery 78: 515–526

de Leval M R, McKay R, Jones M, Stark J, Macartney F J 1981 Modified Blalock-Taussig shunt: use of subclavian artery orifice as flow regulator in prosthetic systemic-pulmonary artery shunts. Journal of Thoracic and Cardiovascular Surgery 81: 112–119

de Leval M, Bull C, Stark J, Anderson R H, Taylor J F N, Macartney F J 1982 Pulmonary atresia with intact ventricular septum: surgical management based on a revised classification. Circulation 66: 272–280

de Leval M, Bull C, Hopkins R, et al 1985 Decision making in the definitive repair of the heart with a small right ventricle. Circulation 72 (Suppl II): II52–II60

Dobell A R C, Bloss R S, Gibbons J E, Collins C E 1981 Congenital valvular aortic stenosis. Journal of Thoracic and Cardiovascular Surgery 81: 916–920

Doty D B, Polonsky D B, Jenson C B 1977 Supravalvular aortic stenosis. Journal of Thoracic and Cardiovascular Surgery 74: 362–371

Doty D B, Marvin W J, Laver R M 1981 Modified Fontan procedure: Methods to achieve direct anastomosis of right atrium to pulmonary artery. Journal of Thoracic and Cardiovascular Surgery 81: 470–475

Ebert P A, Turley K, Stanger P, Hoffman J E, Heymann M A, Rudolph A M 1984 Surgical treatment of truncus arteriosus in the first 6 months of life. Annals of Surgery 200: 451–455

Fontan F, Deville C, Quagebeur J, et al 1983 Repair of tricuspid atresia in 100 patients. Journal of Thoracic and Cardiovascular Surgery 85: 647–660

Glenn W, Patino J 1954 Circulatory bypass of right heart. I. Preliminary observations on direct delivery of vena caval blood into pulmonary artery circulation: azygos vein-pulmonary artery shunt. Yale Journal of Biological Medicine 27:147

Hamilton D I, Sandrasagra F A, Donnelly R J 1978 Early and late results of aortoplasty with a left subclaclavian flap for coarctation of the aorta in infancy. Journal of Thoracic and Cardiovascular Surgery 75: 699–704

Kirklin J W, Blackstone E H, Kirklin J K, Pacifico A D, Aramendi J, Bargeron L M Jr 1983 Surgical results and spectrum of tetralogy of Fallot. Annals of Surgery 198: 251–265

Konno S, Imai Y, Iida Y, Nakajima M, Tatsuno K 1975 A new method for prosthetic valve replacement in congenital aortic stenosis associated with hypoplasia of the aortic valve ring. Journal of Thoracic and Cardiovascular Surgery 70: 909–917

Leanage R, Taylor J F N, De Leval M R, Stark J, Macartney F J 1981 Surgical management of coarctation of the aorta with ventricular septal defect. Multivariate analysis. British Heart Journal 46: 269–277

Liberthson R R, Pennington D G, Jacobs M L, Dagget W M 1979 Coarctation of the aorta: review of 234 patients and clarification of management problems. American Journal of Cardiology 43: 835–840

Litwin S B, Van Praagh R, Bernhard W F 1972 A palliative operatioin for certain infants with aortic arch interruption. Annals of Thoracic Surgery 14: 369–375

Locatelli G, Di Benedetto G, Villani M, Vanini V, Bianchi T, Parenzan L 1979 Transposition of the great arteries. Successful Senning's operation in 35 consecutive patients. Thoracic and Cardiovascular Surgery 27: 120–123

McNicholas K, De Leval M, Stark J, Taylor J F N, Macartney F J 1979 Surgical treatment of ventricular septal defect in infancy. Primary repair versus banding of pulmonary artery and later repair. British Heart Journal 41: 133–138

Monro J L, Brawn W, Conway N 1977 Correction of type B interrupted aortic arch with ventricular septal defect in infancy. Journal of Thoracic and Cardiovascular Surgery 74: 618–623

Moulaert A J, Bruins C C, Oppenheimer-Dekker A 1976a Anomalies of the aortic arch and ventricular septal defects. Circulation 53: 1011–1015

Moulaert A J, Buis-Liem T N, Geldof W C, Rohmer J 1976b The postvalvulotomy propranolol test to determine reversibility of the residual gradient in pulmonary stenosis. Journal of Thoracic and Cardiovascular Surgery 71: 865–868

Muller W H, Dammann J F Jr 1952 The treatment of certain congenital malformations of the heart by creation of pulmonic stenosis to reduce pulmonary hypertension and excessive pulmonary blood flow. Surgery, Gynecology and Obstetrics 95: 213–220

Olin C L, Ritter D G, McGoon D C, Wallace R B, Danielson G K 1976 Pulmonary atresia: surgical considerations and results in 103 patients undergoing definitive repair. Circulation 54 (Suppl III): 35–40

Pacifico A D, Steward R W, Bargeron L M Jr 1983 Repair of transposition of the great arteries with ventricular septal defect by an arterial switch operation. Circulation 68 (Suppl II): 49–55

Panagopoulos P H G, Tatooles C J, Aberdeen E, Waterston D J, Bonham-Carter R E 1971 Patent ductus arteriosus in infants and children. Thorax 26: 137–144

Pennington D G, Liberthson R R, Jacobs M, Scully H, Goldblatt A, Daggett W M 1979 Critical review of experience with surgical repair of coarctation of the aorta. Journal of Thoracic and Cardiovascular Surgery 77: 217–229

Poirier R A, McGoon D, Danielson G K, et al 1977 Late results after repair of tetralogy of Fallot. Journal of Thoracic and Cardiovascular Surgery 73: 900–908

Potts W J, Smith S, Gibson S 1946 Anastomosis of the aorta to a pulmonary artery. Journal of the American Medical Association 132:627

Quaegebeur J M 1986 The arterial switch operation. Rationale, results, perspectives. Chapter 4. The arterial switch operation. An eight year experience. Thesis: Leiden University. Uitgeverij Rozengaard-Deelijk (België). pp 119–176

Quaegebeur J M, Rohmer J, Ottenkamp J et al 1986 The arterial switch operation. An eight-year experience. Journal of Thoracic and Cardiovascular Surgery 92: 361–384

Rashkind W J, Miller W W 1966 Creation of an atrial septal defect without thoracotomy. Journal of the American Medical Association 196: 991–992

Rastan H, Koncz J 1976 Aortoventriculoplasty. A new technique for the treatment of left ventricular outflow tract obstruction. Journal of Thoracic and Cardiovascular Surgery 71: 920–927

Rastelli G C 1969 A new approach to 'anatomic' repair of transposition of the great arteries. Mayo Clinic Proceedings 44: 1–12

Redo S F, Ecker R R 1963 Intrapericardial aortico-pulmonary artery shunt. Circulation 28: 520–524

Reul G J Jr, Kabbani S S, Sandiford F M, Wukasch D C, Cooley D A 1974 Repair of coarctation of the thoracic aorta by patch graft aortoplasty. Journal of Thoracic and Cardiovascular Surgery 68: 696–704

Rowlatt U F, Rimoldi H J A, Lev M 1963 The quantitative anatomy of the normal child's heart. In: Gardner L I (ed) Pediatric clinics of North America, Vol 10, No. 2. Symposium on genetics. Saunders, Philadelphia, p 499–591

Senning A 1975 Correction of transposition of the great arteries. Annals of Surgery 182: 287–293

Somerville J, Ross R 1982 Homograft replacement of aortic root with reimplantation of coronary arteries. Results after one to five years. British Heart Journal 47: 473–482

Stark J 1982 Transposition of the great arteries and left ventricular outflow tract obstruction. In: Moulton A (ed) Current controversies and techniques in congenital heart disease. Appleton Davies, California

Stark J, De Leval M, Waterston D J, Graham G R, Bonham-Carter R E 1974 Corrective surgery of transposition of the great in the first year of life. Journal of Thoracic and Cardiovascular Surgery 67: 673–681

Stefanelli G, Kirklin J W, Naftel D C, et al 1984 Early and intermediate-term (10-year) results of surgery for univentricular atrioventricular connection ('single ventricle'). American Journal of Cardiology 54: 811–821

Stevenson J G, Kawabori I 1984 Noninvasive determination of pressure gradients in children: Two methods employing pulsed Doppler echocardiography. Journal of the American College of Cardiology 3: 179–192

Stewart R W, Kirklin J W, Pacifico A D, Blackstone E H, Bargeron L M Jr 1979 Repair of double-outlet right ventricle. An analysis of 62 cases. Journal of Thoracic and Cardiovascular Surgery 78: 502–514

Studer M, Blackstone E H, Kirklin J W, et al 1982 Determinants of early and late results of repair of atrioventricular septal (canal) defects. Journal of Thoracic and Cardiovascular Surgery 84: 523–542

Trusler G A, Izukawa T 1975 Interrupted aortic arch and ventricular septal defect. Journal of Thoracic and Cardiovascular Surgery 69: 126–131

Van Praagh R, Bernhard W F, Rosenthal A, Parisi L F, Fyler D C 1971 Interrupted aortic arch: surgical treatment. American Journal of Cardiology 27: 200–211

Vosschulte K 1957 Isthmusplastik zur Behandlung dr Aotem Isthmusstenose. Thoraxchirurgie 4:443

Waldhausen J A, Nahrwold D L 1966 Repair of coarctation of the aorta with a subclavian flap. Journal of Thoracic and Cardiovascular Surgery 51: 532–533

Waterston D 1962 Treatment of Fallot's tetralogy in children under one year of age. Rozhl Chir 41:181

Yacoub M H 1979 The case for anatomic correction of transposition of the great arteries. Journal of Thoracic and Cardiovascular Surgery 78: 3–6

Yacoub M H, Radley-Smith R 1984 Anatomic correction of the Taussig-Bing anomaly. Journal of Thoracic and Cardiovascular Surgery 88: 380–388

18

The asymptomatic child with a murmur

The detection of a heart murmur on routine clinical examination (or incidentally during auscultation of the chest because of a respiratory infection or unexplained pyrexia) is probably the commonest cause for referral of a child to the paediatrician or paediatric cardiologist for further assessment of the heart. We will discuss in this chapter the child whose clinical history is essentially summed up as the 'asymptomatic child with a murmur'. Sometimes the 'murmur' is more a click or added sound. All children presenting with any form of additional noise related to the cardiac cycle will therefore be considered.

Murmurs are essentially due to disordered or turbulent flow or to more ordered but non-laminar flow such as vortices. Whatever the precise cause, virtually all *normal* children (or for that matter, all adults) will have a heart murmur when the heart rate is increased (for example, immediately after strenuous exertion or during a high fever). Thus, most children with heart murmurs will have normal hearts!

OVERALL EXAMINATION OF THE CHILD

Physical examination of the cardiovascular system has been discussed in Chapter 8. Full assessment of the cardiovascular system must be made before the importance or otherwise of a murmur can be determined. It should be confirmed that the patient is not cyanosed and does not have clubbing of fingers or toes. There should be no bulging of the sternum, and the respiratory rate must be normal. Pulses must also be normal and equal in upper and lower limbs (coarctation of the aorta must be excluded in all children whose cardiovascular system is examined). Not only should the pulses be normal but the heart rate should be appropriate for the child's age. As previously discussed, tachycardia in itself can produce turbulence within the cardiovascular system and hence produce or accentuate heart murmurs. Murmurs are also a feature of abnormally slow heart rates such as are found in congenital heart (atrioventricular) block (Ch. 11). Palpation of the precordium should be normal, with both a normal parasternal and normal apical impulse. On auscultation it is imperative that heart sounds be listened to and assessed before trying to evaluate murmurs. As discussed in Chapter 8, the second sound is normally split. This normal splitting varies with respiration, the first (aortic) component of the second sound being louder than the second (pulmonary) component. The presence or absence of additional heart sounds, ejection clicks or opening snaps must also be assessed. If present, the extra heart sounds must (if possible) be distinguished from heart murmurs.

Having completed these steps, and having ascertained that a heart murmur is present, certain other of its characteristics must then be established.

CHARACTERISTICS OF MURMURS

First one must decide whether the murmur is systolic, diastolic or continuous. Continuous murmurs are by definition murmurs that start in systole and pass or continue through the second heart sound. They do not have to be heard throughout the whole of systole and diastole. The second feature of note is the intensity of the murmur. Systolic murmurs are usually graded from 1 to 6 (Freeman & Levine, 1933) whereas diastolic murmurs (generally of low intensity) are rated from 1 through 4. Murmurs louder than grade 3 will usually have a structural heart abnormality as their cause. Murmurs of grades 1 to 3 may, depending on their other characteristics, be functional or indicate a cardiac anomaly (see below). Having graded its intensity, the site of maximal intensity is then assessed. All murmurs will have an area where they are loudest. In our unit, the sites of murmurs are indicated according to their relationship to anatomic sites on the chest wall (such as at the second intercostal space just to the left or right of the sternum, or at the cardiac apex, or in the left or right mid-axillary line, as the case may be). We prefer this approach to using terms such as the 'pulmonary' or 'mitral' area. In complex congenital heart disease the latter may be not only inaccurate but positively misleading since the valves may not be in their anticipated sites.

We then turn our attention to the 'contour' of the murmur. Not only should murmurs be assessed as systolic, diastolic or continuous but their timing and pattern within these broad categories should also be established. Systolic murmurs are primarily divided into ejection ('crescendo-decrescendo'), mid-systolic or pan-systolic 'regurgitant' murmurs (Leatham, 1958a, b). They can also be late systolic or plateau-like but finish before the second sound. Diastolic murmurs may occur early, in the middle or late in diastole and can be decrescendo, plateau-like or crescendo in pattern.

The next feature is the pitch of the murmur. Most murmurs in children consist of mixed mid-range frequencies although there are some characteristically high-pitched ('seagull murmur of mitral incompetence') or low-pitched (mid-diastolic murmur of 'mitral stenosis') murmurs. Perhaps included with pitch should be the quality of the murmur. This is described in terms of whether the murmur is 'blowing' with harsh prominent vibrations (accompanied by an easily palpable thrill) or vibratory and buzzing with low pitched vibratory components. Verbal description, however, is a poor substitute for listening. The alternative of phonocardiography for record-keeping requires considerable skill, time and interpretation.

The radiation of the murmur is next considered. The murmur may be transmitted away from the area of maximum intensity in two ways. The first is for the murmur to spread equally in all directions. This occurs particularly when the murmurs are loud. The second alternative is selective radiation along the lines of blood flow. Typical examples are radiation of apical systolic murmurs to the axilla in mitral incompetence and radiation of murmurs due to aortic stenosis from the second right intercostal space into the neck. Two separate murmurs may occasionally be appreciated during the same phase of the cardiac cycle. For instance, valvar pulmonary stenosis may accompany a small ventricular septal defect. Careful auscultation may then demonstrate that the pan-systolic murmur in the fourth/fifth intercostal space just to the left of the sternum decreases as one moves the stethoscope towards the higher intercostal spaces only to become loud again in the second left intercostal space. This should suggest the two separate sources of the murmur, emphasising that attention must be given to the whole precordium and the distribution of murmurs traced carefully.

Finally, careful note is taken of postural changes. Many murmurs, particularly so-called 'innocent murmurs' unassociated with structural heart abnormalities, may be influenced by changes in position of the child.

Significance of the murmur. The first question to be asked in the asymptomatic child referred because of a heart murmur is whether the murmur indicates or reflects the presence of a structural heart abnormality. The alternative is that the child's heart is normal and the murmur is 'innocent'. As has been neatly stated by Anthony et al (1979), innocent murmurs are of no importance except for the confusion that they generate. These authors have distinguished 'innocent' murmurs from 'functional' murmurs, although most would use the terms interchangeably. They defined functional murmurs as the accentuation of 'innocent murmurs' due to increased cardiac output (such as is associated with fever, anxiety, anaemia, exercise or thyrotoxicosis).

INNOCENT MURMURS

All innocent murmurs with one exception are systolic in timing. They are usually short in duration and tend to be mid-systolic. The one innocent murmur that is not systolic but continuous is that of a 'venous hum' due to blood passing from the head and neck veins into the thorax. Several different types of innocent (systolic) murmurs may be heard. They are usually soft, being grade 3 or less in intensity. They are frequently altered by changes in body position and may be reduced or abolished by a Valsalva maneouvre. Implicit in the positive diagnosis of 'innocent murmur' is that the rest of the examination of the cardiovascular system is normal.

The diagnosis of an innocent murmur should be positive rather than being dependent on exclusion. Such positive diagnosis accompanied by reassurance to the parents and discharge of the child is one of the most important activities of the paediatric cardiologist. Specific types of innocent murmurs will now be discussed.

Innocent vibratory murmur (Still's murmur)

This is the commonest of all the innocent murmurs. It is frequently first detected when a child with pyrexia is examined and there is a tachycardia. The murmur is mid-systolic and its site of maximum intensity is the third or fourth intercostal space just to the left of the sternum (Still, 1909). The murmur starts some time after the first heart sound. It is usually low pitched and vibratory in character and is moderately well localised. Occasionally there are some high frequency undertones sharpening the pitch of the murmur. Radiation to the base or apex may be present but the point of maximum intensity is always just to the left of the sternum (or to the right when an otherwise normal heart is right-sided). The murmur is not accompanied by a palpable thrill. Such murmurs may also be detected when children first have a school medical examination at the age of 4 or 5 years. This is probably the time when the murmurs are most prominent. The origin of the murmur is uncertain. It may originate either from acceleration of blood in the left ventricular outflow tract (Wennevold, 1967) or from re-direction of systemic venous return to the outflow tract of the right ventricle (Humphries & McKusick, 1962).

Venous hum

This low frequency continuous murmur is heard maximally in the neck or at the upper right or left sternal border or else at both sites. It results from turbulence of the venous return through the jugular, brachiocephalic and superior caval veins (Potain, 1867). Two peaks of intensity may be present both in systole and diastole. The murmur is easily heard over the base of the heart but becomes inaudible towards the lower left sternal border or the apex. Of all murmurs, this is probably the one most affected by changes in posture. It is loudest with the child in an upright position (either standing or sitting) and often disappears or becomes considerably diminished when the child lies down. Some textbooks suggest that the murmur is best abolished by twisting the neck to either side. We find that adoption of a lying position is a more effective way of abolishing the murmur if it is indeed a venous hum. Exceptionally it is necessary to occlude completely one or both jugular veins by digital pressure in order to abolish the murmur.

Basal ejection systolic murmur

These ejection systolic murmurs are typically heard maximally in the second or third left intercostal space but can occasionally be heard in the second right intercostal space. They may be extremely difficult to distinguish from murmurs due to trivial right or left ventricular outflow tract obstruction. They may also closely resemble the ejection systolic murmur due to excessive flow across the right ventricular outflow tract in patients with atrial septal defects. In the latter case, splitting of the second sound will not vary during inspiration and expiration (Leatham & Gray, 1956), but the murmur in itself may be indistinguishable. In normal individuals small gradients have recently been demonstrated across both right and left ventricular outflow tracts (so-called 'impulse gradients') when catheter-tipped transducers have been used to obtain high fidelity recordings. These murmurs are crescendo-decrescendo in contour (i.e. ejection systolic murmurs), have little radiation and finish well before the second heart sound (Mannheimer, 1940). Very rarely, transmission to the back may be present. As with the majority of innocent murmurs (other than perhaps venous hums) the murmur is accentuated when the cardiac output is increased.

Cardiorespiratory murmur

These are soft and blowing systolic murmurs heard at the apex or between the lower left sternal border and the apex.

They are of varying intensity but occur only during inspiration and can be made to disappear with held expiration. These murmurs require careful differentiation from those due to regurgitation through atrioventricular valves. They are due to segments of lung being intermittently compressed by the heart. Perhaps 'murmur' is an inappropriate term as they are really breath sounds from the compressed lung segments.

Supraclavicular or carotid bruit

A large number of normal children will have short ejection systolic crescendo-decrescendo murmurs over the carotid vessels and in the supraclavicular grooves. These can sometimes be quite loud (up to grade 3) and harsh in quality. As with all murmurs they indicate turbulent flow. In this case, the flow is through the brachiocephalic vessels. Hyperextension of the neck tends to make the murmurs disappear whereas flexion may accentuate them. Unlike the murmurs of arterial valve stenosis, they decrease in intensity below the clavicles.

Basal ejection systolic murmur in the newborn

Neonates frequently have a short early mid-systolic crescendo-decrescendo blowing murmur heard at the base of the heart both to the right and left of the sternum, sometimes with radiation to the axillae. They are usually soft (grade 2/6 maximal intensity) but characteristically they may be heard at the back as well as in the axillae. These murmurs reflect turbulence as a consequence of the dissimilarity in size in the neonate between the pulmonary trunk and the right and left pulmonary arteries (see Ch. 5). The murmur normally disappears by the end of the third or fourth week as the dimensions of the pulmonary arterial pathways rapidly equilibrate.

MURMURS REFLECTING STRUCTURAL HEART DISEASE

Having described the positive clinical features of innocent murmurs, the other way of looking at the diagnostic problem of an asymptomatic child with a heart murmur is to site the murmur and consider the differential diagnosis of murmurs detected.

Systolic murmur

Loud basal systolic murmur

It is essential to confirm that such murmurs are indeed systolic in nature and not continuous. A typical murmur of a persistent arterial duct is dominantly systolic in timing when heard in the neonate or young infant but the murmur just spills through the second sound. If the murmur is indeed harsh and systolic, most frequently it will be ejection in quality and will reflect right or left ventricular outflow tract obstruction. Typically the murmur of aortic stenosis will be maximal in the second right and that of pulmonary stenosis in the second left intercostal spaces. Detailed descriptions of the auscultatory findings in these conditions are presented in the appropriate chapters. Whenever ventricular outflow tract obstruction is suspected, the presence or absence of an ejection click should be sought. In valvar pulmonary stenosis, the ejection click is heard maximally in a similar site to the murmur but will also be audible at the lower left sternal border. The ejection click of valvar aortic stenosis is typically heard at the apex or along the lower left sternal edge (not the second right intercostal space where the murmur is loudest). An aortic ejection click is usually of higher pitch than the first heart sound but may occasionally be confused with the second component of a split first heart sound. The pulmonary ejection click has a higher pitch than the murmur or first heart sound. If the latter is inaudible at the base, the ejection click may at first seem to be the first heart sound. Its higher pitch and clicking quality should differentiate the two. If a click is louder in expiration, it is undoubtedly pulmonary and not aortic. The second heart sound is of major importance in assessing loud basal systolic murmurs. When the two components of the second sound can be easily heard, aortic or pulmonary stenosis is unlikely to be severe. If the second sound is single, this strongly suggests the diagnosis of ventricular outflow tract obstruction.

An electrocardiogram and chest X-ray should be performed in all patients with loud basal systolic murmurs. Pulmonary stenosis which is haemodynamically important will always be accompanied by electrocardiographic evidence of right ventricular hypertrophy. The electrocardiogram may rarely be normal even when there is severe left ventricular outflow tract obstruction. The plain chest radiograph may reveal post-stenotic dilation of the pulmonary trunk or of the ascending aorta and thus help in the differential diagnosis.

Soft basal systolic murmur

Assuming the auscultatory findings to be the only abnormal cardiovascular findings, soft basal systolic murmurs may be innocent. Alternatively, they can suggest mild pulmonary or aortic stenosis, an atrial septal defect or coarctation of the aorta, but still additional abnormalities should be carefully sought. The murmur itself is not as helpful in differential diagnosis as any associated findings. Coarctation of the aorta should be differentiated by comparison of arm and leg pulses and blood pressure measurements in upper and lower limbs. Fixed splitting of the second sound will indicate an atrial septal defect,

although in very young children there may be some uncertainty on the variability of splitting with respiration. As mentioned previously, ejection clicks characterise valvar aortic or pulmonary stenosis even when mild. Bicuspid aortic valves with minimal or no gradient across the left ventricular outflow tract may give rise to soft ejection systolic murmurs in the second right intercostal space. These could easily pass for innocent murmurs, but an apical ejection click will almost invariably be present with the structural anomaly. If the pulses and cardiac impulse are normal and if there are no added sounds, a soft basal systolic murmur is likely to be functional and of no importance.

Loud systolic murmur at lower left sternal border

A loud systolic murmur maximal at the lower left sternal border in an asymptomatic child is most frequently due to a ventricular septal defect. There may or may not be an associated thrill. If the left-to-right shunt is large (which may be the case even in an asymptomatic child) flow across the mitral valve will be increased because of the increased pulmonary venous return. An additional rumbling mid-diastolic murmur will then be present at the apex. Such a murmur should be sought in children suspected of having a ventricular septal defect. Its presence would suggest a pulmonary blood flow at least twice the volume of the systemic flow. Almost more than in any other group, the characteristics of the second sound are of fundamental importance in assessing children with a 'typical' murmur of ventricular septal defect. If the defect is small, the second sound will be normal. If the defect is large the pulmonary component is likely to be accentuated. If there is associated right ventricular outflow tract obstruction, the second sound will be single.

All of these children should have a chest X-ray and electrocardiogram performed. Should there be electrocardiographic evidence of excessive right ventricular hypertrophy in a patient thought clinically to have a ventricular septal defect (assuming the diagnosis to be correct), there must be either associated right ventricular outflow tract obstruction or an elevated pulmonary vascular resistance. This should direct attention back to the second sound. Should the electrocardiogram show disproportionate left ventricular hypertrophy, then subaortic stenosis should be suspected, either alone or in combination with a ventricular septal defect (Smith et al, 1985). One-fifth of patients with subaortic stenosis will have an associated ventricular septal defect and the diagnosis may be impossible to make with certainty on clinical examination. If there is electrocardiographic evidence of disproportionate left ventricular hypertrophy, and cross-sectional echocardiography is not available, then referral for this test is essential in order to evaluate the left ventricular outflow tract.

A certain number of children referred to the paediatric

cardiologist with a provisional diagnosis of ventricular septal defect have, in our experience, turned out to have mitral incompetence. Under these circumstances the murmur is of maximal intensity at the apex rather than just to the left of the sternum. Ventricular septal defect and mitral incompetence may rarely coexist. The majority of children with a loud systolic murmur at the lower left sternal edge and changes on either the electrocardiogram or chest X-ray will require further investigations. Cross-sectional echocardiography will be needed in the first instance and possibly cardiac catheterisation.

Soft systolic murmur at lower left sternal border

A soft systolic murmur at the low or mid-left sternal border may be functional (Still's murmur) or may represent a very small ventricular septal defect. These entities are best differentiated by their particular auditory features. The murmur of a small ventricular septal defect is usually harsher, starts *with* rather than *after* the first sound, and is blowing in quality. Innocent murmurs in particular increase in intensity with increased cardiac output due to pyrexia, anaemia or anxiety. Be the murmur innocent or structural, the second heart sound will be normal.

Apical systolic murmur

Apart from the apical systolic murmur that is present on inspiration but disappears on held expiration (innocent cardiorespiratory murmur – see above), apical systolic murmurs suggest atrioventricular valve incompetence. This is typically mitral but occasionally tricuspid or, in the case of an atrioventricular septal defect, incompetence of the common atrioventricular valve. When pan-systolic, the murmur may result from congenital mitral incompetence. In older children it may be due to acquired rheumatic heart disease. If there is marked mitral regurgitation, the apical impulse will be increased. There will be an accompanying mid-diastolic murmur consequent on the increased left ventricular stroke volume and increased diastolic flow across the mitral valve. Although an accompanying diastolic murmur indicates significant regurgitation (or perhaps mitral stenosis), the loudness or other characteristics of the systolic murmur give little information about the severity of regurgitation. When mitral regurgitation is mild, the chest radiograph and electrocardiogram will be normal. If severe, then cardiomegaly, left atrial enlargement and upper lobe blood diversion will be present (see Ch. 42). The electrocardiogram may also show left atrial hypertrophy with or without left ventricular hypertrophy. An electrocardiogram should always be performed when apical systolic murmurs are present since mitral regurgitation sometimes reflects impaired left ventricular function rather than a primary abnormality of

the valve. Under these circumstances, flat or inverted left-sided T waves may be detected.

Late systolic murmurs suggest mitral valve prolapse (see Ch. 42), especially when accompanied by a mid-systolic click. In our opinion, this anomaly is best diagnosed clinically by the presence of a late systolic murmur, a click or both. Considerable overdiagnosis and unnecessary anxiety may be caused by over-enthusiastic use of, or reliance on, M-mode or even cross-sectional echocardiography.

Diastolic murmurs

An isolated diastolic murmur in an asymptomatic child is rare. The mid-diastolic flow murmur of a large atrial or ventricular septal defect will be accompanied by a more prominent systolic murmur. Apical mid-diastolic murmurs may represent mild mitral stenosis and such children will usually be asymptomatic. Basal early diastolic decrescendo murmurs may be found with mild aortic or pulmonary incompetence. The murmur of aortic regurgitation is high-pitched, decrescendo and maximal along the mid-left sternal border. It is best heard with the child sitting forward with the breath held in full expiration. It is often faint and can easily be missed. Isolated pulmonary regurgitation results in a soft decrescendo early diastolic murmur maximal in the second left intercostal space commencing after the pulmonary component of the second heart sound. It is usually loudest with the child recumbent. Very rarely such a murmur will accompany severe pulmonary hypertension. Then the loud pulmonary component of the second sound with or without an ejection click will be a more prominent sign than the murmur. Any child with a diastolic murmur (even atypical), should have a chest radiograph and an electrocardiogram. A scratchy diastolic murmur may occasionally reflect Ebstein's malformation of the tricuspid valve (see Ch. 30). The electrocardiogram may then show bizarre QRS complexes of right bundle branch block pattern.

Continuous murmurs

Differential diagnosis of continuous murmurs is dealt with in more detail in Chapter 41. As previously discussed the most common continuous murmur heard at the base of the heart is a venous hum (typically under the left clavicle). Failure to abolish a low pitched continuous murmur in the second left intercostal space raises the possibility of a small arterial duct or perhaps other even rarer anomalies (see Ch. 41). Such patients will require further investigation.

Other causes of continuous murmurs include flow through major systemic-pulmonary collateral arteries in pulmonary atresia with ventricular septal defect, through systemic collaterals in coarctation of the aorta, through a ruptured sinus of Valsalva fistula, coronary arteriovenous fistulae or an incompetent truncal valve (to and fro rather than continuous). All illustrate that the remainder of the physical examination is as important as interpretation of the murmur itself in reaching a definitive diagnosis. Again, a chest radiograph and electrocardiogram should be performed in all children in whom a continuous murmur is not abolished by lying down with or without head turning. Further clinical differentiation of this group of conditions can be made using cross sectional echocardiography but most patients will require cardiac catheterisation.

FURTHER INVESTIGATIONS AND IMPLICATIONS OF THE DIAGNOSIS OF AN INNOCENT FUNCTIONAL MURMUR

In view of the high frequency of innocent murmurs in normal children, not all children with a heart murmur can be referred to a specialised paediatric cardiology unit even if such a unit can be found a reasonable distance from where the child lives. In view of the expense, are there clinical reasons for an electrocardiogram and chest X-ray, let alone an echocardiogram? A recent study showed that when made by a trained paediatric cardiologist, the positive diagnosis of either an innocent mumur or no significant heart disease was unlikely to be altered as a consequence of a chest radiograph, electrocardiogram and echocardiogram (Newburger et al, 1983). In the United Kingdom 'experienced consultant paediatrician' could easily be substituted for 'trained paediatric cardiologist'. In practice, the general paediatrician will probably see more children with innocent murmurs than the paediatric cardiologist. Even in Newburger et al's study where the diagnosis was changed to 'definite heart disease', the anomalies found, namely possible cardiomyopathy and probable mitral valve prolapse, in general do not require particular treatment. Patients with a cardiomyopathy and no valve abnormalities do not require antibiotic prophylaxis for dental extractions. Many would not recommend prophylaxis for those with mitral valve prolapse in view of possible complications of antibiotics (Kaplan et al, 1977). This is so even in those where the diagnosis of mitral prolapse is definite on clinical grounds and is not simply made from examination of an echocardiogram. The interpretation of the later is well recognised to be difficult or even dubious (see Ch. 41).

Therefore, if a murmur is positively diagnosed as innocent we do not recommend further investigations.

In conclusion, it is important to stress the truly benign nature of innocent or functional murmurs. When made by a competent observer, diagnosis is found to be correct in 97–100% of patients on follow-up studies (Shapiro, 1939; Marienfeld et al, 1962; Weaver & Walker, 1964). There should be no adverse future indications for life insurance or limitations on employment when a murmur has been positively diagnosed as innocent or functional (Engle, 1977).

REFERENCES

Anthony C L, Arnon R G, Fitch C W 1979 Pediatric cardiology. Medical Examination Publishing Company Inc. 33–40

Engle M A 1977 Insurability and employability: congenital heart disease and innocent murmurs. Circulation 56: 143–145

Freeman A R, Levine S A 1933 The clinical significance of the systolic murmur. A study of 1000 consecutive 'noncardiac' cases. Annals of Internal Medicine 6: 1371–1385

Humphries J O, McKusick V A 1962 The differentiation of organic and 'innocent' systolic murmurs. Progress in Cardiovascular Diseases 5: 152–171

Kaplan E L, Anthony B F, Bisno A, et al 1977 Prevention of bacterial endocarditis. Circulation 56: 139A–143A

Leatham A 1958a Auscultation of the heart. Lancet ii: 703–708

Leatham A 1958b Auscultation of the heart, heart murmurs. Lancet ii: 757–765

Leatham A, Gray I 1956 Auscultatory and phonocardiographic signs of atrial septal defect. British Heart Journal 18: 193–208

Mannheimer E 1940 Callibrated phonocardiography and electrocardiography; clinical-statistical study of normal children and children with congenital heart disease. Acta Paediatrica (Suppl 2) 28: 1–287

Marienfeld C J, Telles N, Silvera J, Nordsieck M 1962 A 20 year follow-up study of 'innocent' murmurs. Pediatrics 30: 42–48

Newburger J W, Rosenthal A, Williams R G, et al 1983 Noninvasive tests in the initial evaluation of heart murmurs in children. New England Journal of Medicine 308: 61–64

Potain S C 1867 Des mouvements et des bruits quise passent dans les veines jugulaires. Bulletins et Memories de la Societie Medicale des Hospitaux de Paris 3: 27–28

Shapiro M J 1939 Follow-up study of systolic murmurs. American Heart Journal 17: 416–422

Smith L D R, Charalambopoulos C, Rigby M L, et al 1985 Discrete sub-aortic stenosis and ventricular septal defect. Archives of Disease in Childhood 60: 196–199

Still G F 1909 Common disorders and disease of childhood. Frowde, Hodder & Stoughton, London

Weaver W F, Walker C H 1964 Innocent cardiovascular murmurs in adult: a 16 year follow-up. Circulation 29: 702–707

Wennevold A 1967 The origin of the innocent 'vibratory' murmur studied with intracardiac phonocardiography. Acta Medica Scandinavica 181: 1–5

Specific Conditions

Atrial isomerism

It has long been recognised that a characteristic constellation of cardiac anomalies accompanies congenital absence of the spleen. As pointed out by Van Mierop et al (1972), absence of the spleen is an obvious autopsy finding which is unlikely to be missed. It is no surprise, therefore, that absence of the spleen was noted as long ago as the 16th century. As discussed by McLean & Craig (1922) and by Gilbert et al (1958), however, it seems most likely that these early cases reported acquired rather than congenital absence, since none were associated with intracardiac malformations. The earliest recorded examples of congenital absence of the spleen are probably those described by Martin and Breschet, both reports appearing in 1826. Multiple spleens occurring as a congenital malformation were first recorded over thirty years previously, by Abernethy in 1793. The significance of these splenic anomalies to the paediatric cardiologist is mainly that they are the harbingers of well-defined syndromes of congenital cardiac disease. It is also pertinent that when the spleen is absent the patient will be more than normally susceptible to infection. But the significance of the cardiac problems has been increased over recent decades by the recognition that the entire body arrangement of patients with the 'splenic syndromes' differs from the usual arrangement (situs solitus) and also from the mirror-image variant (situs inversus). The fact that the organs in patients with asplenia had the basic arrangement of right isomerism, or 'bilateral right sidedness', was first highlighted by Putschar & Mannion (1956). Van Mierop & Wiglesworth (1962) subsequently pointed to the isomerism of the right atrial appendages and sinus nodes. The basic left isomeric nature of patients with polysplenia was then emphasised by Moller and his colleagues (1967). However, despite recognition of isomerism of the organs and atria as the essence of these malformations (which is in contrast to the lateralisation found with usually arranged or mirror-image organs), the cardiac malformations found with these entities have continued to be described under the headings of 'asplenia' and 'polysplenia' (Stanger et al, 1977; Van Praagh, 1977) or else have been grouped together as 'situs ambiguus' (Van Mierop et al, 1972). This is less than ideal at a time when most centres dealing with congenital heart disease use a sequential segmental approach to diagnosis which must start by identification of the arrangement of the atrial chambers. If, in a proportion of cases, this can only be determined by making reference to the state of the spleen, or else is considered to be indeterminate and ambiguous, then sequential analysis in these cases, which are known to be highly complex, is based on a very shaky foundation. But, if the essence of the malformations is indeed isomerism rather than lateralisation, there is nothing ambiguous or uncertain concerning the atrial morphology. Indeed, the isomerism of the bronchial tree was forwarded by Van Mierop et al (1970) as a means of diagnosing these syndromes during life. Yet still they continued to refer to the atrial arrangements as 'asplenia' and 'polysplenia'. Another important pointer to diagnosis during life was the observation by Elliott et al (1968) that the inferior caval vein and the aorta in patients with right isomerism ran on the same side of the spine during their abdominal course. Carefully controlled studies using tomography (Partridge et al, 1975) and high kilovoltage filtered beam radiographs (Deanfield et al, 1980) have corroborated these empirical observations regarding bronchial isomerism. The relationships between the inferior caval vein and the descending aorta were clearly demonstrated ultrasonographically by Huhta et al (1982). The first step in the sequential diagnosis of any patient suspected of having congenital heart disease should, therefore, now be the identification of bodily and atrial arrangement. In this chapter we will describe the morphological and clinical features of the cardiac malformations found in patients with isomeric rather than lateralised organs. The diagnosis of right atrial isomerism then takes with it all the information that would previously have been gleaned from identification of asplenia, and more into the bargain, since not all patients with so-called 'asplenia syndrome' have absent spleens (Layman et al, 1967), although they do have right atrial isomerism (Macartney et al, 1980). Similarly, not all patients with so-called 'polysplenia syndrome' may have multiple spleens but they will certainly have left atrial isomerism.

ANATOMY AND MORPHOGENESIS

Atrial anatomy

The essence of the cardiac malformations is the presence of atrial isomerism. This does not mean that the hearts have two normal right atria (each receiving a superior caval vein, an inferior caval vein and a coronary sinus) or two normal left atria (each receiving four pulmonary veins). Description of atrial isomerism simply means that there is duplication of those parts of the atrial chambers that exhibit the characteristic anatomical features of rightness or leftness. As discussed in Chapter 3, when determining the rightness or leftness of the atrial chambers, it is the morphology of the atrial appendages and their junction with the smooth-walled atrial components which is the defining factor (Fig. 19.1). This is because the venous connexions are variable. For example, the pulmonary veins may be connected to the morphologically right atrium (see Ch. 21). Similarly, although the atrial septum has typical morphologically right and morphologically left sides, it is not always there. It cannot therefore be used as a reliable indicator of rightness or leftness. Thus, the heart with right atrial isomerism will be characterised by the presence of two atrial appendages each with the morphology of the normal right atrial appendage, and each having a broad and extensive junction with the smooth-walled components of the right- and left-sided atrial chambers respectively (Fig. 19.2). In contrast, in the heart showing left atrial isomerism, each of the appendages will have the characteristic morphology of the normal left appendage. Each will have a narrow and constricted junction with the

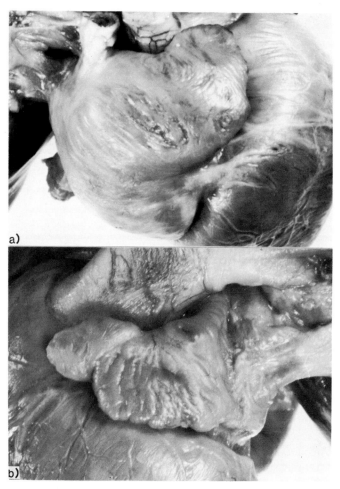

Fig. 19.1 Comparisons of the anatomy of the normal morphologically right (a) and morphologically left (b) atrial appendages.

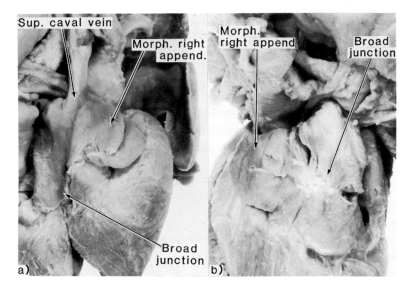

Fig. 19.2 Bilateral appendages of morphologically right type as found in right atrial isomerism.

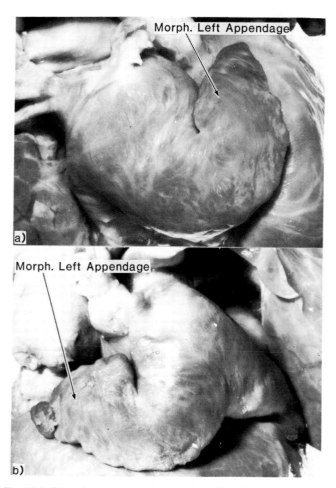

Morph. Left Appendage

a)

Morph. Left Appendage

b)

Fig. 19.3 Bilateral appendages of morphologically left type as found in left atrial isomerism.

smooth-walled atrial components (Fig. 19.3). It was Van Mierop & Wiglesworth (1962) who first wrote in detail on this isomeric nature of the atrial appendages, although Aquilar et al (1956) had previously commented on a case of congenital asplenia that 'two equally prominent auricular appendages were apparent', without specifying their morphological rightness.

As Van Mierop & Wiglesworth (1962) indicated, the major morphological features of rightness of the isomeric appendages are to be found internally. Each appendage is separated along its entire border with the smooth-walled part of the atrium by an extensive junction marked by a prominent terminal crest (Fig. 19.4c). The pectinate muscles occupy the entire lateral wall of the right and left sides of the atrial chambers (Fig. 19.4). The external shape of the appendages is less reliable. Usually morphologically right appendages are triangular but they may form quite a narrow triangle (Fig. 19.4a).

In his first study with Wiglesworth (1962), Van Mierop suggested that the morphologically left atrial appendage had no adequate means of identification. More recently (Van Meirop, 1981) he has described features of morpho-

logical leftness more in keeping with our own experience. We have found it possible in nearly all cases of left isomerism to recognise bilateral morphologically left appendages because of their narrow shape and their constricted junction with the smooth-walled atrial portions. We have noted extensive crenellations along the length of morphologically left appendages. Such crenellations are frequently seen along the base of morphologically right appendages, but not as deep as those seen in left appendages. The left appendages are much more tubular and narrow. The internal architecture of morphologically left appendages is also distinctive (Macartney et al, 1980). The pectinate muscles are not separated from the smooth-walled atrium by a terminal crest and, although the pectinate ridges may extend more laterally than the constricted junction of appendage and atrium, they are more limited in their extent than in morphologically right atrial chambers. By combining the internal and external features of the atrial appendages, we found it possible to identify right and left atrial isomerism and to distinguish these arrangements from hearts with lateralised atria even when we studied each individual atrial chamber in isolation (Macartney et al, 1980).

We have recently encountered several cases having atrial isomerism in which there was broncho-atrial discordance, as first described by Caruso & Becker (1979) (Figs. 19.4, 19.5). The bronchi in our cases were lateralised, having one long and one short bronchus with eparterial and hyparterial relations to the respective branch pulmonary arteries. Nonetheless, it was still possible (applying the principles which define the characteristics of left and right atrial appendages as discussed above) to recognise and diagnose atrial isomerism. The other associated cardiac anomalies found in all cases were as expected for isomerism (see below).

Venous connexions

The connexions of the pulmonary and systemic veins to the smooth-walled components of the right- and left-sided atrial chambers vary considerably in cases with either right or left atrial isomerism. Nonetheless, certain features are so common for each type as to permit their differentiation. It is the connexion of the pulmonary veins which is most reliable in permitting this distinction. In right atrial isomerism, because the morphologically left atrium is lacking, there must, by definition, be anomalous pulmonary venous connexions. Even when all the pulmonary veins connect to one of the morphologically right atrial chambers, be it right- or left-sided, the anatomy is abnormal when compared to the normal connexions of the pulmonary veins to the morphologically left atrium. With such anomalous cardiac connexion, the pulmonary veins crowd together and drain either via a small confluence to the atrial roof (Fig. 19.6a) or else

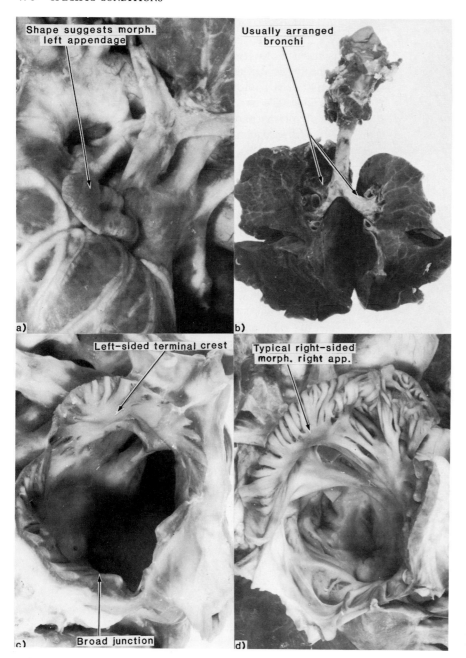

Fig. 19.4 Broncho-atrial discordance in a patient with right atrial isomerism. The bronchi (b) clearly show the usual arrangement (short bronchus to the right – the bronchi are viewed from the front following removal of the heart). At first sight the left-sided appendage also has some appearances of a morphologically left appendage (a). Opening the appendage (c), however, shows that there is a left-sided terminal crest and pectinate muscles as anticipated for a morphologically right appendage. This can be compared with the right-sided appendage (d) which is typical of right morphology. The cardiac anatomy was consistent with right atrial isomerism.

directly into the top of the atrial chamber (Fig. 19.6b). In the normal heart, the pulmonary veins are widely spaced and connect to the posterior corners of the morphologically left atrial chamber. Not all authors recognise that atrial connexion of the pulmonary veins must always be anomalous in right atrial isomerism (Cabrera et al, 1981). Confusion is avoided if it is appreciated that, in the absence of a morphologically left atrium, cardiac connexions of the pulmonary veins are still anomalous even if they are to a left-sided atrium. In the majority of cases, however, such semantic niceties do not arise because the pulmonary veins connect totally to an extracardiac source. The site of anomalous connexion is as varied as in 'isolated'

total anomalous pulmonary venous connexion (see Ch. 21), and the problems of obstruction are the same as with the isolated cases (Macartney et al, 1980; Frescura et al, 1981).

If total anomalous pulmonary venous connexion distinguishes right atrial isomerism, then it is an anomalous connexion of the inferior caval vein which draws attention to the presence of left atrial isomerism. Most frequently the suprarenal segment of the inferior caval vein is totally absent. The abdominal vein continues through either the azygos or hemiazygos system to drain to either the right- or left-sided superior caval vein (Fig. 19.7). To prevent confusion and to clarify descriptions, the term

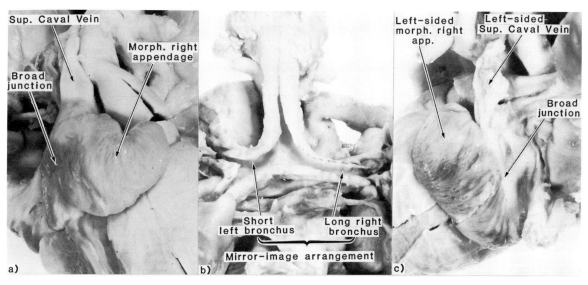

Fig. 19.5 Another example of broncho-atrial discordance. The bronchi (viewed from behind in this instance – b) show mirror arrangement, the short bronchus being left-sided. Both the right (a) and the left (c) appendages, however, are of unequivocally right type, as was their internal morphology. The cardiac anatomy was in keeping with the diagnosis of right atrial isomerism.

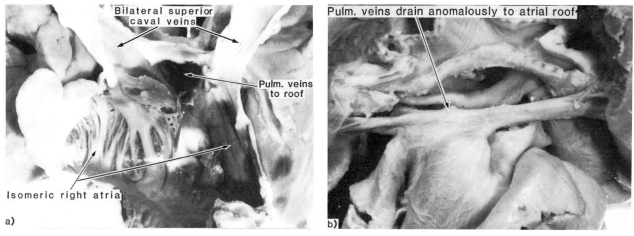

Fig. 19.6 The connexions of the pulmonary veins to the heart in patients with right atrial isomerism. Usually there is total anomalous venous connexion to an extracardiac site. Even when the veins connect to the heart, as in these specimens, they do so in an anomalous fashion. The upper photograph (a) shows the veins draining to a sinus in the atrial roof between bilateral superior caval veins, whilst the lower picture (b) shows all four veins crowding together into the atrial roof.

'azygos' is best restricted to the system of intrathoracic ascending paravertebral veins communicating with the superior caval vein on the right side. 'Hemiazygos' describes the counterpart on the left. These terms can then be used irrespective of the presence of left or right isomerism. It is extremely rare for the hemiazygos system to communicate with the superior caval vein, coronary sinus or atrium in patients without isomerism. Although azygos continuation (in other words, a right-sided channel) has been noted in right isomerism (Freedom & Fellows, 1973; Sapire et al, 1986), to this date, hemiazygos continuation (on the left side) has been reported only in association with left isomerism. In the 11 cases of left isomerism

we studied at autopsy, hemiazygos continuation to a left-sided superior caval vein was present in 6 and connexion to a right-sided vein in 1. Even higher frequencies were noted in the cases studied by Rose et al (1975) and Frescura et al (1981). In those cases in which the inferior caval vein does drain to an atrial chamber, the hepatic veins had been considered to drain separately to the atrial chambers, either unilaterally or bilaterally. More recent experience shows this not to be the case, and a suprahepatic confluent channel has been observed by us in one-third of cases of left atrial isomerism in the case material of the Children's Hospital of Pittsburgh. This is important because the abdominal relationship of the aorta and the inferior caval vein are an excellent guide to the presence of atrial isomerism. In patients with lateralised organs, the aorta lies anterior to the vertebral column, just to the right of the midline with the inferior caval vein slightly anterior and to its right in patients with normal visceral arrangement. The relationship is reversed in mirror-image abdominal visceral arrangement. The inferior caval vein is on the side of the right atrium (see Ch. 3). The hepatic veins always drain via a suprahepatic caval segment even when the abdominal cava is continued via the azygos or hemiazygos systems. The aorta and inferior caval vein are on the same side of the spine, the venous channel being anterior in patients with right atrial isomerism (Elliott et al, 1966). The abdominal vessels are also to the same side of the spine in left isomerism when

there is interruption of the inferior caval vein, this time with the azygos or hemiazygos continuation in posterior position. In most cases, the hepatic veins then drain directly to the atrium rather than via a suprahepatic cava. The difficulty arises in recognising patients with left atrial isomerism in whom there is an inferior caval vein which connects to the atrium. It is suggestive that, in this circumstance, the hepatic veins continue to connect separately to the atrium. If so, then identification of the relationship of the great vessels to each other and the spine together with identification of the connexion of the hepatic veins, either directly into the atrial chambers or to a suprahepatic segment of the inferior caval vein, provides a reliable means of distinguishing non-invasively the presence of right and left atrial isomerism (Huhta et al, 1982). In the single patient reported by Freedom & Fellows (1973) with azygos continuation of the inferior caval vein and 'congenital asplenia' (presumably right atrial isomerism), it was not specified whether the hepatic veins drained directly to the atrium or via a confluent venous channel. In our initial study of right isomerism (Macartney et al, 1980), we found bilateral or straddling drainage of the hepatic veins in 9 of 34 cases, but at that time we did not specify if one side drained via the terminal portion of the inferior caval vein. Re-examination of these cases shows that in most cases the inferior caval vein had been destroyed by the prosector! Inspection of the cases in the cardiopathological museum of the Children's Hospital of Pittsburgh, however, showed that the hepatic veins drained via a common venous channel to the right-sided atrium in one-third of cases, some having azygos or hemiazygos continuation and others not. It would be difficult if not impossible to distinguish

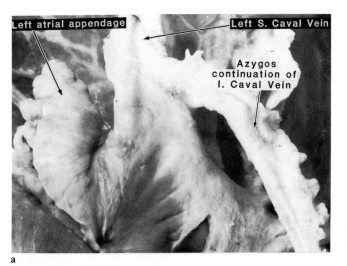

a

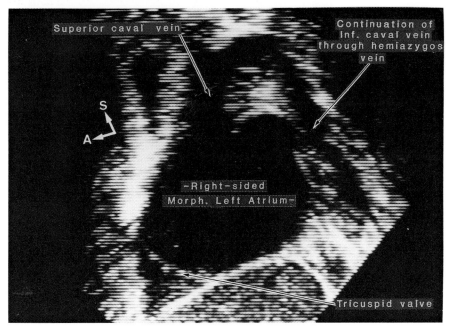

b

Fig. 19.7 Hemiazygos continuation of the inferior caval vein in left atrial isomerism. (a) Shows an anatomic specimen and (b) shows a cross-sectional echocardiogram.

these cases as having isomerism simply by studying the relationships of the abdominal great vessels to the spine.

Coupled with the different pattern of drainage of the pulmonary veins, the inferior caval vein and the hepatic veins, however, it should be possible to distinguish the right and left varieties of atrial isomerism. This is not the case with the connexions of the superior caval veins. Bilateral connexions to the roof of the right- and left-sided atrial chambers can be found in either variety. These connexions are by definition anomalous on each side in left isomerism while in right isomerism they are anatomically normal. Such a bilateral venous connexion is more common in right than left isomerism (53% compared with 18% in our series – Macartney et al, 1980) but the difference between the two groups is not significant. It is much commoner to find a coronary sinus in patients with left isomerism than with right isomerism (Rose et al, 1975). In this respect, it should be noted that Quaegebeur and his colleagues (1979) have considered drainage of a left superior caval vein to the atrial roof along with *absence* of the coronary sinus as the extreme form of 'unroofed coronary sinus'. Others, including ourselves, would expect to find the orifice of the coronary sinus in its anticipated position functioning as an interatrial communication before diagnosing unroofing (see Ch. 22). It is in part because cases with bilateral connexion of superior caval veins directly to the atrial roof were diagnosed as 'unroofed coronary sinus' that the experience of Quaegebeur et al (1979) with this rare anomaly is so extensive! Be that as it may, it is uncommon in our experience and that of Rose et al (1975) and Frescura et al (1981) to find a coronary sinus in right atrial isomerism even when there is only one superior caval vein draining to the atrial chambers.

Atrial septum

The degree of atrial septation also fails positively to discriminate between right and left isomerism (Macartney et al, 1980). In right atrial isomerism, most frequently there is simply a strand of atrial tissue which spans a common atrial cavity (Fig. 19.8d). In only one of the cases we studied (Macartney et al, 1980) was the atrial septum completely lacking, but in three-fifths there was effectively a common atrium. In about a quarter the septum was well-formed superiorly in association with an atrioventricular septal defect (Fig. 19.8c) while in one-tenth the septum was intact or else the oval foramen was probe patent (Figs. 19.8a, b). Rose and her colleagues (1975) gave less precise details of atrial septation, but in their cases one-third showed evidence only of a strand while in the remaining two-thirds there was formation of the superior part of the atrial septum. In their cases with polysplenia (left atrial isomerism), one-third had either a common atrium or else only a strand, while the septum was better formed in the other two-thirds. In our material we also

found an effectively common atrium in one-third. There was an atrioventricular septal defect in nearly half, while the atrial septum was virtually intact in nearly one-fifth.

The atrioventricular junction

As with hearts having lateralised atria, isomeric atrial chambers can each be connected to their own ventricular chamber (biventricular atrioventricular connexion) or else can be connected to only one ventricle (univentricular atrioventricular connexion). When there is a biventricular atrioventricular connexion it is important to describe in detail the ventricular topology. This is because there are two patterns to be found irrespective of whether there is right or left atrial isomerism. In the first pattern, the right-sided atrium (be it of right or left morphology) will be connected to the morphologically right ventricle and the left-sided atrium to the morphologically left ventricle. The ventricular topology will then resemble that found in hearts with usual atrial arrangement and atrioventricular concordance. This is best termed a 'right-hand arrangement' (Fig. 19.9a), and corresponds to the 'd-loop' described by Van Praagh & Vlad (1978). In the second arrangement the right-sided atrial chamber (which again may be of either right or left atrial morphology) will be connected to a morphologically left ventricle and the left-sided atrium will be connected to a morphologically right ventricle. In this second type the ventricular topology is comparable to that almost always found in patients with usually arranged atria and atrioventricular discordance (congenitally corrected transposition). It is a left-hand pattern (Fig. 19.9b) and corresponds to the 'l-loop' initially described by Van Praagh & Vlad (1978). Previously, when discussing the atrioventricular connexions found when each of two isomeric atrial chambers is connected to its own ventricular chamber, we described them as ambiguous (Shinebourne et al, 1976; Tynan et al, 1979). As Thiene has suggested, it is more specific to describe them as isomeric atrial chambers with a biventricular atrioventricular connexion (Thiene & Frescura, 1984), proceeding always to describe the ventricular topology present and, if necessary, any abnormal and unexpected ventricular relationships. Less than half of the cases studied by De Tommasi et al (1981) and Frescura et al (1981) had biventricular atrioventricular connexions. About half had right-hand pattern topology. The frequency of biventricular atrioventricular connexion is much greater in the presence of left atrial isomerism, most usually in association with right-hand pattern ventricular topology (De Tommasi et al, 1981; Frescura et al, 1981).

A univentricular atrioventricular connexion is encountered far more frequently in hearts with right than in left isomerism (Rose et al, 1975; De Tommasi et al, 1981; Frescura et al, 1981). When found, it is almost always due to double inlet ventricle via a common atrioventricular

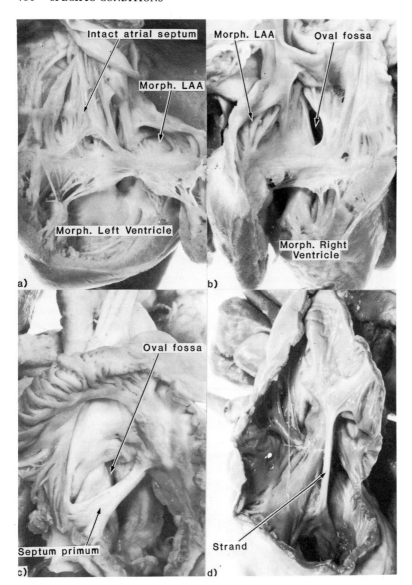

Fig. 19.8 The atrial septum can be variously formed in the presence of atrial isomerism. The upper panels (a & b) show an almost intact septum in a patient with left atrial isomerism, biventricular atrioventricular connexion and left-hand pattern ventricular topology. (c) Shows a well formed septum primum with a subseptal atrioventricular septal defect together with an oval fossa defect in a patient with right atrial isomerism. (d) Shows the more usual pattern in right isomerism where there is simply a septal strand.

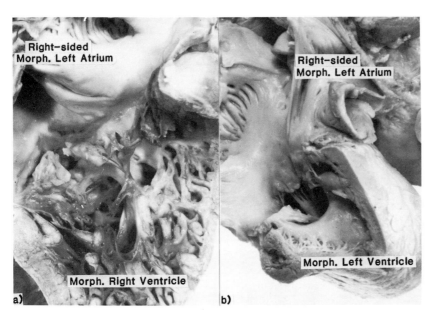

Fig. 19.9 These two photographs show how atrial isomerism and biventricular atrioventricular connexion can exist with either right-hand or left-hand pattern topology. Both hearts have left atrial isomerism. In (a) the right-sided morphologically left atrium connects to a morphologically right ventricle (right-hand pattern). In (b) the right-sided left atrium connects to a morphologically left ventricle (left-hand pattern).

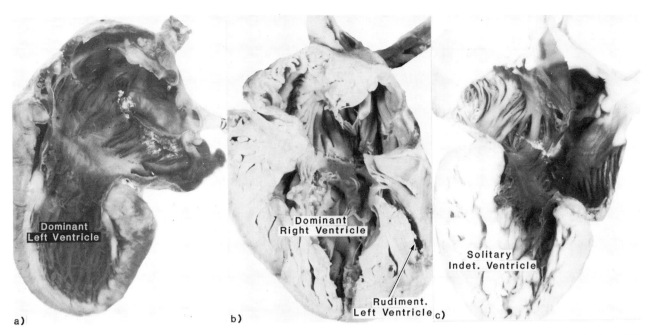

Fig. 19.10 Univentricular connexion via a common valve in three specimens with right atrial isomerism. The connexion is to (a) a dominant left ventricle in the presence of a rudimentary right ventricle (not seen), (b) a dominant right ventricle with a postero-inferior left-sided rudimentary left ventricle, and (c) a solitary indeterminate ventricle.

valve. In over one-third of the hearts studied by De Tommasi et al (1981), the univentricular connexion was to a morphologically right ventricle (Fig. 19.10). A rudimentary left ventricle was discovered in most, usually being left-sided, but in some it was not possible to find a second ventricle. Hearts were also encountered with double inlet to morphologically left and indeterminate ventricles. Among the cases of right isomerism described by Frescura et al (1981), two had absence of the left-sided atrioventricular connexion, the right-sided atrium being connected to a dominant left ventricle. We found a similar arrange-

ment but with the right-sided atrium connected to a dominant right ventricle (Fig. 19.11). Thus, any type of univentricular atrioventricular connexion must be anticipated with any possible ventricular morphology. Although less hearts have left isomerism with univentricular atrioventricular connexion, the same variability must be expected.

As far as the mode of atrioventricular connexion is concerned, the majority of hearts have a common atrioventricular valve, be there a biventricular or a univentricular atrioventricular connexion (Figs. 19.10, 19.12).

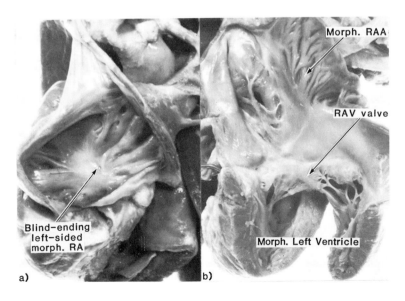

Fig. 19.11 Absence of the left atrioventricular connexion (a) in a patient with right atrial isomerism. The right-sided right atrium is connected to a morphologically left ventricle (b).

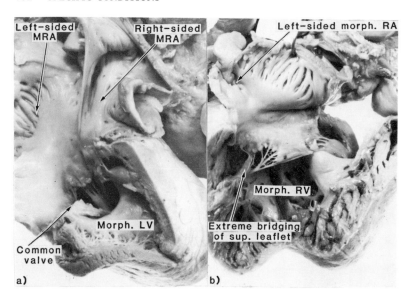

Fig. 19.12 Further photographs of the heart illustrated in Figure 9b showing that the biventricular atrioventricular connexion exists through a common valve orifice. There is an atrioventricular septal defect with extreme bridging of the superior leaflet in the setting of left-hand pattern ventricular topology.

When there is a biventricular connexion, the common valve is found in the setting of an atrioventricular septal defect, and almost always there is extreme bridging of the left anterior leaflet, giving the so-called 'Rastelli type C malformation'. Separate right and left atrioventricular valves are rarely present. 'Clefts' in the right and left valves are then to be expected, but these are no more than the divisions between the superior and inferior components of the two bridging leaflets (see Ch. 24). The finding of two normal and unobstructed valves is rare. In hearts with univentricular connexion and double inlet, a common valve is to be expected irrespective of the morphology of the ventricular chamber connected to the atria (Fig. 19.10). Taken overall, a common atrioventricular junction is to be anticipated, but two normal valves can be found either with right or left atrial isomerism.

As would be expected with such a high incidence of atrioventricular septal defects, the ventricular septum in the majority of hearts with biventricular atrioventricular connexion is deformed in the anticipated fashion. In the cases of right isomerism we studied without an atrioventricular septal defect, ventricular septal defects of perimembranous type were always present, as in the experience of Frescura et al (1981). Cases do exist, however, with an intact ventricular septum, more frequently in patients with left isomerism (Rose et al, 1975; De Tommasi et al, 1981). In all hearts with univentricular atrioventricular connexion, be there right or left isomerism, those with rudimentary ventricles have ventricular septal defects as anticipated for the ventricular morphology present (see Ch. 26).

The ventriculo-arterial junction

Amongst the entire group of hearts with atrial isomerism, there is just as much variability in type and mode of connexion, infundibular morphology and arterial relationships as encountered in congenital heart disease as a whole. Certain patterns, however, occur with significantly different frequencies in the right and left isomeric forms. Pulmonary obstruction or atresia is significantly more common in association with right than with left isomerism (De Tommasi et al, 1981). When there is pulmonary atresia, almost always the pulmonary supply is duct-dependent, although there is no reason why any other source should not be found. Analysis of the ventriculo-arterial junction as a whole (De Tommasi et al, 1981) also showed significant differences. An anterior right-sided aorta and subaortic or bilateral infundibulum were commoner with right isomerism, while ventriculo-arterial concordance was more frequent in left isomerism. Similar findings were recorded by Rose et al (1975) and by Frescura and her colleagues (1981).

The conduction tissues

The morphology of the sinus node reflects the atrial morphology. In right atrial isomerism there are bilateral sinus nodes, each related to the terminal crest and the cavoatrial junction in normal fashion. This finding was first noted by Van Mierop & Wiglesworth (1962) and was confirmed in the more extensive series of Dickinson and his colleagues (1979). In left atrial isomerism there are no terminal crests, and no right atrial appendages. The sinus node cannot therefore occupy its normal position. Indeed, in most of the hearts studied by Dickinson et al (1979) and in hearts we have studied since, it was not possible to identify a sinus node at all, although bilateral nodes were observed in the case reported by Pohanka & Vitek (1978). When Dickinson and his colleagues (1979) did find a node, it was a grossly hypoplastic structure found in the left-sided atrial wall adjacent to the atrioventricular junction.

The atrioventricular conduction tissue disposition reflects both the atrioventricular connexion present and the ventricular topology. When there is a biventricular atrioventricular connexion, the dominant feature is the ventricular topology. A right-hand pattern is associated with an atrioventricular node in its regular position and a posterior penetrating atrioventricular bundle, the axis of conduction tissue being deviated posteriorly as would be expected in presence of an atrioventricular septal defect (Dickinson et al, 1979; Thiene et al, 1981). When there is a left-hand pattern of ventricular topology, there is either an anterior atrioventricular node and conduction system as found typically in corrected transposition, or else a sling of conduction tissue running along the crest of the ventricular septum and connecting regular posterior and anomalous anterior atrioventricular nodes (Anderson et al, 1976; Bharati & Lev, 1978; Frescura et al, 1979; Dickinson et al, 1979; Fig. 19.13). With a univentricular atrioventricular connexion, the ventricular morphology is the domi-

nant feature. When the left ventricle is dominant the node is found in anterior position and the bundle varies in its relationship to the outflow tract of the left ventricle according to the position of the rudimentary right ventricle (see Ch. 26). With connexion to a dominant right ventricle, a regular posterior conduction system is to be expected when the rudimentary left ventricle is left-sided, but an anterior node or sling may be found when the rudimentary left ventricle is right-sided (Essed et al, 1980). A most bizarre disposition of conduction tissues must be expected when there is a solitary and indeterminate ventricle. In the two cases of this type studied by Dickinson et al (1979), slings of conduction tissue were found along the left-sided posterior wall of the atrioventricular junction despite the presence of a solitary ventricle.

Cardiac position

An unusual position of the heart should always alert to the

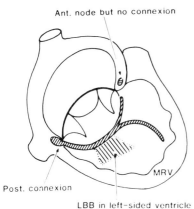

a) Right atrial isomerism
  – right-hand pattern topology

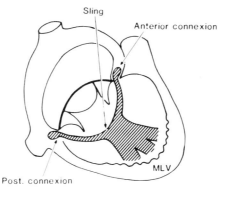

b) Right atrial isomerism
  – left-hand topology

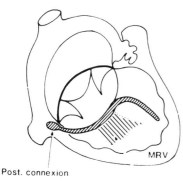

c) Left atrial isomerism
  – right-hand topology

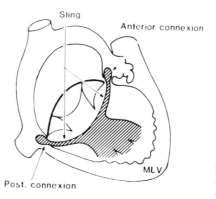

d) Left atrial isomerism
  – left-hand topology

Fig. 19.13 Diagrams illustrating the disposition of the atrioventricular conduction tissues in the cases we have studied histologically with atrial isomerism and biventricular atrioventricular connexion. MRV – morphologically right ventricle; MLV – morphologically left ventricle; LBB – left bundle branch.

presence of isomerism. Analysis of the data from the autopsy series reported by Rose et al (1975), De Tommasi et al (1981), and Frescura et al (1981), demonstrated that the heart was left-sided in about two-thirds, right-sided in one-third and midline in only 2 of 113 cases. A recent review by Sapire et al (1986) of both living patients and necropsy experience indicated a more even distribution of right-sided and left-sided hearts and the same small incidence of a midline heart (1 of 51 cases).

Arrangement of the thoraco-abdominal viscera

Visceral heterotaxy has long been recognised as the hallmark of the 'splenic syndromes'. The disposition of the abdominal organs led Ivemark (1955) to label asplenia as 'a syndrome of visceral symmetry'. Several subsequent authors then pointed to a midline liver as a marker of these 'splenic syndromes' (Forde & Finby, 1961; Lucas et al, 1962). Further experience has shown that this is not the case, and that the abdominal organs are not usually arranged in symmetrical fashion (Shah et al, 1964; Freedom & Fellows, 1973). Our reviews of the material published by the Hektoen Institute group (Macartney et al, 1978) together with our own experience (Macartney et al, 1980) confirms that isomerism cannot be diagnosed from the disposition of the abdominal organs. Of particular note is that, in our 28 cases of right isomerism, in which asplenia would be anticipated, the spleen was absent in only 23. In 10 cases with left isomerism, in which polysplenia is anticipated, multiple spleens were present in only 7, being left-sided in 5 and right-sided in 2 (Macartney et al, 1978). This means that the complex investigations required to establish splenic morphology will provide a relatively poor return in terms of accurate assessment of atrial arrangement. Vaughan et al (1971) stated that, 'Even the patient without heart disease deserves to know whether or not he has multiple splenic lobules'. We wonder why.

The morphology of the thoracic organs, specifically the bronchial tree, is a much better guide to the presence of isomerism. Van Mierop et al (1970) first observed that the bronchial arrangement was asymmetric in patients with lateralised arrangement but symmetrical in patients with isomerism (see: Ch. 3; Fig. 19.5). Finding the long bronchus on the left is therefore indicative of usual arrangement. A right-sided long bronchus indicates mirror-image arrangement, while bilateral long and hyparterial bronchi are indicative of left isomerism and bilateral short eparterial bronchi of right isomerism respectively (Fig. 19.14). The careful radiological studies of Partridge et al (1975) validated this finding and pointed to its value as a reproducable clinical investigation. Not all cases of atrial isomerism, however, have bronchial isomerism. Caruso & Becker (1979) described three cases in which there was discordance between bronchial arrangement and atrial position. We have since observed four similar cases (see Figs. 19.4, 19.5). Nonetheless, the value of examination of the penetrated chest radiograph, or a specially prepared 'filter' film, cannot be overstressed as a step in the evaluation of the infant or child suspected of having atrial isomerism (Deanfield et al, 1980).

Other malformations of the bodily organs occur with some frequency in patients with atrial isomerism. In the cases studied by Freedom (1972), genitourinary anomalies were found in over a quarter including such anomalies as horseshoe kidney, urethral valves, and so on. Other signifi-

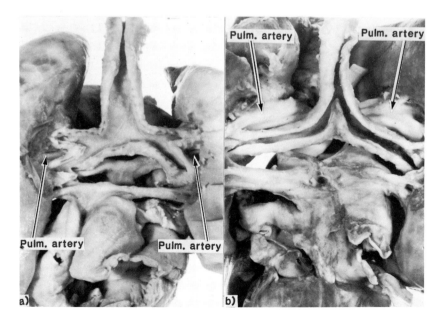

Fig. 19.14 Dissections illustrating the bronchial pattern with (a) right isomerism and (b) left isomerism. Note the different relationship of the lower lobe pulmonary artery to the bronchi.

cant anomalies found in individual patients included tracheo-oesophageal fistula, gall bladder agenesis, annular pancreas and cleft palate. Rose et al (1975) found a similar picture, urinary tract malformations being present in 15% of their patients.

Morphogenesis

Most early studies of the development of the 'splenic syndromes' concentrated their attention upon the spleen, and a most detailed account of the development of the spleen was given by Ivemark (1955). While of undoubted value in terms of knowledge of splenic development, this approach does little to clarify the grossly abnormal cardiac development associated with isomerism. Here, as with the analysis of the heart itself, the significant feature is the isomeric nature of the atrial appendages. As Van Mierop and his colleagues (1972) pointed out, the ventricles develop in series from the inlet and outlet parts of the ventricular 'loop', while the atrial chambers develop in parallel by incorporation of the venous sinus and primary pulmonary vein respectively into the right and left sides of the primitive atrial chamber. It is not surprising, therefore, that the isomeric malformation should produce duplication of the atrial chambers without producing symmetry of the ventricles. On this basis, atrial isomerism is readily understood according to development of the atrial component of the heart tube into either bilateral morphologically right or morphologically left components. Since the primitive atrium forms the vestibules of the definitive atrial chambers together with the atrial appendages, the major feature of atrial isomerism will be a symmetrical development of the atrial appendages. The venous malformations are then equally well explained. With bilateral morphologically right atrial appendages, there will be no focus for growth of the primary pulmonary vein. The intrapulmonary venous plexuses will join up with suitable systemic channels to form total anomalous connexions, or else will connect directly to the atrial chambers to produce an anomalous cardiac connexion. Persistence of the initial bilateral symmetry of the venous sinus accounts for the usual finding of bilateral superior caval veins and absence of the coronary sinus. The bilateral formation of the terminal crests accounts for the development of bilateral sinus nodes. Since the inferior caval vein is able to drain in normal fashion to the right atrium, the hepatic veins will also develop normally. When both the atrial appendages develop morphologically left characteristics, however, the pulmonary vein can develop from either side of the atrium, accounting for the common finding of bilateral pulmonary venous connexions. The presence of two primary pulmonary venous segments presumably 'squeezes' the venous sinus into midline position, but still permits in some cases the persistence of bilateral symmetry. Because the terminal crest develops from the morphologically right side, the superior caval channels will never drain in normal fashion in hearts with left isomerism, and there will be no potential for formation of a normal sinus node. The other effect of this 'squeeze' will be to obliterate the terminal portion of the inferior caval vein, which will then develop alternate routes of drainage via the azygos and hemiazygos systems. The hepatic veins of necessity must then connect themselves directly to the atrial chambers.

Since the ventricles develop in series, they can form in any fashion as occurs in malformations without isomerism. This is reflected in the variation seen in ventricular morphology. The frequent occurrence of a common atrioventricular junction probably reflects the isomeric nature of the atrioventricular vestibules, both developed from the primitive atrial chamber. Although the arterial pole of the heart is also divided in parallel to produce the definitive great arteries, the lack of symmetry in the arterial arrangement probably reflects the haemodynamic effects imposed by the development of the ventricles in series. It is not clear to us why right atrial isomerism should more frequently be associated with a univentricular atrioventricular connexion and with either pulmonary atresia or stenosis.

INCIDENCE AND AETIOLOGY

It is difficult to calculate precisely the incidence of atrial isomerism because until recently it has been described under a bewildering plethora of titles and has been recognised most frequently at autopsy rather than during clinical examination. Nonetheless, estimates based upon the occurrence of the 'splenic syndromes', or of heterotaxia (likely to be under- rather than over-estimates) show that it occurs with significant frequency. In the New England survey (Fyler et al, 1980) 95 of the 2251 presenting infants had heterotaxia. Rose and her colleagues in 1975 discovered 52 cases of polysplenia and asplenia recorded amongst the extensive autopsy records of the Hospital for Sick Children, Toronto. We were able to collect 45 cases from the autopsy collections at Brompton Hospital, Killingbeck Hospital, Leeds, and The Hospital for Sick Children, London, which at that time together probably totalled some 2000 specimens. The degree of potential underestimation of incidence given by these figures is shown by the fact that, when Deanfield and his colleagues (1980) performed filter radiograph on 100 consecutive infants presenting at the Hospital for Sick Children, isomerism was found in 10%. It is also possible that this is an underestimate of the overall population with general isomerism, since some may have bodily isomerism, particularly of left type, without there being any significant cardiac malformation. Only prospective studies using either filtered beam radiography or cross-sectional echocardiography, both now very much feasible propositions (see below), will determine the true incidence of patients with the isomeric forms of bodily arrangement and the percentage of these who have cardiac malformations.

Amongst patients known to have atrial isomerism, there is a tendency for right isomerism to affect males and for left isomerism to affect females. In the patients studied by Rose et al (1975), 60% of those with asplenia, but only 28% of those with polysplenia, were males. In terms of inheritance, some evidence points to atrial isomerism being a simple autosomal recessive trait. In the only family study to date, Rose and her colleagues (1975) found 3 sib pairs in their 60 cases. This gave a recurrence risk of just under 5%, which is much too low for simple autosomal recessive transmission, yet much higher than would be predicted from the multifactorial threshold model. Despite this, both McKusick (1978) and Nora & Nora (1978) list the 'Ivemark syndrome' as an autosomal recessive condition. It may well prove that they are correct, since it is possible that atrial isomerism may be analogous with the animal model provided by the iv/iv mouse (Layton & Manasek, 1980). In this model the homozygotes have disturbed bodily arrangement but only 1 in 5 of these have congenital cardiac lesions and, as in atrial isomerism, these are chiefly atrial anomalies, atrioventricular septal defects and malformations of the ventriculo-arterial junction. If it were found that only a proportion of cases with atrial isomerism presented cardiac malformations, then it too may be inherited in the fashion suggested by McKusick and the Noras. As discussed above, only a prospective study of family members of patients known to have atrial isomerism will resolve this problem. Although the final proof of autosomal recessive inheritance is lacking, other evidence points to the possibility that some cases are inherited as an X-linked disorder. Soltan & Li (1974) found a large kindred in which four males in three sibships had complex cardiac malformations described as 'complex dextrocardia with corrected transposition'. Three sons of a sister, while having no cardiac malformation, did have electrocardiographic evidence of 'malrotation along the sagittal axis'. There have also been several further reports of heart defects in sibs with atrial isomerism, but none involving more than one generation (Badr-El Din, 1962; Simpson & Zellweger, 1973; Chen & Montelione, 1977; Crawfurd, 1978; Katcher, 1980; Zlotgora & Elian, 1981). There are also several reports of parental consanguinity (Schonfeld & Frischman, 1958; Badr-El Din, 1962; Neimann et al, 1966; Katcher, 1980). Campbell (1965) calculated a 5.3% rate of consanguinity in his cases with 'partial situs inversus'. All this points to the fact that there is an increased risk of inheriting atrial isomerism. This should be borne in mind when counselling parents who have produced an infant with isomeric bodily arrangement.

CLINICAL RECOGNITION

There is now no excuse for failing to recognise the presence of atrial isomerism during life (Sapire et al, 1986). In addition to providing a firm base for subsequent sequential diagnosis, this information will also alert the clinician to the likely associated intracardiac lesions, such as total anomalous pulmonary venous connexion with right isomerism and interruption with azygos or hemiazygos continuation of the inferior caval vein with left isomerism. The finding of right isomerism will further alert one to the increased susceptibility to infection known to occur in the absence of the spleen. There are at least two reliable means of detecting atrial isomerism non-invasively which derive from the anatomy discussed above. The first, and most established, is the use of chest radiography, either using the straightforward penetrated chest radiograph (Van Mierop et al, 1970), bronchial tomography (Partridge et al, 1975) or high kilovoltage filtered beam radiograph (Deanfield et al, 1980). The penetrated film has proved unreliable both in our experience and that of others (Vaughan et al, 1971). This is particularly so in small infants, when precision is most needed. Bronchial tomography provides much clearer pictures but involves considerably more irradiation and not infrequently fails to demonstrate the bronchi in tachypnoeic infants because of breathing blur. The filter film technique with high kilovoltage is undoubtedly the best currently available. It was originally developed in Cincinatti by Dunbar (1970) to elucidate the causes of upper respiratory tract obstruction; hence the term 'Cincinatti Film'. On the radiograph, which is exposed with rather less irradiation than a standard chest film, bone detail is effaced to a considerable degree so that soft tissue and gas interfaces in the mediastinum and adjacent lung are readily seen. Exposure time is very short so that breathing blur is no problem. Using this technique, Deanfield et al (1980) obtained adequate bronchial visualisation in 95% of infants studied. It was also possible to recognise the position of the aortic arch from the tracheal indentation it produced and to visualise bronchial compression when present due to enlarged pulmonary arteries. All the required standard information as to heart size and shape, pulmonary vascularity, and so on was retained. Indeed, it can justifiably be asked if the filtered high kilovoltage film is not to be preferred as the standard procedure in the infant suspected of having congenital heart disease! Bronchial isomerism is therefore readily diagnosed from the filtered film. In the patient with either usual or mirror-image arrangement, the ratio of bronchial lengths is always greater than 1.5 (Partridge et al, 1975; Macartney et al, 1978). Finding a ratio of less than 1.5 is diagnostic for isomerism (Fig. 19.15). Usually, once isomerism has been established, the right and left forms can be distinguished simply from their characteristic pattern (Landing et al, 1971). The 'inverted Aries' or

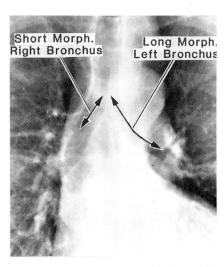

Fig. 19.15 A penetrated radiograph illustrating the usual pattern of bronchial arrangement.

inverted seagull sign is particularly striking for recognition of left bronchial isomerism (Fig. 19.16). Even experienced observers can make errors, however, if they rely on pattern recognition alone. It is therefore pertinent to know that

Partridge et al (1975) showed that morphologically left and morphologically right bronchi could be positively identified with a very small chance of misclassification by relating their absolute length to age. This original method was tedious since it required knowledge of the radiographic magnification. Deanfield et al (1980) showed that the same discrimination could be provided by relating apparent bronchial length to tracheal width, both measured directly from the filtered beam radiograph.

Atrial isomerism can also be identified with almost equal facility using cross-sectional ultrasonography (Huhta et al, 1982). This technique depends on demonstrating the relationship of the aorta and the inferior caval vein to each other and to the spine in short axis sections of the abdomen below the xiphisternum. In the person with normal lateralised bodily arrangement, the inferior caval vein will be identified to the right of the aorta which lies anterior to the vertebral column and the morphologically right atrium will be on the side of the venous channel (Fig. 19.17). The venoatrial connexion can readily be demonstrated by rotating the transducer into long axis and tracing the venous channel, at the same time observing its connexions with the hepatic veins. On occasion an echo-

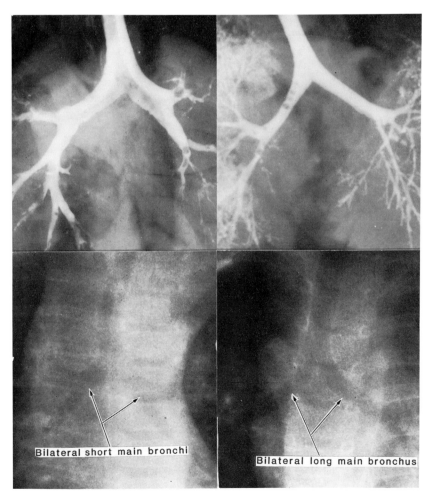

Fig. 19.16 Isomeric bronchial arrangement as shown in the upper panels by contrast bronchiography, and in the lower panels by filter film radiographs. The two left-hand panels show right isomerism and the two-right-hand panels show left isomerism.

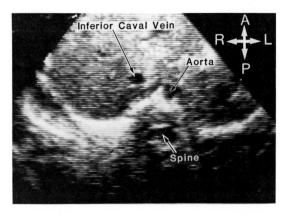

Fig. 19.17 The typical lateralised arrangement of the abdominal great vessels as seen by cross-sectional ultrasonography in a patient with usual atrial arrangement.

free linear space may be seen in normal cases in a position anterior to the aorta, which is suggestive of the inferior caval vein, and which can be traced upwards towards the right atrium. This is the postero-inferior recess of the pleural space and its non-venous identity can be confirmed by inability to trace it inferiorly below the liver.

In patients with right atrial isomerism, the inferior caval vein and the aorta run on the same side of the spine with the vein in anterolateral position (Fig. 19.18), and the hepatic veins drain into the inferior caval vein (Elliott et al, 1966). In contrast, most frequently in patients with left isomerism, there is interruption of the inferior caval vein. The abdominal venous return reaches the heart through the azygos or hemiazygos vein which runs on the same side of the spine as the aorta but in posterior position (Fig. 19.19). Cases having azygos or hemiazygos continuation in presence of usual or mirror-image bodily arrangement can be distinguished from some cases of left isomerism because the hepatic veins drain directly to the atrial chambers with isomerism whereas there is a supra-

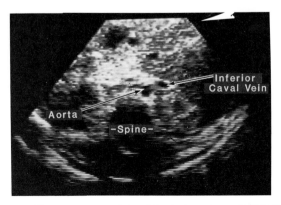

Fig. 19.18 The arrangement of the abdominal great vessels in a patient with right atrial isomerism. Both are to the same side of the spine (the left side) with the caval vein in anterior position.

hepatic inferior caval venous channel in patients with lateralised arrangement. Presence of the hepatic veins with direct atrial connexion also distinguish those cases of left isomerism who possess an abdominal inferior caval vein which is connected to the atrium (Huhta et al, 1982). Not all cases of left isomerism, however, have the hepatic veins connecting directly to the atrial chambers. Nonetheless, the ability in most cases to recognise atrial arrangement by cross-sectional ultrasonography now means that the initial step when investigating an infant suspected of having congenital heart disease should be to direct the sound beam into the abdomen!

CLINICAL FINDINGS

The clinical findings will reflect the associated cardiac lesions so that there are no classical features to be described. Nonetheless, once isomerism has been diagnosed, the clinical findings will often permit the distinction of right and left isomerism. Furthermore, if isomerism has not been diagnosed, the finding of certain features should always direct the physician to identify positively the bodily arrangement.

A high proportion of cases with right isomerism present as neonates with severe cyanosis. This mode of presentation results from the presence of pulmonary atresia or severe pulmonary stenosis in association with defects producing complete mixing of pulmonary and systemic venous blood. The severity of the obstruction to antegrade pulmonary blood flow means that the presence of total anomalous pulmonary venous connexion is almost invariably masked. Most importantly, obstructed pulmonary venous drainage is hardly ever clinically apparent. It will remain masked until pulmonary blood supply is increased by administration of prostaglandins or, catastrophically, by creation of a surgical systemic-pulmonary shunt. In patients with right atrial isomerism, the absence of the spleen in the majority of cases is reflected by the presence of Howell-Jolly or Heinz bodies in the blood (Willi & Gasser, 1955; Lyons et al, 1957). This in itself is not a specific finding since these bodies can be found in the blood of patients with normal spleens (Pearson et al, 1971) and are frequently absent from the blood of patients who have no spleen (Rose et al, 1975). Howell-Jolly bodies have also been reported in the blood of patients with left isomerism (Rodin et al, 1972; Rao & Leonard, 1976).

The clinical findings in left isomerism are non-specific and will simply reflect the associated lesions present. With the non-invasive techniques now available for the reliable recognition of isomerism, there seems to us no justification for invasive studies designed to search for multiple spleens as suggested by Vaughan et al (1971).

The standard chest radiograph gives no positive clues to the presence of isomerism. Once isomerism is diag-

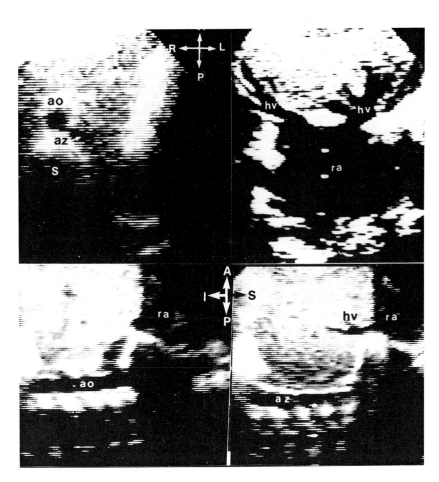

Fig. 19.19 The arrangement of the abdominal great vessels in a patient with left atrial isomerism and hemiazygos continuation of the inferior caval vein. As seen in the upper left-hand panel, both vessels (ao, az) are to the same side of the spine (s) with the vein in posterior position. This is confirmed by the lower panels showing long axis sections. The presence of left isomerism rather than usual arrangement with hemiazygos continuation is demonstrated by showing that the hepatic veins (hv) connect directly to the right-sided morphologically left atrium (ra – upper right panel).

nosed, then the finding of pulmonary oligemia in a cyanosed child favours right isomerism, while the finding of plethora, favours left isomerism.

The electrocardiographic findings are also not specific for diagnosis of isomerism, but once isomerism is identified the pattern present should confirm either right or left isomerism in most cases. In right atrial isomerism the frontal plane P wave axis is usually inferior (Blieden & Moller, 1973) but may be to the left (as with usually arranged atria) or to the right (as with mirror-image atria). About 80% of patients with left isomerism have a superiorly orientated P wave axis. This almost certainly reflects the probable absence or ectopic location of the sinus node (Dickinson et al, 1979). The superiorly orientated P wave axis can also be ascribed to a junctional (nodal) rhythm, especially if the PR interval is very short. This finding is neither highly sensitive nor specific for left atrial isomerism, since we have seen occasional patients with usually arranged or mirror-image atria having this electrocardiographic pattern. Previous authors have noted a relatively high incidence of superior P wave axes in patients with anomalies of systemic venous return, but did not comment as to whether there was left isomerism present (Hancock, 1964; Furuse et al, 1968). The morphology of the QRS complex will reflect the ventricular morphology and will be variable. In view of the association with atrioventricular septal defect, a high proportion of cases will have a superiorly orientated frontal QRS axis.

INVESTIGATION

Ideally the presence of an abnormal atrial arrangement should be made prior to cardiac catheterisation. As we have discussed, this can be accomplished with a high degree of accuracy from cross-sectional ultrasonography or from the radiological anatomy of the bronchi. Where high kilovoltage filter radiography is available, identification of bronchial anatomy presents no problem. As we have seen, ultrasonography is also invaluable, not only in its accepted role of elucidation of the intracardiac anatomy but also in diagnosing positively the existence of abnormal visceral arrangement. This latter feature has been discussed in detail above. In this section, therefore, we will discuss the way in which intracardiac ultrasonography, catherisation and angiocardiography should be performed, secure in the knowledge that isomeric atria exist. The aim of these investigations will be to characterise all the concomitant associated malformations.

Echocardiographic investigation

Potentially it is possible to visualise the atrial appendages echocardiographically and to make an assessment of their morphology. Anatomical sections made to simulate echo-cardiographic views suggest that the morphological differences between the atrial appendages (especially their junction with the atria) are sufficient to determine whether they are of left or right atrial morphology. It is possible in infants with normal atrial arrangement to see both appendages in one sector (Fig. 19.20). The problem arises when the atrial appendages do not lie in their anticipated positions in atrial isomerism. It might be possible to identify each appendage separately and make assessments after both have been visualised. Our experience in trying to locate both atrial appendages in the same sector in larger patients has, to date, not been successful (Sapire et al, 1986). The right atrial appendage-to-right atrial junction is normally retrosternal while the left atrial appendage-to-left atrial junction is quite lateral and somewhat posterior, being hidden behind the lingula of the left lung. The angle subtended by the two appendages is greater than that of most sectors available in cross-sectional ultra-sonographic equipment. It is also extremely difficult to be certain that tangential sections do not artifactually indicate wider or narrower junctions with the atria. In contrast to this uncertainty, the venous connexions can be clearly demonstrated. Thus far normal venous connexions have been the cornerstone of echocardiographic diagnosis of atrial arrangement. The echocardiographic recognition of abnormal venous connexions should therefore immediately raise a high degree of suspicion of atrial isomerism if this is not already known to exist. When one of the superior caval veins drains to the coronary sinus this is not nearly as suggestive of isomerism as when superior caval veins drain bilaterally to the atrial roof. Thus it is important, when bilateral superior caval veins are found, to establish their precise point of junction with the atrium. During the course of this investigation the region of the atrial septum will be studied. If the atrial septum is virtually absent and two caval veins connect to the atrial roof, atrial isomerism is almost certainly present. As we have discussed above, however, it is unlikely that the investigator will have reached this stage without having identified positively the presence of isomerism. Then, if it is known that there is right atrial isomerism, double inlet connexion via a common atrioventricular valve will be anticipated in many cases. If, with this connexion, an interventricular septum is found anterior to the common valve, this indicates double inlet to a left ventricle. An interventricular septum identified posterior to the common valve is diagnostic of a dominant right ventricle, while failure to identify a septum suggests a solitary ventricle of indeterminate type. With a biventricular atrioventricular connexion (each atrium connected to its own ventricular chamber) and a common valve, echocardiographic recognition of ventricular morphology is much less secure than when there are two separate valves. This is because there is no differential attachment of the valves to the septum in presence of a common valve. Almost always with a biventricular connexion, the superior bridging leaflet is free-floating and is attached to apical papillary muscles in both ventricles. The coarse trabeculation of a morphologically right ventricle can, however, often be identified. The site of septal attachments of the inferior bridging leaflet will be a further guide to identification of the morphologically right ventricle.

The common abnormalities of the ventriculo-arterial junction in right isomerism are double outlet right ventricle with pulmonary stenosis or atresia and single outlet of the heart in which no pulmonary outflow can be detected. Ventriculo-arterial discordance was also found with some frequency in right isomerism in the autopsy study of De Tommasi et al (1981), while ventriculo-arterial concordance was relatively common with left atrial isomerism. Echocardiography is of value in the identification of a double outlet connexion, particularly since this is usually associated with a bilateral infundibulum. Equally the presence of a single arterial trunk with pulmonary atresia, ventriculo-arterial discordance or concordance is amenable to echocardiographic diagnosis. The identification and assessment of severity of pulmonary stenosis are much less precise.

Cardiac catheterisation

As with all cardiac catheterisations, the object is a complete delineation of the haemodynamic disturbances. Prior knowledge of the presence of right or left isomerism is invaluable in planning and expediting the procedure. Catheterisation in the presence of left isomerism is most easily performed via the axillary venous approach because of the high incidence of continuation of the inferior caval

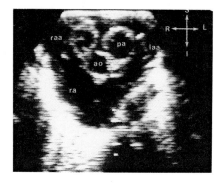

Fig. 19.20 A cross-sectional echocardiogram showing how, in the person with usual atrial arrangement, the morphology of the atrial appendages (raa, lAA) can be distinguished. ra – right atrium; ao – aorta; pa – pulmonary trunk.

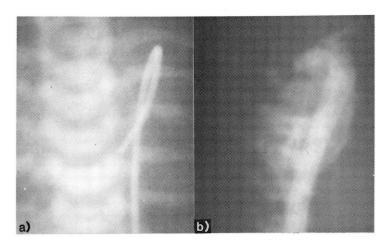

Fig. 19.21 (a) The typical catheter course in a patient with hemiazygos continuation of the inferior caval vein. Contrast has been injected in the vein in (b), confirming its course.

vein via the azygos or hemiazygos venous system. In unexpected cases the operator will recognise the abnormal catheter course when approaching from the leg (Fig. 19.21). Catheterisation can be successfully accomplished through a hemiazygos or azygos continuation, but is more difficult. When there is right atrial isomerism, every attempt should be made to delineate the pulmonary venous connexions because of the high incidence of anomalous drainage, especially the variety in which an anomalous channel passes through the diaphragm and communicates with the inferior caval vein by way of the portal system. If the route of pulmonary venous connexion cannot be established using the saphenous approach, umbilical venous catheterisation should be considered. This is easily performed in a neonate and will identify connexion of the pulmonary veins to the portal system when present. Where possible, the systemic and hepatic venous drainage should also be defined as completely as possible.

In the majority of cases of atrial isomerism, there will effectively be a common atrium. This will usually be manifested by a bidirectional atrial shunt and no pressure difference between the right- and left-sided atrial chambers. Even if there is only a left-to-right atrial shunt, the prevalence of univentricular atrioventricular connexion. double outlet right ventricle or single outlet of the heart leads to evidence of intercirculatory mixing as assessed by arterial Po_2 and its response to inhalation of 100% oxygen (Jones et al, 1976). High right ventricular pressures are usually Po_2 and its response to inhalation of 100% oxygen (Jones et al, 1976). High right ventricular pressures are usually encountered when each atrium is connected to a separate ventricle, either because of obstructed total anomalous pulmonary venous connexion or because of right ventricular outflow tract obstruction.

Angiocardiography

Angiocardiography should elucidate completely the intracardiac anatomy. Because of the complexity of the lesions,

it is sometimes difficult to accomplish this at one 'sitting'. It is therefore important in the sick neonate or infant to concentrate on lesions which may require urgent surgical attention. Thus in right isomerism the demonstration of the route of pulmonary venous return must be established using either pulmonary arterial angiocardiography or, better, by direct injection into the pulmonary veins. When drainage is to the portal vein this can usually be performed via umbilical venous catheterisation (Tynan et al, 1974; Fig. 19.22).

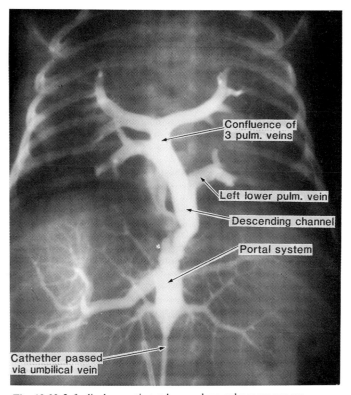

Confluence of 3 pulm. veins

Left lower pulm. vein

Descending channel

Portal system

Cathether passed via umbilical vein

Fig. 19.22 Infradiaphragmatic total anomalous pulmonary venous connexion to the portal system in a patient with right atrial isomerism. The injection was made via a catheter inserted into the umbilical vein.

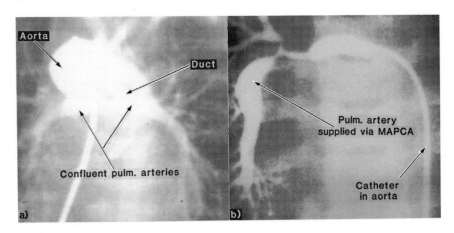

Fig. 19.23 The different types of pulmonary arterial supply which must be demonstrated when present in right atrial isomerism and pulmonary atresia with ventricular septal defect. (a) Shows supply of confluent pulmonary arteries via a duct. (b) Shows supply of the right pulmonary artery via a major aortopulmonary collateral artery (MAPCA).

The presence of pulmonary atresia or severe pulmonary stenosis will be indicated by ventricular angiocardiography. In the case of pulmonary atresia, an aortic injection or selective injection into major systemic-pulmonary collateral arteries may be required to demonstrate the presence and size of central pulmonary arteries (Fig. 19.23). Aortography is also invaluable in the diagnosis or exclusion of coarctation of the aorta, found most usually with the left atrial isomerism. The ventricular injection will indicate ventricular morphology, and show whether there is double inlet ventricle or two separate ventricles each connected to an atrial chamber. It may be difficult to distinguish the detailed anatomy, for example the site, extent and number of ventricular septal defects. This is important. In some cases ventricular septal defects are multiple, while in a minority, usually with left atrial isomerism, the ventricular architecture may be virtually normal. In the more complex cases, because positional anomalies of the heart are more frequent, the initial ventriculogram is often performed with little prior knowledge of the septal orientation. Furthermore this initial ventriculogram is often designed to demonstrate anomalies of the ventriculo-arterial junction. To some extent it is a 'scout' investigation. Before definitive surgery can be performed (see below) detailed ventricular angiocardiograms must be performed in the optimal projections for the heart under study. Correct use of cross-sectional echocardiography will often give enough information to avoid the use of the 'scout' ventriculogram. Not enough stress can be laid on the need to use this form of investigation before embarking on cineangiography. Information concerning rudimentary ventricles can often be better obtained by retrograde arterial catheterisation and injection of contrast in the rudimentary ventricle. This is better than trying to use information from ventriculograms in the dominant ventricle which has been entered through the atrioventricular valves. The first chamber to opacify will be the one in question and will not be obscured by contrast in the dominant ventricle or atria.

At such an investigation the route and connexion of the systemic veins must be established – particularly whether the superior caval veins drain bilaterally to the atrial roof. In left isomerism, or in right isomerism with anomalous pulmonary venous connexion to the atria, the distribution of pulmonary venous orifices must be mapped. Even with the most detailed angiocardiographic study, the precise position of an atrial baffle in complex cases will probably be determined at operation. The precise mode of atrioventricular connexion will be determined by echocardiography, detailed ventricular topology and valve function with angiocardiography, and the precise type of connexion will be established by a combination of the two.

The principles of establishing the ventricular topology and morphology are the same in atrial isomerism as in other conditions. As indicated in the echocardiographic section, double inlet via a common atrioventricular valve may be to a left ventricle with a rudimentary right ventricle, to a right ventricle with a rudimentary left ventricle, or to a solitary indeterminate ventricle. Ventricular topology can only be established by biventricular angiography. When the atria are isomeric it must be remembered that diagnosis of a biventricular atrioventricular connexion does not give the information about ventricular topology that is given by diagnosis of such a connexion with lateralised atria (Anderson & Tynan, 1981).

Once the investigator is aware of the high probability of the existence of isomeric atria, the detailed morphology of the atrial appendages is of little operational significance. The importance of the diagnosis of atrial isomerism is the information it gives concerning the likelihood of associated anomalies of venous connexion, intracardiac anatomy and arterial connexions. Knowledge of the presence of atrial isomerism necessitates complete delineation of these aspects and of the architectural organisation of the ventricular mass before decisions can be made concerning the possibility of definitive surgical treatment.

TREATMENT

The treatment of patients with atrial isomerism will be determined by the severity of associated lesions. Some patients with left atrial isomerism may have no cardiac lesions, and they will require no treatment. Patients with left isomerism in general have less severe malformations than those with right isomerism and hence more chance of corrective surgery. Those with right isomerism will require treatment earlier in life which is more likely to be palliative than corrective. It is axiomatic, however, that each case be treated on its own merits.

Medical management

The severely ill patient requiring medical treatment in infancy will almost certainly have right isomerism, and the lesion producing problems is likely to be severe pulmonary outflow tract obstruction or perhaps obstructed total anomalous pulmonary venous connexion. Prostaglandin therapy to dilate the duct may be indicated (see Ch. 37) followed by a systemic-to-pulmonary shunt. Those with total anomalous pulmonary venous connexion will require open heart surgery. Administration of prostaglandins has also been suggested as a means of unmasking pulmonary venous obstruction. If there is a severe obstruction, dilating a persistently patent duct will result in reversible pulmonary oedema. In our experience it is still possible to induce pulmonary oedema with a surgical shunt even when obstruction has not been unmasked by prostaglandin administration. There is always the danger of severe infection in these patients, since almost always they will have no spleen. The onset of infection should therefore be anticipated and treated accordingly as soon as it is confirmed. The place of prophylactic antibiotics (Waldman et al, 1977) and immunisation against pneumococcus in such cases is not yet established. Apart from these special problems of the severely ill neonate, the medical treatment of other patients with atrial isomerism will be dictated by the associated lesions and symptoms present.

Surgical treatment

Only recently have the complex congenital malformations associated with atrial isomerism been shown to be amenable to surgical correction (Albert et al, 1968; Ando et al, 1976). Surgical treatment, even if only palliative, is possible for most of the combinations usually found with atrial isomerism. Paradoxically, although exceedingly complex malformations are frequent, those anomalies that most usually preclude surgical treatment (such as aortic atresia) are relatively rare.

The patients who can best be considered to have a realistic chance of successful corrective surgery are those with a biventricular atrioventricular connexion. Even in these, the associated malformations may be so severe as to preclude complete correction. At least the presence of two atria, each connected to a separate ventricle, sets the scene for potential correction. When there is a univentricular atrioventricular connexion, with the atrial connected to one ventricle, surgery will be nominally 'corrective' only when there is the possibilty of septating a heart with double inlet left ventricle (McKay et al, 1982). The options offered by the Fontan procedure and its modifications are potentially open to many more patients with atrial isomerism and univentricular atrioventricular connexion. But then the almost universal presence of anomalies of venoatrial connexions will give extra problems (Di Carlo et al, 1983). Only rare cases will prove to be correctable (Girod et al, 1984).

In the analysis of corrective surgery reported by Pacifico et al (1983), only 2 of 17 patients had had previous palliative operations. This points to a high degree of selection in a group where pulmonary atresia or total anomalous pulmonary venous connexion would be anticipated in about half. Furthermore, all were corrected without resort to Fontan-type procedures, although this has been employed in one patient with a biventricular atrioventricular connexion (Gonzalez-Lavin et al, 1977). In the patients corrected by Pacifico and his colleagues (1983), anomalies of venoatrial connexion were found in the majority, but these did not present problems. A suitably tailored atrial baffle was constructed to correct the anomalous connexions, an additional Mustard procedure also being needed in some. Similar procedures had been described previously for isolated patients (Ghosh et al, 1977; Krayenbuhl & Lincoln, 1977; Turley et al, 1981). In terms of the remaining surgery, standard techniques were used to repair each associated defect, modifying them according to the specific anatomy present (Pacifico et al, 1977; Katz et al, 1978; Quaegebeur et al, 1979; Stewart et al, 1979; Pacifico et al, 1980; Kirklin et al, 1981). As might be expected, hospital mortality was greater early in the experience although the mortality was similar with right and left isomerism. It is likely that with increasing experience, and with selection of patients, this improvement will continue. As Pacifico and his colleagues (1983) suggest, 'The surgical team must be experienced with techniques of repair for each defect present and also must have complete and accurate preoperative studies to form a thorough understanding of the anatomy and physiology present in each patient.'

REFERENCES

Abernethy J 1793 Account of two instances of uncommon formations in the viscera of the human body. Philosophical Transactions 83: 59–66

Albert H M, Fowler R L, Glass B A, Yu S K 1968 Cardiac anomalies and splenic agenesis. American Surgeon 34: 94–98

Anderson R H, Tynan M 1981 Sequential chamber localisation. In:

Hamer J, Rowlands D J (eds) Recent advances in cardiology, Vol 8. Churchill Livingstone, Edinburgh, p 265–285

Anderson R H, Smith A, Wilkinson J L 1976 Right juxtaposition of the auricular appendages. European Journal of Cardiology 4: 495–503

Ando F, Shirotani H, Kawai J, et al 1976 Successful total repair of complicated cardiac anomalies with asplenia syndrome. Journal of Thoracic and Cardiovascular Surgery 72: 33–38

Aguilar M J, Stephens H B, Crane J T 1956 Syndrome of congenital absence of the spleen with associated cardiovascular and gastroenteric anomalies. Circulation 14: 520–531

Badr-El Din M K 1962 Syndrome of levocardia, multiple cardiac defects, situs inversus and absent spleen – a case report. American Heart Journal 63: 115–118

Bharati S, Lev M 1978 The course of the conduction system in dextrocardia. Circulation 57: 163–171

Blieden L C, Moller J H 1973 Analysis of the P wave in congenital cardiac malformations associated with splenic anomalies. American Heart Journal 85: 439–444

Breschet G 1826 Memoire sur l'ectopie de appareil de la circulation et particulierement sur celle du coeur. E Duverger, Paris

Cabrera A, Quero M, Pastor E, et al, 1981 Asplenia y polisplenia. Estudio anatomico de 27 casos y revision de la literatura. Revista Latina de Cardiologia 2: 83–98

Campbell M 1965 Causes of malformations of the heart. British Medical Journal 2: 895–904

Caruso G, Becker A E 1979 How to determine atrial situs? Considerations initiated by 3 cases of absent spleen with a discordant anatomy between bronchi and atria. British Heart Journal 41: 559–567

Chen S C, Montelione P L 1977 Familial splenic anomaly syndrome. Journal of Pediatrics 91: 160–161

Crawfurd M D 1978 Renal dysplasia and asplenia in two sibs. Clinical Genetics 14: 338–344

Deanfield J E, Leanage R, Stroobant J, Chrispin A R, Taylor J F N, Macartney F J 1980 Use of high kilovoltage filtered beam radiographs for detection of bronchial situs in infants and young children. British Heart Journal 44: 577–583

De Tommasi S M, Daliento L, Ho S Y, Macartney F J, Anderson R H 1981 Analysis of atrioventricular junction, ventricular mass and ventriculoarterial junction in 43 specimens with atrial isomerism. British Heart Journal 45: 236–247

Di Carlo D, Marcelletti C, Nijveld A, Lubbers L J, Becker A E 1983 The Fontan procedure in the absence of the interatrial septum. Failure of its principle? The Journal of Thoracic and Cardiovascular Surgery 85: 923–927

Dickinson D F, Wilkinson J L, Anderson K R, Smith A, Ho S Y, Anderson R H 1979 The cardiac conduction system in situs ambiguus. Circulation 59: 879–885

Dunbar J S 1970 Upper respiratory tract obstruction in infants and children. American Journal of Roentgenology 109: 227–246

Elliott L P, Cramer G C, Amplatz K 1966 The anomalous relationship of the inferior vena cava and abdominal aorta as a specific angiocardiographic sign in asplenia. Radiology 87: 859–863

Essed C E, Ho S Y, Hunter S, Anderson R H 1980 Atrioventricular conduction system in univentricular heart of right ventricular type with right-sided rudimentary chamber. Thorax 35: 123–127

Forde W J, Finby N 1961 Roentgenographic features of asplenia, a teratological syndrome of visceral symmetry. American Journal of Roentgenology 86: 523–533

Freedom R M 1972 The asplenia syndrome: a review of significant extracardiac structural abnormalities in 29 necropsied patients. Journal of Pediatrics 81: 1130–1133

Freedom R M, Fellows K E Jr 1973 Radiographic visceral patterns in the asplenia syndrome. Paediatric Radiology 107: 387–391

Frescura C, Nava A, Thiene G 1979 Doppia giunzione atrioventricolare specifica in situs ambiguus con asplenia. Giornale Italiano di Cardiolgia 9: 527–531

Frescura C, Marino B, Bosman C, Thiene G 1981 Sindromi asplenica e polisplenica: malformazioni cardiovascolari ed interpretazioni embriogenetiche. In: Progressi in cardiologia pediatrica. Cardiomiopatie e sindromi spleniche. Atti Del X Congresso della Societa Italiana Di Cardiologia Pediatrica. Padova, 2–4 Maggio. Lint, Trieste, p 123–148

Furuse A, Mizuno A, Sato F, Hasegawa T, Kotoda T, Saigusa M 1968 Coronary sinus rhythm in anomalous systemic venous connection. Japanese Heart Journal 9: 200–207

Fyler D C, Buckley L P, Hellenbrand W E, Cohn H E 1980 Report of the New England Regional Infant Cardiac Program. Pediatrics 65 (Suppl): 376–461

Ghosh P K, Donnelly R J, Hamilton D I, Wilkinson J L 1977 Surgical correction of a case of common atrium with anomalous systemic and pulmonary venous drainage. Journal of Thoracic and Cardiovascular Surgery 74: 604–606

Gilbert E F, Nishimura K, Wedum B G 1958 Congenital malformations of the heart associated with splenic agenesis – with a report of five cases. Circulation 17: 72–86

Girod D A, Lima R C, Anderson R H, Ho S Y, Rigby M L, Quaegebeur J M 1984 Double inlet ventricle: Morphologic analysis and surgical implications in 32 cases. Journal of Thoracic and Cardiovascular Surgery 88: 590–600

Gonzalez-Lavin L, Blair T C, Chi S, Sparrow A W 1977 Orthoterminal correction of coexisting d-transposition of the great arteries, subpulmonary stenosis, and a complete form of atrioventricular canal. Journal of Thoracic and Cardiovascular Surgery 73: 694–698

Hancock E W 1964 Coronary sinus rhythm in sinus venosus defect and persistent left superior vena cava. American Journal of Cardiology 14: 608–615

Huhta J C, Smallhorn J F, Macartney F J 1982 Two dimensional echocardiographic diagnosis of situs. British Heart Journal 48: 97–108

Ivemark B I 1955 Implications of agenesis of the spleen in the pathogenesis of conotruncus anomalies in childhood. An analysis of the heart; malformations in the splenic agenesis syndrome, with 14 new cases. Acta Paediatrica Scandinavica 44 (Suppl 104): 1–110

Jones R W A, Baumer J H, Joseph M C, Shinebourne E A 1976 Arterial oxygen tension and the response to oxygen breathing in the differential diagnosis of congenital heart disease in infancy. Archives of Diseases in Childhood 51: 667–679

Katcher A L 1980 Familial asplenia, other malformations and sudden death note. Pediatrics 65: 633–635

Katz N M, Kirklin J W, Pacifico A D 1978 Concepts and practices in surgery for total anomalous pulmonary venous connection. Annals of Thoracic Surgery 25: 479–487

Kirklin J W, Chung G, Pacifico A D, Blackstone E H, Bargeron L M Jr 1981 Repair of A-V canal defects. In: Parenzan L, Crupi G, Graham G (eds) Congenital heart disease in the first three months of life. Casa Editrice Patron, Bologna

Krayenbuhl C U, Lincoln J C R 1977 Total anomalous systemic venous connection, common atrium, and partial atrioventricular canal. Journal of Thoracic and Cardiovascular Surgery 73: 686–689

Landing B H, Lawrence T K, Payne V C, Wells T R 1971 Bronchial anatomy in syndromes with abnormal visceral situs, abnormal spleen and congenital heart disease. American Journal of Cardiology 12: 456–462

Layman T E, Levine M A, Amplatz K, Edwards J E 1967 'Asplenic syndrome' in association with rudimentary spleen. American Journal of Cardiology 20: 136–140

Layton W M, Manasek F J 1980 Cardiac looping in early iv/iv mouse embroys. In: Van Praagh R, Takao A (eds) Etiology and morphogenesis of congenital heart disease. Futura, Mount Kisco, New York, p 109–126

Lucas R V Jr, Neufeld H N, Lester R G, Edwards J E 1962 The symmetrical liver as a roentgen sign of asplenia. Circulation 25: 973–975

Lyons W S, Hanlon D G, Helmholz H R Jr, DuShane J W, Edwards J E 1957 Congenital cardiac disease and asplenia. Report of seven cases. Proceedings of Staff Meetings of the Mayo Clinic 32: 277–286

Macartney F J, Partridge J B, Shinebourne E A, Tynan M J, Anderson R H 1978 Identification of atrial situs. In: Anderson R H, Shinebourne E A (eds) Paediatric cardiology, 1977. Churchill Livingstone, Edinburgh, p 16–26

Macartney F J, Zuberbuhler J R, Anderson R H 1980 Morphological considerations pertaining to recognition of atrial isomerism. Consequences for sequential chamber localisation. British Heart Journal 44: 657–667

McKay R, Pacifico A D, Blackstone E H, Kirklin J W, Bargeron L M Jr 1982 Septation of the univentricular heart with left anterior subaortic outlet chamber. Journal of Thoracic and Cardiovascular Surgery 84: 77–87

McKusick V A 1978 Mendelian inheritance in man, 5th edn. Johns Hopkins University Press, Baltimore

McLean S, Craig H R 1922 Congenital absence of the spleen. American Journal of the Medical Sciences 164: 703–712

Martin M G 1826 Observation d'une deviation organique de l'estomac d'une anomalie dans la situation dans la configuration du coeur et des vaisseaux qui en partent ou qui s'y rendant. Bulletin Société d'Anatomie de Paris 1: 39–43

Moller J H, Nakib A, Anderson R C, Edwards J E 1967 Congenital cardiac disease associated with polysplenia: A developmental complex of bilateral 'left-sidedness'. Circulation 36: 789–799

Neimann N, Pernot C, Gentin G, Vert P, Worms A M 1966 Le syndrome d'Ivemark cardiomyopathie congenitale cyanogene severe heterotaxie thoraco-abdominale complex et asplenie ou polysplenie. Pediatrie 21: 511–532

Nora J J, Nora A H 1978 Genetics and counselling in cardiovascular disease. Charles C Thomas, Springfield, Illinois, p 92

Pacifico A D, Kirklin J W, Blackstone E H 1977 Surgical management of pulmonary stenosis in tetralogy of Fallot. Journal of Thoracic and Cardiovascular Surgery 74: 382–395

Pacifico A D, Kirklin J W, Bargeron L M Jr 1980 Repair of complete atrioventricular canal associated with tetralogy of Fallot or double-outlet right ventricle: report of 10 patients. Annals of Thoracic Surgery 29: 351–356

Pacifico A D, Fox L S, Kirklin J W, Bargeron L M Jr 1983 Surgical treatment of atrial isomerism. In: Anderson R H, Macartney F J, Shinebourne E A, Tynan M (eds) Paediatric cardiology, Vol 5. Churchill Livingstone, Edinburgh, p 223–230

Partridge J B, Scott O, Deverall P B, Macartney F J 1975 Visualization and measurement of the main bronchi by tomography as an objective indicator of thoracic situs in congenital heart disease. Circulation 51: 188–196

Pearson H A, Schiebler G L, Spencer R P 1971 Functional hyposplenia in cyanotic congenital heart disease. Pediatrics 48: 277–280

Pohanka I, Vitek B 1978 The conduction system of the heart in the syndrome of visceral symmetry. Folia Morphologica (Prague) 26: 379–388

Putschar W G J, Mannion W C 1956 Congenital absence of the spleen and associated anomalies. American Journal of Clinical Pathology 26: 429–470

Quaegebeur J, Kirklin J W, Pacifico A D, Bargeron L M Jr 1979 Surgical experience with unroofed coronary sinus. Annals of Thoracic Surgery 27: 418–425

Rao P S, Leonard T 1976 Polysplenic syndrome. Cardiology Digest 11: 14–22

Rodin A E, Sloane J A, Nghiem Q 1972 Polysplenia with severe congenital heart disease and Howell-Jolly bodies. American Journal of Clinical Pathology 58: 127–134

Rose V, Izukawa T, Moes C A F 1975 Syndromes of asplenia and polysplenia. A review of cardiac and non-cardiac malformations in 60 cases with special reference to diagnosis and prognosis. British Heart Journal 37: 840–852

Sapire D W, Ho S Y, Anderson R H, Rigby M L 1986 Diagnosis in life of atrial isomerism: its clinical significance. American Journal of Cardiology 58: 342–346

Schonfeld R, Frischman B 1958 Syndrome of spleen agenesis, defects of the heart and vessels and situs inversus. Helvetica Paediatrica Acta 13: 636–640

Shah K D, Neill C A, Wagner H N, Taussig H B 1964 Radioisotope scanning of the liver and spleen in dextrocardia and in situs inversus with levocardia. Circulation 29: 231–241

Shinebourne E A, Macartney F J, Anderson R H 1976 Sequential chamber localization – logical approach to diagnosis in congenital heart disease. British Heart Journal 38: 327–340

Simpson J, Zellweger H 1973 Familial occurrence of Ivemark's syndrome with splenic hypoplasia and asplenia in sibs. Journal of Medical Genetics 10: 303–304

Soltan H C, Li M D 1974 Hereditary dextrocardia associated with other congenital heart defects: report of a pedigree. Clinical Genetics 5: 51–58

Stanger P, Rudolph A M, Edwards J E 1977 Cardiac malpositions: an overview based on study of sixty-five necropsy specimens. Circulation 56: 159–172

Stewart R W, Kirklin J W, Pacifico A D, Blackstone E H, Bargeron L M Jr 1979 Repair of double-outlet right ventricle. Journal of Thoracic and Cardiovascular Surgery 78: 502–514

Thiene G, Frescura C 1984 Codificazione diagnostica e atlante delle cardiopatie congenite. Edizioni Lint, Trieste, p 43

Thiene G, Wenink A C G, Frescura C, Wilkinson J L, Gallucci V, Ho S Y, Anderson R H 1981 The surgical anatomy of the conduction tissues in atrioventricular defects. Journal of Thoracic and Cardiovascular Surgery 82: 928–937

Turley K, Tarnoff H, Snider R, Ebert P A 1981 Repair of combined total anomalous pulmonary venous connection and anomalous systemic connection in early infancy. Annals of Thoracic Surgery 31: 70–77

Tynan M, Behrendt D, Urquhart W, Graham G R 1974 Portal vein catheterization and selective angiography in diagnosis of total anomalous pulmonary venous connection. British Heart Journal 36: 1155–1159

Tynan M J, Becker A E, Macartney F J, Quero-Jimenez M, Shinebourne E A, Anderson R H 1979 Nomenclature and classification of congenital heart disease. British Heart Journal 41: 544–553

Van Mierop L H S 1981 Morphological characteristics of the atria and their variations, including characteristics in the splenic syndromes. In: Godman M J (ed) Paediatric cardiology, Vol 4. Churchill Livingstone, Edinburgh, Ch 16, p 144–152

Van Mierop L H S, Wiglesworth F W 1962 Isomerism of the cardiac atria in the asplenia syndrome. Laboratory Investigation 11: 1303–1315

Van Mierop L H S, Eisen S, Schiebler G L 1970 The radiographic appearance of the tracheobronchial tree as an indicator of visceral situs. American Journal of Cardiology 26: 432–435

Van Mierop L H S, Gessner I H, Schiebler G L 1972 Asplenia and polysplenia syndromes. Birth Defects: Original Article Series 8: 36–52

Van Praagh R 1977 Terminology of congenital heart disease: glossary and commentary. Circulation 56: 139–143

Van Praagh R, Vlad P 1978 Dextrocardia, mesocardia and levocardia: the segmental approach to diagnosis in congenital heart disease. In: Keith J D, Rowe R D, Vlad P (eds) Heart disease in infancy and childhood. Macmillan, New York, p 638–695

Vaughan T J, Hawkins I F Jr, Elliott L P 1971 Diagnosis of polysplenia syndrome. Diagnostic Radiology 101: 511–518

Waldman J D, Rosenthal A, Smith A L, Shorin S, Nadas A S 1977 Sepsis and congenital asplenia. Journal of Pediatrics 90: 555–559

Willi H, Gasser C 1955 The clinical diagnosis of the triad spleen agenesis, defects of the heart and vessels and situs inversus. Etudes Neonatales 4: 25–66

Zlotgora J, Elian E 1981 Asplenia and polysplenia syndromes with abnormalities of lateralisation in a sibship. Journal of Medical Genetics 18: 301–302

Anomalous systemic venous return

This chapter deals with abnormalities of position and connexion of the major systemic venous channels which drain to the heart, and also with abnormal persistence of the valves of the sinus venosus. Many of these anomalies are incidental findings with little haemodynamic significance. But they may complicate cardiac catheterisation and surgical procedures and may be associated with other more important congenital cardiac anomalies.

A consideration of the morphogenesis of the normal systemic venous system, is helpful in classifying the wide variety of systemic venous anomalies which exist. The embryology of the systemic venous system will therefore be briefly reviewed before considering the individual anomalies and their clinical significance.

MORPHOGENESIS OF THE SYSTEMIC VENOUS SYSTEM

Development of superior caval vein, coronary sinus, and venous valves

Normal venous development is a process of progressive appearance of a series of paired venous structures, development of anastomotic channels between them and the eventual selective regression of certain segments (Figs. 20.1 & 20.2). The sinus venosus, the most proximal portion of the cardiac tube, has right and left sinus horns and empties into the atrial segment of the tube. Three major venous channels drain into the sinus venosus at this stage: the omphalomesenteric (vitelline) veins, the umbilical veins, and the common cardinal veins, the latter entering the sinus horns as the ducts of Cuvier. Each common cardinal vein is formed by the union of the anterior and posterior cardinal veins, which drain the cephalic and caudal regions of the embryo respectively.

Initially the sinus horns and the transverse portion of the sinus venosus are positioned horizontally and lie dorsal to the developing atrium. The left sinus horn and the transverse portion of the sinus venosus become separated from the left side of the atrium by the development of a promi-

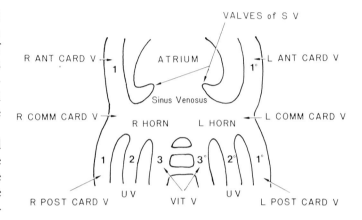

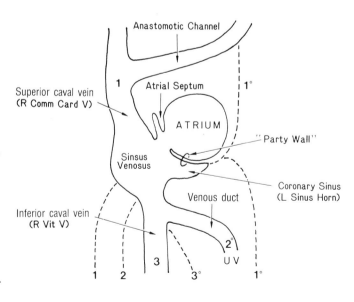

Fig. 20.1 Development of the cephalic portion of the systemic venous system from primitive state of paired cardinal, umbilical and vitelline veins (above) to the most common unpaired adult arrangement (below). Abbreviations: Ant = anterior; Card = cardinal; Comm = common; L = left; Post = posterior; R = right; SV = sinus venosus; UV = umbilical vein, V = vein; Vit = vitelline.

497

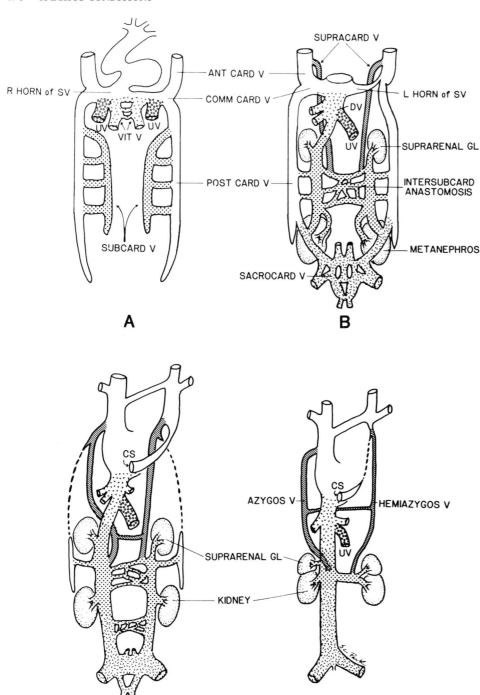

Fig. 20.2 Progression of development of the systemic venous system. (A) 4 mm embryo stage with paired subcardinal veins present. (B) 4 mm stage with appearance of paired sacrocardinal and supracardinal systems. (C) 17 mm stage. (D) Normal term infant's venous pattern showing embryological derivation of structures. GL = gland; CS = coronary sinus; DV = venous duct. Other abbreviations as in Figure 20.1.

nent fold. In addition, anastomotic channels develop between the right- and left-sided venous channels and there is preferential flow to the right-sided structures. There then follows gradual regression of the left-sided vitelline and cardinal veins with increasing prominence of the right sinus horn. The sinus horns and transverse portion of the sinus venosus then shift to the right and become oriented in a more vertical fashion, with the left sinus horn occupying a position which is inferior to the right sinus horn. The

right sinus horn and a part of the transverse portion of the sinus venosus become incorporated into the wall of the right atrium, allowing the future caval veins to connect directly with the right atrium.

A major anastomotic connection between the right and left anterior cardinal veins enlarges and becomes the left brachiocephalic (innominate) vein. The left anterior cardinal vein below this point gradually obliterates. The proximal portion of the left sinus horn persists as the coronary sinus, draining the coronary venous system, and the left duct of Cuvier persists as the ligament or oblique vein of Marshall. The right anterior cardinal vein and the right duct of Cuvier persist as the right superior caval vein.

During the incorporation of the sinus venosus into the right atrium there is an infolding of tissue in the region of the sinu-atrial junction on both the right and left sides. These infoldings are prominent structures during embryonic life, known as the right and left valves of the sinus venosus. The left valve eventually fuses with the atrial septum. The right valve also gradually regresses for the most part, except for inferior portions which persist as valve tissue overlying the orifices of the inferior caval vein (Eustachian valve) and the coronary sinus (Thebesian valve).

A brief note regarding the development of the pulmonary venous system is warranted, considering the occasional coexistence of anomalies of pulmonary and systemic venous drainage. The developing lung is derived from the primitive foregut and shares its early blood supply with the gut via a splanchic plexus. This plexus anastomoses the pulmonary veins and the cardinal venous system. These connexions are lost completely in the normal embryo once the common pulmonary vein is incorporated into the left atrium.

Development of the inferior caval vein

As mentioned above, the first venous channels to appear in the developing embryo are the vitelline, umbilical, and the anterior and posterior cardinal veins. The vitelline system becomes a prominent plexus which includes a vascular network draining the liver. These channels become predominant on the right side of the embryo and maintain their connexion to the right side of the sinus venosus through structures known as the hepatocardiac channels. The right-sided vitelline vein ultimately becomes the terminal or post-hepatic portion of the inferior caval vein.

Initially the umbilical veins are paired structures which lose their connection to the sinus venosus and anastomose to the hepatic sinusoids. The right-sided umbilical vein regresses and the left umbilical vein enlarges to become the only channel bringing blood from the placenta to the embryo. The anastomosis between the left umbilical vein and the hepatocardiac channel becomes the venous duct.

Further changes occur within the developing abdominal region of the embryo. By the 5th week of gestation paired subcardinal veins arise medial to the posterior cardinal veins and serve to drain the urogenital sinuses. The subcardinal veins empty superiorly into the posterior cardinal vein. Anastomotic channels then develop between the two subcardinal veins as well as between the right subcardinal and hepatocardiac channels. It is the right subcardinal vein which becomes predominant and develops into the infrahepatic segment of the inferior caval vein. With continued growth of the trunk of the embryo yet another system of

veins, the sacrocardinal veins, arises dorsal and caudal to the posterior cardinal system. Anastomotic channels between the subcardinal and sacrocardinal systems on the right side will form the renal segment of the inferior caval vein, while the distal portions of the right sacrocardinal vein enlarge and become its most inferior portion. Concomitant with these developments of the paracardinal systems, the posterior cardinal veins themselves gradually involute except for their most proximal portions. As this involution is occurring a supracardinal venous system develops. These channels drain into the terminal portions of the posterior cardinal veins and persist as the azygos and hemiazygos veins, on right and left sides respectively.

The fully developed inferior caval vein is thus formed from four right-sided embryologic structures. The terminal suprahepatic portion is derived from the right vitelline vein. The infrahepatic segment arises from the right subcardinal vein, the renal segment from the anastomotic channels between the subcardinal and sacrocardinal veins, and the most inferior segment from the right sacrocardinal vein. The azygos veins are derived from the supracardinal system.

Development of atrial isomerism

The venous development discussed thus far has presumed the development of anastomotic channels and connexion of the sinus venosus to the right-sided atrium. It is this process which produces the morphologically right atrium, which contains the entirety of the sinus venosus. The left side of the atrium together with the developing pulmonary veins becomes the morphologically left atrium. Concomitant with these changes the body of the primitive atrium buds out its appendages. The one from the systemic side assumes its typically triangular shape and incorporates the cephalic part of the valve of the sinus venosus to form the terminal crest (crista terminalis). The appendage growing from the pulmonary side is much narrower and has no relation with the valves of the sinus venosus. It therefore lacks a terminal crest. All of this depends upon development of a left-sided to right-sided anastomosis. Should the anastomosis develop in right-sided to left-sided fashion, then the left-sided atrium will incorporate the sinus venosus and become the morphologically right atrium while the right-sided atrium becomes the morphologically left atrium. This produces the mirror-image atrial arrangement usually termed 'situs inversus'.

However, in certain circumstances the lateralisation process does not occur and the sinus venosus retains its bilateral symmetry. This lack of lateralisation occurs in two forms. In the one, the valves of the sinus venosus are incorporated bilaterally along with development of right-sided structures. This 'squeezes-out' the anlagen of the primary pulmonary vein so that there is no atrial site for pulmonary venous drainage. Right atrial isomerism therefore has bilateral sinus horns together with bilateral systemic venous drainage, as well as anomalous pulmonary venous drainage. In the other pattern there is bilateral growth of morphologically left structures. Thus the pulmonary venous component predominates and squeezes out the sinus venosus. The major systemic venous channels then make anomalous connexions to these left atrial chambers. The common cardinal veins are more successful in this respect, tending to enter the atrial roof on each side in absence of a terminal crest ('crista terminalis'). The hepatic veins also enter the atrium directly, often bilaterally. The venous return from the lower body usually continues through the supracardinal azygos system and drains to one or other of the anterior cardinal veins (interruption of the inferior caval vein). In those cases with left isomerism in which the inferior caval vein does achieve a direct atrial connexion, it does so separately from the hepatic veins.

CLASSIFICATION

An organised classification of venous anomalies can be most easily achieved by using anatomic rather than embryologic subdivisions (Table 20.1). Within this framework we can then consider aberrations of development in the superior and inferior caval veins and the coronary sinus, as well as total anomalous systemic venous connexion and abnormal persistence of the valves of the sinus venosus. Prevalence, pathophysiology, clinical and laboratory findings, and management will be discussed where appropriate for each anomaly.

ANOMALIES OF THE SUPERIOR CAVAL VEIN

Left superior caval vein draining to the systemic venous atrium

Bilateral superior caval veins

A left-sided superior caval vein draining to the coronary sinus is the most common systemic venous anomaly and results from persistence of the left anterior cardinal vein. This lesion has been noted in 0.3% of autopsied patients in the general population (Geissler & Albert, 1956), but occurs in 2–4.4% of patients with congenital heart disease (Campbell & Deuchar, 1954; Fraser et al, 1961; Cha & Khoury, 1972). A left-sided superior caval vein usually co-exists with a right-sided superior caval vein. An innominate vein connects these two structures in three-fifths of cases and its size varies inversely with that of the left vein (Winter, 1954). The left vein is located anteriorly to both the aortic arch and the left pulmonary artery. It then passes inferiorly, accepts the hemiazygos vein, descends medially into the posterior atrioventricular groove and runs into the coronary sinus, passing between the left pulmonary veins and the left atrial appendage (Fig. 20.3).

Table 20.1 Classification of systemic venous anomalies

Anomalies of the superior caval vein
  Left superior caval vein to right atrium
    — Bilateral superior caval veins
    — Absent right superior caval vein
    — Left superior caval vein with localised coronary sinus defect
  Left superior caval vein to left atrium
  Levoatrial cardinal vein
  Right superior caval vein to left atrium
  Superior caval vein accepting pulmonary veins
  Aneurysm of superior caval vein
Anomalies of the inferior caval vein
  Absence of the infrahepatic segment of the inferior caval vein with azygous continuation
  Inferior caval vein to left atrium
  Inferior caval vein accepting pulmonary veins
  Miscellaneous anomalies
Anomalies of the coronary sinus
Total anomalous systemic venous connexion
Anomalies of the valves of the sinus venosus

The presence of a left-sided superior caval vein does not affect cardiac hemodynamics. It is usually noted as an incidental finding at cardiac catheterisation. Certain clinical findings may suggest its presence. Colman (1967) described the presence of excessive jugular venous pulsations on the left side as a clinical clue. Chest radiographs may suggest the diagnosis if a left superior paramediastinal 'crescent' of water density is present (Cha & Khoury, 1972). Electrocardiograms show a leftward P wave axis in 35% (Momma & Linde, 1969) to 70% (Hancock, 1964) of patients. This abnormal P wave axis has been referred to as 'coronary sinus rhythm' (Scherf & Harris, 1946; Hancock, 1964), and may be a result of persistence of left-sided embryonic pacemaker tissue (Patten, 1956). More likely it indicates that the patients have had unrecognised left atrial isomerism.

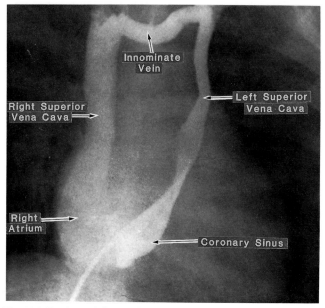

Fig. 20.3 Persistent left superior caval vein draining to the coronary sinus with a bridging innominate vein present.

Both M-mode and cross-sectional echocardiography (Snider et al, 1979; Hibi et al, 1980) demonstrate enlargement of the coronary sinus in the presence of a persistent left superior caval vein. M-mode recordings typically show a dense echo posterior to the mitral valve at the level of the atrioventricular junction and a posterior echo-free space behind the left ventricle which represents the enlarged coronary sinus. On a cross-sectional echocardiogram, the enlarged coronary sinus is best seen in the parasternal long-axis view and is represented by a distinct circular echo-free structure lying posterior to the left atrium in the atrioventricular groove. This finding may also be seen with total anomalous pulmonary venous connexion to the coronary sinus.

At the time of cardiac catheterization an innominate vein should be looked for routinely; its absence is highly suggestive of the presence of a left superior caval vein. If present, the catheter usually passes easily into the enlarged coronary sinus and then into the left caval vein. If the left atrium is visualised during the course of angiography, a dilated coronary sinus may cause an unusual indentation in its inferior border (Owen & Urquhart, 1979).

The presence of a left superior caval vein may make cardiac catheterisation or transvenous pacemaker insertion technically difficult or impossible if a left arm approach is used. At the time of an open heart procedure, a left superior caval vein may be managed by temporary occlusion or by ligation if the venous pressure proximal to the clamp does not rise above 30 mmHg (De Leval et al, 1975). Alternatively, the vessel may require direct cannulation, usually through the right atrium and coronary sinus.

In addition to coronary sinus rhythm, investigators have recently noted the coexistence of fatal arrhythmias and pre-excitation in some patients with a persistent left superior caval vein (James et al, 1976; Davis et al, 1981). Anderson & Latham (1971) described normal cellular morphology of the atrioventricular node in patients with this venous malformation but noted that the atrioventricular node had deviated from a horizontal to a vertical position. Pathologic examination of the conduction system in two patients with left-sided superior caval veins who died presumed arrhythmic deaths showed dispersion of the specialised conduction tissue in a fetal pattern (James et al, 1976). Davis et al (1981) recently reported that the prevalence of pre-excitation was 10 times greater in patients with persistent left superior caval vein than in the general population.

Absent right superior caval vein

Complete absence of the right superior caval vein occurs occasionally in the presence of a left vein draining to the coronary sinus. In this situation the left vein receives a right-sided innominate vein. The right superior caval vein may be represented by a vestigial fibrous cord in the anatomic specimen (Karnegis et al, 1964). This anomaly re-

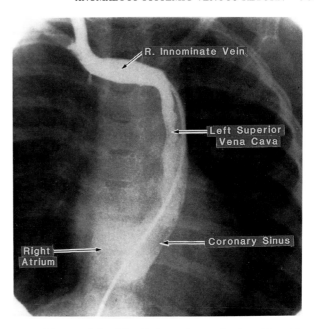

Fig. 20.4 Absence of the right-sided superior caval vein, with a right innominate vein and persistence of the left superior caval vein.

sults from complete involution of the right anterior cardinal vein. Lenox and colleagues (1980) collected 60 cases of absent right superior caval vein from the literature through 1980, and added an additional seven cases from the Children's Hospital of Pittsburgh. This represented an incidence of 0.1% of patients undergoing cardiac catheterisation. Clinical diagnosis may be suggested if the chest radiograph shows absence of the right parasternal shadow of a right superior caval vein. This diagnosis has occasionally been made by radionuclide angiocardiography (Stevens & Mishkin, 1975), but is usually made at cardiac catheterisation (Fig. 20.4). Arrhythmias are not uncommon with this condition and include atrioventricular block, ventricular ectopy, atrial fibrillation, and sinus node dysfunction (Camm et al, 1979; Lenox et al, 1980). If a permanent pacemaker is required, an implanted epicardial system is preferred.

At open heart surgery the left superior caval vein must be cannulated carefully to avoid damage to the area about the coronary sinus which could cause postoperative arrhythmias. Ligation of the left sided superior caval vein must be avoided (DeLeval et al, 1975; Lenox et al, 1980).

Left superior caval vein with coronary sinus atrial septal defect

A defect in the common wall between the left atrium and coronary sinus is a rare anomaly and is usually associated with a persistent left superior caval vein (McCotter, 1916; Mankin & Burchell, 1953; DeLeval et al, 1975; Lee & Sade, 1979). A spectrum of deficiencies can result from maldevelopment in this region. If the deficiency of the common wall is localised there is merely a partial 'unroofing' of the coronary sinus, causing it to communicate with the left atrium. If the deficiency is more marked, the left vein connects directly to the left atrium near the appendage; this is usually associated with an interatrial communication in the usual position of the coronary sinus. (This developmental complex of Raghib et al (1965) is discussed in greater detail below.) A localised coronary sinus defect in association with a left superior vein draining to the coronary sinus may be associated with a physiologic left-to-right shunt from left atrium through the coronary sinus to the right atrium. This may produce physical findings consistent with an atrial septal defect, but would usually be dominated by the clinical findings of the associated congenital heart defects.

Definitive preoperative diagnosis of a localised coronary sinus defect may be quite difficult, but is suggested by a catheter pass from the right atrium into the coronary sinus and then into the left atrium. A contrast injection in the left superior vein may reveal simultaneous filling of both atria. Operative recognition of this defect may also be difficult and has resulted in failure to correct an intra-atrial shunt. The defect is difficult to visualise at the time of surgery because of its location in the left atrium. A suspicion of a coronary sinus defect should be raised if a left superior caval vein is identified and close inspection of the coronary sinus should be made. During cardiopulmonary bypass, the presence of oxygenated blood draining from the coronary sinus suggests the possibility of this anomaly (Lee & Sade, 1979). Options for surgical correction include ligation of the left vein with patching of either the unroofed coronary sinus or the coronary sinus orifice itself. The latter approach creates a small right-to-left shunt since the coronary veins drain to the left atrium postoperatively. If the left vein cannot be ligated, the defect in the roof of the coronary sinus must be closed directly or the flow must be channelled into the right atrium (Lee & Sade, 1979).

Left superior caval vein draining to the left atrium

A persistent left superior caval vein connects to the left atrium in 8% of cases (Lucas & Schmidt, 1977). Patients with this anomaly often have complex congenital cardiac defects (Campbell & Deuchar, 1954). Bilateral superior caval veins with the left vein draining to the left-sided atrium are usually seen with right or left atrial isomerism ('splenic' syndromes) (Ruttenberg et al, 1964; Macartney et al, 1980). Raghib et al (1965) described a developmental complex consisting of left caval connexion to the left atrium, absence of the coronary sinus, and a posteriorly and inferiorly positioned atrial septal defect distinct from the ostium primum variety. In addition, there are case reports of patients with isolated drainage of the left superior caval vein to the left atrium with no associated defects

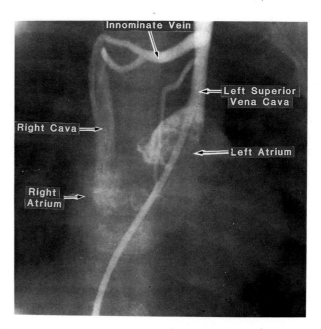

Fig. 20.5 Left superior caval vein connecting to the left atrium associated with a right vein connecting to the right atrium.

(Fig. 20.5), with either right-to-left shunting (Tuchman et al, 1956; Sherafat et al, 1971; Ezekowitz et al, 1978; Konstam et al, 1979) or left-to-right shunting simulating an atrial septal defect (Blank & Zuberbuhler, 1968).

In patients with right or left atrial isomerism, bilateral superior caval veins usually enter into the respective sides of a common atrium and there is considerable venous mixture at atrial level. Associated defects include complex forms of pulmonary atresia, pulmonary stenosis, abnormal ventriculo-arterial connexion, common atrioventricular valves, and anomalous pulmonary venous drainage. Visceral heterotaxia with bilaterally symmetrical lungs and asplenia or polysplenia are anticipated. This represents a developmental complex with embryologically primitive development and a tendency towards bilateral right- or left-sidedness. These patients are usually recognised in the immediate newborn period as having complex cyanotic heart disease, and their left superior caval vein draining to the left-sided atrium is an incidental finding.

Patients with an isolated left superior caval to left atrial connexion usually have a right-to-left shunt (Tuchman et al, 1956). If a sizeable innominate vein connects the two caval veins, there may be a left-to-right shunt instead, simulating an interatrial septal defect. Usually individuals with the left superior caval vein connected to the left atrium are mildly cyanotic and polycythemic. They are minimally symptomatic and may not present for evaluation until adulthood. Cardiac examination, chest radiograph and electrocardiogram are usually normal. A diagnosis of polycythemia rubra vera has been entertained in some of these patients. Occasionally left ventricular hypertrophy and cardiomegaly are present due to the increased left ventricular volume load. The diagnosis can be made non-invasively with radionuclide angiocardiography (Ezekowitz et al, 1978; Konstam et al, 1979).

Connexion of the left superior caval vein to the left atrium predisposes a patient to paradoxical emboli and brain abscess formation (Raghib et al, 1965; Sherafat et al, 1971). Although the anomaly is compatible with survival into the sixth decade, patients probably have at least mild functional impairment, and surgical intervention is indicated once the diagnosis is made. Surgical correction may consist of simple ligation if an adequate bridging innominate vein is present. If not, the left superior caval flow can be baffled or directly transposed to drain to the right atrium, with repair of the associated defects (Lee & Sade, 1979).

Levoatrial cardinal vein

Ed·vards & DuShane (1950) described an anomalous venous connexion between the left atrium and the left innominate vein in a patient with mitral atresia which they termed the levoatrial cardinal vein. This vessel is thought to result from failure of regression of the early connexions between the pulmonary venous and cardinal venous systems in the setting of pulmonary venous obstruction. It differs from a persistent left superior caval vein in that it ascends dorsal to the left pulmonary artery. Similar cases have been described subsequently (Taybi et al, 1965), including a case where the anomalous connexion existed directly between a pulmonary vein and the innominate vein (Lucas et al, 1962). This is a rare abnormality in which the clinical presentation is dominated by the association with atrioventricular valve atresia (Fig. 20.6).

Right superior caval vein draining to the left atrium

Anomalous drainage of the right superior caval vein into the left atrium has been reported rarely as an isolated anomaly. This anomaly is thought to result from malposition of the right horn of the sinus venosus in a leftward and cephalic direction, so that the dominant superior caval vein connects to the left rather than to the right atrium (Kirsch et al, 1961). There is a right-to-left shunt of approximately 30% of systemic venous return (Kirsch et al, 1961), and patients are usually cyanotic. The degree of desaturation may be so mild that these patients escape diagnosis until adulthood (Park et al, 1973; Ezekowitz et al, 1978). They may have normal auscultatory findings but often have electrocardiographic evidence of left ventricular hypertrophy and mild polycythemia consistent with chronic systemic desaturation. A non-invasive diagnosis has been made by nuclear angiography in two adult patients (Park et al, 1973; Ezekowitz et al, 1978) but cardiac

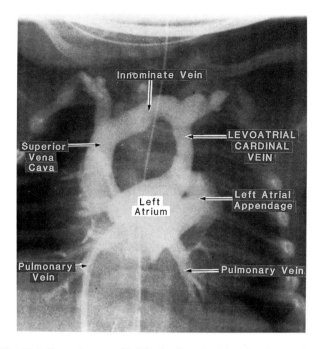

Fig. 20.6 Cineangiogram with injection into the left atrium in a patient with mitral atresia. The only route of egress of contrast is through a levoatrial cardinal vein which connects to the innominate vein.

catheterisation would be necessary to rule out any associated congenital lesions. An arm approach is necessary to visualise the anomalous connexion. Complete surgical correction has been achieved either by anastomosing the anomalous vein to the right atrium (Kirsch et al, 1961) or by pericardial patch diversion of the caval blood flow to the right atrium (Ezekowitz et al, 1978).

Drainage of a right superior caval vein into both atria was recently described for the first time in the English language (Shapiro et al, 1981). In this anomaly, the right-sided pulmonary veins also drained into the superior caval vein which then connected through separate channels into both atria. The left atrium received most of this venous return and the atrial septum was intact. Surgical repair was achieved by diverting all of the system venous return to the right atrium and allowing the pulmonary venous return to traverse the channel which drained to the left atrium. Five similar cases have been reported in the foreign language literature. Paradoxical embolisation with transient hemiparesis was described in the case reported and is a potential complication in any patient with the right superior caval vein connecting to the left atrium.

Superior caval vein receiving pulmonary veins

Anomalous pulmonary venous connections to a right or left-sided superior caval vein may occur as a result of persistence of anastomotic channels between the pulmonary

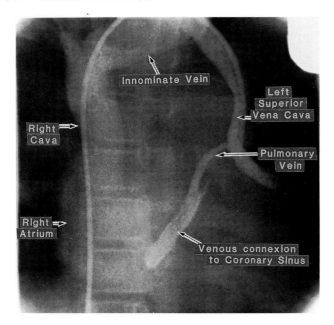

Fig. 20.7 Partial anomalous left pulmonary venous connexion to a left superior caval vein which drains to both coronary sinus and to the innominate vein.

venous and cardinal venous systems (Fig. 20.7). These anomalies are described in greater detail in Chapter 21.

Aneurysm of the superior caval vein

Discrete areas of dilation of the superior caval vein may occur as isolated abnormalities in asymptomatic patients. The term 'aneurysm' is usually reserved for arterial structures, but has been applied to discrete areas of dilation of the superior caval vein. This term is probably more appropriate than that of 'varix' which implies a twisted conformation. Most aneurysms of the superior caval vein have been described in adults, although Franken (1972) reported a 9-year-old patient with this defect. A diagnosis is usually made after a routine chest radiograph demonstrates an incidental finding of a right-sided anterosuperior mediastinal mass. There is no evidence of tracheal compression and the mass has been noted to be larger when the patient is lying supine (Bell et al, 1970; Franken, 1972).

It is presumed that these defects are of a congenital nature and possibly due to an inherent weakness in the venous structure. Patients are not symptomatic and there are no findings on physical examination which would suggest the diagnosis. The differential diagnosis is that of an anterior mediastinal mass and a definitive diagnosis can be made by a nuclear scan or venography. Serial radiographs have shown that these defects do not enlarge significantly with time and surgical intervention is not indicated (Bell et al, 1970; Franken, 1972). A few patients have been reported who developed pulmonary emboli during manipulations of the aneurysm. Rupture of the aneurysm has not been reported.

ANOMALIES OF THE INFERIOR CAVAL VEIN

Absence of the hepatic segment of the inferior caval vein with azygos continuation

The most common venous anomaly involving the inferior caval vein is absence of its infrahepatic segment with azygos continuation to the superior caval vein (Fig. 20.8). The dilated azygos system serves as the major channel of systemic venous return from the lower half of the body. Only the hepatic veins continue to drain to the right atrium. This defect results from failure of the right subcardinal vein to develop properly and to anastomose with the right vitelline vein, leading to enlargement of the right supracardinal vein and providing continuation of systemic venous return to the developing superior caval vein.

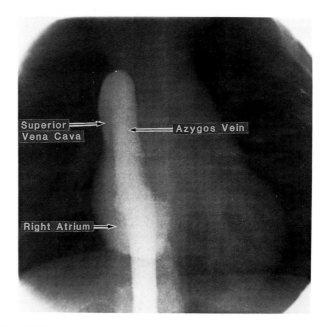

Fig. 20.8 Injection of contrast media into the inferior caval vein near the level of the kidneys demonstrates absence of its infrahepatic segment with azygos continuation to the superior caval vein.

Azygos continuation is seen in 0.6% of patients with congenital heart disease (Anderson et al, 1961). It is frequently associated with complex cyanotic lesions and bears a striking relationship to left atrial isomerism (polysplenia syndrome) (Anderson et al, 1961; Freedom & Ellison, 1973). Strictly speaking, the anomalous vein in cases with left atrial isomerism is a hemiazygos vein, but it is convenient to term it the azygos vein (Fig. 20.9). The enlarged vein may be visible in a frontal chest radiograph as a prominent rounded structure of water density in the right upper perihilar region. Absence of the usual inferior caval shadow on a lateral view may also aid in making a diagnosis, as long as a good inspiration film is obtained, the oesophagus is not filled with barium, and the patient does not have marked

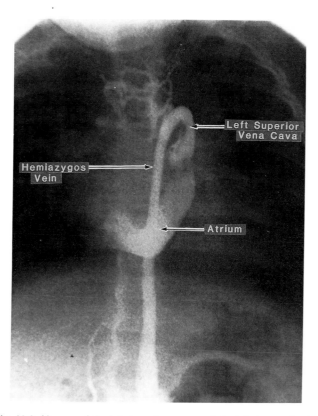

Fig. 20.9 Absence of the infrahepatic segment of the inferior caval vein with hemiazygos continuation to a left-sided atrium in a patient with left atrial isomerism.

increase in pulmonary vascular markings (Heller et al, 1971). Electrocardiograms have been noted to show 'coronary sinus rhythm' or leftward superior P wave axis in a large percentage of these patients who also had left atrial isomerism (polysplenia syndrome – Freedom & Ellison, 1973). Garcia et al (1981) reported six patients with absence of the inferior caval vein with left isomerism who developed complete atrioventricular block.

The presence of this anomaly makes cardiac catheterisation from the lower extremity more difficult, but it can usually be accomplished using a balloon catheter. When the caval vein is cannulated at the time of open heart surgery, care must be taken that the tip of the cannula lies on the cardiac side of the entrance of the azygos vein. The hepatic veins can usually be cannulated as a single vessel (DeLeval et al, 1975). The major significance of this anomaly lies in its association with complex cardiac defects and in the technical difficulty which can accompany cardiac catheterisation.

Inferior caval vein connected to the left atrium

A small number of case reports exist of connexion of the inferior caval vein directly to the left atrium, both with an intact atrial septum (Gardner & Cole, 1955; Meadows,

1961) and with an atrial septal defect (Kim et al, 1971). A distinction must be made between actual connexion to the left atrium and an inferior caval vein which overrides a low-lying atrial septal defect and allows functional drainage of inferior caval blood flow to the left atrium.

This lesion leads to an obligatory right-to-left shunt similar to that seen with superior caval connexion to the left atrium. Patients are usually cyanotic with associated nail-bed clubbing and polycythemia. Electrocardiograms may be normal or show left ventricular hypertrophy and left atrial enlargement. The chest radiograph is not diagnostic. A definitive diagnosis is made by cardiac catheterisation (Fig. 20.10), although it should be possible to diagnose this lesion by nuclear angiography.

These patients may survive into adult life with minimal symptoms but are prone to paradoxical embolization. The defect is amenable to surgical repair (Black et al, 1964; Kim et al, 1971).

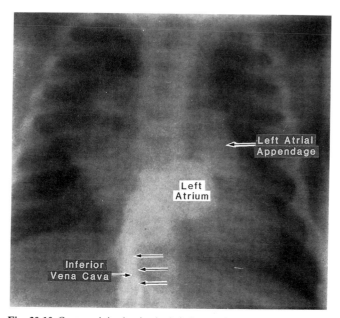

Fig. 20.10 Contrast injection in the inferior caval vein illustrating connexion to the left atrium.

Inferior caval vein accepting pulmonary veins

Total anomalous pulmonary venous connexion below the diaphragm is a well-known entity and is described in detail in Chapter 21. Partial connexion of the pulmonary veins to the inferior caval vein occurs and is frequently associated with the scimitar syndrome. This developmental complex, initially described by Neill et al (1960), consists of hypoplasia of the right lung, anomalous systemic arterial supply to part of the right lung, a right-sided heart, and anomalous pulmonary venous connexion from the right lung through a 'scimitar' vein to the region of the junction of the right atrium and inferior caval vein. The scimitar vein is classically seen as a crescentric density in the right lower lung field in a frontal view chest radiograph. Morbidity may arise from chronic infection in the abnormal lung, increased pulmonary blood flow due to anomalous pulmonary venous connexion, pulmonary venous obstruction, and respiratory insufficiency. Pneumonectomy has been necessary in some of these patients.

Mardini et al (1981) recently reported a case of anomalous left pulmonary venous connexion to the inferior caval vein with associated hypoplasia of the left lung and considered this an example of left-sided scimitar syndrome. The left pulmonary veins connected to both the inferior caval vein and to the innominate vein through a pericardiophrenic vein.

Miscellaneous anomalies of the inferior caval vein

A variety of minor abnormalities of the inferior caval vein have been documented in the general population and have no definite relationship to other congenital cardiac lesions. These include duplication of the inferior caval vein below the level of the renal veins, left-sided inferior caval vein, and circumaortic renal collar. These anomalies can be easily explained by variation in the pattern of regression and anastomosis of the many embryologic structures which contribute to the development of the inferior caval vein. They have no haemodynamic significance but may be of importance when surgical procedures are necessary in the retroperitoneal area (Babaian & Johnson, 1979).

The hepatic veins normally connect to the inferior caval vein but have been reported to connect directly to the left atrium through a separate orifice in a patient with a partial atrioventricular septal defect (DeLeval et al, 1975). This patient underwent reimplantation of the vein into the right atrium.

Complete absence of the inferior caval vein with systemic venous return from the lower extremities flowing entirely through the paravertebral venous plexus and the azygos and hemiazygos systems was reported by Milner & Marchan (1980). It is unlikely that this represents a congenital anomaly and may have been due to a venous thrombosis from a prior pelvic staphylococcal infection.

ANOMALIES OF THE CORONARY SINUS

Several systemic venous anomalies that involve alterations in normal coronary sinus anatomy have already been discussed. These include the various degrees of 'unroofing' of the coronary sinus in association with a left superior caval vein connected directly to the left atrium. In addition, Mantini et al (1966) and Allmendinger et at (1974) reported isolated defects between the left atrium and coronary sinus which resulted in left-to-right atrial shunting without an

interatrial septal defect. These cases did not include a persistent left superior caval vein.

Varying degrees of coronary sinus hypoplasia have also been reported, in which some of the cardiac veins drain separately through dilated Thebesian veins directly into the atria. Other rare anomalies include connexion of the hepatic veins to the coronary sinus, coronary artery to coronary sinus fistula (Mantini et al, 1966) and coronary sinus connexion to the inferior caval vein (Sherman, 1963). It is unusual for anomalies of the coronary sinus to occur as isolated defects and it should be noted that any enlargement of this structure should raise a suspicion of an anomalous systemic or pulmonary venous channel draining through it.

TOTAL ANOMALOUS SYSTEMIC VENOUS CONNEXION

Pearl & Spicer (1980) reported a case of total anomalous systemic venous connexion in which there was absence of the right superior caval vein and of the infrahepatic segment of the inferior caval vein with hemiazygos continuation to a left superior caval vein and then into the left atrium. There was also connexion of the hepatic veins to the left atrium and complete absence of the interatrial septum. This patient was cyanotic and had a short systolic ejection murmur along the right sternal border. He underwent surgical repair at 8 years of age at which time the atria were partitioned to correct venous return, with a pericardial patch placed at the time of atriotomy closure to enlarge the right atrium. This report was the ninth case in the world literature of total anomalous sytemic venous connexion and also reviewed the previously reported cases. The typical anatomic features included the presence of a hypoplastic right atrium, a large interatrial communication, and normal pulmonary artery pressures. They varied in the combination of systemic venous structures present, but shared in having all systemic veins draining to the left atrium. Cardiac catheterisation was necessary for diagnosis and surgical correction has been feasible (De Leval et al, 1975; Pearl & Spicer, 1980). Nodal rhythms have been noted postoperatively in some patients. It is likely that many of these patients have left atrial isomerism.

ANOMALIES OF THE VALVES OF THE SINUS VENOSUS

The valves of the sinus venosus are prominent structures during early embryologic development but later regress. The right venous valve nearly divides the right atrium into two portions early in development but later involutes. Its cephalic portion becomes incorporated into the terminal crest and its caudal portion becomes the Eustachian and

Thebesian valves. The left venous valve becomes incorporated into the atrial septum. Yater (1929) undertook the first comprehensive review of variation in venous valves in the normal heart. Persistence of these valves varied from small remnants to semilunar membranes with and without fenestrations. Sometimes they were completely absent, the Eustachian valve being lacking in 14% and the Thebesian valve in 11% of the hearts examined. In 2% of the cases the Eustachian and Thebesian valves were formed by a single membrane. 2.5% contained Chiari's networks of fine or coarse fibrous strands in the right atrium, extending from the terminal crest to either the Thebesian or Eustachian valves. These networks are usually not of haemodynamic significance, although an early report described a death due to embolization of a thrombus formed on the network (Chiari, 1897). Pathological persistence of the venous valves may produce partial or complete division of the right atrium into a venous sinus, accepting some or all of the systemic veins, and a true right atrium including the right atrial appendage and tricuspid valve. In the most complete form of this anomaly the right venous valve persists as a muscular membrane dividing the right atrium into a venous sinus which accepts the superior and inferior caval veins and the coronary sinus, and a true right atrium communicating with the venous sinus by fenestrations in the persistent venous valve. The venous sinus is also in communication with the oval foramen which allows the potential for right-to-left shunting of systemic venous blood to the left atrium. At least six patterns of division of the right atrium by the venous valves have been described (Rossall & Caldwell, 1957; Kauffman & Anderson, 1963; Lucas

& Schmidt, 1977). There is a striking association of pathological persistence of the right-sided venous valves with hypoplasia of the right ventricle and pulmonary arteries, probably because reduced flow through the tricuspid valve leads to failure of proper development of the right-sided cardiac structures (Doucette & Knoblich, 1963). Major haemodynamic consequences are right-to-left shunting at atrial level and decreased pulmonary blood flow.

Systemic venous obstruction may also be a haemodynamic consequence of these anomalies and has been reported in a 19-year-old patient with symptoms of obstruction of the inferior caval vein (Rossall & Caldwell, 1957). Jones & Niles (1968) reported a case of tricuspid atresia with a redundant sinus venosus valve which caused intermittent obstruction by a 'spinnaker formation.' This was ultimately fatal due to obstruction of the obligatory interatrial communication.

Echocardiography may demonstrate abnormal persistence of a systemic venous valve in the right atrium (Battle-Diaz et al, 1979). The finding of an echo-dense structure in the right atrium could suggest the diagnosis of a right atrial myxoma. However, discovery of this finding in a neonate would make the diagnosis of a persistent right venous valve more likely. Cardiac catheterisation may lead to a diagnosis but exact definition of the abnormal venous valve may not be possible without direct visualisation, either at surgery or autopsy.

Although the spectrum of persistence of the sinus venosus valves is very broad, haemodynamically significant persistence is quite rare.

REFERENCES

Allmendinger P, Dear W E, Cooley D A 1974 Atrial septal defect with communication through the coronary sinus. The Annals of Thoracic Surgery 17: 193–196

Anderson R C, Adams P, Burke B 1961 Anomalous inferior vena cava with azygos continuation (infrahepatic interruption of the inferior vena cava). The Journal of Pediatrics 59: 370–383

Anderson R H, Latham R A 1971 The cellular architecture of the human atrioventricular node, with a note on its morphology in the presence of a left superior vena cava. Journal of Anatomy 109: 443–455

Babaian R J, Johnson D E 1979 Major venous anomalies complicating retroperitoneal surgery. Southern Medical Journal 72: 1254–1258

Battle-Diaz J, Stanley P, Kratz C, Fouron J C, Guerin R, Davignon A 1979 Echocardiographic manifestations of persistence of the right venous valve. The American Journal of Cardiology 43: 850–853

Bell M J, Gutierrez J R, DuBois J J 1970 Aneurysm of the superior vena cava. Radiology 95: 317–318

Black H, Smith G T, Goodale W T 1964 Anomalous inferior vena cava draining into the left atrium associated with intact interatrial septum and multiple pulmonary arteriovenous fistulae. Circulation 29: 258–267

Blank E, Zuberbuhler J R 1968 Left to right shunt through a left atrial left superior vena cava. The American Journal of Roentgenology, Radium Therapy and Nuclear Medicine 103: 87–92

Camm A J, Dymond D, Spurrell R A J 1979 Sinus node dysfunction associated with absence of right superior vena cava. British Heart Journal 41: 504–507

Campbell M, Deuchar D C 1954 The left sided superior vena cava. British Heart Journal 16: 423–439

Cha E M, Khoury G H 1972 Persistent left superior vena cava. Radiology 103: 375–381

Chiari H 1897 Ueber Netzbildungen in rechten Vorhufe des Herzens. Beitrage zur pathologischen Anatomie und zur allgemeinen Pathologie 22: 1–10

Colman A L 1967 Diagnosis of left superior vena cava by clinical inspection, a new physical sign. American Heart Journal 73: 115–120

Davis D, Pritchett E L C, Klein G J, Benson D W, Gallagher J J 1981 Persistent left superior vena cava in patients with congenital atrioventricular preexcitation conduction abnormalities. American Heart Journal 101: 677–679

Doucette J, Knoblich R 1963 Persistent right valve of the sinus venosus; So-called cor triatriatum dextrum: review of the literature and report of a case. Archives of Pathology 75: 105–112

Edwards J E, DuShane J W 1950 Thoracic venous anomalies; I. Vascular connection of the left atrium and the left innominate vein (levoatriocardinal vein) associated with mitral atresia and premature closure of the foramen ovale (case 1). Archives of Pathology 49: 517–528

Ezekowitz M D, Alderson P O, Bulkley B H, et al 1978 Isolated drainage of the superior vena cava into the left atrium in a 52-year-old man. Circulation 58: 751–756

Franken E A 1972 Idiopathic dilatation of the superior vena cava. Pediatrics 49: 297–299

Fraser R S, Dvorkin J, Rossall R E, Eidem R 1961 left superior vena cava; a review of associated congenital heart lesions, catheterization data and roentgenologic findings. American Journal of Medicine 31: 711–716

Freedom R M, Ellison R C 1973 Coronary sinus rhythm in the polysplenia syndrome. Chest 63: 952–958

Garcia O L, Mehta A V, Pichoft A, et al 1981 Left isomerism and complete atrioventricular block: A report of six cases. The American Journal of Cardiology 48: 1103–1107

Gardner D L, Cole L 1955 Long-term survival with inferior vena cava draining into left atrium. British Heart Journal 17: 93–97

Geissler W, Albert M 1956 Persistierende linke obere Hohlvene und mitral Stenose. Zeitshrift fur die Gesamte inhere Medizin und ihre Grenzgebiete 11: 865–874

Hancock E W 1964 Coronary sinus rhythm in sinus venosus defect and persistent left superior vena cava. The American Journal of Cardiology 14: 608–615

Heller R M, Dorst J P, James A E, Rowe R D 1971 A useful sign in the recognition of azygos continuation of the inferior vena cava. Radiology 101: 519–522

Hibi N, Fukui Y, Nishimura K, Miwa A, Kambe T, Sakamoto N 1980 Crosssectional echocardiographic study on persistent left superior vena cava. American Heart Journal 100: 69–76

James T N, Marshall T K, Edwards J E 1976 Desubitaneis mortibus XX. Cardiac electrical instability in the presence of a left superior vena cava. Circulation 54: 689–697

Jones R N, Niles N R 1968 Spinnaker formation of sinus venosus valve; case report of a fatal anomaly in a ten-year-old boy. Circulation 38: 468–473

Karnegis J N, Wang Y, Winchell P, Edwards J E 1964 Persistent left superior vena cava, fibrous remnant of the right superior vena cava and ventricular septal defect. The American Journal of Cardiology 14: 573–577

Kauffman S L, Anderson D H 1963 Persistent venous valves, maldevelopment of the right heart and coronary artery-ventricular communications. American Heart Journal 66: 664–669

Kim Y S, Serrato M, Long D M, Hastreiter A R 1971 Left atrial inferior vena cava with atrial septal defect. Annals of Thoracic Surgery 11: 165–170

Kirsch W M, Carlsson E, Hartmann A F 1961 A case of anomalous drainage of the superior vena cava into the left atrium. Journal of Thoracic and Cardiovascular Surgery 41: 550–556

Konstam M A, Levine B W, Strauss H W, McKusick K A 1979 Left superior vena cava to left atrial communication diagnosed with radionuclide angiography and with differential right to left shunting. The American Journal of Cardiology 43: 149–153

Lee M E, Sade R M 1979 Coronary sinus septal defect; surgical considerations. Journal of Thoracic and Cardiovascular Surgery 78: 563–569

Lenox C C, Zuberbuhler J R, Pane S C, 1980 Absent right superior vena cava with persistent left superior vena cava: Implications and management. The American Journal of Cardiology 45: 117–122

de Leval M R, Ritter D G, McGoon D C, Danielson G K 1975 Anomalous systemic venous connection; surgical considerations. Mayo Clinic Proceedings 50: 599–610

Lucas R V, Schmidt R E 1977 Anomalous venous connections, pulmonary and systemic. In: Moss A J, Adams F H, Emmanoulides G C (eds) Heart Disease in infants, children, and adolescents, 2nd Edn. Williams & Wilkins, Baltimore, Ch 27, p 437–470

Lucas R V, Lester R G, Lillehei C W, Edwards J E 1962 Mitral atresia with levoatriocardinal vein; a form of congenital pulonary venous obstruction. The American Journal of Cardiology 9: 607–613

Macartney F J, Zuberbuhler J R, Anderson R H 1980 Morphological considerations pertaining to recognition of atrial isomerism. Consequences for sequential chamber localization. British Heart Journal 44: 657–667

McCotter R 1916 Three cases of the persistence of the left superior vena cava. Anatomical Record 10: 371–383

Mankin H T, Burchell H B 1953 Clinical considerations in partial anomalous pulmonary venous connection: report of two unusual cases. Proceedings of the Staff Meetings of the Mayo Clinic 28: 463–472

Mantini E, Grondin C M, Lillehei C W, Edwards J E 1966 Congenital anomalies involving the coronary sinus. Circulation 33: 317–327

Mardini M K, Sakati N A, Nyhan W L 1981 Anomalous left pulmonary venous drainage to the inferior vena cava and through the pericardiophrenic vein to the innominate vein: left-sided scimitar syndrome. American Heart Journal 101:860–862

Meadows W R 1961 Isolated anomalous connection of a great vein to the left atrium. Circulation 24, part 1: 669–676

Milner L B, Marchan R 1980 Complete absence of the inferior vena cava presenting as a paraspinous mass. Thorax 35: 798–800

Momma K, Linde L M 1969 Abnormal rhythms associated with persistent left superior vena cava. Pediatric Research 3: 210–216

Neill C A, Ferencz C, Sabiston D C, Sheldon H 1960 The familial occurrence of hypoplastic right lung with systemic atrial supply and venous drainage: 'scimitar syndrome.' Bulletin of the Johns Hopkins Hospital 107: 1–21

Owen J P, Urquhart W 1979 The left atrial notch; A sign of persistent left superior vena cava draining to the right atrium. British Journal of Radiology 52: 855–861

Park H M, Smith E T, Silberstein E B 1973 isolated right superior vena cava draining into left atrium diagnosed by radionuclide angiography. Journal of Nuclear Medicine 14: 240–242

Patten B M 1956 The development of the sinoventricular conduction system. University of Michigan Medical Bulletin 22: 1–21

Pearl W R, Spicer M J 1980 Total anomalous systemic venous return. Southern Medical Journal 73: 259–261

Raghib G, Ruttenburg H D, Anderson R C, Amplatz K, Adams P Jr, Edwards J E 1965 Termination of left superior vena cava in left atrium, atrial septal defect, and absence of coronary sinus; a developmental complex. Circulation 31: 906–918

Rossall R E, Caldwell R A 1957 Obstruction of inferior vena cava by a persistent eustachian valve in a young adult. Journal of Clinical Pathology 10: 40–45

Ruttenberg H D, Neufeld H N, Lucas R V Jr, et al 1964 Syndrome of congenital cardiac disease with asplenia; distinction from other forms of congenital cyanotic cardiac disease. The American Journal of Cardiology 13: 387–406

Scherf D, Harris R 1946 Coronary sinus rhythm. American Heart Journal 32: 443–456

Shapiro E P, Al-Sadir J, Campbell N P S, Thilenius O G, Anagnostopoulos C E, Hays P 1981 Drainage of right superior vena cava into both atria; review of the literature and description of a case presenting with polycythemia and paradoxical embolization. Circulation 63: 712–717

Sherafat M, Friedman S, Waldhausen J A 1971 Persistent left superior vena cava draining into the left atrium with absent right superior vena cava. Annals of Thoracic Surgery 11: 160–164

Sherman F E 1963 An atlas of congenital heart disease. Lea & Febiger, Philadelphia, Ch 3, p 69

Snider A R, Ports T A, Silverman N H 1979 Venous anomalies of the coronary sinus: detection by M-mode, two-dimensional and contrast echocardiography. Circulation 60: 721–727

Stevens J S, Mishkin F S 1975 Persistent left superior vena cava demonstrated by radionuclide angiography: case report. Journal of Nuclear Medicine 16:469

Taybi H, Kurlander G J, Lurie P R, Campbell J A 1965 Anomalous systemic venous connection to the left atrium or to a pulmonary vein. American Journal of Roentgenology, Radium Therapy and Nuclear Medicine 94: 62–77

Tuchman H, Brown J F, Huston J H, Weinstein A B, Rowe G G, Crumpton C W 1956 Superior vena cava draining into left atrium; another cause for left ventricular hypertrophy with cyanotic congenital heart disease. American Journal of Medicine 21: 481–484

Winter F S 1954 Persistent left superior vena cava; survey of world literature and report of thirty additional cases. Angiology 5: 90–132

Yater W M 1929 Variations and anomalies of the venous valves of the right atrium of the human heart. Archives of Pathology 7: 418–441

21

Pulmonary venous abnormalities

This chapter will consider the abnormalities of pulmonary veins and their connexions with systemic veins, with some significant exceptions. The variant of partial anomalous pulmonary venous connexion which so constantly accompanies a sinus venosus atrial septal defect is described in Chapter 22. The anomalous pulmonary venous connexions of any variety which are so commonly associated with atrial isomerism are discussed in Chapter 19, not least because of the particular problems of nomenclature of venous return that arise when isomeric right or left atrial chambers are present. Though divided left atrium may well be considered a pulmonary venous anomaly (Nakib et al, 1967), it is dealt with together with subdivision of the right atrium in Chapter 23.

TOTAL ANOMALOUS CONNEXION

Incidence and aetiology

Total anomalous pulmonary venous connexion without visceral heterotaxy ('asplenia or polysplenia') comprised 2.6% of the patients in the New England Regional Infant Cardiac Program, ranking 12th in frequency and occurring once in 17 000 live births (Fyler et al, 1980).

The incidence of partial anomalous pulmonary venous connexion is more difficult to establish, because anomalous connexion of one vein may be unrecognised either in life or death. Such anomalies were reported in about 1 in 200 routine autopsies by Hughes & Rumore (1944) and Healey (1952). In an extensive surgical and autopsy review. Snellen and colleagues (1968) found that 70% of all cases of anomalous pulmonary venous connexion were of the partial variety. This paper, however, included patients with asplenia and polysplenia. It is impossible to determine in retrospect whether or not atrial isomerism was present.

Earlier reports on total anomalous pulmonary venous connexion stressed the male preponderance in the infra-diaphragmatic variety (Johnson et al, 1958; Lucas et al, 1961; Gathman & Nadas, 1970) and indicated an equal sex incidence in the remaining types (Bonham Carter et al, 1969). In the New England Regional Infant Cardiac Program, 66% of the supracardiac and cardiac types occurred in male infants, while 64% of the infradiaphragmatic type occurred in female infants (Fyler et al, 1980).

Milner and colleagues (1977) collected from the literature 7 reported families where 15 instances of total anomalous pulmonary venous connexion in siblings had occurred. They pointed out that 3 sets of twins (2 identical and 1 non-identical) had been described. In each instance only one twin had been affected. A further example in siblings was documented by Whight and colleagues (1978).

Morphology and morphogenesis

Anatomy

When assessing the morphology of anomalous pulmonary connexions it is necessary to consider several features. First, how much of the pulmonary venous drainage is connected to sites other than the morphologically left atrium? Secondly, do all the anomalously draining veins connect to the same site, and where is the site (or sites) of drainage? Thirdly, is there a stenotic area or region at some point along the route of anomalous drainage? Fourthly, is the anomalous pulmonary venous connexion an isolated malformation, or is it part of a more complex anomaly? Finally, is the cardiac anomaly accompanied by structural malformations of the pulmonary vasculature? Before discussing the variables in each of these features, it is first desirable to clarify our use of the term 'anomalous pulmonary venous connexion'.

We consider a pulmonary vein to be anomalously connected when it is attached to a site other than the morphologically left atrium. In this respect, anomalous pulmonary venous connexion is not synonymous with anomalous pulmonary venous drainage. In some hearts, the pulmonary veins may connect to the left atrium in the presence of mitral atresia and an intact atrial septum. An anomalous venous channel, sometimes termed the 'levoatriocardinal' vein, may then drain the pulmonary venous return to the superior caval vein. In this arrangement therefore, the pulmonary venous *connexions* are normal, but there is anomalous pulmonary venous *drainage*.

The essential anatomy of total anomalous *connexion* as defined above is that all the pulmonary veins connect to a site other than the morphologically left atrium. In the presence of right atrial isomerism it is possible to have all four pulmonary veins connected to the roof of the left-sided atrial chamber. But, because of the absence of any morphologically left atrial structures in this lesion, this will still be considered as a totally anomalous connexion. Since the whole problem of total anomalous pulmonary venous connexion in right atrial isomerism is a special situation, it is discussed in depth in Chapter 19. In this section, we are concerned with total anomalous connexion in the setting of lateralised atrial chambers (usual and mirror-image arrangements).

SITE OF ANOMALOUS CONNEXION.

The major anatomical feature is the site of anomalous drainage. Usually all the pulmonary veins drain to the same site, but mixed total anomalous connexion can occur with different pulmonary veins connecting to separate anomalous sites. It is usual to divide the sites of anomalous connexion into three groups: supracardiac, cardiac and infracardiac. The first two taken together constitute supradiaphragmatic drainage while the infracardiac drainage is at the same time infradiaphragmatic (Fig. 21.1). In each of these different types the anatomic features of therapeutic significance are the precise morphology of the anomalous channel, its proximity to the morphologically left atrium and the presence of obstructive lesions along the pathway. The nature of the pulmonary vasculature is also a major factor in determining the optimal treatment. Extensive studies of the anatomical patterns of total anomalous connexion have been made by Blake and colleagues (1965), by Nakib et al (1967) and by Snellen and colleagues (1968). More exhaustive studies by Bharati & Lev (1973) and Delisle and his colleagues (1976) have confirmed the overall picture emerging from the early studies, as has our own more limited experience. One problem that emerges from the study of these various reports is that cases with isomerism have not previously been distinguished from those without. This must be borne in mind when making comparisons.

The commonest type of anomalous connexion is supracardiac, accounting for nearly half of the cases. Cardiac and infracardiac anomalous connexions account for approximately one-quarter each (bearing in mind the caveats always present when extrapolating from numbers obtained in autopsy studies).

Supracardiac connexion itself can be to the left brachiocephalic (innominate) vein, to the right superior caval vein, to the azygos system of veins or to the left superior caval vein. In the commonest pattern, the four pulmonary veins usually join together in a confluence behind the left atrium, termed the 'horizontal vein' by Delisle et al (1976). From the confluence a vertical vein then runs up to connect with the left brachiocephalic vein. This then runs across to terminate in the right superior caval vein (Fig. 21.2). The course of the vertical vein is vital with regard to obstruction. Usually the vein passes anterior to the left pulmonary artery and this is not associated with obstruction. It is more problematic when the vein passes between the left pulmonary artery and left bronchus (Fig. 21.3): these two structures then form a vice, as elegantly demonstrated by Elliott & Edwards (1962). Post-

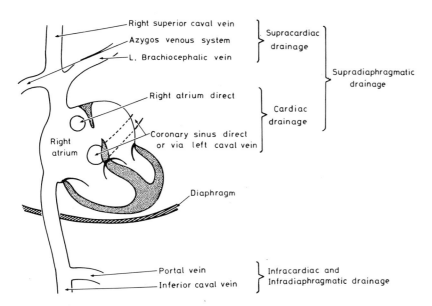

Fig. 21.1 Diagram showing the potential sites of anomalous pulmonary venous connexion and their classification.

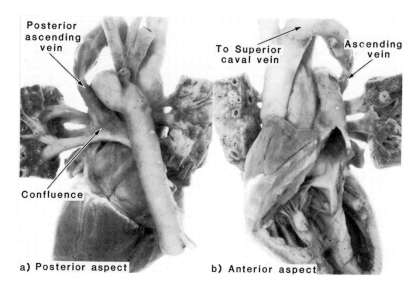

Fig. 21.2 The typical supracardiac 'snowman' type connexion to the superior caval vein seen (a) from behind and (b) from in front. Note the constriction where the ascending vein passes behind the pulmonary arteries. (Photographed and reproduced by kind permission of Dr L. M. Gerlis, Killingbeck Hospital, Leeds, UK.)

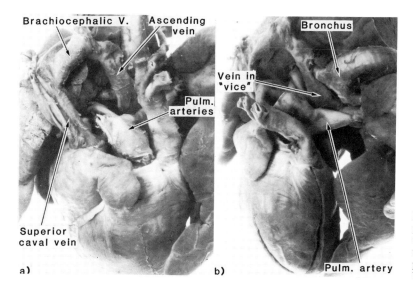

Fig. 21.3 The 'vice' produced when the ascending pulmonary vein passes between the pulmonary arteries and the bronchial tree seen (a) in situ and (b) with retraction of the trachea. (Photographed and reproduced by kind permission of Mrs Audrey Smith, University of Liverpool, UK.)

stenotic dilatation can be found above this site (Kauffman et al, 1962; Delisle et al, 1976). Obstruction with this so-called 'snowman' pattern of anomalous connexion can more rarely occur at the opening of the brachiocephalic vein into the superior caval vein. Nakib et al (1967) have discussed the nature of the vertical vein, pointing out that it has been described as a 'persistent left superior caval vein'. They suggest that this term should only be used when the anomalous venous channel has recognisable components of a left superior caval vein (such as a connexion with the coronary sinus, either via a patent channel or a ligamentous cord) or the site of drainage of an azygos venous channel. The vertical vein can also be part of a left superior caval vein when it communicates directly with the left atrium. It is then also called a 'levo-atriocardinal vein' (Edwards & DuShane, 1950). When the anomalous venous channel has none of these features, it

is an 'anomalous vertical pulmonary vein'. This latter arrangement is by far the commonest finding (Nakib et al, 1967). Snellen et al (1968) suggested that the levoatriocardinal vein could be distinguished because it passed between the left pulmonary artery and left bronchus. As we have seen, this is not the case. A vertical vein can also occupy this position.

The second commonest subtype of supracardiac connexion is directly to the right superior caval vein. Usually with this type the confluence connects directly to the caval vein. Obstruction may occur either at this caval junction or in another vice, this time between the right pulmonary artery and carina (Delisle et al, 1976). Nakib et al (1967) described this type with a vertical vein behind the bronchus. Azygos connexion is usually to the trunk of the vein, but can occur via the hemiazygos system. In this respect, the pattern in which the confluence swings to the

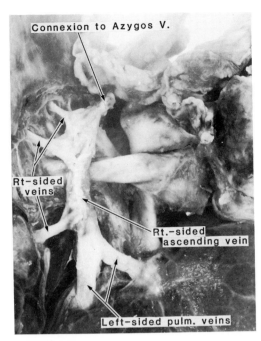

Fig. 21.4 The unusual variant of supracardiac anomalous connexion in which the venous channel crosses the spine and ascends on the right side, connecting in this case to the azygos vein. (Photographed and reproduced by kind permission of Dr L. M. Gerlis.)

right side below the heart can probably be considered as azygos connexion (Fig. 21.4). Both of the cases with azygos drainage reported by Delisle et al (1976) were obstructed. More recently Brenner et al (1983) reviewed the findings of a rare variant of this type in which the ascending right-sided vertical vein was embedded within the right lung. This patient had no spleen.

The cardiac form of anomalous connexion can be found with the pulmonary veins joining the right atrium via the coronary sinus or directly. With connexion via the coronary sinus (Fig. 21.5) there is a problem as to whether this is a cardiac connexion or one via a left superior caval vein. One form of left caval drainage is that of the snowman type. The ascending vein is recognised as being caval because it drains the hemiazygos system (Nakib et al, 1967; their Fig. 7d). But the case of coronary sinus connexion described by the same authors (their Fig. 6) could equally be considered as left caval connexion if the common pulmonary vein between the coronary sinus and the pulmonary confluence were interpreted as being of caval origin. For this reason, it might well be preferable to exclude the left superior caval vein as a site of supracardiac connexion except in cases of mirror-image atrial arrangement. All cases of this type with usual atrial arrangement could be classified adequately as being of snowman or coronary sinus type. In other cases, however, there is no doubt that anomalous connexion is directly to the coronary sinus without an intervening confluent

channel, such as the case illustrated by Blake et al (1965, their Fig. 2D). The cases encountered by Delisle et al (1976) were also presumably of this type, since they commented that there was no horizontal vein present. They pointed out that the coronary sinus itself functioned as a horizontal vein. This facilitated the creation of a large coronary sinus-left atrial window with closure of the orifice of the sinus as a method of surgical treatment (Van Praagh et al, 1972). Obstruction of coronary sinus return is exceedingly rare, although an isolated case has recently been described by Arciniegas and colleagues (1980).

Direct connexion to the morphologically right atrium has been found most frequently in association with other cardiac lesions. Many of the described cases have been associated with atrial isomerism, for example, 4 of the 7 cases of Delisle et al (1976). We will discuss this arrangement in Chapter 19. The other 3 cases described by Delisle et al (1976) were associated with tetralogy of Fallot, complete transposition and double outlet right ventricle, respectively. The importance of these cases is again the lack of either a horizontal vein or an extensive confluence. When a confluence exists, however, so does the possibility of its obstruction at its junction with the right atrium.

The final site of anomalous connexion is both infracardiac and infradiaphragmatic (see Fig. 21.1). In this type the confluence or horizontal vein continues via a descending vertical vein (Fig. 21.6) which passes through the oesophageal orifice of the diaphragm. It then drains through a channel which was part of the venous duct (ductus venosus) in fetal life to terminate in either the portal vein (Fig. 21.7a – common), the inferior caval vein (less common), through both of these or in the gastric veins (Fig. 21.7b – rare). Obstruction is almost universally present with infracardiac connexion because the venous return usually has to pass through the hepatic tissues to reach the systemic veins. Additional discrete stenosis as the vertical vein passed through the diaphragm was noted in 3 of the cases reported by Delisle et al (1976). Furthermore, the vein wall may be abnormally thick and show intimal proliferation (Haworth, 1982).

Excluding the cases of total anomalous pulmonary venous connexion associated with atrial isomerism, a good proportion of the remaining cases have significant associated malformations. In these cases (such as those with abnormal ventriculo-arterial connexions – complete transposition or double outlet right ventricle), the associated abnormality is probably the major lesion. Even when the anomalous connexion is isolated, there is almost always an interatrial communication present so that the venous blood is able to reach the left side of the heart. Delisle et al (1976), however, described a single case with an intact atrial septum as previously had Hastreiter et al (1962).

In any case with total anomalous pulmonary venous connexion, the size of the left atrium and left ventricle are of obvious concern to the surgeon (Parr et al, 1974;

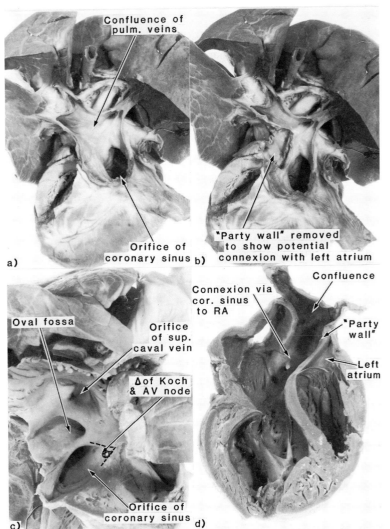

Fig. 21.5 An example of total anomalous pulmonary venous connexion to the coronary sinus. (a & b) A specimen viewed from behind. (b) having had the 'party wall' that initially separated the enlarged coronary sinus from the left atrium removed. (c) The enlarged orifice of the coronary sinus and its proximity to the atrioventricular node. (d) a simulated 'four chamber' section, again demonstrating the 'party wall' between coronary sinus and left atrium. (Photographed and reproduced by kind permission of Mrs Audrey Smith.)

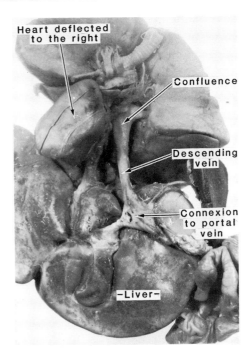

Whight et al, 1978). At first sight, these structures seem small to the morphologist's eye because of the disparate hyperplasia of the right atrium and right ventricle. When Haworth & Reid (1977) measured the inlet-outlet dimensions of the left ventricle, they were normal in 8 of 9 cases, while the left ventricular free wall thickness was normal in all cases. Interestingly, they noted that the right ventricle was dilated and hypertrophied only in cases with supradiaphragmatic venous return.

These excellent studies of Haworth & Reid (1977) and Haworth (1982) were mostly directed at the morphology of the pulmonary vasculature. Here they noted structural changes in all patients studied, including the youngest, who died at 1 day of age. They noted that arterial muscularity increased with age. In anomalous supradiaphrag-

Fig. 21.6 Infradiaphragmatic total anomalous pulmonary venous connexion to the portal vein. (Photographed by kind permission of Dr L. M. Gerlis.)

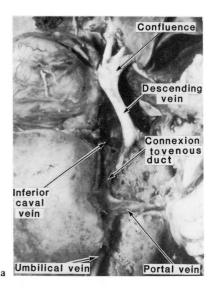

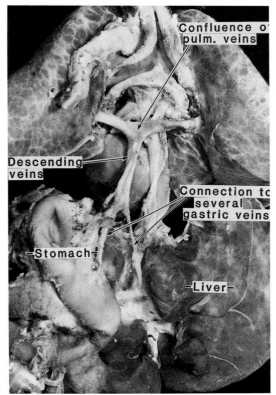

Fig. 21.7 Different sites of infradiaphragmatic anomalous connexion. (a) Connexion to the venous duct (by kind permission of Dr N. Fagg, Guy's Hospital, London, UK) and (b) Multiple small connexions to the gastric veins.

connexion. They too commented on the 'remarkable degree of advanced pulmonary vascular changes found in the entire group, even young infants.' In Haworth's second (1982) study, which was confined to 6 babies who died in the first week of life, the extrapulmonary veins were generally smaller than normal in all. Intimal proliferation was noted in the large pre-acinar veins of 2 of the 6 cases. In no case was it present in all the veins examined. Numerous patent anastomoses between bronchial and pulmonary veins were demonstrated. Some (if not all) these abnormalities had been present during intrauterine life.

Morphogenesis

The development of the pulmonary veins has been extensively studied and there is general agreement concerning the normal mechanism. The pulmonary veins themselves develop along with the growing lung buds. Their union with the morphologically left atrium depends upon growth of the common pulmonary vein from the posterior aspect of the atrial component of the primary heart tube (Aüer, 1948; Neill, 1956; Los, 1968; Van Praagh & Corsini, 1969). After normal fusion, the pulmonary veins are then 'cannibalised' by the atrium to form the normal morphologically left atrial chamber. Total anomalous pulmonary venous connexion is the consequence of failure of development of the common pulmonary vein (Lucas et al, 1962; Delisle et al, 1976). Initially, since the lung buds themselves are derived from the fore-gut, the pulmonary veins have connexions to the systemic venous system. When the common pulmonary vein fails to develop, these anastomoses between pulmonary and systemic venous systems persist and enlarge. An anastomosis with the anterior cardinal systemic venous system then results in supracardiac anomalous connexion. Anastomosis with the sinus venosus produces a cardiac connexion while infradiaphragmatic connexion follows anastomosis with the omphalomesenteric system. As Delisle and his colleagues have indicated (1976), in the strict sense these anastomoses are neither anomalous nor pulmonary, but, if they persist, they certainly result in an anomalous pulmonary venous connexion. Rarely, hearts may be found in which the common pulmonary vein is present, but atretic in its course between the atrium and the pulmonary venous confluence (Lucas et al, 1962). Indeed, sometimes the pulmonary veins may be adjacent to the left atrium with a diaphragm between the two developmental components. An anomalous channel then provides the only route of drainage of pulmonary venous blood. Those hearts, together with the cases described by Lucas et al (1962) and other rare cases discussed by Delisle et al (1976), are readily explained using the developmental hypothesis discussed above.

matic connexion these changes were increased in those cases with low pulmonary flow. The pulmonary veins were arterialised even in the youngest infant. Similar findings were also reported by Newfeld and colleagues (1980) in a larger series of 40 patients. They calculated a pulmonary vascular disease index. This was higher in patients with obstructed as compared to unobstructed anomalous

Pathophysiology

Shunts

There is an obligatory left-to-right shunt, since pulmonary veins return is to the systemic veins or right atrium. A systemic output can only be maintained if there is a right-to-left shunt which is almost always at atrial level. As discussed above, exceptional cases have been described in which the atrial septum was intact. In these cases it is assumed that the right-to-left shunt occurred either at ventricular (Graham et al, 1972; Delisle et al, 1976) or ductal level (Hastreiter et al, 1962).

When the right-to-left shunt is at atrial level, there is a tendency for fetal flow patterns to be maintained by the valve mechanism of the oval foramen (Swan et al, 1956; Gathman & Nadas, 1970). Thus, in the majority of cases of anomalous infradiaphragmatic connexion, the oxygenated blood ascending the inferior caval vein towards the right atrium is directed towards the left atrium. Systemic arterial oxygen saturation is accordingly higher than that in the pulmonary arteries. With an anomalous supracardiac connexion, oxygenated blood tends to be directed down the superior caval vein and through the tricuspid valve. So, in about half of all cases, pulmonary arterial blood is more oxygenated than systemic arterial. In the remaining half, mixing is complete. The same pattern is found for anomalous connexion to the coronary sinus. This is presumably because the orifice of the coronary sinus is directed more towards the tricuspid valve than the oval fossa (Gathman & Nadas, 1970; Shinebourne et al, 1981).

Obstruction to pulmonary venous return

This can occur at any of the sites documented above, within the pulmonary veins at their junction with systemic veins, or in the hepatic sinusoids in the case of connexion to the portal vein when the venous duct is shut. When there is angiographically definable obstruction, the right ventricular pressure is usually suprasystemic (Behrendt et al, 1972); however, there are many infants – particularly those with return to the coronary sinus – in whom (despite absence of angiocardiographic obstruction) the systolic pressure in the two ventricules is more or less equal (Behrendt et al, 1972). Indeed, in one study, no significant difference was found in systolic pressure (measured in either the right ventricle or pulmonary artery) between patients with and without angiographic obstruction in patients with supracardiac or intracardiac connexion (Shinebourne et al, 1981). Pulmonary vascular resistance was calculated in 30 infants who had a right ventricular or pulmonary artery systolic pressure above 70% of aortic or left ventricular systolic pressure. This was above 6 units.m² in 16 and above 8 units.m² in 11 (Shinebourne et al, 1981). This suggests that the main cause of pulmonary hypertension in patients without apparent pulmonary venous obstruction is elevation of pulmonary resistance. This is presumably as a result of the extension of muscle into peripheral arterioles and veins described above (Haworth & Reid, 1977; Haworth, 1982). If this is the cause, the almost invariable fall to normal after successful repair (see below) indicates that it is reversible. Alternatively, at least part of the problem may be due to undetected pulmonary venous obstruction. The contribution of the oval foramen to the problem is controversial. Gathman & Nadas (1970) argued on three grounds that significant obstruction of pulmonary venous return at atrial level was rare. First, patients as a group had similar right atrial pressures whether they were pulmonary hypertensive or not. Second, about a third of pulmonary hypertensive patients had no interatrial pressure gradient at all. In a few, mean left atrial pressure was higher than right. The maximum mean pressure difference in favour of the right atrium was only 7 mmHg. Third, almost all patients with pulmonary vascular obstruction (40/43) also had pulmonary venous obstruction. While these arguments are persuasive as to the unimportant role of the oval foramen in producing pulmonary hypertension, they do not rule out the possibility that a small foramen could limit systemic flow.

Mullins and colleagues (1973) were impressed at the discovery of a small oval foramen in an infant who, shortly before death, was denied balloon atrial septostomy because the atrial pressures were equal. They demonstrated, as had Serratto and colleagues (1968), that interatrial pressure gradients (when they existed) could almost always be abolished by balloon atrial septostomy. They also argued that absence of a pressure gradient between the atria should not be taken to indicate lack of obstruction since atrial compliance is a determinant of atrial pressure. We find this reasoning unpersuasive. To argue, in one breath, that abolition of a pressure gradient indicates that there *was* an obstruction which has been abolished, and in the next breath to say that lack of a gradient does not necessarily mean there is no obstruction, seems to say the least to be inconsistent. Furthermore, whatever the atrial compliances, the *instantaneous* pressure difference across the interatrial communication cannot but be positively correlated with the flow through it, and negatively correlated with its size. *Mean* pressure gradients may well have little to do with the size of the communication, because flow through it varies during the cardiac cycle. We have no information available upon this question. We do know that left ventricular stroke output (and therefore flow through the interatrial communication) is subnormal in about 40% of patients with total anomalous connexion (Graham et al, 1972; Mathew et al, 1977). We also know there is no correlation between left ventricular stroke output and mean interatrial pressure gradient or right ventricular pressure, and that depression of left ventricular stroke output is associated with decrease of left ventricular end-diastolic volume and depression of left ventricular ejection fraction. Unfortunately, we cannot conclude that left ventricular stroke volume is decreased because of the obstruction at the oval foramen. This is because the same depression of left ventricular stroke output was found in a quarter of patients with an atrial septal defect. Flow into the left ventricle in the latter circumstance is certainly not restricted by the size of the interatrial communication (Graham et al, 1972). Mathew and colleagues (1977) found that patients with pulmonary venous obstruction had a lower left ventricular stroke output per m² than those without. They were uncertain as to whether this difference was the result of the pulmonary venous obstruction or of age. By their method, left ventricular stroke output per m² is lower in normal neonates than in normal older infants. Similar findings were reported by Hammon and colleagues (1980).

Consequences of pulmonary venous obstruction

When pulmonary venous return is unobstructed, right ventricular diastolic pressure is low and right ventricular compliance relatively high. Blood returning to the right atrium tends therefore to enter the right ventricle rather than the left atrium. Pulmonary blood flow tends greatly to exceed systemic blood flow. Right ventricular end-diastolic and stroke volumes are considerably increased in consequence (Mathew et al, 1977; Hammon et al, 1980). Since mixing of pulmonary and systemic venous blood is complete (apart from the minor degrees of streaming alluded to above), right atrial (and therefore systemic arterial) blood is rather well oxygenated. Its oxygen saturation may reach into the low nineties.

Pulmonary venous obstruction raises pulmonary venous pressure. Pulmonary oedema is produced if it is sufficiently severe, though bronchopulmonary venous anastomoses may relieve this to some degree. Pulmonary arterial pressure is raised even above systemic pressure in severe cases, and pulmonary blood flow is reduced. The right ventricle therefore becomes pressure rather than volume overloaded (Mathew et al, 1977; Hammon et al, 1980). Systemic arterial oxygen saturation may then fall into the twenties. The depression of systemic arterial saturation (and possibly also output) results in tissue hypoxaemia and metabolic acidosis. These effects of pulmonary venous obstruction are compounded by the changes in small pulmonary veins and arteries already described, which may further increase pulmonary vascular resistance.

In the occasional patient who survives infancy without severe pulmonary venous obstruction, late pulmonary vascular obstructive disease may develop as in atrial septal defect. The effects are the same as that of pulmonary venous obstruction except that no pulmonary oedema occurs.

Presentation and clinical symptomatology

As long ago as 1962, Hastreiter and colleagues recognised that the main determinant of the clinical picture was the presence of pulmonary venous obstruction. Thus, for each of the ensuing sections relating to the clinical picture, patients will be arbitrarily divided into those with and without pulmonary venous obstruction. Some patients with only modest pulmonary venous obstruction fall between the two groups and exhibit features of both.

Patients *with severe pulmonary venous obstruction* present in the first week or two of life with obvious cyanosis and difficulties with feeding and respiration. Early reports suggested that neonates with anomalous infradiaphragmatic connexion were particularly liable to develop cyanosis and dyspnoea during feeding. The explanation offered was the increased pulmonary venous obstruction produced by compression from the oesophagus as the two pass side-by-side through the oesophageal opening of the diaphragm (Lucas et al, 1961). This clinical feature is so common in patients with any cyanotic heart disease that we doubt its diagnostic value. In contrast to what is observed in the respiratory distress syndrome, grunting respiration is very rarely seen in obstructed return. Pointers to respiratory distress syndrome rather than total anomalous pulmonary connexion are maternal diabetes, prematurity, Caesarian section, and very early onset of respiratory difficulties. Any or all of these can, however, happen with the anomalous pulmonary venous connexion. A unique mode of presentation, haematemesis, was described in one patient with infradiaphragmatic return to the left gastric vein (Laurence & Brown, 1960).

Patients *without severe pulmonary venous obstruction* tend to present in heart failure at 2–3 months of age. They have a history of feeding difficulties and sometimes chest infections. Cyanosis is not a symptom.

Clinical findings

Patients *with severe pulmonary venous obstruction* are sick neonates with obvious or severe cyanosis. Skin mottling is frequently superimposed, reflecting poor peripheral perfusion and metabolic acidosis. Tachypnoea is usually marked, though respiration is quiet. Hepatomegaly is occasionally considerable, particularly when drainage is to the portal vein. The peripheral pulses are often somewhat weak. The precordium is quiet. On auscultation there are usually no murmurs. If a murmur exists it is usually unimpressive and mid-systolic. Occasionally a venous hum is heard in the region where pulmonary venous return is obstructed, e.g. under the left clavicle in anomalous connexion via a left vertical vein. The first heart sound is single and the second heart sound is variously described as exhibiting 'physiological' or 'fixed' splitting (Gathman

& Nadas, 1970). The pulmonary component is accentuated and a fourth heart sound may be heard. Rarely, the second heart sound appears single.

When seen from the end of the bed, patients *without severe pulmonary venous obstruction* resemble patients with large ventricular septal defect. They are scrawny and tachypnoeic with respiratory indrawing and tachypnoea. The presence of cyanosis can certainly be missed if the infant is examined in a poor light. Even in a good light, it may not be detected. There is usually hepatomegaly and rfor rales may well be heard in the lungs.

The peripheral pulses are normal to small and the precordium overactive, but without any thrill. On auscultation the first heart sound is normal, usually with wide fixed splitting of the second heart sound. There is an ejection systolic murmur in the pulmonary area due to excessive flow through the pulmonary valve. A mid-diastolic murmur is usually heard at the lower left sternal border, representing excessive flow through the tricuspid valve.

Patients without pulmonary venous obstruction very occasionally survive infancy without heart disease being detected. Such cases present as a typical 'secundum' atrial septal defect with the added features of mild cyanosis and clubbing.

Investigations

Chest radiography

Newborns *with severe pulmonary venous obstruction* have an extremely characteristic chest X-ray with a small or normal sized heart combined with 'ground-glass' lung fields (Lucas et al, 1961; Hastreiter et al, 1962). Kerley B lines are occasionally seen (Robinson et al, 1969) (Fig. 21.8). These appearances are sometimes confused with respiratory distress syndrome. The latter diagnosis can easily be made in most cases because of the more patchy distribution of changes in the lung fields. Furthermore, obliteration of part or all of the cardiac silhouette and the appearance of an air bronchogram (both highly characteristic of respiratory distress syndrome) are rare in total anomalous pulmonary venous connexion.

Patients *without severe pulmonary venous obstruction* have enlarged hearts because of the right ventricular volume overload together with 'ground-glass' lung fields. The pulmonary trunk becomes prominent in older patients, as does the left vertical vein when this is the site of the anomalous venous connexion. This gives rise to the 'snowman' appearance, known to almost every paediatrician and also described as the 'W. C. Fields heart'. This is now of mainly historical importance because patients usually have their defect corrected before the 'snowman' has time to appear, usually in the second year of life (Bonham Carter et al, 1969). Less than one-third of infants with supracardiac anomalous connexion exhibit the 'snowman' (Behrendt et al, 1972). Exceptionally the 'snowman' has been seen at 3 months of age (Gathman & Nadas, 1970).

Electrocardiography

The electrocardiogram shows right axis deviation with a clockwise frontal plane loop and right ventricular hypertrophy. V_1 usually shows an rsR^1 pattern though a qR is seen in 40% of cases. The latter might be thought to indicate the presence of more severe pulmonary hypertension, but there is poor correlation between the two

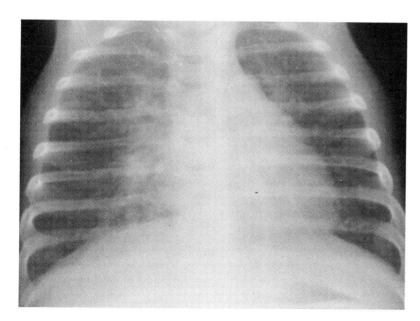

Fig. 21.8 Plain chest X-ray in obstructed total anomalous pulmonary venous drainage, to demonstrate the ground glass appearance of both lung fields.

(Gathman & Nadas, 1970). Disturbances of conduction are rare. Under 1 month of age, only 14% of patients have right atrial hypertrophy, whereas this is seen in 74% between 1 and 3 months and in 90% over 3 months. Patients with pulmonary venous obstruction, who present younger, are much less likely to have right atrial hypertrophy than those without pulmonary venous obstruction.

Echocardiography

M-mode echocardiography is of very limited value in diagnosing total anomalous connexion (Sahn et al, 1979). As in atrial septal defect, there is right ventricular dilation with paradoxical septal movement (Tajik et al, 1972). Both these features may be absent in newborns with pulmonary venous obstruction (Godman et al, 1974; Shiu et al, 1981). The left atrium is small, in contrast to its size in atrial septal defect, but there may be difficulty in defining its extent. This is because in anomalous connexion to the coronary sinus, the anterior margin of that structure often appears as a highly mobile line within the left atrium, lying behind the echoes from the posterior aortic wall and aortic leaflet of the mitral valve (Orsmond et al, 1978; Aziz et al, 1978). Orsmond and colleagues (1978) claimed that the motion of this echo was different from that produced by coronary sinus enlargement resulting from its connexion to a persistent left superior caval vein. Most authorities would not be so confident on this point. In addition to enlargement of the coronary sinus in a particular subgroup of patients, it is sometimes possible to visualise the pulmonary venous confluence as an echo-free space behind the left (Paquet & Gutgesell, 1975) and right (Aziz et al, 1978) atria. It is not possible to recognise individual pulmonary veins. Furthermore, the position of

the pulmonary venous confluence is such that frequently it will not be seen in either of the above positions (Aziz et al, 1978). In one patient with infradiaphragmatic connexion, an echo-free space was shown *not* to be the pulmonary venous confluence (Mortera et al, 1977).

A further problem with recognition of total anomalous connexion with M-mode techniques is that a spurious echo line is frequently seen within the left atrium in patients with normal pulmonary venous connexion. Pulsed Doppler echocardiography is useful in distinguishing between true and spurious echoes in this area. If the echo is spurious, the Doppler signal will be similar on both sides of the line. If the echo does represent a structure, then, as the sampling volume is moved from one side of the echo to the other, there will be an abrupt change in Doppler signal (Stevenson et al, 1979). Pulsed Doppler is also valuable in detecting connexion to a vertical vein. Venous flow *towards* the suprasternal transducer is then detected to the left of the aorta (Skovránek et al, 1980). A persistent left superior caval vein draining to the coronary sinus would produce flow *away from* a suprasternal transducer.

Cross-sectional echocardiography is the definitive non-invasive method of diagnosis. It is possible in infants under 3 months of age with normally connected pulmonary veins to image at least one vein connected to the left atrium in 94% of cases, and at least two in 77% (Sahn et al, 1979). Correlative anatomic studies suggest that the subcostal and apical approaches image the normal left lower and right upper pulmonary veins, whilst the suprasternal approach, given a good window, can demonstrate all four. Hence *failure* to demonstrate any pulmonary vein connected to the left atrium should lead to an assiduous search for the key positive feature required for diagnosis. This is the pulmonary venous confluence, which was recognised in 21

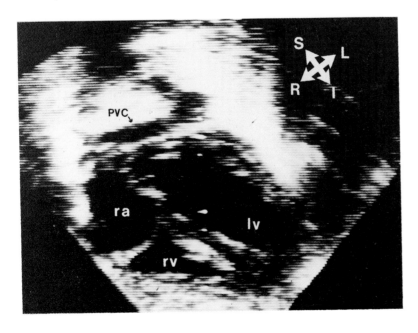

Fig. 21.9 Supracardiac total anomalous pulmonary venous connexion, seen in subcostal four chamber cut. Note the pulmonary venous confluence (PVC) lying behind the left atrium and above it, passing superiorly as it goes to the left. I – inferior; L – left; lv – left ventricle; R – right; ra – right atrium; rv – right ventricle; S – superior. (Reproduced by kind permission of Churchill Livingstone from: Rowlands D J (ed) Recent advances in cardiology, Vol 9.)

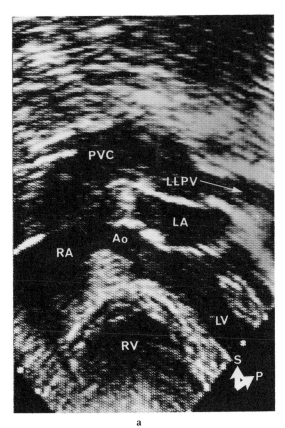

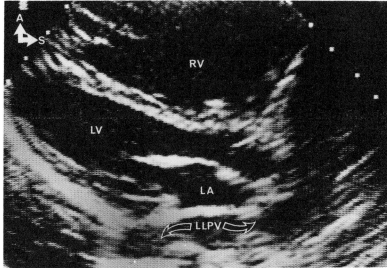

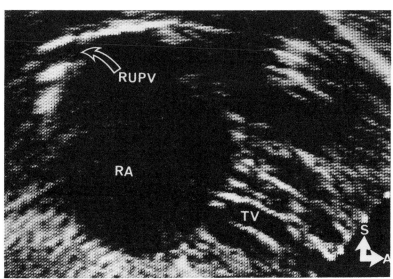

Fig. 21.10 Total anomalous pulmonary venous connexion to the right atrium. (a) Subcostal paracoronal section shows left lower pulmonary vein (LLPV) returning, not to the left atrium (LA), but to the pulmonary venous confluence (PVC). Note the enlargement of the right atrium (RA) and right ventricle (RV). (b) In a parasternal long axis cut, the failure of the left lower pulmonary vein to enter the left atrium is also seen, and the right ventricle clearly compresses the left ventricle (LV). (c) In this detail of a subcostal oblique four chamber section, obtained very posteriorly, the right upper pulmonary vein (RUPV) is returning to the right atrium. Some tricuspid tension apparatus (TV) is seen. A – anterior; Ao – aorta; P – posterior; S – superior.

out of 23 patients studied by Smallhorn and colleagues (1981). It was found in each one of 12 patients where the suprasternal approach with a 5 mHz transducer was used. It should be noted that in many cases of connexion to the coronary sinus the confluence *is* the coronary sinus. In four-chamber cuts from the precordial, subcostal and apical approaches, the confluence can be seen as an echo-free non-pulsatile region beyond and clearly separate from the left atrium (Figs. 21.9, 21.10a). Care should be taken to distinguish this confluence from the right pulmonary artery. This latter originates from the pulmonary trunk, is more anterior, and is usually pulsatile. These four-chamber views also demonstrate the size of the interatrial communication. A characteristic picture of the confluence is obtained from the suprasternal approach, whence the four converging pulmonary veins usually appear in the form of a cross (Smallhorn et al, 1981) (Fig. 21.11). The confluence is occasionally a longer channel, and even more rarely, may be somewhat removed from the left atrium. Once having been discovered, the connexion of the confluence to the systemic venous circulation must be determined.

A *descending* vein, as found in anomalous infradiaphragmatic connexion, can sometimes be seen descending from the confluence from the suprasternal approach (Fig. 21.11b). Much more commonly, the descending vein is found by placing the transducer so as to obtain a subcostal long axis cut of the aorta or inferior caval vein and then scanning from left to right (Smallhorn et al, 1981; Lam et al, 1984). The descending vein is recognised as a channel penetrating

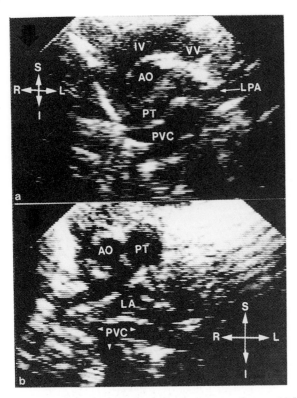

Fig. 21.11 Suprasternal views of pulmonary venous confluence. (a) In this section, the cruciate appearance of the pulmonary venous confluence (PVC) is rather well seen. However, its continuation with the vertical vein (VV) is not seen. (b) In this heart, the pulmonary venous confluence is connected to a descending vein, suggesting total anomalous pulmonary venous connexion to the portal vein. AO – aorta; I – inferior; IV – innominate vein; L – left; LA – left atrium; LPA – left pulmonary artery; PT – pulmonary trunk; R – right; S – superior.

the diaphragm (Fig. 21.12). It is distinguished from the aorta both by its lack of pulsation and lack of connexion to the superior mesenteric artery. It is differentiated from the inferior caval and hepatic veins by its failure to enter one or other atrium and the fact that it runs up behind the heart, where branching can sometimes be recognised (Fig. 21.13). If the site of termination is the portal vein, the descending vein often appears as a finger pointing anteriorly from the oesophageal hiatus towards the hepatic portal (Fig. 21.14). These discriminating features are sufficient in our experience. If doubt persists, then the inferior caval vein can be distinguished from a descending pulmonary vein by its opacification following injection of microbubbles into a leg vein (Snider et al, 1982). Alternatively pulsed Doppler can be used to show that the descending pulmonary vein contains non-pulsatile blood moving inferiorly (Cooper et al, 1984).

A *left vertical* vein is best seen from the suprasternal approach whence its connexion with the innominate vein is easily visualised (Fig. 21.15). The vertical vein can usually be traced to the confluence, particularly since its initial upward course and the confluence can often be seen in subcostal cuts (Fig. 21.16). If the connexion cannot be seen, then Doppler velocimetry or injection of contrast bubbles into the left arm will demonstrate the direction of flow in the vertical vein.

If neither an ascending or descending vein is identified, then the anomalous connexion is most likely either to the coronary sinus or directly to the right atrium. If it is to the *coronary sinus*, then that structure (best identified in cross-section in a precordial long axis cut within the left atrioventricular groove) will be enlarged and will bulge anterosuperiorly into the left atrium. Great care must be taken to distinguish enlargement of the coronary sinus due to its connexion to a left superior caval vein, and its enlargement due to connexion to pulmonary veins. This is best achieved by obtaining a subcostal four chamber cut and tilting the transducer posteriorly. The inferior margin of the coronary sinus thus imaged corresponds to the atrioventricular junction. If the superior margin lies more

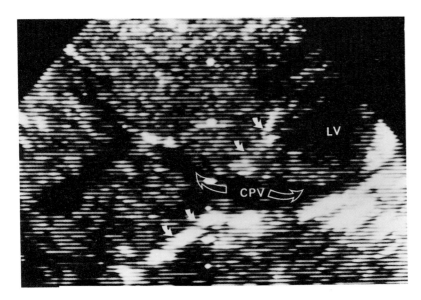

Fig. 21.12 Subcostal long axis section in patient with total anomalous pulmonary venous connexion to portal vein. Note the common pulmonary vein (CPV), identified as such because of its lack of pulsation in real-time, its penetration of the diaphragm (solid white arrows), and its passage immediately behind the heart, of which only the left ventricle (LV) can be seen. An azygos continuation would run much further posteriorly.

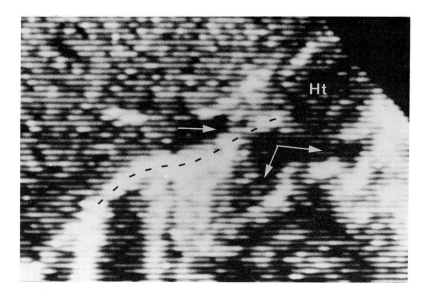

Fig. 21.13 Subcostal long axis section in total anomalous pulmonary venous connexion to portal vein. In this picture, from the same patient as Figure 21.12, the actual point of penetration of the common pulmonary vein through the diaphragm (dotted line) is not seen, but bifurcation of the structure above the diaphragm demonstrates clearly that this is a pulmonary vein, and not a systemic vein or artery. Ht – heart.

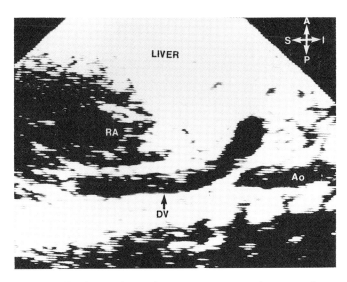

Fig. 21.14 Total anomalous pulmonary venous connexion to portal vein. In this subcostal long axis section, the descending vein (DV) passes anteriorly as it travels inferiorly, moving forward towards the porta hepatis. Thus it is distinguished from both the inferior caval vein and the aorta (Ao). A – anterior; I – inferior; P – posterior; RA – right atrium; S – superior. (Reproduced by kind permission of Churchill Livingstone from Rowlands D J (ed) Recent advances in cardiology, Vol 9.)

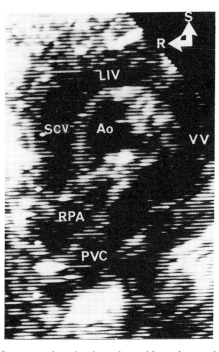

Fig. 21.15 Suprasternal section in patient with total anomalous pulmonary venous connexion to a vertical vein. In this particular patient, the whole of the sweep of pulmonary venous return from pulmonary venous confluence (PVC) via the vertical vein (VV), the left innominate vein (LIV) and the superior caval vein (SCV) is displayed. The venous channel, running around the aorta (Ao) gives the appearance of an ear. R – right; RPA – right pulmonary artery; S – superior.

or less parallel to it, this suggests connexion to a left superior caval vein. If, on the other hand, the superior margin bulges superiorly, then connexion to pulmonary veins should be suspected. This should be sought by making small tilting and rotational movements of the transducer (Fig. 21.17). Anomalous connexion to the *right atrium* may be diagnosed if there is no ascending or descending vein, the coronary sinus is of normal size, and the confluence can be followed to its site of entry to the right atrium (see Fig. 21.10).

Stark and colleagues 1982 reported successful repair of total anomalous pulmonary venous connexion in 6 young infants without previous cardiac catheterisation. Thus, our experience suggests that skilled use of cross-sectional echocardiography avoids the need for cardiac catheterisation in the majority of patients. Huhta and

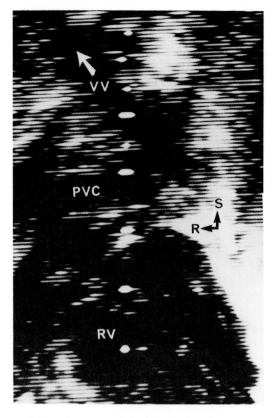

Fig. 21.16 Subcostal paracoronal cut in total anomalous pulmonary venous connexion to a left vertical vein. While this picture on its own would not be diagnostic and suprasternal views would also be required, the connexion of the pulmonary venous confluence (PVC) to the vertical vein (VV) can be rather clearly seen. R – right; RV – right ventricle; S – superior.

colleagues (1985) reported 97% sensitivity and 99% specificity for the technique in diagnosing total anomalous pulmonary venous connexion. Mixed total anomalous pulmonary venous return cannot always be recognised, but then such cases are not always diagnosed by angiocardiography.

Characteristically, the right ventricle is enlarged in total anomalous pulmonary venous connexion. Oliveira Lima and colleagues (1983) found that the greater the ratio between right and left ventricular diameters on echocardiography, the less likely was the patient to survive operation. The method of determining this ratio was curious in that it was either obtained from standard M-mode echocardiography (which would correspond to a precordial long axis cut) or from an apical four chamber cut (which would be in an entirely different plane) or from both.

As always, if the clinical and cross-sectional echocardiographic findings are not typical for the condition, cardiac catheterisation should be performed without hesitation.

Cardiac catheterisation

This will document the pathophysiology already indicated. The site of pulmonary venous obstruction is probably the most interesting information that can be obtained from cardiac catheterisation. It should be remembered, however, that passage of a catheter across the obstruction will temporarily make it worse. Since obtaining the information demands advancing the catheter through an abnormally positioned vein, the safest approach is first to determine the site of the vein. This can be done either by cross-sectional echocardiography or by pulmonary arteriography (see below). Vertical veins can be entered with ease using a suitably curved catheter. If necessary, a guide-

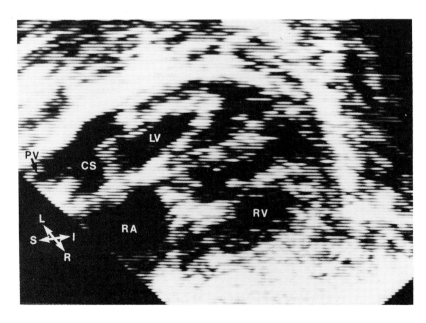

Fig. 21.17 Oblique subcostal four chamber cut in total anomalous pulmonary venous connexion to the coronary sinus (CS). Note the pulmonary vein (PV) returning to the coronary sinus. The left atrium is not in the picture. The right ventricle (RV) is much larger than the left ventricle (LV). (Reproduced by kind permission of Churchill Livingstone from Rowlands D J (ed) Recent advances in cardiology, Vol 9.) I – inferior; L – left; R – right; RA – right atrium; S – superior.

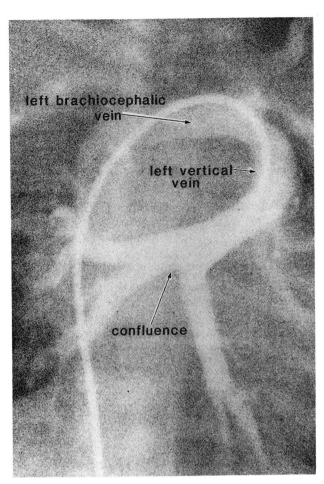

Fig. 21.18 Frontal vein of selective pulmonary vein injection in total anomalous pulmonary venous connexion to a left vertical vein.

wire can be used, passing the catheter from below through the right atrium and via the right superior caval and brachiocephalic veins (Fig. 21.18) (Behrendt et al, 1972). When return is to the coronary sinus, this structure may be entered in the usual fashion. It is usually a simple matter to enter the pulmonary confluence when it connects either to the right atrium or to the right superior or inferior caval veins. In the special case of anomalous connexion to the portal vein, the umbilical vein is the approach of choice (Tynan et al, 1974) since no-one has reported success in traversing the venous duct from the inferior caval vein. In any case, this structure has often closed by the time the patient is catheterised. The catheter should not be left in position for long, as pulmonary venous pressure can rise as high as 50 mmHg if it is not removed at once (Nickerson et al, 1979).

Angiocardiography

It is not easy to demonstrate well the detailed anatomy of the route of anomalous return by angiocardiography. This is probably why relatively little has been published on the subject. In theory, selective pulmonary venous injection is the method of choice. In practice, it is often a frustrating experience because of the refusal of contrast medium to reflux into pulmonary veins against the current unless there is severe pulmonary venous obstruction. The pulmonary venous injection in obstructed connexion to the portal vein published by Tynan and colleagues (1974) shows superb opacification of the pulmonary veins. In contrast, on injection into the coronary sinus (for example) it is rare to see opacification of pulmonary veins even if all are connected to it.

Pulmonary arteriography works well if there is just the right amount of pulmonary venous obstruction. If this is too severe (and particularly if the duct is patent), it may be impossible to demonstrate the pulmonary veins because of loss of contrast medium into the systemic circulation. This happens despite the use of large doses of rapidly injected contrast medium and filming for 20 seconds or more.

By contrast, if there is no pulmonary venous obstruction, pulmonary blood supply may be so high that serious dilution of contrast medium prevents optimal visualisation of the pulmonary veins. Mixed anomalous connexion may be missed because of inadequate definition and simultaneous opacification of all the cardiac chambers. Selective left or right pulmonary arterial injection may improve recognition of the drainage sites in mixed return. Pulmonary arterial wedge injection (Bargeron, personal communication) may be even better.

The appearance of the *vertical vein* is characteristic (Fig. 21.18), as is the typical site of obstruction half way along its course – usually where the vertical vein passes between the 'haemodynamic vice' between the left pulmonary artery and left main bronchus, and also the appearance of anomalous connexion to the *portal vein* (Fig. 21.19). In this condition the pulmonary venous confluence, instead of being horizontal, tends to be vertical. This gives the picture poetically termed 'the tree in winter' (Kawashima et al, 1977). Differentiation between infradiaphragmatic connexion to the portal and hepatic veins is not difficult if selective pulmonary vein injections are made in the latter (Fig. 21.20). When the anomalous connexion is to the azygos or right superior caval vein (Fig. 21.21), the course of the common pulmonary vein is frequently tortuous. Drainage to the coronary sinus is recognised by the 'golf-ball' appearance of the dilated coronary sinus in the frontal projection (Rowe et al, 1961). Initial opacification of the cardiac silhouette occurs at its most posterior point in the lateral projection, contrast medium thereafter flowing downwards and forwards along the coronary sinus into the right atrium (Fig. 21.22). Anomalous connexion to the right atrium is usually diagnosed by recognising that diffuse right atrial opacification (Rowe et al, 1961) precedes left atrial opacification, but for none of the reasons listed above.

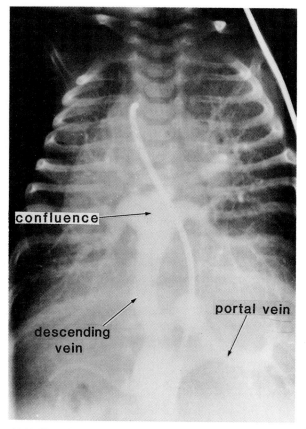

Fig. 21.19 Frontal view of pulmonary arteriogram in patient with total anomalous pulmonary venous connexion to the portal vein. The catheter in the left-sided inferior caval vein and the heart lying to the right, together with the presence of total anomalous pulmonary venous connexion strongly suggest right atrial isomerism, which was indeed present in this patient.

Differential diagnosis

Much of this has already been discussed, and will not be repeated. As we shall see, pulmonary vein atresia presents as total anomalous connexion with severe pulmonary venous obstruction. The two conditions may be indistinguishable prior to surgery when no common pulmonary vein is seen either on cross-sectional echocardiography or angiocardiography.

Unobstructed connexion has to be distinguished from other conditions producing heart failure, mild cyanosis and cardiomegaly with pulmonary plethora and right ventricular hypertrophy. The most important of these is complete transposition with large ventricular septal defect in which the second heart sound is commonly single. Common atrium is easily distinguished by the electrocardiogram, which is typical of an atrioventricular septal defect (a superior counterclockwise frontal plane QRS loop). Total anomalous connexion to the left vertical vein has to be distinguished from levoatriocardinal vein in association with mitral atresia and intact atrial septum (see below). In both conditions pulmonary veins flow to a confluence which empties via a left vertical vein. In the case of levoatriocardinal vein, the confluence is the left atrium. The pulmonary veins are normally connected.

Course and prognosis

With medical treatment alone, 75% of all children with total anomalous pulmonary venous connexion uncomplicated by heterotaxy are dead by their first birthday

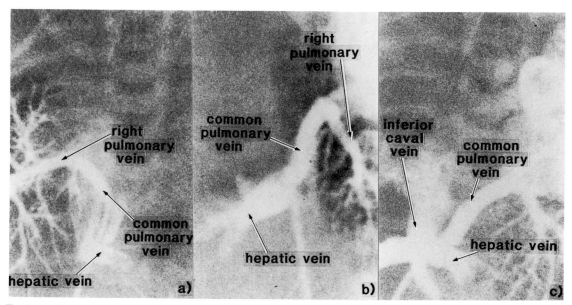

Fig. 21.20 Total anomalous pulmonary venous connexion to the hepatic vein. Panels (a) and (c) are frontal projections, and (b) is a lateral projection of panel (a). The secure identification of the hepatic vein, and its differentiation from other venous structures are obtained by comparing panels (a) and (b). Having done this, it is possible to identify the inferior caval vein in panel (c). It is also possible to recognise that right and left pulmonary veins drain into a common pulmonary vein seen in the frontal projection in both (a) and (c).

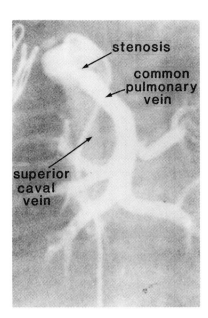

Fig. 21.21 Total anomalous pulmonary venous connexion to the right superior caval vein. Note that the pulmonary venous confluence is vertical rather than horizontal, and that there is a stenosis followed by a post-stenotic dilation of the vein just before it enters the right superior caval vein.

(Bonham Carter et al, 1969). It is of interest that this poor survival in a series of 58 patients occurred despite the fact that only 5 had infradiaphragmatic anomalous connexion. Of 25 patients with pulmonary venous obstruction treated medically, only 2 survived their first year (Gathman & Nadas, 1970).

Medical treatment

Resuscitation of the critically ill neonate and treatment of congestive heart failure are carried out as for any other duct-independent congenital heart defect.

Balloon atrial septostomy

Balloon atrial septostomy undoubtedly produces clinical improvement in the short-term in some patients. It seems to be impossible to identify in advance those patients who will benefit (Serratto et al, 1968; Mullins et al, 1973). It has been recommended as a procedure to 'buy time' so as to operate on the baby at a size when immediate surgical risk is lower. The generally bad prognosis for this disease on medical treatment, together with recent improvements in surgical results even at very young ages, militate strongly against this expectant policy – more so if the objective is to postpone surgery for a year or more.

Balloon atrial septostomy is technically more difficult than in complete transposition because two methods normally used to check that the catheter is in the atrium do not apply. The left atrial saturation is not higher than

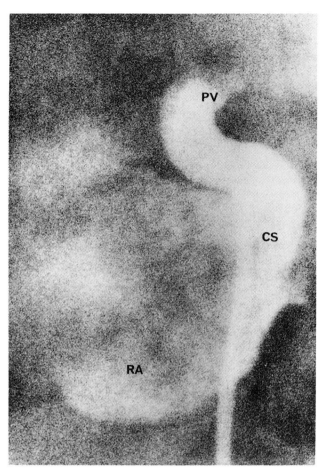

Fig. 21.22 Total anomalous pulmonary venous connexion to the coronary sinus, as seen in the lateral projection. A selective injection has been made into a pulmonary vein (PV). This drains right to the back of the heart, into a channel which can readily be identified as the coronary sinus (CS). This in turn enters the right atrium (RA).

the right, and pulmonary veins cannot be entered from the left atrium. Even using biplane screening, it can be difficult to distinguish a catheter positioned in the left atrium from one in a dilated coronary sinus. Injection of contrast medium through a double lumen catheter is probably the safest conventional method of catheter localisation available, though cross-sectional echocardiography (Allan et al, 1982) is a simpler and more accurate method.

Given the additional complexity of the procedure, is balloon atrial septostomy worth performing? Our belief is that it is not. The interatrial communication is rarely if ever the main cause of the patient's problems, which are best dealt with by immediate surgery. Gathman & Nadas (1970) argued against balloon atrial septostomy on similar grounds, as did Sade and colleagues (1975). Nonetheless, there are two excellent reports of results of cardiac surgery where balloon septostomy is advocated. On closer examination, the grounds for this advocacy do not appear firm. For example, Whight and colleagues (1978) stated that, 'Most infants with non-obstructive TAPVC who were younger than four months of age underwent balloon atrial septostomy, irrespective of the presence or absence of an interatrial gradient'. The definition of 'non-obstructive' is unclear, but seems to have been made on the basis of angiocardiography. Moreover, out of the 13 patients without obstruction who presented below four months of age, only 8 had a septostomy. Turley and colleagues (1980) stated (without giving evidence) that balloon atrial septostomy at cardiac catheterisation can often result in improvement in patients with supracardiac or intracardiac connexion. They then went on to recommend that 'correction should be initiated at the earliest presentation of symptoms', which hardly gives the infant much time to benefit from the septostomy!

Where surgical facilities are suboptimal, balloon atrial septostomy probably does more good than harm. Where surgical facilities are excellent, balloon atrial septostomy is of marginal benefit, if any. We doubt that this question will ever be satisfactorily resolved, given the rarity of the lesion and the widely differing surgical approaches used even in the best centres.

Surgical treatment

Total anomalous pulmonary venous connexion was the first condition in which the necessity of open heart repair in infancy was forced upon surgeons as a result of the appalling natural history, the lack of any adequate alternative by way of palliation, and the potential for excellent long-term results if immediate survival could be achieved. The early results in infancy inevitably involved a high mortality (Cooley et al, 1966: Mustard et al, 1968; Behrendt et al, 1972; Mullins et al, 1973). These included operations in which an anastomosis between the pulmonary venous confluence and the left atrium was created, but the interatrial communication was not closed, and the common pulmonary vein, if obstructed, was not ligated (Mustard et al, 1968: Behrendt et al, 1972). Though subsequent spontaneous closure of the interatrial communication was documented in some patients (Silove et al, 1972), this staged approach is now rarely used. At that time, only isolated reports of successful repair of

infradiaphragmatic connexion had appeared. Over the last decade or so, surgical results have greatly improved. There has been some debate as to whether age or site of connexion is the most important determinant of operative survival. Table 21.1 shows that most deaths occur in patients under a month or over three months of age. Table 21.2 demonstrates that patients with cardiac connexions have the best prognosis, possibly because they have the lowest incidence of pulmonary venous obstruction. The preoperative condition of the patient is probably the most important risk factor. This is demonstrated by the statistically significant association of postoperative death with preoperative ventilation (Katz et al, 1978) and preoperative metabolic acidosis in patients with infradiaphragmatic connexion (Bove et al, 1981). Since there is very little that medical treatment can offer in patients with severe pulmonary venous obstruction, these results certainly argue for prompt referral and surgery – as soon as possible after diagnosis. This should be done preferably without making the patient even sicker by angiocardiography.

In those rare patients who for one reason or another arrive having survived their first year on medical treatment, surgical results are excellent. Gomes and colleagues (1970) reported only 3 operative deaths in 44 patients older than one year for the entire period 1956–1968.

The inaccessibility of the pulmonary venous confluence behind the heart has meant that a bewildering variety of different surgical approaches has been tried. Repair of anomalous connexion to the coronary sinus involves cutting it back into the left atrium and repairing the atrial septum in such a way as to leave the opening in the coronary sinus on its left side. Drainage to the right atrium or lower right superior caval vein can be achieved by shifting the atrial septum to its right side, or creating a prosthetic tunnel to lead pulmonary venous blood to the left atrium. The opening between confluence and right atrium may need to be enlarged. When connexion is to other sites, the confluence must either be reached by dislocating the cardiac apex forwards, by incising posterior pericardial attachments on the right so as to elevate the heart and caval veins and retract them to the left, by approaching through the transverse sinus, or by cutting

Table 21.1 Results of repair of total anomalous pulmonary venous connexion in infancy, by age

Report	Date of operation	Age (months) hospital mortality							
		<1		>1<3		>3<6		>6<12	
Katz et al, 1978	1974–1977	3/9	(33%)	0/6	(0%)	1/3	(33%)	0/1	(0%)
Whight et al, 1978	1969–1976	2/8	(25%)	0/5	(0%)	1/6	(17%)	0/4	(0%)
Turley et al, 1980	1975–1979	2/12	(17%)	1/5	(20%)	0/3	(0%)	0/2	(0%)
Dickinson et al, 1982	1970–1981	2/13	(16%)	2/17	(12%)			4/14	(29%)
Totals:		9/42	(21%)	3/33	(9%)			6/33	(18%)

Table 21.2 Results of repair of total anomalous pulmonary venous connexion in infancy, by site

Report	Date of operation	Hospital deaths and anatomic type							
		Supracardiac		Intracardiac		Infracardiac		Mixed	
Turley et al, 1980	1975–1979	0/9	(0%)	1/6	(17%)	2/6	(33%)	0/1	(0%)
Whight et al, 1978	1969–1976	2/5	(40%)	0/16	(0%)	1/6	(17%)	0/1	(0%)
*Hammon et al, 1980	1969–1979	3/12	(25%)	0/6	(0%)	2/5	(40%)	0/2	(0%)
Bove et al, 1981	1971–1979	15/35	(43%)	3/16	(19%)	8/20	(40%)	0/2	(0%)
Dickinson et al, 1982	1970–1981	3/22	(14%)	2/8	(25%)	1/9	(11%)	2/5	(40%)
Totals:		23/83	(28%)	6/52	(12%)	14/46	(30%)	2/11	(18%)

* one patient was 13 months old

through the right atrial septum and posterior left atrial wall (Katz et al, 1978). A confluence connected to a left vertical vein can also be approached from a left thoracotomy extended trans-sternally (Di Eusanio et al, 1978). Whatever the approach, the objective must be to create as wide an anastomosis as possible between the confluence and the left atrium. Because one patient developed acute liver necrosis after repair of infradiaphragmatic return with ligation of the descending vein (Applebaum et al, 1975), some surgeons recommend leaving this vein unligated. After repair, flow through this high resistance pathway will be negligible (Jegier et al, 1967; Katz et al, 1978).

The late results of repair are in general excellent (Macartney et al, 1980). There have, however, been occasional reports of late pulmonary venous obstruction. This may be at the site of anastomosis (Cooley et al, 1966; Breckenridge et al, 1973; Katz et al, 1978). In the case of connexion to the coronary sinus, stenosis has also been reported at the orifice created between coronary sinus and left atrium (Whight et al, 1978; Dickinson et al, 1982). Obstruction has also been reported of the Dacron baffle used to redirect veins draining to the right atrium towards the left atrium (Dickinson et al, 1982).

On the other hand, some causes of late pulmonary venous obstruction may not be the result of technical error, but of congenital abnormalities of pulmonary veins (Haworth, 1982). Whight and colleagues (1978) report one case of stenosis at the junction between the pulmonary venous confluence and the coronary sinus. More common has been ostial stenosis of one or more pulmonary veins (Friedli et al, 1971; Whight et al, 1978; Katz et al, 1978; Fleming et al, 1979; Bove et al, 1981; Dickinson et al, 1982). Either or both of these problems may have existed unrecognised prior to surgery. The diagnosis is probably best made by selective pulmonary vein angiography, or failing that, by pulmonary artery wedge injection (Bini & Bargeron, 1982). These findings emphasise once again the need for careful follow-up of all patients following cardiac surgery.

Incorporation of the pulmonary veins into the left atrium seems to have restored left atrial volume to normal in most of a small number of patients studied. Seven patients with a preoperative small left ventricular end-diastolic volume who survived operation have been re-studied. In one the volume was unchanged, while in the remainder it had become normal (Graham et al, 1972; Mathew et al, 1977; Whight et al, 1978; Hammon et al, 1980). In five patients a subnormal preoperative left ventricular ejection fraction become normal after operation (Hammon et al, 1980). Arrhythmias are rare, though the electrocardiograms continue to show an rsR^1 in V_2. The chest X-ray returns to normal in 90% of patients and 93% have a normal resting pulmonary artery pressure. Out of 15 patients, 10 showed a resting gradient of 3–7.5 mmHg between the mean wedged pulmonary capillary and the left ventricular end-diastolic pressures. This was primarily due to a slower y descent and a higher v point in the wedge pressure than in the left atrial pressure. In only one of these was there thought to be significant venous obstruction (Whight et al, 1978). Pulmonary artery pressure returns to normal even in patients with infradiaphragmatic connexion (Bove et al, 1981).

These results emphasise that total anomalous pulmonary venous connexion is a gratifying lesion to treat. There are few other cardiac lesions where the results are so bleak without surgery, and so good in the long run when it is successful.

COMMON PULMONARY VEIN ATRESIA

Morphology and morphogenesis

Anatomy

As we have discussed briefly in the previous sections, the essence of this anomaly is absence of functional connexion between the pulmonary veins and the morphologically left atrium (Lucas et al, 1962). The normally formed pulmonary veins converge immediately behind the left atrium to form a venous confluence which has either no outlet or a very limited outlet for pulmonary venous return. In the three cases described by Lucas, atretic strands connected to the right atrium in one patient, the left atrium in another and passed along the oesophagus in the third. In two further cases described by Nakib et al (1967), strands ran along the oesophagus in one and minute strands connected with the paratracheal venous plexuses in the other. We have seen a case which can be compared to this group. The pulmonary veins connected to the left atrium with an imperforate diaphragm between the two and a small anomalous strand connected to the superior caval vein. The embryology has been discussed in the previous section.

Pathophysiology

There is no direct route for blood to enter either the left atrium or any systemic vein, and yet patients have lived for up to a month with this condition (Lucas et al, 1962). How oxygen reaches the systemic arteries is uncertain. One suggested route is via bronchopulmonary venous anastomoses to the pleurohilar bronchial veins which drain into the azygos, hemiazygos and brachiocephalic veins. Alternatively, blood could reflux from pulmonary capillaries into pulmonary arteries, and hence pass through bronchopulmonary arterial anastomoses and bronchial arteries into the systemic circuit (Ledbetter et al, 1978). In one of the earliest cases described (Lucas et al, 1962) a dilated right bronchial vein connecting with dilated oesophageal venous channels was found at autopsy.

The elevated pulmonary capillary pressure causes pulmonary oedema. Excess oedema fluid may escape through dilated lymphatics, which have frequently been described in this condition (Lucas et al, 1962; Rywlin & Fojaco, 1968; Hawker et al, 1972; Ledbetter et al, 1978) and indeed in obstructed total anomalous pulmonary venous connexion (Haworth, 1982).

Clinical presentation

The age at presentation, clinical findings, electrocardiogram and chest X-ray are all described as for total anomalous connexion with severe pulmonary venous obstruction. Echocardiographic findings have not been reported in this condition, but one would anticipate demonstration of a pulmonary venous confluence with no onward venous channel on cross-sectional echocardiography.

Cardiac catheterisation and angiocardiography

Characteristically, there is severe pulmonary hypertension with more-or-less constant, low arterial oxygen saturation in all vessels and cardiac chambers.

Pulmonary angiography often fails to show any pulmonary veins at all, though the confluence can sometimes be recognised (Hawker et al, 1972; Ledbetter et al, 1978). This condition can be easily confused with total anomalous pulmonary venous connexion with extreme pulmonary venous obstruction.

Management

There is no medical treatment. Surgical repair up until 1982 was attempted without success (Hawker et al, 1972), although one successful operation reported for 'infra-diaphragmatic TAPVC' (Friedli et al 1971) may well, on review, have been for atresia of the common pulmonary vein. Khonsari and colleagues (1982) reported successful repair in a 7-day-old, and provided a useful review of the literature.

PARTIAL ANOMALOUS PULMONARY VENOUS CONNEXION

Morphology

Partial anomalous connexion exists where one or more of the pulmonary veins are connected to the morphologically left atrium while the rest are connected to a systemic vein or the right atrium. The varieties of partial return are legion. It may be restricted to part of one lung (partial unilateral anomalous connexion). All of one lung may drain anomalously (complete unilateral anomalous connexion). Part of both lungs may drain anomalously (partial bilateral anomalous connexion) or finally all of one lung and part of the other may be connected to anomalous systemic sites (partial unilateral connexion together with complete unilateral connexion). The sites of anomalous connexion can be to any of those discussed for total anomalous connexion. As with total anomalous connexion, all the anomalously connected veins may drain to the same site or there may be mixed drainage. Obstructed drainage has not been described in the partial form. By describing the amount of lung connected anomalously and the site and drainage and the presence of associated lesions, it is possible to describe clearly all the bewildering complex variations tabulated by Snellen and his colleagues (1968), partial anomalous connexion accounting for 70% of their extensive series.

Some associations with partial anomalous drainage are so frequent to warrant special consideration. The association with 'sinus venosus' atrial septal defect of anomalous drainage of the right pulmonary veins is described in Chapter 22. A situation which could be interpreted as unilaterally complete anomalous drainage with left atrial isomerism is described in Chapter 19. The so-called 'scimitar syndrome' (Neill et al, 1960) is so particular and characteristic a form of partial anomalous drainage that it deserves special consideration. In this lesion, shown by Neill and her colleagues to be familial, the lower lobe of the lung is hypoplastic and is supplied with arterial blood from the descending aorta. Its pulmonary venous return is connected to the inferior caval vein. Recognition of the anomaly itself far antedates the realisation that the anomalous venous channel produced a scimitar-shaped shadow on chest radiography. Park (1912), for example, noted the association with 'dislocation of the heart simulating dextrocardia'. Nonetheless it is undoubtedly the exotic likening of the radiographic appearance to the scimitar by Neill et al (1960) which gives the malformation its aura of excitement and mystery.

Embryology

Presumably the common pulmonary vein in this anomaly will have made connexion only with part of the intrapulmonary venous plexus. Anastomoses between the unconnected pulmonary segments and the systemic venous plexuses persist and develop. However, there is no doubt that very bizarre patterns of drainage do occur which present a challenge to the embryologist, as discussed by Blake et al (1965). This re-emphasises the inadvisability of basing descriptions of congenitally malformed hearts on embryologic hypotheses.

Pathophysiology

Because pulmonary venous obstruction has not been recognised with partial anomalous venous connexions, the haemodynamic effects are entirely the result of an obligatory left-to-right shunt through the anomalously connected segments of lung. No right-to-left shunt occurs as a result of the anomalous connexion. In older patients with pulmonary vascular obstructive disease, a right-to-left shunt can occur through an associated atrial septal defect (Hickie et al, 1956).

When partial anomalous pulmonary venous connexion occurs in association with atrial septal defect, as it does more often than not (Snellen et al, 1968), it is difficult to separate the haemodynamic effects of the two. We shall henceforth consider the pathophysiology only of cases with an intact atrial septum.

When there is complete anomalous connexion of one lung, be it right or left, the left-to-right shunt is usually greater than 50%. In other words, more blood flows through the anomalously connected lung than would be the case if it were normally connected (Frye et al, 1968). The reason for this is almost certainly that pulmonary venous return is to the systemic side of the circulation which has a lower mean pressure than the left atrium. When calculations of pulmonary vascular resistance are made correcting for the proportion of blood flow which would normally go to the anomalously connected lobe or lobes, it appears that this resistance is the same in the normally and anomalously connected regions of lung (Alpert et al, 1977). Thus, it is not the vascular resistance

which determines preferential flow to the anomalously connected lobe or lobes.

The left-to-right shunt at atrial level has the same consequences on the right heart and pulmonary circulation as does an atrial septal defect (see Ch. 22). Pulmonary hypertension is rare, except in some infants with scimitar syndrome who exhibit arterial, but not venous muscularity in both lungs (Haworth et al, 1983).

Presentation and symptoms

Presentation is as for secundum atrial septal defect (see Ch. 22) except that some asymptomatic patients may present with an unexpected abnormality on chest X-ray (see below). Presentation with heart failure in infancy rarely, but definitely occurs, as with interatrial defects at the oval fossa (Frye et al, 1968).

Physical findings

The physical signs in patients with an associated atrial septal defect are as for atrial septal defect (see Ch. 22).

The physical signs in patients with intact interatrial septum are as for atrial septal defect with left-to-right shunt of comparable size except that the second heart sound, though widely split, often varies normally with respiration (McCormack et al, 1960; Frye et al, 1968). Sinus arrhythmia is common. This is presumably because changes in intrathoracic pressure affect the atria to different degrees as they do in normal individuals. This contrasts with what happens in the presence of a large atrial septal defect (see Ch. 22). Thus, if a patient has the pulmonary ejection systolic murmur of an atrial septal defect and yet has physiological splitting of the second heart sound, the diagnosis is highly likely to be partial anomalous connexion with intact atrial septum.

Investigations

Chest radiography

The general appearances of the heart and pulmonary vessels will be exactly as for an atrial septal defect with a comparable left-to-right shunt. But the anomalous pulmonary vein may also be evident. A 'snowman' appearance would suggest return to the left vertical vein, whilst in older patients with return to the inferior caval vein the anomalous pulmonary vein is always visible (Hickie et al, 1956; Frye et al, 1968). We have already highlighted the importance of this appearance as seen in the 'scimitar' syndrome (Neill et al, 1960). The hypoplasia of the right lung, pulmonary sequestration and secondary dextrocardia usually accentuate the 'scimitar' in the frontal projection of the right lung. It is formed by the anomalous right pulmonary vein (Fig. 21.23), though in infants rotation of

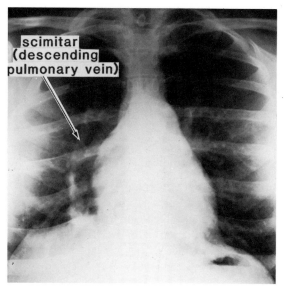

Fig. 21.23 Scimitar syndrome. In this plain chest radiograph there is only mild hypoplasia of the right lung, so the bulk of the heart is still in the left chest. (Original photograph kindly supplied by Dr Simon Rees.)

the heart to the right may completely obscure the scimitar (Haworth et al, 1983). Exceptionally, such a scimitar may be formed by a common right pulmonary vein which descends towards the diaphragm, but ascends to connect normally to the left atrium (Morgan & Forker, 1971).

Electrocardiography

When the partial anomalous connexion is associated with a secundum atrial septal defect, or the atrial septum is intact and the anomalous connexion is supracardiac or to the right atrium, the electrocardiogram is identical to that of a secundum atrial septal defect. Specifically, V_1 shows an rsr[1] or rsR[1] (rarely a QR) pattern in V_1. Partial return to the inferior caval vein with intact atrial septum is characterised by a terminal s[1] or S wave in V_1 (Frye et al, 1968).

Echocardiography

M-mode echocardiography shows the same features as a secundum atrial septal defect with comparable shunt (Tajik et al, 1972). Contrast echocardiography during cardiac catheterisation is of some value. If contrast injected into a pulmonary vein appears *only* in the right heart, this suggests that the vein drains anomalously (Danilowicz & Kronzon, 1979).

Partial anomalous venous connexion is the Achilles heel of the cross-sectional echocardiographer, particularly when associated abnormalities mask its clinical effects. There are two problems. First, even when all four pulmonary veins

are normally connected, they may not be imaged. In particular, fusion of two pulmonary veins on one side into a common pulmonary vein may not be recognised, though it is a common normal variant. Secondly, the great clue to the diagnosis of *total* anomalous pulmonary venous connexion, namely a pulmonary venous confluence, is almost invariably missing in partial anomalous connexion. In short, partial anomalous venous connexion can be positively and reliably diagnosed, particularly if it is via a left vertical vein, but it can rarely, if ever, be ruled out. Surgeons should be aware of this.

Cardiac catheterisation and angiocardiography

Cardiac catheterisation will document the pathophysiology already described. Entry to the anomalous veins may be achieved as for total anomalous connexion.

To demonstrate drainage *outside* the heart, pulmonary arteriography and selective pulmonary venous angiograms may be performed as for total anomalous connexion (Figs. 21.24, 21.25a). In the case of the scimitar syndrome, selective injection of the systemic arterial supply to the lungs is also essential (Fig. 21.25b). To demonstrate partial anomalous connexion *to the right atrium* it is essential to profile the atrial septum. Unless this is done it is not possible to say either from catheter course or contrast flow whether the vein enters the right atrium direct, or whether the catheter has entered the pulmonary vein having first crossed an atrial septal defect. Demonstration of the atrial septum is best achieved by injecting

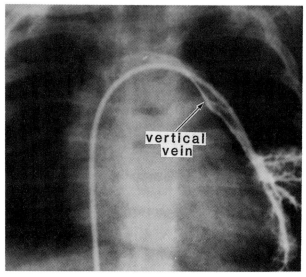

Fig. 21.24 Partial anomalous pulmonary venous connexion to a left vertical vein. Note that on this picture alone it would be impossible to rule out total anomalous pulmonary venous connexion, since by this technique, it is impossible to guarantee retrograde opacification of all pulmonary veins. (Original photograph kindly supplied by Dr Robert Freedom.)

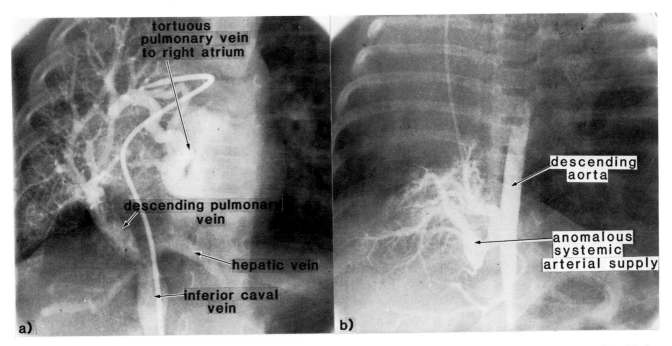

Fig. 21.25 Selective angiography in the scimitar syndrome displayed in the frontal projection. (a) This is a pulmonary arteriogram, filmed in its late stages so as to demonstrate that the pulmonary veins return by two routes to the heart – one a tortuous vein to the right atrium, and one a descending pulmonary vein to the inferior caval vein. (b) A selective injection into a branch of the descending aorta demonstrates the anomalous systemic arterial supply.

into the right upper pulmonary vein in the 30° left anterior oblique projection with 45° of caudocranial tilt (see Ch. 22). This works because contrast medium runs down the upper interatrial septum, thus producing a marked difference in opacification between the two atria. When the right lower pulmonary vein is injected in the same projection, the atrial septum is usually not seen nearly as well. Hence anomalous connexion of the right lower pulmonary vein to the right atrium may be difficult to demonstrate.

Differential diagnosis

The main differential diagnosis is secundum atrial septal defect, which has been discussed at length already. In most cases, particularly when associated with atrial septal defect, it really does not matter if the anomalous connexion is not diagnosed preoperatively, since surgery can easily be adjusted accordingly. Thus invasive investigation of typical secundum atrial septal defect is not justified simply to rule out partial anomalous pulmonary venous connexion (which in any case can be difficult). The only possible exception is complete connexion of the left pulmonary veins to a vertical vein. This then involves a rather more complex operation (see below) than atrial septal defect closure or diversion of other forms of partial anomalous connexion.

Anomalous connexion of one pulmonary vein may give no more than an unimpressive systolic murmur, and therefore be confused with a normal heart. Even if this error is made the patient will not suffer, since the haemo-

dynamic consequences are trivial and there is no risk of bacterial endocarditis.

An associated connecting vein between left upper pulmonary and innominate veins (see below) usually gives rise to a venous hum, whereas partial anomalous connexion to a vertical vein usually does not. There is no connexion between the left atrium and the vertical vein in partial anomalous connexion.

Course and prognosis

This is probably similar to isolated secundum atrial septal defect with a comparable left-to-right shunt. Pulmonary vascular obstructive disease is rare, but undoubtedly occurs (Saalouke et al, 1977).

In the particular case of complete anomalous connexion of the veins from one lung there is a risk that if the respiratory function of the normally connected lung is compromised, death may result. The only fully saturated pulmonary venous blood will then be recirculated to the lung (Conant et al, 1947).

Medical management

This is as for any atrial septal defect, and rarely necessary.

Surgical treatment

Surgical repair is recommended if the pulmonary/systemic

flow ratio is greater than 2 : 1. The techniques are broadly similar to those already described for total anomalous connexion. In the case of supracardiac or infracardiac drainage, complete unilateral anomalous connexion will not be associated with a confluence behind the left atrium. This complicates repair. When the right veins are connected to the superior or inferior caval veins or to a hepatic vein, it is usually possible to create a tunnel within the caval vein and right atrium so as to direct blood to the left atrium. Direct anastomosis of the right pulmonary vein to the left atrium has also been achieved (Frye et al, 1968; Murphy et al, 1971).

The usual method of repair of complete unilateral connexion of the lung to a left vertical vein is to connect the common left pulmonary vein to the amputated stump of the left atrial appendage (Kirklin, 1953). On the grounds that this kind of anastomosis, like all venous anastomoses, is liable to late stenosis, Ports and colleagues (1979) have advocated dividing the vertical vein and incising it longitudinally to form a 'cobra-head' which is then anastomosed to the left atrium in between the left atrial appendage and the entrance of the right pulmonary vein. The circumference of this oblique anastomosis is clearly much larger than the circumference of the vein.

Repair of partial anomalous pulmonary venous return should be carried out electively before a child goes to school. The mortality is less than 1%. The long-term results of venous anastomosis should be followed with care, but we have been unable to find them documented.

ANOMALOUS PULMONARY/SYSTEMIC COLLATERAL VEIN AND LEVOATRIOCARDINAL VEIN

These conditions are frequently found in association with more serious causes of obstruction of pulmonary venous return, such as an intact atrial septum with either left atrioventricular valve atresia, aortic stenosis or aortic atresia, and divided left atrium (cor triatriatum) (Nakib et al, 1967; Beckman et al, 1975; Thilenius et al, 1976). They act as 'safety-valves' enabling pulmonary venous return to escape to the systemic circulation.

Under these circumstances the clinical presentation will be dominated by the lesion causing pulmonary venous obstruction. The presence of anomalous pulmonary/systemic venous collaterals or levoatriocardinal vein will emerge as a chance finding on angiocardiography or (as yet only in theory) on cross-sectional echocardiography. At first glance, levoatriocardinal vein, or an anomalous collateral vein between the left upper pulmonary and brachio-cephalic veins, may be mistaken for total anomalous connexion to the left vertical vein (Fig. 21.26). In both instances pulmonary venous blood returns to a 'confluence' which then drains via a vertical vein. In anomalous

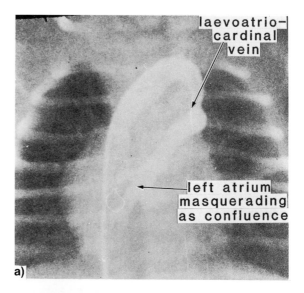

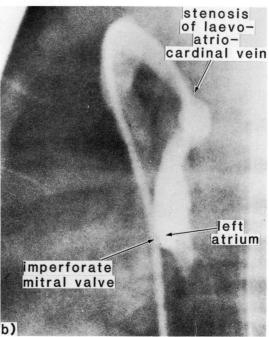

Fig. 21.26 Levoatriocardinal vein in association with imperforate mitral valve. (a) On the basis this frontal angiocardiogram alone, it would be impossible to distinguish this condition from total anomalous pulmonary venous connexion to a left vertical vein. (b) The lateral angiocardiogram in this patient demonstrates that the apparent confluence is in fact the left atrium, and that there is also a bulging structure which is an imperforate mitral valve. To make absolutely certain of the diagnosis, it would be desirable to obtain a selective left ventricular angiocardiogram to demonstrate the imperforate mitral valve from the other side.

connexion to the left vertical vein, the confluence is distinct from the left atrium. In these other conditions the 'confluence' *is* the left atrium. Confusion of these two entities is potentially disastrous (Beckman et al, 1975; Macartney et al, 1976).

The commonest anomalous pulmonary/systemic venous connexion is one which runs from the left upper pulmonary vein to the innominate vein. This can occur as an isolated abnormality, giving rise to a characteristic, if exceptionally rare, clinical picture (Zuberbuhler & Shinebourne, 1979). Patients present without symptoms, but with a venous hum under the left clavicle. Unlike the benign systemic venous hum at the same site, no amount of movement of the head or compression of jugular veins will abolish it.

Cardiac catheterisation and angiocardiography demonstrate precisely the same findings as in partial anomalous connexion to a vertical vein, *except* that the left upper pulmonary vein can be entered in a normal fashion from the left atrium. When contrast medium is injected into the left pulmonary artery, all contrast medium in the left upper pulmonary vein may appear to enter the vertical vein rather than the left atrium. This is because systemic venous pressure is lower than left atrial pressure. On the other hand, if a left atrial injection is performed, opacification of the vertical vein occurs. It is important to recognise this condition and to ensure that there is no stenosis of the pulmonary vein between the vertical vein and left atrium. If so, treatment simply consists of ligation of the vein without cardiopulmonary bypass or, in theory, balloon embolization.

STENOSIS OR ATRESIA OR INDIVIDUAL PULMONARY VEINS

Anatomy

There are two different types of stenosis of individual pulmonary veins (Nakib et al, 1967). The first type is characterised by hypoplasia of one or more of the veins. The narrowing involves the affected vein for a variable distance in both its intra- and extrapulmonary portions. The second variety is due to narrowing of one or more of the veins at its junction with the left atrium, and is termed 'localised pulmonary venous stenosis'. The distinction between these two may be less clear than previously imagined. Driscoll and colleagues (1982) described a case where localised stenosis was relieved temporarily by balloon dilation, but diffuse hypoplasia was found at autopsy. They suggested that dilatation of the vein upstream to the stenosis had masked the underlying hypoplasia.

It is only when several veins are involved that the condition becomes clinically manifest. In the 5 cases encountered by Nakib et al (1967), 2 were of the hypoplastic variety and 3 of the localised type, but in only 2 of the whole series were multiple veins affected. More recently Bini and her colleagues (1984) have encountered 4 cases in which all four pulmonary veins were stenosed at their junction with the left atrium. Such annular fibrotic

stenosis of the pulmonary venous ostia was also described by Edwards (1960), but the constrictions extended into the veins, and were considered to be congenital in origin. Marked secondary changes were observed in the lungs in this case. Shone and his colleagues (1962), however, pointed out that pulmonary venous stenosis could also be due to acquired causes such as constrictive pericarditis, mediastinitis, pulmonary tuberculosis or tumour invasion.

Pathophysiology

Stenosis or atresia of a single (not common) pulmonary vein unassociated with other severe cardiac anomalies has not to our knowledge been described. Most commonly, both pulmonary veins (or the common pulmonary vein on one side) are affected. Just under half the patients described have had other congenital heart defects, varying from simple (atrial septal defect) to complex (left atrioventricular valve atresia) (Driscoll et al, 1982). Pulmonary venous pressure becomes elevated on that side as a result. Pulmonary arterial hypertension ensues, though this is not always severe. In the case of unilateral pulmonary vein atresia (or severe stenosis) pulmonary blood flow will be largely or completely diverted to the contralateral lung. The result is that the pulmonary artery on the obstructed side may be unusually small and there will be none of the usual signs of pulmonary venous hypertension (Binet et al, 1972; Nasrallah et al, 1975). The greater the number of pulmonary veins obstructed, and the more severe the obstruction, the more severe will be the pulmonary hypertension. Elevation of right ventricular end-diastolic pressure may result in a right-to-left shunt through the foramen ovale (Shone et al, 1962).

Presentation and clinical symptomatology

Lesions of a single pulmonary vein might well be asymptomatic and not produce problems. When sufficient veins are affected, patients usually present in early infancy, though sometimes presentation is delayed until early childhood. Dyspnoea and repeated pulmonary infections with failure to thrive are the rule (Bini et al, 1984). Many patients have haemoptysis, and occasionally cyanosis (Sade et al, 1974; Kingston et al, 1983).

Clinical findings

Patients generally look unwell, with tachypnoea, indrawing and occasional cyanosis. There are frequently râles in the chest, and sometimes evidence of right heart failure (Contis et al, 1967). One patient had signs of right pleural effusion (Nasrallah et al, 1975). Murmurs are usually unimpressive, and the heart sounds unremarkable apart from accentuation of pulmonary closure and occasionally, a pulmonary ejection click.

Investigation

Electrocardiography

Right atrial and right ventricular hypertrophy without left-sided changes are almost invariably found (Bini et al, 1984).

Chest radiography

This is the single most helpful non-invasive investigation. Although the chest radiograph may be normal in the early stages (Binet et al, 1972), marked abnormality is the rule. The heart is usually normal in size or slightly enlarged, with prominence of the pulmonary trunk. The lungs show a reticular appearance or ground-glass opacification with or without Kerley B lines in the region of the obstructed vein or veins. There may be hypoplasia of the lung on the affected side. Thus the regional nature of the abnormality is the key to the diagnosis except when all the pulmonary veins are affected (Swischuk & L'Heureux, 1980). It is important to realise that when unilateral pulmonary vein stenosis or atresia is associated with left-to-right shunt, preferential flow to the contralateral lung occurs. If there are no specific indicants of pulmonary venous hypertension on the ipsilateral side, the appearance may be misinterpreted as being due to pulmonary artery stenosis.

Radionuclide angiography

Lung scans following injection of labelled pertechnetate show reduced or absent perfusion in the region of lung drained by the vein or veins which are obstructed (Sade et al, 1974). In two cases, ventilation on the affected side was said to be reduced (Nasrallah et al, 1975; Kingston et al, 1983).

Cardiac catheterisation

This documents the pathophysiology described. Provided that the pulmonary vein is not atretic, it is helpful to record withdrawal traces from pulmonary veins to left atrium, though care should be employed in interpreting the findings. In neonates particularly, pressure gradients may be found in normal pulmonary veins because the veins are not much larger than the catheter. If the left atrium cannot be entered or the pulmonary veins are atretic, pulmonary capillary wedge pressures should be recorded in upper and lower regions of both lungs, preferably simultaneous with a left-ventricular end-diastolic or left atrial pressure (Presbitero et al, 1983). It should be remembered that a normal wedge pressure does not necessarily rule out pulmonary vein stenosis (Geggel et al, 1984). This is because when a catheter is wedged in a pulmonary arteriole, the capillary, venule and vein beyond it act as an extension of the catheter, which may therefore reflect left atrial pressure rather than pulmonary venous pressure proximal to the stenosis.

Angiocardiography

Pulmonary angiocardiography will show slow clearance of contrast medium from one lung in the case of unilateral pulmonary vein stenosis. If this is sufficiently severe or the pulmonary veins are atretic, the contrast medium may well run to-and-fro into the pulmonary artery on that side

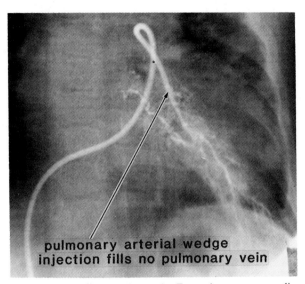

Fig. 21.27 Left pulmonary vein atresia. Even when contrast medium is injected in a pulmonary arterial wedge position, no pulmonary venous opacification occurs. Original photograph supplied by Dr Geoffrey Watson.

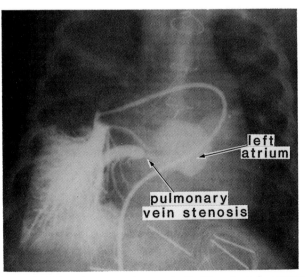

Fig. 21.28 Right pulmonary vein stenosis. In this patient, in contrast to the one in Figure 21.27, pulmonary arterial wedge injection demonstrates well the right lower pulmonary vein and a severe stenosis as it enters the left atrium. (Original photograph supplied by Dr Robert Freedom.)

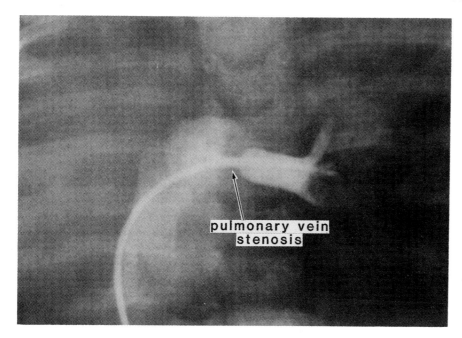

pulmonary vein stenosis

Fig. 21.29 Selective pulmonary vein injection to demonstrate left pulmonary vein stenosis. (Original photograph kindly supplied by Dr Robert Freedom.)

without ever opacifying the pulmonary veins (Fig. 21.27) (Binet et al, 1972; Nasrallah et al, 1975). Pulmonary arteriography does not demonstrate the precise anatomy of pulmonary vein stenosis at all well. Pulmonary arterial wedge angiography may well do better (Fig. 21.28) (Bini & Bargeron, 1982). Selective pulmonary vein injection, if possible, is greatly preferable (Fig. 21.29) (Driscoll et al, 1982).

Diagnosis

Stenosis or atresia of one or two pulmonary veins

This must be distinguished from pulmonary infection, which is far commoner. Lack of fever, elevation of sedimentation rate, leucocytosis, and response to antibiotics all should lead to the suspicion of pulmonary vein stenosis.

Stenosis or atresia of most or all pulmonary veins

This must be distinguished from other causes of generalised elevation of pulmonary venous pressure. The absence of severe cardiomegaly distinguishes pulmonary vein obstruction from left ventricular disease and mitral regurgitation. Mitral stenosis and supravalvar mitral ring almost always exhibit diastolic murmurs and are easily recognisable on cross-sectional echocardiography, as is cor triatriatum. Total anomalous pulmonary venous connexion and common pulmonary vein atresia only present a problem in cyanotic patients, and echocardiography demonstration of a pulmonary venous confluence will rule out stenosis or atresia of individual pulmonary veins.

The most likely disease to cause confusion is pulmonary veno-occlusive disease. Here, however, the pulmonary capillary wedge pressure is usually normal, and no obstruction can be demonstrated in the main pulmonary veins either by pressure measurements or angiocardiography. Pulmonary veno-occlusive disease has not been described in young infants.

Course and prognosis

Without surgical treatment patients will die before reaching adulthood, and frequently much sooner (Sade et al, 1974; Driscoll et al, 1982).

Medical treatment

Standard antifailure treatment will relieve the patient's immediate problem, but may not be effective for long.

Surgical treatment

There is no effective treatment of long segment atresia or severe pulmonary vein hypoplasia except pneumonectomy when the disease is unilateral, and the objective is to cure massive haemoptysis (Nasrallah et al, 1975; Swischuk & L'Heureux, 1980).

Localised atresia or stenosis has been successfully treated in a few instances by patch onlay grafting (Binet et al, 1972; Presbitero et al, 1983), side-to-end anastomosis of the vein to the left atrium (Sade et al, 1974) or excision of an obstructing membrane at the pulmonary vein/left atrial junction (Kawashima et al, 1971). Overall, the prognosis when at least half the veins are stenosed is grim. Bini et al (1984) described 8 patients treated surgically with 5 early and 3 late deaths.

An alternative technique, which might obviate the need for surgery, is venous dilation with a Gruntzig balloon catheter provided that the vein is wide enough to admit the catheter. This was originally applied to a 32-year-old women first during operation and subsequently after transseptal puncture. The patient died 9 months later, but no autopsy was carried out (Massumi et al, 1981). The authors diagnosed her condition as pulmonary veno-occlusive disease without lung biopsy and in the presence of localised stenoses in all four pulmonary veins, which is idiosyncratic. Subsequently, discrete congenital stenoses were dilated in three children. The results were disappointing in that there was recurrence in one patient, death from staphylococcal sepsis in another, and haemodynamic improvement in the short-term with no symptomatic benefit in the third (Driscoll et al, 1982). Lock and colleagues (1984) similarly reported no success in five patients. It seems that neither surgery nor balloon angioplasty have much to offer in this condition.

PULMONARY VARIX

This is a rare anomaly, presenting as a mass in the lung on routine chest X-ray, usually between the fourth and sixth decades. It has been found in patients as young as 7 years. It is usually observed in the right upper pulmonary lobe. The differential diagnosis includes all other space-occupying lesions, but can be established by pulmonary angiography. Treatment consists of observation. If the size increases, surgical treatment of associated lesions causing pulmonary venous hypertension or possibly lobectomy is indicated. Death due to rupture has been reported (Klinck & Hunt, 1933; Perret & Fortelius, 1961; Moro et al, 1978).

REFERENCES

Allan L D, Leanage R, Wainwright R, Joseph M C, Tynan M 1982 Balloon atrial septostomy under two dimensional echocardiographic control. British Heart Journal 47: 41–43

Alpert J S, Dexter L, Vieweg W V R, Haynes F W, Dalen J E 1977 Anomalous pulmonary venous return with intact atrial septum. Diagnosis and pathophysiology. Circulation 56: 870–875

Appelbaum A, Kirklin J W, Pacifico A D, Bargeron L M Jr 1975 The surgical treatment of total anomalous pulmonary venous connection. Israel Journal of Medical Sciences 11: 89–96

Arciniegas E, Henry J G, Green E W 1980 Stenosis of the coronary sinus ostium. An unusual site of obstruction in total anomalous pulmonary venous drainage. Journal of Thoracic and Cardiovascular Surgery 79: 303–305

Aüer J 1948 The development of the human pulmonary vein and its major variations. Anatomical Record 101: 581–594

Aziz K U, Paul M H, Bharati S, Lev M, Shannon K 1978 Echocardiographic features of total anomalous pulmonary venous drainage into the coronary sinus. American Journal of Cardiology 42: 108–113

Beckman C B, Moller J H, Edwards J E 1975 Alternate pathways to pulmonary venous flow in left-sided obstructive anomalies. Circulation 52: 509–516

Behrendt D M, Aberdeen E, Waterson D J, Bonham Carter R E 1972 Total anomalous pulmonary venous drainage in infants. I. Clinical and hemodynamic findings, methods, and results of operation in 37 cases. Circulation 46: 347–356

Bharati S, Lev M 1973 Congenital anomalies of the pulmonary veins. Cardiological Clinics 5: 23–41

Binet J P, Bouchard F, Langlois J, Chetochine F, Conso J F, Pottemain M 1972 Unilateral congenital stenosis of the pulmonary veins. Journal of Thoracic and Cardiovascular Surgery 63: 397–402

Bini R M, Bargeron L M J 1982 Visualization of pulmonary vein obstruction by pulmonary artery wedge injection. Pediatric Cardiology 2: 161–162

Bini R M, Cleveland D C, Ceballos R, Bargeron L M Jr, Pacifico A D, Kirklin J W 1984 Congenital pulmonary vein stenosis. American Journal of Cardiology 54: 369–375

Blake H A, Hall R J, Manion W C 1965 Anomalous pulmonary venous return. Circulation 32: 406–414

Bonham Carter R E, Capriles M, Noe Y 1969 Total anomalous pulmonary venous drainage. A clinical and anatomical study of 75 children. British Heart Journal 31: 45–51

Bove E L, de Leval M R, Taylor J F N, Macartney F J, Szarnicki R J, Stark J 1981 Infradiaphragmatic total anomalous pulmonary venous drainage; surgical treatment and long term results. Annals of Thoracic Surgery 31: 544–550

Breckenridge I M, Oelert H, Graham G R, Stark J, Waterson D J 1973 open-heart surgery in the first year of life. Journal of Thoracic and Cardiovascular Surgery 65: 58–64

Brenner J I, Bharati S, Berman M A, Lev M 1983 Rare type of intrapulmonary drainage of one lung by the other with total anomalous pulmonary venous return. Journal of the American College of Cardiology 2: 1174–1177

Conant J S, Kurland L T, Dale G 1947 Pulmonary tuberculosis associated with anomalous common left pulmonary vein entering the left innominate vein. Journal of Thoracic and Cardiovascular Surgery 16: 422–426

Contis G, Fung R H, Vawter G F, Nadas A S 1967 Stenosis and obstruction of the pulmonary veins associated with pulmonary artery hypertension. American Journal of Cardiology 20: 718–724

Cooley D A, Hallman G L, Leachman R D 1966 Total anomalous pulmonary venous drainage. Correction with the use of cardiopulmonary bypass in 62 cases. Journal of Thoracic and Cardiovascular Surgery 51: 88–102

Cooper M J, Teitel D F, Silverman N H, Enderlein M A 1984 Study of the intradiaphragmatic total anomalous pulmonary venous connection with cross-sectional and pulsed Doppler echocardiography. Circulation 70: 412–416

Danilowicz D, Kronzon I 1979 Use of contrast echocardiography in the diagnosis of partial anomalous pulmonary venous concention. American Journal of Cardiology 43: 248–252

Delisle G, Ando M, Calder A L, et al 1976 Total anomalous pulmonary venous connection: report of 93 autopsied cases with emphasis on diagnostic and surgical considerations. American Heart Journal 91: 99–122

Dickinson D F, Parimelazhagan K M, Tweedle M C K et al 1982 Total anomalous pulmonary venous connection. Repair using deep hypothermia and circulatory arrest in 44 consecutive infants. British Heart Journal 48: 249–54

Di Eusanio G, Sandrasagra F A, Donnelly R J, Hamilton D I 1978 Total anomalous pulmonary venous connection (Surgical technique, early and late results). Thorax 33: 275–282

Driscoll D J, Hesslein P S, Mullins C E 1982 Congenital stenosis of individual pulmonary veins: clinical spectrum and unsuccessful treatment by transvenous balloon dilatation. American Journal of Cardiology 49: 1767–72

Edwards J E 1960 Congenital stenosis of pulmonary veins. Pathologic and developmental considerations. Laboratory Investigation 9: 46–66

Edwards J E, DuShane J W 1950 Thoracic venous anomalie. I. Vascular connection between the left atrium and the left innominate vein (levoatriocardinal vein) associated with mitral atresia and premature closure of the foramen ovale (case 1). II. Pulmonary veins draining wholly to the ductus arteriosus (case 2). Archives of Pathology 49: 517–537

Elliott L P, Edwards J E 1962 The problem of pulmonary venous obstruction in total anomalous pulmonary venous connection to the left innominate vein (editorial). Circulation 25: 913–915

Fleming W H, Clark E B, Dooley K J, et al 1979 Late complications following surgical repair of total anomalous pulmonary venous return below the diaphragm. Annals of Thoracic Surgery 27: 435–439

Friedli B, Davignon A, Stanley P 1971 Infradiaphragmatic anomalous pulmonary venous return. Surgical correction in a newborn infant. Journal of Thoracic and Cardiovascular Surgery 62: 301–306

Frye R L, Krebs M, Rahimtoola S H, Ongley P A, Hallerman F J, Wallace R B 1968 Partial anomalous pulmonary venous connection without atrial septal defect. American Journal of Cardiology 22: 242–250

Fyler D C, Buckley L P, Hellenbrand W E, Cohn H E 1980 Report of the New England Regional Infant Cardiac Program. Pediatrics 65 (Suppl): 376–461

Gathman G E, Nadas A S 1970 Total anomalous pulmonary venous connection. Clinical and physiologic observations of 75 pediatric patients. Circulation 42: 143–154

Geggel R L, Fried R, Tuuri D T, Fyler D C, Reid L M 1984 Congenital pulmonary vein stenosis: Structural changes in a patient with normal pulmonary artery wedge pressure. Journal of the American College of Cardiology 3: 193–199

Godman M J, Tham P, Kidd B S L 1974 Echocardiography in the evaluation of the cyanotic newborn infant. British Heart Journal 36: 154–166

Gomes M M R, Feldt R H, McGoon D C, Danielson G K 1970 Total anomalous pulmonary venous connection. Surgical considerations and results of operation. Journal of Thoracic and Cardiovascular Surgery 60: 116–122

Graham T P Jr, Jarmakani J M, Canent R V J 1972 Left heart volume characteristics with a right ventricular volume overload. Total anomalous pulmonary venous connection and large atrial septal defect. Circulation 45: 389–396

Hammon J W Jr, Bender H W J, Graham T P J, Boucek R J J, Smith C W, Erath H G 1980 Total anomalous pulmonary venous connection in infancy. Ten years experience including studies of postoperative ventricular function. Journal of Thoracic and Cardiovascular Surgery 80: 544–581

Hastreiter A R, Paul M H, Molthan M E, Miller R A 1962 Total anomalous pulmonary venous connection with severe pulmonary venous obstruction. A clinical entity. Circulation 25: 916–928

Hawker R E, Celermajer J M, Gengos D C, Cartmill T B, Bowdler J D 1972 Common pulmonary vein atresia. Premortem diagnosis in two infants. Circulation 46: 368–374

Haworth S G 1982 Total anomalous pulmonary venous return. Prenatal damage to pulmonary vascular bed and extrapulmonary veins. British Heart Journal 48: 513–524

Haworth S G, Reid L 1977 Structural study of pulmonary circulation and of heart in total anomalous pulmonary venous return in early infancy. British Heart Journal 39: 80–92

Haworth S G, Sauer U, Buhlmeyer K 1983 Pulmonary hypertension in scimitar syndrome in infancy. British Heart Journal 50: 182–189

Healey J E 1952 An anatomic survey of anomalous pulmonary veins: their clinical significance. Journal of Thoracic Surgery 23: 433–444

Hickie J B, Gimlette T M D, Bacon A P C 1956 Anomalous pulmonary venous drainage. British Heart Journal 18: 365–377

Hughes C W, Rumore P C 1944 Anomalous pulmonary veins. Archives of Pathology 37: 364–366

Huhta J C, Gutgesell H P, Nihill M R 1985 Cross sectional echocardiographic diagnosis of total anomalous pulmonary venous connection. British Heart Journal 53: 525–534

Jegier W, Charrette E, Dobell A R C 1967 Infradiaphragmatic anomalous pulmonary venous drainage. Normal hemodynamics following operation in infancy. Circulation 35: 396–400

Johnson A L, Wiglesworth F W, Dunbar J S, Siddoo S, Grajo M 1958 Infradiaphragmatic total anomalous pulmonary venous connection. Circulation 340–347

Katz N M, Kirklin J W, Pacifico A D 1978 Concepts and practices in surgery for total anomalous pulmonary venous connection. Annals of Thoracic Surgery 25: 479–487

Kauffman S L, Ores C N, Andersen D H 1962 Two cases of total anomalous pulmonary venous return of the supracardiac type with stenosis stimulating infradiaphragmatic drainage. Circulation 25: 376–382

Kawashima Y, Ueda T, Naito Y, Morikawa E, Manabe H 1971 Stenosis of pulmonary veins. Report of a patient corrected surgically. Annals of Thoracic Surgery 12: 196–202

Kawashima Y, Matsuda H, Nakano S, et al 1977 Tree-shaped pulmonary veins in infracardiac total anomalous pulmonary venous drainage. Annals of Thoracic Surgery 23: 436–441

Khonsari S, Saunders P W, Lees M H, Starr A 1982 Common pulmonary vein atresia. Importance of immediate recognition and surgical intervention. Journal of Thoracic and Cardiovascular Surgery 83: 43–48

Kingston H M, Patel R G, Watson G H 1983 Unilateral absence or extreme hypoplasia of pulmonary veins. British Heart Journal 49: 148–153

Kirklin J W 1953 Surgical treatment of anomalous pulmonary venous connection. Mayo Clinic Proceedings 28: 476–479

Klinck G H J, Hunt H D 1933 Pulmonary varix with spontaneous rupture and death: report of a case. Archives of Pathology 15: 227–237

Lam J, Naeff M S J, Lubbers W J, Nijveld A 1984 2D echocardiographic diagnosis of total anomalous pulmonary venous connection of the infradiaphragmatic type. European Heart Journal 5: 842–845

Laurence K M, Brown R J K 1960 Total anomalous drainage of the pulmonary veins into the left gastric vein. British Heart Journal 22: 295–299

Ledbetter M K, Wells D H, Connors D M 1978 Common pulmonary vein atresia. American Heart Journal 96: 580–586

Lock J E, Bass J L, Castaneda-Zuniga W, Fuhrman B P, Rashkind W J, Lucas R V Jr 1984 Dilation angioplasty of congenital or operative narrowings of venous channels. Circulation 70: 457–464

Los J A 1968 Embryology. In: Watson H (ed) Paediatric cardiology. Lloyd-Luke, London, p1–28

Lucas R V Jr, Adams P J, Anderson R C, Varco R L, Edwards J E, Lester R G 1961 Total anomalous pulmonary venous connection to the portal venous system: A cause of pulmonary venous obstruction. American Journal of Roentgenology 86: 561–575

Lucas R V Jr, Woolfrey B F, Anderson R C, Lester R G, Edwards J E 1962 Atresia of the common pulmonary vein. Pediatrics 29: 729–739

Macartney F J, Bain H H, Ionescu M I, Deverall P B, Scott O 1976 Angiocardiographic/pathologic correlations in congenital mitral valve anomalies. European Journal of Cardiology 4: 191–211

Macartney F J, Taylor J F N, Graham G R, de Leval M, Stark J 1980 The fate of survivors of cardiac surgery in infancy. Circulation 62: 80–91

McCormack R J M, Marquis R M, Julian D G, Griffiths H W C 1960 Partial anomalous pulmonary venous drainage and its surgical correction. Scottish Medical Journal 5: 357–381

Massumi A, Woods L, Mullins C E, Nasser W K, Hall R J 1981 Pulmonary venous dilatation in pulmonary veno-occlusive disease. American Journal of Cardiology 48: 585–589

Mathew R, Thilenius O G, Replogle R L, Arcilla R A 1977 Cardiac function in total anomalous pulmonary venous return before and after surgery. Circulation 55: 361–370

Milner S, Levin S, Marchand P E, Hitchcock F 1977 Total anomalous pulmonary venous drainage in sibs (letter). Archives of Disease in Childhood 52: 984

Morgan J R, Forker A D 1971 Syndrome of hypoplasia of the right lung and dextroposition of the heart: 'scimitar sign' with normal pulmonary venous drainage. Circulation 43: 27–30

Moro C, Marin E, Sanchez A, Solozabal J 1978 Pulmonary varix: report of a case with additional anomalies of the vascular pulmonary tree. American Heart Journal 95: 243–246

Mortera C, Tynan M, Goodwin A W, Hunter S 1977 Infradiaphragmatic total anomalous pulmonary venous connection to portal vein. Diagnostic implications of echocardiography. British Heart Journal 39: 685–687

Mullins C E, El-Said G M, Neches W H, et al 1973 Balloon atrial septostomy for total anomalous pulmonary venous return. British Heart Journal 35: 752–757

Murphy J W, Kerr A R, Kirklin J W 1971 Intracardiac repair for anomalous pulmonary venous connection of right lung to inferior vena cava. Annals of Thoracic Surgery 11: 38–42

Mustard W T, Kean W J, Trusler G A 1968 Transposition of the lesser veins (total anomalous pulmonary venous drainage). Progress in Cardiovascular Diseases 11: 145–155

Nakib A, Moller J H, Kanjuh VI, Edwards J E 1967 Anomalies of the pulmonary veins. American Journal of Cardiology 20: 77–90

Nasrallah A T, Mullins C E, Singer D, Harrison G, McNamara D G 1975 Unilateral pulmonary vein atresia: diagnosis and treatment. American Journal of Cardiology 36: 969–973

Neill C A 1956 Development of the pulmonary veins with reference to the embryology of anomalies of pulmonary venous return. Pediatrics 18: 880–887

Neill C A, Ferencz C, Sabiston D C, Sheldon H 1960 The familial occurrence of hypoplastic right lung with systemic arterial supply and venous drainage 'scimitar syndrome'. Johns Hopkins Medical Journal 107: 1–15

Newfeld E A, Wilson A, Paul M H, Reisch J S 1980 Pulmonary vascular disease in total anomalous pulmonary venous drainage. Circulation 61: 103–109

Nickerson B G, Sahn D J, Goldberg S J, Allen H D 1979 Hazards of inadvertent umbilical venous catheterization in a patient with anomalous pulmonary venous drainage: a case report. Pediatrics 63: 929–931

Oliveira Lima C, Valdes-Cruz L M, Allen H D, et al 1983 Prognostic value of left ventricular size measured by echocardiography in infants with total anomalous pulmonary venous drainage. American Journal of Cardiology 51: 1155–1159

Orsmond G S, Ruttenberg H D, Bessinger F B, Moller J H 1978 Echocardiographic features of total anomalous pulmonary venous connection to the coronary sinus. American Journal of Cardiology 41: 597–601

Paquet M, Gutgesell H 1975 Echocardiographic features of total anomalous pulmonary venous connection. Circulation 51: 559–605

Park E A 1912 Defective development of the right lung due to anomalous development of the right pulmonary artery and vein, accompanied by dislocation of the heart simulating dextrocardia. Proceedings of the New York Pathological Society 12: 88–93

Parr G V S, Kirklin J W, Pacifico A D, Blackstone E H, Lauridsen P 1974 Cardiac performance in infants after repair of total anomalous pulmonary venous connection. Annals of Thoracic Surgery 17: 561–573

Perret L, Fortelius P 1961 Ruptured aneurysm of a pulmonary vein. Acta Tuberculosea Scandinavian 41: 53–55

Ports T A, Turley K, Brundage B H, Ebert P A 1979 Operative correction of total left anomalous pulmonary venous return. Annals of Thoracic Surgery 27: 246–249

Presbitero P, Bull C, Macartney F J 1983 Stenosis of pulmonary veins with ventricular septal defect. A cause of premature pulmonary hypertension in infancy. British Heart Journal 49: 600–603

Robinson A E, Chen J T T, Bradford W D, Lester R G 1969 Kerley B lines in total anomalous pulmonary venous connection below the diaphragm (Type III). American Journal of Cardiology 24: 436–440

Rowe R D, Glass I H, Keith J D 1961 Total anomalous pulmonary venous drainage at cardiac level. Angiocardiographic differentiation. Circulation 23: 77–80

Rywlin A R, Fojaco R M 1968 Congenital pulmonary lymphangiectasis associated with a blind common pulmonary lymphangiectasis associated with a blind common pulmonary vein. Pediatrics 41: 931–934

Saalouke M G, Shapiro S R, Perry L W, Scott L P 1977 Isolated partial anomalous pulmonary venous drainage associated with pulmonary vascular obstructive disease. American Journal of Cardiology 39: 439–444

Sade R M, Freed M D, Matthews E C, Castaneda A R 1974 Stenosis of individual pulmonary veins. Review of the literature and report of a surgical case. Journal of Thoracic Cardiovascular Surgery 67: 953–962

Sade R M, Williams R G, Castaneda A R 1975 Corrective surgery for congenital cardiovascular defects in early infancy. American Heart Journal 90: 656–664

Sahn D J, Allen H D, Lange L W, Goldberg S J 1979 Cross-sectional echocardiographic diagnosis of the sites of total anomalous pulmonary venous drainage. Circulation 60: 1317–25

Serratto M, Bucheleres H G, Bicoff P, Miller R A, Hastreiter A R 1968 Palliative balloon atrial septostomy for total anomalous pulmonary venous connection in infancy. Journal of Pediatrics 73: 734–739

Shinebourne E A, Del Torso S, Miller G A H, Jones O D H, Capuani A, Lincoln C 1981 Total anomalous pulmonary venous drainage (TAPVD): medical aspects and surgical indications. In: Parenzan L, Crupi G, Graham G (eds) Congenital heart disease in the first 3 months of life. Medical and surgical aspects. Casa Editrice Patron, Bologna, p 447–59

Shiu M F, Miles M, Silove E D 1981 Significance of normal septal motion in total anomalous pulmonary venous drainage. British Heart Journal 46: 389–93

Shone J D, Amplatz K, Anderson R C, Adams P J, Edwards J E 1962 Congenital stenosis of individual pulmonary veins. Circulation 26: 574–581

Silove E D, Behrendt D M, Aberdeen E, Bonham Carter R E 1972 Total anomalous pulmonary venous drainage. II. Spontaneous functional closure of interatrial communication after surgical correction in infancy. Circulation 46: 357–367

Skovránek J, Tuma S, Urbancova D, Samanek M 1980 Range-gated pulse Doppler echocardiographic diagnosis of supracardiac total anomalous pulmonary venous drainage. Circulation 61: 841–847

Smallhorn J F, Sutherland G R, Tommasini G, Hunter S, Anderson R H, Macartney F J 1981 Assessment of total anomalous pulmonary venous connection by two-dimensional echocardiography. British Heart Journal 46: 613–623

Snellen H A, Van Ingen H C, Hoefsmit E C M 1968 Patterns of anomalous pulmonary venous drainage. Circulation 38: 45–63

Snider A R, Silverman N H, Turley K, Ebert P A 1982 Evaluation of infradiaphragmatic total anomalous pulmonary venous connection with two-dimensional echocardiography. Circulation 66: 1129–1132

Stark J, Smallhorn J, Huhta J et al 1982 Surgery for congenital heart defects diagnosed with real-time echocardiography. Circulation 66 (Suppl II): 30

Stevenson J G, Kawabori I, Guntheroth W G 1979 Pulsed Doppler echocardiographic detection of total anomalous pulmonary venous return: resolution of left atrial line. American Journal of Cardiology 44: 1155–1158

Swan H J C, Toscano-Barboza E, Wood E H 1956 Hemodynamic findings in total anomalous pulmonary venous drainage. Proceedings of the Staff Meetings of the Mayo Clinic 31: 177–182

Swischuk L E, L'Heureux P L 1980 Unilateral pulmonary vein atresia. American Journal of Roentgenology 135: 667–672

Tajik A J, Gau G T, Ritter D G, Shattenberg T T 1972 Echocardiographic pattern of right ventricular diastolic overload in children. Circulation 46: 36–43

Thilenius O G, Bharati S, Lev M 1976 Subdivided left atrium: an expanded concept of cor triatriatum sinistrum. American Journal of Cardiology 37: 743–752

Turley K, Tucker W Y, Ullyot D J, Ebert P A 1980 Total anomalous pulmonary venous connection in infancy: influence of age and type of lesion. American Journal of Cardiology 45: 92–97

Tynan M, Behrendt D, Urquhart W, Graham G R 1974 Portal vein catheterization and selective angiography in diagnosis of total anomalous pulmonary venous connexion. British Heart Journal 36: 1155–1159

Van Praagh R, Corsini I 1969 Cor triatriatum: pathologic anatomy and a consideration of morphogenesis based on 13 postmortem cases and a study of normal development of the pulmonary vein and atrial septum in 83 human embryos. American Heart Journal 78: 379–405

Van Praagh R, Harken A H, Delisle G, Ando M, Gross R E 1972 Total anomalous pulmonary venous drainage to the coronary sinus. Journal of Thoracic and Cardiovascular Surgery 64: 132–135

Whight C M, Barratt-Boyes B G, Calder A L, Neutze J M, Brandt P W T 1978 Total anomalous pulmonary venous connection. Long-term results following repair in infancy. Journal of Thoracic and Cardiovascular Surgery 75: 52–63

Zuberbuhler J R, Shinebourne E A 1979 Diagnosis and treatment of left atrial to left superior vena caval shunt (abstract). European Journal of Cardiology 10: 311–312

Atrial septal defect

Atrial septal defect is an important congenital cardiac anomaly, both because it is relatively common and because it is more nearly completely correctable than most other cardiac malformations. The diagnosis of an atrial septal defect may be difficult and often there is no suspicion of organic heart disease during infancy and early childhood. The lack of early symptoms and the subtlety of the physical findings tend to delay the diagnosis, sometimes until well into adult life or even until middle or old age. If the left-to-right shunt is large, however, a firm clinical diagnosis can usually be made on the basis of a meticulous cardiac physical examination and a chest radiograph. In some cases the physical examination and/or the chest X-ray may be equivocal. Under these circumstances, cardiologists have been understandably reluctant to subject an apparently healthy asymptomatic child or young adult to invasive study. The newer non-invasive techniques, particularly echocardiography, have made this much less of a clinical problem. They have reduced the need for the annual visits, which charted the emergence either of a more typical picture of atrial septal defect or a functional murmur.

INCIDENCE

Feldt et al (1971) reported a 7% incidence of atrial septal defect among all congenital cardiac anomalies, while Nakamura et al (1964) noted a somewhat higher incidence of 10%. Atrial septal defects accounted for 11% of a series of 15 004 children with congenital heart disease seen at the Toronto Hospital for Sick Children (Keith, 1978). The actual incidence depends, in part, upon one's definition of an atrial septal defect. In an autopsy series it may be difficult to distinguish between cases with an actual 'defect' in the region of the oval fossa and a probe patent foramen ovale in which the flap of the foramen had been competent, with the atrial communication being only potential. The incidence of a probe patent foramen ovale itself has been reported to be from 20–25% (Bedford et al, 1941). The variable prevalence of atrial septal defect in different clini-

cal series is related to the age distribution within the series. A series of infants and young children will have a relatively low prevalence of a clinically apparent interatrial communication as the primary defect, while a series of adults with congenital heart disease will have a high prevalence of atrial septal defect. This is due both to the attrition of patients with other severe and life-threatening defects and because of the frequent delay in diagnosis of an atrial defect until young adulthood. The prevalence also depends upon whether clinically unimportant interatrial communications accompanying more serious defects are included in the series.

The prevalence of clinically significant interatrial communications can perhaps best be judged by the relative frequency of the necessity for surgical closure. During the last 12 years, 2198 infants and children under the age of 18 years have been operated upon for congenital heart disease at the Children's Hospital of Pittsburgh. In 249 (11%) an atrial septal defect was the sole or the most important anomaly. In another 270 (12%) surgical closure of an atrial septal defect was done during repair of another more important anomaly.

During the same period 627 infants and children with congenital heart disease came to autopsy. Of these, none died because of an atrial septal defect but 143 (23%) had an interatrial communication that was incidental or of secondary importance.

An atrial septal defect is generally thought to be more common in females, a 2 : 1 female/male ratio being reported by Weidman et al (1957). Zaver & Nadas (1965), on the other hand, reported a slight male predominence.

Etiology

There are no known intra-uterine events which predispose to an atrial septal defect and most cases occur sporadically with no family history of congenital heart disease. There is a significant familial incidence when the atrial septal defect is associated with certain skeletal abnormalities of the forearm and hand (Holt & Oram, 1960) or with prolongation of the PR interval. In the latter complex, Bizarro et al (1970) reported a nearly 50% incidence of atrial septal defect in subsequent siblings or progeny. There is also occasionally a familial incidence without these associated skeletal or conduction abnormalities. In our own series of 249 patients undergoing repair of an atrial septal defect over the last 12 years, there have been 3 cases in which close relatives have been known to have an atrial septal defect. Two were sisters and one was the daughter of a man with a surgically repaired atrial septal defect.

MORPHOLOGY AND CLASSIFICATION

The accurate classification of atrial septal defects is important, not because the location of the defect alters haemodynamics, but rather because of differences in the incidence of associated anomalies and differences in techniques of surgical repair. It is obviously important for the surgeon in planning repair to be aware of the anomalously connecting pulmonary veins which accompany a sinus venosus defect or of the atrioventricular valve abnormalities which go with an 'ostium primum' defect (atrioventricular septal defect). As an extreme example, it may be difficult to recognise a coronary sinus defect as *an interatrial communication* and not simply as a large coronary sinus if the diagnosis has not been established before surgery.

Understanding the morphology and classification of interatrial communications demands a thorough knowledge of the anatomy and extent of the atrial septum since some of the defects which permit interatrial shunting of blood are outside the confines of the atrial septum. The septum has quite different characteristics on its right and left sides. When the right atrium is opened through a wide incision, a large expanse of atrial 'septum' is seen between the orifices of the superior and inferior caval veins and the attachment of the septal leaflet of the tricuspid valve (Fig. 22.1a). In actuality, only a small part of this area separates the cavities of the two atrial chambers (Fig. 22.1b), namely the floor of the fossa ovalis and its muscular margins (the limbus fossae ovalis).

The superior limbus, often called the 'septum secundum', is made up in its larger part of an infolding of atrial wall between the base of the superior caval vein and the insertion of the right pulmonary veins to the left atrium. This is the area known to surgeons as 'Waterston's groove'. A substantial cleavage plane extends down to the margin of the fossa which can be opened by external dissection. The internal aspect of this groove is the prominent muscle bundle which separates the fossa from the orifice of the superior caval vein. The part of the limbus immediately adjacent to the fossa is a true septal structure. More anteriorly the margin of the limbus continues as a septal structure, but its larger part is the anterior atrial wall overlying the aortic root. Postero-inferiorly the fossa ovalis be-

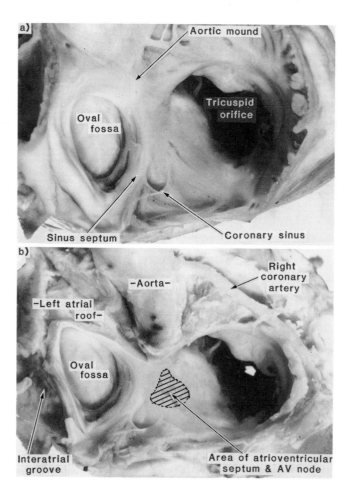

Fig. 22.1 A dissection showing the extent of the true interatrial septum (a) Shows the intact walls of the right atrium. (b) The same specimen after removal of all that tissue which is not part of the septum. Note also the area inferiorly occupied by the atrioventricular septum.

comes directly continuous with the wall of the inferior caval vein. Antero-inferiorly the morphology is more complicated, since the fossa is separated from the orifice of the coronary sinus by the sinus septum. Through the sinus septum runs the tendon of Todaro, one of the important landmarks of the triangle of Koch. The tendon is the continuation of the commissure of the Eustachian and Thebesian valves and inserts medially into the central fibrous body. The parts of the sinus septum and limbus between the tendon and the margin of the fossa are true septal structures since they separate the right and left atrial cavities. The muscular structure between the mouths of the inferior caval vein and the coronary sinus is not septal, but is rather the free wall of the right atrium. The part of the atrial wall between the tendon of Todaro and the septal leaflet of the tricuspid valve is an atrioventricular rather than an interatrial septal structure. This is because the tricuspid valve is attached to the septum more apically than the mitral valve, so the septum between them separates the right atrium from the left ventricle (see Ch. 24). Thus, only the

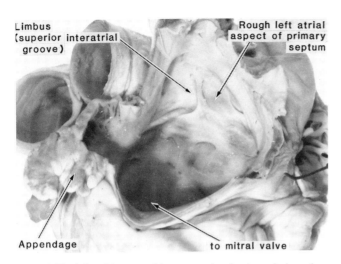

Fig. 22.2 The left atrial aspect of the septum showing its typical rough appearance.

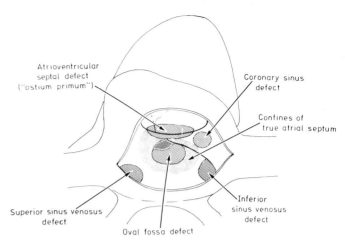

Fig. 22.3 Diagram showing the traditional division of 'atrial septal defects'. As shown, all of these except those within the oval fossa are outside the confines of the interatrial septum. Thus, although they permit unequivocal interatrial shunting and are interatrial communications, they are not strictly 'atrial septal defects'.

thin translucent floor of the fossa ovalis (septum primum) together with the margins of the limbus immediately adjacent to the fossa are true interatrial septal structures.

When viewed from the left atrial aspect, the morphology is far less complex. The floor of the fossa is smooth but in its anterosuperior margin it is roughened and wrinkled (Fig. 22.2). Only a small part of this anterior region is septum, the rest being the area where the septum primum is fused with the anterior atrial wall.

It is on the basis of this septal morphology that we should categorise interatrial communications. Traditionally, atrial septal defects are divided into 'primum' and 'secundum' types (Bedford, 1960) together with sinus venosus defects (Ross, 1956; Davia et al, 1973) and those found at the site of the coronary sinus (Raghib et al, 1965) (Fig. 22.3). Although some may consider it an unnecessarily pedantic point, we consider it important to state that only 'secundum' defects within the confines of the fossa ovalis are true atrial septal defects. Furthermore, these so-called 'secundum defects' result from deficiency of the embryologic septum primum (floor of the fossa ovalis). But the other defects do unequivocally permit interatrial shunting, so they must also be considered.

The so-called 'ostium primum defect' is an atrioventricular septal defect in which the fused bridging leaflets are displaced into the ventricular cavity. In many cases most of the interatrial communication is actually below the level of the normal atrioventricular junction and there is little or no deficiency of atrial septum. Because the underlying anatomy of these defects is that of the atrioventricular septal defect, they will be considered further in the chapter exclusively devoted to that anomaly (see Ch. 24). The sinus venosus defect is usually found in the mouth of the superior caval vein and occasionally in the mouth of the inferior caval vein. In such cases, the limbus fossae ovalis is intact and these defects are almost always associated with

anomalous attachment of right pulmonary veins. The coronary sinus defect is at the anticipated site of the coronary sinus and permits interatrial shunting because of the absence of the common wall normally present between the coronary sinus and left atrium. This type of defect is almost always associated with drainage of the left superior caval vein to the roof of the left atrium between the appendage and the openings of the left pulmonary veins.

With this introduction, we will now describe these defects in more detail.

Defects within the fossa ovalis

Fossa ovalis defects are by far the most common type of interatrial communication and are true atrial septal defects. Usually they are termed 'secundum' defects, but when using this term it must be remembered that the appellation is justified because the defect is present at the site of the embryonic *ostium* secundum, not because of deficiency of the *septum* secundum. (As noted above, the septum secundum is largely the interatrial fold.) The 'secundum' defect results from deficiency, perforation, or complete absence of the floor of the fossa, which is formed by the embryonic septum primum. It should be remembered that in one-quarter of normal individuals the upper border of the septum primum fails to fuse with the left atrial aspect of the 'septum secundum', even though it overlaps the limbus (Edwards, 1960). This is termed a 'probe patent foramen ovale' and, since left atrial pressure is normally higher than right, it does not permit interatrial shunting under ordinary circumstances.

There is a spectrum of defect size, depending on the degree of deficiency of the septum primum. The least severe type of fossa ovalis defect is caused by failure of the

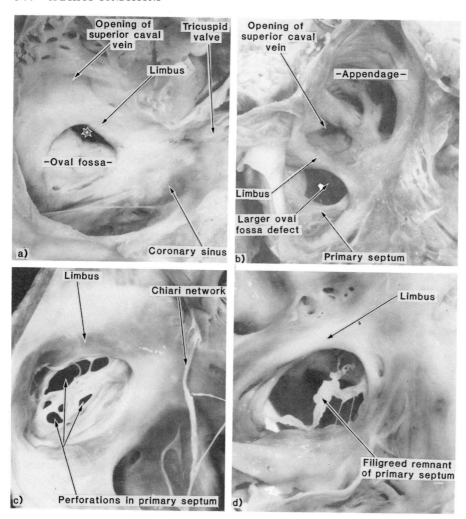

Fig. 22.4 The degrees of deficiency of the flap valve of the oval fossa which produce atrial septal defects of different dimensions and form. Note the remnants of the valves of the venous sinus (Chiari network) visible in (c).

septum primum to overlap entirely the left atrial margin of the limbus (Fig. 22.4a). The septum may be more deficient (Fig. 22.4b) or may become perforate, the perforations being either single or multiple (Fig. 22.4c). Alternatively, the larger part of the septum may disappear, with the fossa itself being criss-crossed by filigreed remnants of the septum (Fig. 22.4d). When the deficiency is marked it extends towards the mouth of the inferior caval vein, which may then open in part to the left atrium. In the most extreme form of fossa ovalis defect the limbus becomes effaced so that the defect extends from the openings of the caval veins and coronary sinus to the septal attachment of the tricuspid valve. It is important to distinguish this latter anomaly from an atrioventricular septal defect with a nearly absent atrial septum. In addition to a small rim of inferior limbus persisting in the fossa ovalis defect, the valve morphology will distinguish the two types. In the fossa ovalis type the left atrioventricular valve is of typical mitral morphology whereas in an atrioventricular septal defect it has a characteristic trileaflet morphology (see Ch. 24).

When defects are present within the confines of the fossa they do not alter the basic disposition of either the sinus or atrioventricular nodes. When the inferior limbus is effaced, however, the node will of necessity be confined to the narrow strip of myocardium between the edge of the defect and the septal attachment of the tricuspid valve. This will still be within the triangle of Koch, but the triangle itself will be narrow. Apart from this circumstance, the morphology of the atrioventricular junctional area will be normal in the presence of septal defects within the fossa ovalis.

Although these defects may exist in isolation, they also occur in combination with many other congenital cardiac malformations.

Sinus venosus defects

The essence of the so-called 'sinus venosus defect' is that it exists outside the confines of the fossa ovalis, usually in the mouth of the superior caval vein (superior defect) but occasionally in the orifice of the inferior caval vein (inferior defect) (Fig. 22.3). Morphological descriptions of these

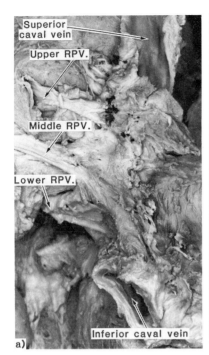

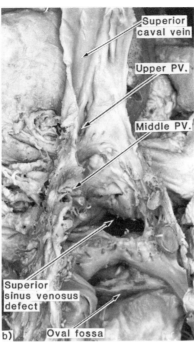

Fig. 22.5 The typical pattern of a sinus venosus defect with anomalous connexion of the right pulmonary veins. (a) The external aspect. (b) The internal appearance. Note that the defect is outside the confines of the true atrial septum (the oval fossa) and that the superior caval vein rides the interatrial wall, being connected to both right and left atrial chambers.

defects are scant and most are based on surgical observations (Davia et al, 1973). In the case of a superior sinus venosus defect, the superior caval vein typically overrides a defect above the superior limbus of the fossa ovalis. In the limited number of cases we have studied there was always associated anomalous insertion of right pulmonary veins into the wall of the superior caval vein (Fig. 22.5). Indeed, conceptually it is necessary to expect that the pulmonary veins will attach to the superior caval wall to provide a conduit whereby the blood can shunt between the atrial chambers (Fig. 22.6). Thus, the defect has a well-circumscribed inferior margin, the superior limbus of the fossa ovalis, but does not have a roof, the superior vena cava being attached in part to the right atrial wall and in part to the anomalous confluence of the right pulmonary veins (Fig. 22.5). Usually the lower right pulmonary vein inserts into the left atrial wall, the middle pulmonary lobe

vein drains into the area of the defect and the upper right pulmonary vein drains into the superior caval vein. Although cases without anomalous pulmonary venous drainage are described in surgical series it is hard to see how a superior sinus venosus defect could exist without there being an anomalous attachment of the right pulmonary veins to the superior caval wall. It is certainly possible, however, that the mal-attached pulmonary veins, together with that part of the superior caval vein, would continue to drain directly to the left atrium.

The presence of a superior sinus venosus defect should not markedly affect the site of the sinus node, which is found lateral to the superior cavoatrial junction, lying immediately subepicardially within the terminal sulcus. Thus, a patch placed to close the defect should not jeopardise the sinus node. Because of the overriding of the superior caval vein and the usual presence of anomalous pulmonary veins, it may not be possible to patch the defect so that normal pulmonary venous return is restored without narrowing the superior caval pathway. In these circumstances it may be difficult if not impossible to widen the caval vein without putting either the sinus node or its vascular supply at risk, since the artery to the node may pass either in front of or behind the cavoatrial junction to enter the node (Anderson et al, 1979). It is also necessary to avoid the lateral part of the terminal sulcus since this is always the site of the sinus node.

Inferior sinus venosus defects are far less common and it seems likely that they too should be associated with an anomalous attachment of the right pulmonary veins. In the solitary example we have studied anatomically the right lower pulmonary vein was anomalously attached to the wall

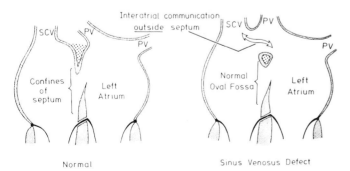

Fig. 22.6 Diagram showing how a sinus venosus defect is outside the confines of the atrial septum, existing because the biatrial connexion of either the superior caval or a pulmonary vein provides an extracardiac interatrial communication.

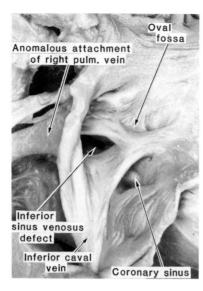

Fig. 22.7 An inferior sinus venosus defect which is outside the confines of the oval fossa. It exists because of the biatrial connexion of the inferior caval vein.

of the inferior caval vein. A defect existed behind the fossa ovalis and allowed the pulmonary veins to drain to the left atrium (Fig. 22.7). Closure of such a defect should jeopardise neither the sinus nor the atrioventricular node. Inferior sinus venosus defects should be distinguished from defects within the oval fossa which extend towards the mouth of the inferior caval vein.

Coronary sinus defects

The constellation of anomalies consisting of a defect at the site of the orifice of the coronary sinus, absence of the coronary sinus itself and connexion of a persistent left superior caval vein to the left atrial roof was first described by Raghib and his colleagues (1965). In essence the anomaly represents total absence of the common wall which normally exists between a persistent left superior caval vein and coronary sinus and the left atrium, so that the orifice of the coronary sinus becomes an interatrial communication and the persistent caval vein drains to the left atrium. A lesser degree of this malformation consists of fenestration (unroofing) of the coronary sinus (Freedom et al, 1981). In some examples of the coronary sinus acting as an interatrial communication, filigreed remnants of the atrial wall persist between the orifice of the coronary sinus and the termination of the left caval vein in the left atrium (Fig. 22.8). More commonly there is no tissue separating the coronary sinus, left caval vein and left atrium. The coronary sinus opening is usually large. Indeed, in one heart we have studied the sinus septum was also deficient so that the coronary sinus defect was confluent with an inferior sinus venosus defect. In another heart, the coronary sinus orifice was of normal dimensions yet, because of total unroofing of the coronary sinus, it was still the site of an interatrial communication (Fig. 22.9). This unroofing of the coronary sinus with an interatrial communication at the coronary sinus orifice and a left caval vein entering the left atrium must be distinguished from bilateral superior caval

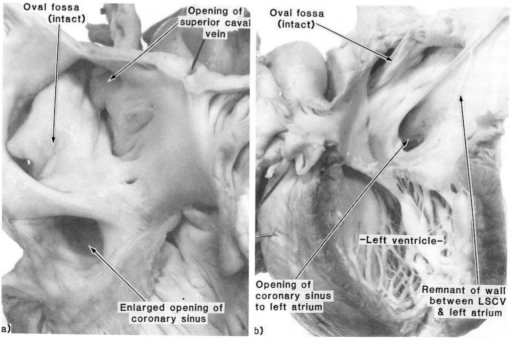

Fig. 22.8 A coronary sinus interatrial communication. (a) Shows the enlarged orifice of the coronary sinus. (b) Shows how this functions as an interatrial communication because of unroofing of the party wall between the persistent left superior caval vein and the left atrium. The left superior caval vein (LSCV) is connected to the left atrial roof between the left pulmonary veins and the appendage.

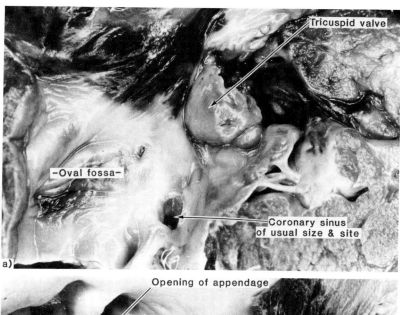

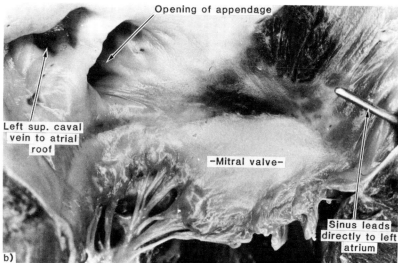

Fig. 22.9 A coronary sinus interatrial communication in which the orifice of the sinus is of usual size – seen from the right atrium in (a). (b) The connexion of a persistent left superior caval vein to the roof of the left atrium and a probe through the orifice of the coronary sinus communicating directly with the cavity of the left atrium.

veins in the presence of atrial isomerism (Macartney et al, 1980). In the latter anomaly, the coronary sinus never forms and the caval veins retain their embryological bilateral symmetry. In the case of an unroofed coronary sinus, the sinus forms initially but the wall between it and the left atrium subsequently resorbs. When a coronary sinus defect is large its anterior margin encroaches on the triangle of Koch and approximates the area of the atrioventricular node. Care must therefore be taken when the defect is closed. It should be noted that in the operating room a coronary sinus defect may be difficult to recognise *as an interatrial communication*, appearing to be simply the coronary sinus itself.

Morphogenesis of interatrial communications

During normal development the embryonic septum primum grows down to divide the primitive atrium, eventually fusing with the atrioventricular endocardial cushions and closing the primary foramen. Its top edge then breaks down to form the secondary foramen, the upper edge of the remaining primary atrial septum being overlapped by the infolding of the atrial roof which forms the superior limbus of the fossa ovalis (the so-called 'septum secundum'). Failure of normal development of the atrioventricular junction prevents the lower edge of the primary septum from fusing with the ventricular septum and results in the so-called 'ostium primum defect'. This is in reality an atrioventricular septal defect and is described further in Chapter 24. It is maldevelopment of the primary atrial septum itself, after it has fused with the ventricular septum, which results in defects within the fossa ovalis. This can either be due to deficiency of its superior edge, so that it no longer overlaps the superior limbus, or breakdown of the septum to a greater or lesser degree, resulting in the various types of perforate or fenestrated fossa ovalis defects (Fig. 22.4). In the most severe fossa ovalis defects the limbus also becomes effaced. Sinus venosus defects are best explained on the basis that the right pulmonary veins are abnormally attached to the wall of either the superior or inferior caval veins (Fig. 22.6). Resorption of the abnormal wall thus formed between pulmonary and caval veins will then produce a defect outside the margins of the fossa ovalis. Finally, as discussed above, the coronary sinus defect is best explained on the basis of unroofing of the coronary sinus in the presence of a persistent left superior caval vein (Fig. 22.8).

ASSOCIATED ANOMALIES

Cardiac

Certain cardiac and vascular anomalies have been reported to occur more frequently in patients with an atrial septal defect than in the general population. Atrioventricular valve abnormalities are part of atrioventricular septal defects and will be considered in Chapter 24. They are less common with other varieties of interatrial communication but do occur. A prolapsing mitral valve, for instance, was found in 17% of patients reported by Leachman et al (1976). The incidence in our operated series was only 3%. The true incidence is hard to determine since the criteria for diagnosing prolapse are different in different institutions.

Anomalous pulmonary venous connexion is a relatively common associated finding in patients with an atrial septal defect, particularly the sinus venosus variety. The overall incidence in our series of operated patients was 14% (83% of those with a sinus venosus defect compared to only 3% of those with a secundum defect).

An atrial septal defect may coexist with a ventricular septal defect, duct or coarctation of the aorta. The true incidence is hard to determine since each of these defects may lead to increased left atrial pressure and size and the interatrial communication may be due to incompetence of the flap of a stretched foramen ovale. Although a small right ventricular outflow tract gradient is common in patients with an atrial septal defect, the pulmonary stenosis is usually functional and related to increased flow. Organic pulmonary stenosis was uncommon in our series of operated patients, occurring in only 14 of 249 (6%).

Non-cardiac anomalies

The association of Down's syndrome with 'primum' (atrioventricular septal) defects is well known and occurred in 23% of patients operated on for such defects in our own institution. The incidence of Down's syndrome was only 4% in our operated series with atrial septal defect. The skeletal anomalies of the syndrome reported by Holt & Oram (1960) and the electrophysiologic abnormalities in the cases of Bizzaro and his colleagues (1970) are examples of non-cardiac anomalies which occur in a few patients. As

with associated cardiac malformations, non-cardiac anomalies are relatively rare in patients with an atrial septal defect.

PATHOPHYSIOLOGY

The pathophysiology of an atrial septal defect is related to the magnitude and direction of blood shunting across the interatrial communication. There is usually a substantial left-to-right shunt across the defect, resulting in a high pulmonary/systemic flow ratio. The primary determinants of the amount of shunting are the size of the defect and the relative inflow resistance, or compliance, of the ventricles. The latter factor is greatly influenced by pulmonary vascular resistance. The compliance of the right and left atria themselves may also play a role, but this has been difficult to prove. As with a ventricular septal defect, the site of the defect in the atrial septum does not influence the magnitude of flow across it, although relative contributions to the shunt from the individual pulmonary veins do vary depending on the location of the defect.

Effect of defect size

The size of the interatrial communication is an important determinant of the magnitude of the shunt. Because of the lower pressures involved, an atrial defect tends to be larger than a ventricular defect with a shunt of similar magnitude. Most clinically recognised atrial septal defects are essentially non-restrictive and approximate the area of the mitral valve orifice. The defect imposes no more restriction to flow across it than does the mitral valve and there is at most a small pressure gradient between the left and right atria. If the defect is smaller and restrictive the pulmonary blood flow will be limited by the defect size and the pulmonary/systemic flow ratio usually will be less than 2 : 1. There is no doubt that many small atrial septal defects escape clinical detection because a limited left-to-right shunt is haemodynamically well-tolerated and causes no abnormalities in the physical examination.

In some cases the interatrial communication may be due to incompetence of the valve of the foramen ovale rather than an actual deficiency of the atrial septum. This incompetence can lead to considerable left-to-right shunting when there are associated abnormalities that lead to increased left atrial pressure. Mitral stenosis, dysfunctional left ventricle, aortic stenosis, coarctation of the aorta, systemic hypertension, duct and ventricular septal defect are examples. If the primary defect leading to volume or pressure overload of the left atrium can be corrected, the valve may become competent and the atrial shunt will then disappear. Some otherwise normal infants may have left-to-right atrial shunting due to transient incompetence of the valve of the foramen ovale (Rudolph, 1974).

Effect of ventricular compliance

If the atrial defect is non-restrictive the magnitude of the shunt will be directly related to the relative resistance to filling offered by the right and left ventricles. The inflow resistance of a ventricle is related to its distensibility, or compliance, which is largely related to its muscle mass. The muscle mass and hence the compliance of the right ventricle is influenced by pulmonary vascular resistance and therefore undergoes predictable postnatal changes. At birth, right and left ventricular compliances are approximately equal and there is little shunting across an atrial defect in either direction. Pulmonary vascular resistance and pressure generally undergo their normal dramatic fall over the first days of life in patients with an atrial septal defect. This is true even in a patient with a large defect, since the pulmonary vascular bed is never exposed to high systemic arterial pressure as it is with a large ventricular septal defect or aorticopulmonary communication. It takes several months, however, before the right ventricular muscle mass decreases relative to the left ventricular muscle mass and a normal adult relationship between the two ventricles is reached. Thus, a significant left-to-right shunt is not expected until several months of age. Pulmonary artery pressure at this stage is almost always normal. Although patients with an atrial septal defect have a normal regression of pulmonary vascular resistance they are susceptible to a secondary increase in resistance if pulmonary blood flow remains high for many years, usually several decades (Weidman et al, 1957; Rudolph, 1974; Keith, 1978). As pulmonary vascular resistance rises, the pulmonary artery pressure also increases. This causes right ventricular hypertrophy with a concomitant decrease in compliance which leads to less left-to-right shunting. As right ventricular compliance approaches that of the left ventricle there is little shunting across the atrial septal defect. If right ventricular compliance exceeds that of the left ventricle a right-to-left atrial shunt results, since the atria will empty preferentially into the more easily filled left ventricle.

If there is associated severe pulmonary stenosis, hypertrophy of the right ventricle will occur and the resulting decreasing compliance of this chamber may eventually lead to right-to-left shunting across an atrial septal defect. A right-to-left atrial shunt may also be caused by tricuspid stenosis.

In addition to changes in right ventricular compliance, abnormal filling characteristics of the left ventricle can also influence the magnitude of the atrial shunt. Filling of the left ventricle is impaired by mitral stenosis or any abnormality that leads to increased end diastolic pressure in the left ventricle. This may result in marked accentuation of the left-to-right shunt across the atrial defect.

Cardiac response to atrial septal defect

The usual haemodynamic characteristics of an uncomplicated atrial septal defect are a large left-to-right shunt and normal pulmonary artery pressure. Flow across the defect is phasic and occurs predominantly in late ventricular systole and early diastole (Levin et al, 1968). Numerous studies have documented that a majority of patients with a typical secundum atrial septal defect have a small right-to-left shunt that occurs mainly from streaming of a portion of the return from the inferior caval vein directly across the defect into the left atrium (Swan et al, 1954; Weidman et al, 1957). This small shunt is not detectable by oximetry (i.e. there is no systemic desaturation) but it can be demonstrated by indicator-dilution techniques (Swan et al, 1954) and by contrast echocardiography (Seward et al, 1975).

The contribution of the pulmonary venous return from each lung to the total left-to-right shunt is unequal. In a typical large secundum defect, 80% of the pulmonary venous return from the right lung shunts left-to-right, in contrast to the 20–40% of the pulmonary venous return from the left lung (Swan et al, 1956a, b; Weidman et al 1957; Rudolph, 1974). In a sinus venosus defect the right upper and/or middle lobe pulmonary veins provide most of the shunted blood. This preferential shunting from the right lung does not occur to any great extent with an ostium primum interatrial communication.

A large left-to-right shunt at the atrial level leads to enlargement of both the right atrium and right ventricle (Graham et al, 1973). The left atrium is of normal size despite the increased pulmonary venous return since the atrial septal defect allows its decompression. Left ventricular dimensions are usually normal although some studies have shown left ventricular end-diastolic volume to be less than normal (Popio et al, 1975).

Systemic cardiac output is almost always normal in children. Exercise tolerance is quite good, probably because the cardiovascular response to exercise favours a decrease in the magnitude of the atrial shunting. The afterload on the left ventricle is decreased by the drop in systemic vascular resistance that attends exercise, tending to facilitate left ventricular filling. The increased cardiac output also augments systemic venous return, competitively filling the right atrium at the expense of shunting across the defect. In contrast to the situation in childhood, systemic cardiac output has been found to be decreased in up to 50% of patients with an atrial septal defect who are greater than 18 years of age (Craig & Selzer, 1968). Numerous studies in adults have shown significant left ventricular dysfunction which may persist even after surgical correction (Flamm et al, 1970; Epstein et al, 1973; Popio et al, 1975).

Despite the greatly increased pulmonary blood flow, pulmonary artery pressure is rarely elevated in children and pulmonary vascular resistance is quite low, frequently less than 1 Wood unit (Nadas & Fyler, 1972). The incidence of pulmonary hypertension in children less than 20 years old is approximately 5% in most studies, and increases to 20% in the 20–40 age range and 50% in patients greater than 40 years of age (Weidman et al, 1957; Bedford & Sellors, 1960; Campbell, 1970; Keith, 1978). The incidence of increased pulmonary vascular resistance also increases with age (Craig & Selzer, 1968; Hamilton et al, 1979) but severe elevation of resistance and Eisenmenger's reaction is unusual, occurring in 6% of patients (Wood, 1958). With severe elevation of pulmonary vascular resistance, right ventricular hypertrophy may increase and compliance decrease sufficiently that cyanosis results from reversal of the atrial shunt. This suggests that there is a slowly progressive development of pulmonary vascular disease in patients with an atrial septal defect, presumably resulting from increased pulmonary blood flow over many years. Heath & Edwards (1958) described changes in the pulmonary vascular bed consistent with this hypothesis, including a predominance of intimal fibrosis and endothelial proliferation with less medial muscular hypertrophy than is seen in patients with ventricular septal defects. There are many aspects of the clinical spectrum, however, that are not explained by this simplistic scheme. Although it is uncommon, some children with isolated atrial septal defects do have pulmonary hypertension. On the other hand, there are adults who live into their sixth and seventh decades with large pulmonary blood flow who have normal pulmonary vascular resistance and pulmonary artery pressure (Craig & Selzer, 1968; Nasrallah et al, 1976). Therefore, there must be individual variation of pulmonary vascular reactivity to various noxious stimuli (e.g. increased pulmonary blood flow, increased pressure, etc.) that is as yet poorly understood.

The chronic right ventricular volume overload caused by an atrial septal defect is generally well-tolerated for many years, particularly when there is no associated elevation of pulmonary artery pressure. Symptoms of congestive heart failure rarely occur before the fourth or fifth decades but have been reported to be present in approximately 35% of adult patients greater than 40 years of age (Craig & Selzer, 1968; Hamilton et al, 1979). Rarely an isolated atrial septal defect may cause congestive heart failure in infancy (Hoffman et al, 1972; Hunt & Lucas, 1973).

Another cardiac consequence of the long-standing left-to-right shunt is the occurrence of atrial arrhythmias, particularly atrial flutter and fibrillation. They presumably result from chronic stretching of the atria and occur most commonly in patients greater than 40 years of age. Hairston et al (1974) found a 24% incidence of these arrhythmias in patients between 45 and 65 years of age, while a 38% incidence has been reported in patients over 60 years (Nasrallah et al, 1976). As with the other complications associated with atrial septal defects, atrial arrhythmias rarely occur in childhood. Recent studies, however, have shown that electrophysiologic studies can demonstrate a

high incidence of subclinical sinus node dysfunction and atrioventricular conduction disturbances in children prior to operative intervention (Clark & Kugler, 1982; Bolens & Friedli, 1984; Ruschhaupt et al, 1984).

CLINICAL FINDINGS

Presentation

Mild dyspnoea on exertion and/or easy fatigue are the most common early symptoms of an interatrial communication. They are usually not present during infancy and childhood, or may be appreciated only in retrospect after a diagnosis of congenital heart disease has been made. Not infrequently, parents report increased activity and vigour after repair, even though they had considered their child to be asymptomatic prior to surgery. Rarely infants less than one year of age may present with congestive heart failure due to an isolated atrial defect. Some children have an increased number of respiratory infections. Symptoms become much more common in the fourth or fifth decade for reasons already discussed. Some patients even with a large atrial septal defect may be in their sixth or seventh decades before dyspnoea on exertion, easy fatigue or frank congestive heart failure occur, and some remain free of disabling symptoms throughout life.

Physical examination

The general physical examination is usually normal, although there is a tendency toward a slender build (Fig. 22.10). Associated non-cardiac abnormalities are uncommon in individuals with a secundum- or sinus venosus-

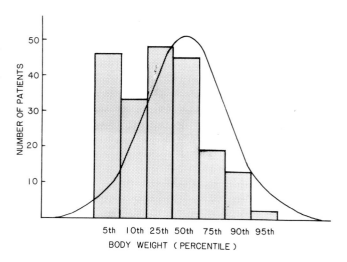

Fig. 22.10 Graph showing the weight percentiles of patients undergoing surgical repair of an atrial septal defect at the Children's Hospital of Pittsburgh. The normal distribution of weight is indicated by the solid line and that in the patients by the bars. The patient distribution is skewed toward the lower percentiles.

type atrial septal defect, Zaver & Nadas (1965) noting only a 4% incidence in a series of 298 patients. Skeletal anomalies of the forearm and hand do occur occasionally and the resulting syndrome (Holt & Oram, 1960) may be inherited. Non-cardiac anomalies much more commonly accompany ostium primum defects; notable examples include Down's syndrome (Park et al, 1977) and the visceral anomalies typically present with atrial isomerism (Macartney et al, 1980).

The jugular venous pulse is usually normal, as are blood pressure and peripheral arterial pulses. A left parasternal lift is often present but precordial motion is normal in some patients, especially if the left-to-right shunt is not large. Cyanosis is not part of the clinical picture of an uncomplicated interatrial communication but can occur under certain circumstances, for example with virtual absence of the interatrial septum or anomalous systemic venous connexion to the left atrium.

The heart sounds are almost always abnormal in a patient with an atrial septal defect and it is difficult to entertain a clinical diagnosis of this anomaly with a completely normal sound pattern. The first sound at the low left sternal border is usually accentuated because of a prominent tricuspid valve closure component (Lopez et al, 1962). The increased diastolic flow across the tricuspid valve tends to keep the leaflets widely open until ventricular systole begins and the wider excursion of the leaflets prior to coaptation may explain the loudness of the closure sound. Alternatively, the wide-open position of the leaflets may result in closure which is slightly late. It therefore occurs during the more steeply rising portion of the ventricular pressure curve and causes a more forceful coaptation. The second sound is characteristically widely and 'fixedly' split, with little or no variation in the width of the split during the respiratory cycle. Fixed splitting may be appreciated during quiet respiration or by listening during held expiration. The latter technique has the advantage of eliminating breath sounds during auscultation and probably is the more sensitive method. If an individual with a normal heart is asked to 'breathe all the way out and then stop breathing', the second sound will be single for 1–3 beats and will then become split, the splitting gradually widening over the next several beats (Fig. 22.11a). In contrast, the second sound of a patient with an atrial septal defect is split at the end of expiration and the degree of splitting does not vary during held expiration (Fig. 22.11b).

The normal inspiratory exaggeration of splitting is supposedly related to the augmentation of systemic venous return induced by the negative intrathoracic pressure of inspiration. The increased right ventricular filling prolongs ejection, leading to a delayed pulmonary valve closure which is then separated from the aortic closure sound. Several reasons for the lack of respiratory variation in splitting in patients with an interatrial communication have been suggested. The most widely accepted explanation postulates a reciprocal relationship of changes in pulmonary and systemic venous return with respiration (Aygen & Braunwald, 1962). In this formulation, inspiration increases systemic but reduces pulmonary venous return, resulting in reduced flow across the atrial defect. Expiration reduces systemic but augments pulmonary venous return, leading to increased defect flow. The result is a nearly constant influx of blood to the right atrium and hence to the right ventricle. The right ventricular stroke volume is therefore constant and both the ejection time and time of closure of the pulmonary valve are unchanged throughout the respiratory cycle. An alternative explanation relates the delayed closure to a separation of the right ventricular and pulmonary artery pressure curves rather than to prolongation of ventricular systole, which rarely occurs. The pulmonary artery curve is typically delayed and the incisura, corresponding to pulmonary valve closure, 'hangs out' beyond the descending ventricular pressure curve (Shaver et al, 1975). This delay in the pulmonary artery curve is thought to be due to an increased capacitance of the pulmonary arteries and a consequent 'laxity' in the system in a patient with a large atrial shunt. The inertia of the blood entering the pulmonary artery following ventricular systole thus briefly sustains blood flow in the pulmonary artery and delays valve closure. In such a 'loose' system respiratory variation in venous return has relatively little effect on the timing of valve closure. Whatever the actual genesis of fixed splitting it is a most valuable sign of a large left-to-right shunt at the atrial level.

The murmurs associated with an atrial septal defect are typically soft and may be absent in infancy and early childhood, explaining the relative lateness of diagnosis in most individuals with this congenital cardiac anomaly. It is extremely uncommon for a murmur to arise at the site of the interatrial communication itself, since there is usually little or no gradient across the defect. Instead, the murmurs are generated by rapid blood flow through the right heart and the pulmonary arterial bed. Almost all individuals with a clinically recognisable atrial septal defect have a crescendo-decrescendo systolic murmur at the high left sternal border, related to rapid flow across the pulmonary valve. The murmur is usually soft and a murmur of greater than a grade III/VI intensity should suggest the possibility of accompanying pulmonary stenosis. (It is easy to overestimate the severity of right ventricular outflow tract obstruction; even a loud systolic murmur may be generated at a very mildly stenotic pulmonary valve. A gradient of as much as 40 torr may be associated with only minimal pulmonary stenosis, the gradient being exaggerated by the increased blood flow). A similar systolic murmur is usually audible in the axillas and over the posterior thorax and is generated by rapid blood flow through the pulmonary arteries.

Most individuals with a large left-to-right shunt through an interatrial communication also have a soft mid-diastolic murmur at the low left sternal border. This murmur is always subtle and is almost never recognised unless one

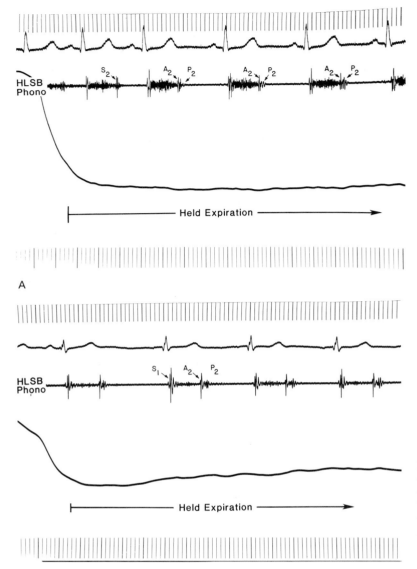

Fig. 22.11 High left sternal border phonocardiogram during held expiration. Respiration is indicated by the solid line. (a) Normal splitting. The second heart sound is single on the first beat and subsequent beats show gradually increasing splitting. (b) Fixed splitting. The second heart sound is split on the first beat and there is only trivial widening of the split with subsequent beats. A₂ – aortic valve closure sound; HLSB phono – high left sternal border phonocardiogram; P₂ – pulmonic valve closure sound; S₁ – first heart sound.

specifically listens for it. The murmur is that of relative tricuspid stenosis and is generated by rapid flow across a normal tricuspid valve. Unlike the murmur of organic or relative mitral stenosis, the murmur is not low pitched and 'rumbling'. Rather, it is of medium pitch and is often 'scratchy'. There is always an audible gap between the second heart sound and the murmur. None of the murmurs associated with an atrial septal defect are affected significantly by the phase of respiration or by position.

Although the murmurs just described arise at a distance from the defect, under certain circumstances a murmur may be generated at the defect itself. The prerequisite is a relatively large gradient across the interatrial septum. Such a gradient occurs only if the defect is small and restrictive and if left atrial pressure is higher than normal, usually because of mitral stenosis (Ross et al, 1963) or

mitral atresia (Zuberbuhler et al, 1975). The murmur is continuous, since under these circumstances left atrial pressure exceeds right atrial pressure throughout the cardiac cycle. The murmur is usually soft and maximal near the lower sternum. Rarely, the murmur is loud with an accompanying thrill and may have a 'roaring' quality.

The physical findings associated with an atrial septal defect are greatly altered by the appearance of pulmonary vascular disease. With an increase in right ventricular pressure the left parasternal lift may become more pronounced. An elevation of pulmonary artery pressure tends to close the pulmonary valve earlier as the typical 'loose' system of an uncomplicated atrial defect becomes more 'tight' and the 'hang out' interval decreases. The elevated pulmonary artery diastolic pressure also contributes to earlier pulmonary closure. The second heart sound, therefore, becomes narrowly split or single as long as right ventricular function is not severely impaired. If right ventricular contractility is sufficiently diminished, pulmonary valve closure will be delayed by a prolonged ejection time and the second heart sound again becomes widely split. Splitting of the second heart sound in an individual with an atrial septal defect and pulmonary hypertension thus depends on right ventricular function. It is narrow or absent as long as right ventricular function is normal and is wide if right ventricular function is compromised.

With an increase in pulmonary vascular resistance, pulmonary blood flow decreases and the systolic and diastolic murmurs associated with rapid blood flow in the right heart and pulmonary arteries disappear. If pulmonary hypertension is severe, new murmurs of pulmonary and tricuspid regurgitation may occur. The murmur of hypertensive pulmonary regurgitation is typically high pitched and decrescendo and is maximal at the high and mid left sternal border. This murmur is usually clinically indistinguishable from the murmur of aortic regurgitation unless the second heart sound is widely split and it can be appreciated that the diastolic murmur begins with the second (pulmonary) component. The murmur of tricuspid regurgitation is high pitched and systolic and is usually maximal at the low left sternal border. It may be either early or pansystolic and may increase in intensity with inspiration (Carvallo's sign – Rivero-Carvallo, 1946).

INVESTIGATION

Electrocardiographic findings

The electrocardiographic features of an atrial septal defect are stereotyped in childhood (Fig. 22.12), but similar findings may be present in normal children or in individuals with other conditions which cause right ventricular volume overload. Normal sinus rhythm is almost invariably present in childhood, but atrial flutter or fibrillation is seen with increasing frequency after 40 years of age. First degree atrioventricular block has been reported to occur in 10–36% of patients (Nadas & Fyler, 1972; Keith, 1978). The P wave morphology is normal in secundum defects, but in nearly 50% of sinus venosus-type defects the frontal plane P wave axis is less than 15 degrees, suggesting a low atrial focus (Davia et al, 1973). In children, the frontal plane QRS axis is almost always in the range of 90–170 degrees, but in the adult the axis may shift leftward to the 70–90 degree range. Although left axis deviation occurring in the setting of an atrial shunt strongly suggests the presence of an ostium primum type of defect, approximately 5% of secundum and sinus venosus defects have this axis (Nadas & Fyler, 1972; Davia et al, 1973). Mild to moderate right ventricular hypertrophy is present in more than 85% of cases and is usually manifested by an RSR' pattern in the right precordial leads. The R or R' wave rarely exceeds 15 mm unless significant elevation of pulmonary vascular resistance and pulmonary artery pressure are present

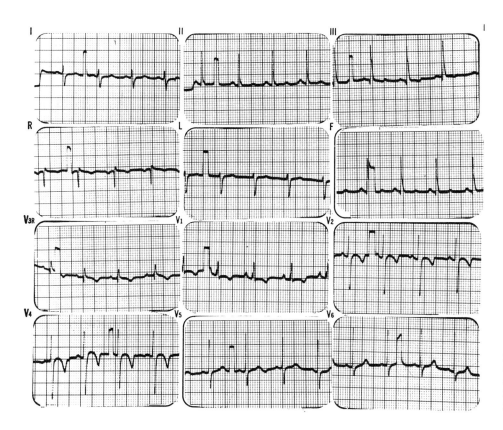

Fig. 22.12 Surface electrocardiogram from a child with a secundum atrial septal defect. There is right axis deviation and mild right ventricular hypertrophy manifested by an RSR' pattern in the right precordial leads.

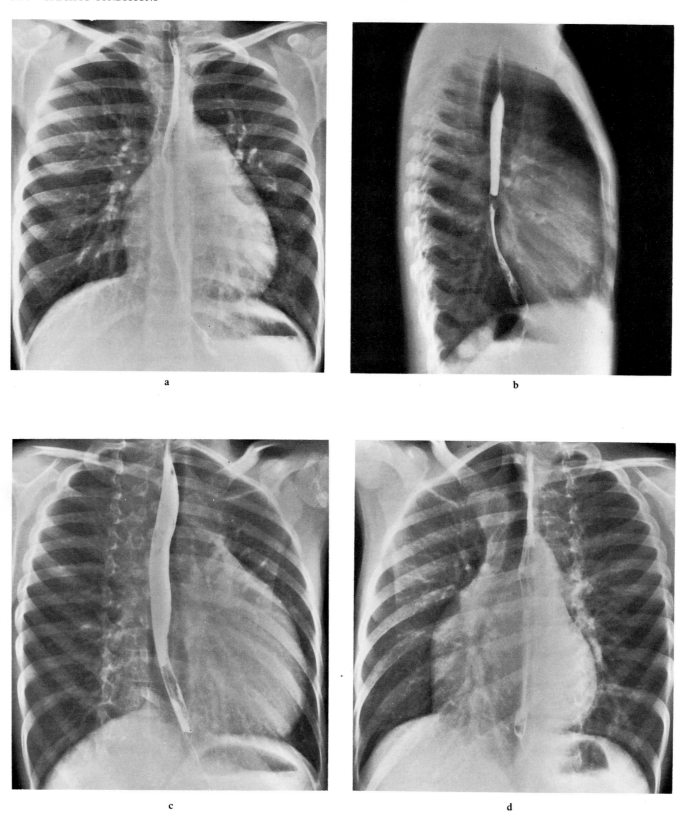

Fig. 22.13 Chest radiograph of a patient with an atrial septal defect. (a) Frontal view. There is cardiomegaly and pulmonary vascular markings are increased. The main pulmonary artery is large and the aortic knob is not apparent. (b) Lateral view. There is no oesophageal deviation to suggest left atrial enlargement. (c) Right anterior oblique view. No evidence of left atrial enlargement but the cardiac shadow approaches the left thoracic wall, suggesting right ventricular enlargement. (d) Left anterior oblique view.

(Rudolph, 1974; Hamilton et al, 1979). The QRS duration is either normal or mildly prolonged (less than 0.11 seconds). Complete right bundle branch block is very rare in childhood, but occurs in nearly half of patients greater than 60 years of age (Nasrallah et al, 1976).

Radiological findings

The chest radiograph shows mild to moderate cardiomegaly in the majority of cases but 10–15% of patients have a normal heart size even when a large left-to-right shunt is present (Hamilton et al, 1979; Young, 1973). However, whether or not the heart is enlarged there is almost always an abnormal contour, with a large right atrium, right ventricle and pulmonary trunk segment and a diminutive aorta (Fig. 22.13). Pulmonary vascular markings are usually increased when the pulmonary/systemic flow ratio is 2 : 1 or greater but the vascularity correlates poorly with the magnitude of the shunt (Rees et al, 1972). Once pulmonary vascular disease develops, the typical findings of Eisenmenger's syndrome may be present, with aneurysmal dilation of the proximal pulmonary arteries and distal tapering of the vessels. In patients with a sinus venosus defect, there may be localised dilation of the proximal superior caval vein at the entrance of the anomalous pulmonary veins, giving the appearance of a higher than normal vascular pedicle in the right hilum. In the majority of patients with this type of defect, however, the radiologic findings are identical to those of a typical secundum defect.

Echocardiographic findings

The classic M-mode echocardiographic findings of an atrial septal defect are nearly always present when there is a large left-to-right shunt (Fig. 22.14). Right ventricular dimensions are increased and, in most cases, there is flattened or

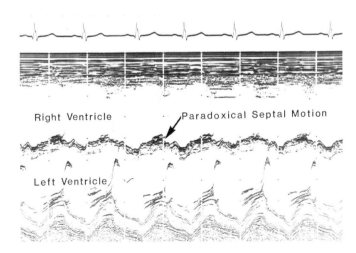

Right Ventricle

Paradoxical Septal Motion

Left Ventricle

Fig. 22.14 M-mode echocardiogram showing an enlarged right ventricle and paradoxical septal motion.

paradoxical septal motion (Meyer, 1977; Meyer et al, 1972; Tajik et al, 1972). An M-mode echocardiogram can be extremely valuable in evaluating a patient with subtle physical findings and a borderline electrocardiogram and chest radiograph. Although the typical echocardiographic features are usually present with a large flow atrial septal defect, they are by no means specific as they merely reflect right ventricular volume overload. Partial or total anomalous pulmonary venous return, pulmonary regurgitation and tricuspid regurgitation can cause identical echocardiographic findings.

Cross-sectional echocardiography has proven to be much more specific and the various types of atrial septal defects can often be identified (Bierman & Williams, 1979). The atrial septum can be visualised in both the apical and subcostal four chamber views. The former view is not as reliable as the latter because there may be artefactual echo 'drop out' simulating an atrial septal defect. The subcostal view allows imaging in a plane perpendicular to the atrial septum and can reliably define the site and approximate size of the defect. A secundum defect is seen in the central portion of the septum while the sinus venosus and ostium primum defects are seen in the superior and inferior portions of the septum, respectively (Fig. 22.15). Furthermore, pulmonary veins can usually be well visualised in these views and anomalous connexions identified, as, for example, in the sinus venosus defect (Nasser et al, 1981). Both M-mode and cross-sectional studies are helpful in diagnosing associated abnormalities such as mitral valve prolapse.

Nuclear angiography

First pass radionuclide angiography has been used to detect and quantitate left-to-right shunts in children (Ginzton et al, 1984). Flow determinations by this technique have correlated well with values obtained by oximetry during cardiac catheterisation. Maltz & Treves (1973) have shown that shunts with pulmonary/systemic flow ratios between 1.2 : 1 and 3 : 1 can be accurately quantitated. Nuclear studies cannot, however, localise an intracardiac shunt. Equilibrium blood pool gated scans may be of value in assessing right and left ventricular function.

Cardiac catheterisation

Cardiac catheterisation continues to be the most sensitive means of detecting an atrial septal defect and the most precise method of quantitating the left-to-right shunt and measuring intracardiac and pulmonary artery pressures. When the fernoral vein approach is used the catheter almost always passes easily through the mid portion of the atrial septum into the left atrium when a fossa ovalis defect is present. An attempt should be made to enter the pulmonary veins to confirm normal drainage to the left atrium.

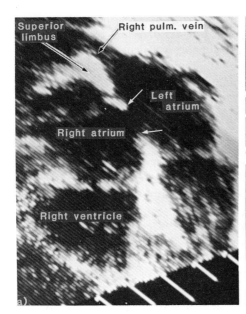 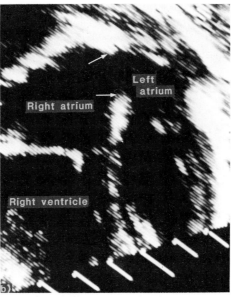

Fig. 22.15 Cross-sectional echocardiograms of atrial septal defects in the subcostal view. (a) Secundum type showing a defect in the mid portion of the atrial septum. (b) Sinus venosus type with a defect in the superior portion of the septum.

An ostium primum defect may be recognised by a lower than usual pass from the right atrium to the left atrium. It is usually easier to enter the left ventricle and more difficult to enter the pulmonary veins when this type of interatrial communication is present. A sinus venosus defect is sometimes quite difficult to traverse when the approach through the inferior caval vein is used. Considerable probing around the superior portion of the atrial septum in the region of the superior cavoatrial junction may be needed to cross the defect. The lateral border of the proximal superior caval vein and right atrium should be explored for possible anomalous return of the right upper or middle lobe pulmonary veins, particularly if a sinus venosus defect is suspected.

The hallmark of an atrial shunt is a step-up in oxygen saturation of at least 5% from the superior caval vein to the right atrium. If the saturation in the superior caval vein is abnormally high (greater than 85%), anomalous pulmonary venous return must be considered and saturations should be obtained from the left brachiocephalic, right subclavian and right internal jugular veins. Anomalies other than an atrial septal defect that result in an increased oxygen saturation in the right atrium include isolated partial anomalous pulmonary venous return, a ventricular septal defect associated with tricuspid insufficiency, a left ventricular to right atrial shunt and a ruptured aortic sinus of Valsalva aneurysm into the right atrium. Another potential pitfall in the use of oximetry for diagnosis is the fact that streaming of oxygenated blood directly across the tricuspid valve can occur so that a step-up in oxygenation is not evident proximal to the right ventricle. This is much more likely to occur with an ostium primum defect. Even when there is a step-up in oxygenation in the right atrium there may be a further step-up in the right ventricle with an isolated atrial septal defect. Samples from the left side of the circulation are fully saturated. The pulmonary to systemic flow ratio can be calculated using the oximetry data and the Fick principle. This ratio is 2 : 1 or greater in 70% of clinically recognised defects (Hamilton et al, 1979).

Mean right atrial pressure is generally normal, but the magnitude of the V wave is usually equal to that of the A wave (loss of normal A wave predominance). Phasic and mean pressures are commonly equal in the two atria if there is a large atrial septal defect, but there may be up to a 3 torr mean gradient across the defect. Right ventricular and pulmonary artery pressures are almost always normal in childhood but pulmonary hypertension may develop with increasing age (Bedford & Sellors, 1960). An occasional infant with a large atrial shunt has elevated pulmonary artery pressure (Hunt & Lucas, 1973). Pulmonary vascular resistance is usually normal or low (i.e. 1 Wood unit or less) in children, but may be elevated in adults. Severe elevation of pulmonary vascular resistance (Eisenmenger's reaction) is uncommon even in older patients, occurring in only 6% of individuals with an atrial septal defect (Wood, 1958). In some patients the large pulmonary blood flow causes a 10–30 torr peak systolic gradient across a normal pulmonary valve and/or a 10–15 torr systolic gradient between the main and branch pulmonary arteries (Weidman et al, 1957; Nadas & Fyler, 1972; Rudolph, 1974). Left atrial pressure is usually somewhat lower than normal and left ventricular pressure is normal.

Indicator dilution studies may be useful in qualitatively and quantitatively evaluating a left-to-right shunt at atrial level. The pulmonary/systemic flow ratio calculated from indicator dilution curves correlates well with that obtained by oximetry (Jarmakani, 1977). Selective pulmonary artery injections of indicator may suggest the presence of partial anomalous pulmonary venous return by showing variable shunt magnitudes and/or appearance times from various portions of the lungs (e.g. a delay in the appearance of indicator injected into the right middle lobe artery if its vein drains directly to the right atrium). It must be emphasised that *functional* return to the right atrium does not imply anatomic *connexion* to the right atrium, since there may be remarkable streaming from normally connected veins. Cardiac output may be determined by injecting indicator into the left ventricle and sampling from the aorta.

Angiocardiography

A left ventriculogram should always be performed in patients with an atrial septal defect to rule out an atrioventricular septal defect, mitral valve prolapse, mitral insufficiency, left ventricular dysfunction or a ventricular septal defect. We usually prefer the anteroposterior and lateral views if a ventricular septal defect is not suspected, as this best demonstrates the 'goose-neck' deformity of the left ventricular outflow tract and 'cleft' left atrioventricular valve of an atrioventricular septal defect. A right ventricular or pulmonary artery injection in the anteroposterior and lateral views defines pulmonary arterial anatomy and pulmonary venous return and allows assessment of the magnitude of the atrial shunt during the levophase. A right ventriculogram has the advantage of demonstrating right ventricular size as well as tricuspid valve competency and pulmonary valve anatomy. The pulmonary arteriogram has the advantage of avoiding arrhythmia at the time of the injection and sometimes allows better definition of the pulmonary venous return. We have found that the right upper pulmonary vein injection in the four chamber view described by Bargeron et al (1977) is particularly helpful in confirming normal drainage of this vein and may delineate the location and size of the atrial defect (Fig. 22.16). Any anomalously draining pulmonary veins that are entered by the catheter should be selectively visualised.

DIAGNOSIS

The diagnosis of an atrial septal defect can be made with virtual certainty when the classical findings of a high left sternal border systolic ejection murmur, wide and fixed splitting of the second heart sound and a medium pitched mid diastolic murmur at the low left sternal border are associated with typical radiographic and electrocardiographic findings. A sinus venosus defect with partial anomalous pulmonary venous return cannot usually be differentiated clinically from a secundum defect, but a low atrial rhythm and/or an unusual shadow in the upper right hilum or the proximal superior caval vein on the chest radiograph should lead one to suspect its presence. Left axis deviation on the electrocardiogram, with or without a mitral insufficiency murmur at the apex, makes the diagnosis of an ostium primum defect very likely. Non-invasive studies such as radionuclide angiography and echocardiography can be used to confirm the presence of a large left-to-right shunt with right ventricular volume overload. The defect itself can often be visualised on the cross-sectional echocardiogram. Several recent reports have shown that uncomplicated secundum and sinus venosus atrial septal defects with confirmatory non-invasive studies can be

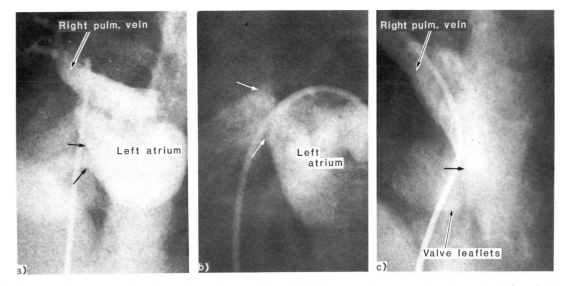

Fig. 22.16 Pulmonary vein angiograms in patients with atrial septal defects. (a) Right upper pulmonary vein angiogram in the four chamber view with a secundum defect. There is shunting across the mid portion of the atrial septum. (b) Left upper pulmonary vein angiogram in the left anterior oblique view with a sinus venosus defect. The shunting is present across the superior portion of the defect. (c) Right upper pulmonary vein angiogram in the four chamber view with an ostium primum defect. There is shunting across the atrioventricular septal defect. A common atrioventricular junction is present that is partitioned into separate left and right orifices.

safely operated upon without routine preoperative catheterisation (Freed et al, 1984; Shub et al, 1985). Although partial anomalous pulmonary venous connexion may be undetected or sinus venosus defects occasionally misclassified, this has not resulted in increased morbidity during operative repair. Currently at our institution we do not recommend routine catheterisation for patients with uncomplicated atrial septal defects, but reserve this study for those cases with atypical clinical or laboratory findings.

Several common conditions must be considered in the differential diagnosis of a soft systolic ejection murmur at the upper left sternal border, including a functional murmur, mild valvar pulmonary stenosis and pulmonary artery stenosis. A functional murmur is distinguished by an otherwise normal cardiovascular examination. Mild valvar pulmonary stenosis virtually always is accompanied by an early systolic ejection sound and the murmur becomes strikingly louder with exercise. Pulmonary artery stenosis has very prominent radiation of the systolic murmur to the back. These latter two anomalies have normal splitting of the second heart sound, lack a diastolic murmur at the low left sternal border and usually do not have evidence of right ventricular overload on the echocardiogram.

Certain other abnormalities must be considered when a systolic ejection murmur at the upper left sternal border is associated with a medium pitched diastolic murmur at the low left sternal border. Ebstein's malformation usually has other abnormalities of the sound pattern including a widely split first sound (sail sound) and/or a gallop and can be definitively diagnosed by echocardiography. Congenital pulmonary stenosis and regurgitation may prove difficult to distinguish from an atrial septal defect on clinical grounds, but the diastolic murmur is best heard higher along the left sternal border and becomes louder in the recumbent position. Congenital tricuspid stenosis produces a diastolic murmur similar to that present with a large atrial defect. This anomaly is quite rare and should be apparent on the echocardiogram. A left ventricular to right atrial shunt is another unusual entity that may be considered in the differential diagnosis, but the systolic murmur is loud and pansystolic and quite different from the systolic ejection murmur associated with an atrial defect. Partial anomalous pulmonary venous return without an associated atrial septal defect is a rare anomaly and in most cases requires cardiac catheterisation for diagnosis. Total anomalous pulmonary venous return without obstruction may at times present similar findings to a large atrial septal defect. The anomalous drainage may be evident on the cross-sectional echocardiogram, and the presence of a higher than expected haemoglobin for the patient's age may suggest mild systemic desaturation. A common atrium may be associated with an atrioventricular septal defect and is usually apparent on the echocardiogram. Occasionally a functional mid-diastolic murmur at the left sternal border is audible that is not associated with any structural heart disease

(Liebman et al, 1968). Another entity that may be confused is the straight back syndrome, with its systolic ejection murmur at the upper left sternal border and large pulmonary trunk segment on the chest radiograph. The lack of the normal thoracic kyphosis on the lateral chest radiograph is diagnostic.

COURSE AND PROGNOSIS

An isolated interatrial communication, even a large one, is usually well tolerated for many years (Campbell, 1970). As has been noted, symptoms are usually minimal or absent during infancy and childhood. This is because the right ventricle is well adapted to a pure volume overload (Rushmer, 1958) and secondary pulmonary hypertension is usually a late complication.

In the usual atrial septal defect the appearance of a large left-to-right shunt is delayed until the right ventricular hypertrophy present at birth regresses and right ventricular compliance decreases. The pulmonary vascular bed thus has time to mature and can accept a large blood flow without an increase in pressure. In the absence of pulmonary hypertension, pulmonary vascular disease either fails to develop or follows an indolent course.

Symptoms tend to occur earlier and to be more severe when there is an associated anomaly, particularly one which tends to impede left atrial emptying through the mitral valve. Examples include left ventricular outflow tract obstruction, coarctation of the aorta, primary left ventricular myocardial disease and mitral stenosis. (Lutembacher's syndrome refers to the combination of an atrial septal defect and mitral stenosis. It now seems to be quite uncommon, probably because of a decreasing incidence of rheumatic heart disease and because of early surgical closure of atrial septal defects.) Non-obstructive associated anomalies may also lead to early congestive heart failure. Infants with both interatrial and interventricular communications are likely to be symptomatic because atrial shunting across even a small defect may be greatly augmented by the increased left atrial pressure associated with a ventricular septal defect.

If impedence to left atrial emptying is markedly increased and is present before the pulmonary vascular bed has had an opportunity to mature, the fetal pulmonary vascular pattern tends to persist, exaggerating the degree of pulmonary hypertension. Under these circumstances, signs of severe and rapidly progressive congestive heart failure may occur. An example is the infant who has both a severe coarctation of the aorta and an interatrial communication. The left ventricular dysfunction engendered by the coarctation raises left atrial pressure and may produce a torrential left-to-right interatrial shunt and severe congestive heart failure which can be effectively treated only by correcting the coarctation.

Occasionally, infants with isolated and uncomplicated atrial septal defects may be symptomatic and experience congestive heart failure (Hoffman et al, 1972; Hunt & Lucas, 1973). It is not clear how these infants differ from asymptomatic ones, although it has been postulated that an atrial septal defect is usually small in infancy and grows large enough to produce symptoms only later in life. According to this formulation, the occasional infant with a large defect is the one who has symptoms early. It is much more likely, however, that a left-to-right shunt large enough to produce symptoms during infancy is due to some unrecognised increased impedance to flow into the left ventricle, such as some subtle alteration in left ventricular compliance or an abnormality of the mitral apparatus (Weinberg et al, 1966). Perhaps the situation is analogous to the older individual with an atrial septal defect which has been well tolerated for several decades who develops a larger left-to-right shunt and becomes symptomatic following the appearance of left ventricular dysfunction, whether it be induced by systemic hypertension, coronary artery disease or some primary myocardial abnormality.

Secondary pulmonary hypertension does eventually appear in some patients with an atrial septal defect and is an important factor in the development of both the cyanosis and congestive heart failure which can complicate the course of the anomaly. The addition of a pressure load may compromise right ventricular function and lead to frank congestive heart failure, or to right-to-left shunting through the atrial defect even in the absence of overt failure. Cyanosis which appears only with congestive heart failure tends to disappear after treatment with diuretics or cardiotonic agents, while cyanosis occurring in the absence of failure tends to be permanent and is an important sign of irreversible pulmonary vascular disease. Although a trivial degree of right-to-left shunting occurs in many individuals with an interatrial communication (Swan et al, 1954), sufficient shunting to produce recognisable cyanosis is distinctly unusual in an uncomplicated atrial defect. If the atrial septum is rudimentary or entirely absent some right-to-left shunting is usual and there may be mild cyanosis. Anomalies of systemic venous return are not common but may be responsible for cyanosis in an occasional patient with atrial septal defect. Drainage of a persistent left superior caval vein to the left atrium is part of the developmental complex described by Raghib et al (1965) and is associated with an interatrial communication which is the orifice of the coronary sinus. Inferior caval venous drainage may be anatomically or functionally anomalous, with flow to the left atrium or to both atria. This most commonly occurs when there is no inferior rim of the interatrial defect and the inferior caval vein overrides the interatrial septum, but has also been reported with defects in the fossa ovalis.

Spontaneous closure of an atrial septal defect is much less common than spontaneous closure of a defect in the interventricular septum. However, several authors have reported such closure, including Keith (1978), who documented closure in 3% of 445 patients with catheter-proven atrial septal defects. Hoffman et al (1972), Mody (1973) and, more recently, Cockerham et al (1983), showed that spontaneous closure occurs in up to 50% of infants with atrial septal defects discovered within the first year of life.

Atrial arrhythmias are relatively uncommon in children with atrial septal defects but they tend to become more common with advancing age (Campbell, 1970; Saksena & Aldridge 1970; Hairston et al, 1974; Nasrallah et al, 1976). Atrial flutter or fibrillation occurs frequently in older individuals with a large left to right shunt and an enlarged right atrium.

Rarely, paradoxical embolism may occur, with a clot from the pelvic or leg veins crossing the defect and entering the systemic circulation. ('Paradoxical' refers to the passage of a clot from right to left atrium when a predominant left-to-right shunt is present. As has been discussed above, a small right-to-left shunt is not uncommon in patients with an atrial septal defect and may be augmented during a Valsalva manoeuvre or a Valsalva equivalent such as straining at stool.) Infectious endocarditis is a very rare complication of an atrial septal defect unless there is an associated anomaly which predisposes to endocarditis (Zaver & Nadas, 1965).

Natural history studies in patients with atrial septal defects who have not undergone surgical correction suggest an average life expectancy between 36 and 49 years (Cosby & Griffith, 1949, Moss & Siassi, 1971; Campbell, 1970) although longevity was much greater in the absence of pulmonary hypertension (Dalen et al, 1967). Because the data from these studies were largely gathered in an era when associated rheumatic mitral valvar disease was more common, they probably do not accurately reflect the life expectancy of an individual with an isolated atrial septal defect today. Although symptoms are very uncommon in the first several decades of life, approximately two-thirds of patients greater than 40 years of age will have one or more of the complications discussed above (e.g. congestive heart failure, pulmonary hypertension, atrial arrhythmias or paradoxical emboli) (Keith, 1978).

MANAGEMENT

As has been noted, symptoms rarely occur in children with an atrial septal defect. Medical management with digitalis and diuretics is indicated in the occasional infant who presents with congestive heart failure, since several studies have shown that many of these children will have spontaneous closure of the defect or, at least, will have abatement of their symptoms (Cayler, 1967; Hoffman et al, 1972; Hunt & Lucas, 1973, Mody, 1973). Surgical intervention is clearly indicated in all children with large left to right shunts (i.e. pulmonary/systemic flow ratio 2 : 1 or greater) to prevent eventual pulmonary hypertension, congestive heart failure and atrial arrhythmias. When the defect is small and the flow ratio is less than 1.5 : 1, surgery is not indicated, since late sequels are rare and life expectancy probably normal. With borderline shunts (i.e. flow ratio between 1.5 and 2.0), a tricuspid flow murmur, right ventricular enlargement on the echocardiogram, radiographic findings and the size of the defect on angiocardiography should all be considered in the decision regarding surgical intervention. There is no evidence to suggest that there is any risk to the patient in delaying surgery for several years in the hope that the magnitude of the shunt may decrease. The only contraindication to surgery is pulmonary vascular disease, evidenced by marked elevation of pulmonary vascular resistance (i.e. greater than 8 index units) (Rudolph, 1974). Dalen et al (1967) showed a high operative mortality and decreased life expectancy in patients who underwent surgical repair of an atrial septal defect in the face of pulmonary vascular disease.

The timing of elective surgery does not seem to be crucial, but we recommend correction between four and six years of age. The risk of cardiopulmonary bypass is low at this age and there seems to be a psychological advantage in accomplishing repair prior to the school years. There are also emotional benefits with the child being old enough to communicate with family and staff about the hospitalisation and surgery. Earlier surgical intervention is indicated if there is marked cardiomegaly, growth failure or congestive heart failure. Although marked impairment of growth is only rarely seen in childhood, a postoperative growth spurt can be expected (Cohn et al, 1967).

Open heart repair of atrial septal defects has been carried out with excellent success for many years and the operative mortality is now less than 1% in centres experienced in congenital heart disease. The surgical approach to secundum defects consists of either direct suture or patch closure, depending on the size of the opening. When a sinus venosus defect is present a patch is necessary and can usually be placed so as to close the interatrial communication and, at the same time, redirect anomalously draining pulmonary veins into the left atrium. Perioperative complications are rare and include the post-pericardiotomy syndrome and transient arrhythmias. Air embolisation is an uncommon but tragic complication that is more likely when a right lateral thoracotomy is used, since this approach makes air evacuation more difficult. Obstruction at the superior caval vein may rarely occur following repair of a sinus venosus defect.

The long-term results of surgery are excellent and re-sidual shunts are very rare. Complete resolution of cardiomegaly on the chest radiograph and of right ventricular hypertrophy on the electrocardiogram are expected. However, a long term follow-up of 71 postoperative patients by Young (1973) demonstrated persistent radiographic cardiac enlargement in 30% of patients. Of the 8 patients with residual cardiomegaly who were recatheterised, 5 were found to have normal haemodynamics and 3 had elevation of right atrial and right ventricular end diastolic pressures. Meyer et al (1982) recently demonstrated persistent right ventricular enlargement by echocardiography in 80% of 51 children followed up to 5 years postoperatively.

Arrhythmias, including supraventricular tachycardia and atrioventricular conduction disturbances, occasionally persist after repair of atrial septal defects (Young, 1973; Clark & Kugler, 1982). Those patients with sinus venosus defects appear to be more at risk than those with secundum defects. Clark et al (1975) reported long-term sinus node dysfunction in 40% of patients following repair of sinus venosus defects and 16% of postoperative patients with secundum atrial defects. We found that 29% of patients at the Children's Hospital of Pittsburgh with sinus venosus defects had persistent sinus node dysfunction after surgery. This was manifested by a low atrial pacemaker in 6 patients, and severe bradycardia-tachycardia syndrome which required a permanent pacemaker and drug therapy in another patient. Although it has been presumed that these postoperative arrhythmias result from intra-operative damage to nodal or conduction tissue, numerous recent studies have demonstrated that intracardiac electrophysiology may detect a high preoperative incidence of sinus node dysfunction in patients with secundum atrial septal defects (Clark & Kugler, 1982; Bolens & Friedli, 1984; Ruschhaupt et al, 1984).

Because bacterial endocarditis is so rare with isolated secundum atrial septal defects, antibiotic prophylaxis is not generally considered necessary pre- or postoperatively (Zaver & Nadas, 1965; Kaplan et al, 1977).

Transcatheter closure of atrial septal defects has been successfully accomplished in humans (Mills & King, 1976; Rashkind & Cuaso, 1977). In view of the superb results and minimal risks of open heart repair of atrial septal defects this is currently not a recommended alternative to surgery in most patients.

In summary, an atrial septal defect is an important congenital cardiac anomaly because it is relatively common and because its surgical treatment is so successful. An individual born with this cardiac malformation when suitably treated should be able to enjoy a normal life expectancy free from cardiovascular morbidity.

REFERENCES

Anderson K R, Ho S Y, Anderson R H 1979 The location and vascular supply of the sinus node in the human heart. British Heart Journal 41: 28–32

Aygen M M, Braunwald E 1962 The splitting of the second heart sound in normal subjects and in patients with congenital heart disease. Circulation 25: 328–345

Bargeron L M, Elliott L P, Soto B, Bream P R, Currey G C 1977 Axial angiography in congenital heart disease. Section I. Concept, technical and anatomical considerations. Circulation 56: 1075–1083

Bedford D E 1960 The anatomical types of atrial septal defect: Their incidence and clinical diagnosis. American Journal of Cardiology 6: 558–574

Bedford D E, Sellors T H 1960 Atrial septal defect. In: Jones A M (ed) Modern trends in cardiology. Butterworths, London, p 138

Bedford D E, Papp C, Parkinson J 1941 Atrial septal defect. British Heart Journal 3: 37–68

Bierman F Z, Williams R G 1979 Subxiphoid two-dimensional imaging of the interatrial septum in infants and neonates with congenital heart disease. Circulation 60: 80–90

Bizarro R O, Callahan J A, Feldt R H, Kurland L T, Gordon H, Brandenburg R O 1970 Familial atrial septal defect with prolonged atrioventricular conduction: A syndrome showing the autosomal dominant pattern of inheritance. Circulation 41: 677–683

Bolens M, Friedli B 1984 Sinus node function and conduction system before and after surgery for secundum atrial septal defect: an electrophysiologic study. American Journal of Cardiology 53: 1415–1420

Campbell M 1970 Natural history of atrial septal defect. British Heart Journal 32: 820–826

Cayler G C 1967 Spontaneous functional closure of symptomatic atrial septal defects. New England Journal of Medicine 276: 65–73

Clark E B, Kugler J D 1982 Preoperative secundum atrial septal defect with coexisting sinus node and atrioventricular node dysfunction. Circulation 65: 976–980

Clark E B, Roland J A, Varghese P J, Neill C A, Haller J A 1975 Should the sinus venosus type ASD be closed? A review of the atrial conduction defects and surgical results in twenty-eight children (Abstr). American Journal of Cardiology 35:127

Cockerham J T, Martin T C, Gutierrez F R, Hartmann A F Jr, Goldring D, Strauss A W 1983 Spontaneous closure of secundum atrial septal defect in infants and young children. American Journal of Cardiology 52: 1267–1271

Cohn L H, Morrow A G, Braunwald E 1967 Operative treatment of atrial septal defect: Clinical and haemodynamic assessment in 175 patients. British Heart Journal 29: 725–734

Cosby R S, Griffith G C 1949 Interatrial septal defect. American Heart Journal 38: 80–89

Craig R J, Selzer A 1968 Natural history and prognosis of atrial septal defect. Circulation 37: 805–815

Dalen J E, Haynes F W, Dexter L 1967 Life expectancy with atrial septal defect: Influence of complicating pulmonary vascular disease. Journal of American Medical Association 200: 442–446

Davia J E, Cheitlin M V, Bedynek J L 1973 Sinus venosus atrial septal defect: Analysis of fifty cases. American Heart Journal 85: 177–185

Edwards J E 1960 Congenital malformations of the heart and great vessels. A. Malformations of the atrial septal complex. In: Gould S E (ed) Pathology of the Heart, 2nd Edn. Charles C. Thomas, Springfield, p 260–293

Epstein S E, Beiser G D, Goldstein R E, Rosing D R, Redwood D R, Morrow A G 1973 Hemodynamic abnormalities to mild and intense upright exercise following operative correction of an atrial septal defect or tetralogy of Fallot. Circulation 47: 1065–1075

Feldt R H, Avasthey P, Yoshimasu F, Kurland L T, Titus J L 1971 Incidence of congenital heart disease in children born to residents of Olmsted County, Minnesota, 1950–1969. Mayo Clinic Proceedings 46: 794–799

Flamm M D, Cohn K E, Hancock E W 1970 Ventricular function in atrial septal defect. American Journal of Medicine 48: 286–294

Freed M D, Nadas A S, Norwood W I, Castaneda A R 1984 Is routine preoperative cardiac catheterization necessary before repair of secundum and sinus venosus atrial septal defects? Journal of American College of Cardiology 4: 333–336

Freedom R M, Culham J A G, Rowe R D 1981 Left atrial to coronary sinus fenestration (partially unroofed coronary sinus). Morphological and angiocardiographic observations. British Heart Journal 46: 63–68

Ginzton L E, French W, Mena I 1984 Combined contrast echocardiographic and radionuclide diagnosis of atrial septal defect: accuracy of the technique and analysis of erroneous diagnosis. American Journal of Cardiology 53: 1639–1642

Graham T P, Jarmakani J M, Atwood G F, Canent R V 1973 Right ventricular volume determinations in children. Normal values and observations with volume and pressure overload. Circulation 47: 144–153

Hairston P, Parker E F, Arrants J E, Bradham P R, Lee W H 1974 The adult atrial septal defect: Results of surgical repair. Annals of Surgery 179: 533–547

Hamilton W T, Haffajee C I, Dalen J E, Dexter L, Nadas A S 1979 Atrial septal defect secundum: Clinical profile with physiologic correlates in children and adults. In: Roberts W C (ed) Congenital heart disease in adults. F.A. Davis Company, Philadelphia, p 267–277

Heath D, Edwards J E 1958 The pathology of hypertensive pulmonary vascular disease. Circulation 18: 533–547

Hoffman J I E, Rudolph A M, Danilowicz D 1972 Left to right atrial shunts in infants. American Journal of Cardiology 30: 868–875

Holt M, Oram 1960 Familial heart disease with skeletal malformations. British Heart Journal 22: 236–242

Hunt C E, Lucas R V 1973 Symptomatic atrial septal defect in infancy. Circulation 47: 1042–1048

Jarmakani J M 1977 Cardiac catheterization. In: Moss A J, Adams F H, Emmanouilides G C (eds) Heart disease in infants, children and adolescents 2nd Edn. Williams & Wilkins Baltimore, p 116–117

Kaplan E L, Anthony B F, Gijno A, et al 1977 American Heart Association report. Prevention of bacterial endocarditis. Circulation 56: 139A–143A

Keith J D 1978 Atrial septal defect: Ostium secundum, ostium primum and atrioventricularis communis (common AV canal). In: Keith J D, Rowe R D, Vlad P (eds) Heart disease in infancy and childhood, 3rd Edn. Macmillan, New York, p 380–404

Leachman R D, Cokkinos D V, Cooley D A 1976 Association of ostium secundum atrial septal defects with mitral valve prolapse. American Journal of Cardiology 38: 167–169

Levin A R, Spach M S, Boineau J P, Canent R V, Capp M P, Jewett P H 1968 Atrial pressure-flow dynamics in atrial septal defects (secundum type). Circulation 37: 476–488

Liebman J, Sood S 1968 Diastolic murmurs in apparently normal children. Circulation 38: 755–762

Lopez J F, Linn H, Shaffer A B 1962 The apical first heart sound as an aid in the diagnosis of atrial septal defect. Circulation 26: 1296–1301

Macartney F J, Zuberbuhler J R, Anderson R H 1980 Morphological considerations pertaining to recognition of atrial isomerism. Consequences for sequential chamber localization. British Heart Journal 44: 657–667

Maltz D L, Treves S 1973 Quantitative radionuclide angiography. Determination of Qp/Qs in children. Circulation 47: 1049–1056

Meyer R A 1977 Pediatric echocardiography. Lea & Febiger, Philadelphia, p 145–163

Meyer R A, Schwartz D C, Benzing G III, Kaplan S 1972 The ventricular septum in right ventricular volume overload. American Journal of Cardiology 30: 349–353

Meyer R A, Korfhagen J C, Corvitz W, Kaplan S 1982 Long-term follow-up study after closure of secundum atrial septal defect in children: An echocardiographic study. American Journal of Cardiology 50: 143–148

Mills N L, King T D 1976 Non-operative closure of left-to-right shunts. Journal of Thoracic and Cardiovascular Surgery 72: 371–378

Mody M R 1973 Serial hemodynamic observations in secundum atrial septal defect with special reference to spontaneous closure. American Journal of Cardiology 32: 978–981

Moss A J, Siassi B 1971 The small atrial septal defect – operate or procrastinate? Journal of Pediatrics 79: 854–857

Nadas A S, Fyler D C 1972 Pediatric cardiology. Saunders, Philadelphia, p 317–334

Nakamura F F, Hauck A J, Nadas A S 1964 Atrial septal defects in infants. Pediatrics 34: 101–106

Nasrallah A T, Hall R J, Garcia E, Leachman R D, Cooley D A 1976 Surgical repair of atrial septal defect in patients over 60 years of age. Long term results. Circulation 53: 329–331

Nasser F N, Tajik A J, Seward J B, Hagler D J 1981 Diagnosis of sinus venosus atrial septal defect by two-dimensional echocardiography. Mayo Clinic Proceedings 56: 568–572

Park S C, Mathews R A, Zuberbuhler J R, Rowe R D, Neches W H, Lenox C C 1977 Down syndrome with congenital heart malformation. American Journal of Diseases of Children 131: 29–33

Popio K A, Gorlin R, Teicholz L E, Cohn P F, Bechtel D, Herman M V 1975 Abnormalities of left ventricular function and geometry in adults with an atrial septal defect. Ventriculographic, hemodynamic and echocardiographic studies. American Journal of Cardiology 36: 302–308

Raghib G, Ruttenberg H D, Anderson R C, Amplatz K, Adams P Jr, Edwards J E 1965 Termination of left superior vena cava in left atrium, atrial septal defect, and absence of coronary sinus. A developmental complex. Circulation 31: 906–918

Rashkind W J, Cuaso C C 1977 Transcatheter closure of atrial septal defect in children (Abstr). Proceedings of the Association of European Pediatric Cardiology 13:49

Rees A, Farro O, Rodriguez R 1972 Phonocardiographic, radiological and haemodynamic correlation in atrial septal defect. British Heart Journal 34: 781–786

Rivero-Carvallo J M 1946 New diagnostic sign of tricuspid insufficiency. Archivas del Instituto de Cardiologia de Mexico 16: 531–539

Ross D N 1956 The sinus venosus type of atrial septal defect. Guy's Hospital Reports 105: 376–381

Ross J J, Braunwald E, Mason D T, Braunwald N S, Morrow A G 1963 Interatrial communication and left atrial hypertension. A cause of continuous murmur. Circulation 28: 853–860

Rudolph A M 1974 Congenital diseases of the heart. Year Book Medical Publishers, Chicago, p 239–264

Ruschhaupt D G, Khoury L, Thilenius O G, Replogle R L, Arcilla R A 1984 Electrophysiologic abnormalities of children with ostium secundum atrial septal defect. American Journal of Cardiology 53: 1643–1647

Rushmer R F 1958 Work of the heart. Modern Concepts of Cardiovascular Disease 27: 473–477

Saksena F B, Aldridge H E 1970 Atrial septal defect in the older patient. A clinical and hemodynamic study in patients operated on after age 35. Circulation 42: 1009–1020

Seward J B, Tajik A J, Spangler J G, Ritter D N 1975 Echocardiographic contrast studies. Initial experience. Mayo Clinic Proceedings 50: 163–169

Shaver J A, O'Toole J D, Curtiss E I, Thompson M E, Reddy P S, Leon D F 1975 Second heart sound: The role of altered greater and lesser circulation. Physiologic principles of heart sounds and murmurs. American Heart Association Monograph No. 46, American Heart Association, New York

Shub C, Tajik A J, Seward J B, Hagler D J, Danielson G K 1985 Surgical repair of uncomplicated atrial septal defect without 'routine' preoperative cardiac catheterisation. Journal of American College of Cardiology 6: 49–54

Swan H J C, Burchell H B, Wood E H 1954 The presence of venoarterial shunts in patients with interatrial communication. Circulation 10: 705–713

Swan H J C, Hetzel P S, Wood E H 1956b Quantitative estimation by indicator-dilution technics of contribution of blood to the left-to-right shunt in atrial septal defect. Circulation 14: 212–220

Tajik A J. Gau G T, Ritter D G, Schattenberg T T 1972 Echocardiographic pattern of right ventricular diastolic volume overload in children. Circulation 46: 36–43

Weidman W H, Swan H J C, DuShane J W, Wood E H 1957 A hemodynamic study of atrial septal defect and associated anomalies involving the atrial septum. Journal of Laboratory and Clinical Medicine 50: 165–185

Weinberg M, Miller R A, Hastreiter A R, Raffensperger J G, Fell E H, Bucheleres HgG 1966 Congestive heart failure in children with atrial septal defect. Journal of Thoracic and Cardiovascular Surgery 51: 81–87

Wood P 1958 The Eisenmenger syndrome or pulmonary hypertension with reversed central shunt. British Medical Journal 2: 701–709

Young D 1973 Later results of closure of secundum atrial septal defect in children. American Journal of Cardiology 31: 14–22

Zaver A G, Nadas A S 1965 Atrial septal defect – secundum type. Circulation 31–32, Suppl III: 24–32

Zuberbuhler J R, Lenox C C, Park S C, Neches W H 1975 Continuous murmurs in the newborn. Physiologic principles of heart sounds and murmurs. American Heart Association Monograph No. 46, American Heart Association, New York

23

Partitioning of atrial chamber ('cor triatriatum')

Partitioning of one of the atrial chambers is a rare but important malformation in as much as untreated severe symptoms or death may ensue. When recognised and operated upon, life expectancy may be normal. Either the morphologically right or morphologically left atrium can be divided by fibromuscular partitions into two compartments. Division of the morphologically left atrium is by far the commonest type. When used in isolation, the term 'cor triatriatum' almost always refers to the divided left atrium, but it is more accurate to describe either 'cor triatriatum sinister' or 'dexter', or, for those who prefer the vernacular, to speak either of a 'partitioned left' or 'partitioned right' atrium. The condition is exceedingly rare. A partitioned atrium was the rarest lesion bar one in the files of the Hospital for Sick Children, Toronto (less than 0.1% – Rowe, 1978). Nonetheless, the malformations are sufficiently well circumscribed to warrant their own chapter.

PARTITIONED MORPHOLOGICALLY LEFT ATRIUM

Morphology and morphogenesis

Church (1868) is usually credited as being the first to describe partitioning of the left atrium. According to Perloff (1978), division of the chamber was commented upon by Andral in 1829, while it was Borst (1905) who coined the term 'cor triatriatum'. Since then there have been several classifications, not all of which are restricted to cases which represent a congenitally partitioned atrial chamber. James (1962) included in his grouping examples of total anomalous pulmonary venous connexion to the coronary sinus together with aneurysms of the atrial septum, neither of which would generally be considered as partitioning of the left atrium. Thilenius et al (1976) proposed an expanded concept which included rare cases reported in the literature with atresia of the coronary sinus orifice and anomalous pulmonary venous connexion to a midline additional chamber, which then drained to the morphologically right atrium. They also described a

further solitary case coexisting with mitral atresia in which there was a midline atrial compartment which received neither systemic nor pulmonary veins. As they indicated, it is as well to be aware of these variants. There is little doubt, however, that almost all cases encountered in clinical practice will be of 'classical' type. It is this anomaly ('cor triatriatum sinister') with which we shall mainly be concerned in the remainder of this chapter, although we shall add a brief note on the salient features of the rarer types.

In the typical example, an obliquely orientated fibromuscular partition divides the morphologically left atrium into a proximal chamber which is connected to the pulmonary veins and a distal chamber in communication with the atrial appendage and the mitral vestibule (Fig. 23.1). These chambers have been described in various ways, such as 'superior' and 'inferior', 'upper' and 'lower', 'common pulmonary venous' and 'left atrial', and 'accessory' and 'left atrial chambers'. The terms 'proximal' and 'distal' have themselves been used with opposite meanings by different groups. Despite this, we concur with Thilenius et al (1976) that it is sensible to name the chambers according to the direction of blood flow, and we are therefore following their precedent.

Although the usual examples all have the oblique dividing partition, there is considerable variability within this basic pattern. The significant variations are the size of the communication between the proximal and distal chambers, the site of an interatrial communication (if present), and the connexion of the pulmonary veins, although any other associated malformation can coexist. The size of the communication between the left atrial chambers was the basis of Loeffler's categorisation (1949). There is a spectrum of size from non-restrictive (which is rare) to the more usual arrangement in which it is a pinhole meatus (Fig. 23.2). Usually the communication is single, but multiple orifices between the parts of the atrium have been described (Niwayama, 1960). The atrial septum is intact in up to half the cases. When present, a septal defect is almost always within the oval fossa. It most

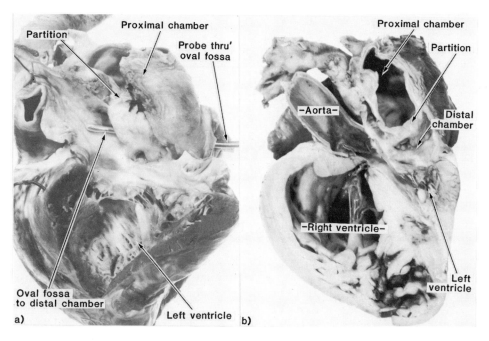

Fig. 23.1 An example of 'classical' partitioned left atrium (cor triatriatum sinister). (a) Shows the heart viewed obliquely from behind while (b) is a simulated 'four chamber plus aortic root' cut of the same heart.

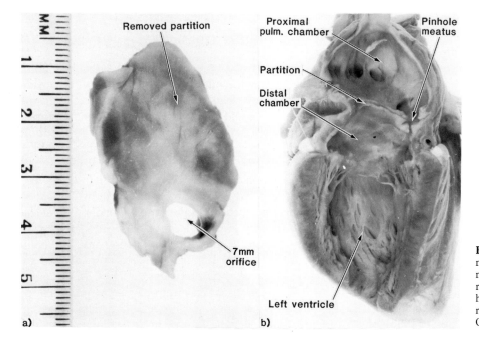

Fig. 23.2 The size of the hole in the dividing membrane can vary markedly. (a) Shows a meatus of reasonable size in a partition removed at surgery, while (b) shows a pinhole in an autopsy specimen. (Figure 23.2b is reproduced by kind permission of Dr L. M. Gerlis, Killingbeck Hospital, Leeds, UK.)

frequently communicates with the distal left atrial chamber. In the series reported by Thilenius and his colleagues (1976), about one-quarter of their 'classical' cases had the atrial septal defect communicating with the proximal chamber. This is not to suggest that this variant had not been described before, since Somerville (1966) and others had discussed the effect of a right atrial communication with the proximal chamber. It is, nonetheless, surprising that so many of the Chicago series should exhibit this variant. It is also possible to find the partitioning membrane crossing the oval fossa when the latter

is intact. In his excellent review, Niwayama (1960) cites three examples. Although usually at the oval fossa, rare cases have been described where the communication with the distal chamber is an atrioventricular rather than an atrial septal defect (Thilenius et al, 1979). This has been found with a common atrioventricular orifice (Thilenius et al, 1976 – case 19); with separate right and left valve orifices ('primum atrial septal defect') (Thilenius et al, 1976 – case 4; Marin-Garcia et al, 1975 – case 10) and with a so-called 'transitional type' (Marin-Garcia et al, 1975 – case 8). It is significant that in case 4 of Thilenius et al

(1976), the ostium primum defect to the distal chamber coexisted with a 'secundum' defect to the proximal chamber. In the cases with common orifice and so-called 'transitional anatomy', the atrial septum was said to be absent. It is also noteworthy that one case of partitioned left atrium was found in the setting of an atrioventricular septal defect with intact septal structures (Silverman et al, 1984). Just as the morphology of the interatrial communications can vary, so can their size. This feature was the basis of the classification of Gasul et al (1966).

The pulmonary veins usually connect to the proximal left atrial chamber, but many types of partial anomalous venous connexion can be found. This is shown by the exceedingly complex categorisation designed by Thilenius et al (1976) to cope with this variability. We prefer to account for these uncommon associated lesions in descriptive fashion. Any other lesion can coexist with a partitioned left atrium, including such complex malformations as mitral atresia (Marin-Garcia et al, 1975 – case 9), discordant atrioventricular connexion (Marin-Garcia et al, 1975 – case 12) and the examples of atrioventricular septal defect discussed above.

The histological structure of the dividing membrane was extensively reviewed by Niwayama (1960), who added further details from his own cases. In essence the septum is made up of myocardium, said by Niwayama (1960) to be continuous with the posterior wall of the proximal chamber. Hagenauer (1931) had commented upon the double nature of this wall, showing how in his case there was a second layer continuous with the muscular wall of the distal chamber. This fact was later verified and expanded by Van Praagh & Corsini (1967). They used the histological arrangement as evidence in favour of their 'entrapment hypothesis' of morphogenesis (see below). They emphasised the endothelial and fibrous components of the membrane, as had others previously (Niwayama, 1960). Niwayama also indicated how calcium deposits had been observed in selected cases.

Before leaving our description of 'classical' cor triatriatum, it is pertinent to consider briefly the system of categorisation of Marin-Garcia et al (1975). They distinguished diaphragmatic, hour-glass and tubular types, basing their division on the concept that the anomaly represented improper absorption of the common pulmonary venous component of the developing left atrium. Thus, only their diaphragmatic type corresponds to the 'classical' subdivided left atrium discussed above. In their hour-glass type there is a constriction between a pulmonary venous confluence and the rest of the left atrium, while in the tubular type the pulmonary confluence itself forms the area of potential stenosis. When stenotic, these lesions certainly have much in common haemodynamically with the classical type of divided left atrium. Anatomically, however, they seem more akin to stenosis of the common pulmonary vein. Certainly they will pose different prob-

lems for surgical correction from the 'classical' lesion (see below).

Usually the right side of the heart is considerably hypertrophied in presence of a partitioned left atrium. In keeping with this (as with other cases of obstructed pulmonary venous return), there are marked changes within the lungs. According to Niwayama (1960), these were first mentioned by Palmer (1930). The changes were studied in detail by Edwards and his colleagues (1951), who found varicose dilation of the alveolar capillaries and concentric medial thickening of the pulmonary arterioles with luminal narrowing. A prominent inner elastic membrane was noted in the muscular pulmonary arteries. Becu and his colleagues (1955) subsequently noted prominent dilation of the pleural lymphatics.

Morphogenesis

It has generally been accepted that divided left atrium of the classical type occurs because of failure of absorption of the common pulmonary vein into the left atrium. This so-called 'malincorporation concept' was popularised by Loeffler (1949), Griffith in 1903 having observed 'failure in the complete amalgamation of that part of the atrium which is said to be derived from the confluent portions of the pulmonary veins and that derived from the left-hand division of the common auricle of the embryonic heart.' The malincorporation hypothesis supplanted other theories based on overgrowth of the valve of the oval foramen or displacement of the primary pulmonary vein. Paradoxically, the malincorporation hypothesis itself more readily explains the hour-glass and tubular anomalies of Marin-Garcia and his colleagues (1975). It was dissatisfaction with the malincorporation and malseptation hypotheses which directed Van Praagh & Corsini (1969) towards their 'entrapment' concept. This stated that, during its development, the primary pulmonary vein was caught in a vice between the left sinus horn and the rest of the venous sinus. As evidence for their concept they cited the five layers to be seen histologically within the dividing partition. This entrapment concept accounts well for the classical type. It less readily explains the variant in which the atrial septal defect, unequivocally at the oval fossa, communicates with the proximal chamber (Thilenius et al, 1976). It is possible to combine concepts of malseptation with the entrapment hypothesis to account for these variants. As Thilenius et al (1976) comment, however, all these theories are of necessity speculative.

Incidence and aetiology

Rowe (1978) observed that partitioning of the left atrium was the second rarest individual lesion recorded in the files of the Hospital for Sick Children, Toronto. It represented less than 0.1% of their case load. Only 4 examples were found in nearly 4000 catheterisations performed at the Brompton Hospital from 1970–1982 (Ostman-Smith et al, 1984). In the review of Niwayama (1960), it was observed to affect males more frequently than females (in the ratio of 3 : 2). Only 4 out of the 10 'classical' variants were males in the autopsy series of Marin-Garcia et al (1975), while 17 of the 23 cases described by Thilenius et al (1976) were males. Taken overall, this indicates male preponderance, but the precise figures are not certain. There has been no observed aetiology for the lesion.

Presentation and clinical features

The age and mode of presentation relate to the tightness of the communication between the proximal and distal chambers. Usually there is tight stenosis and the patients present in infancy or early childhood with dyspnoea and frequent respiratory infections. Frequently they are considered to have primary pulmonary disease. The patients may not present until adult life when the communication is restrictive. The presenting feature is then usually dyspnoea on effort but may be frank haemoptysis. The cases presenting earlier do so with tachypnoea and cyanosis as in total anomalous pulmonary venous connexion. When cyanosis is present this usually represents a right-to-left shunt from the right atrium through an oval foramen or atrial septal defect to the atrial side (distal chamber) of the partitioned left atrium. The combination with partial anomalous pulmonary venous connexion does not usually give cyanosis and may alleviate the obstructive symptoms (Somerville, 1966).

The clinical signs are dominated by evidence of pulmonary venous congestion and pulmonary hypertension. When the communication between the proximal and distal chambers is absent (or small), the child, or frequently infant, will be breathless at rest and will have subcostal recession. The child will be pale and sweating, with tachycardia, and extreme breathlessness on feeding, but usually will remain fully saturated. There is a right ventricular heave and, on auscultation, the pulmonary component of the second sound is almost always accentuated with or without a pulmonary ejection click. No murmurs may be heard, although an apical diastolic murmur may simulate mitral stenosis. A soft, blowing systolic murmur may represent secondary tricuspid regurgitation in severe cases. Occasionally the apical murmur is continuous or the early diastolic murmur of pulmonary incompetence secondary to pulmonary hypertension may be heard. The signs of congestive heart failure are found when this supervenes, including crepitations in the lungs and a palpable liver. These effects of pulmonary hypertension are alleviated when there is partial anomalous pulmonary venous connexion.

Investigations

Chest radiography

The routine chest radiograph usually reveals cardiomegaly and shows the presence of pulmonary venous obstruction. The so-called 'staghorn' or 'butterfly wing' sign is seen because of prominent venous engorgement of the upper pulmonary veins. Pulmonary arterial hypertension is reflected by a prominent pulmonary knob. Enlargement and hypertrophy of the proximal left atrial chamber results in posterior deviation of the oesophagus (as seen in the barium swallow) and the finding of a double density shadow at the right cardiac border.

Electrocardiography

Right ventricular hypertrophy is almost invariably present. The frontal mean QRS axis is usually between +120 and +140 degrees. Apart from broad P waves which are sometimes present (as a consequence of right atrial hypertrophy), the rhythm and remainder of the electrocardiographic pattern are usually within normal limits.

Echocardiography

It is now well established that diagnosis can be made either by M-mode or by cross-sectional (Figs. 23.3, 23.4) echocardiography, the latter being the definitive investigation (Ostman-Smith et al, 1984). The M-mode findings are of an abnormal echo recorded on the left atrial aspect of the mitral valve along with findings of right ventricular overload. The position of the abnormal echo is further from

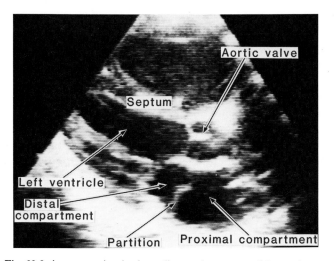

Fig. 23.3 A cross-sectional echocardiogram in parasternal long axis section showing the dividing partition within the left atrium. (Reproduced by kind permission of Dr S. C. Park, Children's Hospital of Pittsburgh, USA.)

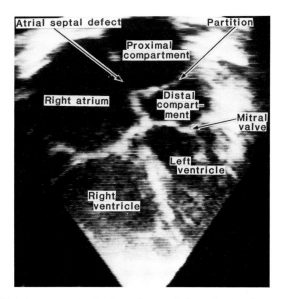

Fig. 23.4 A cross-sectional echocardiogram in four chamber long axis plane showing the dividing partition in the left atrium. (Reproduced by kind permission of Dr S. C. Park, Children's Hospital of Pittsburgh, USA.)

the valve than with supravalvar stenosing left atrial ring (Lundstrom, 1972). The linear appearance of the partition in no way resembles the more 'cloud-like' echoes found with a left atrial myxoma (Popp & Harrison, 1969). The finding of a normal mitral valve echo excludes mitral stenosis. Cross-sectional echocardiography permits direct visualisation of the obstructive membrane (Ostman-Smith et al, 1984). The site of interatrial defects should be discernible if present. If making the diagnosis with M-mode techniques alone, it should be borne in mind that in some normal patients an echo-dense line may be found in the middle of the left atrium when the sound beam is angulated laterally and cephalad. The addition of cross-sectional techniques should exclude these 'false-positives'. In their absence, it is questionable if patients should be submitted to surgery on M-mode evidence alone.

Catheterisation and angiography

The haemodynamic findings can be highly suggestive of the usual form of divided left atrium. An elevated pulmonary arterial wedge pressure is found in the presence of normal pressure tracings in the distal left atrial chamber recorded by entry via the right atrium and an oval foramen or septal defect. It is not always possible, however, to enter the latter chamber. If a conclusive diagnosis has been obtained echocardiographically, it is questionable if septal puncture (McGuire et al, 1965) is justified in order simply to verify the normal pressure in the distal left atrium. It may be possible, however, to enter the distal chamber retrogradely to obtain this information (Brickman et al,

1970). These typical findings will not be found when the oval fossa communicates with the proximal atrial chamber. A high left atrial pressure will then be recorded (Niwayama, 1960) and the diagnosis must be made from angiocardiography. This is usually done by selective pulmonary arterial injection. There is prolonged opacification of the proximal chamber on the follow-through. The obstructing diaphragm is seen in profile as an oblique linear translucency (Fig. 23.5). The distal chamber can be seen to contract vigorously during atrial systole while the proximal chamber tends to contract poorly. The partition can be seen to move towards the mitral valve in ventricular diastole but straightens after closure of the valve (Ellis et al, 1964). Clearer definition is obtained if it is possible to inject directly within the distal chamber (Perry et al, 1967; Brickman et al, 1970). This part of the left atrium is small and outlined superiorly by the straight contour of the partition. This appearance may also be seen during left ventricular angiocardiography should ectopic beats produce mitral regurgitation (Miller et al, 1964; Girod & Kurlander, 1966).

Differential diagnosis

In infants and children this lesion has to be distinguished from other causes of pulmonary venous obstruction. It may be difficult to differentiate total anomalous pulmonary venous connexion from pulmonary venous obstruction, since the conditions have similar clinical, radiological and electrocardiographic findings. A proportion of cases of divided left atrium will be fully saturated while breathing 100% oxygen, in contrast to cases of total anomalous pulmonary venous connexion. The two are readily distinguished, however, by both echocardiography and catheterisation, even when the partitioned left atrium is itself associated with partial anomalous pulmonary venous connexion. Rowe (1978) indicated that there may be other problems in diagnosis (in particular, stenosis of a common pulmonary vein). Although included in Marin-Garcia's categorisation (1975), the latter lesion is not usually considered as a 'classical' divided left atrium. As Rowe (1978) discussed, the other conditions to be distinguished in infancy and childhood are congenital stenosis of individual pulmonary veins, atresia of the common pulmonary vein, supravalvar stenosing ring of the left atrium, congenital mitral stenosis and perhaps endocardial fibroelastosis with severe aortic stenosis. All of these are causes of pulmonary venous congestion in a fully saturated child. In addition to these cardiac lesions, it should be remembered that a partitioned left atrium can readily be mistaken for primary lung disease and vice-versa. As with all clinical diagnosis, a high index of suspicion is important. The diagnosis of divided left atrium is probable if the patient is fully saturated with signs of pulmonary hypertension,

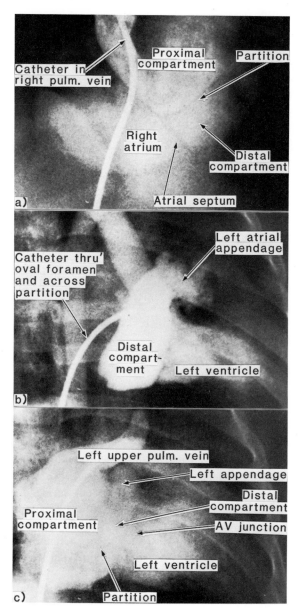

Fig. 23.5 A series of projections of angiograms taken from a patient with the 'classical' variety of divided left atrium. (a) A four chamber projection following injection into the right upper pulmonary vein. It fills the proximal chamber. (b) A right anterior oblique projection following the injection of contrast into the distal compartment of the divided left atrium. (c) Also taken in right anterior oblique projection, showing the site of the dividing partition following an injection into the left upper pulmonary vein. (Angiograms reproduced with kind permission of Dr S. C. Park, Children's Hospital of Pittsburgh.)

pulmonary venous congestion in the chest radiograph and an echocardiogram showing a normal mitral valve. In older patients there is a quite different differential diagnosis. Rheumatic mitral stenosis or left atrial tumour or thrombus are then the most likely alternatives (Lucas & Schmidt, 1968).

Treatment

The only appropriate treatment is surgical. The dividing partition is resected on cardiopulmonary bypass. This is usually achieved via a right atrial incision, visualising the partition through the oval foramen or an atrial septal defect. An approach via the left atrium is recommended in older patients by some (Richardson et al, 1981). Medical treatment is indicated initially for those patients in heart failure, but only until the diagnosis is made. Surgery should have every chance of success. There was only 1 death in the 15 patients operated at the Hospital for the Sick Children, Great Ormond Street, and the Brompton Hospital (Stark & de Leval, 1983; Ostman-Smith et al, 1984). The prognosis is excellent in the patients who survive operation. Pulmonary arterial changes have been reversible in those patients studied postoperatively (Anderson & Varco, 1961; Gialloreto & Vineberg, 1962).

RARER VARIANTS OF PARTITIONED LEFT ATRIUM

In their expanded concept, Thilenius and his colleagues (1976) described a single case encountered clinically and abstracted several other cases from the literature which could not adequately be categorised within the 'classical' concept. So far, we are unaware of any other workers who have encountered hearts of this type, but the possibility must exist. The feature distinguishing their exceptional case (and the others culled from previous reports) was the position of the distal atrial chamber. In the usual type, the distal chamber is funnel-shaped and situated basally. The coronary sinus empties normally within the morphologically right atrium. In their exceptional case, the systemic and pulmonary veins entered the morphologically right and left atrial chambers respectively in normal fashion. The coronary sinus also drained normally to the right atrium. But there was an additional midline proximal chamber which was not connected to any venous structures. It communicated via the oval fossa with the morphologically right atrium and via another communication with the distal left atrium. The chamber was demonstrated by angiography via the oval fossa. Mitral atresia was also present and this dominated the clinical picture. It is difficult to assess the possibility of such hearts existing without mitral atresia, since then the interposed third atrial chamber would significantly interrupt the circulation during fetal life. Thus the clinical significance of this variant remains to be established.

The essential feature of the unusual group of hearts which Thilenius and his colleagues garnered from the literature was atresia of the normal coronary sinus ostium with total or anomalous connexion of the pulmonary veins to the proximal atrial chamber. The proximal chamber was said to be wedge-shaped and again was located in the midline adjacent to the inferior part of the atrial septum. In these hearts the oval fossa was always in communication with the distal chamber and the coronary sinus itself was rudimentary. According to Thilenius et al (1976), such hearts had been described by Lam et al (1962), by Wedemeyer et al (1970), and by Patten & Taggart (1929). 8 such examples had been recorded by these authors, 6 in the series of Lam and his colleagues (1962). From the clinical point of view, these hearts resemble most closely total anomalous pulmonary venous connexion to the coronary sinus. The proximal atrial chamber in each case communicated not with the distal left atrium but with the morphologically right atrium. They would, therefore, probably present as obstructed total anomalous pulmonary venous connexion. Indeed, unless the atretic orifice of the coronary sinus was itself recognised, the cases would probably be diagnosed as total anomalous venous connexion. The surgical treatment is certainly as for the latter anomaly. Although in terms of categorisation these hearts are appropriately considered as partitioned left atria, in practical terms they can be grouped with anomalous pulmonary venous connexion (see Ch. 21).

PARTITIONING OF THE MORPHOLOGICALLY RIGHT ATRIUM

Division of the morphologically right atrium is considerably rarer than of the left. Most recorded examples have been presented as case reports subsequent to diagnosis at autopsy (Doucette & Knoblich, 1963; Kauffman et al, 1962; Jones & Niles, 1968; Runcie, 1968). Since then Verel et al (1970) diagnosed a case during life while Hansing et al (1972) similarly reported successful diagnosis together with surgical repair. All of these examples were due to persistence of the embryonic valves of the venous sinus ('sinus venosus'). The dividing partition is therefore placed between the venous sinus and the distal part of the right atrium (which is comprised of vestibule and appendage). Doucette & Knoblich (1963) designed a categorisation to distinguish different morphological types according to the precise valvar structure involved. This hardly seems justified with such a rare lesion and it is of little clinical significance. The embryonic valvar structures (whose significance during fetal life is to direct the richly oxygenated inferior caval blood across to the left atrium and thence to the aorta) normally regress in late fetal life and early childhood. They persist only as the Eustachian and Thebesian valves (valves of the inferior caval vein and coronary sinus respectively). These valves can retain their fetal proportions in abnormal conditions and then divide the right atrium. Most examples have coexisted with atresia or stenosis of the pulmonary valve or else with tricuspid atresia. The haemodynamic effect of the partition itself is then of little significance, since the blood is required to cross the oval fossa and the persistent valves augment this flow pattern. The lesion is of more significance when the tricuspid and pulmonary valves are patent. Then the valve can become aneurysmal and protrude into the right ventricle like a windsock. Jones & Niles (1968) graphically likened this variant to a spinnaker sail. Surgical removal of this type is essential. A further variant has also been reported where the partition does not stretch between the venous sinus and the rest of the right atrium but instead forms a supratricuspid valve ring (Folger, 1968). Nakano corrected surgically one example of this type (1973).

REFERENCES

Anderson R C, Varco R L 1961 Cor triatriatum: successful diagnosis and surgical correction in a 3-year-old girl. American Journal of Cardiology 7: 436–440

Andral G 1829 Precis d'anatomie pathologique. Cited by Perloff. 2: p 313

Becu L M, Tauxe W N, DuShane J W, Edwards J G 1955 Anomalous connection of pulmonary veins with normal pulmonary venous drainage. Report of case associated with pulmonary venous stenosis and Cor Triatriatum. American Archives of Pathology 59: 463–470

Borst M 1905 Ein Cor triatriatum. Verhandlung der Deutschen Pathologischen Gesellschaft 9: 178–191

Brickman R D, Wilson H, Zuberbuhler J R, Bahnson H T 1970 Cor triatriatum. Clinical presentation and operative treatment. Journal of Thoracic and Cardiovascular Surgery 60: 523–530

Church W S 1868 Congenital malformation of the heart: abnormal septum in left auricle. Transactions of the Pathological Society of London 19: 188–190

Doucette J, Knoblich R 1963 Persistent right valve of the sinus venosus. Archives of Pathology 75: 105–112

Edwards J E, DuShane J W, Alcott D L, Burchell H E 1951 Thoracic venous anomalies. III. Atresia of the common pulmonary vein, the pulmonary veins draining wholly into the superior vena cava (Case 3). IV. Stenosis of the common pulmonary vein (Cor triatriatum). American Archives of Pathology 51: 446–460

Ellis K, Griffiths S P, Jesse M J 1964 Diagnosis of cor triatriatum by left ventricular angiocardiography. Report of a case. American Journal of Roentgenology 92: 669–675

Folger G M Jr 1968 Supravalvular tricuspid stenosis. Association with developmental abnormalities of the right heart and derivatives of the sixth aortic arch. American Journal of Cardiology 21: 81–87

Gasul B M, Arcilla R A, Lev M 1966 Heart disease in children. Lippincott, Philadelphia, p 869–881

Gialloreto O P, Vineberg A 1962 A case of cor triatriatum studied 5 years after surgery. American Journal of Cardiology 9: 598–602

Girod D, Kurlander G J 1966 Diagnosis of cor triatriatum by left ventricular angiocardiography. Report of a case. Diseases of the Chest 50: 535–538

Griffith T W 1903 Note on a second example of division of the cavity of the left auricle into two compartments by a fibrous band. Journal of Anatomy and Physiology 37: 255–257

Hagenauer J 1931 Die Pathogenese einer seltenen Herzmissbildung (Cor triatriatum), Frankfurter Zeitschrift fur Pathologie 41: 332–356

Hansing C E, Young W P, Rowe C C 1972 Cor triatriatum dexter. Persistent right sinus venous valve. American Journal of Cardiology 30: 559–564

James T N 1962 Classification of triatrial hearts. Anatomical Record 143: 79–91

Jones R N, Niles N R 1968 Spinnaker formation of the sinus venosus valve. Circulation 38: 468–473

Kauffman S L, Ores C N, Anderson D H 1962 Two cases of total anomalous pulmonary venous return of the supracardiac type with stenosis simulating infradiaphragmatic drainage. Circulation 25: 376–382

Lam C R, Green E, Drake E 1962 Diagnosis and surgical correction of two types of triatrial heart. Surgery 51: 127–137

Loeffler E 1949 Unusual malformation of the left atrium pulmonary sinus. Archives of Pathology 48: 371–376

Lucas R V Jr, Schmidt R E 1968 Anomalous venous connections, pulmonary and systemic. In: Moss A J, Adams F (eds) Heart disease in infants, children and adolescents. Williams & Wilkins, Baltimore, p 702–707

Lundstrom N R 1972 Ultrasound cardiographic studies of the mitral valve region in young infants with mitral atresia, mitral stenosis, hypoplasia of the left ventricle and cor triatriatum. Circulation 45: 324–334

McGuire L B, Nolan T B, Reeve R, Dammann J F Jr 1965 Cor triatriatum as a problem of adult heart disease. Circulation 31: 263–272

Marin-Garcia J, Tandon R, Lucas R V Jr, Edwards J E 1975 Cor triatriatum: study of 20 cases. American Journal of Cardiology 35: 59–66

Miller G A H, Ongley P A, Anderson M W, Kincaid O W, Swan H J C 1964 Cor triatriatum. Hemodynamic and angiographic diagnosis. American Heart Journal 68: 298–304

Nakano S 1973 Surgical treatment of cor triatriatum. Japanese Journal of Thoracic Surgery 25: 541–547

Niwayama G 1960 Cor triatriatum: review. American Heart Journal 59: 291–317

Ostman-Smith I, Silverman N H, Oldershaw P, Lincoln C, Shinebourne E A 1984 Cor triatriatum sinistrum. Diagnostic features on cross sectional echocardiography. British Heart Journal 51: 211–219

Palmer G A 1930 Cardiac anomaly (so-called double left auricle). Report of a case. American Heart Journal 6: 230–236

Patten B M, Taggart W B 1929 Unusual type of triatrial heart. Archives of Pathology 8: 894–905

Perloff J K 1978 The clinical recognition of congenital heart disease. Saunders, Philadelphia, p 163–170

Perry L W, Scott L P III, McClenathan J E 1967 Cor triatriatum: Preoperative diagnosis and successful surgical repair in a small infant. Journal of Pediatrics 71: 840–847

Popp R L, Harrison D C 1969 Ultrasound for diagnosis of atrial tumour. Annals of Internal Medicine 71: 785–787

Richardson J V, Doty D B, Siewers R D, Zuberbuhler J R 1981 Cor triatriatum (subdivided left atrium). Journal of Thoracic and Cardiovascular Surgery 81: 232–238

Rowe R D 1978 Anomalies of venous return. In: Keith J D, Rowe R D, Vlad P (eds) Heart disease in infancy and childhood. Macmillan, New York, p 577–583

Runcie J 1968 A complicated case of cor triatriatum dexter. British Heart Journal 30: 729–731

Silverman N H, Ho S Y, Anderson R H, Smith A, Wilkinson J L 1984 Atrioventricular septal defect with intact atrial and ventricular septal structures. International Journal of Cardiology 5: 567–572

Somerville J 1966 Masked cor triatriatum. British Heart Journal 28: 55–61

Stark J, de Leval M 1983 In: Surgery for congenital heart disease. Grune & Stratton, New York, p 246–251

Thilenius O G, Bharati S, Lev M 1976 Subdivided left atrium: an expanded concept of cor triatriatum sinistrum. American Journal of Cardiology 37: 743–752

Thilenius O G, Vitullo D, Bharati S, et al 1979 Endocardial cushion defect associated with cor triatriatum sinistrum or supravalve mitral ring. American Journal of Cardiology 44: 1339–1343

Van Praagh R, Corsini I 1969 Cor triatriatum: pathologic anatomy and a consideration of morphogenesis based on 13 postmortem cases and a study of normal development of the pulmonary vein and atrial septum in 83 human embryos. American Heart Journal 78: 379–405

Verel D, Pilcher J, Hynes D M 1970 Cor triatriatum dexter. British Heart Journal 32: 714–716

Wedemeyer A L, Lucas R V, Castaneda A R 1970 Surgical correction in infancy of an unusual form of triatrial heart. Journal of Thoracic and Cardiovascular Surgery 59: 685–690

24

Atrioventricular septal defects

There is a group of lesions unified by the anatomy of their abnormal atrioventricular junction. Usually termed 'endocardial cushion defects' or 'atrioventricular canal malformations', they have in common a defect at the site of the normal atrioventricular septum. This is the case whether they are found with separate right and left atrioventricular valves ('ostium primum atrial septal defect') or a common valve orifice ('complete atrioventricular canal'). For this reason we describe them here as 'atrioventricular septal defects' (Becker & Anderson, 1982).

PREVALENCE AND AETIOLOGY

Atrioventricular septal defects form 3% of all congenital heart defects, the male : female ratio being 1.1 : 1 (Keith, 1978). There is a strong association with Down's syndrome (see Ch. 2), in that about a third of patients with Down's syndrome have an atrioventricular septal defect with common orifice, and 5% an 'ostium primum atrial septal defect' (Rowe & Uchida, 1961). Contrariwise, a high proportion of all patients with atrioventricular septal defects have Down's syndrome. Emanuel and colleagues (1968) found this proportion to be one-third, whereas in the Liverpool population study (Dickinson et al, 1981) all patients with common atrioventricular orifice also had Down's syndrome. This close association with trisomy 21 argues against the usual multifactorial model put forward to explain the inheritance of congenital heart disease (Burn, 1983). So do the four siblings reported by Yao and colleagues in 1968 (all of whom were born of normal parents and yet had 'ostium primum' defects), and the large pedigree reported in which atrioventricular septal defect behaved like an autosomal dominant trait (O'Nullain et al, 1977). Sanchez-Cascos (1978) found recurrence in 14 of 161 first degree relatives (8.7%), and Emanuel and colleagues (1983) found a recurrence risk in the offspring of parents with atrioventricular septal defects of 9.6%, or 13.4% if only female propositi were considered. This is much higher than in other defects.

ANATOMY

The basic morphology of the atrioventricular junction

The basic malformation underscoring the group of lesions is within the atrioventricular junction. By 'atrioventricular junction' we mean the area of the heart where the atrial myocardium is contiguous with the ventricular myocardium. The two segments of myocardium are separated from one another throughout the junction by the fibro-fatty atrioventricular groove ('sulcus') and the atrioventricular fibrous plane ('annulus fibrosus'), except in the region of the penetrating atrioventricular bundle. In the normal heart, the junction as thus defined can then be subdivided into the right and left parietal components (which surround the tricuspid and mitral orifices respectively) together with a septal component between the orifices. The morphology of the normal junction is such that the septal component is relatively small. This is because the left ventricular outflow tract and the aortic valve ring are wedged between the diverging antero-superior limbs of the mitral and tricuspid orifices (Fig. 24.1). In the upper left-hand quadrant (as viewed from below – Fig. 24.1) of the left atrioventricular orifice, there is no contiguity between atrial and ventricular myocardium. This is the area of aortic-mitral valvar fibrous continuity. The right and left margins of this region of valvar fibrous continuity are thickened to form the central fibrous body and the left fibrous trigone respectively. There are other aspects of the area which are pertinent to the morphology of atrioventricular septal defects. In the normal septal area of the atrioventricular junction, small as this area may be, the septal leaflet of the tricuspid valve is attached at a considerably more apical level than is the mitral valve leaflet (Fig. 24.2). Because of this, the plane of the septal atrioventricular junction slopes from the mitral attachment above to the tricuspid attachment lower down. Between the two, a part of the septum is interposed between the left ventricular and the right atrial chambers. This is the atrioventricular *muscular* septum (Fig. 24.2b), which must be distinguished from the atrioventricular *membranous*

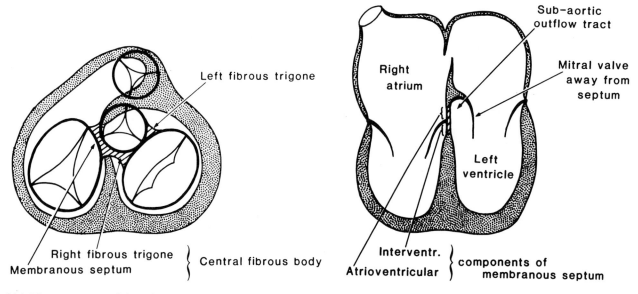

Fig. 24.1 The arrangement of the valve rings and septal structures in the normal heart as seen in the short axis section viewed from beneath (left) and in 'four chamber' section (right).

septum (Fig. 24.2a). The latter, together with the interventricular membranous septum, is an integral part of the central fibrous body. This structure forms the right wall of the left ventricular outflow tract and interposes between the outflow tract and the right heart chambers.

Because of its 'wedged' position, the subaortic outflow tract lifts the 'septal' quadrant of the mitral valve leaflets away from the septum. In contrast, in the tricuspid orifice the leaflet is attached to the inlet septum over a considerable area. This anatomy is pertinent to the naming of the valve leaflets (Fig. 24.3). In the mitral orifice, the leaflets are divided by obliquely orientated anterolateral and posteromedial commissures into a short and square leaflet (best termed the aortic leaflet, but often termed the 'anterior leaflet') and a more extensive, but narrower mural leaflet, the latter being subdivided into a variable number

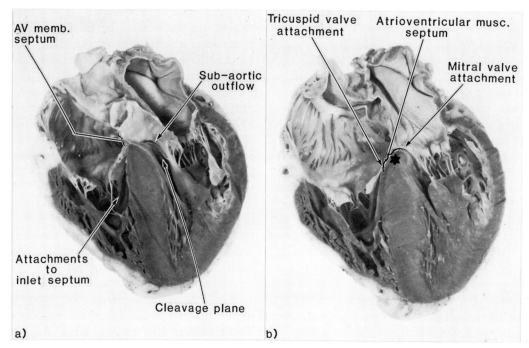

Fig. 24.2 Simulated 'four chamber' sections in long axis through a normal heart showing (a) the atrioventricular membranous and (b) the atrioventricular muscular septal structures.

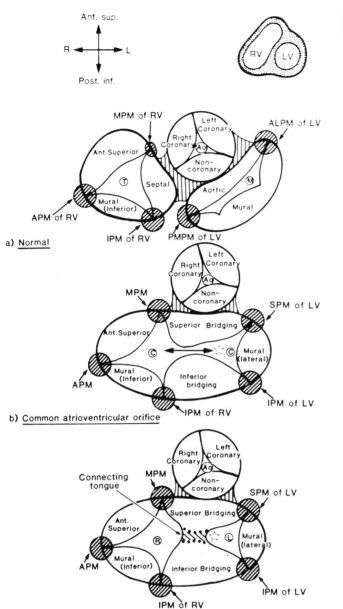

a) Normal

b) Common atrioventricular orifice

c) Separate right and left atrioventricular orifices

Fig. 24.3 Diagrammatic representation of the arrangement of the valve rings as viewed from beneath (see insets for orientation), comparing the leaflet arrangements and papillary muscle positions in (a) normal, (b) atrioventricular septal defects with common orifice, and (c) atrioventricular septal defects with separate right and left atrioventricular orifices. Abbreviations: A – anterior; Ant – anterior; Ao – aorta; C – common; I – inferior; L – lateral; L – left; M – medial; M – mitral; P – posterior; PM – papillary muscle; R – right; S – superior; T – tricuspid. Where a letter is used twice, its position makes it obvious whether it refers to a valve (e.g. 'M' for mitral valve) or a position (e.g. 'M' for medial).

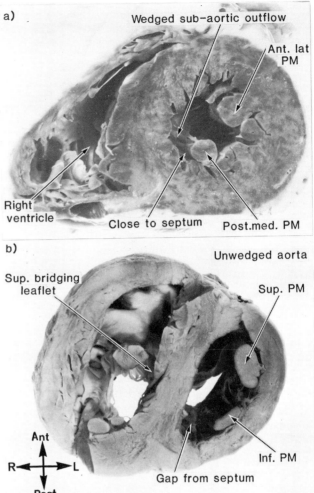

Fig. 24.4 The ventricular mass viewed from below in short axis section and showing the different orientation of the left ventricular papillary muscles (PM) in (a) the normal and (b) an atrioventricular septal defect.

of scallops, usually three. The paired left ventricular papillary muscles supporting the commissures are similarly positioned obliquely within the ventricle in anterolateral and posteromedial position (Fig. 24.4a). The tricuspid valve has three commissures. They are located in antero-

septal, anterolateral and inferior position. The anteroseptal commissure is supported by the medial papillary muscle (of Lancisi) and the septal leaflet swings 'round the corner' from the region of the membranous septum to reach it (see Ch. 25). From this small muscle the extensive antero-superior leaflet, interposed between inlet and outlet portions of the right ventricle, reaches across to the large anterior papillary muscle. From the anterior muscle the mural or inferior leaflet extends to the inferior papillary muscle, which is frequently indistinct. Then, between it and the medial papillary muscle, numerous small muscles usually anchor the septal leaflet of the tricuspid valve directly to the inlet part of the muscular septum.

The final feature of normal morphology which is pertinent to a study of atrioventricular septal defects concerns the ventricular mass rather than the junction. In the normal heart, the distance from the attachment of the mitral valve at the crux to the ventricular apex (the inlet dimension) is much the same as the distance from the ventricular apex to the attachment of the aortic valve to the outlet muscular septum (the outlet dimension).

The basic morphology of atrioventricular septal defects

The morphology of an atrioventricular septal defect departs significantly from the normal in terms of five of the features enumerated above. First, there is a defect at the anticipated site of the muscular and atrioventricular septal structures of the normal heart. This is found irrespective of whether there is a common atrioventricular orifice or separate right and left orifices (Fig. 24.5). Because of this septal defect, there is no contiguity between atrial and ventricular septal structures. This is responsible for the second feature, namely the presence of a common atrioventricular junction, again irrespective of whether there is a common orifice or separate right and left orifices. Thus, instead of finding the 'spectacle' arrangement of right and left atrioventricular junctions as seen in the normal heart (Fig. 24.3a), there is an ovoid common junction (Figs. 24.3b,c, 24.6). The third feature different from the normal also contributes to the ovoid appearance of the common atrioventricular junction. Irrespective of the number of valve orifices, the left ventricular outflow tract is no longer wedged between the left and right atrioventricular orifices as seen in the normal heart. Instead the aortic valve is anterosuperior to the common junction (Fig. 24.6). Although there is aortic-atrioventricular valve continuity in atrioventricular septal defects, and although the ends of the area of continuity are strengthened to form left and right fibrous trigones, the morphology of the

trigones is in no way comparable with the normal heart (see Fig. 24.3). The right trigone may interpose between left ventricular outflow tract and right atrium and form an atrioventricular fibrous septum (Piccoli et al, 1979a), but this structure cannot be compared with the normal atrioventricular membranous septum.

Since there is a common atrioventricular junction which lacks any septal atrioventricular contiguity, the fourth feature is the arrangement of the valve leaflets guarding the junction. The valve leaflets of atrioventricular septal defects *cannot* be interpreted or understood in terms of the normal mitral and tricuspid valves. The valve has five basic leaflets. These five leaflets, seen to their best advantage in an atrioventricular septal defect with common orifice (Fig. 24.3b), may be so arranged as to divide the orifice into separate right and left atrioventricular components (Fig. 24.3c). But, even when there are separate right and left atrioventricular orifices ('ostium primum atrial septal defects'), the atrioventricular junction is still common to both (Fig. 24.6b) and has the valve arranged in basic five-leaflet fashion, albeit divided into a trifoliate left valve and a quadrifoliate right valve by a connecting tongue of valve tissue (Fig. 24.3c). Additionally there is a fundamental difference from the normal in the arrangement of the left ventricular papillary muscles. The paired muscles remain, but instead of being in anterolateral and posteromedial position (Fig. 24.4a), they are located one in front of the other (Fig. 24.4b; Carpentier, 1978). Frequently they may be even more abnormally positioned, particularly the superior muscle which may be located so as to compromise the left ventricular outflow tract (Piccoli et al, 1982; Chin et al, 1983) or else be the solitary muscle producing a

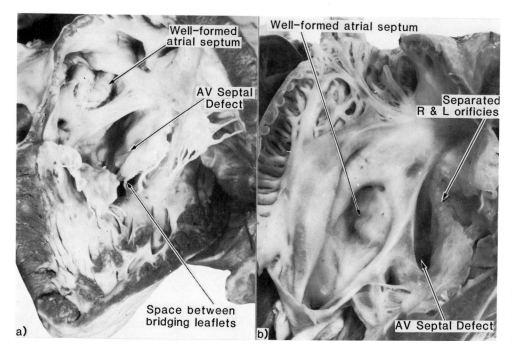

Fig. 24.5 Atrioventricular (AV) septal defects (a) with common valve orifice and (b) with separate right (R) and left (L) valve orifices. Both are viewed from the right side following an incision through the inferior part of the right atrioventricular junction. Note that the defects are at the site of the normal atrioventricular septal structures and that the atrial septum is well-formed in both, extending down to the level of the atrioventricular junction.

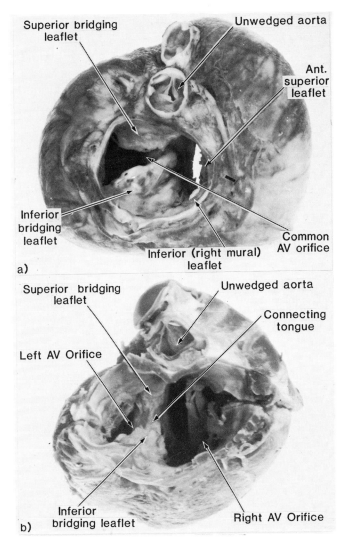

Fig. 24.6 Dissected atrioventricular junctions viewed from above with (a) a common atrioventricular (AV) orifice and (b) separate right and left atrioventricular orifices.

'parachute' arrangement (David et al, 1982). The arrangement of the right ventricular muscles is comparable with the normal heart, being in medial, anterior and inferior position (Fig. 24.3c). But the position of the medial papillary muscle is itself variable, this variability forming the basis for one subcategorisation of atrioventricular septal defects with common orifice (see below).

Five papillary muscles supporting commissural chords must produce the basic arrangement of five valve leaflets. Three of the leaflets are confined to one or other of the ventricles, one being in the left and two in the right. The left mural leaflet, much less extensive than the mural leaflet of the normal mitral valve (Penkoske et al, 1985), extends between the superior and inferior left ventricular papillary muscles. The anterosuperior and right mural leaflets are confined to the right ventricle and basically conform to their pattern in the normal heart. In contrast, the two remaining leaflets have no counterpart in the normal heart. They extend between a left ventricular and a right ventricular papillary muscle. As such, they are anchored in both ventricles, the leaflets themselves crossing the septum. Sometimes they cross to a limited extent, and in other cases are firmly attached to the septum at the crossing point. Nonetheless, since they extend between right and left ventricular papillary muscles, they can conveniently be called 'bridging' leaflets. The division between the left ventricular components of these bridging leaflets is, to all intents and purposes, a commissure (Carpentier, 1978). It is not supported by a papillary muscle, but neither are commissures in arterial valves (Anderson et al, 1985). The left valve, therefore, is a trifoliate valve (Carpentier, 1978). The space between the leaflets is most frequently termed a 'cleft' in the anterior or aortic leaflet of the mitral valve. There is no way that the aortic leaflet of a normal mitral valve can be cloven to replicate this septal commissure of the trifoliate left valve of an atrioventricular septal defect (Becker & Anderson, 1982). Surgeons should appreciate that the division between the left ventricular components of the bridging leaflets (be there a common orifice or separate right and left orifices) is part of the communication between left atrium and left ventricle (Fig. 24.7; Frater, 1965; Van Mierop & Alley, 1966). Closing this space at surgery can

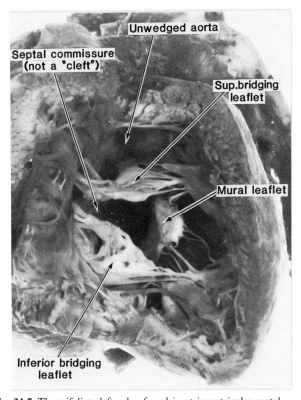

Fig. 24.7 The trifoliate left valve found in atrioventricular septal defects as seen from the apex of the left ventricle. The so-called 'cleft' is the division between the left ventricular components of the bridging leaflets and functions as a commissure.

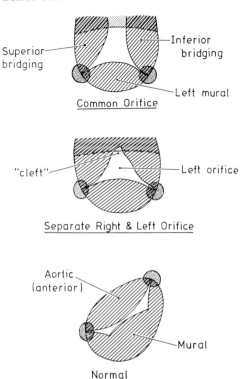

Fig. 24.8 The difference between the leaflet arrangements of the left valve in atrioventricular septal defects. The valves are drawn as they would be seen by surgeon at operation through a right atriotomy.

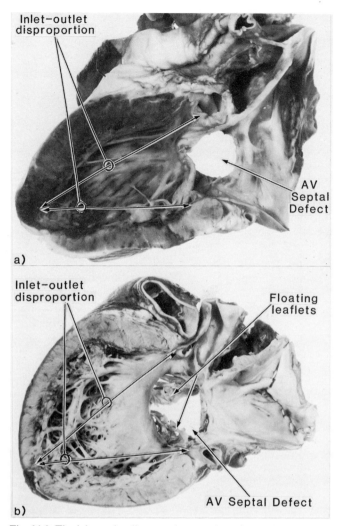

Fig. 24.9 The inlet-outlet disproportion seen in atrioventricular septal defects with (a) only the potential for interatrial shunting (ostium primum atrial septal defect) and (b) with common orifice and the potential for both atrial and ventricular shunting.

never produce a valve which resembles the normal mitral valve (Fig. 24.8).

The final alteration in morphology which characterises an atrioventricular septal defect lies in the architecture of the ventricular mass. In the normal heart, left ventricular inlet and outlet dimensions are the same. In atrioventricular septal defects the outlet dimension is considerably greater than that of the inlet (Fig. 24.9). Whether this is because the inlet is shorter than normal (Blieden et al, 1974) or the outlet is longer is inconsequential. Probably it is a combination of the two (Van Mierop, 1977; Piccoli et al, 1979a). Suffice it to say that the disproportion between inlet and outlet dimensions is readily apparent, and is within the same range be there a common atrioventricular orifice or separate right and left orifices (Piccoli et al, 1979a; Penkoske et al, 1985). If the valve leaflets are removed from an atrioventricular septal defect, it is not possible to judge simply from examination of the ventricular mass the type of atrioventricular septal defect which was initially present (Becker & Anderson, 1982). The specific type depends on the one hand on the morphology of the atrioventricular valve leaflets and on the other hand on the level of shunting through the atrioventricular septal defect. These features together serve to subclassify the group of lesions unified because of the basic atrioventricular septal defect.

Subcategorisation of atrioventricular septal defects

Some distinguish the types of atrioventricular septal defect according to whether or not a ventricular septal defect is present, in other words according to the level of shunting (Brandt et al, 1972). More usually (Wakai & Edwards, 1956, 1958; Campbell & Missen, 1957; Somerville & Jefferson, 1968) the hearts are subclassified depending upon whether there is a common atrioventricular orifice ('complete' form – see Fig. 24.3b) or whether the valve leaflets are joined by a connecting tongue in the plane of the ventricular septum to produce separate right and left atrioventricular orifices ('partial' form – see Fig. 24.3c). Both of these features are significant and should be described, as should other factors such as the relationship of the atrioventricular junction to the atrial and ventricular chambers ('dominance') and the presence of associated malformations.

Level of shunting through the atrioventricular septal defect

As described, the essence of the whole group is a hole in the area which, in the normal heart, is occupied by the atrioventricular muscular and membranous septal structures. The hole produced is unequivocally an atrioventricular septal defect. When it is small, it may occupy an area no bigger than that usually occupied by the atrioventricular septal structures (see Fig. 24.5). This points to the paradox of the conventional description of an atrioventricular septal defect with separate right and left atrioventricular orifices as an ostium primum *atrial* septal defect. In a small defect, as has been emphasised by several earlier investigators, the entirety of the hole is on the *ventricular* aspect of the atrioventricular junction. Usually the defect is larger than the area of the normal atrioventricular septum because of coexisting deficiencies of the atrial septum, the ventricular septum or both. But whatever its size, the level of shunting through the defect depends on the relationship of the bridging leaflets and the septal structures. When the bridging leaflets are connected to each other by a tongue and both leaflets and tongue are firmly attached to the crest of the *ventricular* septum, then shunting through the defect occurs at *atrial* level (Fig. 24.10 – upper right). Should the bridging leaflets and the connecting tongue (if present) be attached to the underside of the *atrial* septum, however, then the shunting would be at *ventricular* level (Fig. 24.10 – lower left). If, in contrast, the leaflets were attached to neither the atrial nor the ventricular septal crests, there would be the potential for both atrial and ventricular shunting through the septal defect (Fig. 24.10 – lower right). The extent of ventricular shunting will vary, depending on the degree to which the superior or inferior bridging leaflets are tethered to the septum, and to the connecting tongue if there are separate right and left atrioventricular orifices. By separating the feature of the attachment of leaflets and tongue to the septum, it is possible to avoid the need to designate a 'transitional' or 'intermediate' category of defects. This convention is responsible for considerable confusion. Wakai & Edwards (1956, 1958) used these terms to describe those hearts in which the bridging leaflets approached each other, but were not joined by a connecting tongue although both leaflets were firmly attached to the septum. In these hearts there is a common orifice, but all the shunting is effectively at atrial level. Brandt and his colleagues (1972) used the term 'transitional' to described those hearts with separate right and left atrioventricular orifices which had the potential for interventricular communication between the underside of the leaflet tissue separating the valve orifices and the ventricular septum. Yet others (Bharati et al, 1980) constructed a formidable alphanumeric system to combine these features. We avoid the need to enter this arena simply by describing separately the arrangement of the valve orifices

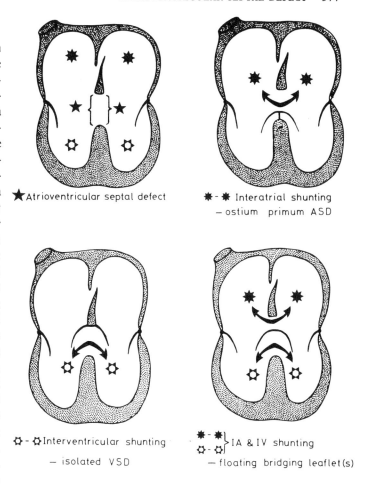

★ Atrioventricular septal defect

✳ - ✳ Interatrial shunting
— ostium primum ASD

✿ - ✿ Interventricular shunting
— isolated VSD

✳ - ✳
✿ - ✿ } IA & IV shunting
— floating bridging leaflet(s)

Fig. 24.10 The level of shunting through an atrioventricular septal defect (upper left) depends upon the attachment of the bridging valve leaflets and the connecting tongue (if present) to the septal structures. See text for further discussion. (Reproduced by kind permission of the publishers from Anderson, Becker, Lucchese, Meier, Rigby and Soto (1983) The Morphology of Congenital Heart Disease. Castle House Publications, Tunbridge Wells, UK.)

(separate or common) and the level for potential shunting (atrial level, ventricular level or both). Nonetheless, there is no doubt that two types of atrioventricular septal defect are so frequent that they stand out as special entities within the overall group, namely, those with separate right and left valve orifices and primarily interatrial shunting ('ostium primum atrial septal defect') and those with a common valve orifice ('common atrioventricular canal'). Further subcategories are to be found in each of these types, along with the third type, in which there is only the capacity for interventricular shunting in a heart with all the anatomical stigmata of an atrioventricular septal defect. We will therefore describe these types and subtypes in more detail before going on to consider the features of chamber dominance and associated malformations which are common to the group of atrioventricular septal defects as a whole.

Types of atrioventricular septal defect

'Ostium primum atrial septal defect'

The features of these hearts is that the superior and inferior bridging leaflets are themselves fused together by a connecting tongue to form separate right and left atrioventricular orifices (Fig. 24.11). The leaflet tissue is usually firmly adherent to the ventricular septum (Fig. 24.10 – upper right). The greater majority have a so-called 'cleft' left atrioventricular valve. The 'cleft' is in reality, a functional commissure in the trifoliate left valve. The atrioventricular septal defect extends between the lower edge of the atrial septum and the atrial surface of the fused bridging leaflets. The size of the defects depends upon the degree of associated deficiency of the atrial septum. When the atrial septum is well-formed, the defect occupies an area no larger than that of the normal atrioventricular septal structures. In contrast, when the atrial or ventricular septal structures are themselves deficient, the defect may be huge. If the atrial septum is totally lacking, there may be a common atrium with separate right and right atrioventricular valve orifices. It follows that different defects of the atrial septum (patent oval foramen, defects within the oval fossa, sinus venosus defect) can all coexist with an atrioventricular septal defect. As we have already discussed, although the valve morphology found most frequently with an 'ostium primum atrial septal defect' is described as a 'cleft mitral valve', this is a mismoner. The significance to the surgeon of not closing the 'cleft' has been emphasised previously (Frater, 1965; Van Mierop & Alley, 1966; Carpentier, 1978). Despite this there seems to be an amazing reticence to accept the triofoliate

morphology of the left valve and, instead, a comparably surprising desire to compare it with the normal mitral valve (see Fig. 24.8). The right atrioventricular valve is essentially a four-leaflet structure and may on occasion have a division between the right ventricular components of the bridging leaflets. On other occasions the two components may be fused and liberated from the septum producing a true 'septal' leaflet. More usually neither of these arrangements is found. Instead the connecting tongue and the superior bridging leaflet are turned in and are attached to the ventricular septum (Fig. 24.12) so that there is no free leaflet tissue in this superior part of the septal component of the right atrioventricular valve (McGoon et al, 1983; Penkoske et al, 1985).

Usually in the atrioventricular septal defect with separate valve orifices, the bridging leaflets are themselves firmly attached to the ventricular septum. When the leaflets are not thus attached, there is an interventricular communication between the underside of the leaflet tissue and the crest of the septum. Such a communication tends to be small, admitting only a probe (Fig. 24.13a). Frequently these interchordal spaces are multiple. Rarely the bridging leaflets and the connecting tongue may float freely, dividing the atrioventricular septal defect into sizeable atrial and ventricular components (Fig. 24.13b).

Rarely an ostium primum defect may be found which lacks any 'cleft' between the left ventricular components of the bridging leaflets. This is the variant which Goor & Lillehei (1975) have termed the 'corrected' defect. It has all the stigmata of an atrioventricular septal defect except that the left valve has bi- rather than trifoliate configuration. The leaflet tissue continues to bridge, however, and becomes confluent with that of the right valve. The left ventricular outflow tract is typical for an atrioventricular septal defect.

We have gone to some length to indicate that the division between the left ventricular components of the bridging leaflets of atrioventricular septal defects is not a cleft in a normal mitral valve (Anderson et al, 1985). But hearts certainly do exist with normal septal structures, a normal left ventricular outflow tract and a normal ventricular mass in which the only lesion is a division in the aortic (anterior) leaflet of the mitral valve (see Ch. 43). These are not atrioventricular septal defects. They should not be categorised along with atrioventricular septal defects in the way suggested by Di Segni & Edwards (1983). The features which permit differentiation of the isolated mitral cleft from an atrioventricular septal defect have been well described by Smallhorn et al (1982a, b, c). They were confirmed by the measurements of Penkoske et al (1985). Although we illustrated an example of a so-called 'isolated cleft' in an atrioventricular septal defect with intact septal structures (Piccoli et al, 1979a), subsequent examination revealed that the heart had initially possessed an ostium primum defect which had been surgically closed! The

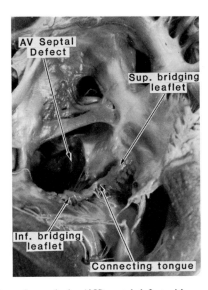

Fig. 24.11 An atrioventricular (AV) septal defect with separate valve orifices produced by a connecting tongue joining the bridging leaflets along the crest of the ventricular septum ('ostium primum atrial septal defect').

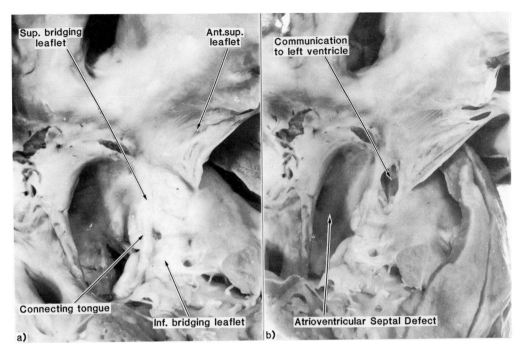

Fig. 24.12 An atrioventricular septal defect with separate valve orifices ('ostium primum atrial septal defect') in which the right atrioventricular valve 'septal' leaflet (a) is simply the connecting tongue and the superior bridging leaflet turned in and attached to the septum. (b) Removal of these structures produces a communication with the left ventricle.

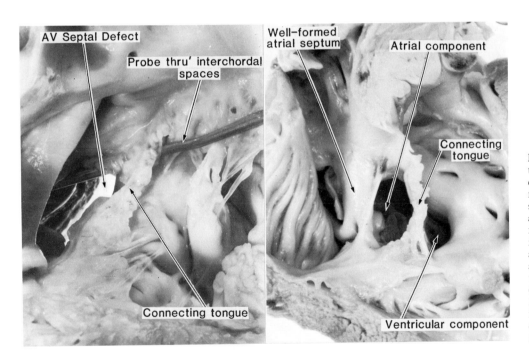

Fig. 24.13 The varying size of the interventricular communication which can be found in atrioventricular (AV) septal defects with separate right anad left valve orifices. (a) A further view of the heart illustrated in Fig. 24.11 in which a probe has been passed through a small interchordal space beneath the superior bridging leaflet. (b) In contrast, the bridging leaflets and the connecting tongue float freely and divide the septal defect into interatrial and interventricular compartments.

endothelialisation of the patch was not noticed during our initial study. Since then, however, we have seen an atrioventricular septal defect with all the morphological features, including a trifoliate left valve, but with intact septal structures (Fig. 24.14; Silverman et al, 1984). It is this latter type of heart which should be considered as a 'forme fruste' of an atrioventricular septal defect, not the isolated mitral cleft as promoted by Di Segni & Edwards (1983).

Atrioventricular septal defects with shunting at ventricular level

The so-called 'isolated atrioventricular canal' type of ventricular septal defect is another source of confusion. Examples are to be found with all the morphological features of an atrioventricular septal defect in which the bridging leaflets are attached to the underside of the atrial septum. In our experience such hearts are rare, although

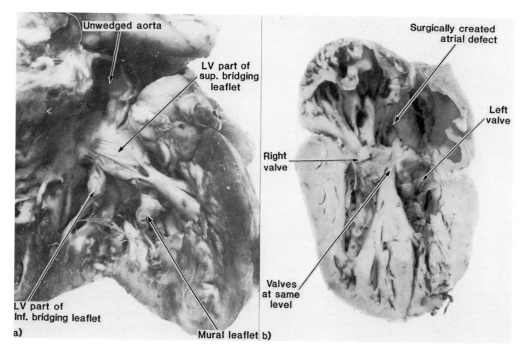

Fig. 24.14 An atrioventricular septal defect with intact atrial and septal structures. (a) The typical trifoliate left valve and unwedged subaortic outflow tract. (b) The valve leaflets attached to the contiguous atrial and ventricular septal structures at the same level (no atrioventricular septum). The defect within the atrial septum was surgically created.

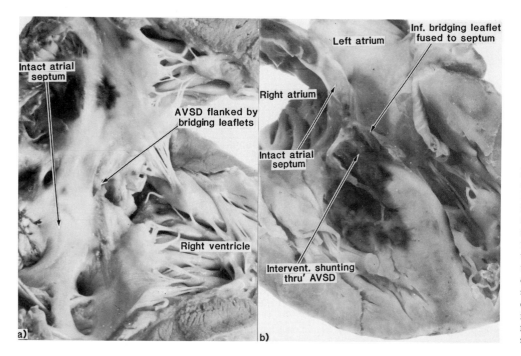

Fig. 24.15 Atrioventricular septal defects with common valve orifice, but with the potential only for interventricular shunting. (a) The right-sided chambers. Note the superior bridging leaflet extending through the septal defect. The valve leaflets co-apt against the underside of the atrial septum during ventricular diastole. (b) A similar heart cut in simulated 'four chamber' section showing the inferior bridging leaflet which is firmly adherent to the atrial septum.

they can be found with common orifice (Fig. 24.15) or separate right and left atrioventricular valves. The hearts with the potential only for interventricular shunting through the atrioventricular septal defect have all the expected morphological stigmata of the overall group. But many more hearts are described using this term which have no features of an atrioventricular septal defect. Most prove to be no more than perimembranous ventricular septal defects extending into the inlet septum (Moulaert,

1978; Soto et al, 1980; Milo et al, 1980). Several authorities (Neufeld et al, 1961; Rastelli et al, 1968b; LaCorte et al, 1976) describe the defect found with a straddling tricuspid valve as an 'atrioventricular canal' type of defect. This is fallacious and potentially misleading. In an atrioventricular septal defect, the ventricular septum (although scooped out and to this extent deficient) usually runs to the crux of the heart. Because of this, the atrioventricular conduction tissues arise from the regular atrioventricular node albeit deviated in postero-inferior direction. The distinguishing feature of nearly all hearts with straddling right-sided tricuspid valves is that the inlet muscular septum does not extend to the crux. The atrioventricular conduction tissues then arise from an anomalous node (Milo et al, 1979). It is vital to distinguish the defect in hearts with straddling tricuspid valves from atrioventricular septal defects (see Ch. 28). Very rarely atrioventricular septal defects with common orifice can be found with the septum deviated from the crux as in straddling tricuspid valve (Pillai et al, 1985). In these the ventricular conduction axis arises from an anomalous posterolateral node.

Atrioventricular septal defect with common valve orifice

The distinguishing feature of these hearts is that the common atrioventricular junction is guarded by a common five-leaflet atrioventricular valve. As in the variant with separate right and left valves, the size of the atrial defect can vary from being huge (common atrium) to the situation in which the lower edge of the atrial septum reaches down to the plane of the atrioventricular junction. At first sight it may be difficult to recognise the common orifice in the latter variety. Although there is an atrioventricular communication during ventricular diastole (when the valve leaflets are open), this can be completely obliterated during systole. More usually the atrial septum is not so well-formed. Then there is a gap between the septum and the atrial surface of the bridging leaflets. Oval fossa and sinus venosus defects may coexist. The conventional subdivision of atrioventricular septal defects with common orifice depends on the papillary muscle attachment of the superior bridging leaflet, but this should not obscure the significant variability to be found in the arrangement of the inferior bridging leaflet. The variability of the superior leaflet was first noted and highlighted by Rastelli and colleagues (1966). They described three major types. In the first, the bridging leaflet was mostly contained in the left ventricle and was usually tightly tethered to the crest of the ventricular septum (Fig. 24.16a). Its commissure was supported by the medial papillary muscle. In the second type the

leaflet extended more into the right ventricle, not being attached to the ventricular septum, but being attached to an anomalous right ventricular papillary muscle (Fig. 24.16b). In the final type the free-floating bridging leaflet extended even further into the right ventricle and

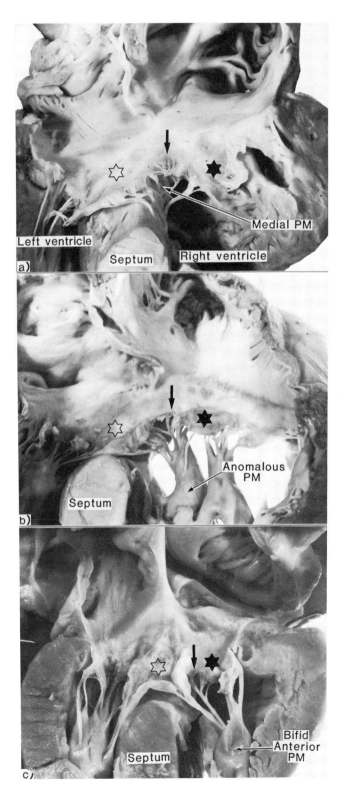

Fig. 24.16 The Rastelli classification of hearts with common atrioventricular orifice depends on the extent to which the superior bridging leaflet is committed to the right ventricle. (a) A so-called 'type A'. There is minimal bridging and the commissure between the superior bridging leaflet (open star) and the antero-superior leaflet of the right ventricle (solid star) is supported by the medial papillary muscle. (b) Type B. There is increased bridging, a concomitant diminution in size of the anterosuperior leaflet and the commissure is supported by an anomalous right ventricular papillary muscle. The medial papillary muscle is absent. (c) The sequence continues in the type C, where the commissure, together with the supero-inferior commissure, is supported by the bifid anterior papillary muscle (PM). The medial papillary muscle is again absent. The superior bridging leaflet is no more divided in the type A than in the type C.

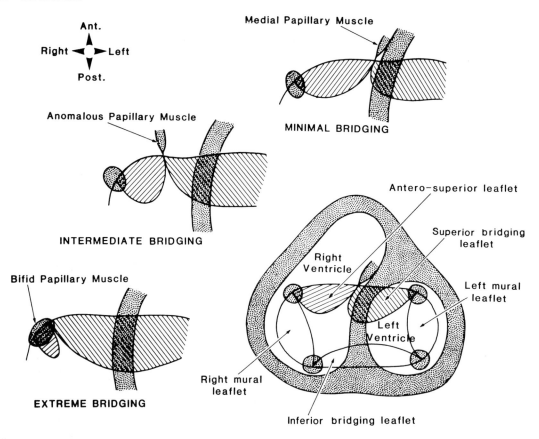

Fig. 24.17 A diagrammatic representation of the anatomy illustrated in Fig. 24.16, showing how the degree of bridging of the superior leaflet varies according to the position of the commissure between the anterosuperior and superior bridging leaflets.

was attached to the anterior papillary muscle (Fig. 24.16c). Some subsequent investigators (Ugarte et al, 1976) were unable to confirm all of Rastelli's observations, in particular the existence of their second variety (so-called 'Rastelli types B'). We (Piccoli et al, 1979b) endorsed completely Rastelli's observations, but disagreed in the interpretation of the findings along the lines suggested by Ugarte et al (1976). Rastelli and colleagues (1966) argued that, in their type A, the 'anterior leaflet' was cleft, whereas in their type B and C it was undivided. Overall they interpreted the results in terms of a quadrifoliate atrioventricular valve. Our observations (Piccoli et al, 1979b) and those of Ugarte et al (1976) had indicated that the leaflet was as undivided in type A as in the other types (Fig. 24.17). The only difference was in the amount by which the superior bridging leaflet was committed to the right ventricle. The division between the two superior valve segments in the type A malformation, interpreted by Rastelli et al (1966) as a cleft, is supported by the normally positioned medial papillary muscle of the right ventricle (Anderson et al, 1985). Indeed, when viewed from the right ventricular outlet, it is indistinguishable from the normal antero-septal tricuspid valve commissure. Although not commented upon by Rastelli et al (1966), there is equal variability in

the arrangement of the inferior bridging leaflet. This relates not so much to the extent of bridging, since almost always it extends well into both ventricles, as to its tethering. Sometimes, it is divided by a well-formed raphe which is firmly attached to the ventricular septum. In other hearts it is tethered by chords as it crosses the septum, while in others it floats quite freely (Penkoske et al, 1985).

The left ventricular outflow tract

By virtue of its anterior and unwedged position, the left ventricular outflow tract is particularly susceptible to obstruction. This is true irrespective of whether there is a common orifice or separate right and left valves. On anatomic examination the tract almost always seems narrowed (Fig. 24.18). The length of the outflow tract and the extent of the narrowing is more marked in defects with the superior bridging leaflet firmly fused to the septal crest ('ostium primum' defects) (see Fig. 24.9) (Ebels et al, 1986). This potential obstruction is not reflected by pressure measurements during life. It is additional lesions compromising an already narrow channel which are responsible for haemodynamically significant obstruction,

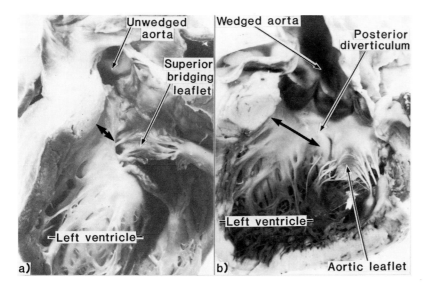

Fig. 24.18 The capacious outflow tract of the wedged subaortic area of the normal heart (b) compared with the intrinsically narrow outflow tract of an atrioventricular septal defect (a).

or alternatively the effect of surgery (Lappen et al, 1983). Any of the lesions which produce subaortic stenosis in the normal heart can produce similar problems with even greater facility in atrioventricular septal defects (Piccoli et al, 1982). These lesions are septal bulging, subaortic diaphragmatic or tunnel lesions (Lappen et al, 1983), anomalous insertion of left ventricular papillary muscles (Chin et al, 1983) and 'fibrous tissue tags'. The 'fibrous tissue tags', although frequently termed 'endocardial cushion tissue' (Gomes et al, 1980), almost certainly have nothing to do with the embryonic endocardial cushions (see Ch. 4). They originate from the fibrous tissue which abounds in the outflow tract, and can take origin from the partially formed interventricular membranous septum, from the anterior bridging leaflet tissue or from anomalous fibrous tissue.

Atrioventricular conduction tissues in atrioventricular septal defect

The atrioventricular conduction tissues have the same basic disposition in all types of atrioventricular septal defects. They have been well described by Lev (1958), and Feldt and colleagues (1970). Our own observations (Thiene & Anderson, 1978; Wenink et al, 1978; Thiene et al, 1981) endorse these earlier findings. The basic problem relates to the lack of the atrioventricular septal structures, this being the area of the normal heart when the atrioventricular node becomes the penetrating atrioventricular bundle. Because of the atrioventricular septal defect, the inferior limb of the atrial septum makes contact with the ventricular septum only at the crux. It is only at the crux, therefore, that the atrioventricular conduction axis can penetrate. The entire nodal area is displaced posteriorly and inferiorly. Although demarcated by a well-formed triangle (Fig. 24.19), this nodal triangle is not the same as the normal triangle of Koch. Nonetheless, it does provide

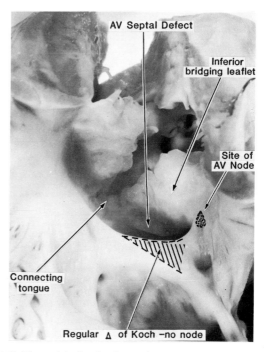

Fig. 24.19 The nodal triangle of an atrioventricular septal defect with separate right and left valve orifices compared with the regular triangle of Koch. The conduction axis penetrates at the apex of the nodal triangle (see Figs. 24.20, 24.21). The specimen is orientated as would be seen by the surgeon at operation.

a guide to the site of the penetrating bundle. From this posteriorly deviated penetrating bundle, an elongated non-branching bundle runs either on the crest of the inlet septum or to its left side, being covered by the inferior bridging leaflet. The bundle branches are found more posteriorly than in the normal heart. Only the right bundle branch extends along the crest in the bare area found in the presence of a common orifice (Fig. 24.20). In hearts with separate orifices this part of the axis is covered over

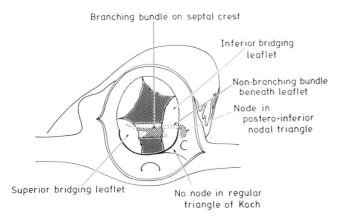

Fig. 24.20 A representation of the disposition of the conduction axis in an atrioventricular septal defect with a common valve orifice. The drawing represents the view of the surgeon approaching through the right atrium.

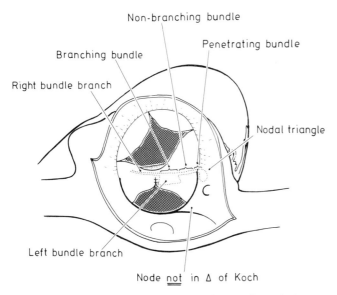

Fig. 24.21 The conduction tissue disposition in an atrioventricular septal defect with separate right and left valve orifices ('ostium primum atrial septal defect'). The orientation is the same as Fig. 24.20.

by the connecting tongue of leaflet tissue (Fig. 24.21). Because of the anterior position of the left ventricular outflow tract, the left bundle branch is less at risk during surgical relief of any outflow tract obstruction than in the normal heart.

Associated malformations

Any lesion can coexist with an atrioventricular septal defect if it is anatomically possible. We have already mentioned some of the more frequent, notably atrial septal malformations and left ventricular outflow tract obstructions. Common atrioventricular valves can be found with any heart with two atrioventricular connexions (that is,

with double inlet ventricle, discordant or ambiguous atrioventricular connections as well as with a concordant atrioventricular connexion). But the anatomy is quite different in double inlet (see Ch. 26) and discordant (see Ch. 35) connexions as compared with that in a concordant atrioventricular connexion. For this reason we prefer not to categorise common orifice found with these other connexions along with atrioventricular septal defects. Thus, we reserve the term 'atrioventricular septal defect' for those hearts with biventricular atrioventricular connexions. Atrioventricular septal defects in these settings usually have concordant ventriculo-arterial connexions, but they can be found with other ventriculo-arterial connexions. Complete transposition is rare, but it is by no means uncommon to find double outlet right ventricle, particularly when there is atrial isomerism (see Ch. 36). Of the other associated lesions, tetralogy of Fallot or pulmonary stenosis are particularly important, as is presence of a second muscular ventricular septal defect. Because of the frequent left ventricular obstruction, coarctation is a particularly common accompaniment.

Chamber dominance

Most usually in atrioventricular septal defects, be there separate right and left valves or a common orifice, the right and left atrioventricular junctions are of comparable diameter and the ventricles are of similar size. This usual variety can therefore be described as the balanced form. Bharati & Lev (1973) pointed out the significant variations that exist when the common atrioventricular junction is committed primarily to the right ventricle (right ventricular dominance) or to the left ventricle (left ventricular dominance – Fig. 24.22). The right ventricular dominant form is always associated with clinically significant hypoplasia of left ventricular and aortic structures. The left ventricular dominant type almost always has right ventricular and pulmonary arterial hypoplasia. Although the distinction is sometimes difficult, right ventricular dominant atrioventricular septal defects should be distinguished from hearts with common orifice and double inlet right ventricle. Similarly left ventricular dominance should be differentiated from double inlet left ventricle via a common valve (Smallhorn et al, 1981). In this respect it is particularly important to recognise those hearts with common orifice which are intermediate between true double inlet left ventricle and atrioventricular septal defects. These are the hearts with malalignment of the inlet septum which are analogous to straddling tricuspid valve (Pillai et al, 1984). Because of the malaligned inlet septum they have an anomalous posterolateral conduction tissue axis. Ventricular dominance is now well recognised. The concept of chamber dominance can equally be extended to the atria. With ventricular dominance, either the entire right or left side of the heart is predominant. In the arrangement of

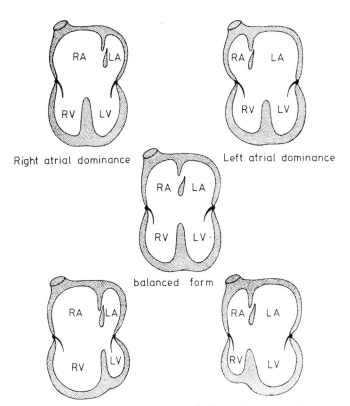

Fig. 24.22 The communication between the atrial (RA, LA) and the ventricular (RV, LV) chambers can vary markedly between different atrioventricular septal defects. Usually the junction is equally shared, giving a balanced pattern. However, there may be dominance of either the right or left sides of the heart. The concept of dominance can be extended to include those hearts in which either the right or left atrium is dominant and the only exit for the non-dominant atrium is through the atrioventricular septal defect.

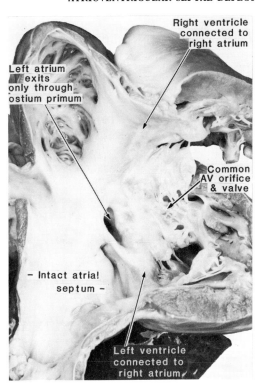

Fig. 24.23 The atrioventricular junction is an atrioventricular septal defect with common valve orifice and right atrial dominance. The common valve is equally shared between the ventricles, but is connected almost exclusively to the right atrium. The only exit from the left atrium is via the atrioventricular septal defect ('ostium primum'). (Photographed and reproduced by kind permission of Dr J. R. Zuberbuhler, Children's Hospital of Pittsburgh.)

atrial dominance, the common atrioventricular junction is equally shared by the ventricles, but is exclusively connected either to the right or left atrium (Fig. 24.22). The only exit for the other atrium is through the 'ostium primum atrial septal defect' (Fig. 24.23). The term 'double outlet atrium' (Horiuchi et al, 1976) may be appropriate in this context, but not in the absence of an atrioventricular septal defect (Alizivatos et al, 1985). We believe it also makes sense to consider these as atrioventricular septal defects with right or left atrial dominance.

MORPHOGENESIS

Almost all the literature concerning the morphogenesis of atrioventricular septal defects has taken as its starting point the assumption that the atrioventricular endocardial cushions contribute markedly to the formation of both the definitive septal structures and also to the atrioventricular valve leaflets (Van Mierop, 1970). It is because of these assumptions that the term 'endocardial cushion defect' has

enjoyed such widespread popularity. Regrettably the concepts underscoring this approach do not bear rigorous examination, either from the stance of embryological evidence or of the anatomy of the definitive lesions. It is very attractive to argue that complete failure of fusion of the endocardial cushions will result in a 'complete' defect. Partial failure of fusion could then, arguably, result in the 'ostium primum atrial septal defect' and, at the same time, account for the 'cleft in the anterior leaflet of the mitral valve'. But something much more fundamental must happen to produce an atrioventricular septal defect. We have already seen how the anatomy of atrioventricular septal defects is different from the normal in more respects than a simple hole in the septum and a 'cleft' in the anterior leaflet of the mitral valve. Indeed, the very fact that isolated clefts in the aortic leaflet of the mitral valve do exist, but have totally different anatomy from atrioventricular septal defects, is very strong evidence that the abnormal development is more than simple failure of fusion of the embryonic endocardial cushions.

It is very likely that an initial failure of fusion of the cushions is the first step in the production of an atrioventricular septal defect. But the cushions do not go on to produce the valve leaflets and the septal structures.

Valve leaflet formation is a very late developmental event, a fact well known to German embryologists and anatomists in the nineteenth century (Bernays, 1876; Gegenbaur, 1885). Thus, the abnormal atrioventricular valve leaflets in atrioventricular septal defects will be produced and sculpted from the abnormal ventricular mass of this lesion. It is therefore necessary to look for the mechanism which results in the development of a common atrioventricular junction with an unsprung aorta. This is where it is important to understand the real function of the atrioventricular endocardial cushions. They act as the forerunner of the atrioventricular valves in early development and serve to glue together the central point of the developing atrioventricular junction. Having glued together the superior and inferior aspects of the junction, the aortic outflow tract can then be incorporated into the developing left ventricle (see Ch. 4). The leaflets of the mitral and tricuspid valves are then subsequently delaminated from the ventricular walls or sculpted from the primary fold in the setting of a normally wedged subaortic outflow tract (Wenink & Gittenberger de Groot, 1985). If the endocardial cushions do not fuse together, then this focal point for subsequent development of the ventricles is lost. The atrioventricular junction will not grow in 'spectacle' fashion. Instead, its superior and inferior margins will spring apart. Additionally it will not be possible for the subaortic outflow tract to be incorporated into the developing left ventricle in wedged position. Thus, the initial failure of fusion of the endocardial cushions will produce the basic ventricular mass of an atrioventricular septal defect. The maldevelopment will also explain the presence of the basic septal defect itself. This is because, in the normal, the fusing cushions also provide the focal point for appropriate development and alignment of the atrial and ventricular septal structures. The precise type of atrioventricular septal defect will then depend upon the way in which the atrioventricular valve leaflets are delaminated and developed from the abnormal ventricular mass. In summary, although the initial insult resulting in an atrioventricular septal defect almost certainly is failure of fusion of the endocardial cushions, it is simplistic to suggest that the septal defect and valve malformations all result from failure of the development of tissue of 'cushion origin'. As far as we are aware, there is no evidence from embryology to support this popular notion, but a lot of evidence which negates it (Allwork, 1982; Wenink & Gittenberger de Groot, 1985).

PATHOPHYSIOLOGY

Atrial shunting

There is almost always an atrial component of the defect, across which there is a left-to-right shunt. In about a third of patients, even those with separate right and left valves,

there is also a very small right-to-left shunt (Park et al, 1976). In the case of a common atrium, more right-to-left atrial shunting occurs. This is both because of lack of a septum and because of the high incidence of anomalous systemic venous connexions. Particularly in cases with atrial isomerism, the blood from the left superior caval vein, instead of flowing into the coronary sinus and thence into the right atrium, empties directly into the left upper corner of the atrium. Coronary venous blood drains by tiny veins directly into the atrium. Bidirectional shunting at atrial level produces complete mixing of pulmonary and systemic venous return in about half of the patients (Rastelli et al, 1968c). In the extremely rare variant characterised by right atrial dominance, malalignment of the atrial septum with the ventricular septum results in a considerable right-to-left shunt at atrial level (Corwin et al, 1983; Alizivatos et al, 1985).

Ventricular shunting

If there is a large ventricular component of the defect, the direction of flow through it will depend upon resistance to outflow from the two ventricles. Thus, subaortic stenosis or coarctation will favour left-to-right shunting whereas right ventricular outflow tract obstruction and pulmonary vascular obstructive disease will favour right-to-left shunting. When none of these complicating factors is present, the shunt is left-to-right, as in simple ventricular septal defect.

Volume loading

An atrial left-to-right shunt produces right ventricular volume overload, whereas a ventricular shunt in this direction primarily overloads the left ventricle (Culpepper et al, 1978). In patients with a common valve orifice, volume overload of the left ventricle is much more marked than that of the right (Thanopoulos et al, 1978).

Valve leaflets guarding the atrioventricular junction are usually incompetent, be there a common orifice or separate ones. Thus, left and right atrioventricular valve regurgitation occur, with the former usually being more important because of its effect upon the systemic ventricle. This regurgitation produces further volume overloading of the ventricles. A depressed left ventricular ejection fraction has been found by some authors (Thanopoulos et al, 1978) but not by others (Culpepper et al, 1978; Jarmakani et al, 1978).

It is convenient to separate septal defects from valve regurgitation in order to understand the pathophysiology better. In reality, they are inseparable. For example, the regurgitant jet through the left atrioventricular valve frequently is directed toward the right atrium, thereby having a similar haemodynamic effect to a left ventricular/right atrial fistula. If there were such a thing as a pure shunt from left ventricle to right atrium in an atrioventricular septal defect, it would be obligatory (Rudolph, 1970), since it would not depend on pulmonary vascular resistance. Excessive flow through the left and right components of the atrioventricular valve occurs both because of the left-to-right shunts and the valvar regurgitation.

Pressure loading

The right ventricular pressure is most commonly elevated because of a large ventricular component of the defect. Right ventricular hypertension, however, is very occasionally due to an associated partition within the left atrium (Thilenius et al, 1976) or double outlet right atrium with an obstructive interatrial communication (Alizivatos et al, 1985). It also occurs in some patients with isolated ostium primum defects, presumably secondary to left atrioventricular valve regurgitation (Brandt et al, 1972; Macartney et al, 1979). An alternative explanation for pulmonary hypertension is the presence of an obligatory left ventricular to right atrial shunt (Rudolph, 1970). As there is usually no right ventricular outflow tract obstruction, right ventricular hypertension leads to pulmonary hypertension. This in turn sets the stage for the development of pulmonary vascular obstructive disease. Newfeld and colleagues (1977) found grade IV Heath & Edwards (1958) changes in a 10½-month-old infant with a common valve orifice. The youngest patient with an isolated ventricular septal defect who had such severe changes was 22 months old. The general tendency, however, was for patients with atrioventricular septal defects and common orifice to have pulmonary vascular disease of a similar severity at a given age to those with large isolated ventricular septal defects. After the age of 2 years, the majority had pulmonary vascular disease of grade III–V, though this group may have been selected by virtue of having had an autopsy. The distribution of lesions within the lung has been shown by serial sections to be more like that found in complete transposition than ventricular septal defect (Haworth, 1984). A large component of the resistance is due to strategically placed proximal rather than distal lesions.

It is of some interest that, in patients with atrioventricular septal defects, there was a very poor correlation between measured pulmonary vascular resistance and the degree of histological pulmonary vascular disease (Newfeld et al, 1977). This suggests temporary rather than permanent elevation of pulmonary vascular resistance under the conditions of cardiac catheterisation. This in turn may explain the difference of opinion as to whether Down's syndrome predisposes patients with atrioventricular septal defects to the development of pulmonary vascular disease. Newfeld and colleagues (1977), on the basis of histology, felt that it did not. In contrast, Chi & Krovetz (1975) provided convincing evidence that, in patients with similar cardiac defects, pulmonary hypertension and elevated pulmonary vascular resistance were commoner in those with Down's syndrome. These divergent observations could be reconciled if one argued that patients with Down's syndrome (who have a strong tendency to upper airways obstruction) were more susceptible to alveolar hypoventilation during cardiac catheterisation than otherwise normal patients. Alveolar hypoventilation would undoubtedly raise pulmonary vascular resistance (Macartney et al, 1969).

PRESENTATION AND SYMPTOMATOLOGY

Patients with large ventricular components, severe left atrioventricular valve regurgitation, significant left ventricular hypoplasia or complicating associated lesions such as coarctation of the aorta present with severe heart failure in early infancy. If the ventricular component was the only problem, there would be a 'latent' period of 2–3 months after birth before presentation. Unfortunately, the other problems listed frequently result in severe failure in the first month of life. Patients without these complicating factors may well escape detection of heart disease in infancy. They then present with an incidental murmur or, in the case of a common atrium, with mild cyanosis.

CLINICAL FINDINGS

Infants in heart failure mimic patients with a large isolated ventricular septal defect, except that they may present earlier. The peripheral pulses are usually normal, but sometimes reduced in the presence of severe uncompensated failure or left ventricular hypoplasia (Freedom et al, 1978). The precordium is active. A systolic thrill, maximal at the lower left sternal border, suggests the presence of interventricular shunting. The first heart sound is normal, whereas the second is usually widely split, and may or may not vary with respiration. The sound of pulmonary valve closure is accentuated. The pan-systolic murmur at the lower left sternal border usually radiates much better toward the axilla than in isolated ventricular septal defect because of the associated left atrioventricular valve regurgitation. Equally, the mid-diastolic murmur due to excessive forward flow through the left atrioventricular valve is not localised as in ventricular septal defect. Because of associated excessive flow through the right atrioventricular valve, it is also well heard at the lower left sternal border. Cyanosis is not usually present at this age; if it is, it is the result of pulmonary venous desaturation, a common atrium, or right atrial dominance.

Older asymptomatic children present in the same way as do children with other forms of atrial septal defect (see Ch. 22). For some reason, the anticipated apical pan-systolic murmur is not found unless left atrioventricular valve regurgitation is severe. A patient who appears to have an atrial septal defect uncomplicated except by mild cyanosis probably has a common atrium or right atrial dominance.

Infancy is occasionally uneventful, particularly in those patients with Down's syndrome. The patient then presents later in childhood with the Eisenmenger syndrome. Cyanosis is present, and the systolic and diastolic murmurs noted above are usually reduced or absent. A murmurless heart is less likely than in, say, ventricular septal defect, because of atrioventricular valve regurgitation. Pulmonary valve closure is even more accentuated, and the second heart sound may become single. An early diastolic murmur of pulmonary regurgitation may supervene.

INVESTIGATIONS

Chest radiography

The heart and aortic arch are usually on the left. There is generalised cardiac enlargement in proportion to the volume overload of the two ventricles. Because of the valvar regurgitation present, the heart may be enlarged even in the absence of a left-to-right shunt. In other words, cardiac enlargement may be present even when there is severe right ventricular outflow tract obstruction or pulmonary vascular obstructive disease. The pulmonary trunk is prominent and peripheral vasculature engorged except in the presence of right ventricular outflow tract obstruction. High kilovoltage filtered beam chest radiography (Deanfield et al, 1980) may show left bronchial isomerism. If so, interruption of the inferior caval vein, common atrium, or both should be suspected (Macartney et al, 1980b).

Electrovectorcardiography

A highly distinctive pattern of abnormalities is present (Toscano-Barbosa et al, 1956). The P wave axis is usually normal, except in the presence of left isomerism when a superior P wave axis is usually found (Ongley et al, 1976). Left atrial hypertrophy and less commonly, right atrial hypertrophy, are found in about 20% of patients. First degree heart block was found in 93% of patients with common orifice and 70% of patients with separate right and left atrioventricular valves (Ongley et al, 1976). The superiorly orientated frontal QRS loop is manifested by dominant S waves in leads III and aVF. When the frontal QRS loop is displayed or constructed, it is seen to be counterclockwise (see Ch. 11). The further the mean axis is deviated upwards and to the right, the more likely is there to be a common valve orifice. The initial portion of the QRS loop is directed downward and to the right in 93% of cases. This characteristic feature separates atrioventricu-

lar septal defects quite well from those other lesions with a superiorly orientated, counter-clockwise frontal plane loop (such as complete transposition with ventricular septal defect or double outlet right ventricle with subpulmonary defect, each with or without pulmonary stenosis or coarctation). Tricuspid atresia is easily distinguished by the lack of right ventricular forces in the precordial leads. In atrioventricular septal defects a delay in right ventricular depolarisation is almost invariable, indicating right ventricular volume overload. A qR pattern in the right precordial leads in the presence of an otherwise typical electrocardiogram suggests left ventricular hypoplasia (Freedom et al, 1978) though it also occurs in 20% of patients with common orifice without other complicating features (Ongley et al, 1976). The superiorly orientated frontal axis frequently prevents left ventricular hypertrophy from manifesting itself on the precordial leads. Prolongation of the QRS interval occurs in 60% of patients with common orifice and 38% with separate right and left valve orifices (Ongley et al, 1976).

Echocardiography

M-mode echocardiography shows enlargement of the right ventricle. Left ventricular enlargement is also seen in the presence of interventricular shunting or left atrioventricular valve regurgitation. There is paradoxical septal motion in presence of separate valve orifices ('ostium primum defects') provided that left atrioventricular valve regurgitation is not too severe. Prolonged diastolic septal apposition of the superior leaflet of the left atrioventricular valve and marked reduplication of its systolic image are also characteristic features. No atrial septum is seen on scanning from the right to the left valve. On scanning in the long axis of the heart, the left valve is seen to be situated more anteriorly than normal. A ventricular septal defect may be identified if present. Apparent movement of valve leaflet tissue across the septum strongly suggests a common orifice (Williams & Rudd, 1974; Pieroni et al, 1975). Sometimes, however, the valve tissue *appears* to move across the septum when there are separate right and left valves (Hagler, 1976). The distinction between a common valve and separate right and left orifices is made more readily from the subcostal window (Sutherland et al, 1980; Fernandez Aceytuno et al, 1982). A ventricular component is likely to be present when a large atrioventricular valve is seen to occupy completely the space between the anterior and posterior heart walls, straddling a ventricular septum which is visualised when scanning the ventricular cavity. On scanning from the common valve to the aorta, the right component of the valve appears close to the aortic valve. When no ventricular component is present, two atrioventricular orifices are seen separated by a septum.

Cross-sectional echocardiography is diagnostic (Hagler

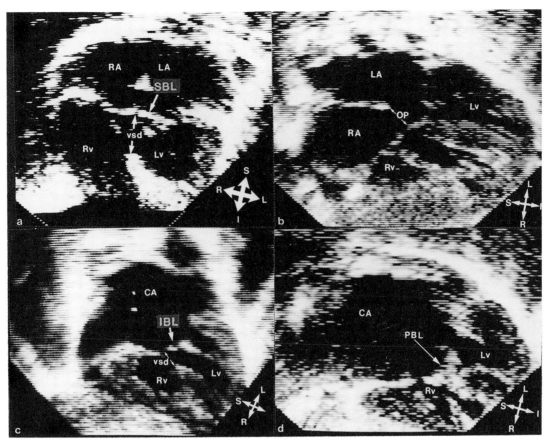

Fig. 24.24 (a) Foreshortened apical four chamber cut in patient with common atrioventricular orifice. The superior bridging leaflet (SBL) is attached to the crest of the interventricular septum, but there is an interventricular communication (vsd) between the chords. (b) Subcostal four chamber cut to demonstrate two atrioventricular valves at the same level beneath 'ostium primum atrial septal defect' (OP). (c) Subcostal four chamber cut showing ventricular component (vsd) beneath inferior bridging leaflet (IBL). (d) In this patient the inferior bridging leaflet (IBL) is firmly attached to the interventricular septum. CA – common atrium; I – inferior; L – left; LA – left atrium; Lv – left ventricle; R – right; RA – right atrium; Rv – right ventricle; S – superior.

et al, 1979; Smallhorn et al, 1982a,c). Apical and subcostal four chamber cuts demonstrate absence of the atrioventricular septum. This is shown either by the bridging leaflets crossing the ventricular septum when a ventricular component is present (Figs. 24.24a, 24.25, 24.26) or else by origin of leaflets at the same level from the crest of the ventricular septum (Fig. 24.24b,d). Demonstration of an atrioventricular septum producing offsetting of the atrioventricular valves makes the diagnosis of atrioventricular septal defect untenable. On the other hand, lack of atrioventricular valve offsetting is seen in a number of conditions which are not atrioventricular septal defects (such as double inlet ventricle, perimembranous inlet ventricular septal defect and straddling tricuspid valve; Smallhorn et al, 1982b). Thus, further information is required to establish the diagnosis of atrioventricular septal defect. Almost always it will be possible to demonstrate an 'ostium primum' septal defect (Figs. 24.24, 24.25, 24.27) or a common atrium (Figs. 24.24c,d, 24.28) on four chamber views. Such a defect never has atrial septal tissue in its floor

(except occasionally at its extreme postero-inferior and antero-superior margins). This feature becomes most important when one considers the (admittedly rare) combination of absence of one atrioventricular connexion with straddling of the other atrioventricular valve (Ho et al, 1982) in association with a large atrial septal defect at the oval fossa. Unless the presence of atrial septal tissue between the absent connexion and the straddling valve is recognised, this condition may easily be confused with atrioventricular septal defect.

Rarely, the interatrial septum in atrioventricular septal defects extends down to the level of the atrioventricular junction and either fuses with (Fig. 24.26a) or is in systolic contact with (Fig. 24.25) the bridging leaflets. In such cases there is usually a ventricular communication beneath the leaflets, but the appearances are easily confused with those of a perimembranous inlet ventricular septal defect. A prominent distinguishing feature then becomes the recognition of bridging leaflets from the subcostal window (Fig. 24.26b).

An equally important key, however, is the appearance

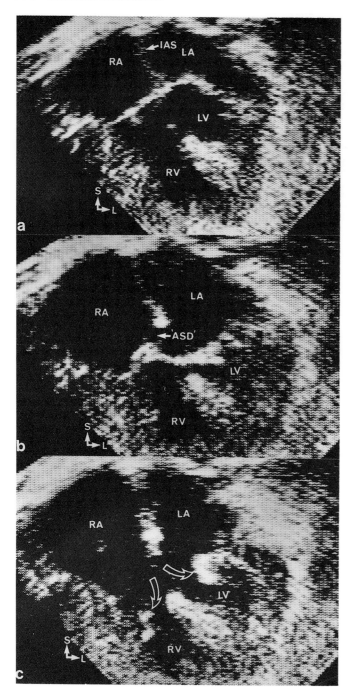

Fig. 24.25 Series of apical four chamber cuts in patient with common atrioventricular orifice. (a) In systole, the superior bridging leaflet contacts the interatrial septum (IAS), giving the impression that the interatrial septum is intact. (b) In early diastole, the superior bridging leaflet moves away from the lower margin of the interatrial septum, leaving an interatrial communication ('ASD'). (c) Later in diastole, the free floating superior bridging leaflet has moved out of the plane of the transducer, leaving only the mural leaflets (curved white arrows). L – left; LA – left atrium; LV – left ventricle; RA – right atrium; RV – right ventricle; S – superior.

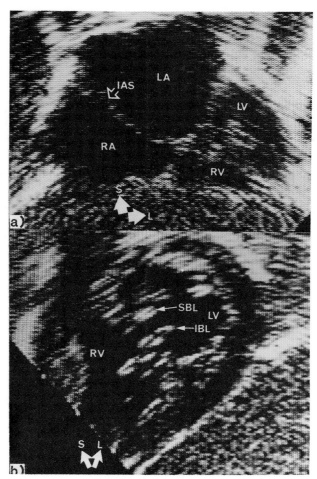

Fig. 24.26 Atrioventricular septal defect with intact atrial septum. (a) Subcostal four chamber view with transducer directed well posteriorly. Note the intact interatrial septum (IAS) on this frame. The only clue to the presence of an atrioventricular septal defect would be the fact that both atrioventricular valves are at the same level, but this is by no means specific for atrioventricular septal defect. (b) Subcostal oblique short axis cut. Note the superior (SBL) and inferior (IBL) bridging leaflets, which in real-time are easily distinguishable from the ventricular septum. These establish the diagnosis of an atrioventricular septal defect. L – left; LA – left atrium; LV – left ventricle; RA – right atrium; RV – right ventricle; S – superior.

of the left atrioventricular valve, particularly as seen in precordial short axis scans from the aortic root to the left ventricle (Fig. 24.29, 24.30). In perimembranous inlet ventricular septal defect, the left valve is a normal mitral valve. As the transducer moves down from the aortic valve, so it cuts the 'anterior' leaflet of the mitral valve over the quite broad area of mitral/aortic continuity. The normal anterior leaflet then appears as a very solid structure bowing slightly into the left ventricular outflow tract. As the scan is continued inferiorly, so the typical fish-mouth appearance of the valve appears (Ch. 12). A cleft in the otherwise normal anterior mitral leaflet, pointing toward the left ventricular outflow tract is *not* a feature of atrioventricular septal defects (Fig. 24.29 – lower panel) (Smallhorn et al, 1982a,b,c, see Ch. 43).

If a similar scan is attempted in an atrioventricular septal defect, none of the above features are recognised. The area of aortic/left atrioventricular valve continuity is

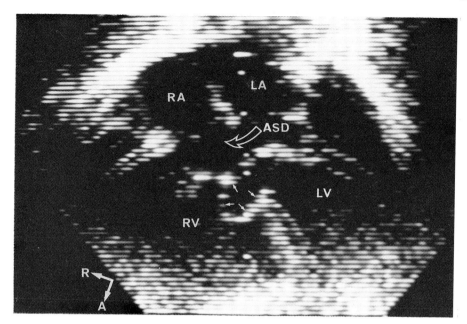

Fig. 24.27 Atrioventricular septal defect with no ventricular component in apical four chamber cut. The pocket of valve tissue (small white arrows) bulging from the left to right ventricle, gives the erroneous impression that there is an interventricular communication. In fact, the only communication present between the sides of the heart is the atrial component (ASD). A – anterior; LA – left atrium; LV – left ventricle; R – right; RA – right atrium; RV – right ventricle.

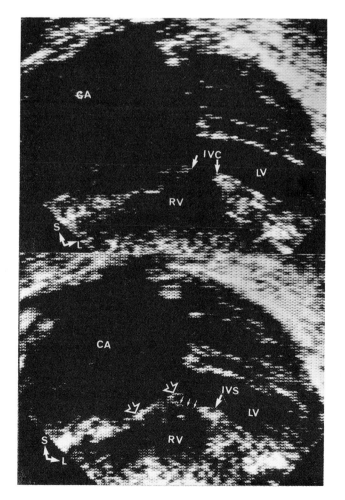

much attenuated. Instead of a bifoliate valve with a solid anterior leaflet which forms the back wall of the left ventricular outlet, a trifoliate valve is seen (Fig. 24.29 – upper panel). Furthermore, transducer rotation more or less into a sagittal plane is required before this trifoliate valve is seen to best advantage. This is because of displacement of the right margin of the left atrioventricular valve down the septum (Beppu et al, 1980). The so-called 'cleft in the anterior mitral leaflet' points not to the left ventricular outflow tract, but to the right ventricle (Fig. 24.30) (Smallhorn et al, 1982a). Accessory chords may be seen running from the 'cleft' (in fact the functional commissure between the superior and inferior bridging leaflets) to the ventricular septum. They form one potential substrate for left ventricular outflow tract obstruction (Fig. 24.31).

The abnormal unwedged position of the aorta relative to the atrioventricular junction is so central to the nature of atrioventricular septal defects that abnormalities in this region can be observed with the transducer in almost any position. For example, a normal four chamber aortic root cut cannot be obtained from either apical or subcostal windows (Sutherland et al, 1982). Instead, from subcostally, a goose-neck deformity can be demonstrated which is comparable to the structure so familiar to angiocardiog-

Fig. 24.28 Subcostal four chamber cuts of patient with common atrium and interventricular communication at different times during the cardiac cycle. In (a) there is clearly an interventricular communication (IVC) beneath the inferior bridging leaflet, shown with hollow white arrows in (b). In (b) the interventricular communication appears to be closed because the cut has gone through a chorda (small white arrows) connecting the inferior bridging leaflet to the interventricular septum (IVS). CA – common atrium; L – left; LV – left ventricle; RV – right ventricle; S – superior.

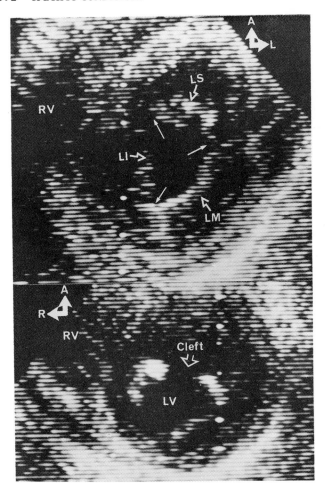

Fig. 24.29 Comparison between the trifoliate valve of an atrioventricular septal defect and an isolated mitral valve cleft. Upper panel shows clearly a trifoliate left atrioventricular valve with three commissures (long white arrows). These separate the left inferior (LI), the left superior (LS) and the left mural (LM) leaflets of the left atrioventricular valve. Lower panel in contrast, an isolated cleft is clearly in addition to a normal bileaflet mitral valve. Further cuts in these patients would demonstrate that the commissure between the left superior and left inferior leaflets of the left atrioventricular valve and atrioventricular septal defect points to the right atrium and right ventricle, whereas the cleft in a normal mitral valve points towards the left ventricular outflow tract. A – anterior; L – left; LV – left ventricle; R – right; RV – right ventricle.

raphers (Yoshida et al, 1980) (Fig. 24.32). The abnormal relationship of the left atrioventricular valve to the septum means that, in parasternal long axis cuts in diastole, what may at first sight be interpreted as anterior mitral leaflet lies much further anteriorly than usual. If the transducer is angulated slightly medially, this leaflet may be seen to cross the septum where there is a ventricular communication above it. Diastolic apposition of the left superior leaflet to the septum is normal. If it persists in systole this is strongly suggestive of potential or actual left ventricular outflow tract obstruction (Lappen et al, 1983). As has been pointed out (Piccoli et al, 1982), 'the morphology existing in atrioventricular septal defects is just sufficient to satisfy the needs for outflow from the left ventricle. Anything which compromises the morphology further might rapidly produce symptomatic obstruction'. Potential left ventricular outflow tract obstruction of this type may well be haemodynamically undetectable preoperatively. It can be unmasked by operative repair of the defect (Taylor & Somerville, 1981; Ben-Shachar et al, 1981; Lappen et al, 1983). Short and long axis views of the left atrioventricular

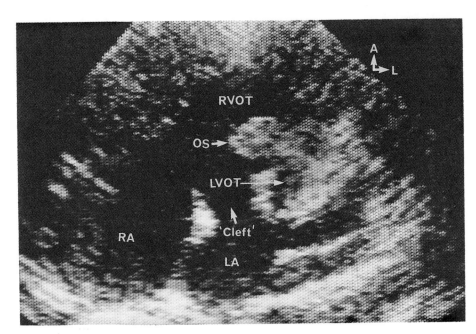

Fig. 24.30 Oblique short axis cut of left ventricular outflow tract in a patient with a common atrioventricular orifice. During diastole, the 'cleft' opens towards the right atrium (RA) and right ventricular outflow tract (RVOT). It does not open towards the left ventricular outflow tract (LVOT). A – anterior; L – left; LA – left atrium; OS – outlet septum; RA – right atrium.

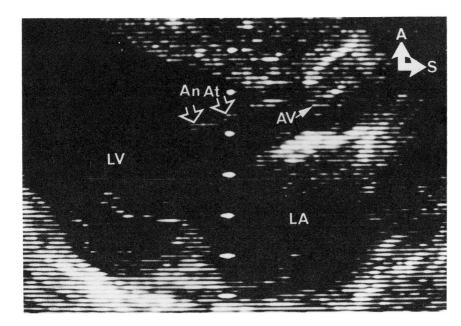

Fig. 24.31 Slightly oblique parasternal long axis cut of patient with common atrioventricular orifice. Note the anomalous attachment (AnAt) of the left atrioventricular valve to the septum, producing potential left ventricular outflow tract obstruction. A – anterior; AV – aortic valve; LA – left atrium; LV – left ventricle; S – superior.

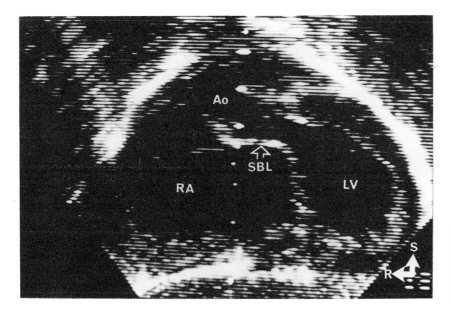

Fig. 24.32 Subcostal long axis view of left ventricle in patient with atrioventricular septal defect. Note the goose-neck deformity of the left ventricular outflow tract, produced by the superior bridging leaflet (SBL). LV – left ventricle; R – right; RA – right atrium; S – superior.

valve may also demonstrate that it has a double orifice (Warnes & Somerville, 1983). Chin and colleagues (1983) have described how the abnormal position of the papillary muscles in atrioventricular septal defects may be recognised in subcostal short axis cuts of the left ventricle. According to their account (which does not square well with anatomic observations), the anterolateral papillary muscle is displaced posteriorly from its normal position, while the posteromedial papillary muscle is in its usual site. More recently, Ebels and his colleagues (1985) have performed similar measurements which provide results more in keeping with the anatomic studies. They have shown also that the presence of regurgitation through the left valve may be correlated with the position of the commissure between the inferior bridging and left mural leaflet along with the dimensions of the latter leaflet. Equally importantly, subcostal short axis cuts demonstrate abnormalities such as single or triple papillary muscle, which appear to increase surgical mortality by increasing left ventricular inflow obstruction.

Having established the presence of an atrioventricular septal defect, two features are important for subcategorisation. On the one hand, it is necessary to establish whether the bridging leaflets are separate and discrete structures (common orifice) or whether they are joined to one another by a connecting tongue (separate right and left atrioventricular orifices). On the other hand, it is necessary to determine the level of shunting through the atrioventricular septal defect. This depends on whether the bridging leaflets are attached to or apposed to the underside of the atrial septum (ventricular shunting alone), whether they are attached to the crest of the ventricular septum (atrial shunting alone) or whether they 'float' (ventricular and atrial shunting). The rare finding of an atrioventricular septal defect with only the potential for ventricular shunting has already been discussed, along with the features which permit its differentiation from an isolated perimembranous inlet ventricular septal defect. The potential for atrial and ventricular shunting, or for atrial shunting alone, must be judged with reference to both the superior and inferior bridging leaflets.

The presence of a ventricular component between the superior bridging leaflet and the crest of the septum is best assessed from somewhat foreshortened apical four chamber cuts (see Fig. 24.24a). When no ventricular component is present, the leaflet tissue on either side may spring directly from the septum. Alternatively, an impenetrable raphe consisting of fused chords may interpose between the conjoined leaflets and the crest of the septum. Sometimes this raphe is bowed so far from left to right that it appears as a pocket of tissue bulging into the right ventricle (see Fig. 24.27). When such a pocket is present, its mouth takes the form of a gap between the superior bridging leaflet and the septum. At first sight this may be confused with an interventricular communication. In cases of doubt, contrast echocardiography with injection into the left ventricle will demonstrate accumulation of bubbles within the pocket with no passage of bubbles from the left to the right ventricle. If the raphe is not impenetrable, but contains interchordal spaces, these constitute an interventricular communication. This is usually seen with a

common valve orifice and minimal bridging of the superior leaflet (Rastelli type A) (see Fig. 24.24a). With increasing degrees of bridging, so the insertion of the chords from the superior bridging leaflet moves from the crest of the ventricular septum to its right side (Rastelli type B) and so on down to a papillary muscle at the apex of the right ventricle or on its free wall (Rastelli type C). If a transducer without a good near field is used, it may be impossible to demonstrate an apical papillary muscle. Nonetheless, the 'free-floating' superior bridging leaflet will still be obvious, appearing like a bucket handle in systole and flying out of the plane of the transducer in diastole (see Fig. 24.25).

A similar analysis of the inferior bridging leaflet can be made from the subcostal window (see Fig. 24.24c,d). The transducer is first directed well posteriorly, so that virtually only the atria are seen. Anterior angulation then brings the crux of the heart into view. Still further anterior tilting demonstrates the interventricular septum and inferior bridging leaflet. Sometimes movement of the heart makes an interventricular defect appear and disappear at different times in the cardiac cycle (Fig. 24.28).

Sometimes a ventricular component is recognisable beyond one or both of the bridging leaflets and yet a constant blob of tissue is seen separating the two atrioventricular orifices. This represents a tongue of tissue joining the two bridging leaflets. Such an appearance is characteristic of atrioventricular septal defect with separate right and left valve orifices together with a ventricular component.

Four chamber cuts also permit easy recognition of left or right ventricular or atrial dominance (Figs. 24.33, 24.34), and of common atrium (see Figs. 24.24c, d,

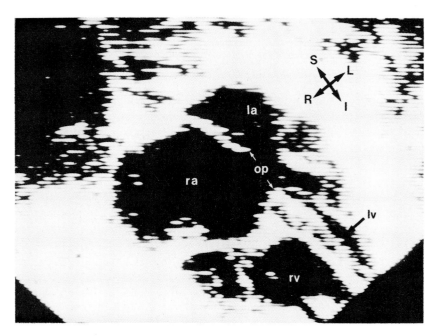

Fig. 24.33 Subcostal four chamber cut of atrioventricular septal defect with dominant right ventricle. Note that the interventricular septum is well aligned with the interatrial septum. I – inferior; L – left; la – left atrium; lv – left ventricle; op – ostium primum atrial septal defect; R – right; ra – right atrium; rv – right ventricle; S – superior.

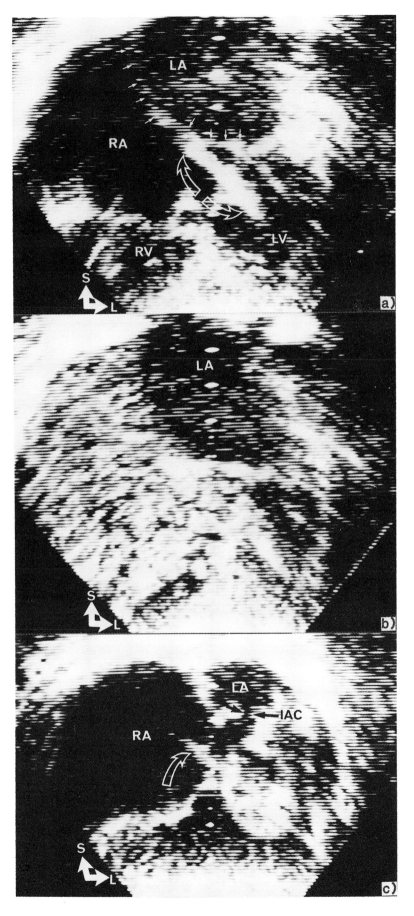

Fig. 24.34 Atrioventricular septal defect with dominant right atrium (double outlet right atrium). Apical four chamber sections. (a) The interatrial septum (small white arrows), separates the left (LA) and right (RA) atria. In this view no interatrial communication is seen. A catheter (curved white arrows) has been passed from the right atrium directly into the left ventricle (LV). (b) On injection of contrast bubbles, there is dense opacification of the left ventricle, and because of regurgitation of the left atrioventricular valve, the right atrium, but the left atrium is spare. (c) With the transducer angulated somewhat more posteriorly, the interatrial communication (IAC) can now be seen, but was obviously obstructed. The catheter (curved white arrow) is still visible. L – left; LV – left ventricle; RA – right atrium; RV – right ventricle; S – superior.

24.28). Demonstration of a strand of tissue between ostium primum and oval fossa atrial septal defects is typical of right atrial isomerism. Recognition of common atrium or a strand of this type should prompt the investigator to assess atrial arrangement and hepatic venous connexions with particular care, and to demonstrate or rule out a persistent left superior caval vein (see Ch. 19).

The assessment of *infundibular* anomalies requires a slightly different approach in hearts *with* as opposed to those *without* atrioventricular septal defects (Macartney et al, 1984). To begin with, it is unusual in hearts with associated infundibular stenosis (Figs. 24.35b, 24.36) to see overriding of the aorta in parasternal long axis sections (Fig. 24.35a). Instead, it is usually possible to demonstrate continuity between the anterior wall of aorta and the interventricular septum, as in cases where there is no infundibular stenosis (Fig. 24.35a). Thus origin of both great arteries anterior to the superior bridging leaflet in parasternal long axis cuts indicates double outlet right ventricle

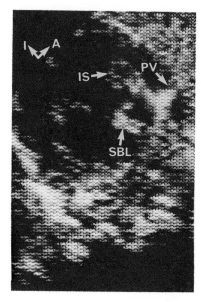

Fig. 24.36 Atrioventricular septal defect with infundibular and pulmonary valve (PV) stenosis. In this high precordial cut, mid-way between a long and short axis, the infundibular septum (IS) is clearly encroaching on the right ventricular outflow tract. A – anterior; I – inferior; SBL – superior bridging leaflet.

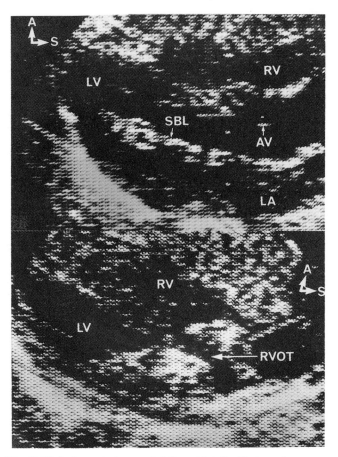

Fig. 24.35 Atrioventricular septal defect with infundibular and pulmonary valve stenosis. (a) In this parasternal long axis section, note that there is no apparent overriding of the aortic valve (AV). (b) As the transducer is rotated towards the short axis view, so the narrow right ventricular outflow tract (RVOT) is seen. A – anterior; LA – left atrium; LV – left ventricle; RV – right ventricle; S – superior; SBL – superior bridging leaflet.

(Fig. 24.37). What may be misinterpreted as anterior mitral valve leaflet in such cuts is the right portion of the superior bridging leaflet.

There is another key to the understanding of infundibular anomalies in presence of atrioventricular septal defects. This is the descent of the outlet septum (as seen from subcostally) onto the superior bridging leaflet so as to separate the two outflow tracts (Fig. 24.38). Should these outflow tracts be connected to inappropriate great arteries, there will be a discordant ventriculo-arterial connexion (transposition) (Fig. 24.39). If, on the other hand, there is outlet extension of the defect, there will be communication with both outflow tracts, double outlet right ventricle (Fig. 24.40) being the most common result. One method, when using this 'cut', of distinguishing double outlet right ventricle from tetralogy of Fallot is to draw lines under both arterial valves and drop perpendiculars down to the ventricles. The arterial valve 'belongs' to the ventricle this perpendicular enters. Thus a method which does not work for standard double outlet right ventricle seems reliable when used in hearts with an atrioventricular septal defect (Macartney et al, 1984).

In one variety of double outlet right ventricle with atrioventricular septal defect, the outlet septum encroaches upon the subaortic rather than the subpulmonary infundibulum (Fig. 24.41). The correct echocardiographic diagnosis of common atrioventricular orifice with corrected transposition has also recently been reported (Cloez et al, 1983). Here the clue was the moderator band in the left-sided ventricle. The level of attachment and morphology

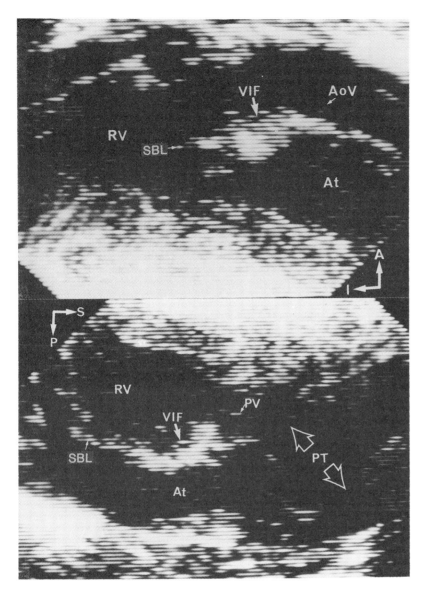

Fig. 24.37 (a) Atrioventricular septal defect with double outlet right ventricle. In this parasternal long axis view of the right ventricle (RV), the aortic valve (AoV) is seen originating from the right ventricle, above the ventriculo-infundibular fold (VIF). (b) With slight rotation of the transducer, the pulmonary valve (PV) is also seen to originate from the right ventricle (RV) and leads to the pulmonary trunk (PT). Note that both great arteries originate anterior to the superior bridging leaflet (SBL) which would not be the case were there ventriculo-arterial concordance. However, it is difficult to know on these views along whether the cut really is going through the right rather than the left ventricle. A – anterior; At – common atrium; I – inferior; P – posterior; S – superior.

of the 'septal' leaflets are of no value in assessing ventricular morphology in atrioventricular septal defects.

Range-gated Doppler velocimetry is useful in detecting the direction and degree of atrioventricular regurgitation.

As should be clear, cross-sectional echocardiography demonstrates everything that angiocardiography does and more. Thus in many circumstances there is no indication for cardiac catheterisation prior to surgery. This applies particularly to two groups, young infants with severe heart failure and older asymptomatic patients without a ventricular component. If there is any clinical suggestion of elevation of pulmonary vascular resistance in either group, however, cardiac catherisation is indicated.

Radionuclide imaging

Radionuclide imaging has no useful diagnostic role in this condition unless it is in demonstrating anomalies of systemic venous connexion.

Magnetic resonance imaging

Magnetic resonance imaging provides images similar to those of short axis echocardiographic sections (Jacobstein et al, 1985), but at much greater expense.

CARDIAC CATHETERISATION AND ANGIOCARDIOGRAPHY

These investigations are chiefly indicated when there is doubt about the level of pulmonary vascular resistance, if the non-invasive findings are atypical, if multiple associated anomalies are demonstrated, or if it is felt necessary

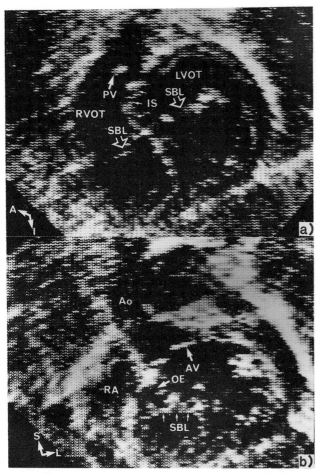

Fig. 24.38 Subcostal paracoronal sections in patient with common atrioventricular orifice. (a) In this cut, the infundibular septum (IS) separates left (LVOT) and right (RVOT) ventricular outflow tracts, above the superior bridging leaflet (SBL). (b) With slight clockwise rotation of the transducer, the ascending aorta (Ao) is seen to originate above the left ventricle and aortic valve (AV), and there is slight outlet extension (OE) of the ventricular component of the defect. A – anterior; I – inferior; L – left; PV – pulmonary valve; RA – right atrium; S – superior.

to exclude the presence of a small duct. The haemodynamic abnormalities found will be as already documented and will normally be indistinguishable from those of an atrial septal defect with or without an associated ventricular septal defect. The only unusual feature is the low course of the catheter across the atrial defect (Wakai et al, 1956). It is important to measure the left ventricular and systemic arterial pressures simultaneously. Otherwise, minor degrees of left ventricular outflow tract obstruction (which may later become more significant) will be missed (Taylor & Somerville, 1981; Lappen et al, 1983).

Angiocardiography

The best known angiocardiographic abnormality is also the one whose interpretation has proved so difficult. It is seen on the frontal projection of the left ventriculogram (Fig. 24.42). In diastole, the left ventricular outflow tract appears scooped out to give a classical 'goose-neck' deformity (Baron et al, 1964). The neck of the goose consists of densely opacified contrast medium above the superior bridging leaflet, between it and the left margin of the aortic valve (Fig. 24.43a). It is the wedged position of the aortic root which normally prevents contrast medium from becoming densely opacified at this point in hearts without atrioventricular septal defects (Fig. 24.43b). The fact that the left atrioventricular valve faces more leftward than usual elongates this band of dense opacification which is the left ventricular outflow tract. The goose-neck deformity depends upon the left ventricular origin of the aorta. If there is double outlet right ventricle the goose-neck will either be atypical (Fig. 24.44) or unrecognisable. But whatever the arterial connexion, a second abnormality – that of the body of the goose (Blieden et al, 1974) – will be present. To understand its genesis, it is essential to distinguish between the free wall and septal (if any) attachments of the left atrioventricular valve (Fig. 24.45). The line of attachment of the left component of the atrioventricular valve to the left ventricular free wall (i.e. its annulus), when traced inferomedially in diastole, runs straight across, more or less horizontally, to the right margin of the left ventricular cavity. This is in contrast to its usual upward curve to the right margin of the aortic valve (Macartney et al, 1979). This abnormal free wall attachment (present in all types of atrioventricular septal defect) reflects the 'sprung' nature of the atrioventricular junction and results in left ventricular inlet/outlet disproportion. It is characteristically smooth in outline.

By contrast, the scooped-out septum (once universally thought to be the cause of the goose-neck deformity in all varieties of atrioventricular septal defects (see e.g. Tenckhoff & Stamm, 1973; Acerete et al, 1978), can only be visualised angiocardiographically when contrast medium becomes trapped on one side of leaflet tissue while non-opacified blood enters the left ventricle on the other. Those conditions pertain only when leaflet tissue is firmly attached to the septum, that is in defects with no ventricular component (Macartney et al, 1979). Under these circumstances the septal attachments of the bridging leaflets (which usually form part of the annulus of the left atrioventricular valve) appear as sharp lines, puckered because of the numerous short chords which bind them to the septum. They are separated by the 'cleft', which apppears as a protodiastolic line of non-opacified blood (Fig. 24.42 – left panel). Because the edges of the 'cleft' are usually thickened, they also appear as a non-opacified line during systole (Rastelli et al, 1967). Thus, in defects with separate right and left valves, two separate geese, together with their necks, may be seen. A smooth goose is formed by the free wall portion of the annulus of the left atrioventricular valve. A puckered one is also present, formed by

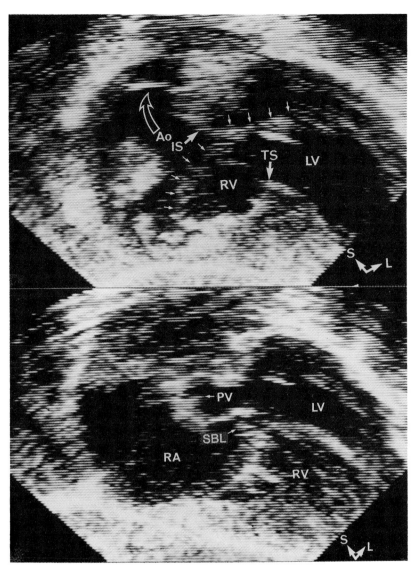

Fig. 24.39 Subcostal paracoronal sections of heart with common atrioventricular orifice and ventriculo-arterial discordance. In this heart, the infundibular septum (IS) separates the left and right ventricular outflow tracts just as in Figure 24.38, but the aorta (Ao) originates from the right ventricle (RV), and the pulmonary valve (PV) lies above the left ventricle (LV). (a) The small white arrows indicate the superior bridging leaflet and the trabecular septum (TS) separates the left (LV) and right (RV) ventricles. (b) The infundibular septum, to the left of the pulmonary valve inserts into the superior bridging leaflet (SBL). L – left; RA – right atrium; S – superior.

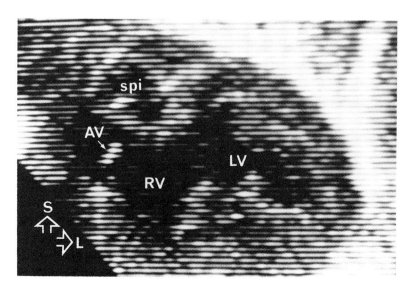

Fig. 24.40 Atrioventricular septal defect with double outlet right ventricle. In this subcostal paracoronal section, the aortic valve (AV) lies obviously above the right ventricle (RV). The subpulmonary infundibulum (spi) is walled off from the interventricular communication much as in classical double outlet right ventricle with subaortic ventricular septal defect and without atrioventricular septal defect. L – left; LV – left ventricle; S – superior.

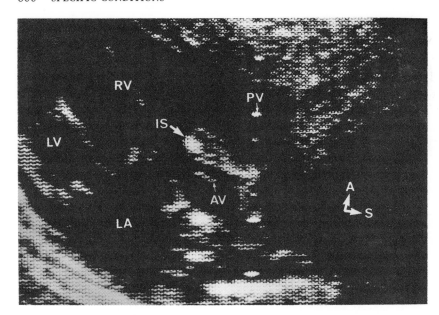

Fig. 24.41 Oblique parasternal long axis cut in patient with common atrioventricular orifice, double outlet right ventricle, and displacement of the infundibular septum (IS) into the left ventricular (LV) outflow tract. Note the wide open right ventricular outflow tract leading up to the pulmonary valve (PV). A – anterior; AV – aortic valve; LA – left atrium; RV – right ventricle; S – superior.

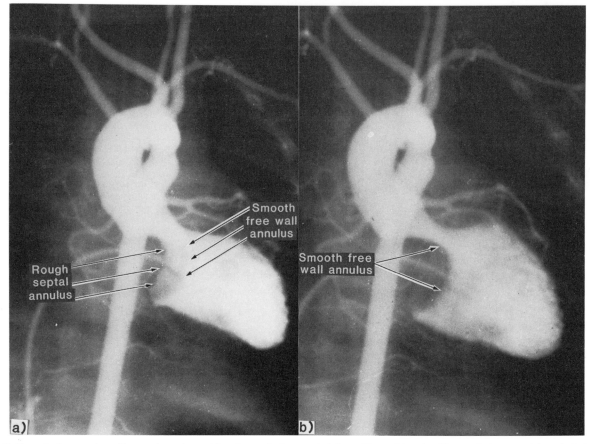

Fig. 24.42 Frontal plane angiocardiogram in patient with atrioventricular septal defect with partitioned orifices and aberrant right subclavian artery. Both pictures show diastolic frames, but in (b), only the smooth portion of the annulus, being that related to the left ventricular free wall, is demonstrated. In (a), the smooth portion of the annulus is still seen, albeit somewhat fainter, and in addition, the rather rough portion of the left atrioventricular valve annulus where the left atrioventricular valve is bound down to the septum is seen. In this panel, immediately below the catheter is seen a non-opacified line corresponding to leaflet thickening on either side of the 'cleft'. Thus, in (a), two 'goose-necks' and therefore two 'geese' are seen.

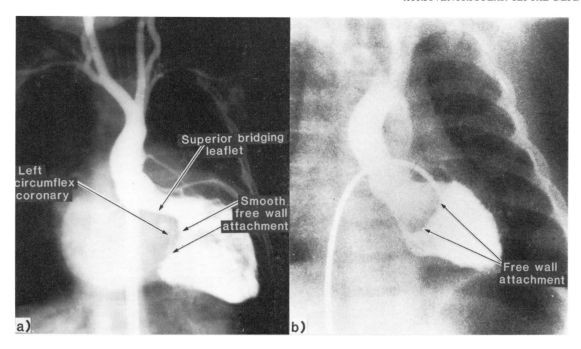

Fig. 24.43 Comparison of the angiographic appearances of the left atrioventricular valve in atrioventricular septal defect and the mitral valve in a normal left ventricle, as seen from the frontal projection. (a) In atrioventricular septal defect, the goose-neck consists of heavily opacified blood lying above the superior bridging leaflet. The smooth attachment of the left atrioventricular valve is shown to be its free wall attachment, because of its close relation to the course of the left circumflex coronary artery lying in the left atrioventricular groove. (b) When the aorta originates normally from the left ventricle, in its wedged position, there is no superior bridging leaflet for contrast to pass above, and therefore no goose-neck. The free wall attachment is well seen, but contrast its course with that seen in (a).

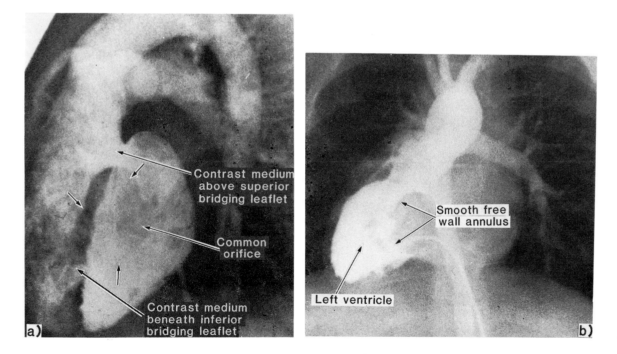

Fig. 24.44 Atrioventricular septal defect with double outlet right ventricle, right-sided heart and right atrial isomerism. (a) A common orifice is seen overriding the septum. Both great arteries clearly originate from the right ventricle. (b) The heart is in the right chest and the apex is to the right. Notice that the left ventricle is the mirror image of a normal left ventricle. The smooth free wall annulus of what is known to be the common atrioventricular orifice is seen, but note that there is no obvious goose-neck deformity, since the aorta originates from the right ventricle. Note also juxtaposition of the descending aorta and the inferior caval vein (shown by the catheter course), indicating right atrial isomerism.

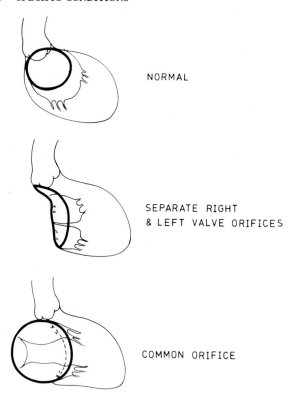

NORMAL

SEPARATE RIGHT & LEFT VALVE ORIFICES

COMMON ORIFICE

Fig. 24.45 Diagram to demonstrate the differing appearances of the atrioventricular valve annuli in normal hearts, those with partitioned atrioventricular orifices and those with a common atrioventricular orifice. For further explanation, see text.

the septal portion of its annulus (Fig. 24.42). In defects with common orifice, only the smooth free wall attachment is seen (Fig. 24.45; Macartney et al, 1979). More informative projections for left ventriculography are the left and

right anterior oblique ones (Brandt et al, 1972; Macartney et al, 1979) which may be modified, if so desired, by caudocranial angulation (Macartney et al, 1979; Soto et al, 1981; Nath et al, 1984). The 'four chamber' and 'long axis' views of the left ventricle are nothing more than 45° and 60° left anterior oblique projections with 30° of caudocranial tilt. The elongated right anterior oblique projection is nothing more than a 30° right anterior oblique projection with 30° of caudocranial tilt. The appearances of right and left anterior oblique views will therefore be discussed first, and then the effects of caudocranial tilt will be considered.

In left anterior oblique projections, whether there is a common orifice (Fig. 24.46 – left panel) or separate right and left orifices (Fig. 24.47), the left atrioventricular component of the valve is seen to arise along a broad front from the septum in diastole. By contrast, in the normal heart in this projection the mitral annulus chastely 'kisses' the septum, only contacting it immediately beneath the aortic valve (Fig. 24.46 – right panel). In the right anterior oblique projection, the muscular atrioventricular septum is normally seen to separate the mitral and aortic valves. In atrioventricular septal defects, its absence is manifested by the fact that the superior bridging leaflet swings from the aortic valve (Brandt et al, 1972). The same abnormality has been described in right ventricular angiocardiograms in patients with associated tetralogy of Fallot (Nath et al, 1984). As the right anterior oblique projection separates the right ventricular outflow tract from the atria, it is the best view for detecting immediate right ventricular filling after a left ventricular injection, this in itself indicating an interventricular communication.

Interventricular communications are more directly seen on the left oblique projection, in which either the entire

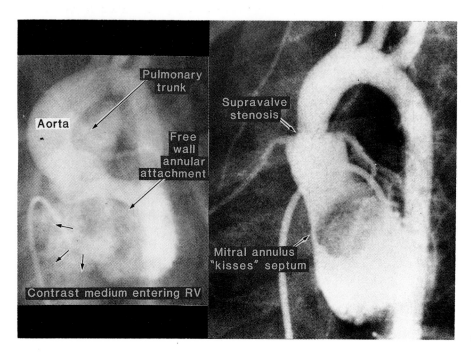

Aorta

Pulmonary trunk

Free wall annular attachment

Supravalve stenosis

Mitral annulus "kisses" septum

Contrast medium entering RV

Fig. 24.46 Comparison of left anterior-oblique projections of left ventricular angiocardiograms in patients with and without atrioventricular septal defect. Left panel: note the contrast medium crossing from left-to-right ventricle, and the way in which the left atrioventricular valve embraces the septum. Right panel: by contrast, the normal mitral annulus only kisses the septum. This patient had idiopathic hypercalcaemia syndrome.

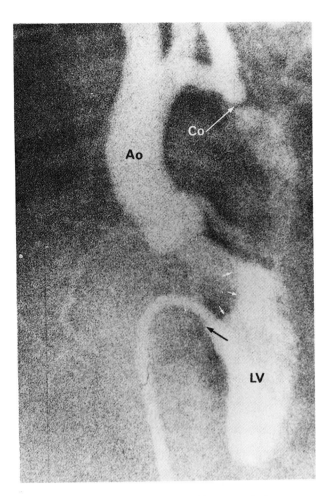

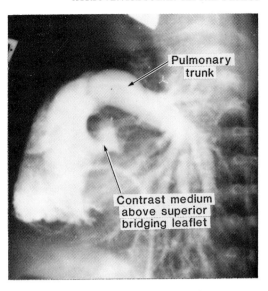

Fig. 24.48 Atrioventricular septal defect with ventricular component. In this patient with pulmonary vascular obstructive disease, the elevated pulmonary vascular resistance produced a right-to-left shunt of blood above the superior bridging leaflet on a right ventricular angiocardiogram. In the presence of obstruction to right ventricular outflow of one kind or another, the ventricular component of the defect is often better seen on a right than a left ventricular angiocardiogram.

Fig. 24.47 Atrioventricular septal defect with no ventricular component and coarctation of the aorta. Left ventriculogram in left anterior oblique projection with caudocranial tilt. Note the smooth free wall annulus (small white arrows) and the way in which the left atrioventricular valve embraces the septum. No contrast medium passes to the right ventricle beneath the inferior bridging leaflet (black arrow). Ao – aorta; Co – coarctation; LV – left ventricle.

common valve is seen in diastole as a relatively non-opacified, circular or more triangular orifice overriding the ventricular septum (Fig. 24.44), or else contrast medium is seen to pass in systole above the superior (Fig. 24.46 – left panel), or beneath the inferior bridging leaflets. When there is a right-to-left shunt at ventricular level, these signs may be better seen on a right than a left ventricular angiocardiogram (Fig. 24.48). Adding caudocranial tilt to the left anterior oblique view profiles the interatrial septum much better, and also elongates the otherwise foreshortened interventricular septum (Fig. 24.46). This may be important, because if the ventricular component is large, the left anterior oblique projection without caudocranial tilt may not demonstrate the ventricular septum at all. In general, the less foreshortening of the ventricular septum the better, because this increases the chance of demonstrating a muscular trabecular ventricular

septal defect and separating it from the atrioventricular septal defect. Lengthening of the subaortic outflow tract by caudocranial tilt also improves demonstration of left ventricular outflow tract obstruction due to a discrete shelf, fibromuscular tunnel or accessory valve tissue (Figs. 24.49, 24.50) (Gow et al, 1984). The only disadvantage of adding caudocranial tilt to the left anterior oblique projection is that it obscures somewhat the passage of contrast medium above the superior bridging leaflet. Addition of caudocranial tilt to the right anterior oblique projection has little effect. Discriminant function analysis of angiocardiographic features together with the right ventricular systolic pressure resulted in a correct distinction of cases with separate right and left valve orifices from those with common orifice in 92% of cases (Macartney et al, 1979). It is not possible reliably to recognise the insertion of tension apparatus by angiocardiography (Soto et al, 1981). The angiocardiographic appearances of double orifice of the left atrioventricular valve have been described (Warnes & Somerville, 1983), but we have not found them either sensitive or specific.

Once the characteristic appearance of a common atrioventricular orifice is imprinted in the memory, it becomes easy to recognise even in the presence of discordant ventriculo-arterial connexions, be this associated with a concordant (Fig. 24.51) or discordant (Fig. 24.52) atrioventricular connexion.

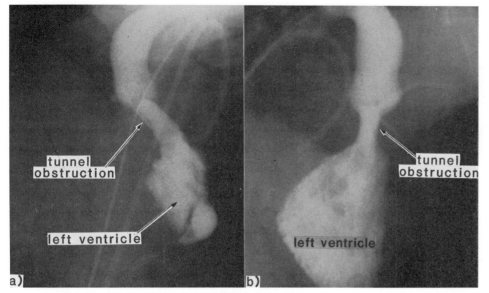

Fig. 24.49 Atrioventricular septal defect with no ventricular component and tunnel left ventricular outflow tract obstruction. (Both original photographs are reproduced with kind permission of Dr Robert Freedom). (a) Left anterior oblique projection with caudocranial tilt demonstrates the narrow left ventricular outflow tract in systole. (b) The tunnel obstruction is also well seen in diastole in the right anterior oblique equivalent projection.

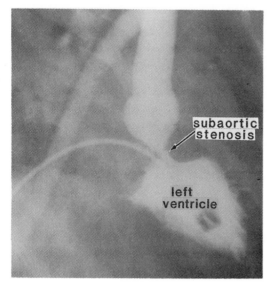

Fig. 24.50 Atrioventricular septal defect with no ventricular component and more discrete subaortic stenosis (compare Figure 24.49). During systole, the subaortic stenosis is well seen in the right anterior oblique projection with caudocranial tilt. (The original photograph is reproduced by kind permission of Dr Robert Freedom.)

NATURAL HISTORY

The prognosis without surgery relates to whether there are separate right and left valves, orifices ('ostium primum defect') or a common orifice. When shunting is exclusively at atrial level the outlook for patients initially is good. In contrast, the long-term survival of patients with common atrioventricular orifice without surgery is, in general, very poor. Berger and colleagues (1979), in an actuarial analysis of the age at death in autopsied patients, showed that only 54% of infants could be expected to survive six months, 35% one year, and only 4% five years. This dismal outlook without surgery was also found in a review of the status of heart in unoperated patients by Somerville and colleagues (1981). During the first year of life, 55% either died or had important medical problems, the majority being related to severe associated defect and intractable cardiac failure without associated respiratory problems. Subsequent morbidity and mortality were associated with the development of pulmonary vascular disease or serious arrhythmia. Unlike in isolated ventricular septal defect, there is no evidence of either spontaneous closure or reduction in the importance of the haemodynamic defect with medical treatment.

A contrary view of the natural history of patients with common atrioventricular orifice comes from data on 47 patients with Down's syndrome in whom the decision not to operate was taken at one year of age. Only four late deaths occurred over a follow-up period of up to 27 years (Bull et al, 1985). This approximates the expected survival in patients with Down's syndrome without heart disease (Fabia & Drolette, 1970). The patients described by Berger and colleagues (1979) were selected by death and autopsy, whereas it seems probable that some selection by survival occurred in the Brompton study.

The truth must lie somewhere between these extremes. By their first birthday, 14% of the patients with Down's syndrome reported by Bull et al (1985) had already died, excluding a few who were offered banding of the pulmonary trunk or complete repair; this is a figure far lower than the autopsy data indicate. Furthermore, an unknown, but probably high, number never reached the referring hospital (Sondheimer et al, 1985).

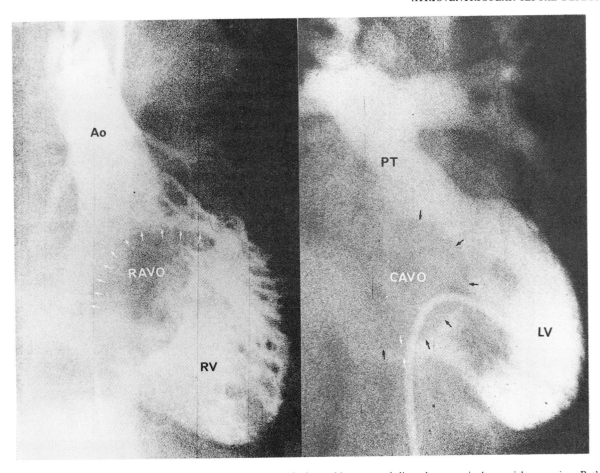

Fig. 24.51 Atrioventricular septal defect with right-hand pattern ventricular architecture and discordant ventriculo-arterial connexion. Both are frontal plane projections. The left-hand panel is of a right ventricular injection and the right-hand panel is of a left ventricular injection. Each injection shows different portions of the annulus of the common atrioventricular orifice (CAVO) which is therefore labelled the right atrioventricular orifice (RAVO) in the left-hand panel. In the right-hand panel a jet of contrast medium (white arrows) is seen passing below the inferior bridging leaflet from left-to-right ventricle. There is an obvious discordant ventriculo-arterial connexion. Ao – aorta; LV – left ventricle; PT – pulmonary trunk; RV – right ventricle.

A large majority of patients remain well in infancy. Intractable cardiac failure at this age is always invariably due to left atrioventricular valve regurgitation. After the first decade, however, there is a progressive increase in the incidence of complications. By the age of 40, only a few patients are well. This deterioration is largely due to the development of arrhythmias, pulmonary vascular disease being uncommon (Somerville et al, 1981).

TREATMENT

Medical

Heart failure and associated respiratory infections need the usual medical treatment (see Ch. 16). Acute administration of hydrallazine has been shown to reduce the left-to-right shunt in the majority of infants with atrioventricular septal defects, but there have been no reports of its value when used chronically (Artman et al, 1984).

Infants who do not respond to anti-failure therapy require surgical treatment. The argument for a prolonged trial of medical treatment before undertaking surgery is less strong than in isolated ventricular septal defect, since there is a strictly limited chance of spontaneous cure or reduction in importance of the atrioventricular septal defect.

Surgical

Interventricular communication absent

Most patients without an interventricular communication survive infancy without requiring surgery. In the massive series reported by Studer and colleagues (1982), only 6% of 140 patients without a ventricular component or major associated anomaly required operation within the first year of life. This was in contrast to 37% of 97 patients who had a ventricular component, but no other associated anomaly (P<0.001). Patients in the first year of life with intractable failure (but no interventricular communication) almost by definition have severe left atrioventricular valve regurgi-

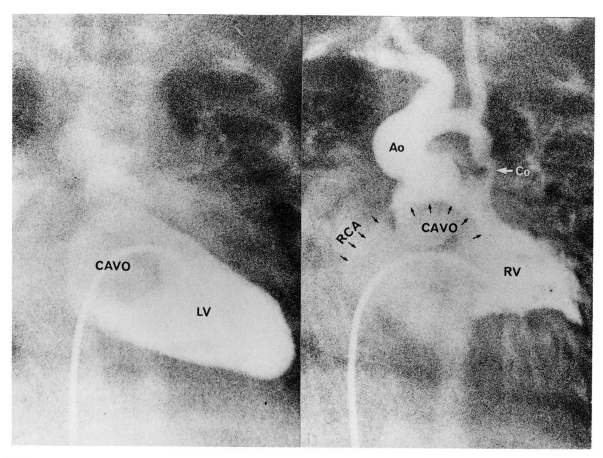

Fig. 24.52 Common atrioventricular orifice with left-hand pattern of ventricular topology and ventriculo-arterial discordance. Both are frontal plane projections. In the left-hand panel, contrast medium is injected into a typical smooth walled boot-shaped left ventricle (LV). In the right-hand panel, contrast medium is injected into a typical coarsely trabeculated triangular right ventricle (RV). Different portions of the common atrioventricular orifice (CAVO) are seen in both projections. The right coronary artery (RCA) marks the right side of the common atrioventricular orifice from externally. Ao – aorta; Co – coarctation.

tation which will not be improved by banding of the pulmonary trunk. There is no alternative to attempting complete repair in such patients. But severe left atrioventricular valve regurgitation is not only a risk factor for operative and late death, but also for the requirement of reoperation on the left atrioventricular valve (Studer et al, 1982). The majority of patients with separate right and left atrioventricular orifices and no more than mild pulmonary hypertension may undergo elective repair just before they begin school. In those patients with a pulmonary/systemic flow ratio less than 2:1, however, and without significant cardiomegaly or left atrioventricular valve regurgitation, there is no need for operation. This is particularly so in that repair being elective does not mean that it is trivial and comparable with repair of an atrial septal defect (see Ch. 22).

Though complete heart block should never be produced by a surgeon who understands the course of the conduction system, it still occasionally happens. It is worthy of note, therefore, that there are at least two ways of avoiding the need to cross the conduction tissue axis. The first is to place the atrial patch so as to leave the coronary sinus draining to the left atrium. The second is to place all the sutures in the leaflet tissue of the *left* atrioventricular valve. The other important surgical decision concerns the repair of the left atrioventricular valve. Although both Frater (1965) and Van Mierop & Alley (1966) pointed to the potential anatomical disadvantage of closing the 'cleft', most surgeons have produced excellent results by approximating the edges of the left ventricular components of the bridging leaflets. The problem is that, although this procedure usually avoids postoperative valve regurgitation, it does so at the expense of narrowing the orificial area of the left valve. With this in mind, Carpentier (1978) revisited the concept of the trifoliate left valve. He recommended repair on the basis of considering the so-called 'cleft' as the commissure between the left ventricular components of the bridging leaflets. He postulated that closure of this structure was needed only to the extent of preventing postoperative regurgitation. As yet, no data are available comparing repair in trifoliate fashion with the classical approach in a controlled trial. Multivariate analysis suggested in one series that failure to do a three leaflet repair was a risk factor for valve repair failure, and possibly for operative death (Rizzoli et al, 1984). In some cases, however, left atrioventricular valve regurgitation may be impossible to avoid whichever technique is used. Left atrioventricular valve replacement may then be necessary either at the time of repair (Castaneda et al, 1971; Taguchi et al, 1968) or at later reoperation (McMullan et al, 1973). It is then important to appreciate the morphology of the left ventricular outflow tract and to understand how easy it is to produce postoperative obstruction in a previously unrestricted channel (Ebels et al, 1985). The hospital mortality for repair of 'ostium primum' defects was 7.9% between 1964 and 1972 in 101 patients undergoing operation at the Mayo Clinic (McMullan et al, 1973). Of these, 3 deaths occurred in infants. Studer and colleagues (1982) reported 5 deaths out of 140 patients without associated anomalies (3.6%) operated upon between 1967 and 1982. Lincoln, in a smaller series of patients undergoing operation at the Brompton Hospital over a ten year period, had an operative mortality of 3% and a late mortality of 4% (Pillai et al, 1986).

The presence of a common atrium does not affect the indications for surgery. But when there is atrial isomerism, the frequently associated anomalous systemic venous connexions may require modifications of standard cannulation and/or baffle procedures in the atrium to ensure that the systemic veins drain appropriately (Huhta et al, 1982).

Interventricular communication present

There is an argument for banding of the pulmonary trunk in this group, particularly in those with little or no atrioventricular valve regurgitation. Most workers have abandoned this procedure because of its poor immediate (Somerville et al, 1967; Newfeld et al, 1977; Cooper et al, 1979) and late (Macartney et al, 1980a) results. There is suggestive, though not conclusive, evidence that pulmonary artery banding can produce both right and left ventricular

hypoplasia in patients with atrioventricular septal defects (Fisher et al, 1984). In fairness, as has so often happened in the past, the results of banding have improved once primary repair in infancy has been embarked upon by a few centres. Silverman and colleagues (1983) recently reported only one hospital death (4.7%) among 21 patients with atrioventricular septal defect and common valve undergoing banding between 1974 and 1982. Of these infants, 4 had gone on to complete repair, all of them surviving. These results are certainly impressive when set against previous experience. They were achieved despite moderate to severe left atrioventricular valve regurgitation in 4 patients. The true significance of this report will not emerge until all patients have undergone complete repair. The case put forward by Williams and colleagues (1983) for individualised surgical management (banding in infants under 4–5 kg and primary repair thereafter) is also based upon good results with both forms of treatment.

Table 24.1 presents the results of repair of uncomplicated atrioventricular septal defects with common orifice at various ages from various centres. In the first year of life the mean hospital mortality from these various results is 20%. The figures as presented do not reflect the very dramatic recent improvement that has been experienced in some centres. For example, the mortality reported by Chin et al (1982) for the period January 1978 to June 1980 was 1/21 (4.8%). Studer and colleagues (1982), by using multivariate logistic regression, were able to demonstrate a mortality as of 1982 of 5–13% for patients with common valve orifice who were in New York Heart Association class III on presentation. The precise estimate depended on the degree of atrioventricular valve regurgitation. The same authors showed that when all other risk factors are taken into account (which cannot be done in a simple portrayal like Table 24.1), age at operation has not been an incremental risk factor since 1976. This seems to be the strongest argument of all in favour of primary repair in infancy.

When all atrioventricular septal defects were taken

Table 24.1 Hospital mortality for uncomplicated atrioventricular septal defects with common orifice at various ages.

	Age (years)	Era	Operations	Deaths	%
Culpepper et al (1978)	0–1	1974–1978	12	4	33
Cooper et al (1979)	0–1	1975–1977	6	1	17
Mair & McGoon (1977)	0–1	1972–1975	5	1	20
Mavroudis et al (1982)	0–1	1975–1981	37	9	24
Bender et al (1982)	0–1	1977–1981	24	2	8
Chin et al (1982)	0–1	1975–1980	29	6	21
Abruzzese et al (1983)	0–1	1977–	25	4	16
Stewart et al (1979)	1–2	1975–	4	0	0
McMullan et al (1972)	>3	1963–1972	27	2	7

together, multivariate logistic analysis identified several risk factors for hospital death. These were – an earlier date at operation, increasing severity of preoperative atrioventricular valve incompetence, increasing disability at time of presentation, and the presence of an interventricular communication or an accessory valve orifice. This particular analysis did not include information from preoperative cardiac catheterisation. There was also a strong association between hospital death and major associated lesions such as tetralogy of Fallot or double outlet right ventricle. When information from angiocardiograms was included, it emerged that right and left ventricular dominance were also incremental risk factors. These authors did not look at the effect of pulmonary vascular resistance. This is unfortunate, because two other groups (Mavroudis et al, 1982; Abruzzese et al, 1983) had found that elevation of pulmonary vascular resistance by no more than 4–5 units.m^2 was sufficient to raise hospital mortality. Interestingly, the multivariate analysis performed by Rizzoli and colleagues (1984) showed that elevation of pulmonary vascular resistance was an incremental risk factor additional to those discovered by Studer and colleagues (1982). Another suggested risk factor which has not been subjected to statistical analysis is the presence of additional ventricular septal defects not detected by angiocardiography (Chin et al, 1982). It should be noted that the technique for angiocardiography used in this study did not include axial views.

All these risk factors pre-exist in the patient and cannot be changed at the time of operation. A hot debate rages about which precise method of surgical repair should be used, but there is no clear evidence to support any view. The arguments centre around two questions. First, should the superior and inferior bridging leaflets be divided when necessary to insert the atrioventricular patch, as originally advocated by Rastelli and colleagues (1968a)? If not, a two-patch technique is employed in which the ventricular patch is inserted beneath and attached to the bridging leaflets, followed by the atrial patch which is sewn to the ventricular patch, thus sandwiching leaflet tissue securely between the two patches. This is said to reduce the incidence of leaflet dehiscence, which features as a rare problem in all series (Katz et al, 1981). The second problem relates to the treatment of the left atrioventricular valve. Should the aim of treatment be to produce a competent, non-stenotic trifoliate structure (Carpentier, 1978) or to try and replicate a normal mitral valve? The confusion over these two questions is compounded by the recent advocacy of an 'endocardial cushion prosthesis' with horizontal wings as well as a vertical patch for repair of complete defects (Kawashima et al, 1983). The only point of general agreement among surgeons is that the underlying anatomy of the leaflets in atrioventricular septal defects is so variable that an individual approach to the problem of repair must be made in each patient.

Repair in the presence of major associated lesions

Patients with right ventricular outflow tract obstruction, (either due to associated tetralogy of Fallot or else the presence of double outlet right ventricle) should have systemic-pulmonary shunts as a first-stage operation for relief of cyanotic spells or significant cyanosis at any time within the first two or three years of life. This conservative policy is dictated by the relatively high risk of complete repair of these complex lesions (Sridaromont et al, 1975). This relates principally to the difficulty of both successfully dividing the common valve *and* creating an unobstructed pathway from the left ventricle to the aorta. In these particular cases, use of a two-patch technique (one to close the atrial component and the other to direct blood flow to the aorta) may partly explain improved recent results (Bastos et al, 1978; Binet et al, 1980; Pacifico et al, 1980; Arcineagas et al, 1981). Nonetheless, the Mayo Clinic team have continued to repair associated tetralogy of Fallot with a single patch and reported two hospital deaths from 12 patients in the last 10 years (Uretzky et al, 1984). Successful repair of a patient with discordant ventriculoarterial connexion, subpulmonary stenosis and a common atrioventricular orifice has been achieved by over-sewing the 'tricuspid' half of the valve, closing the atrial defect and inserting a right atrial/pulmonary artery conduit (Gonzalez-Lavin et al, 1977). More recently, successful repair of the same lesion has been reported in a more definitive way (Alfieri & Plokker, 1982). A two-patch technique was used, with the atrial patch forming a Mustard baffle. A valved conduit was used to bypass left ventricular outflow tract obstruction.

Subaortic stenosis associated with atrioventricular septal defect (usually without interventricular communication) often becomes manifest after an initial apparently successful repair of an 'ostium primum' atrial septal defect (Taylor & Somerville, 1981; Lappen et al, 1983). The treatment is excision in the first instance (Spanos et al, 1977), but the risk of recurrence appears high.

The *long-term results* of repair of these defects are largely dependent on the degree of preoperative pulmonary vascular disease, the extent of 'cure' of left atrioventricular valve regurgitation (Studer et al, 1982), and the integrity of the conduction system. Late heart block of all degrees has been described (McMullan et al, 1973; Culpepper et al, 1978) as well as atrial flutter (Rastelli et al, 1968c), and fibrillation. To what extent these arrhythmic complications are the *result* of surgery is unclear, since the same complications occur in patients who are not treated surgically (Somerville, 1965). Down's syndrome is not a risk factor for hospital death, but it is a significant incremental risk factor for late postoperative death (Studer et al, 1982).

In their useful report of postoperative cardiac catheterisation in patients with common valve orifice, Culpepper et al (1978) reported one patient operated upon at 14 months with quite severe elevation of pulmonary vascular resistance preoperatively who showed no fall at postoperative catheterisation. In patients operated on below this age, elevated preoperative resting pulmonary vascular resistance invariably fell to normal postoperatively. Progressive pulmonary vascular disease leading to death following satisfactory repair of patients with common orifice (Lillehei et al, 1969) and those with common atrium, but without interventricular component (Rastelli et al, 1968c) has been reported.

When the severe preoperative abnormalities of the atrioventricular valves are considered, it is remarkable how completely regurgitation through the left atrioventricular valve can be abolished (Braunwald & Morrow, 1966; Griffiths et al, 1969). An apical systolic murmur postoperatively does not necessarily indicate regurgitation, though it may reflect the development of subaortic stenosis (Taylor & Somerville, 1981; Lappen et al, 1983). This is particularly important since M-mode and cross-sectional echocardiography in a group of 64 patients who had had defects without ventricular components repaired showed 3 with frank left ventricular outflow tract obstruction and the potential for such obstruction in many more (Ebels et al, 1984). 28% of patients showed premature aortic valve closure, and these had a significantly higher rate of narrowing of the left ventricular outflow tract in systole than the remainder.

Actuarial survival for all patients with atrioventricular septal defects was 95% at 6 years in those without failure of left atrioventricular repair, as compared with 33% at 5 years when such failure occurred. 88% of all cases were in New York Heart Association functional class I and 11% in class II (Studer et al, 1982). Unfortunately little or no objective information as to the exercise capacity of these patients exists in the literature, particularly for those patients with common valve orifice.

Repair of cardiac defects associated with Down's syndrome

In Britain there is no statutory requirement to operate upon patients with Down's syndrome. This leaves the doctor and parents free to decide what to do in the best interests of the child. This is never a straightforward matter, particularly in a society where, if the child outlives the parents, he or she is unlikely to find care outside an institution.

The physician is obliged, as ever, to present the facts about survival with and without operation as honestly as he or she can. As has been pointed out, survival without operation once the child reaches 1 year of age is surprisingly high (Bull et al, 1985). As (or even more) important is that the physician be prepared to listen to the parents' feelings on the matter, and particularly to be sensitive to the music behind the words. Parents may in their heart feel one thing, and express quite another with their lips. When the physician has sensed as best he or she can what it is that the parents are really asking for, he should recommend firmly that particular course. To make firm recommendations without listening to the parents is crass. To leave the decision entirely to them is cruel. If the above policy is adopted, no harm is done if the decision turns out to have been the right one. If the decision appears later to have been wrong, the burden of guilt felt by the parents may be colossal if they feel they and they alone were responsible. The clinician needs broad shoulders under these circumstances, but, being more accustomed to living with tragedy than the parents, should better be able to face up to apparent failure.

REFERENCES

Abruzzese P A, Livermore J, Sunderland C O, et al 1983 Mitral repair in complete atrioventricular canal. Ease of correction in early infancy. The Journal of Thoracic and Cardiovascular Surgery 85: 388–395

Acerete F, Herraiz Sarachaga I, Quero Jimenez M, Delgado J A, Knapp K, Moreno Granados F 1978 Atrioventricular canal malformations – anatomo-angiocardiographic correlations. In: Anderson R H, Shinebourne E A (eds) Paediatric cardiology 1977. Churchill Livingstone, Edinburgh, p 448–458

Alfieri O, Plokker M 1982 Repair of common atrioventricular canal associated with transposition of the great arteries and left ventricular outflow obstruction. The Journal of Thoracic and Cardiovascular Surgery 84: 872–875

Alizivatos P, Anderson R H, Macartney F J, Zuberbuhler J R, Stark J 1985 Atrioventricular septal defect with balanced ventricles and malaligned atrial septum: Double outlet right atrium. Report of 2 cases. The Journal of Thoracic and Cardiovascular Surgery 89: 295–297

Allwork S P 1982 Anatomical-embryological correlates in atrioventricular septal defect. British Heart Journal 47: 419–429

Anderson R H, Zuberbuhler J R, Penkoske P A, Neches W H 1985 Of clefts, commissures and things. The Journal of Thoracic and Cardiovascular Surgery 90: 605–610

Arciniegas E, Hakimi M, Farooki Z W, Green E W 1981 Results of total correction of tetralogy of Fallot with complete atrioventricular canal. The Journal of Thoracic and Cardiovascular Surgery 81: 768–73

Artman M, Parrish M D, Boerth R C, Boucek R J Jr, Graham T P Jr 1984 Short-term hemodynamic effects of hydralazine in infants with complete atrioventricular canal defects. Circulation 69: 949–954

Baron M G, Wolf B S, Steinfeld L, Van Mierop L H S 1964 Endocardial cushion defects. Specific diagnosis by angiocardiography. American Journal of Cardiology 13: 162–175

Bastos P, De Leval M, Macartney F, Stark J 1978 Correction of type C atrioventricular canal associated with tetralogy of Fallot. Thorax 33: 646–648

Becker A E, Anderson R H 1982 Atrioventricular septal defects. What's in a name. The Journal of Thoracic and Cardiovascular Surgery 83: 461–469

Bender H W, Hammon J W Jr, Hubbard S G, Muirhead J, Graham

T P 1982 Repair of atrioventricular canal malformation in the first year of life. The Journal of Thoracic and Cardiovascular Surgery 84: 515–522

Ben-Shachar G, Moller J H, Castaneda-Zuniga W, Edwards J E 1981 Signs of membranous subaortic stenosis appearing after correction of persistent common atrioventricular canal. American Journal of Cardiology 48: 340–344

Beppu S, Nimura Y, Sakakibara H, et al 1980 Mitral cleft in ostium primum atrial septal defect assessed by cross-sectional echocardiography. Circulation 62: 1099–1107

Berger T J, Blackstone E H, Kirklin J W, Bargeron L M Jr, Hazelrig J B, Turner M E Jr 1979 Survival and probability of cure without and with operation in complete atrioventricular canal. Annals of Thoracic Surgery 27: 104–111

Bernays A C 1876 Entwicklungsgeschichte der Atrioventrikularklappen. Morphologie Jahrebuch 2: 479–518

Bharati S, Lev M 1973 The spectrum of common atrioventricular orifice (canal). American Heart Journal 86: 553–561

Bharati S, Lev M, McAllister H A J J, Kirklin J W 1980 Surgical anatomy of the atrioventricular valve in the intermediate type of common atrioventricular orifice. The Journal of Thoracic and Cardiovascular Surgery 79: 884–889

Binet J P, Losay J, Hvass U 1980 Tetralogy of Fallot with type C complete atrioventricular canal: surgical repair in three cases. The Journal of Thoracic and Cardiovascular Surgery 79: 761–764

Blieden L C, Randall P A, Castaneda A R, Lucas R V, Edwards J E 1974 The 'goose neck' of the endocardial cushion defect: anatomical basis. Chest 65: 13–17

Brandt P W T, Clarkson P M, Neutze J M, Barratt-Boyes B G 1972 Left ventricular cineangiography in endocardial cushion defect (persistent common atrioventricular canal). Australasian Radiology 16: 367–376

Braunwald N S, Morrow A G 1966 Incomplete persistent atrioventricular canal: operative methods and the results of pre- and postoperative hemodynamic assessments. The Journal of Thoracic and Cardiovascular Surgery 51: 71–80

Bull C, Rigby M L, Shinebourne E A 1985 Should management of complete atrioventricular canal be influenced by coexistent Down syndrome. Lancet 1: 1147–1149

Burn J 1983 Congenital heart defects – the risks to offspring. Archives of Disease in Childhood 58: 947–948

Campbell M, Missen G A J 1957 Endocardial cushion defects: common atrioventricular canal and ostium primum. British Heart Journal 19: 403–418

Carpentier A 1978 Surgical anatomy and management of the mitral component of atrioventricular canal defects. In: Anderson R H, Shinebourne E A (eds) Paediatric cardiology 1977. Churchill Livingstone, Edinburgh, p 477–486

Castaneda A R, Nicoloff D M, Moller J H, Lucas R Jr 1971 Surgical correction of complete atrioventricular canal utilizing ball-valve replacement of the mitral valve. Technical considerations and results. The Journal of Thoracic and Cardiovascular Surgery 62: 926–931

Chi T P L, Krovetz L J 1975 The pulmonary vascular bed in children with Down syndrome. Journal of Pediatrics 86: 533–538

Chin A J, Keane J F, Norwood W I, Castaneda A R 1982 Repair of complete common atrioventricular canal in infancy. The Journal of Thoracic and Cardiovascular Surgery 84: 437–445

Chin A J, Bierman F, Sanders S P, Williams R G, Norwood W I, Castaneda A R 1983 Subxiphoid 2-dimensional echocardiographic identification of left ventricular papillary muscle anomalies in complete common atrioventricular canal. American Journal of Cardiology 51: 1695–1699

Cloez J L, Ravault M C, Worms A M, Marcon F, Pernot C 1983 Complete atrioventricular canal defect associated with congenitally corrected transposition of the great arteries: two-dimensional echocardiographic identification. Journal of the American College of Cardiology 1: 1123–1128

Cooper D K C, de Leval M R, Stark J 1979 Results of surgical correction of persistent complete atrioventricular canal. The Thoracic and Cardiovascular Surgeon 27: 111–115

Corwin R D, Singh A K, Karlson K E 1983 Double-outlet right

atrium: a rare endocardial cushion defect. American Heart Journal 106: 1156–1157

Culpepper W, Kolff J, Lin C-Y, Vitullo D, Lamberti J, Arcilla R A, Replogle R 1978 Complete common atrioventricular canal in infancy – Surgical repair and postoperative hemodynamics. Circulation 58: 550–558

David I, Castaneda A R, Van Praagh R 1982 Potentially parachute mitral valve in common atrioventricular canal. The Journal of Thoracic and Cardiovascular Surgery 84: 178–186

Deanfield J E, Leanage R, Stroobant J, Chrispin A R, Taylor J F N, Macartney F J 1980 Use of high kilovoltage filtered beam radiographs for detection of bronchial situs in infants and young children. British Heart Journal 44: 577–583

Dickinson D F, Arnold R, Wilkinson J L 1981 Congenital heart disease among 160480 liveborn children in Liverpool 1960 to 1969. Implications for surgical treatment. British Heart Journal 46: 55–62

Di Segni E, Edwards J E 1983 Cleft anterior leaflet of the mitral valve with intact septa. A study of 20 cases. American Journal of Cardiology 51: 919–926

Ebels T, Meijboom E J, Anderson R H, et al 1984 Anatomic and functional 'obstruction' of the outflow tract in atrioventricular septal defects with separate valve orifices ('Ostium primum atrial septal defect'): an echocardiographic study. American Journal of Cardiology 54: 843–847

Ebels T, Ho S Y, Anderson R H, Meijboom E J, Eijgelaar A 1986 The surgical anatomy of the left ventricular outflow tract in atrioventricular septal defect. Annals of Thoracic Surgery 41: 483–488

Emanuel R, Nichols J, Anders J M, Moores E C, Somerville J 1968 Atrioventricular defects – a study of 92 families. British Heart Journal 30: 645–651

Emanuel R, Somerville J, Inns A, Withers R 1983 Evidence of congenital heart disease in the offspring of parents with atrioventricular defects. British Heart Journal 49: 144–147

Fabia J, Drolette M 1970 Life tables up to age ten years for mongols with and without congenital heart defect. Journal Mental Deficiency Research 14: 235–242

Feldt R H, DuShane J W, Titus J L 1970 The atrioventricular conduction system in persistent common atrioventricular canal defect: correlations with electrocardiogram. Circulation 42: 437–444

Fernandez Aceytuno A M, Bethencourt Gonzales A, Macaya Miguel C, Tynan M, Anderson R H 1982 Subxiphoid M-mode echocardiography in atrioventricular defects. Pediatric Cardiology 3: 119–125

Fisher E A, Doshi M, DuBrow I W, Silverman N, Levitsky S 1984 Effect of palliative and corrective surgery on ventricular volumes in complete atrioventricular canal. Pediatric Cardiology 5: 159–166

Frater R W M 1965 Persistent common atrioventricular canal. Anatomy and function in relation to surgical repair. Circulation 32: 120–129

Freedom R M, Bini M, Rowe R D 1978 Endocardial cushion defect and significant hypoplasia of the left ventricle: a distinct clinical and pathological entity. European Journal of Cardiology 7: 263–281

Gegenbaur C 1885 In: Lehrbuch der Anatomie des Herzen. Wilhelm Engelmann, Leipzig, p 639

Gomes A S, Nath P H, Singh A, Lucas R V, Amplatz K, Nicoloff D M, Edwards J E 1980 Accessory flap like tissue causing ventricular outflow obstruction. The Journal of Thoracic and Cardiovascular Surgery 80: 211–216

Gonzalez-Lavin L, Blair T C, Chi S, Sparrow A W 1977 Orthoterminal correction of coexisting d-transposition of the great arteries, subpulmonary stenosis, and a complete form of atrioventricular canal. The Journal of Thoracic and Cardiovascular Surgery 73: 694–698

Goor D A, Lillehei C W 1975 Atrioventricular canal malformations. In: Congenital Malformations of the Heart. Grune & Stratton, New York, p 132–153

Gow R M, Freedom R M, Williams W G, Trusler G A, Rowe R D 1984 Coarctation of the aorta or subaortic stenosis with atrioventricular septal defect. American Journal of Cardiology 53: 1421–1428

Griffiths S P, Ellis K, Burris J O, Blumenthal S, Bowman F O Jr, Malm J R 1969 Postoperative evaluation of mitral valve function in ostium primum defect with cleft mitral valve (partial form of atrioventricular canal). Circulation 40: 21–29

Hagler D J 1976 Echocardiographic findings in atrioventricular canal defect. In: Feldt R H (ed) Atrioventricular canal defects. Saunders, Philadelphia, p 87–109

Hagler D J, Tajik A J, Seward J B, Mair D D, Ritter D G 1979 Real-time wide-angle sector echocardiography: atrioventricular canal defects. Circulation 59: 140–150

Haworth S G 1984 Pulmonary vascular disease in different types of congenital heart disease. Implications for interpretation of lung biopsy findings in early childhood. British Heart Journal 52: 557–571

Heath D, Edwards J E 1958 The pathology of hypertensive pulmonary vascular disease. A description of six grades of structural changes in the pulmonary artery with special reference to congenital cardiac septal defect. Circulation 18: 533–547

Ho S Y, Milo S, Anderson R H, et al 1982 Straddling atrioventricular valve with absent atrioventricular connection. Report of 10 cases. British Heart Journal 47: 344–352

Horiuchi T, Saji K, Osuka Y, Sato K, Okada Y 1976 Successful correction of double outlet left atrium associated with complete atrioventricular canal and 1-loop double outlet right ventricle with stenosis of the pulmonary artery. The Journal of Cardiovascular Surgery 17: 157–161

Huhta J C, Smallhorn J F, Macartney F J, Anderson R H, De Leval M 1982 Cross-sectional echocardiographic diagnosis of systemic venous return. British Heart Journal 48: 388–403

Jacobstein M D, Fletcher B D, Goldstein S, Riemenschneider T A 1985 Evaluation of atrioventricular septal defect by magnetic resonance imaging. American Journal of Cardiology 55: 1158–1161

Jarmakani J M, George B, Wheller J 1978 Ventricular volume characteristics in infants and children with endocardial cushion defects. Circulation 58: 153–157

Katz N M, Blackstone E H, Kirklin J W, Bradley E L, Lemons J E 1981 Suture techniques for atrioventricular valves. The Journal of Thoracic and Cardiovascular Surgery 81: 528–536

Kawashima Y, Matsuda H, Hirose H, Nakano S, Shimazaki Y, Miyamoto K 1983 Surgical treatment of complete atrioventricular canal defect with an endocardial cushion prosthesis. Circulation 68 (Suppl II): 139–143

Keith J D 1978 Prevalence, incidence and epidemiology. In: Keith J D, Rowe R D, Vlad P (eds) Heart disease in infancy and childhood, 3rd Edn. Macmillan, New York, p 3–13

LaCorte M A, Fellows K E, Williams R G 1976 Overriding tricuspid valve: echocardiographic and angiocardiographic features. 8 cases of ventricular septal defect of atrioventricular canal type. American Journal of Cardiology 37: 911–919

Lappen R S, Muster A J, Idriss F S, et al 1983 Masked subaortic stenosis in ostium primum atrial septal defect: recognition and treatment. American Journal of Cardiology 52: 336–340

Lev M 1958 The architecture of the conduction system in congenital heart disease. I. Common atrioventricular orifice. Archives of Pathology 65: 174–191

Lillehei C W, Anderson R C, Ferlic R M, Bonnabeau R C Jr 1969 Persistent common atrioventricular canal. Recatheterization results in 37 patients following intracardiac repair. The Journal of Thoracic and Cardiovascular Surgery 57: 83–94

Macartney F J, Panday J, Scott O 1969 Cor pulmonale as a result of chronic nasopharyngeal obstruction due to hypertrophied tonsils and adenoids. Archives of Disease in Childhood 44: 585–592

Macartney F J, Rees P G, Daly K, et al 1979 Angiocardiographic appearances of atrioventricular defects with particular reference to distinction of ostium primum atrial septal defect from common atrioventricular orifice. British Heart Journal 42: 640–656

Macartney F J, Taylor J F N, Graham G R, De Leval M, Stark J 1980a The fate of survivors of cardiac surgery in infancy. Circulation 62: 80–91

Macartney F J, Zuberbuhler J R, Anderson R H 1980b Morphologic considerations pertaining to recognition of atrial isomerism. Consequences for sequential chamber localisation. British Heart Journal 44: 657–667

Macartney F J, Rigby M L, Anderson R H, Silverman N H 1984

Cross-sectional anatomy of infundibular anomalies associated with atrioventricular septal defects, as displayed by cardiac ultrasound. (abstract). Pediatric Cardiol 5:230

McGoon D C, Puga F J, Danielson G K 1983 Atrioventricular canal. In: Sabiston D C, Spencer F C (eds) Gibbon's surgery of the heart. Saunders, Philadelphia, p 1051–1066

McMullan M H, McGoon D C, Wallace R B, Danielson G K, Weidman W H 1973 Surgical treatment of partial atrioventricular canal. Archives of Surgery 107: 705–710

McMullan M H, Wallace R B, Weidman W H, McGoon D 1972 Surgical treatment of complete atrioventricular canal. Surgery 72: 905–912

Mair D D, McGoon D C 1977 Surgical correction of atrioventricular canal during the first year of life. American Journal of Cardiology 40: 66–69

Mavroudis C, Weinstein G, Turley K, Ebert P A 1982 Surgical management of complete atrioventricular canal. The Journal of Thoracic and Cardiovascular Surgery 83: 670–679

Milo S, Ho S Y, Macartney F J, et al H 1979 Straddling and overriding atrioventricular valves: morphology and classification. American Journal of Cardiology 44: 1122–1134

Milo S, Ho S Y, Wilkinson J L, Anderson R H 1980 The surgical anatomy and atrioventricular conduction tissues of hearts with isolated ventricular septal defects. The Journal of Thoracic and Cardiovascular Surgery 79: 244–255

Moulaert A J 1978 Anatomy of ventricular septal defect. In: Anderson R H, Shinebourne E A (eds) Paediatric cardiology 1977. Churchill Livingstone, Edinburgh, p 113–124

Nath P H, Soto B, Bini R M, Bargeron L M Jr, Pacifico A D 1984 Tetralogy of Fallot with atrioventricular canal. An angiographic study. The Journal of Thoracic and Cardiovascular Surgery 87: 421–430

Neufeld H N, Titus J L, DuShane J W, Burchell H B, Edwards J E 1961 Isolated ventricular septal defect of the persistent common atrioventricular type. Circulation 23: 685–696

Newfeld E A, Sher M, Paul M H, Nikaidoh H 1977 Pulmonary vascular disease in complete atrioventricular canal defect. American Journal of Cardiology 39: 721–726

O'Nullain S, Hall J G, Stamm S J 1977 Autosomal dominant inheritance of endocardial cushion defect. Birth Defects 13(3A): 143–147

Ongley P A, Pongpanich B, Spangler J G, Feldt R H 1976 The electrocardiogram in atrioventricular canal. In: Feldt R H (ed) Atrioventricular canal defects. Saunders, Philadelphia, p 51–75

Pacifico A D, Kirklin J W, Bargeron L M Jr 1980 Repair of complete atrioventricular canal associated with tetralogy of Fallot or double-outlet right ventricle: report of 10 patients. Annals of Thoracic Surgery 29: 351–356

Park J M, Ritter D G, Mair D D 1976 Cardiac catheterisation findings in persistent common atrioventricular canal. In: Feldt R H (ed) Atrioventricular canal defects. Saunders, Philadelphia, p 76–86

Penkoske P A, Neches W H, Anderson R H, Zuberbuhler J R 1985 Further observations on the morphology of atrioventricular septal defects. The Journal of Thoracic and Cardiovascular Surgery 90: 611–622

Piccoli G P, Gerlis L M, Wilkinson J L, Lozsadi K, Macartney F J, Anderson R H 1979a Morphology and classification of atrioventricular defects. British Heart Journal 42: 621–632

Piccoli G P, Wilkinson J L, Macartney F J, Gerlis L M, Anderson R H 1979b Morphology and classification of complete atrioventricular defects. British Heart Journal 42: 633–639

Piccoli G P, Ho S Y, Wilkinson J L, Macartney F J, Gerlis L M, Anderson R H 1982 Left-sided obstructive lesions in atrioventricular septal defects. An anatomic study. The Journal of Thoracic and Cardiovascular Surgery 83: 453–460

Pieroni D R, Homcy E, Freedom R M 1975 Echocardiography in atrioventricular canal defect. A clinical spectrum. American Journal of Cardiology 35: 54–58

Pillai R, Ho S Y, Anderson R H, Shinebourne E A, Lincoln C 1984 Malalignment of the interventricular septum with atrioventricular septal defects: its implications concerning conduction tissue disposition. The Thoracic and Cardiovascular Surgeon 33 32: 1–3

Pillai R, Ho S Y, Anderson R H, Shinebourne E A, Lincoln J C R 1986 Ostium primum atrioventricular septal defect – An anatomical and surgical review. Annals of Thoracic Surgery 41: 458–461

Rastelli G C, Kirklin J W, Titus J L 1966 Anatomic observations on complete form of persistent common atrioventricular canal with special reference to atrioventricular valves. Mayo Clinic Proceedings 41: 296–308

Rastelli G C, Kirklin J W, Kincaid O W 1967 Angiocardiography of persistent common atrioventricular canal. Mayo Clinic Proceedings 42: 200–209

Rastelli G C, Ongley P A, Kirklin J W, McGoon D C 1968a Surgical repair of the complete form of persistent common atrioventricular canal. The Journal of Thoracic and Cardiovascular Surgery 55: 299–308

Rastelli G C, Ongley P A, Titus J L 1968b Ventricular septal defect of atrioventricular canal type with straddling right atrioventricular valve and mitral valve deformity. Circulation 37: 816–825

Rastelli G C, Rahimtoola S H, Ongley P A, McGoon D C 1968c Common atrium: anatomy, hemodynamics, and surgery. The Journal of Thoracic and Cardiovascular Surgery 55: 834–841

Rizzoli G, Mazzucco A, Brumana T, et al 1984 Operative risk of correction of atrioventricular septal defects. British Heart Journal 52: 258–265

Rowe R D, Uchida I A 1961 Cardiac malformation in mongolism: a prospective study of 184 mongoloid children. American Journal of Medicine 31: 726–735

Rudolph A M 1970 The changes in the circulation after birth. Their importance in congenital heart disease. Circulation 41: 343–359

Sanchez-Cascos A 1978 The recurrence risk in congenital heart disease. European Journal of Cardiology 7: 197–210

Silverman N, Levitsky S, Fisher E, DuBrow 1, Hastreiter A, Scagliotti D 1983 Efficacy of pulmonary artery banding in infants with complete atrioventricular canal. Circulation 68 (Suppl II): 148–153

Silverman N H, Ho S Y, Anderson R H, Smith A, Wilkinson J L 1984 Atrioventricular septal defect with intact atrial and ventricular septal structures. International Journal of Cardiology 5: 567–572

Smallhorn J F, Tommasini G, Macartney F J 1981 Two-dimensional echocardiographic assessment of common atrioventricular valves in univentricular hearts. British Heart Journal 46: 30–34

Smallhorn J F, de Leval M, Stark J, et al 1982a Isolated anterior mitral cleft. Two dimensional echocardiographic assessment and differentiation from 'clefts' associated with atrioventricular septal defect. British Heart Journal 48: 109–116

Smallhorn J F, Sutherland G R, Anderson R H, Macartney F J 1982b Cross-sectional echocardiographic assessment of conditions with atrioventricular valve leaflets attached to the atrial septum at the same level. British Heart Journal 48: 331–341

Smallhorn J F, Tommasini G, Anderson R H, Macartney F J 1982c Assessment of atrioventricular septal defects by two dimensional echocardiography. British Heart Journal 47: 109–121

Somerville J 1965 Ostium primum defect: factors causing deterioration in the natural history. British Heart Journal 27: 413–419

Somerville J, Jefferson K 1968 Left ventricular angiocardiography in atrioventricular defects. British Heart Journal 30: 446–457

Somerville J, Agnew T, Stark J, Waterston D J, Aberdeen E, Bonham Carter R E, Waich S 1967 Banding of the pulmonary artery for common atrioventricular canal. British Heart Journal 29: 816–828

Somerville J, Revel-Chion R, Van Der Cammen T, Presbitero P 1981 Atrioventricular defects – natural and unnatural history. In: Godman M J (ed) Paediatric cardiology 4. Churchill Livingstone, Edinburgh, p 404–416

Sondheimer H M, Byrum C J, Blackman M S 1985 Unequal cardiac care for children with Down's syndrome. American Journal of Diseases of Children 139: 68–70

Soto B, Becker A E, Moulaert A J, Lie J T, Anderson R H 1980 Classification of ventricular septal defects. British Heart Journal 43: 332–343

Soto B, Bargeron L M Jr, Pacifico A, Vanini V, Kirklin J W 1981 Angiography of atrioventricular canal defects. American Journal of Cardiology 48: 492–499

Spanos P K, Fiddler G I, Mair D D, McGoon D C 1977 Repair of atrioventricular canal associated with membranous subaortic stenosis. Mayo Clinic Proceedings 52: 121–124

Sridaromont S, Feldt R H, Ritter D G, Davis G D, McGoon D C, Edwards J E 1975 Double-outlet right ventricle associated with persistent common atrioventricular canal. Circulation 52: 933–942

Stewart S, Harris P, Manning J 1979 Complete endocardial cushion defect. Operative technique and results. The Journal of Thoracic and Cardiovascular Surgery 78: 914–919

Studer M, Blackstone E H, Kirklin J W, et al 1982 Determinants of early and late results of repair of atrioventricular septal (canal) defects. The Journal Thoracic and Cardiovascular Surgery 84: 523–542

Sutherland G R, Van Mill G J, Anderson R H, Hunter S 1980 Subxiphoid echocardiography – a new approach to the diagnosis and differentiation of atrioventricular defects. European Heart Journal 1: 45–53

Sutherland G R, Godman M J, Smallhorn J F, Guiterras P, Anderson R H, Hunter S 1982 Ventricular septal defects. Two dimensional echocardiographic and morphological correlations. British Heart Journal 47: 316–328

Taguchi K, Sasaki N, Okii Y, Matsuura Y, Hirao M 1968 Surgical experience with persistent common atrioventricular canal in a series of eighty-two patients. Particular consideration on the correction of valve incompetence and deficiency of the ventricular septum. The Journal of Thoracic and Cardiovascular Surgery 55: 501–517

Taylor N C, Somerville J 1981 Fixed subaortic stenosis after repair of ostium primum defects. British Heart Journal 45: 689–697

Tenckhoff L, Stamm S J 1973 An analysis of 35 cases of the complete form of persistent common atrioventricular canal. Circulation 48: 416–427

Thanopoulos B D, Fisher E A, DuBrow I W, Hastreiter A R 1978 Right and left ventricular volume characteristics in common atrioventricular canal. Circulation 57: 991–995

Thiene G, Anderson R H 1978 The conducting tissues in atrioventricular canal malformations. In: Anderson R H, Shinebourne E A (eds) Paediatric cardiology 1977. Churchill Livingstone, Edinburgh, p 437–447

Thiene G, Wenink A C G, Frescura C, et al 1981 The surgical anatomy of the conduction tissues in atrioventricular defects. The Journal of Thoracic and Cardiovascular Surgery 82: 928–937

Thilenius O G, Bharati S, Lev M 1976 Subdivided left atrium: an expanded concept of cor triatriatum sinistrum. American Journal of Cardiology 37: 743–752

Toscano-Barbosa E, Brandenburg R U, Burchell H B 1956 Electrocardiographic studies of cases with intracardiac malformations of the atrioventricular canal. Proceedings of the Staff Meetings of the Mayo Clinic 31: 513–523

Ugarte M, De Salamanca F E, Quero M 1976 Endocardial cushion defects. An anatomical study of 54 specimens. British Heart Journal 38: 674–682

Uretzky G, Puga F J, Danielson G K, et al 1984 Complete atrioventricular canal associated with tetralogy of Fallot. Morphological and surgical considerations. The Journal of Thoracic and Cardiovascular Surgery 87: 756–766

Van Mierop L H S 1970 Pathology and pathogenesis of the common cardiac malformations. In: Brest A N, Downing D (eds) Cardiovascular clinics 21. Davis, Philadelphia, p 27–60

Van Mierop L H S 1977 Pathology and pathogenesis of endocardial cushion defects. Surgical implications. In: Davila J C (ed) Second Henry Ford Hospital International Symposium on Cardiac Surgery. Appleton-Century-Crofts, New York, p 201–207

Van Mierop L H S, Alley R D 1966 The management of the cleft mitral valve in endocardial cushion defects. Annals of Thoracic Surgery 2: 416–423

Wakai C S, Edwards J E 1956 Developmental and pathologic considerations in persistent common atrioventricular canal. Proceedings of the Staff Meetings of the Mayo Clinic 31: 487–500

Wakai C S, Edwards J E 1958 Pathologic study of persistent common atrioventricular canal. American Heart Journal 56: 779–794

Wakai C S, Swan H J C, Wood E H 1956 Hemodynamic data and findings of diagnostic value in nine proved cases of persistent common atrioventricular canal. Proceedings of the Staff Meetings of the Mayo Clinic 31: 500–508

Warnes C, Somerville J 1983 Double mitral valve orifice in atrioventricular defects. British Heart Journal 49: 59–64

Wenink A C G, Gittenberger de Groot A C 1985 The role of atrioventricular endocardial cushions in the septation of the heart. International Journal of Cardiology 8: 25–44

Wenink A C G, Anderson R H, Thiene G 1978 The conducting system in hearts with atrioventricular canal malformations. In: Van Mierop L H S, Oppenheimer-Dekker A, Bruins C L D (eds) Embryology and teratology of the heart and the great arteries. Leiden University Press,The Hague, p 55–61

Williams R G, Rudd M 1974 Echocardiographic features of endocardial cushion defects. Circulation 49: 418–422

Williams W H, Guyton R A, Michalik R E, et al 1983 Individualized surgical management of complete atrioventricular canal. The Journal of Thoracic and Cardiovascular Surgery 86: 838–844

Yao J, Thompson M W, Trusler G A, Trimble A S 1968 Familial atrial septal defect of the primum type: a report of four cases in one sibship. Canadian Medical Association Journal 98: 218–219

Yoshida H, Funabashi T, Nakaya S, Maeda T, Taniguchi N 1980 Subxiphoid cross-sectional echocardiographic imaging of the 'goose-neck' deformity in endocardial cushion defect. Circulation 62: 1319–1323

25

Ventricular septal defect

Defects in the interventricular septum can occur as isolated anomalies or in association with many other defects. They are found as integral parts of the tetralogy of Fallot, double outlet ventricles and most cases of common arterial trunk. They occur as a component of atrioventricular septal defects and are frequently encountered in association with complete and congenitally corrected transposition, pulmonary atresia and coarctation of the aorta. Even when found as 'isolated' defects, complicating associated abnormalities are encountered such as persistence of the arterial duct, aortic or mitral regurgitation, or acquired subvalvar pulmonary stenosis. In this chapter we will consider only isolated ventricular septal defect but included in the discussion will be these last-mentioned complicating lesions.

Although defects in the interventricular septum were recognised previously, it is with the name of Henri Roger (1879) that the anomaly is historically linked. It was Roger who recognised that isolated ventricular septal defect produced a typical murmur and was consistent with prolonged life and good health.

PREVALENCE

Without question, isolated ventricular septal defect is the most common congenital cardiac malformation, if we exclude the two-leaflet aortic valve and prolapse of the mitral valve (Roberts, 1984). It is difficult to obtain an accurate assessment of prevalence, since most individuals with an isolated ventricular septal defect, being asymptomatic, are not candidates for cardiac catheterisation and angiography. Thus, in the majority, there is no objective proof of the presence of a defect, although this may well change with the advent of cross-sectional echocardiography. Certainly the high rate of spontaneous closure which is known to occur (French, 1918; Weber, 1918; Evans et al, 1960) means that autopsy data underestimate the incidence of the defect. In series depending heavily on clinical observation, the estimated prevalence varies from

1.35–2.94 per 1000 live births (Carlgren, 1959; Hoffman & Rudolph, 1965; Mitchell et al, 1971; Hoffman & Christianson, 1978).

MORPHOLOGY AND CLASSIFICATION

Classifications of isolated ventricular septal defect have been many and varied, ranging from the simple 'high' and 'low' (Lev, 1959) to the exceedingly complex nosology derived from embryologic premises by Goor et al (1971). What should be expected from a classification of ventricular septal defects? Certainly it should communicate the position of the defect within the ventricular septum. Knowledge of the structures forming the margins of the defect is equally important. If, at the same time, the system can convey inferential information about the proximity of the defect to the atrioventricular conduction tissue axis and the likelihood of the defect closing spontaneously, then most necessary facts have been supplied. The system proposed by Soto et al (1980) satisfies these needs, and it is the classification we have employed. It is as amenable to use by the echocardiographer (Sutherland et al, 1982) or the angiographer (Soto et al, 1978) as by the morphologist. It is of particular value to the surgeon, since it conveys knowledge of the likely disposition of the conduction tissue (Milo et al, 1980).

The system is based upon the premise that, viewed descriptively, the ventricular septum has three muscular components and is completed by a fourth fibrous component, the membranous septum. The three muscular components are the inlet septum, separating the ventricular inlets, the apical trabecular septum between the ventricular trabecular components, and the outlet (or infundibular) septum between the ventricular outlets (Fig. 25.1). To an extent, this division is simplistic in the setting of the normal heart. This is because the 'inlet' septum separates mostly the inlet of the right ventricle from the outlet of the left by virtue of the wedge position of the sub-aortic outflow tract and because the 'outlet'

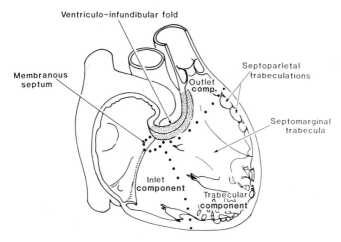

Fig. 25.1 Diagram showing the basic descriptive components of the ventricular septum as viewed from the right ventricular aspect, along with other important right ventricular landmarks. In many respects, diagrams such as this are simplistic. For example, only a small part of the subpulmonary infundibulum labelled 'outlet septum' is truly an interventricular septal structure. Nonetheless, this is the area occupied by defects between the outlet components when they are present. The normal therefore serves as the framework for description of the abnormal, recognising that they are rarely identical in all respects.

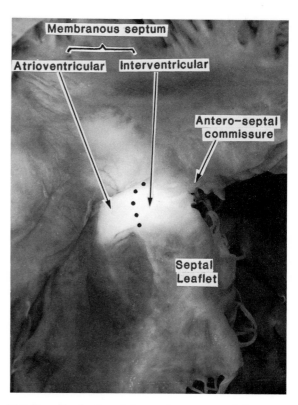

Fig. 25.2 Transillumination of the membranous part of the septum (which is viewed from the right) shows how it is divided by the attachment of the septal leaflet of the tricuspid valve. Note that the antero-septal commissure is lateral to the membranous septum ('round the corner'). (Prepared and reproduced by kind permission of Professor A. E. Becker, University of Amsterdam, The Netherlands.)

muscular septum is barely represented in the normal heart. Nonetheless, it provides the needed point of departure for simple description of septal defects.

Other features of this normal anatomy, however, warrant further consideration in the context of isolated ventricular septal defects. Because the tricuspid valve attaches to the ventricular septum at a more apical level than the mitral valve, part of the inlet muscular septum is normally positioned between the right atrium and the left ventricle – the atrioventricular muscular septum. This septum is usually present in most isolated ventricular septal defects. The attachment of the tricuspid valve across the area of membranous septum in the normal heart divides this fibrous portion into atrioventricular and interventricular components (Fig. 25.2). The size of these two components varies markedly from heart to heart. In the infant heart the interventricular component is usually either small or non-existent (Allwork & Anderson, 1979). In hearts with ventricular septal defects, the atrioventricular component of the membranous septum is almost invariably present in some form or other. The interventricular component may be present as an intact structure. Even when a defect abuts on the central fibrous body, the interventricular membranous septal remnant is frequently present as a ridge or sheet-like fold of fibrous tissue. The antero-septal commissure of the tricuspid valve, supported by the medial papillary muscle, is usually 'round the corner' (Fig. 25.2) from the central fibrous body. The septal leaflet of the tricuspid valve then overhangs the interventricular component of the normal membranous septum like a curtain (Figs. 25.2, 25.3). Frequently in

normal hearts the septal leaflet is divided, a 'cleft' running up to the area of the central fibrous body and dividing the leaflet into superior and inferior components.

Basic classification of ventricular septal defects

The basic division of ventricular septal defects is into those defects which have entirely muscular rims (muscular defects) or those in which part of the rim of the defect is made up of valve leaflet tissue and its attachments (Fig. 25.4). The latter group is by far the commonest. It can be further subdivided into a group in which the valve tissue is that of the aortic valve at its attachment to the central fibrous body (membranous septum) and another group in which the aortic valve is in fibrous continuity with the pulmonary valve. The defects in which the aortic valve and central fibrous body form part of the rim of the defect are most frequently referred to as 'membranous' defects. But this nomenclature implies that the defect results from absence of the interventricular component of the membranous septum, and this is rarely the case. Usually the interventricular membranous septum is present as a fold of tissue in the fibrous rim of those defects. As Becu et al (1956) indicated, the defects are

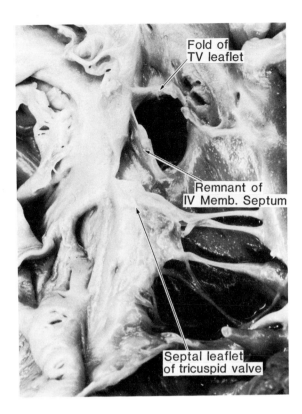

Fold of
TV leaflet

Remnant of
IV Memb. Septum

Septal leaflet
of tricuspid valve

almost always of considerably greater area than that normally occupied by the interventricular membranous septum. For these reasons we prefer to describe them as *perimembranous* defects. Since the attachments of the aortic valve always form part of the fibrous rim of a perimembranous defect, these defects are of necessity subaortic (Fig. 25.5a). The morphologist, however, introduces a potential area of confusion when he describes all perimembranous defects as being 'subaortic'. His viewpoint can be from the left ventricle, and then the defect unquestionably is beneath the aortic valve (Fig. 25.5a). But so, relatively speaking, are all other defects of the ventricular septum. Furthermore, to the echocardiographer, it is more natural to describe a defect with overriding of the aorta as being 'subaortic' (Capelli et al, 1983). This is because, when the valve is closed, the leaflets form the roof of the defect

Fig. 25.3 A perimembranous ventricular septal defect in which the septal leaflet of the tricuspid valve has been reflected to show the remnant of the interventricular membranous septum. Note also the fibrous fold attached to the valve leaflet in the roof of the defect. (Photographed and reproduced by kind permission of Dr J. .R. Zuberbuhler, University of Pittsburgh, USA.)

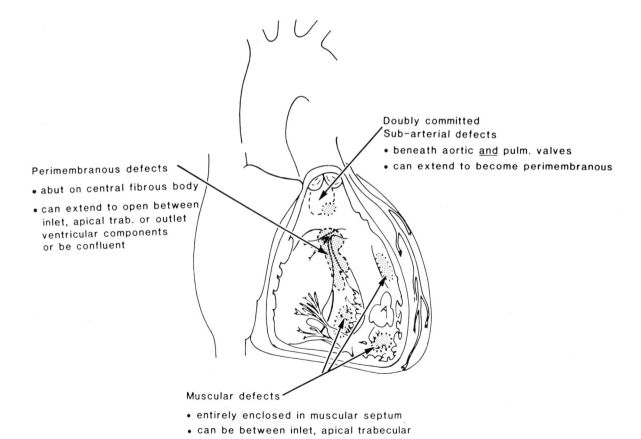

Perimembranous defects
• abut on central fibrous body
• can extend to open between inlet, apical trab. or outlet ventricular components or be confluent

Doubly committed
Sub-arterial defects
• beneath aortic <u>and</u> pulm. valves
• can extend to become perimembranous

Muscular defects
• entirely enclosed in muscular septum
• can be between inlet, apical trabecular or outlet ventricular components

Fig. 25.4 Diagram showing the basic categorisation of ventricular septal defects according to the morphology illustrated in Figure 25.1.

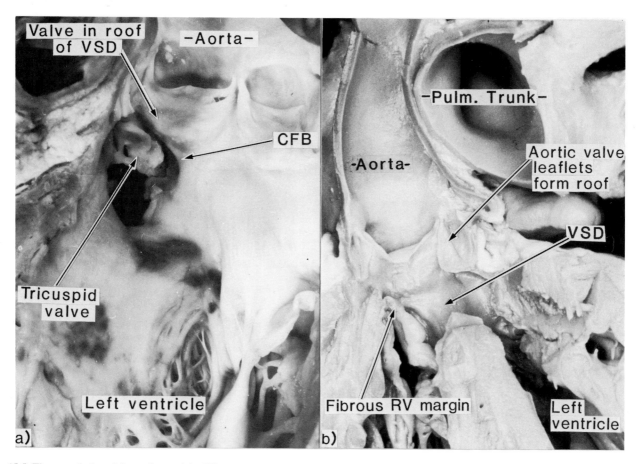

Fig. 25.5 The term 'subaortic' may be used in different ways by different disciplines. As the morphologist views all perimembranous defects from the left ventricle (a) they are seen to be roofed by the area of fibrous continuity between aortic, mitral and tricuspid valves – thus being 'subaortic' although the aortic valve is connected almost exclusively to left ventricular structures. The echocardiographer, in contrast, may reserve the term 'subaortic' for those in which the crest of the septum is overridden by the aortic valve (b). In this heart, the morphologist would describe the fibrous right ventricular aspect as the ventricular septal defect, which would still be considered as being 'subaortic'. (Figure 25.5b is reproduced by kind permission of Dr J. R Zuberbuhler, Children's Hospital of Pittsburgh, USA.)

(Fig. 25.5b). It is important, therefore, to appreciate that the aortic valve attachment is part of the rim of a perimembranous defect. A further group of subaortic defects is those in which the aortic valve in continuity with the pulmonary valve forms the rim of the defect. These defects are not only subaortic, but also subpulmonary. They are therefore called 'doubly committed subarterial' defects. Thus, in terms of their rims, ventricular septal defects may be perimembranous, muscular or doubly committed subarterial (Fig. 25.4). The first two groups can then be still further subdivided depending upon whether they extend or are located so as to open into the inlet, the apical trabecular or the outlet components of the morphologically right ventricle (Table 25.1).

Perimembranous ventricular septal defects

These defects, often called 'membranous defects', have in common the feature that the aortic valve at its attachment to the central fibrous body forms the upper margin of their right ventricular border, a feature paradoxically seen best from the left ventricle (Fig. 25.5). But their extent can vary markedly (Fig. 25.6). Hardly ever in autopsy series are defects described in which the area is so small as to be due simply to absence of the interventricular membranous septum. More usually the defect results from deficiency of the adjacent muscular septum. The part of the septum most deficient forms the basis for subclassification.

When the defect extends to communicate mostly with the inlet of the right ventricle, then the aortic valve and central fibrous body form the anterior part of the right ventricular margin of the defect. The postero-inferior part is roofed by a conjoined area of mitral to tricuspid continuity. The area of atrioventricular muscular septum is correspondingly reduced. When viewed from the right ventricle, the defect is curtained from view by the septal leaflet of the tricuspid valve. The medial papillary muscle is located anteriorly and cephalad to the defect (Fig. 25.6a). Sometimes these defects are termed the 'isolated atrioventricular canal' type (Neufeld et al, 1961).

Table 25.1 Classification of ventricular septal defects.

Perimembranous* (abut on area of continuity between atrioventricular and arterial valves)
— opening into inlet of right ventricle
— opening towards apex of right ventricle
— opening into outlet of right ventricle
— confluent defects

Muscular* (surrounded by muscle of ventricular septum)
— in inlet septum
— in apical trabecular septum
— in outlet septum
— multiple
— co-existing with perimembranous defect

Doubly committed and juxtaarterial (roofed by arterial valves in fibrous continuity)
— with muscular postero-inferior rim
— extending to become perimembranous

* Muscular and perimembranous defects can coexist with malalignment of septal structures

This term can be confusing. Sometimes the perimembranous inlet defect can extend so far posteriorly as to reach the crux. The heart will then have a common atrioventricular junction, a three-leaflet left valve and all the other stigmata of an atrioventricular septal defect (see Ch. 24). More frequently the defect affects only part of the inlet septum. The left valve is a typical mitral valve and the anatomic features of an atrioventricular septal defect are not present. Furthermore, perimembranous inlet defects are anatomically distinct from atrioventricular septal defects with a common valve but with the defect being confined to the ventricular septum. Hearts with tricuspid valves straddling a defect in the inlet septum are distinct from both these groups (Milo et al, 1979). For these reasons, the implication that any inlet septal defect can be termed an 'isolated atrioventricular canal type' (Neufeld et al, 1961; Titus & Rastelli, 1976; LaCorte et al, 1976) is misleading. We believe that the term is best avoided.

More frequent perimembranous defects are those in which the general axis of the defect is towards the cardiac apex. Then, although adjacent areas of inlet and outlet septa are deficient, it is mostly the trabecular septum which is lacking. In these trabecular perimembranous defects, the medial papillary muscle of the tricuspid valve tends to be located towards the apex of the defect itself (Fig. 25.6b). Frequently the septal leaflet of the tricuspid valve is cleft. If the two components of the valves are at all bound down to the defect margins, then left ventricular to right atrial shunting can occur through the cleft in the tricuspid valve. Although such shunts are frequently stated to be due to absence of the atrioventricular membranous septum, the latter mechanism is much more unusual as the cause of a cleft. The key to differentiation of the two types is the attachment of the septal leaflet of the tricuspid valve (Fig. 25.7).

The third type of perimembranous defect is the one which extends so as to open between the ventricular outlet components. The feature of these defects is that the medial

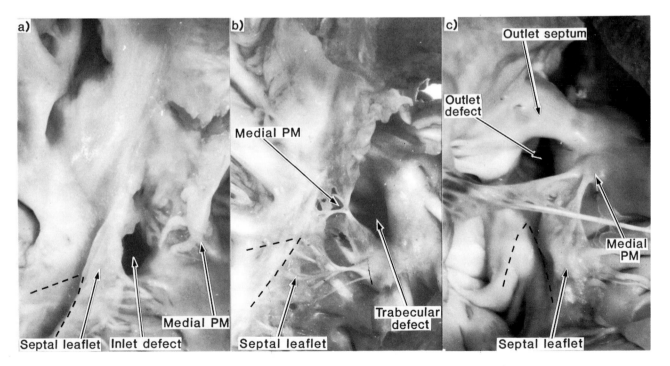

Fig. 25.6 Three different variants of perimembranous defects viewed from the right ventricular aspect. All are roofed by the central fibrous body. The defect in (a) however, extends to communicate mostly between the inlets; that in (b) extends to the apex of the ventricle ('trabecular'); that in (c) opens mostly between the outlet components. Note the differing relationship of the medial papillary muscle (PM) to the various defects.

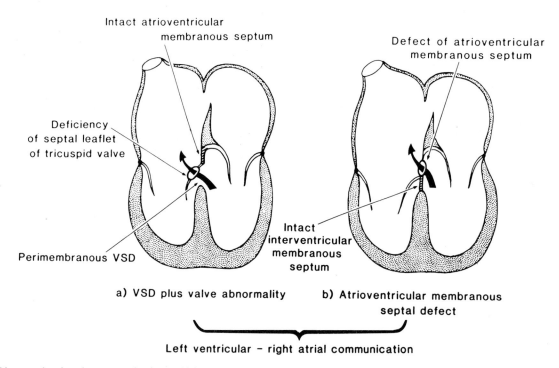

Fig. 25.7 Diagram showing the two mechanisms which produce a left ventricular-right atrial communication. The possibility shown in (a) – a tricuspid valve lesion coexisting with a perimembranous ventricular septal defect (VSD) – is the more common. Isolated defects of the atrioventricular membranous septum (b) are described mostly in the surgical literature. These are *not* examples of the lesions we term 'atrioventricular septal defects' because, of necessity for a left ventricular-right atrial communication, the aortic valve must occupy its usual 'wedge' position. In keeping with this, the left valve is a normal mitral valve.

papillary muscle is related to the postero-inferior rim (Fig. 25.6c). The outlet septum may simply be deficient or can be malaligned relative to the trabecular septum. When there is malalignment of the outlet septum, then either the aortic valve or the pulmonary valve overrides. A malalignment outlet defect with aortic overriding is closely related to tetralogy of Fallot (see Ch. 32). The distinction between them depends upon the infundibular morphology. When the pulmonary valve overrides, there is deviation of the outlet septum into the left ventricular outflow tract (Becu et al, 1955). This usually produces marked subaortic obstruction. These defects tend to be associated with aortic arch malformations, either severe tubular hypoplasia or arch interruption between the brachiocephalic and common carotid arteries (Van Praagh & McNamara, 1968; Moulaert et al, 1976; Ho et al, 1983; Kutsche & Van Mierop, 1984). Oftentimes a perimembranous defect can extend so that it opens into both the inlet and outlet components of the right ventricle. These are much more common than pure 'trabecular' lesions and are best described as confluent defects (Fig. 25.8; Ueda & Becker, 1985).

Fig. 25.8 The right ventricular aspect of a defect which extends to communicate between the inlets and outlets and extends out also towards the ventricular apex. These are best termed 'confluent defects'. (Photographed and reproduced by permission of Dr J. R. Zuberbuhler, University of Pittsburgh, USA.)

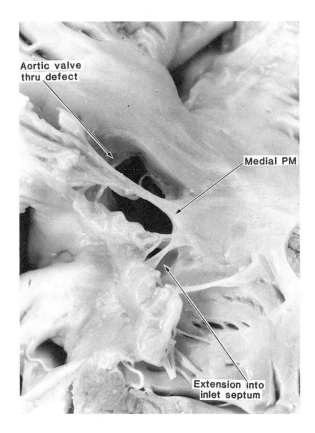

Irrespective of whether a perimembranous defect extends to open between the inlet, trabecular or outlet ventricular components (or is confluent), the basic distribution of the atrioventricular conduction tissues is the same. There are, however, important subtle differences between the three subtypes. In the normal heart the penetrating component of the atrioventricular conduction axis passes through the central fibrous body to branch on the septal surface of the left ventricular outflow tract. Since the central fibrous body forms the postero-inferior margin of perimembranous defects, this will be the site of penetration of the axis. The landmark of the atrioventricular node, as in the normal heart, is the apex of the triangle of Koch. When the defect is between the inlet components, the triangle may itself be displaced posteriorly.

Nonetheless the apex of the triangle (and hence the site of the penetrating bundle) will be normally positioned. When the axis has penetrated through the central fibrous body it is generally related to the postero-inferior rim of the perimembranous defect (Truex & Bishof, 1958; Lev, 1960; Titus et al, 1963). But the precise relationship of its non-branching component to the septal crest depends upon the type of defect (Milo et al, 1980). It is much closer to the crest in a defect between the inlet components. It becomes more remote as the defect extends to open between the outlets (Fig. 25.9). Very occasionally the branching bundle may be positioned astride the septum in an outlet defect, but this is an exceptional finding (Titus et al, 1963; Anderson et al, 1977).

Because perimembranous defects are closely related to

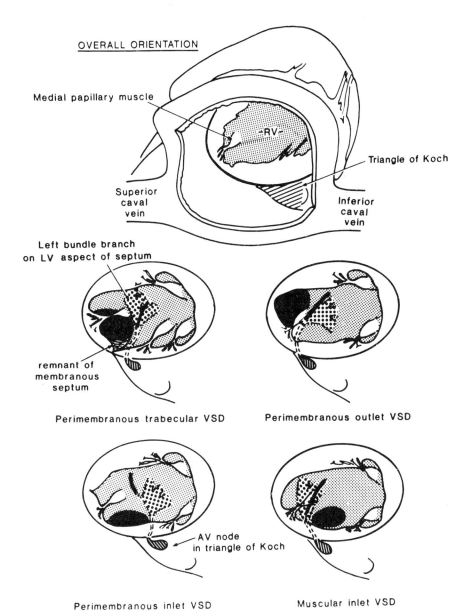

Fig. 25.9 The overall relationship of the conduction axis is illustrated in perimembranous defects and contrasted with the arrangement in a muscular inlet defect (lower right-hand panel). The axis is carried on the left ventricular aspect of the septum, i.e. it is mostly in a safe position except where it is related to the rim of the defect.

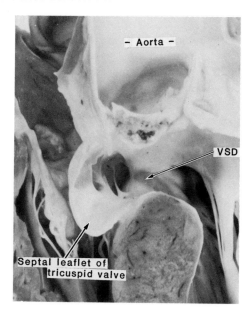

Fig. 25.10 This perimembranous defect, seen in four chamber section, has been closed by plastering down of the septal leaflet of the tricuspid valve. (Photographed and reproduced by kind permission of Professor M. J. Davies, St George's Hospital, Tooting, London, UK.)

the septal leaflet of the tricuspid valve, there is always the possibility that they may be closed because of plastering down of the leaflet across the defect (Fig. 25.10). The most likely defects to close in this fashion are small inlet or trabecular defects. Defects between the outlet components, particularly when complicated by malalignment, are unlikely to close by this mechanism. Neither are extensive inlet defects. Another closely related mechanism of closure is aneurysmal enlargement of fibrous tissue tags in the environs of the defect. Although often described as 'aneurysm of the membranous septum' (Varghese & Rowe, 1969), it is unusual for the membranous septal remnant to be involved. In most cases the grape-like lesions are sculpted from the tricuspid valve leaflets (Chesler et al, 1968). Sometimes the tags are more extensive hammock-like lesions with chordal attachments to the septum. In other cases, the aneurysmal tags can be found plastered across the defect and almost closing it (Fig. 25.11). The defects most likely to be closed by aneurysmal transformation of tricuspid tissue tags are trabecular or small inlet perimembranous defects (Somerville, 1979; Anderson et al, 1983; Beerman et al, 1985). The incidence and importance of aneurysms of the membranous septum (referred to as 'pseudoaneurysms') in the natural history of isolated perimembranous ventricular septal defects has recently been reviewed (Ramaciotti et al, 1986). Their report indicates that the presence of a 'pseudoaneurysm' means there is a better chance of spontaneous closure of the defect, better clinical improvement and less necessity for surgical closure of the defect than when it is absent.

Aneurysmal prolapse of the right aortic valve leaflet can be found with perimembranous defects, particularly outlet defects when the infundibular septum is markedly deficient. Prolapse of the non-coronary leaflet is also described (Van Praagh & McNamara, 1968; Tatsuno et al, 1973). Rarely such a prolapse may produce partial or complete plugging of the defect and result in spontaneous closure (Moss & Siassi, 1970).

In all of these possible mechanisms of closure or diminution in size, contraction and fibrosis around the edges of the defect are contributory, while they also provide a possible nidus for development of infective endocarditis.

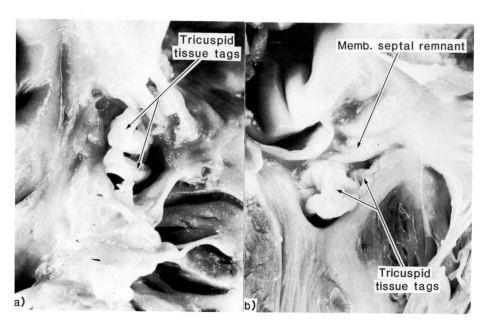

Fig. 25.11 A perimembranous defect almost closed by formation of tissue tags from the leaflets of the tricuspid valve, and viewed from the right (a) and left (b) ventricular aspect. Note that the tags do *not* originate from the remnant of interventricular membranous septum. (Photographed and reproduced by kind permission of Dr J. R. Zuberbuhler, Children's Hospital of Pittsburgh, USA.)

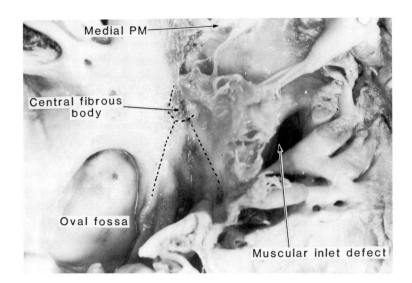

Fig. 25.12 A muscular inlet defect viewed from its right ventricular aspect. The central fibrous body is normally formed.

Muscular defects

Defects with entirely muscular rims can exist anywhere in the septum. Basically they can be subdivided into those in the inlet, trabecular, or outlet components. Muscular defects themselves can be multiple, particularly when in the trabecular septum, or can coexist with perimembranous or juxtaarterial defects.

Inlet muscular defects are largely covered by the septal leaflet of the tricuspid valve (Fig. 25.12). When they are towards the crux, there is no difficulty in distinguishing muscular from perimembranous inlet defects. When the muscular inlet defect is close to the central fibrous body, differentiation is more difficult. The key is that, in the muscular defect, a muscular bar (which may be quite small) separates the septal leaflets of the mitral and tricuspid valves (Fig. 25.13a). These are in fibrous continuity in a perimembranous defect between the inlet components (Fig. 25.13b). This difference is crucial. In the muscular defect the ventricular conduction tissue axis passes above or anterosuperior to the defect (to the left hand as viewed by the surgeon – see Fig. 25.9d). It is always beneath (or postero-inferior) to a perimembranous defect (to the right hand as viewed by the surgeon – see Fig. 25.9a–c). The branching portion of the atrioventricular conduction axis is therefore related to the opposite quadrant of a muscular inlet defect as compared to a perimembranous defect.

Trabecular muscular defects are frequently large holes which tend to be found to one or other side of the septomarginal trabeculation. These large trabecular muscular defects can be multiple. Not infrequently a single opening (as viewed from the left ventricular aspect) is crossed by the trabeculation to produce two openings when viewed

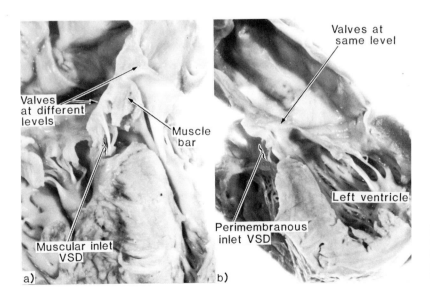

Fig. 25.13 Four chamber sections illustrating the different formation of the atrioventricular muscular septum which is the key to distinction of a muscular inlet defect (a) from a perimembranous defect between the ventricular inlet components (b).

from the right ventricle. Many smaller trabecular muscular defects give the so-called 'swiss-cheese' septum. These may be particularly difficult to define in the autopsy specimen. Although the atrioventricular conduction axis is itself unrelated to trabecular muscular defects, the distal bundle branches may pass through the defect, producing 'pseudo-bifurcations' on the floor of the hole (Latham & Anderson, 1972). Whether or not heart block produced by 'tracking' along the fibrous sheaths of the conduction fascicles could occur from a trabecular defect is undecided. It seems unlikely, since there is no reported incidence of heart block following their repair.

Outlet or infundibular muscular defects are small and usually single (Fig. 25.14a) although they can coexist with other defects. Their superior rim is the outlet septum (often attenuated) while the inferior muscular rim which separates the defect from the membranous septum is formed by fusion of the posterior limb of the septomarginal trabecula with the ventriculo-infundibular fold. This muscle rim separates the conduction tissue axis from the crest of the septum, thus providing protection from surgical damage (Fig. 25.14b). This type of defect has been termed an 'intracristal' defect (Rosenquist et al, 1973). Muscular outlet defect is more explicit. Small muscular defects probably close spontaneously simply by growth of the muscular septum surrounding them. Anatomical studies in themselves cannot provide unequivocal evidence of closure of muscular defects. Such evidence can only be provided by serial studies using angiography or echocardiography. Some muscular defects are seen at autopsy with fibrous rims, supporting another mechanism of spontaneous closure.

Doubly committed juxtaarterial defects

Doubly committed juxtaarterial defects are sometimes called 'supracristal' defects. Exactly the same problems of nomenclature beset this group of defects as beset the muscle bundles in the tetralogy of Fallot – Which bundle is the crista? If we examine a so-called 'infracristal defect' (see Fig. 25.6), it is termed 'infracristal' because it is *below* the outlet septum. It is above the posterior limb of the septomarginal trabeculation, which is separate from the ventriculo-infundibular fold because there is tricuspid to aortic valvar continuity. The essence of the 'supracristal' defect is virtual absence of the outlet septum, there being continuity between the facing leaflets of the aortic and pulmonary valves. Those who term this defect 'supra-cristal' do so because the defect is above the posterior limb of the septomarginal trabeculation, which happens in these cases to be fused with ventriculo-infundibular fold (Fig. 25.15b). Thus, both 'infra-' and 'supra-' cristal defects are above the same structure, the posterior limb of the septomarginal trabeculation. It is the nature of the 'crista' that has changed rather than the margin of the defect. As with the muscular outlet defect, the fusion of the ventriculo-infundibular fold and the septomarginal trabeculation separates tricuspid and aortic valves and distances the conduction tissue axis from the edge of the defect. Occasionally the juxtaarterial defect can extend to become perimembranous (Fig. 25.15b). Then the conduction tissue is more likely to be at risk, although even in perimembranous outlet defects it is usually some distance from the crest of the septum (Milo et al, 1980). This defect is termed 'juxtaarterial' because it is directly related to *both* aortic and pulmonary valves. Indeed, it is because of this

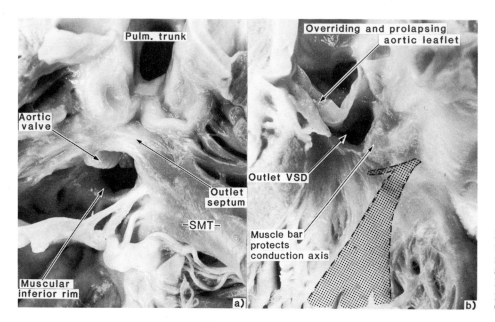

Fig. 25.14 A muscular defect between the ventricular outlets seen (a) from the right and (b) from the left ventricular aspects. Note the prolapsing aortic valve leaflet and the muscular rim which protects the conduction axis (superimposed in b).

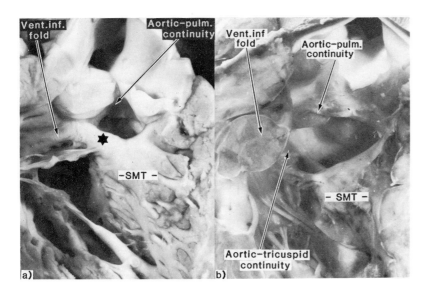

Fig. 25.15 Doubly committed juxtaarterial defects are distinguished because the roof is made up of continuity between aortic and pulmonary valves. They can have (a) muscular postero-inferior rims or (b) extend to become perimembranous. SMT – septomarginal trabeculation.

that both arterial valves frequently override the septum, giving a series of anomalies whose end-point is double outlet left ventricle (Ueda & Becker, 1986). Such hearts with doubly committed juxta-arterial defects and over-riding of both arterial valves have been termed 'double outlet both ventricles' (Brandt et al, 1976). It is because the aortic valve is unsupported by the outlet septum that prolapse of the aortic leaflet is so frequent with the juxtaarterial defect. Nonetheless aortic prolapse can also lead to valve insufficiency with a perimembranous defect (Van Praagh & McNamara, 1968; Tatsuno et al, 1973).

Morphogenesis

As described in Chapter 4, normal closure of the embryonic interventricular communication is dependent upon normal connexion of the inflow portion to the right ventricle and the subaortic outflow tract to the left ventricle. Thereafter the communication is closed by tissue derived from various sources (see Ch. 4 for details). It is *not* closed by the interventricular membranous septum. At the stage at which the interventricular communication is closed, the septal leaflet of the tricuspid valve is not yet formed and so there is no interventricular component. Perimembranous defects *cannot* be explained simply on the basis of failure of the interventricular component of the membranous septum to close the interventricular foramen. It is more likely that there is deficiency of the muscular septum in the environs of the closing plug of tissue, which is consequently of insufficient area or volume to effect closure. Deficiency of the different areas of the muscular septum would then account for the diversity in position and orientation of perimembranous defects.

Muscular defects are more easily explained. It is now established that the muscular septal components are derived from different morphogenetic sources (see Ch. 4). Furthermore, the primordia of the inlet and trabecular septa are produced by coalescence of embryonic trabeculations. Muscular defects could therefore result either from failure of the trabeculations to coalesce – this giving the swiss-cheese septum when extensive – or from failure of fusion of the different components of the muscular septum. For example, failure of fusion of the outlet septum with the trabecular septum and the septomarginal trabeculation gives a good explanation for the outlet muscular defect. The doubly committed juxtaarterial defect, in contrast, is well-explained simply on the basis of failure of formation of the outlet components of the muscular septum.

PATHOPHYSIOLOGY

The pathophysiology of ventricular septal defect is determined by the size of the defect and the state of the pulmonary vascular resistance. The site of the defect within the septum has little influence. Between them, these two features govern the direction and magnitude of flow through the defect, and thus the clinical features and symptomatology.

The effect of defect size

The size of the defect is dominant. Below a critical size, the defect itself presents a resistance to flow through it. This controls the magnitude but not the direction of the shunt. Above this critical size, there is no appreciable resistance to flow. Both magnitude and direction of flow are then determined by the level of pulmonary vascular resistance. There is little 'hard' data concerning this critical size. Some authorities (Rudolph, 1974; Graham et al, 1977) have made statements unsupported by scientific investigation to the effect that defects smaller than the aortic orifice are restrictive. In this respect, Sherman (1963) in his atlas of congenital heart disease pointed out that three-quarters of the defects seen in autopsied hearts from children are less than 75% of the diameter of the aorta. Perhaps more importantly, he noted that the older the patients the smaller were the defects observed. Lucas et al (1961) attempted to quantitate the critical size itself by comparing the diameter of the defect with body surface area. They found the critical size to be a defect whose diameter was 1 cm/m^2 body surface area. This corresponds to an orificial area of approximately $0.8 \text{ cm}^2/\text{m}^2$. Defects having ratios smaller than this were restrictive and produced minor or no haemodynamic changes. This suggests that the critical size is smaller than the aortic orifice, since a normal aortic orifice is calculated to be approximately $2.0 \text{ cm}^2/\text{m}^2$ body surface area. In practice, the judgement of defect size is generally made on haemodynamic grounds. When there are left-to-right shunt and no other associated anomalies such as pulmonary stenosis, a large defect is one which permits equalisation of systolic pressures in the two ventricles and in the aorta and the pulmonary trunk: in other words it is unrestrictive. Since right and left ventricles do not contract exactly simultaneously, there is always some inequality in the ventricular pressures. Thus, throughout the greater part of systole the pressure difference will promote left-to-right shunting. In 'isovolumic' relaxation, right-to-left shunting probably occurs. This is cleared by the subsequent diastolic left-to-right shunt unless right ventricular ejection is obstructed (Levin et al, 1967).

A restrictive defect is then one in which right ventricular and pulmonary arterial systolic pressures are lower than those in the left ventricle and aorta. The size of such defects may vary from those which are just restrictive (i.e. allowing some elevation of right-sided pressures) to small defects in which the right-sided pressures are normal. In effect, therefore, defects can be grouped into two categories: restrictive and unrestrictive. In the restrictive group there is a continuum of size between those large enough to allow a quite serious haemodynamic disturbance and those so small that there is only a small left-to-right shunt with normal right-sided pressures.

The effects of pulmonary vascular resistance

The effect of pulmonary resistance on the flow through restrictive defects is always secondary to the defect size. The smaller the defect, the lower the flow through it. In unrestrictive defects the pulmonary vascular resistance (and, to a lesser extent, systemic vascular resistance) is the controlling factor. When the pulmonary vascular resistance is low, the flow through the defect (and thus pulmonary blood flow) will be high. Usually it is more than three times as high as the systemic blood flow. Such a high pulmonary blood flow is not present at birth. It takes a finite time for the pulmonary resistance to fall from high intra-uterine to the normal postnatal levels. It is possible that the major fall is accomplished in the normal infant by 1–2 weeks of age (Dawes, 1968; Rudolph, 1970).

This fall may be delayed in patients with a large ventricular septal defect and be limited in its extent. Structural factors which contribute to this include limited postnatal lung growth and limitation of the number of intra-acinar blood vessels. In addition there is hypertrophy of the muscular coat of the intra-acinar arteries and veins (Wagenvoort et al, 1961; Naeye, 1966; Haworth et al, 1977; see Ch. 6). It is not entirely clear why lung growth and lung blood vessel proliferation are limited, but muscular hypertrophy of the blood vessels is probably secondary to the increased pulmonary flow. Such a high pulmonary blood flow leads to a high left atrial pressure which is known to cause pulmonary vasoconstriction in experimental animals (Rudolph, 1965). If the vasoconstriction is maintained, vascular muscular hypertrophy will presumably occur.

This delay in fall of the pulmonary resistance means that the maximum haemodynamic effects of an unrestrictive defect may not be reached for some weeks after birth. The time and course and the extent of the fall in pulmonary resistance are all variable. The maximum flow through the defect, however, is usually achieved between 1 and 6 weeks of age. The maximum fall in resistance is usually enough to allow a very high pulmonary blood flow but may be so limited that little flow occurs through the defect. Such patients may escape detection until the effects of severe pulmonary vascular disease are apparent.

Once having fallen to its lowest value, pulmonary vascular resistance may increase again with the development of the pathological changes of pulmonary vascular disease (Haworth et al, 1977; Rabinovitch et al, 1978). This usually occurs only in patients with a high pulmonary arterial pressure from birth and thus is almost confined to those with an unrestrictive defect. As the resistance rises, shunt flow decreases. When pulmonary vascular resistance exceeds that in the systemic circuit, the flow through the defect will change from left-to-right to right-to-left. Thus the level of resistance determines the direction of shunt flow. Secondary effects of severe pulmonary vascular disease include enlargement of the right ventricle, the pulmonary trunk and the 'annular' attachments of the leaflets of the pulmonary valve. These may cause detectable but usually haemodynamically insignificant pulmonary regurgitation.

When defects are restrictive, there is wide spectrum of restrictiveness. In many the defect is so small that the pulmonary vascular resistance has little or no effect on the magnitude of flow through it. In others the defect is restrictive (not allowing equalisation of pressures between the two ventricles) but is big enough to permit a significant elevation of right ventricular and pulmonary arterial pressures. In these defects the level of pulmonary vascular resistance will play a significant (albeit subordinate) role in controlling the magnitude of pulmonary blood flow. Between the two extremes of restrictive defects there is a continuum of defect size and therefore of pathophysiological effects.

The effect of pulmonary outflow tract obstruction

The above discussion has presumed an unobstructed pulmonary outflow tract. If there is coexisting right ventricular outflow tract obstruction (either valvar or subvalvar) then the resistance to ejection from the right ventricle will have a similar effect to elevation of the pulmonary vascular resistance. The flow through an unrestrictive defect (and thence pulmonary blood flow) will be limited in proportion to the severity of the obstruction. In restrictive defects, obstruction to the right ventricular outflow will result in elevation of right ventricular pressure again in proportion to the severity of obstruction. The right ventricular pressure in extreme cases may come to exceed that in the left ventricle. As in unrestrictive defects, pulmonary outflow tract obstruction in the larger of the restrictive defects will also have a limiting effect on the magnitude of flow. There will be a reversal in the direction of the shunt in all cases where right ventricular pressure exceeds that in the left ventricle. Although pulmonary valvar obstruction may be present unequivocally from birth, subvalvar obstruction can be acquired.

The cardiac response to ventricular septal defect

The cardiac effects of a ventricular septal defect depend initially on the magnitude of pulmonary blood flow. With a large pulmonary blood flow (usually in non-restrictive defects) left atrial and left ventricular end-diastolic volumes are increased and left ventricular muscle mass is always increased (Jarmakani et al, 1969). Pressure-volume studies of the left ventricle demonstrate the marked increase in left ventricular work imposed by a large defect (Jarmakani et al, 1968). This necessitates left ventricular hypertrophy as a compensatory mechanism. With a very large pulmonary blood flow there is also an increase in right ventricular dimensions. Because of the elevated right ventricular pressure, there will be an even more marked increase in right ventricular work. This results in additional right ventricular hypertrophy. This hypertrophic response may be one mechanism for the development of subvalvar pulmonary stenosis.

Left ventricular work is increased with restrictive defects in relation to the pulmonary blood flow but the right ventricle is relatively spared. Thus, left ventricular hypertrophy occurs but with little increase in right ventricular size or muscle mass. With elevation of pulmonary vascular resistance or with development of right ventricular outflow obstruction, left ventricular work is diminished because of the decrease in pulmonary blood flow. The elevation of right ventricular pressure results in right ventricular hypertrophy which dominates the picture.

The pathophysiological effects of a ventricular septal defect can, in three situations, result in congestive cardiac failure. The first is an unrestrictive defect with high pulmonary blood flow when the compensatory mechanisms are insufficient to provide an adequate systemic blood flow under all circumstances. These mechanisms include recruitment of all sarcomeres to operate at their optimal end-diastolic length, muscular hypertrophy of right and left ventricles and increased catecholamine drive to the ventricles. These circumstances are usually reached before the age of 6 months. The second situation occurs much later. It is encountered when the right ventricular myocardium has undergone degenerative changes occurring as a consequence of long-term ejection against high resistance. This is found with pulmonary vascular disease and prolonged and severe right ventricular outflow tract obstruction. The final situation is when a ventricular septal defect is complicated by aortic regurgitation. This imposes a further volume load on the left ventricle. It results in cardiac failure when it is severe enough to outstrip the compensatory mechanisms as discussed above. It is most frequently seen in older children and adults.

CLINICAL FEATURES

Presentation

Ventricular septal defects are rarely, if ever, detectable at birth, since it takes a few weeks for the pulmonary vascular resistance to fall from the high intra-uterine levels. Fetal levels of pulmonary vascular resistance are high enough to limit the flow through even an unrestrictive defect to levels insufficient to provide an audible murmur. Thus it is rare for a ventricular septal defect to be diagnosed at routine postnatal examination on the first day of life. If a defect is diagnosed in the neonatal nursery, it is almost invariably during examination of the baby just prior to the mother's discharge. Even at the end of the first week of life, when many murmurs are detected, it is rare for the pulmonary vascular resistance to have fallen sufficiently for the patient to be symptomatic. Symptoms, when they occur, are related to the high pulmonary blood flow. Diminished lung compliance and elevation of the left atrial pressure due to high pulmonary blood flow initially causes tachypnoea. This progresses with the onset of congestive cardiac failure to dyspnoea on effort. This is manifested when the baby feeds. In a typical unrestrictive or large restrictive defect, the parents are likely to complain that their baby takes progressively longer to feed over the first month or two of life. Feeding leads to rapid exhaustion of the baby. Not only is it prolonged, but it does not provide sufficient caloric intake for weight gain. With the development of severe cardiac failure, the baby will become obviously dyspnoeic even at rest. Intercostal, subcostal and supraclavicular recession are then readily seen. This increased work of respiration imposes an increased requirement for energy. This is not satisfied because of the difficulty of feeding. Failure to thrive due to inadequate caloric intake ensues. Failure to thrive is, indeed, an alternative mode of presentation in infancy. It occurs in those babies with defects large enough to allow high pulmonary blood flow but in which the defect size or level of pulmonary vascular resistance prevents the development of intractable congestive cardiac failure. Another association with high pulmonary blood flow is an increased susceptibility to respiratory infection. The parents may complain that their baby has frequent 'chesty' colds. It may be during such an episode that a murmur is noted and that cardiac failure is precipitated.

A small and restrictive defect may be detected at any age by the discovery of a murmur. But such a defect will rarely if ever cause symptoms. When a defect is found in this fashion after the age of 1 year, it is highly unlikely that in itself it will ever cause congestive cardiac failure. No such assurance can be given when discovered in early infancy.

There is a further small group of patients with ventricular septal defect who escape detection in infancy. They present with diminished effort tolerance and cyanosis during middle childhood or adolescence. These patients usually have severe pulmonary vascular disease. Even careful history-taking fails to elicit evidence of symptoms during infancy. It is probable that at no stage did their pulmonary vascular resistance fall to levels permitting a left-to-right shunt flow sufficient to allow recognition of the defect.

Another alternative and rare presentation is with respiratory symptoms because of bronchial compression due to grossly enlarged pulmonary arteries. Typically it is the right middle lobe bronchus which is compressed, but the left main and upper lobe bronchi may also be involved (Stanger et al, 1969). This presentation is most frequently seen in patients with severe pulmonary vascular disease.

Thus, ventricular septal defects rarely if ever present in the first days of life. In small restrictive defects, presentation is by the incidental discovery of a murmur, the patient remaining asymptomatic. In large but restrictive defects and in unrestrictive defects, the initial finding may be a murmur but symptoms rapidly ensue. It may be the symptoms of dyspnoea and failure to thrive which call attention to the heart. In rare cases presentation occurs only with the recognition of a right-to-left shunt in those cases with irreversible vascular disease, and these cases may also present because of respiratory problems.

Physical signs

The appearance of the patient is again dependent on the magnitude of flow through the defect. Those with small and restrictive defects are generally entirely normal. With large restrictive defects but without frank congestive cardiac failure, patients tend to be small and thin for their age with evidence of dyspnoea such as intercostal recession. Chronicity is suggested by a depression at the insertion of the diaphragm. This depression is at the site described by Harrison (a Lincolnshire general practitioner, 1766–1838) as a late effect of rickets (Bailey & Clain, 1954). There will also be bulging of the left chest indicating cardiomegaly. With large unrestrictive defects, similar appearances of more severe degree will be seen without the evidence of chronicity. Cyanosis will not be seen except in those older patients with severe pulmonary vascular disease or severe right ventricular outflow tract obstruction.

On palpation, a systolic thrill is felt in almost all patients, localised to the second, third and fourth intercostal spaces at the left sternal border. If the thrill is maximal in the first intercostal space or higher, and yet the auscultatory features are otherwise typical of a ventricular septal defect, this suggests the presence of a doubly committed and juxtaarterial defect (Steinfeld et al, 1972). Only when the defect flow is very small will this sign be lacking. With small restrictive defects there are usually no other palpable abnormalities. When the defect is large with a high flow, the cardiac impulse will be hyperdynamic and the thrill may be more widespread. In presence of severe pulmonary vascular disease a localised left parasternal heave of right ventricular type and a palpable second sound are the striking features. The peripheral pulses are normal. Abnormalities such as a high volume pulse or absent femoral pulse should suggest an associated arterial duct or coarctation respectively.

The most typical auscultatory finding, namely the loud pan-systolic murmur localised to the second and third left intercostal spaces, was not accepted as being due to a ventricular septal defect at Roger's initial presentation to the Academie de Medicine (1879). This murmur is typical of all ventricular septal defects with a left-to-right shunt even when they are small and restrictive. The murmur starts with the first sound and continues up to the second sound. If the murmur starts with the first heart sound but stops short of the second, it is suggestive of the defect being a small muscular one closing in late systole. It is said that a pan-systolic murmur may continue past the aortic component of the second heart sound (Harris et al, 1976). This is rarely appreciated by the ear. Similarly, the ear usually does not detect any variation in the intensity of the murmur although phonocardiography does show that the murmur is loudest during mid-systole. When pulmonary blood flow is limited by pulmonary resistance, the systolic murmur is abbreviated and may be completely absent. In such cases an early diastolic murmur of pulmonary regurgitation may be heard as well as a pulmonary click. In cases where the pulmonary blood flow is high, the flow through the mitral valve is sufficient to produce a mid-diastolic murmur at the apex. The presence of this murmur is taken to indicate that pulmonary blood flow is more than twice the systemic flow. In patients with no other signs of pulmonary vascular disease the appearance of a high-pitched early diastolic murmur is highly suggestive of the onset of aortic regurgitation.

In the absence of pulmonary vascular disease, the heart sounds appear normal. It is claimed that the second heart sound is widely split, with delay of its pulmonary component (Graham et al, 1977). In our experience, although seen on phonocardiography, it is rarely appreciated on auscultation. In patients with pulmonary hypertension, the pulmonary second sound is louder. In severe cases the increased intensity is easy to detect. In less severe cases the fact that the second heart sound is audibly split at the apex indicates that the pulmonary component is louder than normal. Development of this finding during follow-up should alert one to the possibility that pulmonary vascular disease is developing. The second heart sound becomes single once severe pulmonary vascular disease has developed (Sutton et al, 1968).

Electrocardiographic findings

The electrocardiographic features are not specific for ventricular septal defect. As may be expected, they do reflect the haemodynamic status. So, in patients with large unrestrictive defects presenting with a high pulmonary blood flow in infancy, there will be a normal sinus rhythm (probably with tachycardia), a frontal QRS axis within the normal range for age, and biventricular hypertrophy. Finding a superior axis suggests either multiple defects (Fox et al, 1978), an atrioventricular septal defect or that an isolated perimembranous defect excavates the inlet portion of the ventricular septum. Tall T waves over the right precordial leads in infancy strongly suggest that the right ventricular pressure is at systemic levels. Cardiac rhythm and the QRS axis are usually normal in large restrictive defects after the first few months of life. The QRS pattern is that of left ventricular dominance with deep Q waves over the left chest leads indicating left ventricular volume overload. In small restrictive defects the electrocardiogram may be entirely normal.

In the early months of life serial electrocardiograms provide more prognostic information than a single tracing. Large unrestrictive defects maintain the biventricular QRS morphology while the smaller defects show the normal diminution of right ventricular forces with age. At any age the presence of pulmonary vascular disease or severe right ventricular outflow tract obstruction is reflected by right without left ventricular hypertrophy and right axis deviation. Should aortic regurgitation complicate a small ventricular septal defect or, alternatively, occur in a patient with established right ventricular outflow obstruction, then the changes of left ventricular volume overload will come to dominate the picture.

Radiological findings

Once more these changes reflect the haemodynamic state. In the first days of the life the chest X-ray is usually entirely normal. With the development of left-to-right shunting the lung fields become plethoric. When the pulmonary blood flow is large (as in unrestrictive defects) cardiomegaly is noted and pulmonary plethora is marked. The cardiac contour in such infants has no specific features. When defects are restrictive with only mild elevation of the pulmonary blood flow, the chest X-ray may always appear normal.

The development and progression of pulmonary vascular disease is reflected in diminution of the peripheral pulmonary vascular shadows, leading to the classical 'pruning' of the peripheral pulmonary arteries seen best in older children and adults. This is accompanied by progressive overall reduction in heart size as the pulmonary blood flow falls, but with characteristic enlargement of the pulmonary knob. When right ventricular outflow tract obstruction occurs, there is reduction in both central and peripheral pulmonary artery shadowing and enlargement of the pulmonary trunk is rare. When complicated by aortic regurgitation, there will be progressive enlargement of the heart with the cardiac contour suggesting left ventricular dominance.

Echocardiographic findings

The present generation of real-time cross-sectional echocardiographic machines permit demonstration of the actual defect in the majority of cases (Bierman et al, 1980; Cheatham et al, 1981; Van Mill et al, 1981; Sutherland et al, 1982; Capelli et al, 1983). Not only do they show the presence of a defect, but also permit its accurate localisation. Furthermore, because the defect can usually be identified in more than one 'cut', its size can be estimated. A perimembranous defect is recognised in long axis, four chamber and short-axis views. Perimembranous defects opening to the inlet of the right ventricle are recognised by cuts through the ventricular inlet portions (Fig. 25.16) while defects between the outlets are best seen on subcostal cuts tracking from four chamber to outlet planes (Fig. 25.17). Muscular inlet defects are best seen in the four chamber cuts, either from apical or subcostal approaches (Fig. 25.18). Large trabecular muscular defects are identified in four chamber and short axis planes (Fig. 25.19), while outlet muscular defects are identified

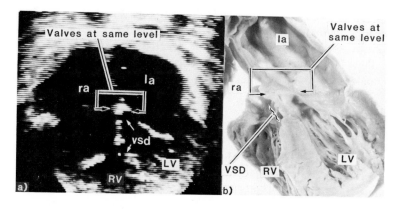

Fig. 25.16 A perimembranous defect between the inlet components is characterised by fibrous continuity between the mitral and tricuspid valves roofing the defect. This feature removes the usual off-setting of the valve attachments. The cross-sectional echocardiographic four chamber section is compared with a heart from a different patient sectioned in similar fashion.

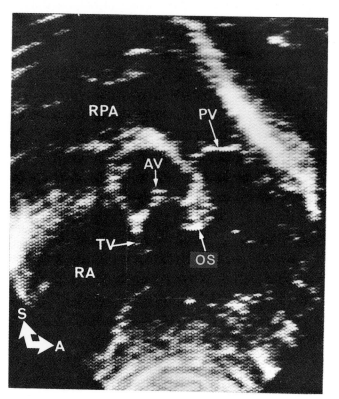

from long axis or subcostal approaches. Small or multiple trabecular muscular defects are those least likely to be visualised. Doubly committed juxtaarterial defects are recognised because of the continuity of aortic and pulmonary valves in the roof of the defect and are seen in long axis (Fig. 25.20), short axis and subcostal oblique views (Fig. 25.21). If present, prolapse of the aortic valve leaflets will be visualised (Fig. 25.22). By rotating the transducer it is also possible to show whether a doubly committed juxtaarterial defect is perimembranous or is separated from the central fibrous body by a muscular rim. Cross-sectional echocardiography also demonstrates the proximity of the defect to structures which may close it, such as aneurysmal formation of tricuspid tissue tags or tricuspid valve leaflet tissue across the defect (Fig. 25.23). Identification of the site of the ventricular septal defect at

Fig. 25.17 A perimembranous outlet defect seen in an oblique subcostal paracoronal cut. The outlet septum (OS) is seen as a right ventricular structure and part of the aortic valve (AV) overrides the remainder of the septum, which is not visualised. The section therefore gives the impression of double outlet right ventricle, but the aortic valve is mostly connected to the left ventricle. RA – right atrium; PV – pulmonary valve; RPA – right pulmonary artery; TV – tricuspid valve.

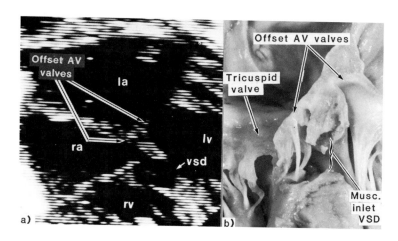

Fig. 25.18 A four chamber cross-sectional echocardiogram in a muscular inlet defect showing the normal off-setting of the atrioventricular (AV) valves. It is compared with a comparable anatomic section of a heart from a different patient.

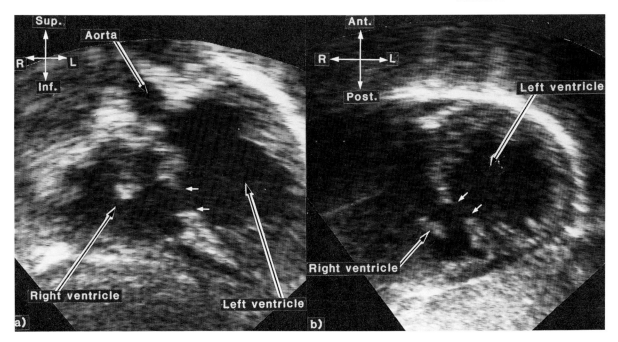

Fig. 25.19 A four chamber section (a) rotating into short axis (b) illustrating a muscular defect in the apical trabecular septum (between white arrows). (Reproduced by kind permission of Dr G. R. Sutherland, Wessex Cardiothoracic Centre, Southampton, UK.)

initial examination will for the first time provide hard evidence about the rate of spontaneous closure for different types of defects in different sites (Sutherland et al, 1987a, b).

In addition to these specific diagnostic findings, the echocardiograph also reflects the haemodynamic state. Left atrial and left ventricular dilation are easily seen in infants with a high pulmonary blood flow, the left ventricle being hyperdynamic. These changes are appreciated during cross-sectional echocardiography but can be quantified by M-mode techniques. With large unrestrictive defects there will be a concomitant increase in right ventricular dimensions, while in small restrictive defects the ventricular size and performance may be normal. Further insight into the physiological state is obtained by studying pulmonary valve motion. With a high pulmonary flow but a low pulmonary vascular resistance the motion is normal, but when there is a high pulmonary vascular resistance, the valve closure line is flattened and the a-dip disappears. The onset of aortic regurgitation is indicated by the appearance of diastolic vibration of the mitral valve, best appreciated on the M-mode tracing. In these cases the cross-sectional echocardiogram may show the abnormalities of the aortic valve responsible for the regurgitation. For example, a prolapsing aortic leaflet may be demonstrated (Fig. 25.22), or alternatively perforations and vegetations associated with infective endocarditis may be identified.

Peripheral injection of contrast material adds little to the basic diagnosis of ventricular septal defect, but when a right-to-left shunt is present the contrast material will be seen appearing in the aorta using both cross-sectional and M-mode techniques. Doppler techniques permit diagnosis of a ventricular septal defect and provide important haemodynamic data. The diagnosis can be made on the basis of abnormal jugular venous blood flow (Kalmanson et al, 1974). A more reliable method is to detect the turbulent flow across the defect within the ventricles (Stevenson et al, 1978). This technique is accurate in nine-tenths of cases, and careful technique permits the jet to be 'tracked' across the ventricle. Better still, the precise position of the defect may be demonstrated by duplex colour-coded Doppler/cross-sectional imaging (Ortiz et al, 1985). The maximum velocity in the jet can be measured reliably with continuous wave Doppler when guided by cross-sectional imaging. The pressure gradient which can then be estimated correlates well with that measured by invasive studies (Valdes-Cruz et al, 1983; Colo et al, 1982).

Nuclear angiography

First pass studies demonstrate the presence of a left-to-right or a right-to-left shunt and permit quantitation of the systemic-pulmonary flow ratio (Gates et al, 1973; Alderson et al, 1975). Gated blood-pool scans allow assessment of left ventricular size and performance, but do not differentiate the different sites or type of defect. They should prove to be of value in the long-term post-operative assessment, particularly when performed in association with an exercise or stress-testing protocol.

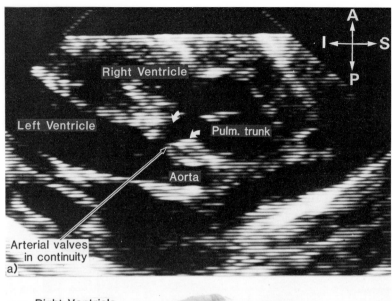

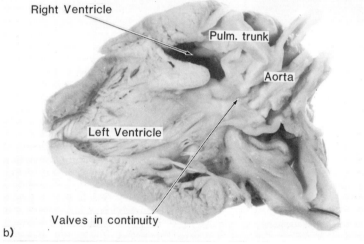

Fig. 25.20 A doubly committed juxtaarterial defect seen in long axis parasternal section (a) with a comparable anatomic section in a heart from a different patient (b).

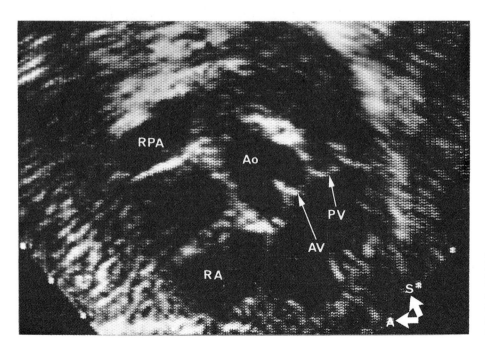

Fig. 25.21A doubly committed juxtaarterial defect seen in subcostal oblique paracoronal section, the aortic arch and pulmonary valves (AV, PV) are seen in fibrous continuity, but the septum is not visualised. RPA – right pulmonary artery; RA – right atrium; AO – aorta.

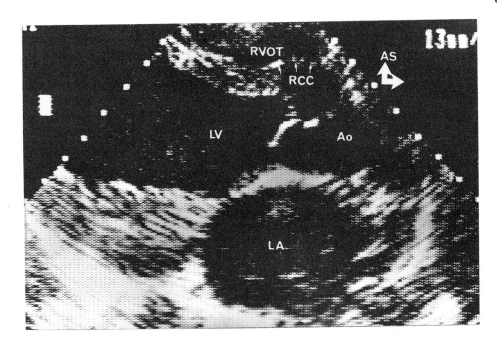

Fig. 25.22 This parasternal long axis section of a doubly committed juxtaarterial defect shows prolapse of the right coronary leaflet (RCC) of the aortic (Ao) valve into the right ventricular outflow tract (RVOT) LV – left ventricle; LA – left atrium.

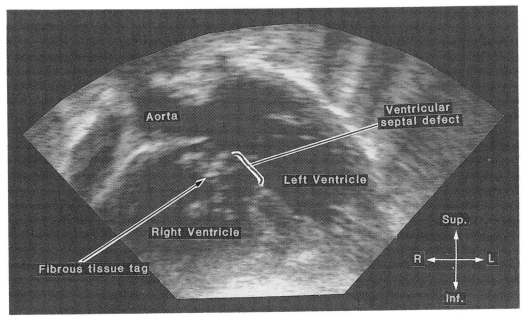

Fig. 25.23 This four chamber section shows a fibrous tissue tag from the tricuspid valve partially closing a perimembranous ventricular septal defect. (Reproduced by kind permission of Dr G. R. Sutherland, Wessex Cardiothoracic Centre, Southampton, UK.)

Cardiac catheterisation

This technique is an essential part of the assessment of large restrictive and unrestrictive defects. It makes possible the measurement of intracardiac pressures, particularly the pulmonary arterial pressure, and the assessment of pulmonary blood flow. From this information it is possible to calculate the pulmonary vascular resistance. In addition it provides confirmation that the defect is interventricular by the detection of a step-up in oxygen saturation at ventricular level or the passage of the catheter from right ventricle to left ventricle or aorta. If a ventricular septal defect is modified by tricuspid valve abnormalities to function as a left ventricular-right atrial shunt, then the step-up in oxygen saturation will be detected in the right atrium. This will also be detected when a ventricular septal defect coexists with an atrial septal defect or when there is an atrioventricular septal defect. Cardiac catheterisation provides further information about the associated defects. For example, passage of the catheter from the pulmonary

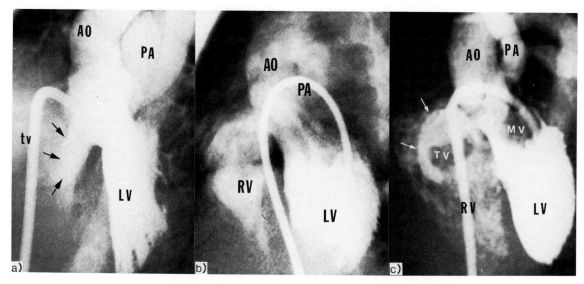

Fig. 25.24 The different types of perimembranous defect as seen in long axial projection of a left ventricular injection. (a) Shows a defect between the inlet components, (b) shows a small trabecular defect, and (c) shows a defect extending into the outlet component. TV – tricuspid valve; MV – mitral valve; RV – right ventricle; LV – left ventricle; Ao – aorta; PA – pulmonary trunk. (Reproduced by kind permission of Dr B. Soto, University of Alabama in Birmingham, USA.)

trunk to the descending aorta indicates the presence of a communication between these two arteries, usually an arterial duct.

The findings at catheterisation reflect the pathophysiology. Unrestrictive defects with a high pulmonary blood flow have similar pressures in right and left ventricles. With an unobstructed right ventricular outflow and a low pulmonary vascular resistance the pulmonary arterial systemic pressure will be similar to that in the aorta. The diastolic and mean pulmonary arterial pressures, however, will be lower than aortic pressures. In those cases, a high pulmonary blood flow will be measured oximetrically or by dye-dilution curves. In large but restrictive defects, the right ventricular and pulmonary arterial pressures will be lower than those in the left ventricle and aorta.

Angiocardiography

This is directed to anatomical delineation of the defect itself and to the diagnosis or exclusion of associated abnormalities. Left ventricular angiocardiograms are mandatory for anatomical diagnosis, although the efficacy of cross-sectional echocardiography may, in the future, reduce the need for these studies. When they are performed, it is best to choose an axial oblique projection (Bargeron et al, 1977; Elliott et al, 1977; Soto et al, 1978; Green et al, 1981). The long axis view is the best one for demonstration of the different types of perimembranous defect (Fig. 25.24; Santamaria et al, 1983). Doubly committed juxtaarterial defects will also be shown on this view, but demonstration of the lack of tissue separating the defect from the pulmonary valve requires a right anterior oblique projec-

tion (Fig. 25.25). The long axis view is again best for muscular trabecular defects (Fig. 25.26). A muscular inlet defect is well demonstrated by the four chamber view (Fig. 25.27a) while a muscular outlet defect is profiled in the long axial projection (Fig. 25.27b). If there is doubt about the site of the defect, the long axis view is helpful because inlet septal defects appear behind the line of the anterior portion of the trabecular septum. Careful examination of the angiocardiograms should always be under-

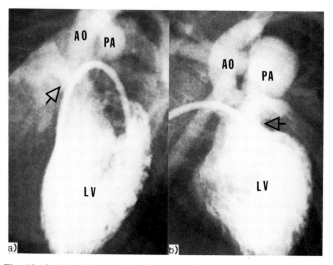

Fig. 25.25 A doubly committed juxtaarterial defect (arrow) as seen (a) in long axial and (b) right anterior oblique projection of a left ventricular injection. Abbreviations as for Figure 25.24. (Reproduced by kind permission of Dr B. Soto, University of Alabama in Birmingham, USA.)

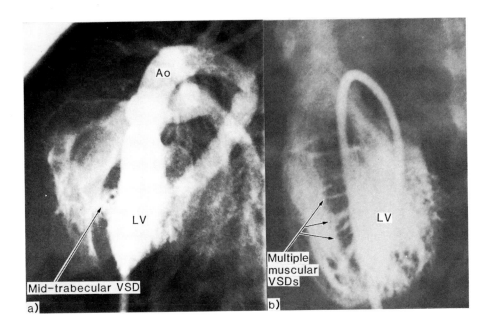

Fig. 25.26 Long axial projections of left ventricular injections showing (a) a solitary and (b) multiple muscular defects of the apical trabecular septum. (Reproduced by kind permission of Dr B. Soto, University of Alabama in Birmingham, USA.)

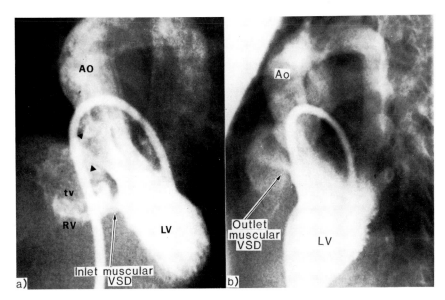

Fig. 25.27 Long axial projections of left ventricular injections showing (a) an inlet muscular and (b) an outlet muscular defect. Abbreviations as in Figure 25.24. (Reproduced by kind permission of Dr B. Soto, University of Alabama in Birmingham, USA.)

taken to exclude mitral regurgitation. In patients with pulmonary hypertension, a persistent arterial duct must be excluded. Frequently this is possible on the axial oblique left ventricular injection. When this is not the case, aortography must be performed. A similar approach is also necessary to exclude associated aortic coarctation. Retrograde aortography is important when aortic regurgitation is suspected. Right ventricular angiography is indicated when right ventricular outflow obstruction is found on cardiac catheterisation (Pongiglione et al, 1982). This is best performed in the 45° head-up position in the anteroposterior and lateral projections. Right ventricular angiography (or recirculation pictures from a right-sided injection) have little or no place in the investigation of an isolated ventricular septal defect.

Left ventricular angiograms can be used for quantitative assessment of left ventricular function. Left ventricular end-diastolic volume is usually increased and the ejection fraction is normal or increased. These indices have prognostic significance but rarely if ever will the decision whether or not to correct be influenced by these findings.

DIAGNOSIS

Until recently the definitive diagnosis of isolated ventricular septal defect depended upon cardiac catheterisation and angiocardiography. Now the diagnosis can be made with certainty in the majority of cases using cross-sectional echocardiography. In many instances, however, the diagnosis can be made from purely clinical evidence supported by the electrocardiogram and the chest X-ray. Thus, in an asymptomatic child over the age of 1 year, the typical physical signs taken together with the chest X-ray and electrocardiogram permit a confident diagnosis. This is not the case in infancy, particularly early infancy. Then a ventricular septal defect is frequently a component of a more complex heart lesion. It may be difficult on clinical grounds alone to be certain whether the defect is isolated. For example, when a ventricular septal defect occurs in the setting of complete transposition, the pulmonary blood flow may be so high that cyanosis is not clinically apparent. Yet the thrill and murmur and the radiographic and electrocardiographic features may be compatible with an isolated lesion. In such cases the blood gas response to inhalation of 100% oxygen (Jones et al, 1976) may indicate that the malformation is a complex one. Occasionally this test is misleading, particularly when the ventricular septal defect is accompanied by a common arterial trunk. Echocardiography is invaluable in differentiating isolated defects from more complex anomalies and should therefore be performed in all symptomatic infants suspected to have ventricular septal defect. Nowadays the role of cardiac catheterisation is limited to the assessment of the appropriateness of treatment and the complete elucidation of very complex malformations. Although the clinical features may leave the diagnosis of isolated ventricular septal defect in doubt, the investigations when expertly performed leave little possibility of alternative diagnosis. The only possible area of confusion is a ventricular septal defect so large that only a rim of septal tissue can be identified separating portions of the ventricles of distinctive right and left pattern. This condition is frequently misdiagnosed as double inlet to a solitary indeterminate ventricle. Although on angiocardiographic or echocardiographic grounds it may be suspected that a rim of ventricular septum is present, this can only be confirmed by direct inspection (see Ch. 26).

COURSE AND PROGNOSIS

The majority of patients with isolated ventricular septal defect live normal lives both in terms of duration and quality (Weidman et al, 1977a, b). Approximately 50–60% close spontaneously (Alpert et al, 1973; Corone et al, 1977). This usually happens during the first 5 years of life but spontaneous closure can occur at any age. As the defect becomes smaller, the murmur is said to lose its pansystolic nature, becoming shorter and decrescendo. These changes have value in predicting those defects which are about to close (Moss & Siassi, 1970). Of those patients whose defect persists, most lead normal active lives with very little risk of a cardiac death before the age of 40 years (Corone et al, 1977).

A small number of infants, perhaps 10–15%, develop congestive cardiac failure requiring medical treatment (Keith, 1978). This almost invariably occurs during the first 6 months of life. Many of these children do not survive longer than 6 months unless surgical treatment is performed. Some, however, are adequately controlled on medical treatment and do not require surgery as a life-saving procedure. Such infants frequently have pulmonary hypertension as a consequence of their large defects and are at risk for the development of pulmonary vascular disease. They form the only reliably identifiable group of the 3–6% of all cases who develop this complication. Any infant with pulmonary hypertension persisting through the early months of life is likely to develop pulmonary vascular disease. This is established and irreversible in the majority before the age of 1 year. Patients who have experienced little or no fall in pulmonary vascular resistance after birth form the remainder of the high risk subjects. Tragically this latter group may escape detection until cyanosis supervenes. It is important to recognise that irreversible and progressive pulmonary vascular disease is present in the affected patients long before they become cyanosed. The prognosis of patients with ventricular septal defect and pulmonary vascular disease is poor, but survival into adult life is common: death usually occurs before 40 years of age. In female patients with pulmonary vascular disease, pregnancy poses a particular risk. This is because blood loss of moderate degree, as may occur at delivery, can precipitate an irreversible low output state. Women with this condition should therefore be advised to avoid pregnancy. If they do not heed this advice, a difficult choice is necessary, since termination of pregnancy also carries a significant risk. On balance, unwanted pregnancies should be terminated. If the patient strongly wishes to continue, with careful supervision many can deliver safely (Szekely & Snaith, 1974).

Two other complications of isolated ventricular septal defect may cause death before the age of 40 years. The first is development of aortic regurgitation (Keane et al, 1977). The reported incidence varies between 1 and 5% (Moss & Siassi, 1970). It occurs most usually either when the defect is doubly committed and juxtaarterial or when the defect is perimembranous (Van Praagh & McNamara, 1968). It can also occur in the presence of muscular outlet defects when the infundibular septum is hypoplastic (Tatsuno et al, 1973). Almost always it is the right coronary aortic leaflet which prolapses through the defect. In perimembranous defects the non-coronary leaflet also may be involved. It is often recommended that surgical treatment be offered as soon as significant aortic regurgitation is recognised (Treasure et al, 1971). But it is now known that in the majority of patients the condition is well tolerated during childhood. Occasionally, heart failure, refractory to medical treatment, occurs in children, but it is more frequently encountered during adult life.

The second complication is infective endocarditis. The incidence is approximately 1–2 per 1000 patient years (Shah et al, 1966; Keith, 1978; Gersony & Hayes, 1977), representing a risk of approximately 1 in 10 of developing infective endocarditis before the age of 70 (Keith, 1978). It is, however, more likely that infective endocarditis will be contracted after the age of 20 years than in childhood or adolescence. The size of defect has no influence on the incidence of the complication (Gersony & Hayes, 1977). Most patients who nowadays develop infective endocarditis are successfully treated. The lifetime risk of dying from infective endocarditis occurring in the setting of isolated ventricular septal defect has been computed to be of the order of 2–3% (Keith, 1978). Surgical closure of defects does not eliminate the chance of contracting this infection. Indeed, it may initiate it (Gersony & Hayes, 1977; Keith, 1978). Avoidance of infective endocarditis cannot therefore be proposed as an indication for the surgical closure of ventricular septal defects.

MANAGEMENT

When a patient presents in early infancy, the outcome is always in doubt. Thus, an asymptomatic infant presenting with a murmur at 1 month of age may be in intractable heart failure by the age of 3 months. Similarly, spontaneous closure of ventricular septal defect may occur even when the defect has been large enough to cause heart failure in infancy. The prognosis must always, therefore, be guarded during the first few months of life. Asymptomatic infants should be closely followed with echocardiographic assessment of the anatomy and pulmonary valve motion. Those remaining asymptomatic with no signs or investigations suggesting pulmonary hypertension require no treatment. They should take no precautions other than prophylactic measures against infective endocarditis. These infants have small restrictive defects. Infants with congestive cardiac failure severe enough to suggest that surgical treatment may be necessary should have a complete haemodynamic assessment. Initially they should be treated medically. If the heart failure is intractable to medical treatment, then surgical intervention is indicated. These infants usually have unrestrictive defects. Intractability of the heart failure is judged to be present when, despite maximal medical treatment with diuretics and digoxin, the infant requires nasogastric tube feeding.

Infants responding to medical treatment may have unrestrictive defects, but usually have large restrictive ones. In either event the pulmonary arterial pressure will be elevated in early infancy. In those with initially large but restrictive defects, it may fall to nearly normal values by the age of 6–9 months. If the pulmonary arterial pressure does not fall, the patient must be considered to be at risk for the development of irreversible pulmonary vascular disease. Therefore, any infant with previously measured pulmonary hypertension (or with clinical, electrocardiographic, echocardiographic or radiological evidence suggestive of pulmonary hypertension) should have a complete haemodynamic assessment 6–9 months of age. If the pulmonary arterial systolic pressure is 75% of the systemic, and there is still a left-to-right shunt, surgery is indicated for the prevention of pulmonary vascular disease. If the pulmonary arterial pressure is lower, conservative management should be continued. A basic assumption behind this policy is that pulmonary vascular disease can be prevented or reversed in its early stages. It is not certain that this is possible in all cases. The above recommendations give the best chance of achieving this aim at present. It must be borne in mind that, in some cases, this policy will result in defects being closed which would have closed spontaneously (Blackstone et al, 1976) with the attendant surgical risks. At present the balance of the risks between corrective and expectant management appears to favour correction. If and when more precise ways of predicting reversibility and irreversibility of pulmonary vascular disease are developed, this policy will be modified accordingly.

It is rare for surgery to be required with an isolated defect after the age of 1 year. Occasional patients who have escaped detection with a large left-to-right shunt and cardiomegaly may need surgical closure in childhood.

Aortic regurgitation, when it occurs, may be sufficiently severe to cause cardiomegaly or heart failure. In the latter instance surgery should be performed at any age. If frank heart failure is not present it is best to defer surgery until adolescence or adult life, since prosthetic aortic valve replacement may be required. Severe right ventricular outflow tract obstruction develops in between 5 and 10% of patients (Kaplan et al, 1963; Nadas & Fyler, 1968). It always requires surgical treatment. Corrective surgery should be performed if possible. The best results are probably obtained between 2 and 5 years of age.

Surgical management

When surgery is required as a life-saving procedure in early infancy, there are two options. The first is to perform a palliative operation (banding of the pulmonary trunk) followed by correction at a later age. The second is to perform primary closure. Although there is no consensus regarding the optimum, there is now a tendency for primary closure to be performed with greater frequency than banding. The choice depends upon the expertise of the medical and surgical teams involved, and in some cases on the anatomy of the defect or defects.

Banding of the pulmonary trunk is a safe and effective palliative procedure (Stark et al, 1970). But when assessing the risk, account must be taken of the cumulative risk of palliation and subsequent correction. In the best hands this should be below 10% (Seybold-Epting et al, 1976; Turina, 1978). Banding, however, does have its complications, particularly the development of subvalvar pulmonary obstruction. This may contribute to the development of cyanosis with its attendant risks which will make definitive surgery a more complex undertaking. It is therefore advisable that the corrective operation should not be delayed beyond the second year of life. Patients with ventricular septal defect who have had banding of the pulmonary trunk also have an unduly high incidence of subaortic stenosis (Freed et al, 1973). Whether this is because the presence of the subaortic stenosis means that banding was more likely to be needed, or because banding has a tendency to cause subaortic stenosis is still not quite clear. In many centres banding is the preferred operation in small infants with multiple ventricular septal defects and in those with inlet septal defects where primary closure would carry a significant risk of damage to the atrioventricular valve tension apparatus. Banding is rarely if ever indicated in patients beyond the age of 6 months.

Closure of an isolated ventricular septal defect can be performed as an emergency in the first 6 months of life – in the best centres with mortality rates comparable with the cumulative mortality rates of the two-stage approach (Agosti & Subramanian, 1975; Barratt-Boyes et al, 1976; Blackstone et al, 1976; Rein et al, 1977; McNicholas et al, 1978, 1979; Macartney et al, 1980). The operation can be performed using a ventriculotomy, or by a transatrial approach. The applicability of the transatrial approach depends upon the size of the defect. Doubly committed juxtaarterial defects and multiple defects present particular difficulties. Nothing is lost, even in these cases, by carrying out an initial transatrial exploration, since this allows accurate placement and therefore limits the extent of the necessary ventricular incision (Lincoln, 1978). An apical left ventriculotomy may be the best approach for multiple defects (Singh et al, 1977; Griffiths et al, 1981).

Elective surgery for ventricular septal defect should aim to be corrective. Patients surviving the first 6 months of life with persisting pulmonary hypertension should have primary closure of the defect before the age of 1 year. The possible routes for closure are the same as those for emergency treatment. Similarly, those with a large left-to-right shunt who have escaped detection or for other reasons have survived the first year of life should be corrected at the first opportunity. In all patients the only direct contraindication to surgery is established and severe pulmonary vascular disease. The initial assessment of pulmonary vascular disease is made from the haemodynamic data. Patients with a calculated pulmonary vascular resistance greater than 8 units/.m² are generally considered inoperable. In those with calculated resistances of between 4 and 8 units, it is not possible to say whether the pulmonary vascular disease has become irreversible: more information must be provided to permit rational decisions in these

cases. The administration of 100% oxygen during the cardiac catheterisation nearly always produces a fall in calculated pulmonary vascular resistance. The greatest fall occurs in the patients with the highest pulmonary vascular resistance when breathing room air. Patients with undoubtedly severe pulmonary vascular disease retain measurable reactivity in their pulmonary vasculature (Morrison & Macartney, 1979). In the presence of severe pulmonary vascular disease, therefore, the demonstration of reactivity is not necessarily an index of operability. This casts doubt on the value of this test in the assessment of operability in patients with less severe elevation of pulmonary vascular resistance. Administration of 100% oxygen may be helpful in patients with pulmonary venous desaturation, since it should reverse the transient hypoxic vasoconstrictor response. Indeed, if such patients have a restrictive ventricular septal defect, administration of 100% oxygen can cause a prompt drop in pulmonary arterial pressure from systemic levels. In doubtful situations, a lung biopsy may provide useful information (Rabinovitch et al, 1978). It has been proposed (Nihill et al, 1978) that pulmonary wedge angiography can provide similar information to the lung biopsy about the state of the pulmonary arteries. The claims made for this technique have yet to be validated.

Elective surgery is also required when subvalvular pulmonary stenosis is present. Resection of the obstructing muscle will be necessary at the time of closure. The presence of aortic regurgitation poses greater problems. It has been suggested that closure of the defect in itself may limit the valvar regurgitation, this being most effective in doubly committed juxtaarterial defects (Keane et al, 1977). Indeed, there is a case to be made for closing all doubly committed juxtaarterial defects as soon as they are diagnosed, even in those rare instances where there is neither congestive cardiac failure nor high pulmonary arterial pressure. Once aortic regurgitation has developed, it is rarely possible in our experience to avoid a direct attack upon the aortic valve. Initially this may be conservative, and good reports have been reported in the short and immediate term (Spencer et al, 1962; Trusler et al, 1973). But aortic valve replacement has been recommended as the best initial form of treatment, particularly when the aortic valve leaflets are deformed (Somerville et al, 1970). The balance of the evidence, however, leads us to recommend an initial conservative approach wherever possible, with replacement only where this has failed or is impossible.

Course after surgery

The majority of patients are considerably improved following corrective surgery. The clinical condition of approximately half the patients is graded as good or excellent on follow-up examination. Of the remaining patients, very few are still classified as poor, whereas such a classification is frequent prior to surgery (Weidman et al, 1977a, b). A significant cause of morbidity and mortality is pulmonary vascular disease. When this is established it usually progresses inexorably despite a corrective operation. To a great extent this complication is avoided by early corrective surgery (Sigmann et al, 1977). Late postoperative exercise testing should provide objective data on cardiac performance after correction. Available evidence again confirms the advantage of early surgery (Maron et al, 1973).

Disturbances of cardiac rhythm occur in a small proportion of patients following corrective surgery (approximately 5% – Weidman et al, 1977a), approximately 2% suffering complete heart block. Even with precise knowledge of the conduction tissues, surgical heart block does still occur. This frequently requires the insertion of an artificial pacemaker, with its attendant morbidity (Ennker et al, 1985). Nonetheless, permanent pacing should certainly be provided if the patient remains in congestive cardiac failure with a slow heart rate. When Stokes-Adams attacks occur, or if 24-hour monitoring of the electrocardiogram demonstrates prolonged period of asystole, episodes of ventricular tachycardia or ventricular fibrillation pacing should be provided even if the patient is asymptomatic. In practice, a slow heart rate of 30–40 beats/min at any time of the day is frequently used as a relative indicator for pacing. It follows then that 24-hour tape monitoring is mandatory in all patients with heart block following surgery for ventricular septal defect. This investigation should be repeated periodically during follow-up. In the absence of symptoms, it should be performed at yearly or 6-monthly intervals. 24-hour tape monitoring should also be performed in patients with postoperative ventricular ectopic beats. There is some suggestive evidence that these, by triggering a life-threatening ventricular arrhythmia, may be responsible for sudden death (Gillette et al, 1977; Schuilenberg, 1981).

Intraventricular conduction disturbances are seen in the majority of patients who have had open heart surgery. Right bundle branch block is certainly seen following repair of ventricular septal defect, be this performed transatrially or by the ventricular route (Lincoln et al, 1978; Friedli, 1981). When this is an isolated phenomenon it is not a prognostic sign. When associated with left axis deviation and a prolonged PR interval (see Ch. 11) it may well be a precursor of late complete heart block, particularly when the postoperative period has been complicated

by a period of transient complete heart block (Krongrad, 1978). In these cases, and in those where the right bundle branch block and left axis deviation are not associated with a prolonged PR interval, intracardiac electrophysiologic studies may assist in predicting the outcome (Friedli, 1981). The prognostic significance of all these changes vis-a-vis sudden unexpected death is at present uncertain (Schuilenberg, 1981). Close surveillance with 24-hour tape monitoring is a wise precaution. As with complete heart block, there are no generally accepted criteria for the insertion of a prophylactic pacemaker.

Crucial to the long-term outcome in patients with intraventricular conduction disturbances is the site of interference with the conduction tissues. If this is central (i.e. within the atrioventricular bundle) the risk of complete heart block is greater than if the damage is solely peripheral (i.e. within the peripheral bundle branches). While intracardiac electrophysiological studies (see Ch. 54) have been suggested as being helpful, this is not always the case (Schuilenberg, 1981). Atrial arrhythmias may occur if there is damage to the sinus node (for instance, during cannulation) but nowadays these are a rare occurrence following surgery for correction of ventricular septal defect.

The other common complication is a residual ventricular septal defect (Weidman et al, 1977a). In general such residual defects are of little haemodynamic significance but occasionally will be large enough for there to be a considerable residual left-to-right shunt. When this results in congestive cardiac failure or persistent cardiac failure, revision of the operation is indicated. The presence of a residual ventricular septal defect reinforces the need for life-long prophylactic measures against infective endocarditis. These measures should be continued even when the operation appears to have been totally successful.

Patients undergoing surgery for ventricular septal defect are at risk for all the complications associated with open heart surgery performed for any reason, including brain damage, renal damage, post-pericardotomy syndrome, pulmonary complications and so on. The majority of patients, however, suffer no ill-effects, are improved and go on to lead normal lives. This they should be encouraged to do. Although it is too early to predict the ultimate life-span of such patients, organisations such as the armed services and the police force can be prevailed upon to accept recruits who have undergone surgical repair of ventricular septal defect.

REFERENCES

Agosti J, Subramanian S 1975 Corrective treatment of isolated ventricular septal defect in infancy. Journal of Pediatric Surgery 10: 785–793

Alderson P O, Jost R G, Strauss A W, Boonvisut S, Markham J 1975 Radionucleotide angiography improved quantitation of left-to-right shunts using area ratio techniques in children. Circulation 51: 1136–1143

Allwork S P, Anderson R H 1979 Developmental anatomy of the membranous part of the ventricular septum in the human heart. British Heart Journal 41: 275–280

Alpert B S, Mellitis E D, Rowe R D 1973 Spontaneous closure of small ventricular septal defects; probability rates in the first five years of life. American Journal of Diseases of Childhood 125: 194–196

Anderson R H, Monro J L, Ho S Y, Smith A, Deverall P B 1977 Les voies de conduction auriculo-ventriculares dans le tetralogie de Fallot. Coeur 8: 793–807

Anderson R H, Lenox C C, Zuberbuhler J R 1983 Mechanisms of closure of perimembranous ventricular septal defect. The American Journal of Cardiology 52: 341–345

Bailey H, Clain A 1954 In: Demonstration of physical signs in clinical surgery. Wright, Bristol, p 149–150

Bargeron L M, Elliott L P, Soto B, Bream P R, Curry G C 1977 Axial cineangiography in congenital heart disease. Section I. Concept, technical and anatomical considerations. Circulation 56: 1075–1083

Barratt-Boyes B G, Neutze J M, Clarkson P M, Shardey G C, Brandt P W T 1976 Repair of ventricular septal defect in the first two years of life using profound hypothermia and total circulatory arrest techniques. Annals of Surgery 184: 376–390

Becu L M, Tauxe W N, DuShane J W, Edwards J E 1955 A complex of congenital cardiac anomalies: ventricular septal defect, biventricular origin of the pulmonary trunk and subaortic stenosis. American Heart Journal 50: 901–911

Becu L M, Fontana R S, DuShane J W, Kirklin J W, Burchell H B, Edwards J E 1956 Anatomic and pathologic studies in ventricular septal defect. Circulation 14: 349–364

Beerman L B, Park S C, Fischer D R, et al 1985 Ventricular septal defect associated with aneurysm of the membranous septum. Journal of the American College of Cardiology 5: 118–123

Bierman F Z, Fellows K, Williams R G 1980 Prospective identification of ventricular septal defects in infancy using subxiphoid two-dimensional echocardiography. Circulation 62: 807–818

Blackstone E H, Kirklin J W, Bradley E L, DuShane J W, Appelbaum A 1976 Optimal age and results in repair of large ventricular septal defects. Journal of Thoracic and Cardiovascular Surgery 72: 661–679

Brandt P W T, Calder A L, Barratt-Boyes B G, Neutze J M 1976 Double outlet left ventricle. Morphology, cineangiography, diagnosis and surgical treatment. American Journal of Cardiology 38: 897–909

Capelli H, Andrade J L, Somerville J 1983 Classification of the site of ventricular septal defect by 2-dimensional echocardiography. The American Journal of Cardiology 51: 1474–1480

Carlgren L-E 1959 The incidence of congenital heart disease in children born in Gothenburg 1941–1950. British Heart Journal 21: 40–50

Cheatham J P, Latson L A, Gutgesell H P 1981 Ventricular septal defect in infancy: detection with two dimensional echocardiography. The American Journal of Cardiology 47: 85–89

Chesler E, Korns M E, Edwards J E 1968 Anomalies of the tricuspid valve, including pouches, resembling aneurysms of the membranous ventricular septum. The American Journal of Cardiology 21: 661–668

Colo J, Stevenson J G, Pearlman A S 1982 A comparison of two dimensional echocardiography and pulsed Doppler for diagnosis of ventricular septal defect (abstract). Circulation 66: 11–232

Corone P, Doyen F, Gaudeau S, Guerin F, Vernant P, Ducam H, Rumeau-Rouquette C, Gaudeul P 1977 Natural history of ventricular septal defect. A study involving 790 cases. Circulation 55: 908–915

Dawes G S 1968 Fetal and neonatal physiology. Year Book Medical Publishers, Chicago, p 95–96

Elliott L P, Bargeron L M, Bream P R, Soto B, Curry G C 1977 Atrial cineangiography in congenital heart disease. Section II. Specific lesions. Circulation 56: 1084–1093

Ennker J, Stegman Th, Luhmer I, Oelert H 1985 Risks and benefits of cardiac pacing in children. International Journal of Cardiology 8: 125–134

Evans J R, Rowe R D, Keith J D 1960 Spontaneous closure of ventricular septal defects. Circulation 22: 1044–1054

Fox K M, Patel R G, Graham G R, Taylor J F N, Stark J, de Leval M, Macartney F J 1978 Multiple and single ventricular septal defects. A clinical and haemodynamic comparison. British Heart Journal 40: 141–146

Freed M D, Rosenthal A, Plauth W H Jr, Nadas A S 1973 Development of subaortic stenosis after pulmonary artery banding. Circulation 47–48 (Supplement III) 7–10

French H 1918 The possibility of a loud congenital heart murmur disappearing when a child grows up. Guy's Hospital Gazette New Series 32:87

Friedli B 1981 Prognostic significance of ventricular conduction abnormalities and extrasystoles after open heart surgery. In: Becker A E, Losekoot T G, Marcelletti C, Anderson R H (eds) Paediatric cardiology, Vol 3. Churchill Livingstone, Edinburgh, p 150–159

Gates G F, Orme H W, Dore E K 1973 Cardiac shunt assessment in children with macroaggregated albumin technetium-99m. Radiology 112: 649–653

Gersony W M, Hayes C J 1977 Bacterial endocarditis in patients with pulmonary stenosis, aortic stenosis or ventricular septal defect. Circulation 56: 1184–1187

Gillette P C, Yeoman M A, Mullins C E, McNamara D G 1977 Sudden death after repair of tetralogy of Fallot. Electrocardiographic and electrophysiologic abnormalities. Circulation 56: 566–571

Goor D A, Lillehei C W, Edwards J E 1971 Ventricular septal defects and pulmonic stenosis with and without dextroposition. Anatomic features and embryologic implications. Chest 60: 117–128

Graham T P, Bender H W, Spach M S 1977 Defects of the ventricular septum. In: Moss A J, Adams F H, Emmanouilides G C (eds) Heart disease in infants, children and adolescents, 2nd Edn. Williams & Wilkins, Baltimore, p 140–161

Green C E, Elliott L P, Bargeron L M Jr 1981 Axial cineangiographic evaluation of the posterior ventricular septal defect. The American Journal of Cardiology 48: 331–335

Griffiths S P, Turi G K, Ellis K, Krongrad E, Swift L H, Gersony W M, Bowman F O Jr, Malm J R 1981 Muscular ventricular septal defects repaired with left ventriculotomy. The American Journal of Cardiology 48: 877–886

Harris A, Sutton G, Towers M 1976 Ventricular septal defect. In: Physiological and clinical aspects of cardiac auscultation. Medi-Cine, London, p 108

Haworth S G, Sauer U, Buhlmeyer K, Reid L 1977 Development of the pulmonary circulation in ventricular septal defect: a quantitative structural study. American Journal of Cardiology 40: 781–788

Ho S Y, Wilcox B R, Anderson R H, Lincoln J C R 1983 Interrupted aortic arch – anatomical features of surgical significance. The Thoracic and Cardiovascular Surgeon 31: 199–205

Hoffman J I E, Rudolph A M 1965 The natural history of ventricular septal defects in infancy. American Journal of Cardiology 16: 634–653

Hoffman J I E, Christianson R 1978 Congenital heart disease in a cohort of 19 502 births with long term follow up. American Journal of Cardiology 42: 641–647

Jarmakani M M, Edwards S B, Spach M S, et al 1968 Left ventricular pressure-volume characteristics in congenital heart disease. Circulation 37: 879–889

Jarmakani M M, Graham J P Jr, Canent R V Jr, Spach M S, Capp M P 1969 Effect of site of shunt on left heart-volume characteristics in children with ventricular septal defect and persistent ductus arteriosus. Circulation 40: 411–418

Jones R W A, Baumer J H, Joseph M C, Shinebourne E A 1976 Arterial oxygen tension and response to oxygen breathing in differential diagnosis of congenital heart disease in infancy. Archives of Diseases in Childhood 51: 667–673

Kalmanson D, Aigueperse J, Veyrat C, Cornec C, Chiche P 1974 Non-invasive technique for diagnosing congenital and acquired ventricular septal defects using directional Doppler ultrasound: correlations with phasic flow velocity patterns of shunt. British Heart Journal 36: 428–445

Kaplan S, Dauod G I, Benzing G, Devine F J, Glass I H, McGuire J 1963 Natural history of ventricular septal defect American Journal of Diseases in Childhood 105: 581–587

Keane J F, Plauth W H, Nadas A S 1977 Ventricular septal defect with aortic regurgitation. Circulation 56: Supp. I.72–I.77

Keith J D 1978 Ventricular septal defect. In: Keith J D, Rowe R D, Vlad P (eds) Heart Disease in Infancy and Childhood. 3rd Edition. Macmillan, New York. p 321–379

Krongrad E 1978 Prognosis for patients with congenital heart disease and postoperative intraventricular conduction defects. Circulation 57: 867–870

Kutsche L M, Van Mierop L H S 1983 Pulmonary atresia with and without ventricular septal defect: a different etiology and pathogenesis for the atresia in the 2 types. The American Journal of Cardiology 51: 932–935

LaCorte M A, Fellows K E, Williams R G 1976 Overriding tricuspid valve. Echocardiographic and angiocardiographic features. 8 cases of ventricular septal defect of atrioventricular canal type. American Journal of Cardiology 37: 911–919

Latham R A, Anderson R H 1972 Anatomical variations in atrioventricular conduction system with reference to ventricular septal defects. British Heart Journal 34: 185–190

Lev M 1959 The pathologic anatomy of ventricular septal defect. Diseases of the Chest 35: 533–545

Lev M 1960 The architecture of the conduction system in congenital heart disease. III. Ventricular septal defect. Archives of Pathology 70: 529–549

Levin A R, Spach M S, Canent R V Jr, et al 1967 Intracardiac pressure-flow dynamics in isolated ventricular septal defect. Circulation 35: 430–441

Lincoln C 1978 Transatrial versus ventricular closure of isolated ventricular septal defect. In: Anderson R H, Shinebourne E A (eds) Paediatric cardiology 1977. Churchill Livingstone, Edinburgh, p 155–162

Lucas R V Jr, Adams P Jr, Anderson R C, Meyne N G, Lillehei C W, Varco R L 1961 The natural history of isolated ventricular septal defect. A serial physiologic study. Circulation 24: 1372–1387

Macartney F J, Taylor J F N, Graham G R, de Leval M, Stark J 1980 The fate of survivors of cardiac surgery in infancy. Circulation 62: 80–90

McNicholas K W, Bowman F O Jr, Hayes C J, Edie R N, Malm J R 1978 Surgical management of ventricular septal defects in infants. Journal of Thoracic and Cardiovascular Surgery 75: 346–353

McNicholas K, de Leval M, Stark J, Taylor J F N, Macartney F J 1979 Surgical treatment of ventricular septal defect in infancy. Primary repair versus banding of pulmonary artery and later repair. British Heart Journal 41: 133–138

Maron B J, Redwood D R, Hirshfeld J W, Goldstein R E, Morrow A G, Epstein S E 1973 Postoperative assessment of patients with ventricular septal defect and pulmonary hypertension. Response to intense upright exercise. Circulation 73: 864–874

Milo S, Ho S Y, Macartney F J, Wilkinson J L, et al 1979 Straddling and overriding atrioventricular valves: Morphology and classification. American Journal of Cardiology 44: 1122–1134

Milo S, Ho S Y, Wilkinson J L, Anderson R H 1980 The surgical anatomy and atrioventricular conduction tissues of hearts with isolated ventricular septal defects. Journal of Thoracic and Cardiovascular Surgery 79: 244–255

Mitchell S C, Korones S B, Berendes H W 1971 Congenital heart disease in 56 109 births. Incidence and natural history. Circulation 43: 323–332

Morrison G W, Macartney F J 1979 Effects of oxygen administration, bicarbonate infusions, and brief hyperventilation on patients with pulmonary vascular obstructive disease. British Heart Journal 41: 584–593

Moss A J, Siassi B 1970 Natural history of ventricular septal defect. Cardiovascular Clinics 2: 140–154

Moulaert A, Bruins C C, Oppenheimer-Dekker A 1976 Anomalies of the aortic arch and ventricular septal defects. Circulation 53: 1011–1015

Nadas A S, Fyler D C 1968 Ventricular septal defect. A review of current thoughts. Archives of Diseases of Childhood 43: 268–282

Naeye R L 1966 The pulmonary arterial bed in ventricular septal defect. Anatomic features in childhood. Circulation 34: 962–983

Neufeld H N, Titus J L, DuShane J W, Burchell H B, Edwards J E 1961 Isolated ventricular septal defect of the persistent common atrioventricular canal type. Circulation 23: 685–696

Nihill M R, Mullins C E, McNamara D G 1978 Visualisation of the pulmonary arteries in pseudotruncus by pulmonary vein wedge angiography. Circulation 58: 140–147

Ortiz E, Robinson P J, Deanfield J E, Franklin R, Macartney F J, Wyse R K H 1985 Localization of ventricular septal defect by simultaneous display of superimposed colour Doppler and cross-sectional echocardiographic images. British Heart Journal 54: 53–60

Pongiglione G, Freedom R M, Cook D, Rowe R D 1982 Mechanism of acquired right ventricular outflow tract obstruction in patients with ventricular septal defect: an angiocardiographic study. American Journal of Cardiology 50: 776–780

Rabinovitch M, Haworth S G, Castaneda A R, Nadas A S, Reid L M 1978 Lung biopsy in congenital heart disease: a morphometric approach to pulmonary vascular disease. Circulation 58: 1107–1121

Ramaciotti C, Keren A, Silverman N H 1986 Importance of pseudoaneurysms of the ventricular septum in the natural history of isolated perimembranous ventricular septal defects. American Journal of Cardiology 57: 268–272

Rein J C, Freed M D, Norwood W I, Castenada A R 1977 Early and late results of closure of ventricular septal defects in infancy. Annals of Thoracic Surgery 24: 19–27

Roberts W C 1984 The 2 most common congenital heart diseases (editorial). The American Journal of Cardiology 53:1198

Roger H 1879 Recherches cliniques sur la communication congenitale des deux coeurs, par innoclusion de septum interventriculaire. Bulletin de l'Academie de Medicin 8: 1077–1085

Rosenquist G C, Sweeney L J, Stemple D R, Christianson S D, Rowe R D 1973 Ventricular septal defect in tetralogy of Fallot. American Journal of Cardiology 31: 749–754

Rudolph A M 1965 The effects of post-natal circulatory adjustments in congenital heart disease. Paediatrics 36: 763–772

Rudolph A M 1970 The changes in the circulation after birth: their importance in congenital heart disease. Circulation 41: 343–359

Rudolph A M 1974 Congenital Diseases of the Heart. Year Book Medical Publishers, Chicago, p 206

Santamaria H, Soto B, Ceballos R, Bargeron L M Jr, Coghlan H C, Kirklin J W 1983 Angiographic differentiation of types of ventricular septal defects. American Journal of Radiology 141: 273–281

Schuilenberg R M 1981 Mechanisms of abnormal impulse formation and conduction. In: Becker A E, Losekoot T G, Marcelletti C, Anderson R H (eds) Paediatric cardiology, Vol 3. Churchill Livingstone, Edinburgh, p 107–121

Seybold-Epting W, Reul G J, Hallman G L, Cooley D A 1976 Repair of ventricular septal defect after pulmonary artery banding. Journal of Thoracic and Cardiovascular Surgery 71: 392–397

Shah P, Singh W S A, Rose V, Keith J D 1966 Incidence of bacterial endocarditis in ventricular septal defects. Circulation 34: 127–131

Sherman F E 1963 An Atlas of Congenital Heart Disease. Lea & Febiger, Philadelphia

Sigmann J M, Perry B L, Behrendt D M, Stern A M, Kirsh M M, Sloan H E 1977 Ventricular septal defect: results after repair in infancy. American Journal of Cardiology 39: 66–71

Singh A K, de Leval M, Stark, J 1977 Left ventriculotomy for closure of muscular ventricular septal defects. Annals of Surgery 186: 577–580

Somerville J 1979 Congenital heart disease – changes in form and function. British Heart Journal 41: 1–22

Somerville J, Brandao A, Ross D N 1970 Aortic regurgitation with ventricular septal defect. Circulation 41: 317–330

Soto B, Coghlan C H, Bargeron L M Jr 1978 Angiography of ventricular septal defects. In: Anderson R H, Shinebourne E A (eds) Paediatric Cardiology 1977. Churchill Livingstone, Edinburgh, p 125–135

Soto B, Becker A E, Moulaert A J, Lie J T, Anderson R H 1980 Classification of ventricular septal defects. British Heart Journal 43: 332–343

Spencer F C, Bahnson H T, Neil C A 1962 The treatment of aortic regurgitation associated with a ventricular septal defect. Journal of Thoracic and Cardiovascular Surgery 43: 222–233

Stanger P, Lucas R V Jr, Edwards J E 1969 Anatomic factors causing respiratory distress in acyanotic congenital cardiac disease: special reference to bronchial obstruction. Pediatrics 43: 760–769

Stark J, Tynan M, Tatooles C J, Aberdeen E, Waterston D J 1970 Banding of the pulmonary artery for transposition of the great arteries and ventricular septal defect. Circulation 41: II.116–129

Steinfeld L, Dimich I, Park S, Baron M G 1972 Clinical diagnosis of isolated subpulmonic (supracristal ventricular septal defect. American Journal of Cardiology 30: 19–24

Stevenson J G, Kawabori I, Dooley T, Guntheroth W G 1978 Diagnosis of ventricular septal defect by pulsed Doppler echocardiography. Sensitivity, specificity and limitations. The American Journal of Cardiology 58: 322–326

Sutherland G R, Godman M J, Smallhorn J F, et al 1982 Ventricular septal defects. Two dimensional echocardiographic and morphologic correlations. British Heart Journal 47: 316–328

Sutherland G R, Godman M J, Hunter S, Keeton B R, Bain H H 1987a The natural history of perimembranous ventricular septal defects – a correlative echocardiographic/haemodynamic study. In press

Sutherland G R, Godman M J, Keeton B R, Burns J 1987b The natural history of ventricular septal defects – a long-term prospective echocardiographic study. In press

Sutton G, Harris A, Leatham A 1968 Second heart sound in pulmonary hypertension. British Heart Journal 30: 743–756

Szekely P, Snaith L 1974 Ventricular septal defect. In: Heart disease and pregnancy. Churchill Livingstone, Edinburgh, p 157

Tatsuno K, Konno S, Sakakibara S 1973 Ventricular septal defect with aortic insufficiency. Angiographic aspects and a new classification. American Heart Journal 85: 13–21

Titus J L, Rastelli G C 1976 Anatomic features of persistent common atrioventricular canal. In: Feldt R H (ed) Atrioventricular canal defects. Saunders, Philadelphia, p 13–35

Titus J L, Daugherty G W, Edwards J E 1963 Anatomy of the atrioventricular conduction system in ventricular septal defect.Circulation 28: 72–81

Treasure R L, Hopeman A R, Jahne E J, Green D C, Czarnecki S W 1971 Ventricular septal defect with aortic insufficiency. Annals of Thoracic Surgery 12: 411–418

Truex R C, Bishof J K 1958 Conduction system in human hearts with interventricular septal defects. Journal of Thoracic Surgery 35: 421–439

Trusler G A, Moes C A F, Kidd B S L 1973 Repair of ventricular

septal defect with aortic insufficiency. Journal of Thoracic and Cardiovascular Surgery 66: 394–403

Turina M 1978 Early closure versus two-stage treatment for ventricular septal defect. In: Anderson R H, Shinebourne E A (eds) Paediatric cardiology 1977. Churchill Livingstone, Edinburgh, p 147–154

Ueda M, Becker A E 1985 Classification of hearts with overriding aortic and pulmonary valves. International Journal of Cardiology 9: 353–360

Valdes-Cruz L M, Horowitz S, Mesel E, et al 1983 A pulsed Doppler echocardiographic method for calculation of pulmonary and systemic flow: accuracy in a canine model with ventricular septal defect. Circulation 68: 597–602

Van Mill G J, Moulaert A, Harinck E 1981 Two-dimensional echocardiographic localisation of isolated ventricular septal defects. In: Hunter S, Hall R (eds) Echocardiography I. Churchill Livingstone, Edinburgh, p 249–265

Van Praagh R, McNamara J J 1968 Anatomic types of ventricular septal defect with aortic insufficiency. American Heart Journal 75: 604–619

Van Praagh R, Bernhard W F, Rosenthal A, Parisi L F, Fyler D C 1971 Interrupted aortic arch: Surgical treatment. American Journal of Cardiology 27: 200–213

Varghese P J, Rowe R D 1969 Spontaneous closure of ventricular septal defects by aneurysmal formation of the membranous septum. Journal of Pediatrics 75: 700–703

Wagenvoort C A, Neufeld H N, DuShane J W, Edwards J E 1961 The pulmonary arterial tree in ventricular septal defect. A quantitative study of anatomic features in fetuses, infants and children. Circulation 23: 740–748

Warden H E, De Wall R A, Cohen M, Varco R L, Lillehei C W 1957 A surgical-pathologic classification for isolated ventricular septal defects and for those in Fallot's tetralogy based on observations made on 120 patients during repair and under direct vision. Journal of Thoracic and Cardiovascular Surgery 33: 21–44

Weber F P 1918 Can the clinical manifestations of congenital heart disease disappear with the general growth and development of the patient? British Journal of Childhood Diseases 15:113

Weidman W H, Blount S G, DuShane J W, Gersony W M, Hayes, C J Nadas A S 1977a Clinical course in ventricular septal defect. Circulation 56: I.56–I.69

Weidman W H, DuShane J W, Ellison R C 1977b Clinical course in adults with ventricular septal defect. Circulation 56: I.78–I.79

Index

Abdominal organ arrangement, atrial isomerism associated, 484–5
Abdominal vessels
development, 499
great, see Great vessels
Abdomino-thoracic exteriorisation of the heart, 1058–9
Absolute refractory period, 238
Acid lipase deficiency, 1250
Acidosis, 383
electrocardiographic features, 302
Acinar arteries
development, 130, 131, 133
in pulmonary hypertension, 141, 147, 148
Acini, structure and function, 123
Acquired heart disease, 151
Action potential(s)
cardiac-, 237–9, 244
fast response, 237–8
recording in different locations, 244
slow response, 237–8
systemic alterations and their effects on, 298–306
ventricular muscle-, 238
Admission to cardiology unit, 1385–9
Adrenal gland tumours
hypertension associated with, 1312–13
surgery, 1313
Adrenal insufficiency, electrocardiographic effects of, 306
Adrenaline, hypertension and, 1312, 1313, see also Noradrenaline
Adrenocortical hypertension, 1311–12
Aetiology of congenital heart disease, 15–39, 42–59
Africa, heart disease in, prevalence, 7
Afterload, 165, 166, 434–5
definition, 165, 434
Age-dependency
aortic coarctation clinical findings, 1095–7, 1105
blood pressure measurements, 1294–6
electrocardiograph waves and intervals, 258–63 passim
heart rate, 257
rheumatic heart disease incidence, 1197–8
surgical risks, 791, 1365
Agromegaly, 1252
Airway
anatomy, 125
compression, 140, 196
damage, 152
obstruction, 152, see also Vascular rings

lung function tests with, 398
presentation with, 196
resistance, measurement, 398–9, 400
Alagile syndrome, 1267–8
Aldosterone levels, hypertension associated, 1307, see also Hyperaldosteronism
Altitude
effects on extra-uterine life, 151
persistent ductus arteriosus associated with, 941
Alveolar oxygen measurement, 399
Alveolar wall arteries, occluded, 137
Amiodarone therapy
in hypertrophic cardiomyopathy, 1149
in pregnancy, 1357
Amoxycillin therapy in endocarditis, 1238–9
Anaemia
haemolytic-, 1268, 1327
iron deficiency, 775
Anaesthesia
antibiotic therapy for patient receiving, 1239
in catheterisation, 365–6
drugs used in, 366
electrocardiographic effects, 304
in pregnancy, 1358
Anastomoses
pulmonary-bronchial arteries, 125
surgical, see Transplants, grafts and anastomoses
Andersen's disease, 1247
Aneuploidy
autosomal, 15–21
defects caused by, 15–22, 941
sex chromosomal, 21–2
Aneurysm
caval vein, 503–4
coronary artery, 1082–3, 1171
ductus arteriosus, 947
electrocardiographic features, 298
pseudo-, 622
sinus of Valsalva, see Sinus of Valsalva
vein of Galen, 202, 1002–4, 1005
ventricular, 298
Aneurysmal (fibrous tissue) tags
septal closure by, 633
valve obstruction by, 622
Angiocardiography/angiography (including ventriculography), 376–7, see also Aortography; Arteriography; Atriography
catheterisation for, see Catheterisation
ciné, 712, 1096, 1147, 1325, 1332, 1335
complications arising, 383

equipment, 363–4
features and findings in
aortic arch defects, 1113–15, 1130, 1131
aortic atresia, 752–4
aortic coarctation, 1096, 1099–1101, 1102
aortic regurgitation, 998, 1212–13
aortic stenosis, 981, 982, 984, 990–1, 992, 994, 995, 1003, 1115, 1210
aorto-left ventricular defect, 998
aortopulmonary window, 925–7, 1001
arteriovenous abnormal connexions, 1012, 1016
atrial chamber partitioning, 567, 568
atrial isomerism, 491, 492
atrial septal defects, 555, 557, 598–603
atrioventricular septal defects, 598–604, 782
brachiocephalic artery, anomalous, 1132, 1133
complete transposition, 846, 848–9, 1069
coronary artery anomalies, 1075–6
corrected transposition, 876–8
criss-cross heart, 1069
diminutive descending aorta, 753
discordant atrioventricular connections, 876–80
double inlet ventricle, 663–7
Ebstein's (and related) malformations, 728–9
endocardial fibroelastosis, 1226–7
endomyocardial fibrosis, 1331, 1332, 1335
Fallot's tetralogy, 784–6
hypertrophic cardiomyopathy, 1147
hypoplastic left heart syndrome, 752–6, 757
mitral valve anomalies, 754, 755, 756, 1033–6, 1048–50, 1202, 1203, 1208
persistent ductus arteriosus, 944
pulmonary atresia, 113, 223, 713, 716–17, 816–23
pulmonary sling, 1134, 1135
pulmonary stenosis, 534, 785, 881, 849, 967–8
pulmonary vascular disease, 146, 534
pulmonary venous anomalies, 491, 523, 533, 534, 535
rheumatic heart disease, 1202, 1203, 1208, 1210, 1212–13, 1214, 1215
sinus of Valsalva aneurysm, 1003, 1007, 1009
straddling atrioventricular valves, 702, 703, 704

Angiocardiography
  features and findings in (*contd.*)
    systemic disease, 1246–68 *passim*
    tricuspid atresia, 221, 689
    tricuspid incompetence, 1214
    tricuspid stenosis, 1215
    truncus arteriosus, 917–21
    tumours, cardiac, 1156
    vascular rings, 1130, 1131
    ventricular hypoplasia, 703
    ventricular septal defects, 631, 634–5,
      816–22, 879, 1115
  principles of, 376–7
  problems, 663
  quantitative, 368–9
  radionuclide, *see* Angiocardiography/
    angiography, radionuclide
  ventricular measurement by, 160, 161, 162,
    170, 173
  wedge, pulmonary vein, 818–19
Angiocardiography/angiography, radionuclide
    (nuclear), 162, 219–24
  features and findings
    atrial septal defects, 555
    complete transposition, 846
    mitral valve anomalies, 1033
    pulmonary atresia, 816
    pulmonary vein atresia/stenosis, 534
    tricuspid atresia, 221, 688
    ventricular septal defects, 631, 816
Angioplasty
  balloon-, 377–8, 971
    in aortic coarctation, 1103–4
  patch-, 1104
  subclavian flap-, 446, 447, 1104
Angiotensin, 1307
  -renin system, 1307, 1310
Antenatal
  heart disease, *see* Pregnancy
  mortality, *see* Mortality
Anti-arrhythmic drugs, 1212–19 *passim, see
    also specific drugs*
  electrocardiographic effects, 302–4
  in pregnancy, 1356–7
Antibiotic therapy
  blind-, 427–9, 1239
  decision theory involving, 427–9
  efficiency, assessment, 1240
  in endocarditis, 1237–8, 1238–40
  in rheumatic disease, 1190, 1191–2
Antibodies, auto-immune, 1336
Anticoagulant therapy in pregnancy, 1357
Antihypertensive drug(s)
  dose, 1314, 1315
  intravenous/intramuscular, 1315
  mode of action, 1314, 1315
  oral, 1314
  side effects, 1314
  therapy, 1305–6, 1314–15
Anti-inflammatory drug therapy, 1192–3
Aorta
  anatomy
    congenital heart disease associated,
      111–13
    neonatal, 111–13
  ascending, diminutive, 738, 984
    angiocardiographic features, 752, 753,
      985
    size, surgical considerations, 759
  ascending, shunts involving, *see* Waterston
    anastomoses
  continuity, restoration, 1116
  descending thoracic

graft to pulmonary trunk, 758, 759
    pressure measurements with hypoplastic
      heart, 749–52
  dilation (surgical), 1103–4
  dissection risks in pregnancy, 1358
  echocardiographic features, 334, 340
    fetal, 353, 354
  left sided, 833, 834, 882, 895–6
  morphogenesis, 111–13, 932
  neonatal
    anatomy, 111–13
    constriction, 1093
  overriding, *see* Aortic overriding
  radiological features, 205
  reconstruction, 1116
  right sided, 834, 835, 892, 893–4, 1127,
    1128
  right ventricular connexions to, 902
  selective injection, 531
Aortic arch
  atresia, 1107, 1126
  double, 932, 1126, 1129, 1130
    surgery, 1131
  echocardiographic features, 353, 845
  interruption, 447, 1106–16
    aetiology, 1106
    associated lesions, 1110
    clinical findings, 1110–11
    fetal, 1107
    incidence, 1106
    isolated, 1109, 1110
    investigations, 1097–1101
    medical management, 1115
  morphogenesis, 1109–10
  morphology, 1107–9
  natural history/course, 1115
  pathophysiology, 1110
  prognosis, 1115
  sites, 1107, 1108, 1123–7
  surgical management, 447, 1115–16
  truncus arteriosus associated, 914, 919,
    923
  types, 447, 1092
  left, 1127, 1128
  morphogenesis, 932, 1123, 1124
  patency, 1126
  position
    diagnostic value, 201
    mal-, 79, 779
    superior, 844, 845
  radiographic features, 205
  right, 779, 932, 1126, 1128, 1131
    associated anomalies, 1127
  tubular hypoplasia of, 1088, 1089, 1092,
    1107
  vascular sling associated features, 1126–7
Aortic atresia, 737
  aetiology, 737
  angiocardiographic features, 753, 754,
    756
  associated conditions, 757
  clinical features/findings, 746
  electrocardiographic features, 748–9
  haemodynamic investigations, 749–52
  incidence, 737
  intrapulmonary artery abnormalities
    associated with, 135–6
  morphogenesis, 744
  morphology, 739–40, 742, 742–3
Aortic coarctation
  abdominal, 1098
  aetiology, 1087
  angioplasty, 1103–4

aortic atresia associated, 741
    aortographic demonstration, 755
  associated anomalies, 1091–2, 1095, 1099,
    1104–5
  clinical features/findings, 1095–7
    age-related, 1095–7, 1104
  complications, 1092
  diagnosis, 1101–2, 1114
  discrete, 1088, 1089
  ductally affected, 940
  echocardiographic features, 603
  hypertension associated with, 1310–11
  investigations, 1097–1101
    invasive, justification, 1099–1101
  isolated, 1101, 1102
  isthmal hypoplasia and, 1101
  lesions producing, 1088–92
    diagrammatic representation, 1088
    shelf-, 1088, 1089, 1090
    waist-, 1088, 1089
  medical management, 1102–3
  morphogenesis, 1092
  morphology, 1087–92
  natural history/course, 11, 1102
  paraductal, 1090
  pathophysiology, 1093–5
  postductal, 1091, 1099
  preductal, 112, 1089, 1099
  pregnancy risks, 1358
  prevalence, 1087
  prognosis, 1102
  pulmonary oedema caused by, 212
  radiographic features, 200, 212, 214, 215
  recurrent/residual, 1103, 1104, 1106
  resected, 1101
  surgical management, 1104–6, 1310
    complications, 1105, 1106
    elective, 1105–6
    non-elective, 1104
  tubular hypoplasia and, 1088, 1089, 1092,
    1107
Aortic connexions in pulmonary atresia,
    800–1
Aortic orifice, transfer of, 95
Aortic overriding, Fallot's tetralogy with,
    771–3
  angiographic features, 786
  electrocardiographic features, 781, 783
Aortic regurgitation, 996–9, 1211–13
  acquired, 997, 998
  aetiology, 996
  clinical features/findings, 991, 1212
  congenital, 997
  incidence, 1211
  investigations, 996–7, 1212–13
  medical management, 1213
  natural history/course, 1211
  physiology, 1211–12
  quantitation, 1213
  rheumatic, 1211–13
  surgical management, 638, 997–8, 1213
  ventricular septal defect associated, 636,
    639
Aortic root
  echocardiographic features, 353, 357,
    358
  growth, measurement, 355
  replacement, 987
  valve atresia and, 744
Aortic stenosis, 977–87, 1209–11
  aetiology, 992–3
  cardiac output in, 415
  classification, 977

Aortic stenosis (*contd.*)
  clinical features/findings, 978, 979, 980,
    981, 982–3, 989, 994, 1210
  critical, 984
    in infancy, 979
  diagnosis, differential, 980, 996
  echocardiographic features, 346, 347, 979,
    980, 983, 989, 990, 994, 1113
  exercise testing in, 397, 415
  intra-pulmonary artery abnormalities
    associated with, 135–6
  investigations, 979, 980, 981, 983–4,
    989–91, 994, 1210
  isolated, 977–8, 1209–10
  medical management, 985, 986, 991
  mild/moderate, 980–1
  morphology/pathology, 978, 979, 987–8,
    993–4, 1197
  natural history/course, 11, 986
  pathogenesis, 988, 993–4
  predictors, 415
  prevalence, 977, 1209–10
  recurrent, 993
  relief, 378
  rheumatic, 1197, 1209–11
  sub (valvar), 459, 583, 604, 987–92
    aortic arch interruption associated with,
      1110, 1113, 1115
    fixed-, 987–92
    membranous, 988, 991
  supra (valvar), 459, 460, 992–6
    angiocardiographic features, 968
  surgical management, 458–9, 981, 985,
    986–7, 991–2, 995–6, 1210–11
  trivial, 980
  valvar, 459, 977–87
Aortic valve, *see also* Valves
  aortic coarctation associated with defects of,
    1091–2
  bicuspid, 980, 980–1, 1091–2
  commisurotomy, 1210
  closure
    aneurysmal, 622
    premature, 990
    timing, 187
  development, 100–1
  domed-, pliable, 981–7
  echocardiographic features, 341–2, 813,
    979, 980, 983, 989, 990
  endocarditis involving, 1231–2, 1233
  leaflet
    echocardiographic features, 633
    lumpy attachments, 978, 984, 985–6
    prolapse, 633
    right, 633
  Marfan's syndrome involving, 1254–5
  notching beneath, 991
  overriding, 340, 341, 813
  regurgitation and incompetence *see* Aortic
    regurgitation
  replacement, 987, 1211, 1213
  right ventricular connexions in Fallot's
    tetralogy, 773
  rings, arrangement, 572
  stenosis, *see* Aortic stenosis
  surgery, 1210, 1255, *see also* Aortic
    regurgitation; Aortic stenosis; Aortic
    valvotomy
Aortic valvotomy, 459, 981, 985, 986–7
  indications, 986–7
  open-, 987
  results, 987
  timing, 985

Aortography
  ascending, 1113–14
  features and findings in
    aortic arch interruption, 1113–14
    aortic atresia, 752–4
    aortic stenosis, 984, 995
    aorto-left ventricular defect, 998
    diminutive descending aorta, 753
    sinus of Valsalva aneurysm, 1003, 1007,
      1009
Aorto-left ventricular defect, 997–8
Aortopulmonary anastomoses/conduits
  obstruction at the site, 806–7
  obstruction within, 807–8
Aortopulmonary collateral arteries, 134–5,
    802, 803–4
  echocardiographic features, 815
  hypoperfusion with, 149
  interconnexions with other arteries,
    821–2
  ligation, 824, 825
  necrosis, 824, 825
  obstruction within, 802
  selective injection, 810, 818
  stenosis, 135
Aortopulmonary septum
  development, 95–7
    mal-, 924
    patterns in different species, 101
Aortopulmonary window
  angiographic features, 925–7, 1001
  aortic arch interruption associated with,
    1110, 1112, 1114
  classification, 924
  clinical features/findings, 925
  diagnosis, differential, 917, 921, 927
  echocardiographic features, 814, 917
  investigations, 925
  medical management, 927
  morphology, 924
  natural history/course, 927
  pathophysiology, 925
  prognosis, 922
  surgical management, 927–8
    considerations, 926–7
Aortoventriculoplasty, 458–9
Argon, cardiac output measurements using,
    406–7
Arrhythmias, 1273–91, *see also*
    Bradyarrhythmias; Tachyarrhythmias
  atrial, *see* Atrial arrhythmias
  drug therapy, *see* Anti-arrhythmic drugs
  fetal
    detection, 359–60
    treatment, 360
  floppy mitral valve associated, 1047, 1051
  persistent, 560
  post-operative, 560, 639, 769, 792–3, 854,
    1279
  in pregnancy, 1356–7
  systematic interpretation, 1273–7
  ventricular, *see* Ventricular arrhythmias
Arrhythmogenic right ventricular dysplasia,
    734, 1287
Arterial blood flow, *see* Arterial circulation
Arterial circulation/blood flow
  detection/measurement, 185
  oxygenation determinants, 839–40
  pulmonary, *see* Pulmonary arteries
  quality testing, 399–400, 414
  sampling, 399, 405, 406
Arterial dilation, generalised, 138–9
Arterial duct, *see* Ductus arteriosus

Arterial junction, development, 95–6
Arterial outflow tract, maldevelopment, 898,
    see also Ventricular outflow tracts
Arterial relationships, 78–9
Arterial switch operation
  diagrammatic representation, 857
  life expectancy estimation, 432, 433
  optimal timing, 431–4
  patient selection, 858, 859–9
  survival curve, 432
  for transposition, 456, 857–9
Arterial trunk
  common
    echocardiographic features, 340, 357,
      358
    magnetic resonance imaging, 230, 231
    pulmonary vessel enlargement associated
      with, 209
    repair, 458
  maldevelopment, 838
  solitary, 804, 805
Arterial valves, *see also specific valve*
  defects in truncus arteriosus, 913, 914
  development, 100–1
Arterial wall motion, 185
Arteries, *see specific type*
Arteriography, *see also*
    Angiocardiography/Angiography
  features and findings in
    coronary artery aneurysms, 1083
    pulmonary venous obstruction, 523, 524
    renal artery stenosis, 1300
  pulmonary, 523, 524, 1033
Arteriohepatic dysplasia, 1267–8
Arteriolar dilator therapy, 438–9
Arteriotomy, repair, 371–2
Arteriovenous fistulas/malformations,
    1010–19
  aetiology, 1011, 1013
  clinical features/findings, 1011–12, 1015
  complications, 1017
  coronary, 715, 1002, 1081–2
  diagnosis, differential, 1012, 1016
  incidence, 1013
  investigations, 1012, 1016
  management, 1012–13, 1017–19
  occlusion, 1017–19
  pathology/pathogenesis, 1010, 1015
  pathophysiology, 1011, 1014–15
  pulmonary, 1013–19
    classification, 1014
  systemic, 1010–12
Arthralgia, poly-, 1189
  management, 1193
Arthritis
  poly-, 1186
    management, 1193
  rheumatoid, 1264
Arthrogryopsis multiplex congenita, 1260
Aschoff body/nodule, 1185
Asia, heart disease in, prevalence, 6–7
Aspartoglycosaminuria, 1250
Aspirin therapy, 1192, 1193
Asplenia, *see* Atrial isomerism
Asthma, exercise induced, 396
Asymptomatic children
  with murmurs, *see* Murmurs
  radiography, 197–8
Atria
  activation, 243, 1274
  arrangement (situs), *see* Situs
  caval vein connexion to, 327, 329, 502–3,
    503, 505

Atria (*contd.*)
  chamber
    echocardiographic examination, 328–30
    partitioning, *see* Atrial chamber
      partitioning
  common
    in conjoined twins, 1061
    echocardiographic features, 589, 591
  contraction, *see* Contraction
  development, 86–9
  enlargement, *see* Atrial enlargement
  left
    catheterisation, 375
    filling defect, 1034, 1035
    growth, 355
    injection, usefulness, 1033–4
    pressure, 375, 1033
    right ventricle communication, 683
  morphological features, 66, 68–70
  polarisation/depolarisation, 245–7, 252
  right
    -left ventricle communication, 619, 620
    oximetry, 556
    pulmonary venous connexion to, 512,
      519, 521, 522, 530
  septum, *see* Atrial septum
  surgical repair routes via, 449–50
  terminology, anatomical, 66, 68–70
Atrial appendage(s)
  bilateral, 474–5, 485
  echocardiographic features, 491
  juxtaposition, 1063–5
    left sided, 1063, 1064, 1065, 1066
    right sided, 1064
  morphogenesis, 485, 499
  morphology, 69, 474–5
Atrial arrhythmias
  aetiology, 550
  fibrillation, 1288
  flutter, 1288
  post-operative, 854
Atrial chamber partitioning (cor
    triatriatum), 563–9
  left, 563–8
    categorisation, 565
    clinical features, 566
    diagnosis, differential, 567–8
    incidence and aetiology, 565–6
    inter-atrial communications, 563–5 *passim*
    intra-atrial communications, 563, 564
    management, 568
    membrane structure, 565
    morphogenesis, 565
    morphology, 563–5
    presentation, 566
    rare variants, 568–9
  right, 569
Atrial conduction system, 235–6
Atrial ectopic rhythm, left, 268
Atrial enlargement
  bi-, 280
  electrocardiographic features, 279–81
  left, 280
  radiographic features, 204
  right-, 279–80
    in pulmonary atresia, 716, 717
Atrial fibrillation, 1288
Atrial flutter, 1288
Atrial hypertrophy, *see* Atrial enlargement
Atrial isomerism (and asplenia/splenic
    syndrome), 473–93
  aetiology, 486
  anatomy, 69, 70, 71, 72, 474–84

atrial appendage juxtaposition with, 1064
atrioventricular septal defect with, 601
clinical features and findings, 486–9
  in conjoined twins, 1061
diagnosis, differential, 882
double outlet ventricle with, 896–7
echocardiographic features, 327–8, 329
electrocardiographic features, 268, 269, 489
incidence, 485–6
inheritance, 487
investigations, 489–91
management, 493
morphogenesis, 485, 499–500
right vs left, 474–84
venous connexions, 475–9, 499–500, 502,
  524
Atrial pacing, 1280, 1281
Atrial redirection procedure, 456
  in complete transposition, 456, 852–6
  patient selection, 859, 860
  timing, 855
Atrial septectomy, *see* Septectomy
Atrial septostomy, *see* Septostomy
Atrial septum
  architecture, 97, 543
    angiographic features, 530–1
    echocardiographic features, 330, 335,
      338–40
  defect(s), 541–60
    aetiology, 541–2
    associated anomalies, 548
    atrial isomerism associated, 479, 480
    cardiac response to, 549–50
    caval vein anomalies associated with,
      501–2, 505
    coronary sinus defect associated with,
      501–2
    classification, 543
    clinical presentation, 550
    deliberate creation of, *see* Septectomy
    diagnosis, 557–8
    incidence, 541
    investigations, 553–7
    isolated, 558–9
    management, 559–60
    morphogenesis, 547–8
    morphology, 542–3
    natural history/course, 10–11, 558–9
    pathophysiology, 548–50
    physical examination, 550–3
    primum type, *see* Ostium primum
    prognosis, 558–9
    pulmonary stenosis associated, 962
    radiographic features, 208, 555
    repair, 380, 448, 449
    secundum type, 531, 543
    size, effect of, 548–9
    spontaneous closure, 558
    symptoms, 559–60
  formation, 86, 87–91 *passim*
Atrial valves, *see specific valve*
Atriography in hypoplastic left heart
    syndrome, 754, 755
Atriopulmonary connexion, surgically created,
    460–1
Atrioventricular block, 1278–81
  complete-, 1279
    congenitally, 1278
    surgically acquired, 1279
  first degree, 1289
  second degree, 1275, 1276, 1290
    type 1 (Wenckebach), 1275, 1276
  trypanosomiasis associated, 1327

Atrioventricular canal
  defects, isolated, 618–19, *see also*
    Atrioventricular septal defects
  development, 90–1
Atrioventricular conduction
  axis, 236–7
  disturbances, 1278–81
  measurement, 1275–6
  pre-exitation, 286–91
Atrioventricular connexion
  absent, 676–9 *passim*, 745
    straddling atrioventricular valve with,
      699, 706, 707–8
  absent left, 71, 72, 335, 481, 706, 707,
    744, 757
    morphology, 745
  absent right, 71, 72, 335, 675
    echocardiographic features, 686
    morphogenesis, 683–4
    morphology, 677, 678–81, 683, 706
  accessory, 288
  ambiguous, 71
  atrial isomerism associated, 479–81, 867,
    1069
  biventricular, 71, 333–5, 479, 480, 482,
    483
    aortic atresia and, 757
  concordant, 71, 269–70, 271, 337
    aortic atresia and, 743
    in pulmonary atresia, *see* Pulmonary
      atresia
    straddling atrioventricular valves with,
      698, 699, 701, 704
    in tricuspid atresia, 677, 681, 682, 687,
      690
  criss-cross heart related to, 1068–70
  discordant, 71, 271–2, 461, 883–4
    aortic atresia and, 744
    concordant ventriculo-arterial connexions
      and, 883
    corrected transposition and, 867–84
    double outlet ventricle and, 883–4, 896,
      908
    single outlet with, 884
    surgical management, 461
  disturbed, recurrence risks in
    sibs/offspring, 35
  double inlet, *see* Double inlet ventricle
  mode of, 73–4, 336–8, 481–2
  surgical manufacture, 460
  transposition related to, 830
  types, 70–2, 333–6, 643
  univentricular, 71–2, 75, 479–81, 483,
    643
    aortic atresia and, 742–3, 757
    atrial arrangement, 643, 644
    diagnosis, differential, 882–3
Atrioventricular dissociation, 248
Atrioventricular junction, 70–2
  in atrial isomerism, 479–82
  connexions at the, *see* Atrioventricular
    connexions
  echocardiographic examination, 320, 333–8
  invagination, 98, 99
  left, atresia/hypoplasia, 737–61 *passim*
  morphogenesis, 90–1, 98, 653–4
  morphology, 571–4, 675–6
  unguarded, 682
Atrioventricular nodes, 236
  anomalies in corrected transposition, 870
  mesothelioma of 1160
Atrioventricular rings, morphogenesis, 102,
  103, 104

Atrioventricular septum
  defects, *see* Atrioventricular septum, defects
  membranous, 571–2, 616
  muscular, 571–2
Atrioventricular septal defects, 571–609 *see also* Atrioventricular canal; Endocardial cushions; Ostium primum
  aetiology, 38–9, 571
  associated malformations, 584
  atrial isomerism associated, 479, 480
  chamber dominance with, 584–5
  classification, 578–85
    sub-, 576; 593–4
  clinical findings, 587–8
  common valve orifice associated with, 574, 575, 576, 580, 581–2, 589, 590, 591, 600, 607–8, 608–9
  complete-, 452
  complete transposition with, 832–3
  definition, 543
  dominant right ventricular form of, 742
  Fallot's tetralogy with, 782
  hypoplastic left ventricle associated with, 742
  inlet/outlet disproportion in, 576
  investigations, 588–603
  medical management, 605
  morphogenesis, 585–6
  morphology, 575–85
  natural history/course, 11, 604–5
  pathogenesis, 38
  pathophysiology, 586–7
  presentation, 587
  prevalence, 571
  pulmonary vascular abnormalities associated with, 142–3
  seperate valve orifices with, 578, 579
  shunting levels through, 577
  surgical management, 451–2, 605–9
    aims, 608
    interventricular communications associated with, 607–8
    long term results, 608
    major lesions associated with, 608–9
    mortality for, 607–8, 609
    risk factors, 608
  symptomatology, 587
Atrioventricular sequential pacing, 1281
Atrioventricular valves, *see also specific valves and* Valves
  atresia, 336, 744
    associated heart patterns, 760
    palliation, 760
    venous anomalies associated with, 503
  common, 73, 335–6, 337, 338, 574, 575, 576
    angiocardiographic features, 600, 602, 603, 667
    in atrial isomerism, 482
    atrioventricular septal defect associated with, 574, 575, 576, 580, 581–2, 589, 590, 591, 600, 607–8, 608–9
    double inlet ventricle with, 666, 667, 698, 699
    echocardiographic features, 589–96 *passim*
    natural history, 604
    Rastelli classification, 581–2
    repair, 452
    stradling of, 698, 699
  corrected transposition associated with defects of, 881–2
  development, 98–100

double inlet ventricle associated with defects of, 648, 649, 665–7
double outlet ventricle associated anomalies of, 895
  echocardiographic features, 330, 331, 332, 336–8, 339, 343, 344, 657–61
  imperforate, 336–7, 675, 681, 740
  incompetence, murmurs associated with, 469
  leaflets
    arrangement, normal, 572–3
    arrangement with atrioventricular septal defect, 575–6, 576
    bridging, 573, 577, 578, 581–2, 589, 594, 608
    five-, 581
    morphogenesis, 99, 586
    naming, 572, 573
  left
    atrioventricular septal defect with, 598, 600
    regurgitation, abolishment, 609
    repair, 606–7
    replacement, 607
  morphological terminology, 68, 72–3
  orifice arrangement, 572–3
    atrioventricular septal defects classified by, 574, 576, 577
  overriding, 73, 333, 338, 700, 703, 704, 705, 905
    left, 704, 705
    right, 703, 704
  regurgitation, detection, 343, 344
  right
    angiocardiographic features, 689, 690
    echocardiographic features, 687
    morphogenesis, 684
    morphology, 675, 677–8, 681–2
  size and tension, determination, 661
  stenosis, severe
    angiocardiographic features, 668
    echocardiographic features, 662
  straddling, 73, 333, 338, 339, 650, 697–719
    absent atrioventricular connexion with, 707–8
    corrected transposition associated, 881–2
    definitions, 697–8
    diagnosis, 699–705, 882
    incidence, 699
    left, 703–5
    morphogenesis, 707, 708–9
    morphology, 699–705
    right, 700–3
    surgery, corrective, 706–7
    surgery, palliative, 705
    ventricular relationships, 699–705
  ventricular commitment of the, 337–8
  ventricular identification by viewing of, 330, 331, 332
Atrium, *see* Atria
Auscultation
  diagnostic value, 185–9
  findings with specific conditions, *see* Murmurs; Sounds
  method, 185–6
Autoimmunity, diseases involving
  endocardial fibrosis, 1336
  endocarditis, 1230
  myocarditis, 1169–71
  rheumatic heart disease, acute, 1183
Autopsies, pulmonary vascular pathology studies using, 127–8

Autosomal defects
  aneuploidy, 15–21
  single gene, 21–4, 25
  syndromes caused by, 47–59 *passim*
Axillary vessels, catheterisation via, 369, 370–2
Axis (mean vector)
  determination, 252–5
  deviation, 254–5

Bacteraemia, 1237–8
  diagnosis, 1237
Bacteria
  endocarditis associated, 1230–1
  rheumatic fever associated, 1179–85
Baffle (repair) operations
  life expectancy estimates, 432, 433
  optimal timing, 429–34
  survival curve, 432
Balloon, oesophageal, uses, 399
Balloon angioplasty, *see* Angioplasty
Balloon atrial septostomy, *see* Septostomy
Balloon catheters, 374, 377–8
  detachable, 379, 1017, 1018
  Gruntzig, 536
  types, 379
  uses, 816, 1114
  visualisation, 1018, 1114
Balloon valvoplasty, *see* Valvoplasty
Banding, *see* Pulmonary arteries; Pulmonary trunk
Becker's muscular dystrophy, 1258
Bed rest for rheumatic heart disease, 1191, 1192, 1193
Beri-beri, 1262–3
Bicuspid valve, *see* Mitral valve
Bifascicular block, 286, 1289
Bilateral conus, 77
Bilharziasis, cardiac signs, 1321–3
Biopsies
  endomyocardial, 375–6
  lung, 127, 141
Blade atrial septostomy, 380–1
Blalock-Hanlon septectomy/operation, 445
Blalock-Taussig shunt/operation, 444
  for Fallot's tetralogy, 788
  modified, 788
  for tricuspid atresia, 691
Bleeding, cyanosis/polycythaemia associated, 775
Blockage, *see* Obstruction
Blood
  cultures, *see* Cultures
  flow/circulation, *see* Circulation
  gas analysis, 365, 399–400
  loss, 382
  mixing, *see* Circulation
  pressure, *see* Pressure
Body size/weight, allowances for
  in exercise testing, 403, 409
  in haemodynamic measurements, 388–90
Bone deformities/abnormalities, heart diseases associated with, 45
Brachial artery pulse in aortic stenosis, 982
Brachial cut-down (catheterisation), 372
Brachiocephalic artery
  aberrant, 1127, 1128
  tracheal compression by, 1132–3
Bradyarrhythmias/bradycardias, 1276–81
  catheter induced, 382
  -tachycardia syndrome, 1277–8

Bradykinin, effects on ductus arteriosus, 937–8
Brain, *see entries under* Cerebral; Neurological
Branchial arch development, 130
  in different species, 101
Breathing, *see* Respiration; Respiratory distress syndrome
Bronchial arteries
  anatomy, 124–5
  circulation, 150
  development, 130
Bronchial circulation
  acquired, 821
  anatomy, 124–5
  angiographic visualisation, 821
  arterial, 150
  pulmonary circulation anastomoses to, 125, 150
  in pulmonary hypertension, 143
  venous, 125
Bronchial morphology, 69, 70
  atrial isomerism associated, 484–5
    radiographic features, 486–7
Bronchial vein anatomy, 125
Broncho-atrial discordance, 475, 476, 477
Bronchogram of absent pulmonary valve, 785
Bronchopulmonary anastomoses, 125, 150
Bruit, supraclavicular and carotid, 467
Bundles
  anatomy
    with double inlet ventricle, 649
    with corrected transposition, 570–1
  branches, *see* Left bundle branch; Right bundle branch
Burns, hypertension associated with, 1314
Bypass surgery, cardiopulmonary
  problems/damage created by, 147, 1369
  in sickle cell haemoglobinopathy, 1328

C-reactive protein, 1183
  test, 1183, 1189
Calcification, coronary artery, 1082, 1227
Cancers, *see* Tumours
Candida, endocarditis associated, 1231, 1237
Captopril therapy, 438
Carbon dioxide
  arterial (Pa_{CO_2}), 405, 406
  mixed venous (Pv_{CO_2}), 405, 406
  production ($\dot{V}CO_2$)
    cardiac output measured from, 405–6
Cardiac action potential, 237–9
Cardiac activity, sequence, recording, *see* Electrocardiography
Cardiac connexions, notation scheme, 228, 229, 230, 231
Cardiac contour, abnormal, differential diagnosis, 197–8
Cardiac cycle, phases, 166–71
Cardiac output ($\dot{Q}$)
  with atrial septal defect, 549
  control, 434
  fetal, neonatal comparisons, 113
  measurement, 225–6, 365, 405–7
    age related to, 411
    definition, 403–4
    by dye dilution, 365, 386–7
    in exercise, 405–7, 411–13
    non-invasive, 395, 402, 405–7
    by thermodilution, 365
Cardiogenesis, 85–105
Cardiomegaly

cardiomyopathy associated, 197, 198, 203
  diagnosis, 197
  pulmonary atresia with, 717
  trypanosomiasis associated, 1325
Cardiomyopathy
  cardiomegaly associated, 197, 198, 203
  chronic, 1324
  drug-induced, 1266–7
  hypertrophic, 1137–50
    aetiology, 1138
    associated conditions, 1138–9
    clinical features/findings, 1141–3
    diagnosis, differential, 1149–50, 1227
    investigations, 1143–7
    management, 1147–9
    obstructive, pregnancy risks, 1359
    pathomorphology, 1139–40
    pathophysiology, 1140–1
    prognosis, 1149
  inherited, 23, 1138
  primary, 1328
  syndromes associated with, 46
  trypanosomiasis associated, 1324
Cardiopulmonary bypass, *see* Bypass surgery
Carditis, pan-, rheumatic, 1184, 1186–8, *see also* Endocarditis; Myocarditis; Pericarditis
  treatment, 1192–3
Carnitine deficiency, 1262
Carotid artery
  catheterisaton, 372
  common
    interruption proximal to, 1125–6
    -subclavian artery, interruption between, 1124–5
Carter effect, definition, 29
Catecholamine production, hypertension associated with, 1312–13
Catheter(s), cardiac
  balloon-, *see* Balloon catheters
  broken, 383
  choice, 373–6
  cobra-, 818
  guide-wires, 375–6
  knotted, 382–3
  manipulation, 373–6
  position, 376
  visualisation/recognition, 343, 344, 375
  Shirley transvalvar-, 374
Catheterisation, cardiac, 363–91
  complications, 368–9, 382–3
  consultation prior to, 1385–9
  costs, 12
  cut-down-, 369–72
  data obtained, 384–91
    calculations made from, 384–5
    in normal children, 388–9
    interpretation of, 390–1
  findings and/or treatment using
    aortic arch interruption, 1112–13
    aortic atresia, 749–52
    aortic coarctation, 1009–101, 1103–4
    aortic regurgitation, 1212–13
    aortic stenosis, 979, 983–4, 1210
    aortopulmonary window, 925–7
    arteriovenous abnormal connexions, 1012, 1016, 1017
    atrial chamber partitioning, 567
    atrial isomerism, 490–1
    atrial septal defects, 555–7
    atrioventricular septal defects, 597–8, 608–9
    complete transposition, 847–8, 850–1

coronary artery anomalies, 1075–6
corrected transposition, 876
double inlet ventricle, 661–3
double outlet ventricle, 904–5
Ebstein's (and related) malformations, 728–9
endocardial fibroelastosis, 1226
Fallot's tetralogy, 782–4
hypoplastic left heart syndrome, 749–52
mitral valve anomalies, 749–52, 1033, 1048–9, 1202, 1208
persistent ductus arteriosus, 944
pulmonary atresia, 717–18, 816, 817, 818, 825, 826
pulmonary stenosis, 880, 967, 969, 972
pulmonary vascular disease, 146
pulmonary venous anomalies, 522–3, 525–6, 531, 533, 534
rheumatic heart disease, 1202, 1208, 1210, 1212–13, 1214, 1215
sinus of Valsalva aneurysm, 1009
systemic disease, 1246–68 *passim*
tricuspid atresia, 688–9
tricuspid stenosis, 1215
truncus arteriosus, 917–21
tumours, cardiac, 1156
ventricular septal defects, 633–4, 847, 879, 905
indicator dilution studies, 386–7, 556–7
in-patient vs out-patient practices, 365
interventional, 377–82, 825
laboratory requirements, 363
mortality risks, 383, 728
necessity, 1099–101
parental adaptation after, 1390–2
percutaneous, 366–9
prelude to, 365–6
premedication, 365–6
repair of incision, 371–2
retrograde, 374
routes/approaches, 366–73
safety measures, 363
$\dot{V}O_2$ measurement during, 404–5
Causes of congenital heart disease, 15–39, 42–59
Caval vein(s)
  arrangement, echocardiography, 327, 328, 329, 478, 487–8
  catheterisation, 501, 505
  connexions/positions
    anomalous, 476–9, 502–3, 503, 505
    to atria, 327, 329, 502–3, 503, 505
  fetal blood flow in, 110–11
  inferior, *see* Caval veins, inferior
  superior, *see* Caval veins, superior
Caval vein(s), inferior, 329
  absent, 506
  in atrial isomerism, 467–9, 487–8
  azygos continuations, 477, 478, 488, 504–5
  connexions, 329
    anomalous, 476–9, 504–6
  hemizygos continuations, 477–9, 488
  hepatic segment, absence, 504
Caval vein(s), superior, 329
  absent, 501
  aneurysm, 503
  in atrial isomerism, 477
  bilateral, 501, 546–7
  connexions, 329, 477
    anomalous, 500–4, 523, 525, 545, 547
  development, 497–9
  left, 500–1, 501–2

Caval vein(s) superior (*contd.*)
  obstruction, post-surgical, 853
  right, 501, 503, 523, 525
Cellular electrophysiology, 237–41
Central nervous system
  electrocardiographic effects of, 304–5
  injury, 305
Centronuclear myopathy, 1259
Cerebral abscess, cyanosis associated, 787
Cerebral embolus, management risks, 423–8
Cerebral haemorrhage, patent ductus
    associated, 948
Chamber, cardiac
  connexions in complete transposition,
    831–4
  dominance, 584–5
  echocardiographic visualisaton, 321, 342
  enlargement/hypertrophy,
    electrocardiographic features, 272–80
  localisation, sequential, 65–8
  volume measurement, 387–8
Charcot-Marie-Tooth disease, 1260–1
Chest pain, presentation with, 197
Child (during illness)
  care, in-patient, 1389
  communication with, 1377–9
    cognitive, 1377–7
    emotional, 1379
    with poor prognosis, 1378
  preferences of, 1400
  preparation of, for procedures and events,
    1378
  psychological aspects, 1373–81
  social aspects, 1385
Chorea (rheumatic-; Sydenham's-; St. Vitus
    dance), 1188
  treatment, 1193
Chromosome defects, *see* Aneuploidy
Chromosome 8, short arm trisomy, 20
Circulation and flow, blood
  arterial, *see* Arterial circulation
  in child with congenital heart disease,
    111–13
  collateral, *see* Collateral arteries
  in complete transposition, 838–9
  development, 85–6, 109–115, 840
  failure, 435–40
    causes, 435
    clinical features, 435–6
    neonate/small infant, 435
    treatment, 437–40
  fetal, 109–11, 113–19, 939
    distribution and control of, 110–11
    organisation, 110
    persistent, 151
    pulmonary atresia affected, 715
  fetal-neonatal switch, 114–19
  functional properties, 434
  measurement, 384–5, 387, *see also* Doppler
    ultrasound
  mixing, 193–4, *see also* Shunts
    in conjoined twins, 1060
    diagnosis, 193–4
    with double inlet ventricles, 654–5
    venous, in tricuspid atresia, 683–4
  neonatal, 111, 115–19, 840, 1093–4
  normal, 838
  pulmonary, *see* Pulmonary circulation
  systemic, 384–5, *see also* Systemic venous
    return
  venous, *see* Venous system
Circumflex (coronary) artery, anomalous
    origin, 1078–9

Clicks, *see* Sounds
Clinical features of cardiac syndromes, 47–59
Clinical presentation of heart disease, 191–8
Coarctation, aortic, *see* Aortic coarctation
Coils, steel, vessel closure using, 379, 825,
    1017, 1019
Collagen synthetic disorders, cardiac signs,
    1253–6
Collateral circulation, 532–3, 1091, 1113
  acquired, 809–10, 811, 820
  aortopulmonary, 802, 803–4
Communication (between people)
  with child, *see* Child
  jargon used in, 1386–7
  with parents on child admission, *see*
    Consultation
Community aspects of child illness, 1381
Complete transposition, *see* Transposition,
    complete
Computerised tomography, cardiac aspects,
    217–18
Conduction
  atrial, 235–6
  atrioventricular, *see* Atrioventricular
    conduction
  intercellular, 240–1
  interventricular, delay, 280–6
  intracellular, 237–40
  Mahaim-, 289–90
  system, *see* Conduction system
Conduction system
  anatomy, 235–7
  atrioventricular axis, 236–7
  defects and disturbances, *see* Conduction
    system defects and disturbances
  development, 102–4
  surgical avoidance, 606
  surgical damage/trauma and post-operative
    problems, 560, 639, 769, 792–3, 854,
    1279, 1369
Conduction system defects and disturbances,
    280–90, 1288–91
  atrial isomerism associated, 482–3
  atrioventricular septal defect associated,
    583–4
  complete transposition associated, 833
  corrected transposition associated, 870–1,
    881
  double inlet ventricle associated, 649,
    650–1, 652
  double outlet ventricle associated, 897–8
  electrocardiographic features, 280–90, *see*
    also Electrocardiography
  Fallot's tetralogy associated, 768, 769
  interventricular, 280–90
    delay, diffuse, 280
    post-operative, 639
  straddling atrioventricular valves, 700–1,
    705
  syndromes associated with, 46
  tricuspid atresia associated, 680, 681
  truncus arteriosus associated, 915
  trypanosomiasis associated, 1324, 1325
  ventricular septal defect associated, 621,
    697–8
Coni's disease, 1247
Conjoined twins, *see* Twins
Connective tissue disease, 1264–6
  electrocardiographic effects, 305–6
Consultation(s), 1385–9
  decision making in, 1390–1, 1400
  deficiencies in, 1386
  difficulties with, 1385

  length, 1387
  post-surgical, 1394
  pre-catheterisation, 1385–9
  questions from parents, 1387, 1391, 1394
Contraceptive pill, *see* Oral contraceptive
Contractility, 165–6
  aortic stenosis and, 415
  definition, 165
  hypertrophic cardiomyopathy effects on,
    1141
  index, 413, 415
Contraction
  atrial, 360, 1291
    premature, 1287, 1291
  ductus arteriosus, 936–7
    factors affecting, 937, 938
  fetal, 360
  ventricular, 1291
    incoordinate-, 171
    isovolumic-, 167
    phase, *see* Systole
    timing, 224
    velocity, 177
  ventricular-atrial comparisons, 360
Contrast media
  echocardiographic use, 342–3, 344
  hazards, 383
  injection, 377, 817, 1033–4
    considerations, 377, 387, 663–6 *passim*
    selective, 666, 808, 810, 818, 1132, 1133
    simultaneous, 718, 809
Conversations with parents/child, *see*
    Communication
Cor pulmonale, 152
Cor triatriatum, *see* Atrial chamber
    partitioning
Cor triloculare biatriatum, *see* Double inlet
    ventricle
Coronary artery
  aberrant course, 1079–81
  aneurysms, 1082–3, 1171
  anomalies and diseases, 1003, 1073–83
    arising from pulmonary trunk, 296–7,
      1002, 1004, 1074–7, 1227
    classification, 1073–4
    clinical features/findings, 1075, 1077–82
      passim, 1083
    complete transposition associated, 833–4,
      835
    corrected transposition associated, 713,
      715
    diagnosis, 1076, 1077–82 *passim*, 1083,
      1227
    Fallot's tetralogy associated, 786
    floppy mitral valve associated, 1041
    investigations, 1075–6, 1077–82 *passim*,
      1083
    medical management, 1076, 1083
    morphogenesis, 1073, 1077–82 *passim*
    morphology, 1073, 1077–82 *passim*
    myocardial infarction caused by, 296–7
    natural history/course/prognosis, 1076,
      1077–82 *passim*
    pathophysiology, 1074, 1077–82 *passim*
    prevalence, 1073
    of the proximal segments, 1078–9
    pulmonary atresia associated, 713, 715
    surgical management, 1076–7, 1082
  calcification, 1082, 1227
  circulation to lung from, 818, 819
  development, abnormal, 715
  fistulous communications, 715, 1002,
    1081–2

Coronary artery *(contd.)*
  injection, 818, 819
  intramural, 1081
  morphology, 1073
  ostial, 1078–9
  relocation, 857, 858
Coronary ostium, left
  atresia, 1077–8
  stenosis, 1077–8
Coronary sinus
  anomalies, 506, 546–7
    angiocardiographic features, 525
    atrial isomerism associated, 479
    atrial septal defect associated, 501–2,
      546–7
    caval vein anomalies associated with, 500
    complete transposition associated with,
      834
    echocardiographic features, 501, 520–1,
      522
    enlargement, detection, 501
    hypoplasia, 506
    morphology, 546–7
    pulmonary vein anomalies associated
      with, 209, 512, 513, 520–1, 522, 525
    unroofing, 546–7
  development, 497–9
  rhythm, 501
Corrected transposition, *see* Transposition,
  corrected
Cost (economic) of congenital heart disease,
  11–13
Course of untreated disease, *see* Natural
  history
Cox proportional hazards method, 1366–7
Coxsackie viruses, rheumatic heart disease
  associated, 1182
Criss-cross hearts, 75, 1065–71
Crista, 77, 78, 766, 767
  defects, 624–5
Cross-sectional echocardiography, *see*
  Echocardiography, cross-sectional
Culture, blood
  endocarditis, infective, diagnosis,
    1236–7
  management decisions involving results of,
    426, 427, 428–9
  negative-, 1237
Current flow, cellular, 239–40
Cushing's syndrome, 1312
Cutix laxa, 1254
Cyanosis, 191–4, *see also* Hypoxia
  atrial septal defect associated, 559
  atrial isomerism associated, 488
  complete transposition associated, 840, 841,
    842
  double outlet ventricle associated, 900
  diagnosing, 183, 191, 843
    differential, 192–4
  during catheterisation, 382
  exercise induced, 397
  Fallot's tetralogy associated, 774
    clinical presentation, 775–7
    effects, 775, 786–7
    relief, 776–6, 787
    hyper-, 777
  hypoplastic left heart syndrome associated,
    746
  murmurs associated with, 1006
  pulmonary atresia associated, 715, 718,
    811, 812
  pulmonary stenosis associated, 964
  tricuspid atresia associated, 684–5

Cyanotic heart disease, 192–4
  definition, 192
  natural history, 10
Cyclo-oxygenase enzymes, 116, 935
Cystic fibrosis, pulmonary hypertension
  associated with, 152–3

Damus-Stansel-Kaye procedure, 859
Deafness, heart defects associated with, 44
Death, child, parental experience, 1380–1
Decision
  making, parental, 1390–1, 1400
  theory, 421–34
  tree(s), 421–9
    complex, 423–9
Dentistry, endocarditis and, 1234, 1237–8,
  1239
Depolarisation
  atrial, 245–7, 252
  cellular, 237–41
  intercellular, 240–1
  ventricular, 242, 248, 249, 252
    abnormal, 252
Depositions, cardiac disease due to, 1263–4
Dermatoglyphics in Down's syndrome, 18
Dermatomyositis, 1170–1
Desoxycorticosteroid levels, hypertension
  associated, 1311–12
Detection of heart disease, frequency, age
  related, 6
Development
  complete transposition effects on, 841–2
  heart, 85–105
Diabetes, 1252
  teratogenicity, 25
Diastole
  pressure in, *see* Pressure
  sounds in, *see* Sounds
  ventricular function in, 172–6, 177, *see also*
    Relaxation
    assessment, 177
Digital vascular imaging, 364
Digitalis (and Digoxin), 302–3
  electrocardiographic effects, 302–3
  interactions, 435
  toxicity, 302–3
  treatment
    in circulatory failure, 435
    controversies, 1282–4
    dose regime, 436, 1356
    in endocardial fibroelastosis, 1227
    in pregnancy, 1356
Digoxin, *see* Digitalis
Dilators
  arteriolar, 438–9
  mixed, 438–9
  vaso-, *see* Vasodilators
  veno-, *see* Venodilators
Dilution curves, 386–7
Dipole concept of cellular current flow,
  239–40
Direct ventricular puncture, 373
Disopyramide, electrocardiographic effects,
  303
Diuretics therapy
  in circulatory failure, 436–7
  complications, 437
  dose regime, 437
  in pregnancy, 1356
  in systemic hypertension, 1314, 1315
Dobutamine therapy, 440

Doctor-parent relations, 1389, *see also*
  Medical profession
Doppler ultrasound/echocardiography, 185,
  347–8, 1346
  clinical applications, 345–8
  continuous, 344–5
  measurements and findings in
    ductus closure, 950
    mitral valve insufficiency, 1032–3
    pulmonary venous abnormalities, 518
    ventricular septal defects, 631
  pulsed-, 344, 518
  quantitative, 347
  range gating in, 344, 345
  transcutaneous, 348
Doty technique, 459, 460
Double inlet ventricle (cor triloculare
  biatriatum), 71, 72, 335, 336, 643–71
  angiocardiographic diagnosis, 663–7
    algorithm for, 664
    hallmark feature, 664
  aortic atresia and, 743
  clinical findings, 655–6
  clinical symptomatology, 655
  common atrioventricular orifice associated
    with, 666, 667, 698, 699
  echocardiographic features, 658–63
  indeterminate (ventricle), 651–2
  investigations, 656–7
  left (ventricle), 645–50
    mitral anomalies associated with, 1025
  medical management, 669
  morphogenesis, 653–5
  morphology, 643–53
  natural history/course, 667–8
  pathophysiology, 654–5
  presentation, 655
  prevalence, 654
  right (ventricle), 650–1
  surgical management, 467, 668–71, 907–8
    corrective, 669–71
    palliative, 668–9
    relative merits, 671
Double outlet ventricles
  angiocardiographic features, 113, 905, 906
  associated defects, 891
    influence of, 899–900
  atrioventricular septal defects associated
    with, 596–7, 599, 600
  classification, 890–8
  clinical presentation, 900
  definition, 889
  diagnosis, differential, 905–7
  discordant atrioventricular connexions with,
    883–4, 896, 908
  double inlet with, 647
  investigations, 900–5
  left, 680, 884, 890, 896–7
  morphogenesis, 898–9
  morphology, 680, 890–8
  pathophysiology, 899
  prevalence, 890
  right, 883–4, 891
    parachute mitral valve with, 1035
    variants, 891–7
  surgical management, 907–8
    palliative, 907
    risk factors, 907, 908
Down's syndrome, 16–18
  atrial septal defects associated with, 548
  atrioventricular septal defect associated
    with, 587
  dermatoglyphics, 18

Down's syndrome (*contd.*)
  facies, 16
  genetic counselling, 19
  karyotype, 16
  management
    repair of cardiac defects, 609
    social/clinical issues of, 1394–5
  mosaic-, 17
  natural history of heart disease, 604
  quality of life, 1401
  translocation-, 17–18
Drug(s), *see also specific types/names of drugs*
  heart disease inducing, 1266–7
  hypertensive, 1314
  pre-catheterisation, 365–6
  teratogenic, 25
  treatment, principles of, 434–40
Duchenne's muscular dystrophy, *see* Muscular
    dystrophy
Ductus arteriosus, 115–17, 931–53
  absence, 932–3
  anatomy, 115–16
  aneurysm, 947
  aortic interruption distal to, 1123–4, 1125
  bilateral, 741, 932
  bradykinin effects, 937–8
  closure
    detection, 950
    late (spontaneous), 945
    natural, 116, 936–7, 950
    over-extensive, 1092
    surgical, 379–80, 445–6, 944–5, 950, 953
  constriction, 1093
  dilatation, 440, 934–5
  echocardiographic visualisation, 340–1, 348,
    847, 943–4, 950
  historical considerations, 931
  importance, 938
  innervation, 934
  ipsilateral, 1126–7, 1127
  left sided, 1126, 1131
  microscopic features, 933
  morphogenesis, 933
  morphology, 933–5
  musculature, 933–4
  patency (drug-maintained), 951–2
  patency (normal/fetally maintained),
    115–16, 935–6
  patency (persistent), 151, 940–8
    aetiology, 940–2
    clinical features/findings, 942–3
    complications, 945–8
    diagnosis, 945
    electrocardiographic features, 294, 943
    incidence, 941–2, 942
    inheritence, 28–30
    investigations, 943
    natural history/course, 10, 945
    pathophysiology, 30, 942–3
    pulmonary vessel enlargement associated
      with, 209
    surgical management, 379–80, 445–6,
      944–5, 950, 953
    wall morphology, 30
  patency (in the premature), 948–51
    clinical features/findings, 948
    investigations, 949
    management, 950–1
    pathophysiology, 949
  pulmonary time-activity curves with, 221
  right sided, 1127, 1128
  role in various malformations, 938–40,
    1092, 1093–4

shunting
    left to right, 949
    right to left, 754
  sling, 1135
  steroid effects, 937
  -subclavian artery, aortic interruption
      between, 1124
  tortuous, 814, 821
Ductus venosus
  anomalous connexions to, 512, 514
  closure, 115
  in heart disease, 115
Dye dilution, measurements by, 386–7,
    556–7
Dying child, parental experience, 1380–1
Dyspnoea, symptomatic relief, 776–7

Ear defects, heart defects associated with, 44
Ear-lobe puncture, 405, 406
Ebstein's anomaly, 720–35
  aetiology, 720
  clinical features/findings, 725
  diagnosis, 729–31
  echocardiographic features, 357, 881
  fetal detection, 723
  hallmark lesion, 724
  imperforate atrioventricular valve with, 681
  incidence, 720
  investigations, 725–9
  management, 729–31
  mitral valve with, 1025, 1026
  morphogenesis, 724
  morphology, 720–4
  natural history/course, 729
  pathophysiology, 724–5
  prognosis, 729
  pulmonary atresia associated with, 713
  severe, 723
Echocardiography (general features), 319–348
  contrast, 342–3, 1015
  cross-sectional, *see* Echocardiography, cross-
      sectional
  doppler, *see* Doppler ultrasound
  during exercise, 413
  features and findings with
    aortic arch interruption, 1111–12,
    aortic coarctation, 1098–9, 1100
    aortic regurgitation, 997, 1212
    aortic stenosis, 346, 347, 979, 980, 983,
      989, 990, 994, 1113, 1210
    aortic valve, endocarditis affected, 1232
    aortopulmonary window, 917, 925
    arteriovenous abnormal connexions, 1012
    atrial appendage juxtaposition, 1065
    atrial chamber partitioning, 566–7
    atrial isomerism, 487–8, 490
    atrial septal defects, 555
    atrioventricular septal defects, 588–97,
      782
    complete transposition, 228–9, 843–7
    conjoined twins, 1062
    coronary artery anomalies, 1075
    corrected transposition, 875–6
    criss-cross heart, 1069
    double inlet ventricle, 657–61
    double outlet ventricle, 902–4, 905
    Ebstein's (and related) malformations,
      726–7, 728
    endocardial fibroelastosis, 1227
    endocarditis, 1232, 1236

exteriorised heart, 1059
    Fallot's tetralogy, 780–2, 783
    heart malposition/abnormal relationships,
      1059, 1062, 1065
    hypertrophic cardiomyopathy, 1144,
      1145, 1146
    hypoplastic left heart syndrome, 748,
      749, 750, 751
    mitral valve anomalies, 905, 1029–33,
      1039, 1047–8, 1201–2, 1208
    myocarditis, 1167–8
    pericarditis, 1173–4
    persistent ductus arteriosus, 943–4, 950
    pulmonary atresia, 716, 717, 812–16
    pulmonary stenosis, 346, 846, 875, 881,
      966–7
    pulmonary venous anomalies, 518–22,
      530
    rheumatic heart disease, 1201–2, 1208
    sinus of Valsalva aneurysm/fistula, 1008
    straddling atrioventricular valves, 701,
      702, 703, 705
    systemic disease, 1246–67 *passim*
    tricuspid atresia, 686–8
    tricuspid stenosis, 1218
    tricuspid incompetence, 1214
    truncus arteriosus, 917
    tumours, cardiac, 1155–6
    ventricular septal defects, 629–31, 632,
      633, 634, 688, 812–16 *passim*, 849,
      879, 1113
  M-mode, *see* Echocardiography, M-mode
  prenatal, 351–61
    false negative diagnosis, 359
    false positive diagnosis, 359
    future value, 361
Echocardiography, cross-sectional, 319–48
  balloon atrial septostomy positioning by,
    851
  cardiac anatomy revealed by, 319–23
  contrast media used in, 342–3, 344
  cuts/section/planes
    coronal, 322, 323
    in fetal cardiac examination, 352
    four chamber, 162, 321, 323, 324, 330,
      331, 332, 342, 352, 357
    long axis, 322, 324, 325, 332, 343
    paracoronal, 325, 326
    parasagittal, 325, 326
    sagittal, 322, 323
    short axis, 320, 321, 323, 326
    subcostal, 322, 325
    two chamber, 324
  examination principles, 322–4
  prenatal, 351–3, 355–6
  structural identification by, 324–42
  ventricular dimensions measured by, 161–2
  views to the heart, 322–4
    windows giving, 322, 323, 324
Echocardiography, M-mode (single beam)
  atrioventricular connexions examined by,
    335, 336, 339, 340
  contrast media used in, 342, 343
  great artery identification by, 341
  limitations, 319
  prenatal, 354, 359–60
  ventricle identification by, 332–3
  ventricular dimensions measured by, 161,
    163
Economic costs of congenital heart disease,
    11–13
Ectopia cordis (exteriorisation of the heart),
    1057–9

Edward's syndrome, 18, 19
Effort tests, *see* Exercise
Ehlers-Danlos syndrome, 1254
Eisenmenger's syndrome in pregnancy,
    1357–8
Ejection
    sounds, *see* Murmurs; Sounds
    ventricular, *see* Ventricles
Electrocardiogram, *see also*
        Electrocardiography
    callibration, 241–2, 309
    derivation of the, 245–52
    normal, 255–67
        adolescent, 256
        neonatal, 256
    paper, 241–2
        drag, 310
    stylus position, 311
Electrocardiography/Electrovectorcardiography,
        235–313, *see also* Electrocardiogram
    children with murmurs, 468, 469
    computer analysis, 242, 243
    features in various diseases/conditions,
        266–306
        aortic coarctation, 1097–8
        aortic regurgitation, 996–7, 1212
        aortic stenosis, 981, 982–3, 986, 989,
            994, 1210
        aortopulmonary window, 925
        arrhythmias/conduction disturbances,
            280–91, 1273–91 *passim*
        arteriovenous abnormal connexions,
            1012, 1015
        atrial enlargement, 279–80
        atrial chamber partitioning, 566
        atrial isomerism, 267–8, 489
        atrial septal defects, 553–5
        atrioventricular septal defects, 588
        complete transposition, 843
        coronary artery anomalies, 296–7, 1075
        corrected transposition, 871–3
        cyanotic heart disease, 193, 194
        double inlet ventricle, 656
        double outlet ventricle, 901
        Ebstein's (and related) malformations,
            725–6
        endocardial fibroelastosis, 1225–6
        Fallot's tetralogy, 780
        heart failure, 195
        hypertrophic cardiomyopathy, 1143–4
        hypoplastic left heart syndrome, 747–9
        infarction, 297–9
        injury, cardiac, 293–7
        ischaemia, 291–3
        malposition of the heart, 266–72
        mitral valve anomalies, 1029, 1200,
            1206–7
        myocarditis, 1166–7
        pericarditis, 294–5, 1173
        persistent ductus arteriosus, 294, 943
        pulmonary atresia, 715–16, 812
        pulmonary hypertension, 1200, 1206
        pulmonary stenosis, 880, 965–6
        pulmonary venous anomalies, 517–18,
            530
        rheumatic carditis, 1188, 1189, 1200,
            1206, 1210, 1212, 1214, 1215
        systemic diseases, 1246–68 *passim*
        tricuspid atresia, 685–6
        tricuspid incompetence, 1274
        tricuspid stenosis, 1215
        truncus arteriosus, 917
        tumours, cardiac, 1155

ventricular hypertrophy, 270, 272–9,
        780, 843, 873, 1143, 1144, 1225–6
    ventricular septal defects, 629, 812, 879
leads, 243–5, 246
    incorrectly positioned, 306–8
    left axis deviation, 873
    malfunctioning system, 309–10
    measurement, 241–2, 1275
        in exercise, 412–13
    patient manipulation during, 308–9
    patient movement during, 308
    planes, 245
    standardisation, 241–2
    waves and intervals, 242–3, 244
        artefacts affecting, 306–13
        differentiating, 264–5
        diseases/conditions affecting, 266–306
        normal values, 277
Electrophysiological studies
    cellular-, 237–41
    invasive, 1275–6, 1283, 1284, 1285
Electrovectorcardiography, *see*
        Electrocardiography
Ellis-van Creveld syndrome, 23
Embolisation of vessels, 378–9, 825, 1017,
        1019
Embolisms, *see also* Thromboses
    air-, 383
    cerebral, management risks, 423–8
    endocarditis associated, 1234
    heart disease associated with, 215
    heart tumour associated, 1153–4
    thrombo-, 215
        prosthetic valve associated, 1037
        pulmonary hypertension associated with,
            153
Embryology of the heart, 85–105
Emery Dreyfuss disease, 1259
Emotions
    in child illness, 1376, 1379
    surgery and its effects on, 1376
End-diastolic pressure, 167, 168
    ventricular, 173–4
End-systolic pressure-volume/dimension
        relations, 170
Endocardial cushion(s)
    development, 90, 96, 98
    fusion, failure, 585, 586, 915
Endocardial fibroelastosis/sclerosis, 1223–7
    aetiology, 1223–4
    cardiomyopathies associated with, 1325
    clinical features, 1225
    diagnosis, differential, 1227
    hypoplastic left ventricle associated, 740,
        741
    incidence, 1223
    investigations, 1225–7
    natural history/course, 1225
    pathogenesis, 1223–4
    pathology/pathophysiology, 1223, 1224–5
    primary, 1223–7
    prognosis, 1227
    pulmonary radiographic features, 214
Endocardial/endomyocardial fibrosis, 1328–6
    aetiology, 1335–6
    bilateral, 1329
    diagnosis, 1333
    epidemiology, 1329
    histological features, 1330
    incidence/prevalence, 1329
    laboratory data, 1333
    management, 1333–5
        comparative studies, 1333–4

pathophysiology, 1331
    prevention, 1336
    signs and symptoms, 1331–3
    treatment-induced, 1266, 1267
    ventricular
        bi-, 1333, 1334, 1335
        left, 1331–2, 1334
        right, 1331, 1334–5
Endocardial outlet
    ridges, 96
    septum, development, 96–7
Endocardiectomy, 1334, 1335
Endocarditis, infective, 1229–41
    aetiology, 1229–31
    clinical features, 1233–6
    diagnosis, 1236–7
    management
        decisions, 423–9
        medical, 1239–40
        surgical, 1240–1
    pathology, 1233
    persistent ductus arteriosus associated,
        947
    prevalence/incidence, 1229, 1231
    prevention, 1238–9
        in pregnancy, 1355–6
    prosthetic valve-, 423–9
    radiographic features associated with, 215
    rheumatic heart disease associated, 1184
    symptoms, 1234–5
    ventricular septal defect associated, 637
Endocardium
    activation, 248, 250
    biopsy, 375–6
    development, 94–6 *passim*
Endocrine disorders
    cardiac involvement, 1252
    hypertension associated, 1311–13
Endomyocardial fibrosis, *see* Endocardial
        fibrosis
Endoscopic forceps, 381
Environmental factors in heart disease, 16,
        28
Eosinophilia, hyper-, endomyocardial fibrosis
        associated with, 1366
Epicardial activation, 248, 250
Epidemiology of heart disease, 30, *see also*
        Incidence
Erythema marginatum, 1188
Erythromycin prophylaxis, 1239
Esophagus, *see* Oesophagus
Ethanolaminosis, 1247
Ethical considerations, 1399–1402
    in catheterisation tests, 389
    in Down's syndrome, 1395
    in exercise testing, 395–6
    four sets of, 1399, 1402
Eustachian valves, development, 87, 506–7
Examination, physical, 184–9
Exercise, 395–417
    advisability with aortic stenosis, 986
    capacity with double inlet ventricle, 655
    hypertension and, 1297
    intolerance, estimating, 396, 414
    performance tests, 395, 396, 397, 401–13
        in children with heart disease, 413–17
        maximum, 401–2, 409–10, 414
        post-aortic coarctation repair, 1106
        simple progressive, 402, 408, 409
        stopping (decided by child), 409–19
        submaximum, 402–4, 410–13
        types, 401–4
    pulmonary reserve for, 395

Experimentation, ethical considerations, 1402
Expiration, *see also* Respiration; Ventilation
  gas measurement, 404
  heart sound features associated with, 186–7
Expired flow-volume loop, 398
Exteriorisation of the heart, *see* Ectopia cordis
Eye defects, heart defects associated with, 43

Fabry's disease, 1251
Facies, abnormal, heart defects associated
  with, 42–3
Facioscapulohumeral muscular dystrophy,
  1258–9
Fainting, *see* Syncope
Fallot's tetralogy, 765–93
  aetiology, 39, 765
  clinical presentation, 775–7
  complications, 786–7
    post-operative, 792
  double outlet ventricle relationship to,
    889–90
  exercise tolerance, 396, 414–15
  hallmark, 765
  incidence/prevalence, 765
  investigations, 779–86
  magnetic resonance imaging in, 229–30
  medical management, 787
  morphogenesis, 774
  morphology, 765–73
  natural history/course, 786–7
  pathophysiology, 774–5
  physical examination, 777–9
  postoperative management, 791–3
  pulmonary hypoperfusion with, 148, 149
  pulmonary radiographic features, 207
  surgical management, 787–93
    choice, 790
    corrective, 453–4, 789–90
    double outlet ventricle relationship to,
      889–90
    measurements for predicting outcome,
      789
    medical management, 787
    palliative, 787, 788–9
    right bundle branch block after, 1289
    risk factors, 790–1
Family
  experience of dying child by, 1380–1
  importance to child of, 1374, 1375
  long term adjustments by, 1381
Family studies
  blood pressure, 1296–7, 1347
  in heart disease aetiology, 28–9, 33–4
Fascicular block, 284–6
  bi-, 286, 1289
  electrocardiographic features, 284–6
  tri-, 286, 1289
Fasciculoventricular conduction, 289–90
Fat, *see* Lipids; Obesity
Fear
  of pain, 1379
  parental, 1389, 1390
Femoral arterial catheterisation
  percutaneous, 366, 368
  cut-down, 369
  complications, 368–9
Femoral pulse, 1093, 1095
Femoral 'triangle', anatomy, 370
Femoral venous catheterisation, percutaneous,
  366–7
  complications, 368

Fetal echocardiography, 351–3, 355–6
Fetus, fate with maternal congenital heart
  disease, 1354
Fibroelastic hamartoma (=fibroma), 1156,
  1157–8
Fibroelastoma (=fibroma), 1156, 1157–8
Fibroelastosis, endocardial, *see* Endocardial
  fibroelastosis
Fibroma, 1156, 1157–8
Fibrosis
  endomyocardial, *see*
    Endocardial/endomyocardial fibrosis
  intimal, pulmonary artery, 138
  post-operative development, 1369
Fibrous tissue tags, *see* Aneurysmal tags
Fick equation, 384
Fick method, indirect, 405–6
Filaria, endomyocardial fibrosis associated
  with, 1336
Financial costs of congenital heart disease,
  11–13
Fistulas
  arteriovenous, *see* Arteriovenous fistulae
  coronary artery, 715, 1002, 1081–2
    surgery, 1082
  pulmonary artery, 1081
  sinus of Valsalva, *see* Sinus of Valsalva
Fits, presentation with, 196
Follow-up
  patients lost to, 1364–5
  postoperative-, 1363–70
Fontan procedure, 443, 462
  mortality, 693
  for tricuspid atresia, 691, 692, 693
Fontan-Kreutzer procedure, evaluation,
  670–1, *see also* Kreutzer procedure
Foramen
  ovale, fetal blood flow across, 109–10
  primary, 91, 92, 93, 94
Forced expired volume, 398
Forced vital capacity, 398
Foreign bodies, removal, 381–2
Formalin infiltration, ductal wall, 952
Fossa ovalis
  defects, 543
    atrial isomerism associated, 480
  morphogenesis, 547, 548
  morphology, 542, 543
45X Turner's syndrome, 21-2, 1087
Freidreich's ataxia, 1259–60
Fucosidosis, 1251
Functional residual capacity, 397
Fungal infections, endocarditis associated,
  425, 426, 1231

α-Galactosidase-A deficiency, 1251
Gangliosidoses, 1251–2
Gases
  blood analysis, 365, 399–400
  exchange, measurement, 404–5, 412
  inert, cardiac output measurement using,
    406–7
Gastric vein, anomalous connexions to, 512,
  514
Gastrointestinal features/findings, *see* Gut
Gaucher's disease, 1250–1
Gene defects (causing heart disease),
  47–59
  polygenic, 26–30, 39
  single, 22–5, 26

Genetic causes of heart disease, 15–30, 31–9
  passim, 47–59
Genetic counselling
  for Down's syndrome, 19
  -figure (%), 35–7
Genitourinary anomalies, heart diseases
  associated with, 45
Gianturco coil, 825
Glenn operation, 691, 789
Glucocorticoids, effects on ductus arteriosus,
  937
Glucosylceramidosis, 1250–1
Glycogen storage disease of the heart,
  1245–7
  cardiomyopathy, associated with, 1138
  diagnosis, differential, 1227
  type II (Pompe's disease), 22, 23, 1246–7
    electrocardiographic features, 289
    heart failure in, 195
  type III-V, 1247
Glycoprotein degenerative disorders, 1249–50
Grafts, *see* Transplants, grafts and
  anastomoses
Gram negative microbes, endocarditis
  associated, 1231
Gram positive microbes, endocarditis
  associated, 1230–1
Great arteries
  echocardiographic features, 340–1
  morphology/arrangement, 76, 110–11, 341
    double inlet ventricle associated, 657
    terminologies used to describe, 68
  neonatal, 111–13
  posterior, abnormal position, 339
  pressure-flow relationship, 169
  relationships between, 78–9
  septal repair via, 451
  transposition, *see* Transposition
Great vessels
  abdominal, arrangement, 69–70
    in atrial isomerism, 488, 489
    echocardiographic examination, 327, 328,
      488, 489
  arteries, *see* Great arteries
Growth
  adaptation to, 395
  charts, cardiac, electrophysiologically
    determined, 354, 355, 356
  complete transposition effects on, 841–2
Gruentzig balloon, 536
Gut
  anomalies, heart diseases associated with,
    45
  radiography, 217

Haemangioma, 1159
Haematocrit level in Fallot's tetralogy, 775
Haemochromatosis, 1263–4
Haemodynamics, 384–91
  calculations, 384–8
  in exercise, 401–13
  findings in, *see also* Catheterisation
    complete transposition, 847–8
    coronary artery anomalies, 1076
    Fallot's tetralogy, 774–5
  normal values, 388–90
  psychological significance, 1373–4
Haemoglobinopathies, sickle cell, *see* Sickle
  cell

Haemosiderosis, 139
Halothane, electrocardiographic effects of, 304
Heart (general features), *see also entries under* Cardiac
abnormal relatonships, 1063–71
anatomy, normal
echocardiographic determination, 319–22
fetal, 351–3
apex, position, 81
diagnostic value, 204, 205
chambers, *see* Chambers
configuration, radiographic determination, 203–5
criss-cross, *see* Criss-cross heart
development, 85–105
disease/defects
acquired, 151
exercise testing, 396–7
psychological aspects, 1373–81
recurrence risks, 35–7
social aspects, 1385–96
syndromes associated with, 42–59
effect of tumours on, 1154
left sided with mirror image arrangement, 1063
malposition (extra-thoracic), *see* Ectopia cordis
malposition (intra-thoracic), 1062–3
atrial isomerism associated, 483–4
electrocardiographic determination, 266–72
positions, possible, 80
radiography, general principles, 202–5, 213
rate
age dependence, 257, 409, 411
in exercise, 409, 410
normal, 256–7, 1276
oxygen consumption related to, 410, 411
right sided, 872, 874, 877, 1062–3
size
changes, conditions causing, 202–3
enlarged, *see* Cardiomegaly
radiographic determination, 202–3
tumours, *see* Tumours
Heart block, *see also* Fascicular block; Left anterior hemiblock; Left posterior hemiblock; Right bundle branch; Left bundle branch
exercise tolerance in patients with, 415
fetal, 360
risks in pregnancy, 1359
surgically caused, 792–3
Heart failure
cause, radiographic diagnoses, 202, 203, 204, 205
clinical presentation, 194–5, 901
congestive, 627
persistent ductus arteriosus associated, 945–6
rheumatic carditis associated, 1187–8
tricuspid atresia associated, 691
double outlet ventricle associated, 901
management, 1193
in pregnancy, 1356
truncus associated, 921–2
Heart sounds, *see* Murmurs; Sounds
Heath and Edward's 1958 classification for pulmonary hypertension, 137–8, 147–8
Heparin, 1357
Hepatic veins
arrangement
in atrial isomerism, 488

echocardiographic determination, 327, 328
pulmonary venous anomalous connexions to, 524
Heredopathic atactica polineuritiformis, 1261
History-taking, 183–4
Hormonal disorders, *see* Endocrine disorders
Hospitalisation, emotional problems, 1376
Humeroperineal myopathy, X linked, 1259
Hunter syndrome, 1248
Hurler-Sheie syndrome, 1248
Hurler's polydystrophy, pseudo-, 1249
Hurler's syndrome, 1247–8
Hydrallazine treatment, 438
Hydrocortisone, effect on ductus arteriosus, 937
Hydroxylase deficiency
11β-, 1311
17-, 1311–12
Hyperaldosteronism
dexamethasone-suppressible, 1312
primary, 1312
Hypercalcaemia, 301
electrocardiographic features, 299, 301
hypertension associated with, 1314
infantile idiopathic (=William's syndrome), 968, 992–3, 1005
physical features, 994
Hypereosinophilia, myocardial fibrosis associated with, 1336
Hyperkalaemia, 299–300
electrocardiographic features, 299–300
Hyperlipoproteinaemia, cardiovascular risks, 1348
Hypermagnesaemia, electrocardiographic features, 301
Hypernatraemia, electrocardiographic features, 302
Hyper-reninism, primary, 1310
Hypertension
coarctation associated, 1310–11
malignant, 1305
post-operative residual, 447, 1105
paradoxical-, 1105
permanent-, 1105
in repair of aortic coarctation, 1105
pulmonary, *see* Pulmonary hypertension
renal, 1300, 1301–2, 1307–10
pathophysiology, 1307–8
persistent, 1308
systemic, *see* Systemic hypertension
other causes, 1314–15
Hypertensive crises, management, 1315
Hyperthyroidism
cardiological involvement, 1253
electrocardiographic effects, 1253
Hypertrophy, *see* Atrial enlargement; Ventricular hypertrophy
Hypocalcaemia, 301
electrocardiographic effects, 299, 301
Hypoglycaemia, 383
electrocardiographic effects, 302
Hypokalaemia, 301
electrocardiographic effects, 299, 300
Hypomagnesaemia, electrocardiographic effects, 301–2
Hyponatraemia, electrocardiographic effects, 302
Hypoplasia (heart)
left, *see* Hypoplastic left heart syndrome
right, imaging, 230–1
Hypoplastic left heart syndrome, 737–61, *see also* Ventricular hypoplasia

clinical features/findings, 745–6
diagnosis, differential, 756, 757
incidence and aetiology, 737–8
investigations, 746–56
morphogenesis, 744–5
morphology, 737–44
surgical management, palliative 756–61
aims, 758
problems, 145
suitability, 758
survival, 761
Hypothermia, 383
electrocardiographic effects, 304
use in surgery, 443, 1328
Hypothyroidism
cardiological effects, 1253
electrocardiographic effects, 306
Hypoxaemia
demonstration, 843
tricuspid atresia associated, 690
Hypoxia
diagnosing cause of, 399
electrocardiographic effects, 302
experimentally induced, 153
Fallot's tetralogy associated, 775
responses to, 775
treatment, 440

Iduronate sulphate deficiency, 1248
Imaging techniques, heart and chest, 202–32, *see also specific techniques*
comparisons, 202, 231–2
Immune-complex, endocarditis associated, 1235–6
Immunisation against streptococci, 1195
Impedence, chest, cardiac output measurement from, 407
In-patient stay, 1388
Incidence (of congenital heart disease), 3–7, 30
definition, 3
during pregnancy, 1353–4
of various forms, 1354
rates
early studies of, 3–4
effects of prenatal death on, 3
intensive studies of 4–5
specific lesions, 5–7
Inclusion cell disease, 1249
Indian children, pulmonary hypertension in, 152
Indomethacin, ductal closure induced by, 950–1
Infarction
myocardial, 296–8
anterolateral, 296
electrocardiographic features in, 294, 296–8
lateral acute, 297
papillary muscle, 297, 741
pseudo-, 298
Infective endocarditis, *see* Endocarditis
Inflammatory disease, *see also* Carditis
non-rheumatic, 1165–76
pan-cardiac, 1185
rheumatic, *see* Rheumatic heart disease
Infundibular
defects/anomalies, 596
double outlet ventricle associated, 892, 293, 897
morphogenesis, 774, 898–9

Infundibular
defects/anomalies (*contd.*)
muscular-, 624
stenosis, 596
morphology, 77–8, 332, 333
pulmonary (valve)
absence, 800, 801
echocardiographic features, 354, 355
maldevelopment, 774
pulmonary atresia associated appearance, 800, 801
radiographic features, 205
stenosis, *see* Pulmonary stenosis
Infundibular (conus) artery, anomalous origin, 1078, 1079
Infundibular septum
displacement, 600
maldevelopment, 899
Infundibular spasm, 777
Infundibulectomy, 789
Inheritance in heart disease, 15–30, 31–9 *passim*, 47–59
Injections, *see* Contrast media
Injury, myocardial, *see* Myocardium
Innominate artery, *see* Brachiocephalic artery
Inotropic agent(s)
selection, 440
therapy, 439–40
Inspection, diagnostic value, 184–5
Inspiration, *see also* Respiration; Ventilation
gas measurement, 404
heart sound features associated with, 186–7
Intelligence
subnormal, heart defects associated with, 42–3
surgical effects on, 1375–6
Intercostal artery, selective injection, 811
Interventricular communications, *see* Ventricular communications
Intestinal anomalies, gastro-, heart disease associated with, 45
Intimal (pulmonary arterial) cellular proliferation, 138
Intimal cushions, ductal, morphogenesis, 934
Intimal fibrosis (pulmonary arterial), 138
Intrapulmonary arteries, *see* Pulmonary arteries
Iron deposition, 1263–4
Ischaemia
electrocardiographic features, 291–3, 294
injury, due to, 294
myocardial, 291–3
coronary artery anomalies associated with, 1074, 1075
renal, 1307
subendocardial, 292
transmural, 292
Isomerism sequence (incomplete situs inversus), 34–8, 38–9, 70
atrial, *see* Atrial isomerism
bronchial, 70
Isoprenaline treatment, 663

J point, 242
depression, 413
elevation, 291
Joint problems
endocarditis associated, 1235
rheumatic disease associated, 1185
Jugular vein catheterisation, 372

Kartagener's syndrome, 34
Kawasaki's disease (Mucocutaneous lymph node syndrome), 297–8, 1082–3, 1169–70
arteriographic features, 1083
electrocardiographic features, 297–8
symptoms, 1171
Kidney, *see entries under* Renal
Konno procedure, 458–9
Kreutzer procedure, 691, 692, 693, *see also* Fontan-Kreutzer procedure
Kugelberg-Welander syndrome, 1261
Kyphoscoliosis, electrocardiographic features, 272

Labour in patients with heart disease, 1355
Laplace relation/law, 164
Left anterior hemiblock
aetiology, 284
electrocardiographic features, 284, 285
Left bundle branch
anatomy, 284
anterior, 284
block, 283–4, 1289–90, *see also* Fascicular block
complete, 283–4, 1289–90
electrocardiographic features, 283–4
incomplete, 284
posterior, 284
Left posterior hemiblock, electrocardiographic features, 284–5
Left ventricular hypertrophy, *see* Ventricular hypertrophy
Lesions, specific, *see also specifically named lesions*
incidence of, 5–7
mortality rate, 9–11
natural history, 9–11
obstructive, predicting gradients across, 347
Levoatrial cardinal vein, 503, 532–3
angiographic features, 532
Lidocaine, electrocardiographic effects, 303
Life expectancy, *see also* Mortality; Survival
in Marfan's syndrome, 1255
in persistent ductus arteriosus, 945
weighted-, 433–4
Limb reduction, heart defects associated with, 44
Lipids, blood
elevated, risk factors, 1347–8
normal values, 1348
Lipomatosis cordis, 731, 732, 733, 734
Liver radiography, 216–17
Lown-Ganong-Levine syndrome, electrocardiographic features, 288–9
Lung
blood supply, *see* Pulmonary circulation
development, effect of hypoperfusion on, 148–9
disease, *see also specific diseases*
chronic, 152–3
exercise testing with, 396–7
pulmonary hypertension in, 152–3
function, 1014
normal, 400–1
testing, 395, 396, 397–400
'ground-glass' appearance, 517
radiographic features, 205–13, 214–15
rheumatic valve disease associated changes, 1197
scanning, radioisotopic, 400, 401

volume
components, 397
developmental changes, 400
reduction, conditions associated with, 149
Lupus erythematosis
neonatal, 1265
systemic, 1169, 1264–5
Lymph node syndrome, mucocutaneous, *see* Kawasaki's disease
Lymphatics, pulmonary, 127
Lymphocytes, T, *see* T cell
Lymphosarcoma, echocardiographic features, 1156

M-mode echocardiography, *see* Echocardiography, M-mode
McArdle's disease, 1247
Magnetic resonance imaging, 225–31
conventional, 225
costs, 231
diagnoses of abnormalities by, 226–31
echoplanar-, 225, 226–31 *passim*
Mahaim conduction, 289–90
Malaria, cardiac signs in, 1323
Malposition of the heart, *see* Heart
Management, 421–40
general principles, 421–34
medical, *see* Medical management
surgical, *see* Surgical management
Mannosidoses, 1250
Marfan's syndrome, 23, 1254–6
definition, 1038
floppy mitral valve associated with, 1040, 1044
inheritance, 23
pregnancy risks, 1358–9
Maroteaux-Lamy syndrome, 1249
Maximum effort/exercise performance tests, 401–2, 409–10, 414
Maximum mid-expiratory flow, 398
Maximum oxygen uptake, *see* Oxygen uptake
Mean vector, *see* Axis
Media, pulmonary
atrophy, 148–9
fibrinoid necrosis, 139
hypertrophy, 138, 141
thickness
changes at birth, 132
in the study of disease, 140, 141, 152
Medical management
aortic arch interruption, 1115
aortic coarctation, 1102–3
aortic stenosis, 985, 986, 991
aortopulmonary window, 927
arrhythmias, 1282–4, 1284, 1284–6, 1286, 1287–8, 1288, 1291
atrial isomerism, 493
atrioventricular septal defects, 605
coronary artery anomalies, 1076, 1083
double inlet ventricle, 668
endocardial fibroelastosis, 1227
endomyocardial fibrosis, 1333–4
endocarditis, infective, 1239–40
Fallot's tetralogy, 787
mitral valve anomalies, 1037, 1208
myocarditis, 1168, 1169, 1169–70, 1171
pericarditis, 1175
persistent ductus arteriosus, 950–1
in pregnancy, 1355, 1355–7, 1359
pulmonary atresia, 718–19, 823
pulmonary stenosis, 969–72
pulmonary venous anomalies, 525–6

Medical management (*contd.*)
  rheumatic heart disease, 1191–3, 1208,
    1210, 1214
  systemic disease, 1246–68 *passim*
  systemic hypertension, 1302, 1306–7, 1311,
    1314–15
  transposition, 429–34, 455–7, 461, 829,
    850–61
  tricuspid atresia, 690–1
  ventricular septal defects, 637
Medical profession
    -child communication, 1374, 1380
    -parent communication, 1380
Medication, *see* Drugs
Mental retardation, heart defects associated
    with, 42–3
Mesothelioma of the atrioventricular node,
    1160
Metabolic disease
  cardiac signs, 1245–56
  electrocardiographic effects of, 306
Mineralocorticoid excess, apparent, 1312
Mirror image arrangement (situs inversus) 34
  abdominal, 207
  atrial, *see* Situs
  electrocardiographic features, 269–71
  incomplete, *see* Isomerism sequence
  of all the organs, 1063
Mitochondrial myopathies, 1261
Mitogen, changes caused by, 145
Mitral annuloplasty, 1209
Mitral arcade, anomalous, 1035, 1036
Mitral atresia
  angiographic features, 754, 755, 756
  clinical features, 746
  haemodynamic investigations, 749–52
  morphology, 739
Mitral insufficiency/incompetence, 1027,
    1204–9
  clinical features/findings, 1028–9, 1205–6
  investigations, 1206–9
  medical management, 1208
  physiology, 1205
  pure, 1028–9
  rheumatic, 1197
  severity, estimation, 1208
  surgical management, 1037, 1209
    indications, 1209
Mitral regurgitation, 1029, 1045, 1205
  detection, 1033, 1035–6, 1208
Mitral ring (annulus), 1042
  angiocardiographic features, 1049
  fulcrum, 1049
  supravalvar
    echocardiographic features, 1032
    management, 1037
    morphology, 1025
Mitral stenosis, 1198–204
  associated conditions, 1203
  clinical features, 1199–200
  investigations, 1200–2
  medical management, 1037
  morphology, 1025
  physiology, 1199
  rheumatic, 1198–204
    pathology, 1196–7
  relief, angioplastic, 378
  surgical management, 378, 1036–8, 1198,
    1203–4
    indications, 1203–4
Mitral valve (general features), *see also*
    Atrioventricular valves; Valves
  annulus/ring, *see* Mitral ring

anomalies/diseases, *see* Mitral valve
    anomalies/diseases
  definition, 74
  development, 98–100
  echocardiographic features, 335, 339
  leaflets, 1042
    defects, *see* Mitral valve
      anomalies/diseases
    mural, 1043–4
  line of closure, 1043
  morphology
    both atrioventricular valves with, 648
    in left ventricular hypoplasia, 739
    normal, 1041–3
  repair, 1038, 1209, *see also various Mitral
    valve anomalies and defects*
  replacement, 1037–8, 1051, 1204, 1207,
    1209
  tension apparatus, 1026–7, 1042–3
    failure, 1044–5
Mitral valve, floppy (syndrome), 1038–51
  aetiology, 1040–1, 1044–5
  associated conditions, 1040–1
  clinical presentation, 1046
  clinical symptomatology, 1046
  definition, 1038–9
  diagnosis, 1039, 1040
  incidence, 1039–40
  inheritance, 1041
  investigations, 1046–50
  management, 1041
  morphogenesis, 1041
  morphology, 1041
  natural history/course, 1050–1
  pathophysiology, 1044–5
    myocardial theory, 1045–6
    valvar theory, 1045
  physical signs, 1046
  prognosis, 1050–1
Mitral valve anomalies/diseases, 1023–51
  aetiology, 1023
  atrioventricular septal defects and, 578,
    578–9
  billowing valve, 1045–6
  buckling valve, 1047, 1048
  cleft, 590, 592, 1025–6, 1031
    isolated, 1025–6, 1030
    types, 1025–6
  clinical features/findings, 1028–9
  diagnosis, differential, 1036
  double orifice, 1026, 1027, 1031
  double outlet ventricle associated, 894, 895
  dysplasia, 1023
  endocardial elastosis associated, 1225
  floppy valve, *see* Mitral valve, floppy
  hammocking, 1047, 1048
  hypoplasia, 1023–7
  imperforate valve, 533, 747, 1025, 1032,
    1034, 1035, 1036–7
    associated defects, 1025
  incidence, 1023
  incompetence/insufficiency, *see* Mitral
    insufficiency
  investigations, 1029–36
  leaflets, 1025–6
    aortic, 1027, 1145–6
    floppy, 1043–5
    motion, abnormal, 1047–8, 1201–2
    prolapse, 1050
  Marfan's syndrome associated, 1254–5
  medical management, 1037
  morphology 1023
  natural history/course, 1036

overriding valve, 704, 905
parachute valve, 1024, 1025, 1030, 1034–5
pathophysiology, 1027–8
prognosis, 1036
prolapsed valve, 1039, 1040, 1041, 1044–5,
    1047, 1048
  aetiology, 1044–5
  angiocardiographic features, 1049–50
  pseudo-, 1049
regurgitation, *see* Mitral regurgitation
rheumatic, 1196–7
small orifice, 1225
stenosis, *see* Mitral stenosis
straddling valve, 702–5, 905
supravalvar ring, *see* Mitral ring
surgical management, 1037–8
systolic anterior motion, 1145–6
of the tension apparatus, 1026–7, 1044–5
Mitral valvotomy, 1037, 1198, 1204
  age distribution, 1198, 1203, 1204
  transventricular closed-, 1204
Moral responsibilities to child, parental
    perception, 1388, 1392, 1393, 1396
Morphogenesis of the heart, 85–105
Morquio's syndrome, 1248–9
Mortality (and survival), *see also* Life
    expectancy; Survival; Survivors
  catheterisation risks, 383
  childhood, 7–9
  complete transposition associated, 849–50
  during management, evaluating probability,
    420–34 *passim*
  endocarditis associated, 1229
  hypertrophic cardiomyopathy associated,
    1149
  pregnant women with heart disease, 1354
  prenatal (stillborn)
    effect on incidence rates, 3
    lesions occurring, distribution of, 5
  rates
    for heart disease, 7–9
    for specific lesions, 9–10
  surgical
    acceptable levels, 422–3, 429–34
    arterial switch operation, 860
    atrial redirection, 860,
    atrioventricular septal repair, 607–8, 609
    corrected transposition, 883
    double outlet ventricle, 907, 908
    endomyocardial fibrosis, 1334
    Fallot's tetralogy, 787, 793
    mitral valve anomalies, 1037, 1204
    pulmonary circulation improvement, 824,
      825
    pulmonary venous anomalous connexion
      repair, 526, 527
    Rastelli operation, 856–7
    truncus arteriosus, 922, 923
    ventricular septal repair, 451, 669–70,
      907
  vs medical mortality, 422–34
  truncus associated, 921
  tumour (cardiac) associated, 1157
Mosaic Down's syndrome, 17
Mother
  during child hospitalisation, 1389
  -infant relationships, 1375, 1392
Mucocutaneous lymph node syndrome, *see*
    Kawasaki's disease
Mucolipidoses, 1249
Mucopolysaccharidoses, 1247–9
Muller handle steerable catheter system,
    374–5

Murmurs, heart, 465–8, 1001–19
  assymptomatic child with a, 195–6,
    465–70
    examination, 465
  Austin-Flint, 1213
    examination, 465
  bruit, 467
  cardiorespiratory, 467
  characteristics, 465–6
  continuous, 189, 465, 469–70, 718,
    1001–19
    acquired, 1006–7
    causes, 1001–7
    specific lesions producing, 1007–19
    types, 1001–7
  contour, 466
  defects/diseases associated with, 467–70
    aortic regurgitation, 996, 1212
    aortic stenosis, 979, 980, 981, 982–3,
      989, 994, 1002, 1210
    aortopulmonary window, 925
    atrial septal defects, 551–2, 557, 558
    complete transposition, 842–3
    double inlet ventricle, 656
    double outlet ventricle, 900–1
    endocarditis, infective, 1235
    Fallot's tetralogy, 777–8, 778–9
    hypertrophic cardiomyopathy, 1143
    mitral valve anomalies, 1028, 1029, 1039,
      1040, 1046, 1187, 1199–200, 1206
    persistent ductus arteriosus, 942–3, 944
    pulmonary atresia, 715, 718, 812
    pulmonary stenosis, 551, 964–5, 969
    rheumatic heart disease, 1186–7,
      1199–200, 1206, 1210, 1212, 1214
    tricuspid valve anomalies, 685, 725, 1214
    truncus arteriosus, 916–17
    tumours, cardiac, 1154
    ventricular septal defects, 628–9, 778,
      812
  diagnosis
    differential, 195–6, 465–70
    investigations following, 470
    value, 188–9, 470
  diastolic, 189
    late, 1213
    sternal border, soft, 551–2
  innocent, 466–7, 470
  intensity/loudness, 188, 189, 465
  location, 189
  pitch, 466
  radiation, 466
  significance, 466
  Still's, 466–7
  systolic, 188–9, 467–8
    apical, 469
    basal, loud, 467–8
    basal, soft, 468
    diastolic, 469
    ejection, 188, 189, 467, 964, 965
    late, 1039, 1040, 1046, 1051
    pan-, 188, 189, 628
    phonocardiogram of, 981
    sternal border, loud, 469–70
    sternal border, soft, 469, 551, 558, 771
  timing and character, 188–9
  to and fro, 1006
  venous hum, 467, 944
  vibratory, 466–7
Muscular dystrophy (with cardiological
  effects), 1256–9
  Becker's, 1258
  childhood, 1257

Duchenne's, 1256–7
  electrocardiographic effects of, 305
  inheritance, 24
  facioscapulohumeral, 1258–9
  myotonic, 1257–9
Mustard procedure, 852–4
  effect, diagrammatic representation,
    853
  risk analysis, 1365
Myocardial fibres, *see also* Ventricular
  fibres
  architecture, 159–60, 171
    abnormal, 1139
  forces developed, 165
  length, 167
  shortening, 165, 169
Myocardial fibrosis, trypanosomal, 1327
Myocardial infarction, *see* Infarction
Myocardial ischaemia, *see* Ischaemia
Myocardial rings, 102–4
Myocardial scintigraphy, *see* Scintigraphy
Myocardiopathy, *see* Cardiomyopathy
Myocarditis, 1165–71
  acute-, 1324
  electrocardiographic features, 294, 295
  generalised autoimmune-, 1169–71
  histological features, 1165
  hypersensitivity-, 1266
  infectious, 1166–9
    bilharzial, 1322–3
    clinical features/findings, 1166
    diagnosis, differential, 1168–9, 1227
    epidemiology, 1166
    investigations, 1166–8
    laboratory findings, 1166
    medical management, 1168
    prevalence, 1168
    prognosis, 1166
    viral, 1166, 1227
  injury due to, 294
  rheumatic heart disease associated,
    1184
  toxic-, 1206
  trypanosomal-, 1324, 1326, 1327
Myocardium
  abnormal
    hypertrophic, *see* Cardiomyopathy
    mitral valve prolapse associated with,
      1045–6
  autoimmunity, 1183
  development, 88, 89, 102–5, 114
  dysfunction, 1284
  fatty infiltration, 731, 732, 733, 734
  function, 114
  injury, 293–6
    electrocardiographic features, 293–6
    subendocardial, 293
    subepicardial, 293
  inlet, undermining, 98, 100
  normal anatomy, 159–60
  stress, 175
    development, 164
    neonatal/small infants, 435
  tumours located in, 1154
  vascularisation, 104–5
  ventricular
    in double inlet ventricle, 649–50
    right, parietal, absence, 732
  wall movement, assessment, 226
Myocytes, hypertrophic, 1140
Myopathies with cardiological effects,
  1256–61
Myoxoma, 1158–9

Natural history
  of heart disease, 7–9
  of specific lesions, 9–11
Neonatal disease, psychological adjustment to,
  1374–5
Neoplasms, *see* Tumours
Nervous system, *see* Central nervous system
Neurofibromatosis, hypertension associated
  with, 1308
Neurological disorders, hypertension
  associated with, 1301, 1314
Neuromuscular disorders, 1246, 1256–61
  electrocardiographic effects of, 305
Newborn, disease in, psychological
  adjustments to, 1374–5
Niemann-Pick disease, 1250
Nifedipine therapy in hypertrophic
  cardiomyopathy, 1149
Nitroprusside (sodium) treatment, 438
Nitrous oxide method of cardiac output
  measurement, 406–7
Nodoventricular conduction, 289–90
Nodules
  Aschoff-, 1185
  subcutaneous, 1189
Noonan's syndrome, 24
Noradrenaline
  plasma levels, post coarctation repair,
    1105
  production, hypertension associated with,
    1312–13
Nuclear cardiology, 219–25, *see also*
  Radionuclide
Nuclear magnetic resonance, *see* Magnetic
  resonance imaging

Obesity, cardiovascular risks, 1348
Obstruction, catheter caused, 382, *see also*
  specific vessels and lesions
Ocular defects, heart defects associated with,
  43
Oesophageal compression, conditions causing,
  1123–35
Oesophography, findings with
  brachiocephalic artery causing tracheal
    compression, 1132, 1133
  double aortic arch, 1129, 1130
  pulmonary sling, 1134–5
  vascular rings, 1129, 1130
Open-heart surgery
  atrial septal repair, 561
  Fallot's tetralogy, 787–8
  sickle cell haemoglobinopathy and, 1327–8
Operations, *see* Surgery
Oral contraceptive
  cardiovascular risks, 1349
  hypertension associated with, 1307, 1349
Organ arrangement, atrial isomerism
  associated, 484–5
Organomegaly, heart defects associated with,
  42
Osteogenesis imperfecta, 1255
Ostium primum, 577, 578–9
  aetiology, 39
  definitions, 543, 547
  diagnosis, 556
  echocardiographic features, 569
  inheritance, 39
  morphology, 543–4, 578
  repair, 451, 452
    mortality, 607

Out-patient stage, consultations during
  post-operative, 1393–4
  pre-operative, 1385–9
Oval foramen, *see* Foramen ovale
Oval fossa, *see* Fossa ovalis
Over-protection, parental, 1376–7
Oximetry, 220, 364
  in complete transposition, 847–8
  pitfalls, 556
  in truncus arteriosus, 918–19
Oxygen
  content/tension (P_{O_2}), 399–400
    developmental changes, 400–1
    ductus arteriosus closure and, 936–7
    fetal, 109–10
  saturation, 384
    with atrial shunts, 556
  uptake/consumption, *see* Oxygen
    uptake/consumption
Oxygen uptake/consumption
  maximum ($\dot{V}_{O_2}$) 401–12 *passim*
    age related, 409, 410–12
    attainment, 401
    gender related, 409
  measurement, 364, 384, 386, 401–12 *passim*
  -work rate relationship, 402, 403
Oxygenation, systemic arterial, determinants,
  839–40

P wave, 243, 244, 245, 247, 259
  artefacts affecting, 311, 312
  diseases/conditions affecting, 266–306
    passim
    arrhythmias, 1276
    atrial enlargement, 279–80
    atrial isomerism, 267–8, 489
  mean vector, 255
  normal shape, 257–8
  U and T wave differentiation from, 265,
    266
Pa_{CO_2}, 405, 406
Pv_{CO_2}, 405, 406
PGE_1/PGE_2, 116, 117, 935, 951–2
PGI_2, *see* Prostacyclin
P_{O_2}, *see* Oxygen
P-P interval, assessment, 1274
P-R interval and segment, 186, 242, 258–9
  diseases/conditions affecting
    rheumatic heart disease, 1189
    Wolff-Parkinson-White syndrome, 287,
      288
P-T interval, *see* T-P interval
Pacemakers, implantable/permanent, 1279,
  1279–81
Pain
  chest, presentation with, 197
  fear of, 1379
Palpation
  diagnostic value, 184–5
  ventricular septal defect findings, 628
Palpitations, presentation with, 197
Papillary muscle
  in atrioventricular septal defects, 573, 574,
    575, 581–2
    echocardiographic features, 593
  hypoplasia, 1023–5
  infarction, 297, 741
    electrocardiographic features, 297
  mitral valve, 1043
    abnormal, 1023–5, 1026–7
  necrosis, 741

Papilloedema, cyanosis associated, 787
Parent
  burden on, 1389, 1401
  during child hospitalisation, 1385–94
  informed refusal by, 1401
  preferences, 1400
  self-help, 1380, *see also* Family
Parietal band, 766, 767
Patau's syndrome, *see* Trisomy 13
Patency, arterial duct, *see* Ductus arteriosus
Patient, *see* Child
Pectus excavatum, electrocardiographic
  features, 272
Peer group relations (parental), 1389
Penicillin, *see also* Amoxycillin
  allergy, alternative therapy, 1239
  therapy in rheumatic heart disease, 1191,
    1193, 1194
Perforation, cardiac, catheter caused, 382
Perfusion, *see* Ventilation
Pericardial effusion
  quantitation, 1174
  trypanosomiasis associated, 1325
Pericardial patch closure, 452
Pericardiotomy, post-, syndrome, 1176
Pericarditis
  bacterial, acute, 1175
  clinical features/findings, 1173
  constrictive, 1175
  electrocardiographic features, 294–5, 1173
    injury due to, 294–5
  investigations, 1172–4
  management, 1175
  pathophysiology, 1171–2
  rheumatic heart disease associated, 1184,
    1188
  viral, 1173
    acute, 1175
Pericardium
  complications following opening of, 1176
  deficiency of, 1059–60
Peroneal muscular atrophy, 1260–1
PGE_1/PGE_2, 116, 117, 935, 951–2
PGI_2, *see* Prostacyclin
Phaeochromocytoma, hypertension associated
  with, 307, 1312–13
Phenylketonuria teratogenicity, 25–6
Phenytoin
  electrocardiographic effects of, 303
  therapy, 1288
Phonocardiograms
  atrial septal defect, 552
  hypertrophic cardiomyopathy, 1142–3
  floppy mitral valve syndrome, 1046
Physical examination, 184–9
Pituitary gigantism, 1252
Placental circulation, removal, 114
Plasma renin, *see* Renin
Plethysmography, uses, 397, 398–9
Plexiform lesions, pulmonary arterial, 139–40
Pneumomediastinum, electrocardiographic
  features, 272
Pneumonectomy, 272
Pneumonia, Pulmonary oedema, differential
  diagnosis, 213
Pneumothorax, electrocardiographic
  features, 272
P_{O_2}, *see* Oxygen
Policy options on child management, 1395–6
Polyarteritis nodosa, infantile, 1083
Polycythaemia, secondary, 775
Polydactyly, heart defects associated with, 44
Polygenic heart disease, 27–30, 39

Polygenic threshold model, 26, 27
  features, 26
Pompe's disease, *see* Glycogen storage disease
  of the heart
Portal vein, pulmonary venous anomalous
  connexion to, 512, 513, 520, 521, 523,
    524
Positions, heart, *see* Heart
Potts anastomosis, 788–9
Pre-exitation syndrome, 286
Pre-load, 165, 166
Prednisolone therapy, 1193
Pregnancy
  fetus during, heart disease in
    detection, 357–60
    high risk groups, 356
    outcome, 356
    screening for, 355–61
  mother during, heart disease in
    incidence, 1353
    management, 1355–9
    natural history, 1353–4
Prenatal heart disease, *see* Pregnancy
Prenatal mortality, *see* Mortality
Pressure, blood
  diastolic, 413, 1294, 1338
    end-, 167–8, 173–4
  familial aggregation, 1296–7, 1347
  fetal, 113
  -flow relations, in great arteries, 168
  measurement, 1293–4
    aortic coarctation associated, 1095
    aortic stenosis associated, 425, 994, 1210
    catheter effected, 364, 384–6
    diagnostic value, 185
    in exercise tests, 413, 415
    hypertrophic cardiomyopathy associated,
      1146
    mitral valve anomaly associated, 1033, 1202
    pulmonary venous obstruction associated,
      515–6
    rheumatic heart disease associated, 1202
    technique, 1293–4
    tricuspid stenosis associated, 1215
    ventricular endomyocardial fibrosis
      associated, 1332, 1333
  normal, 1294–7, 1338–9, 1346
    boys, 1294, 1295, 1338
    girls, 1295, 1338
    in the tropics, 1338–9
  pulmonary arterial, *see* Pulmonary arteries
  salt related, 1349
  systolic, 413, 1294, 1296, 1338
    end-, 170
  tracking, 1296, 1346–7
  variability, 1296
  -volume relations, ventricular, 169–70,
    174–5, 627
Prevalence (of congenital heart disease)
  childhood, 11, 12
  definition, 3
Primary foramen, 91, 92, 93, 94
Primary ring, 103–4
Procainamide
  electrocardiographic effects of, 303
  in pregnancy, 1357
Progeria, 1267
Propanolol
  electrocardiographic effects of, 304
  therapy, 787
Prostacyclin (PGI_2)
  role, 117, 118
  therapy, 438–9

Prostaglandins (PG) *see also* Prostacyclin
 E₁, 116, 117, 935, 951–2
 E₂, 116, 117, 935, 951–2
 F₂, 935
 problems associated with, 952, 1095
 side effects, 952
 therapy, 439
  in atrial isomerism, 493
  ductus patency maintainance, 951–2
  in hypoxia, 441
  indications, 421
  intravenous, 421
Prosthetic valves, *see* Valves
Protection, over-, parental, 1376–7
Pseudo-Hurler polydystrophy, 1249
Pseudo-infarction, 298
Psychological responses, *see also* Child
 to heart disease, 1373–81
 to surgery, 792, 1375–6
Psychotropic drugs, electrocardiographic
   effects of, 304
Pulmonary airways, *see* Airways
Pulmonary arteries, *see also* Pulmonary
   circulation
 absent, 134, 805, 920
 anomalies, 111–13
  Fallot's tetralogy associated, 773, 781,
    783, 784, 785
  hypoplastic left heart syndrome, 741
  truncus arteriosus associated, 915
 banding
  for tricuspid atresia, 691
  for truncus arteriosus, 922
  other syndromes requiring, 758, 760
 bifurcation, 815
 bronchial artery anastomoses, 125, 150
 central
  confluent, 821
  hypoplastic growth potential, 149–50
  injection into, 818
  interconnexion with other arteries, 821–2
  obstructions, 808
 confluence, 802, 803
  angiographic features, 819
 development, 116–19, 130–1, 132–3
  abnormal, 111–13
 dilation, 138–9
 diminutive, surgical choices, 790
 echocardiography, 781, 783, 813–16
 fistulas, 1081
 hypertension, bilharzial, 1321–2
 hypertension associated changes in, 136–44
 injection, selective, 567, 568
 intimal fibrosis, 138
 intra-
  connexion failures, 134–5
  developmental abnormalities, 135
  identification, 129
  interconnexions with other arteries,
    821–2
  obstructions, 808
 intrapericardial, 801–2
 left
  anomalous origin, *see* Pulmonary sling
  tortuous duct supplying, 814
 media, *see* Media
 musculature, 130–1, *see also* Media
  assessment, 129
  in pulmonary hypertension, 138–40, 141,
    142, 151
 number
  assessment, 129
  reduction, 136

plexiform lesions, 139–40
pressure, 551, 552–3
 assessment, 146–7
 curve, 551
right
 anomalous origin, 818
 identification, 815
to right ventricle, surgical connexion, 825
size, quantitation, 781, 783
stenosis, 963, 1005, 1006
 demonstration, 785
supply (to lung)
 in atrial isomerism, 492
 collateral, 802, 803–4, 805, 809–10, 811,
   817, 820
 duplicate, 822
 morphogenesis, 804–6
 multifocal, 803, 804
 optimisation, 823–4
 in pulmonary atresia, 801–4, 805, 806–9
 site of obstruction, 806–9, 822
 sources, 819–22
 unifocalisation, 824
 surgical anastomoses involving, 1135, *see
   also* Waterston anastomoses
 thromboses, 149
 wall structure, 130–1
Pulmonary arteriolar resistance
 in the study of disease, 140, 141
 in truncus arteriosus, 920
Pulmonary arterioles, obstruction, 808–9
Pulmonary arteriovenous malformations, *see*
   Arteriovenous fistulas/malformations
Pulmonary atresia (valvar), *see also* Pulmonary
   vein
 angiographic features, 113, 223, 816–23
 arterial abnormalities associated with,
   111–12, 134–5, 136
 associated conditions, 711
 classification, 711–14, 799–80
 clinical findings, 715, 811–12
 cyanosis associated with, 192–3
 diagnosis, 717, 718, 822
 investigations, 812–16
 medical management, 823
 morphogenesis, 804–7
 morphology, 711–14, 799
 natural history/course, 718–19, 822–3
 pathophysiology, 714–15, 806–10
 presentation, 811
 prevalence, 799
 prognosis, 718–19
 symptomatology, 811
 surgical management, 719
  corrective, 452–3, 454–5, 824–6
  long term results, 826
  palliative, 823–4
  risk factors, 823
 ventricular septal defect with, 135, 799–826
  common settings, 800
Pulmonary blood flow, *see* Pulmonary
   circulation
Pulmonary circulation (and vasculature),
   123–53, *see also* Pulmonary arteries
 angiographic measurements, 220–2, 816–22
 branching patterns, 130
 bronchial circulation anastomosed to, 125
 collateral, 802, 803–4, 809–10, 811, 817,
   820
 control during surgery, 454
 damage, classification, 137–8
 defects and diseases
  haemodynamic measurements, 386

heart sounds associated with, 629
 methods of studying, 127–30, 140–1
 morphometric analysis, 140–1
 pathogenesis, 145–6
 postoperative survival, 147–8, 850
 preoperative assessment, 146–7
 prevention, 148, 637
 radiographic features, 206–13, 629
defects and diseases of, conditions
   associated with
 aortopulmonary window, 926
 atrial isomerism, 488
 atrial septal defects, 550, 552
 atrioventricular septal defects, 587,
   608–9
 complete transposition, 838–9, 841,
   847–8
 Eisenmonger's syndrome, 1357, 1358
 pulmonary atresia, 801–4, 805, 806–9
 tricuspid atresia, 684
 truncus arteriosus, 916, 920
 ventricular septal defects, 626–7, 629,
   637, 638
 development, 116–19, 130–3
  heart disease effects on, 118–19, 141–4
  neonatal, 132–3
  postnatal, 133
  prenatal, abnormal, 133–6
  prenatal, normal, 130–2
 double outlet ventricle associated, 899
 duct dependent, 816, 819, 820, 822, 938–9
  treatment, 951
 enlargement (of vessels), 208–10
 experimental changes in, 153
 in heart disease, 127–30, 133–6, 141–4
 inadequate, relief of, 669
 morphology/anatomy, 123–7
  techniques of analysis, 129–30
 narrowing (of vessels), 206–8
 obstruction to, tricuspid atresia classified
   by, 679
 source in pulmonary atresia, 816–22
Pulmonary commisurotomy, 972
Pulmonary disease, *see also specific diseases*
 circulatory, *see* Pulmonary circulation
 ductal shunting associated with, 949
 parenchymal, cyanosis associated, 192
Pulmonary endothelial cells, role in
   pulmonary vascular disease, 145
Pulmonary function and features, *see* Lung
   and entries under Pulmonary
Pulmonary hypertension, 136–48
 aetiology, 151–3
 atrial septal defect associated, 559
 atrial chamber partitioning associated, 566
 atrial redirection and, 856
 atrioventricular septal defect associated,
   587
 bilharzial, 1321–2
 experimentally induced, 153
 lung disease associated with, 152–3
 management, postoperative, 147–8
 mitral stenosis associated, 1199
 murmurs associated with severe-, 552
 persistent, 151, 152
 persistent ductus arteriosus associated, 946
 primary, 152
 pulmonary vein stenosis/atresia associated,
   533
 rheumatic heart disease associated, 151
 surgically effected, 144–5, 856
 thromboembolic, 153
 venous, radiographic features, 211, 212

Pulmonary hypoperfusion, 148–50
  effect on lung development, 148–9
  palliative surgery, 144, 145
Pulmonary infundibulum, *see* Infundibulum
Pulmonary isomerism in conjoined twins, 1061
Pulmonary lymphatics, 127
Pulmonary oedema
  aetiology, 212
  radiographic features, 210–13, 746, 747
Pulmonary oligaemia, 192–3
Pulmonary outflow tract, *see also* Pulmonary trunk; Pulmonary valve
    obstruction
      double outlet ventricle associated, 897
      effect on ventricular septal defect, 627
    wedging, 869
Pulmonary perfusion, imaging, 222
Pulmonary schistosomiasis, 1321–2
Pulmonary (vascular) sling (distal origin of left pulmonary artery), 816, 1133–5
  diagnosis, 1134–5
  radiographic features, 216, 218
Pulmonary stenosis
  aetiology, 959–60
  angiocardiographic features, 534, 785, 881, 849, 967–8
  atrioventricular septal defects with, 596
  clinical findings, 964–5
  complete transposition associated with, 837
  corrected transposition associated with, 879–80
  diagnosis, 968–9
  double outlet ventricle associated, 892, 895–6
  echocardiographic features, 346, 840, 875, 881, 966–7
  exercise testing in, 397, 416
  Fallot's tetralogy associated, 770–1, 773
  incidence, 959–60
  investigations, 965–8
  medical management, 969–72
  morphology, 961–3
  natural history/course, 11, 969
  pathogenesis, 963
  pathophysiology, 963–4
  prognosis, 969
  radiographic features, 200, 206, 207, 880, 965
  severe, 966
  sites, 959
  sub(valvar)/infundibular, 639, 649, 770–1, 772, 963
    conditions leading to, 836–7
    echocardiographic features, 846, 875, 966–7
  supravalvar, 965
  surgical management, 461, 883, 972–3
    angioplastic, 378
    corrective, 452–3
    elective, 638
    palliative, 378, 972–3
    progress after, 973
    types, 961–3
  valvar, 960–3, 963
    domed-, 960, 961
  ventricular septal defect associated with, 837, 879
Pulmonary time activity curves, 220–2
Pulmonary trunk, *see also* Pulmonary outflow tract
  banding, 144–5, 147, 445, 1105
    in atrioventricular valve atresia, 760

  in hypoplastic left heart syndrome, 758
    value, 607, 637–8
    with ventricular septal defects, 637–8
  connexions, 353, 354
  coronary artery anomalous course from, 1080
  coronary artery anomalous origin from, 296–7, 1074–7, 1227
  development, 132, 133
  dilation, post-stenotic, 962
  echocardiographic features, 340, 343, 353, 356, 357, 358
  graft to descending thoracic aorta, 758, 759
  pressure measurements with hypoplastic left heart syndrome, 749–52
  in pulmonary hypertension, 152
  structure, 146
  hypertension associated arrangement, 874–5
Pulmonary valve, *see also* Valves
  absent, 773, 776, 779, 783, 785
    radiographic features, 216, 780
    surgical risks, 791
  annulus, small, surgical risks, 791
  anomalies associated with pulmonary atresia, 713, 714
  atresia, *see* Pulmonary atresia
  closure, timing, 187
  commisural fusion, 960, 961
    surgery, 972
  dysplasia, 961
    in complete transposition, 832
  imperforate, producing atresia, 800
  infundibula, *see* Infundibula
  normal echocardiographic features, 353, 354
  regurgitation, 553
    murmur of, 553
  stenosis, *see* Pulmonary stenosis
  thickening, echocardiographic features, 966
Pulmonary valvoplasty, 453, 970–2
Pulmonary valvotomy, 452, 453
  for pulmonary stenosis, 972
  for right ventricular outflow tract obstruction, 719
Pulmonary varix, 537
Pulmonary vascular damage, 137–40
Pulmonary vascular disease, *see* Pulmonary circulation
Pulmonary vascular markings associated with-atrial septal defects, 554, 555
  cyanotic heart disease, 193, 779
  Fallot's tetralogy, 779
  pulmonary atresia, 812
Pulmonary vascular resistance
  atrial septal defect effect on, 549, 550
  developmental changes, 116–18, 133
  maternal mortality with elevated, 1354, 1357–8
  measurement, 146–7, 385
  obstructions and, 809
  persistent ductus arteriosus effect on, 946–7
  pulmonary atresia effect on, 809
  shunt produced by, 603
  ventricular septal defect effect on, 626–7
Pulmonary vasculature, *see* Pulmonary circulation
Pulmonary veins
  abnormalities, 511–36
  assessment, 129
  atresia
    clinical features/findings, 528, 533
    common-, 527–8

  diagnosis, 535
  investigations, 528, 534–5
  left-, 534
  management, 528, 535–6
  morphology/morphogenesis, 527–8, 533
  pathophysiology, 528, 533
  progress and prognosis, 534
  single-, 533–6
  atrial connexions, 329
    anomalous, 512, 519, 521, 522, 530
    natural, 329
    surgical, 527
  collateral, anomalous, 532–3
  descending, 519–20, 523
  development, 130, 132, 499, 514
    abnormal, 514
  dilation (surgical), 536
  entrapment, 565
  extra, 137
  horizontal, 511, 512
  injection, selective, 535
  intra-, 130
  malincorporation, 565
  stenosis
    clinical features/findings, 533
    diagnosis, 535
    investigations, 534–5
    left, 535
    management, 535–6
    morphology, 533
    pathophysiology, 533
    progress and prognosis, 535
    right, 535
    single-, 533–6
  vertical, 511–12, 520
  wedge angiography, 818–19
Pulmonary venous confluence
  accessibility, 526–7
  recognition, 518–19, 520, 522
Pulmonary venous congestion, *see* Pulmonary venous obstruction
Pulmonary venous connexions, anomalous, 503–32
  atrial isomerism with, 475–6, 477
  angiocardiography, 491–2
  atrial septal defects with, 548
  partial, 448–9, 528–32
    atrial partitioning with, 565
    to caval vein, 503, 504
    clinical features/findings, 529
    diagnosis, differential, 531
    investigations, 529–31
    morphogenesis, 529
    morphology, 528–9
    natural history/course, 531
    pathophysiology, 529
    prognosis, 531
    repair, 448–9, 531–2
  to sinus venosus, 545, 548
  surgical management, 448–9, 526–7, 531–2
  total, 136, 209, 212, 213, 448, 477, 506, 511–27
    aetiology, 511
    clinical findings, 516
    clinical symptomatology, 516
    diagnosis, 516–24, 569
    incidence, 511
    infracardiac, 448, 512
    infradiaphragmatic, 512, 513, 514, 519, 521
    intracardiac, 448, 512, 518
    investigations, 517–23
    management, 448, 525–7

Pulmonary venous (*contd.*)
 total
  morphology/morphogenesis, 511–14
  pathophysiology, 515–16, 522
  presentation, 516
  progress/prognosis, 524
  repair, 448, 526–7
  site of, 510–14
  supracardiac, 448, 511–12
 venous return obstruction due to, *see*
   Pulmonary venous return, anomalous
Pulmonary venous hypertension, radiographic
  features, 211, 212
Pulmonary venous obstruction/congestion
 atrial chamber partitioning causing, 567–8,
   852–3
 diagnosis, differential, 567–8
 pulmonary venous anomalous connexions
   causing, *see* Pulmonary venous return,
   anomalous
 radiographic features, 1207
Pulmonary venous return, anomalous, 511–36
 obstruction/congestion from, 515–16, 566
  consequences, 516
  late, 527
  severe, 516, 517
Pulmonary vessels, *see* Pulmonary arteries;
   Pulmonary circulation: Pulmonary veins
Pulse
 in aortic arch interruption, 1111
 in aortic coarctation, 1095, 1096, 1097
 in aortic regurgitation, 996
 in aortic stenosis, 982, 994
 diagnostic value, 184, 185, 195
 femoral-, 1093, 1095
  post-catheterisation decreases, 368
 in heart failure, 195
 in hypertrophic cardiomyopathy, 1142
 presentation due to deficient, 196
Purkinje cells
 depolarisation/repolarisation, 238, 251
 ventricular, 251

Q̇, *see* Cardiac output
Q wave, 259
 amplitude, 260
 diseases/conditions affecting, 266–306 *passim*
  corrected transposition, 871–3
  discordant atrioventricular connexions,
   871–3
  myocardial infarction, 296–8
  ventricular hypertrophy, 278–9, 873
Q-OT interval, 266, 267
QRS (complex), 243, 248, 254, 259
 amplitude, 260–2
  lower limit of, 262–3
 artefacts affecting, 306–13
 diseases/conditions affecting, 266–306
   passim
  arrhythmias, 1273–4
  atrioventricular septal defect, 589
  Fallot's tetralogy, 780
  interventricular conduction disturbances,
   281, 282, 283
  left anterior/posterior hemiblocks, 284–5
   Lown-Ganong-Levine syndrome, 288–9
   tricuspid atresia, 685–6
   ventricular hypertrophy, 274
   ventricular septal defect, 629
   Wolff-Parkinson-White syndrome, 287,
    288

 duration, 259, 1276
 mean vector, 252–4, 259, 283–4
 morphology, 259–60
QRS-T angle, 255, 256
Q-T intervals, 265–6, 267
 congenital prolongation, 304–5
 disease, conditions and factors affecting,
   266–306 *passim*
  arrhythmias, 1050, 1051
  central nervous system, 304–5
  mitral valve anomalies, 1050, 1051
Quality of life, 1401
Quinidine, 303
 electrocardiographic effects of, 303
 in pregnancy, 1356
 toxicity, 303

R wave, 242, 248, 259
 amplitude, 260–2, 263
  diseases/conditions affecting, 266–306
   passim
   ventricular hypertrophy, 275, 278
 intervals between, *see* R-R interval
 plus S wave amplitude, 261, 263
R' waves, 259–60
 diseases/conditions affecting, 266–306
   passim
  ventricular hypertrophy, 276
R-R interval, 256
 regularity, assessment, 1273, 1274
R/S ratio, 263
 diseases/conditions affecting, 266–306
   passim
  ventricular hypertrophy, 276
RSR', diseases/conditions affecting, 266–306
   passim
  atrial septal defects, 553
  interventricular conduction defects,
   282–3
  ventricular hypertrophy, 276
Racial groups, incidence of heart disease,
   6–7
Radiation-induced heart disease, 1267
Radiography, chest, 201–17
 features and findings with, 202–13
  abnormal, with asymptomatic child,
   197–8
  aortic arch defects, 1111, 1129, 1130
  aortic coarctation, 212, 1097
  aortic regurgitation, 997
  aortic stenosis, 983, 989, 994
  aorto-left ventricular defect, 997
  aortopulmonary window, 925
  arteriovenous abnormal connexions,
   1012, 1015
  atrial chamber partitioning, 566
  atrial isomerism, 486–7
  atrial septal defects, 208, 555
  brachiocephalic artery, anomalous, 1133
  complete transposition, 209, 210, 211,
   843
  coronary artery anomalies, 1075
  corrected transposition, 873–5
  double inlet ventricle, 656–7
  double outlet ventricle, 902
  Ebstein's (and related) malformations,
   725
  endocardial fibroelastosis, 1226
  Fallot's tetralogy, 779–80
  hypertrophic cardiomyopathy, 1144
  hypoplastic left heart syndrome, 746–7

  mitral valve anomalies, 1029, 1046,
   1200–1, 1207
  myocarditis, 1166, 1167
  pericarditis, 1172–3
  persistent ductus arteriosus, 209, 943
  pulmonary atresia, 717, 812
  pulmonary hypertension, 1200, 1201,
   1322
  pulmonary sling, 1134–5
  pulmonary stenosis, 200, 206, 207, 880,
   965
  pulmonary vascular disease, 146
  pulmonary venous anomalies, 209, 213,
   517, 529–30, 534
  rheumatic heart disease, 1187, 1200–1,
   1207
  systemic disease, 1246–68 *passim*
  truncus arteriosus, 917
  tumours, cardiac, 1155
  vascular rings, 1129, 1130
  ventricular septal defects, 208, 215, 629,
   879
 views, required, 201–2
Radionuclide(s)
 administration, 220
 imaging/scanning, 219–25, *see also specific*
   techniques
  cardiac output measured by, 407
  of lungs, 400, 401
  role, 224–5
  of tumours (cardiac), 1156
Rastelli procedure, 457, 856–7
 diagrammatic representaton, 856
Rebreathing technique, cardiac ouput
   measurements using, 405, 406–7
Receptors
 response to adrenergic stimuli, 439
 types, 439
Recurrence risks in sibs/offspring of heart
   disease, 34, 35–9
Refractory period, action potential, 238
Refsum's disease, 1261
Relaxation (ventricular), 172–7, *see also*
   Diastole
 incoordinate, 175–6
 isovolumic, 172
Renal artery stenosis/obstruction
 ateriography, 1300
 hypertension due to, 1308–9
 investigation, 1308
Renal disease, hypertension associated, *see*
   Hypertension
Renal hypertension, *see* Hypertension
Renal ischaemia
 evidence, 1309
 hypertension generated by, 1307
Renal parenchymal disease, 1309–10
 hypertension associated with, 1309–10
Renin
 overproduction, 1310
 plasma, activity
  coarctation associated, 1094, 1105, 1310
  hypertension associated, 1306, 1307–8,
   1310
Renovascular hypertension, 1308–9
Repolarisation
 atrial, 245–7, 252
 cellular, 237–41
  intercellular, 240–1
  phases, 238
 early- (syndrome), 291
 ventricular, 242–3, 248–51, 252
  abnormal, 252

Research, ethical considerations, 1402
Resistance, circulatory, calculation, 385–6, *see also* Pulmonary vascular resistance; Systemic resistance
Respiration, *see also* Expiration; Inspiration; Ventilation
  effects of aortic arch anomalies, 1128–9
  effects of heart failure, 194
  heart sounds associated with, 186–7
Respiratory distress syndrome
  diagnosis, differential, 212–13
  ductal shunting associated, 949
Resting lung volume, 397
Rhabdomyofibroma (=fibroma), 1156, 1157–8
Rhabdomyoma, 1156–7
  echocardiographic features, 357, 1155
Rheumatic heart disease, 1179–1215
  acute, *see* Rheumatic heart disease, acute
  chronic valvar-, 1195–1215, 1231, *see also specific valve*
    epidemiology, 1195
    pathology, 1196–8
    relative frequencies, 1196
    specific conditions, 1198–1215
  endomyocardial fibrosis and, 1329, 1336
  healing processes, 1195
  pulmonary hypertension in, 151
Rheumatic heart disease, acute, 1179–95
  aetiology, 1180–1
  clinical features/findings, 1186
  diagnosis, 1185–91
    Jones's criteria, 1185, 1186
  epidemiology, 1179–80
  incidence, 1179–80, 1190
    during pregnancy, 1353
  laboratory tests, 1189
  management, 1191–3
  natural history/course, 1190–1
  pathogenesis, 1183–4
  pathology, 1184–5
  prevention, 1193–5
    immuno-1195
    lifetime, 1194–5
    primary, 1193–4
    secondary, 1194–5
  recurrence, 1180, 1190, 1194
Rheumatoid arthritis, 1264
Rib anomalies
  heart disease associated with, 215, 1097
  notching, 1097
Right bundle branch
  anatomy, 237
  block, 280–3, 286, 1289
    cause, 282
    complete, 281–2, 792–3
    electrocardiographic features, 281–3, 286
    incomplete, 282–3
    surgically caused, 792–3
Right heart hypoplasia, imaging, 230–1
Right ventricular hypertrophy, *see* Ventricular hypertrophy
Risk
  factors
    in atrioventricular septal repair, 608
    cardiovascular, in infancy/childhood, 1345–9
    analysis of surgical-, 1365–7
    in systemic hypertension management, 1306, 1307
  ratios, 425–6, 427–8
Rubella
  persistent ductus arteriosus linked to, 941
  teratogenicity, 25

S wave, 242, 248, 259–60
  amplitude, 260–2, 263
  diseases/conditions affecting, 266–306 *passim*
    ventricular hypertrophy, 275–6
S/R ratio, *see* R/S ratio
S-T segment, 242–3, 263–4
  diseases/conditions affecting, 266–306 *passim*, 413
  injuries from various causes, 293–6
ST-T wave changes, aortic stenosis associated, 983
Saint Vitus dance, *see* Chorea
Salicylate therapy in rheumatic heart disease, 1192, 1193
Salt/sodium levels
  cardiovascular risks, 1348
  hypertension associated, 1304–5, 1348
Sandhoff disease, 1252
Sanfillipo syndrome, 1248
Saphenous vein
  catheterisation, 369–70
  graft, 1300
Sarcoidosis, electrocardiographic effects of, 307
Scapuloperoneal myopathy, autosomal dominant, 1258
Schistosomiasis, cardiac signs, 1321–3
Scimitar vein/syndrome, 505–6, 528–9
  angiographic features, 531
  radiographic features, 530
Scintigraphy, 224
  of coronary artery anomalies, 1075
  of hypertrophic cardiomyopathy, 1146
Scoliosis
  kypho-, 272
  pulmonary hypertension associated with, 153
Selenium deficiency, 1261–2
Senning procedure, 455, 854–6
  diagrammatic representation, 855
  risk analysis, 1365
Sensitivity analysis, 423
Septa, *see* Septum
Septal band, 766, 767
  in Fallot's tetralogy, 767
Septal puncture, trans-, 374–5
Septation, *see also specific septa*
  failure, 585–6, 625
  mal-, in Fallot's tetralogy, 774
  natural/developmental, 86–87 *passim*
  surgical, 450–1, 462, 608, 625, 638
Septectomy, atrial, 445
  blade-, 380–1
  for complete transposition, 852
  for double inlet ventricle, 669
  laser-, 381–2
Septostomy, atrial, balloon, 380
  for complete transposition, 850–1
  fossa ovalis rupture following, 832
  postoperative survival, 429, 851
  for pulmonary venous obstruction, 525–6
Septum, *see also specific septa*
  atrial/ventricular malalignment, 870, 871,
  at the atrioventricular junction, 86, 338–40
  formation, *see* Septation
  growth, measurement, 355
  primum
    defect, *see* Ostium primum
    development, 88, 89, 90, 92–3
  repair, *see* Septation
  secundum
    defect, 531, 543
    developmment, 89, 90

structures/components, 92
  arrangement, 92, 573
  notation, 92, 227, 228, 229, 230
Sex chromosome defects
  aneuploidy, 21–2
  gene, single, 24
  syndrome caused by, 47–55 *passim*
Sex differences in R wave amplitude, 263
Sheie syndrome, 1248
Shock, cardiogenic
  management, 436
  presentation with, 196
  types, 436
Shunts
  atrioventricular septal defect associated, 577
  bidirectional, 221, 222, 385
  blood flow measurements, 384–5
  blood oxygen measurements, 399–400
  cavopulmonary, 444–5
  complete transposition associated, 838, 839–40
  definition, 839
  interatrial, surgery for, 451, 452
  left to right cardiac, 195, 219
    angiographic detection/quantitation, 219, 220, 555
    atrial septal defects with, 549–50, 555, 556, 559–60
    pulmonary venous abnormalities with, 515, 529
    ventricular septal defects with, 626
  left to right ductal, 116, 949
  measurement, 226, 408, 1016
  pulmonary, obligatory vs dependent, 119, 226, 408
  pulmonary arteriovenous malformation associated, 1014–15, 1016
  pulmonary venous connexion anomaly associated, 515
  right to left cardiac
    angiographic detection, 220–2
    cyanosis and, 192
    echocardiographic detection, 343
    pulmonary vein abnormalities with, 515
  right to left ductal, 754, 1110
  surgical, injection into, 818 *see also specific procedure*
  surgical intervention, 559–60
  systemic-pulmonary, insertion, 144, 145, 444
    with double inlet ventricle, 669
    murmurs associated, 1006–7
    with pulmonary atresia, 824
  ventricular, inter-, 577, 579–81, 586, 602–3
Sialidosis, 1250
Siblings (of ill child), psychological considerations, 1379–80
Sickle cell haemoglobinopathies
  cardiac problems with, 1268, 1326–8
  clinical types of, 1327
  frequency, 1326–7
  open heart surgery and, 1327
  pathophysiology, 1326
Simpson's rule, 387–8
Sinu-atrial ring, 103
Sinu-atrial septum, development, 86–7
Sinu-atrial valves, development, 97–8
Sinus bradycardia, 1276–7
Sinus node
  activity, recordings, 1275
  defects/dysfunction, 1277
    atrial isomerism associated, 482
  morphology, 235

Sinus of Valsalva
  aneurysm/fistula, 1002, 1003,
    1007–10
    aetiology, 1007
    clinical findings, 1008
    complications, 1007–8
    incidence, 1007
    investigations, 1008–9
    management, 1009–10, 1017–19
    morphology/morphogenesis, 1007–8
    natural history/course, 1009
    pathophysiology, 1008
    prognosis, 1009
  coronary artery anomalous course from,
    1080
  coronary artery anomalous origin from,
    1078–9
Sinus rhythm, 256, 257, 269
  abnormal, 269
Sinus venosus
  defects, 5
    arrhythmias associated with, 560
    inferior-, 545–6
    morphogenesis, 547–8
    morphology, 541, 544–5, 546
    repair, 545
    superior, 544–5
  development, 86–7, 88, 95, 497–9,
    499–500
  valves
    anomalies, 506–7
    development, 499, 506–7
    remnants, 544
Situs (with reference to atrial arrangement),
    65, 68–70, 200–1, 474–9, *see also*
    Atrial isomerism
  in conjoined twins, 1061
  echocardiographic examination, 327–30,
    875
  electrocardiographic determination, 266–8,
    271, 872
  inversus (mirror-image arrangement), 34,
    64, 69, 70, 71, 72, 327, 1063
    atrial appendage juxtaposition and, 1063,
      1064, 1065
    incomplete, *see* Isomerism sequence
    malpositioned heart and, 1063
  solitus (normal arrangement), 69, 327
  transposition related to, 831
  tricuspid valve and, 700–5 *passim*
  univentricular atrioventricular connexions
    and, 644, 645
Size, body, *see* Body size
Skeleton, defects in, heart disease
    associated with, 45
Sleeping sickness
  Gambian-, 1324–6
  Rhodesian-, 1324
Sly syndrome, 1249
Smoking, cardiovascular risks, 1349
Snares, 381
Social aspects of heart disease, 1385–96
  special cases, 1394–5
Sodium, *see* Salt/sodium levels
Sodium nitroprusside therapy, 438
Sounds, heart, *see also* Murmurs
  additional, 188
  clicks, 188
    ejection, 188, 468
    non-ejection, 188, 1039, 1040, 1045,
      1046, 1051
  diagnostic value, 186–9
  diastolic, 187–8, 188

findings with
    aortic stenosis, 979, 980, 982–3, 989
    aortopulmonary window, 925
    atrial septal defects, 551–2
    complete transposition, 842
    corrected transposition, 871
    Fallot's tetralogy, 778, 779
    hypertrophic cardiomyopathy, 1143, 1199
    mitral valve anomalies, 1028, 1029,
      1039–40, 1045, 1046, 1199, 1206
    persistent ductus arteriosus, 942–3
    pulmonary atresia, 813
    pulmonary stenosis, 964–5, 969
    rheumatic heart disease, 1206
    truncus arteriosus, 916
  first-, 186
  fourth-, 188
  second-, 186–7
  systolic, mid-, 188, 1039–40, 1045, 1046,
    1051
  third-, 187–8
Sphingolipidoses, 1250–1
Sphingomyelin lipidosis, 1250
Sphygmomanometer cuff size, 1293, 1295
Spinal muscular atrophy, juvenile, 1261
Splenic syndrome, *see* Atrial isomerism
Squatting, symptomatic relief by, 776–7
Staff, *see* Doctors; Medical profession
Staphylococci, endocarditis associated, 1230
Starling's law, 434
Steel coils, vessel closure using, 379, 825,
    1017, 1019
Stenoses, *see also specific valve/vessel*
  heart sounds diagnostic of, 180
  relief, 378, 379
  ultrasonic detection, 345
Stethoscope, examinations, *see* Auscultation
Still's disease, 1264
Still's murmur, 466–7
Stillborn, *see* Mortality
Straight back syndrome, electrocardiographic
    features, 272
Streaming, effect of, 899–900
Steinert's disease, 1257–8
Steroid therapy
  effects on ductus arteriosus, 937
  rheumatic heart disease, 1192, 1193
Storage diseases with cardiological
    involvement, 1245–52
Streptococci (group A)
  alpha-, 1230
  antigens/immunogens, 1181, 1181–3
  enteric, 1230
  infections
    diagnostic tests, 1180–1, 1181–3, 1189,
      1193–4
    endocarditis associated, 1229, 1230
    recurrence, 1180, 1190, 1194
    rheumatic lever associated with, 1179–85
    symptoms, 1139
    treatment/prevention, 1190, 1191–2,
      1193–5, 1239–40
  infectious carriers, 1195
  proteins/enzymes/products, 1181, 1182
    hypersensitivity, delayed, 1184
    M/M-associated, 1182
    streptolysin O, 1181, 1182, 1183
    streptolysin S, 1183
    toxic-, 1183
  vaccines against, 1195
Stroke volume, ventricular, *see* Ventricles
Subclavian artery
  aberrant, 600, 1109, 1126–7, 1128, 1131

  anomalous course, 1090–1
  anomalous origin, 1107, 1108
  aortic coarctation involving, 1096, 1097
  -common carotid artery, aortic interruption
    between, 1124–5
  -duct, aortic interruption between, 1124
  fistulous communication, 1002, 1004, 1005,
    1012, 1013
  -left coronary artery anastomoses, 1077
  shunt using, *see* Blalock-Taussig shunt
  tortuous dilated, 1002, 1004, 1005, 1012,
    1013
Subclavian flap angioplasty, 446, 447, 1104
Submaximal exercise performance tests,
    402–4, 410–13
Sulcus tissue, echocardiographic features,
    686, 687
Suprasternal puncture, 372–3
Supravalvar mitral ring, *see* Mitral ring
Supraventricular arrhythmias, 881
  tachy-, *see* Ventricular tachycardias
Supraventricular crest, 78
Surgery, 443–62
  corrective, 445–62, 1393–4
  costs, 12
  deciding on, 422–3, 425
  diseases/defects requiring
    aortic arch anomalies, 1115–16, 1131
    aortic coarctation, 1104–6
    aortic regurgitation, 1213
    aortic stenosis, 458–9, 981, 985, 986–7,
      991–2, 1210–11
    aorto-left ventricular defect, 997–8
    aortopulmonary window, 927–8
    arrhythmias, 1279–81, 1288
    atrial chamber partitioning, 568
    atrial isomerism, 493
    atrial septal defects, 559–60
    atrioventricular septal defects, 605–9
    brachiocephalic artery, anomalous,
      1132–3
    complete transposition, *see* Transposition,
      complete
    coronary artery anomalies, 1076–7, 1082
    corrected transposition, 883
    double inlet ventricle, 467, 668–71
    double outlet ventricle, 907–8
    Ebstein's (and related) malformations,
      729–31
    endocarditis, infective, 1240–1
    endomyocardial fibrosis, 1333, 1334–5
    Fallot's tetralogy, 787–93
    hypertrophic cardiomyopathy, 1149
    hypoplastic left heart syndrome, 756–9
    mitral valve anomalies, 1036–8, 1198,
      1203–4, 1208
    persistent ductus arteriosus, 379–80,
      445–6, 944–5, 950, 953
    pulmonary arteriovenous malformation,
      1017
    pulmonary atresia, 719, 823–6
    pulmonary sling, 1135
    pulmonary stenosis, *see* Pulmonary
      stenosis
    pulmonary venous anomalies, 525–6,
      531–2
    rheumatic heart disease, 1203–4, 1208,
      1210, 1213, 1214, 1215
    sinus of Valsalva aneurysm/fistula,
      1009–10
    straddling atrioventricular valves, 705–8
    systemic disease, 1246–68 *passim*
    systemic hypertension, 1300, 1309

Surgery (*contd.*)
  diseases/defects requiring
    tricuspid atresia, 691–3
    tricuspid stenosis, 1215
    tricuspid incompetence, 1214
    truncus arteriosus, 922–3
    tumours, cardiac, 1160–1
    vascular ring, 1131
    ventricular septal defects, *see* Ventricular
      septum, defects
  endocarditis caused by, 1234
  mortality from, *see* Mortality
  new problems created by, 1369
  open heart, *see* Open heart surgery
  palliative, 1393–4
    limitations, 1368
    principles of, 444–5, 447
    and pulmonary hypertesion, 144–5
  parental adaptation after, 1393–4
  in pregnancy, 1355
    preparation for, psychological aspects, 1378
  principles of, 443–62
  residual defects
    intentional, 1368–9
    unintentional, 1368
  results/effects
    functional, 1367–8
    psychological (on child), 1375–6
    sub-optimal long term, 1368–70
  timing, 429–34, 560, 855–6
  transplant, *see* Transplants, grafts and
    anastomoses
  verdict, pronouncing, 1394
Survival, *see also* Life expectancy; Mortality;
    Survivors
  actuarial, calculation, 1365
  of treatment, evaluating probabilities,
    420–34
Survivors from heart disease, *see also* Life
    expectancy; Mortality; Survival
  liveborn, 8
  natural history, 10–11
  postoperative, 1363–70
    complication rate, 1363–5
    with pulmonary hypertension, 147–8
Suture
  continuous, 456
  interrupted positive, 450
  septal, 450, 451
Switch operation, arterial, *see* Arterial Switch
    operation
Sympathetic activity, hypertension associated,
    1304
Sympathomimetic agent(s) therapy, 439–40
  dose regime, 439
Syncope
  aortic stenosis associated, 982
  diagnosis, 183–4
  presentation with, 196–7
Syndromes involving the heart
  aetiology, 47–59
  clinical features, 47–59
  tables listing, 42–59
Systemic alterations
  by tumours, 1153
  effect on electrocardiography, 298–306
Systemic arteriovenous fistulas, 1010–12
Systemic circulation/blood flow
  arterial, *see* Arterial circulation
  in complete transposition, 939–9
  ductus dependent, 838–40
  in Eisenmonger's syndrome, 1357, 1358
  venous, *see* Systemic venous system

Systemic diseases, cardiological responses,
    1245–68
Systemic hypertension, 1293–315
  aetiology, 1298, 1299
  classification, 1298
  clinical features, 1299–1301
  complications, 1299–1301
  definition, 1297
  diagnosis, 1301–2, 1306
  follow-up measurements, 1346
  genetic component, 1304, 1306
  infantile/neonatal, 1302–3
  medical management, 1302, 1306–7
  other causes of, 1314–15
  prediction, 1296
  prevalence, 1298–9, 1302, 1303
  prevention, 1339
  primary (essential), 1298, 1303–7
    pathogenesis, 1303–4
    investigation, 1306
  prognosis, 1302
  risk factor management, 1306, 1339
  screening, 1302, 1346–7
  secondary, 1298, 1307–14
  severe, 1302
  surgical management, 1300, 1309
  tropically occurring, 1338–9
Systemic lupus erythematosus, 1169, 1264–6
Systemic resistance
  in Eisenmonger's syndrome, 1357, 1358
  vascular, 385
Systemic venous return
  connexions and positions, anomalous,
    476–9, 500–7
    in atrial isomerism, 476–9, 499–500
    correction, 852–6
  morphogenesis, 85, 86–7, 497–500
  obstruction, postoperative, 852, 853
Systole
  murmurs/sounds in, *see* Murmurs; Sounds
  ventricular function in, 165–6

T cell deficiency
  monitoring, 1115
  rheumatic heart disease associated, 1183
T wave, 243, 248–50, 251, 264, 265–6
  abnormalities, diseases/conditions associated
    with, 266–306 *passim*
    arrhythmias, 1050–1, 1051
    atrial enlargement, 280
    injuries (from various causes), 293–5
    interventricular conduction defects, 282
    ischaemia, 291–3
    mitral valve anomalies, 1050–1, 1051
    ventricular hypertrophy, 274–5, 278
  artefacts affecting, 311, 312, 313
  changes
    primary/secondary, 291
    functional, 290–1
  genesis, 251, 291
  mean vector, 255
  P and U wave differentiation from, 264–5
  -QRS angle, *see* QRS-T angle
Ta wave, 245, 247
T-P interval/segment, 266, 267
Tachyarrhythmias/tachycardia, *see also*
    Arrhythmias
  -bradycardia syndrome, 1277–8
  catheter induced, 382
  ventricular/supraventricular, *see*
    Ventricular tachycardia

Takayasu arteritis, hypertension associated
    with, 1308
Talking
  to children, 1377
  with parents, *see* Consultation
Taussig-Bing anomaly (=subpulmonary
    ventricular septal defect), 457, 893,
    907–8
Tay-Sachs disease, 1252
Teeth extraction, endocarditis associated with,
    1234, 1237
Tendon of Todaro, development, 87
Teratogens, 25–6
  effect of ductus arteriosus development, 933
Teratoma, 1157
Terminology in paediatric cardiology, 65–80
Tetralogy of Fallot, *see* Fallot's tetralogy
Thebesian valves, 507
Therapy, *see* Management
Thiamine deficiency, 1262–3
Thoracic exteriorisation of the heart, 1057–9
Thoracic gas volume, 39
Thoraco-abdominal viscera arrangement in
    atrial isomerism, 484–5
Thorax radiography, 214–6, *see also*
    Radiography, chest
Thromboembolism, *see* Embolism
Thromboses, *see also* Embolism
  ductus arteriosus, 947–8
  pulmonary artery, 149
  vegetations composed of, 1232, 1233
Thromboxane, role, 936
Thyroid disorders with cardiological effects,
    1253
Timing of treatment, 421–9
  surgical, 429–34, 560, 855–6, 985, 1211
Tobacco, cardiovascular risks, 1349
Tolazine therapy, 438
Tomography, computerised, cardiac aspects,
    217–18
Toxic immunological hypothesis, 1184
Trabecular components, 74
  apical, 67, 68, 449–56, 688
    hypoplasia, 733, 734
    obstruction, 967
  defects, 619, 623–4, 631, 635, 688
    repair, 449–50
  morphology, 67–8
  rudimentary ventricle, 647
  septomarginal, 78, 93
  ventricle identification from, 330, 331, 332
Trachea
  compression, conditions causing, 1123–35
  radiography, 216, 217, 218, 219
Traction, hypertension and, 1297
Transcatheter occlusion of pulmonary
    arteriovenous malformation, 1017–19
Translocation Down's syndrome, 17
Trans-septal puncture, 374–5
Transplantation (cardiac), pulmonary
    hypertension and, 145
Transplants, grafts and surgical anastomoses,
    444–62 *passim*
  aortic, 1116
  arterial, 1077, 1078
  cardiac, 145
  involving coronary arteries, 1077, 1078
Transposition (of the great arteries)
  complete, *see* Transposition, complete
  corrected, *see* Transposition, corrected
  definitions, 76, 79, 829–31
  surgery, 461, 744, 883 *see also*
    Transposition, complete

Transposition, complete
aetiology, 831
aortic atresia and, 743
cardiac effects of, 840–1
clinical features/findings, 842–3
criss-cross heart associated with, 1067, 1068, 1069
diagnosis, 193–4, 228–9, 844, 849
distinction from other transpositions, 829–31
double outlet ventricle associated with, 899
ductal effects on, 940
haemodynamics, 385, 847–8
investigations, 843–7
magnetic resonance imaging, 228–9
medical management, 850
morphogenesis, 838
morphology, 831
other conditions associated with, 1603
pathophysiology, 838–9
postoperative fate, 860
prevalence, 831
pulmonary effects of, 142–3, 840–1
surgical management, 455–7, 850–60
choice, 859–60
corrective/directive, 852–60
palliative, 850–2
timing, 429–34, 855–6
ventricular outflow tract obstruction with, 456–7
ventricular septal defect with, 456–7, 832, 833, 834–6
Transposition, corrected (congenitally), 461, 744
associated malformations/anomalies, 878–82
clinical presentation, 871
criss-cross heart with, 1066–7
definition, 830, 867–8
diagnosis, differential, 882–3
investigations, 871–8
morphology, 868–71
natural history, 868
physiology, 868
prevalence, 868
surgical management, 883
uncomplicated, 868
Trauma, *see* Injury
Treadmill settings and oxygen consumption, 403
Treatment, *see* Management
Triangle of Koch displacement, 621
Tricuspid atresia, 675–93
aetiology, 676–7
atrial appendage juxtaposition with, 1065
classical, 676, 678–81
categorisation, 679
clinical features/findings, 685
definition, 675–6
diagnosis, 689–90
incidence, 676–7
investigations, 685–9
medical management, 690–1
morphogenesis, 682–3
morphology, 675–6, 677–82
pathophysiology, 683–4
postoperative complications, 693
postoperative management, 693
prognosis, 690
radionuclide angiographic features, 221, 688
surgical management, 459–61, 690–3
corrective, 691–3
palliative, 690–1

relative merits, 693
selection criteria, 692
variants, 681–2
Tricuspid incompetence, 1213–14
clinical features/findings, 1213–14
incidence, 1213
management, 1214
Tricuspid stenosis, rheumatic, 1214–15
pathology, 1197
Tricuspid valve, *see also* Atrioventricular valves; Valves
closure, delayed, 726, 727
definition, 74
development, 98–100, 101
fetal, echocardiographic features, 354, 357
leaflet anomalies, 713, 714–15, 731
anterosuperior, displaced, 723, 728
blockage/closure of a defect by, 621–2
complete absence, 732, 733
mural, displaced/malformed, 722, 727
septal, displaced/malformed, 357, 722, 723
septal, absent, 722
leaflet development, 724
lesions/defects/diseases, 347, 731–4
atresia, *see* Tricuspid atresia
corrected transposition associated, 880–1
dysplasia, 731, 880
Ebstein's malformation, *see* Ebstein's malformation
imperforate valve, 690
incompetence, *see* Tricuspid incompetence
pulmonary atresia associated with, 713
regurgitation, 347
septal defects associated with, 619, 620
stenosis, *see* Tricuspid stenosis
straddling valve, 700–2, 705
motion, abnormal, 725
replacement, 731
sounds, 186, 725
surgical repairs effected via, 449, 450
surgical treatment of, 729–31
patient selection, 730
tension apparatus, insertion anomalies, 902, 903, 904
Trifascicular conduction disturbances, 286, 1289
Trisomy 8p syndrome, 20
Trisomy 13 (Patau's syndrome), 18–19
features, 18–19, 20
Trisomy 18 (Edward's syndrome), 18, 19
Trisomy 21, *see* Down's syndrome
Tropics (paediatric cardiology in), 1321–39
congenital heart diseases in, 1337–8
aetiology, 1337
diagnostic problems, 1338
incidence/prevalence, 1337–8
Truncal root, angiography, 918, 919
Truncal valve
incompetence, 921
severe, 922–3
replacement, 922–3
Truncus arteriosus (the structure), development, 95–6
Truncus arteriosus (the syndrome), 913–23
classification, 914
clinical features/findings, 916–17
investigations, 917
medical management, 921–2
morphogenesis, 915
morphology, 913–15
natural history/course, 921

pathophysiology, 915–16
prognosis, 921
surgical management, 920, 922–3
Trypanosomiasis
African, 1324–6, 1327
American, 1323–4
cardiac signs in, 1323–7
Tumours, adrenal, *see* Adrenal gland tumours
Tumours, cardiac, 1153–61
clinical signs/symptoms, 1153–4
electrocardiographic features, 295–6
fetal, 357
incidence, relative, 1153
injury due to, 295–6
intracavitary, 1154
investigations, 1154–7
surgical management, 1160–1
types, 1156–61
benign, 1153, 1156–61
child-, 1153
infant-, 1153
malignant, 1153, 1160
Twin studies of heart defects, 30–3
incidence compared to singletons, 32
Twins
conjoined, 33, 1060–2
anomalous arrangement, 1061
monozygotic, excess of heart defects in, 32–3
Turner's syndrome, 45X-, 21–2, 1087

U wave, 243, 251, 264
disease/conditions affecting, 266–306 *passim*
P and T wave differentiation from, 264–5
Uhl's anomaly, 731–4
Ultrasound, *see* Doppler ultrasound; Echocardiography
Umbilical vessels, catheterisation via, 372
Umbrellas, repairs effected using, 379–80
Univentricular hearts, 67
in atrial isomerism, 479–81, 483
controversial definitions/distinctions/associations, 643, 680–1
types, 643, *see also* Atrioventricular connexions; Double inlet ventricle
Ureteric stone catcher, 381
Urogenital anomalies, heart disease associated with, 45

$\dot{V}CO_2$, *see* Carbon dioxide production
$\dot{V}D$, 408, 412
$\dot{V}E$, 405, 410, 412
$\dot{V}O_2$ *see* Oxygen uptake
Vaccination against streptococci, 1195
Valves (general features), *see also specific valve*
area, measurement, 386
chronic rheumatic disease of, *see* Rheumatic heart disease
common, *see* Atrioventricular valves
echocardiographic examination, 321, 330–3, 334, 335, 337, 341, 343, 344
formation, 97–104
incompetence, measurement, 224, 226, 469
motion, 341
prosthetic
antibiotic prophylaxis, 1239
aortic, 987, 1211, 1213
caged ball, 1213
endocarditis, 423–9

Valves
  prosthetic *(contd.)*
    mitral, 1037–8, 1051, 1204, 1207, 1209
    Starr–Edward's ball, 1209
    tricuspid, 731
    truncal, 922–3
  regurgitation, detection, 343, 344, 345,
      346, 347
  rings, arrangement, 572, 573
  stenosis, *see Stenoses and specific valves*
  straddling, *see Atrioventricular valves and
      specific valves*
Valvoplasty, balloon, 377, 378
  diagrammatic representation, 970
  for pulmonary stenosis, 453, 970–2
Valvotomy, *see specific valve*
Vancomycin, endocarditis prevention with,
    1239
Vascular defects, syndromes associated with,
    46, *see also specific vascular system*
Vascular rings, 1123–33
  classification, 1123–7
  clinical features/findings, 1127
  diagnosis, 1129–30
  incidence, 1123
  investigations, 1129–30
  management, 1130–1
    postoperative, 1131
  morphology, 1123–7
  radiographic features, 216, 217, 218, 219
Vascular slings, *see Pulmonary slings*
Vascular system development, 85–6, *see also
    Circulation*
Vascularisation, myocardial, 104–5
Vasodilators
  developmental roles, 117
  for systemic hypertension, 1302, 1314, 1315
  treatment, 438
    dose regime, 438
Vectorcardiography, *see Electrocardiography*
Vegetations, 1232, 1233
Vein of Galen fistulas/aneurysms, 202,
    1002–4, 1005, 1011, 1012
Venodilator therapy, 438
Venous duct, *see Ductus venosus*
Venous hum, 467, 944
Venous system
  atrial connexions, redirection, 852–6
  mixing, in tricuspid atresia, 683–4
  pulmonary, *see Pulmonary venous system*
  systemic, *see Systemic venous system*
Venous valves, *see Sinus venosus*
Ventilation, *see also Respiration*
  dead space- (V̇D), 408, 412
  measurement, 404
  minute-, (V̇E), 405, 410, 412
  -perfusion
    imbalance shunt, 399–400
    relationships, 408
Ventricle(s) (general features)
  cavity shape, 160–3, 1147, 1148
  cavity size, 160–2
    measurement, 712, 717
    significance of, 163
  compliance, 174–5
    atrial septal defect effects on, 549
  components, 67
  contraction, *see Contraction*
  development (normal), 162–3
  diverticulum of the, 1058
  dominance, 1059
    with atrioventricular septal defect, 584–5
    with pulmonary atresia, 716

ejection, 167–70
  fraction, 163, 222–3
  pre-, period, 167
  time, 168
  velocity, 168–9, 177
enlarged/dilated, 359, *see also Ventricular
    hypertrophy*
  echocardiographic features, 522, 555
  radiographic features, 204
filling, 173–6, 177
functions, 159–77
  with double inlet ventricle, 655
  during development, 113–14
  during diastole, 172–6, 177
  during systole, 165–6
  growth effects, 162–3
  monitoring/assessment, 159–77, 222–4,
      225–6, 388, 413
  surgically impaired, 854
  in tricuspid atresia, 684
hypoplasia, *see Hypoplastic left heart
    syndrome; Ventricular hypoplasia*
identification, echocardiographic, 330–3
inlet/outlet portion, *see Ventricular inlets;
    Ventricular outlets*
inverted-, 870
left, 67
  contractility theory of disease in, 166
  filling, 173
  response to ventricular septal defect, 627
  -right atrium communication, 619, 620
  mass, *see Ventricular mass*
  mature, 93–4
  morphology, 67, 68
    atrial arrangements associated with, 72
    in atrial isomerism, 485, 492
  position, electrocardiographic
      determination, 268–71
  pressure
    fall, rate, 172–3
    loading with atrioventricular septal
        defects, 587
    -volume relations, 169–70, 174–5, 627
  repolarisation/depolarisation, *see
      Depolarisation; Repolarisation*
right, 67
  dysplasia, 731, 732, 733, 734, 1287
  left atria communication, 683
  pulmonary artery surgical connexion to,
      825
  size, in pulmonary atresia, 711–12, 717
rudimentary, 68, 75
  definition, 698
  left, 650–1
  right, 645–50 *passim*, 680, 1059
septal repair via, 450–1, 451
solitary, *see Univentricular hearts*
stroke volume, 163, 167–8, 407
  age related, 411–12
  pulmonary vein abnormality related,
      515–16
supero-inferior, 1070–1
terminology used to describe, 66–8, 70–9
    passim
topology and relationships, 74–6, 269–71
  atrial isomerism associated, 479, 492
  atrioventricular septal defect associated,
      605, 606
  corrected transposition associated, 881
  criss-cross heart associated, 1067–70
  straddling atrioventricular valve
      associated, 700–5
trabeculations, *see Trabeculations*

volume/dimensions
  loading, 586–7
  measurement, 160–1, 223, 225–6, 356,
      387, 388
  -pressure relations, 169–70, 174–5
wall, *see Ventricular walls*
Ventricular aneurysm, 298
Ventricular arrhythmias
  brady-, *see also Ventricular bradycardia*
  mitral valve anomaly associated, 1047, 1051
  tachy-, *see Ventricular tachycardia*
  treatment caused, 382, 639, 793
Ventricular communication (inter-), *see also
    Shunts; Ventricular septum, defects*
  closure
    natural, 90–95 *passim*
    surgical, 10, 461, 638
  echocardiographic features, 591, 904
  morphogenesis, 94, 95
  obstructive, 648
  surgery with, 607–8
Ventricular endomyocardial fibrosis, *see
    Endocardial fibrosis*
Ventricular enlargement, *see Ventricles;
    Ventricular hypertrophy*
Ventricular exclusion procedure, 670–1
Ventricular fibre architecture, 159–60 *see also
    Myocardial fibres*
  abnormal, 160
Ventricular hypertrophy, *see also
    Cardiomyopathy*
  assessment, 129–30, 164
  bi-, 279
  diastolic dysfunction associated with, 174–5
  electrocardiographic features, 270, 272–9,
      780, 843, 873, 1143, 1144, 1225–6
  Fallot's tetralogy associated, 708
  left, 162, 276–9, 985
  mitral valve regurgitation associated, 1211
  pulmonary stenosis associated, 961–2,
      963–4
  right, 129–30, 152, 273–6, 780
  trypanosomiasis associated, 1325
Ventricular hypoplasia
  left, 737, *see also Hypolastic left heart
      syndrome*
    atrioventricular septal defect associated
        with, 742
    morphology, 738–41
  right
    imaging, 230–1, 703
    management, 452–3
Ventricular inlet(s)
  components, 67, 68
  defects, *see Ventricular inlet defects*
  development, 91–5, 98–9
  septum, 92, 333, 334, 615–16
    morphology/morphogenesis, 91–5,
        615–16
  myocardium, undermining, 98, 100
  trabeculations, 98–9
Ventricular inlet defect(s)
  double-, *see Double inlet ventricle*
  Fallot's tetralogy with, 770, 771
  overriding, 698
  septal
    atrialisation, 726–7
    complete transposition with, 836
    corrected transposition with, 878–9
    muscular, 451, 623, 631, 635, 770, 771
    perimembranous, 590, 619–20, 630, 634,
        701, 770, 771, 878, 879
Ventricular inversion, 75

Ventricular 'loop', 74, 75
Ventricular mass, 163–4
  architecture
    atrioventricular septal defect associated,
      573–4, 576
    normal, 573–4
    pulmonary atresia associated, 800–1
  definition, 66–7
  echocardiographic features, 321, 573
Ventricular muscle repolarisation, 248–51, *see
  also specific muscle*
Ventricular outflow tract(s)
  with common atrioventricular orifice, 592
  'goose neck' deformity, 593, 598, 600, 601
  maldevelopment, 838
  musculature, terminological description,
    766–7
  normal, 766
  obstruction, *see* Ventricular outflow tract
    obstruction
Ventricular outflow tract obstruction
  clinical presentation at birth, 775–6
  demonstration, 717, 718, 983
  hypertrophic cardiomyopathy associated,
    1140–1, 1148
  left, 457, 458–9, 1227, *see also* Aortic
    stenosis
    atrioventricular septal defect associated
      with, 582–3, 604
    complete transposition associated, 456–7,
      836–7
    corrected transposition associated with,
      879–80
    diagnosis, differential, 1227
    effect, 841
    repair, 854
    site, bedside signs, 978
    subaortic, 990
  minimal, 776
  moderate, 775–6
  right, 453–5
    atrioventricular septal defect with, 608
    Fallot's tetralogy and, 765–7, 768, 769,
      770, 771, 774–6
    hypertrophic cardiomyopathy with, 1148
    pulmonary atresia with, 711, 715, 718,
      813
    treatment/repair, 453–5, 456–7, 719, 789
    ventricular septal defect with, 454–5
  severe-, 775
Ventricular outlet(s)
  components, 67, 68
  defects/obstruction, *see* Double outlet
    ventricles; Ventricular outflow tract
    obstruction; Ventricular outlet defects
  development, 91–5
  morphology, 77–8
  musculature, 79, 766, 767
  ridges, 94
  septum, 94, 96–7, 333, 334, 616
    defects, *see* Ventricular outlet defects,
      septal
    surgical deviation, 856
Ventricular outlet defect(s), septal, *see also*
  Double outlet ventricles
  absence, 770
  complete transposition associated, 834–5,
    836, 837
  deviation and hypertrophy, 770, 772, 801,
    837
  Fallot's tetralogy associated, 766–70 *passim*
  muscular/infundibular, 624, 635, 688, 767,
    846, 849

  perimembranous, 619–20, 630
Ventricular pacing, 1280
Ventricular puncture, direct, 373
Ventricular septum
  components, 92, 333, 615–16
  defects, *see* Ventricular septum, defects
  development, 91–5
  echocardiographic features
    cross-sectional, 321, 333, 334, 335,
      358–9
    M-mode, 332, 333
  inlet/outlet portions, *see* Ventricular inlet
    defects; Ventricular outlet defects
  membranous, 321, 333, 335, 616
  morphology, 615–16
Ventricular septum, defects, *see also* Fallot's
  tetralogy; Ventricular communication;
  Ventricular inlet defects; Ventricular
  outlet defects
  aortic arch interruption with, 1108, 1115
  aortic atresia associated with, 756
  aortic coarctation with, 1091, 1095, 1099,
    1100, 1104–5, 1116
  aortic stenosis with, 978, 980–1
  atrial isomerism with, 482
  atrial septal defects associated with, 548
  cardiac response to, 627
  classification, 615, 616–18, 619
  clinical presentation, 627–8
  closure
    hazards, 690
    spontaneous, 10
  complete transposition with, 456–7, 832,
    833, 834–6
  conduction axis arrangement, 621
  confluent, 620
  corrected transposition associated with,
    878–9
  diagnosis, 635–6
  double inlet ventricle with, 652–3, 655,
    663–7
  double outlet ventricle with, 890, 891,
    892–4, 897
  doubly committed, 895, 1109
  doubly committed subarterial/juxtaarterial,
    617, 618, 619, 625–6, 769, 770
    angiocardiographic features, 634
    echocardiographic features, 632, 633
  Fallot's tetralogy with, 767–70, 779
  fetal, 358–9
  infundibular, 742
  investigations, 629–35
  large/huge, 652–3
    symptoms, improvement with time, 779
  medical management, 637
  morphogenesis, 625
  morphology, 617–25
  multiple, 895
  murmurs with, 468–9
  muscular, 616, 617, 623–4, 625
    angiocardiographic features, 635
    echocardiographic features, 631, 688
    inlet/outlet, *see* Ventricular inlet defects;
      Ventricular outlet defects
    trabecular, 623–4, 631, 635, 688
  muscular rims with, 769
  natural history/progress, 10, 636–7, 690
  neonatal events, 118, 119
  non-committed, 457–8, 895
  pathophysiology, 625–7, 634, 806
  perimembranous, 358, 449, 450, 451, 454,
    616–17, 618–22, 625
    angiocardiographic features, 634, 849

  echocardiographic features, 630, 633
    inlet/outlets, *see* Ventricular inlet defects;
      Ventricular outlet defects
    trabecular, 619
    variants, 619, 634
  physical signs, 628–9
  postoperative management, 638–9
  pressure calculations with, 347
  prevalence, 615, 799
  prognosis, 637–8
  pulmonary atresia with, *see* Pulmonary
    atresia
  pulmonary vascular abnormalities associated
    with, 134, 135, 141–2, 143, 208
  residual, 639
  restrictive, 626, 627, 628
  size of, effect, 625–6
  subaortic, 457, 617–18, 893, 894, 895–6,
    907, 1109
    obstruction of, relief, 669
  subpulmonary, 457, 893, 907–8
  supracristal, 625–6
  surgical management, 637–9, 907–8
    corrective, 449–51, 454, 455, 456–7,
      457–8, 461, 638–9, 854, 856–7, 883
    palliative, 454–5, 637
    problems created by, 1369
  thickening/hypertrophy/bulging, 836, 978,
    980–1, 990, 1139, 1144, 1145
  tricuspid atresia associated with, 678, 688
  truncus arteriosus associated, 914
Ventricular tachycardia, 1286–8, *see also*
  Ventricular arrhythmias
  catheter induced, 382
  management, 1287–8
  restrictice, 908
  supra-, 382, 1281–6
    in the child, 1284
    chronic, 1284–6
    infantile, 1282–4
    treatment, 1282–4, 1284
Ventricular walls, *see also* Ventricular septum
  hypertrophy, pulmonary stenosis associated,
    962
  motion, 169
    incoordinate, 171
    regional, 171
  stress, 164
  thickness
    measurement, 163–4, 226, 356
    significance, 164–5
    normal vs transpositional heart, 833
Ventriculo-arterial connexions, 76–7
  atrial isomerism associated, 490
  concordant, 648, 653
    atrioventricular discordant connexions
      and, 883
    surgical management, 461
    tricuspid atresia with, 678, 679, 680,
      684, 687, 689
  criss-cross heart related to, 1069
  discordant, 599, 605, 606, 646, 659
    angiographic features, 848
    aortic atresia with, 743, 744
    corrected transposition with, 867
    echocardiographic features, 844, 846, 876
    incidence, 867
    surgical management, 461
    tricuspid atresia with, 679–80, 684, 687,
      690
  disturbed/abnormal, recurrence risks in
    sibs/offspring, 35
  modes of, 65, 77

Ventriculo-arterial (*contd.*)
　transposition related to, 830
　types of, 867
Ventriculo-arterial junction, 76–9
　atresia/hypoplasia of the, 737–61 *passim*
　atrial isomerism and the, 482
　connexions at the, *see* Ventriculo-arterial
　　connexions
　echocardiographic features, 341–2
Ventriculo-infundibular fold, 78, 915
Ventriculography, *see* Angiocardiography
Ventriculotomy
　damage caused by, 792–3
　left, 451
　transverse, 7
Venturi effect, 1233
Verapamil
　electrocardiographic effects, 304
　therapy
　　for hypertrophic cardiomyopathy, 1149
　　intravenous, 1284
　　for supraventricular tachycardia, 1284

Viruses
　endocarditis associated, 1233
　myocarditis associated, 1166, 1227
　rheumatic heart disease associated, 1182
Viscera arrangement, atrial isomerism
　　associated, 484–5
Visiting the child, 1389
Vital capacity, 397
　forced-, 398
Vitamin B_1 deficiency, 1262–3

Warfarin therapy, 1357
Waterston anastomosis, 145, 444
　in Fallot's teralogy, 788
William's syndrome, 968, 992–3, 1005
Wolff-Parkinson-White (WPW) syndrome,
　　288, 881, 1286
　atrial fibrillation in, 1289
　electrocardiographic features, 287, 288,
　　1283

electrophysiological features, 1283
　natural history, 1286
　treatment, 1282–3, 1289
Work load/capacity, 396
　maximum, height relationship to, 408, 412
Work rate-oxygen uptake relationship, 402,
　　403
WPW syndrome, *see* Wolff-Parkinson-White
　　(WPW) syndrome

X-linked defects, *see* Sex chromosome defects
X-linked humeroperineal myopathy, 1259

Yeast infections, endocarditis associated,
　　1231, 1237

Zygosity, heart defects in twins related to, 32